MEDICAL CODING

A Journey

BETH A. RICH, B.S., CPC-H

Pittsburgh Technical Institute
Oakdale, Pennsylvania

Boston   Columbus   Indianapolis   New York   San Francisco   Upper Saddle River   Amsterdam
Cape Town   Dubai   London   Madrid   Milan   Munich   Paris   Montreal   Toronto
Delhi   Mexico City   São Paulo   Sydney   Hong Kong   Seoul   Singapore   Taipei   Tokyo

Publisher: Julie Levin Alexander
Publisher's Assistant: Regina Bruno
Editor-in-Chief: Marlene McHugh Pratt
Executive Editor: Joan Gill
Development Editor: Alexis Breen Ferraro, iD8-TripleSSS Media Development LLC
Associate Editor: Bronwen Glowacki
Editorial Assistant: Stephanie Kiel
Director of Marketing: David Gesell
Marketing Manager: Katrin Beacom
Senior Marketing Coordinator: Alicia Wozniak
Managing Production Editor: Patrick Walsh
Production Liaison: Julie Boddorf
Production Editor: Kelly Ricci
Senior Media Editor: Matt Norris
Media Project Manager: Lorena Cerisano
Manufacturing Manager: Lisa McDowell
Creative Director: Andrea Nix
Senior Art Director: Maria Guglielmo
Interior Designer: Christina Cantera
Cover Designer: Christina Cantera
Cover Photo: gornjak/Shutterstock.com
Composition: Aptara®, Inc.
Printing and Binding: Courier Kendallville
Cover Printer: Lehigh-Phoenix Color/Hagerstown

Text design graphic images used by permission of gornjak/Shutterstock, Max Krasnov/Shutterstock, zentilia/Shutterstock, and Orla/Shutterstock.

Library of Congress Cataloging-in-Publication Data

Rich, Beth A.
  Medical coding : a journey / Beth A. Rich.
    p. ; cm.
Includes bibliographical references and index.
ISBN 978-0-13-254177-0
I. Title.
[DNLM: 1. Clinical Coding—methods. 2. Disease—classification. WX 173]
616.001'2—dc23

                 2012019314

10 9 8 7 6 5 4 3 2 1

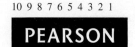

ISBN-13: 978-0-13-254177-0
ISBN-10:   0-13-254177-7

This book is dedicated to you, the coding student, here to learn medical coding to further your career. May this book provide you with the knowledge that you need to be successful. I wish you the best of luck in your future! You can do it!

"Throw back the shoulders, let the heart sing, let the eyes flash, let the mind be lifted up, look upward and say to yourself . . . Nothing is impossible!"—Norman Vincent Peale

This book is also dedicated to the memory of my grandmother, Susan Morabito, who remains a source of inspiration to me, and my stepfather, Joseph Hoffman, whose wise advice I will always remember. They continue to live on in my heart and in the hearts of others whose lives they have so poignantly influenced.

Brief Contents

Contents

Section III ICD-9-CM and ICD-10-CM Coding 187

Section VII Radiology, Pathology and Laboratory, Medicine, and Coding with HCPCS 947

Thank you for choosing *Medical Coding: A Journey*, a comprehensive textbook for learning and assigning diagnosis and procedure codes, including code sets that all U.S. healthcare providers and insurance companies are required to use.

This textbook is designed for beginning coding students, starting with basic concepts and continuing to build on the knowledge learned throughout subsequent chapters. Students who need to learn medical coding as a career choice or learn it for only part of their jobs will benefit from this easy-to-read textbook. It includes medical terminology definitions and pronunciation guides, introductions to numerous medical specialties to provide the background information necessary to better understand coding, and start-to-finish explanations of a variety of conditions, diseases, and disorders, along with descriptions of many types of medical procedures. There are also detailed discussions on anatomy and physiology to help the student better prepare for coding diagnoses and procedures. Examples, photos, and guidelines walk students through each step of the coding process. Unique exercises available in the textbook, *MyHealthProfessionsLab*, or the instructor's manual use video, chart audits, online research, and medical record interpretation to reinforce coding skill and accuracy.

The textbook also covers current healthcare issues affecting medical coding and insurance reimbursement, regulations concerning medical records, including the electronic health record, and privacy regulations. There is discussion about medical coding careers, an exploration of how medical coding jobs are different from other positions in healthcare, and an explanation of how medical coding fits into the entire revenue cycle because revenue is what helps healthcare providers remain financially viable. The text examines where medical coders work, what career options are available to them, and what it takes to become certified in the profession.

The conversational style of this book speaks directly to students and makes no assumptions about students' previous knowledge. There is a walkthrough of each step of the coding process explaining medical procedures and conditions, using coding examples and *Take-a-Break* coding exercises featuring realistic physician and hospital settings. Current references to Medicare coverage and reimbursement make the book up-to-date. In-text learning aids include helpful photos, diagrams, tables, bulleted or numbered steps, coding guidelines, and coding hints, as well as coding manual Index entries of where to locate codes for specific diagnoses and procedures.

The text reviews coding diagnoses and procedures using the following code sets: the International Classification of Diseases, 9th Revision, Clinical Modification (ICD-9-CM) for diagnoses and inpatient hospital procedures; International Classification of Diseases, 10th Revision, Clinical Modification (ICD-10-CM) (draft version) for diagnoses; and International Classification of Diseases, 10th Revision, Procedure Coding System (ICD-10-PCS) for procedures (the code sets that will eventually replace ICD-9-CM), Current Procedural Terminology, 4th Edition (CPT-4) for professional services and procedures, and the Healthcare Common Procedure Coding System (HCPCS) for supplies, equipment, and medications.

TEXTBOOK ORGANIZATION

The text is divided into eight sections:

Section 1: Introduction to Medical Coding contains two chapters. The first introduces the student to the field of medical coding and examines how coding differs from billing, and the second chapter covers the various coding systems, or code sets, along with types of medical records, and privacy and security rules governing patient information.

Section 2: Introduction to ICD-9-CM and ICD-10-CM Coding teaches the student ICD-9-CM diagnosis coding, including coding conventions and General Coding Guidelines, and Diagnostic Coding and Reporting Guidelines for Outpatient Services. This section also teaches ICD-10-CM diagnosis coding, incorporating ICD-10-CM coding exercises into subsequent chapters.

Section 3: ICD-9-CM and ICD-10-CM Coding teaches the student how to assign diagnosis codes for patients who do not have current medical problems, such as patients who are seeing a physician to have an annual examination. The section also covers diagnosis codes for accidents, injuries, burns, infectious diseases, circulatory system disorders, tumors, complications of pregnancy and childbirth, and conditions involving the blood, nervous system, skin, and musculoskeletal system. This section also covers inpatient diagnosis coding, Medicare reimbursement for inpatient and outpatient services and procedures, and coding inpatient hospital procedures.

Section 4: CPT-4 and HCPCS Coding, and Coding with Modifiers introduces the student to coding professional services and procedures using the CPT-4 code set, assigning HCPCS codes for supplies and equipment, and assigning modifiers to codes. CPT-4 exercises throughout the text build on the student's diagnosis coding skills by requiring both a procedure code and diagnosis code for real-world exercises.

Section 5: Evaluation and Management (E/M) Coding and Anesthesia Coding walks the student through the complexities of coding professional services under evaluation and management, using a step-by-step approach to continue to build coding skills. The section also covers the specialty of anesthesia, which has unique coding requirements.

Section 6: Surgery Coding contains an introductory chapter to orient the student to coding surgical procedures and then covers coding for procedures in each specialty in the same order that the CPT-4 manual presents the specialties.

Section 7: Radiology, Pathology and Laboratory, Medicine, and Coding with HCPCS covers background information about radiology, pathology, and laboratory specialties and coding procedures for all of them, as well as a variety of other specialties and procedures covered under the Medicine chapter in the CPT-4 manual. A chapter is devoted to a better understanding of HCPCS codes and how to assign them, along with numerous exercises.

Section 8: Professionalism introduces the student to the importance of professionalism in a coding career and how to handle interactions with patients, including steps for dealing with an angry or upset patient.

Appendices contain instructions for accessing coding guidelines for ICD-9-CM, ICD-10-CM, and ICD-10-PCS, and documentation guidelines used to assign evaluation and management (E/M) codes. Appendices also include differences between the ICD-9-CM and ICD-10-CM code sets, normal lab values for numerous tests that patients receive, normal vital signs, and modifiers used for HCPCS codes.

UNIQUE FEATURES

Consistent pedagogical elements appear throughout the text and in the supplemental material to facilitate instruction and learning.

- **Learning Objectives**—A list of the primary skills students should have after completing the chapter appears at the beginning of each chapter.
- **Key Terms and Abbreviations**—A list of the important terms students need to know. These terms appear in boldface type and are defined at their first appearance in the chapter. They also appear in the comprehensive glossary at the end of the book.

- **Medical Terminology**—Medical terms that students may be unfamiliar with appear in blue font and are defined at their first appearance in the chapter. Pronunciations are provided in the margins.

- An **Introduction** for each chapter alerts the student to information that will be covered in the chapter and how best to prepare to learn it.

- **Detailed anatomy and physiology discussions** orient the student to various body systems' structures and functions before the student learns how to code diagnoses and procedures for those body systems.

- **Detailed exercises** for both ICD-9-CM and ICD-10-CM, and HCPCS, and CPT-4 outline real-world scenarios, complete with physician names and specialties, patients' names and conditions, and procedures that the physician performs.

- **Workplace IQ Exercises** present a realistic scenario and ask students to problem-solve and incorporate the higher levels of Bloom's Taxonomy.

- **Destination: Medicare Exercises** ask students to go to Medicare's website to research coding, billing, and reimbursement regulations from manuals and provider guides. Medicare is the largest payer in the U.S., and learning Medicare regulations is imperative to successful coding.

- **Pointers from the Pros** provides interviews with healthcare professionals who hold a variety of positions to offer the student real-world advice for handling many types of workplace situations.

- **Interesting Facts** give the student the opportunity to learn more about a given topic in each chapter.

- **Colored photos and anatomy diagrams** illustrate various conditions, procedures, and anatomy and physiology discussions.

- **A Look Ahead to ICD-10-CM Exercises** are found in every chapter that covers ICD-9-CM, giving students practice assigning diagnosis codes from the new code set.

- A **Chapter Review** provides students with 10 multiple-choice questions to review chapter content and 10 coding exercises to further expand the coding skills they learned in the chapter.

- **Video Pit Stop Exercises** (found in the Instructor's Manual) direct students to watch different types of videos—surgery, computer-based training, and healthcare topics—and code the patient's diagnosis and procedure.

- **Medical Record Interpretation Exercises** (found on *MyHealthProfessionsLab*) ask students to tie together all of the information they have learned by reviewing an actual medical record and interpreting the meaning of the physician's documentation—including the patient's diagnoses and why the physician performed specific services and procedures.

- **Chart Auditing Exercises** (found on *MyHealthProfessionsLab*) direct students to review diagnosis and procedure codes for accuracy and determine the rationale of code assignments.

SUPPLEMENTS PACKAGE/ANCILLARY MATERIALS

For the Student

- ***MyHealthProfessionsLab for Medical Coding: A Journey*** includes Pretests and Posttests to assess the skills the student learns in each chapter, as well as thousands of coding practice exercises.

MyHealthProfessionsLab™

For the Instructor
- MyTest
- PowerPoint Lecture Notes
- Image Library PowerPoint slides
- Instructor's Manual

About the Author

Beth A. Rich is a seasoned writer with several years of experience writing for newspapers and healthcare newsletters, with numerous articles published, accomplishing much of the work while working full-time in the healthcare industry. She also worked as an instructional designer for a national insurance company and national online curricula publisher, writing software and work processes training manuals for instructors and students. While she was working in healthcare, she wrote numerous healthcare training manuals for hospitals, a healthcare consulting firm, and physician practices. The topics of the training manuals included functions of practice management and hospital software; processes of patient access, charge entry, insurance and patient billing, payment applications, credit and collections, and medical transcription; accounts payable; marketing; customer service; and conducting consulting presentations.

Ms. Rich has over 20 years of broad-based healthcare experience working for numerous healthcare specialties and settings, including acute care, skilled nursing, mental health, dental, pharmacy, and rehabilitation. She started in healthcare while she was a freshman in college, working part-time at a community mental health center in the business office. After that, she held various positions in billing and coding and worked her way up to management. She spent several years managing patient access and patient financial services, in addition to managing a customer service call center, for hospitals and large physician groups with multiple locations. She also managed medical chart auditing, medical coding, facilities management, accounts payable, and marketing. Her project management experience includes overseeing all operations for opening new outpatient facilities, creating new departments, and overseeing training and processes for implementing and converting physician and hospital software systems.

Several years ago, Ms. Rich transitioned from management to healthcare consulting and teaching. She was a senior consultant for a national healthcare consulting firm, working with physician groups and hospitals to conduct revenue cycle reviews, medical coding reviews, pricing audits, software integration analyses, and charge description master reviews to ensure accurate charging, coding, billing, and collections. Her teaching experience includes working in both the corporate setting and for postsecondary schools. In the corporate setting, Ms. Rich developed numerous training programs and oversaw trainers for creating a new customer service call center for a retail and mail order pharmacy, and for creating credit and collections divisions for hospitals and physician groups. Her role included training staff and overseeing trainers in patient access, medical coding, order entry, billing and collections, payment applications, and financial reporting. She has worked as an adjunct instructor for postsecondary schools for 10 years.

For the past 7 years, Ms. Rich has worked as a medical instructor for Pittsburgh Technical Institute (PTI) in Oakdale, Pennsylvania. She is the lead coding instructor, creating online and on-ground curricula for coding certification and national coding exam preparation programs. In addition to teaching beginning, intermediate, and advanced medical coding courses, Ms. Rich also teaches coursework in insurance billing, reimbursement, and regulations, insurance and patient collections, revenue cycle processes, practice management software, and medical records. Her courses also cover electronic health records, charge description master, medical office management, medical transcription, patient relations/customer service, professionalism, and job readiness, including job interviews, resume preparation, and work performance. While she was at PTI, Ms. Rich was nominated for the Pennsylvania Association of Private School Administrators (PAPSA) teaching award.

Ms. Rich has a Bachelor of Science degree in English/writing and is a Certified Professional Coder-Hospital (CPC-H) through the American Academy of Professional Coders (AAPC), of which she is an active member. She is also a member of the American Health Information Management Association (AHIMA) and the Healthcare Financial Management Association (HFMA).

Acknowledgments

The author would like to thank the following people for all of their help during this project:

- Bryan Martin, my husband, my soul mate, for his steadfast faith, caring, understanding, sacrifices, and devotion, the quintessential husband and housecarl, who selflessly agreed to embark on this journey with me. I could not have done it without him.
- Mary Hoffman, my mother, for always supporting me, especially when the going got tough and for her willingness to help me review chapters.
- Jim Yohe, my father, for cheering me on and for his promise to alert the news media when the book is published.
- My family, for all of their encouragement.
- Deborah Sulkowski, Medical Department Chair, Pittsburgh Technical Institute, for her patience, flexibility, and belief in my abilities.
- Chris Ringer, Medical Coding Instructor, Pittsburgh Technical Institute, for her expert advice, guidance, and contributions.
- Leslie Meckling, Classroom Assistant, for all of her help, positive attitude, and sense of humor, enabling me to laugh at seemingly humorless situations.
- My students, who encouraged me and influenced how and why I wrote this book, providing me with countless experiences to share with others.
- My colleagues at Pittsburgh Technical Institute for their support, including the medical coding instructors who contributed to this book. I can now respond to the question that everyone has continued to ask me, "Is the book done yet?" with an enthusiastic "Yes!"
- All of the healthcare professionals who agreed to interviews and those who contributed their writing expertise, including the following writers:

Gina Augustine, MLS, RT, RHIT, CPC, CPC-H, CPhT
Teresa Barbour, RN, CPC
Lorraine M. Papazian-Boyce, MS, CPC
Regina Glenn, PhD, RHIA, CCS
Ruth McClellan, CPC
Kimberly Norris, AAB, BSM, CPC, NCICS
Kimberly Renk, RN, BSN, CPC, CPMA
Christine Ringer, CPC
Steven Smith, MSA, CPC
Margie Stackhouse, RHIA, CPC
Peter Viola, MBA, RHIA
Patricia Zubritzky, CPC, CPAM

Finally, I would like to thank Wendy DiLeonardo, Career Account Manager of Pearson Education, for suggesting that I write a book, and Joan Gill, Executive Editor, Pearson Education, for giving me the opportunity to do so.

The author and publisher wish to thank the following reviewers, all of whom provided valuable feedback and helped to shape the final text:

Kelly M. Anastasio, CPC, CPC-H,
  CPC-I, CPC-C
Certified Professional Medical Coding
  Instructor
Medical Coding Academy, CT

Lori Bentley, RMA, CMRS
Allied Health Instructor
Remington College, TN

Monica Carmichael
Director of Allied Health
Miller-Motte Technical College, SC

Michelle Cranney, MBA, RHIT, CCS-P, CPC
Program Director, Health Sciences
Virginia College, VA

Janet A. Evans, RN, MBA, MS, CCS, CPC-I
Coding Program Coordinator
Burlington County College, NJ

Susan Holler, MSEd, CMBS, CMRS
Allied Health Instructor
Bryant and Stratton College–Southtowns, NY

Jennifer Holmes
Curriculum Development Specialist
Concorde Career Colleges, Inc., KS

Lorretta K. Lassiter-Belton, CCS, BSBA
Medical Billing and Coding Coordinator
Centura College, SC

Cindy McPike, AA, BS, JD, CPC
Lead Instructor, Medical Billing and
  Coding Specialist Program
Medtech College, IN

Kim Smith Norris, CPC, NCICS,
  AAB, BSM
Academic Program Director, Medical
  Insurance, Billing and Coding
Everest University, FL

Le'Cheryl Purnell
Medical Billing and Coding
  Coordinator
Centura College/Charleston, SC

Barbara L. Rutigliano, MS, CPC,
  CIRCC, RT(R)
Instructor
Goodwin College, CT

Debra Steele, Occupational
  Education and Technology/PhD
Instructor
University of Arkansas, Fort
  Smith, OK

A Journey Through Medical Coding

Learning Objectives

After completing this chapter, you should be able to

- Spell and define the key terminology in this chapter.
- Describe the subsection Surgery—Respiratory system.
- Discuss how to code from the subheading Nose.
- Identify how to use the codes in the subheading Accessory Sinuses.
- Explain how to code from the subheading Larynx.
- Define how to use the codes in the subheading Trachea and Bronchi.
- Describe how to code in the subheading Lungs and Pleura.

• **Learning Objectives** open each chapter and provide a list of the primary skills that students should have after completing the chapter.

• **Key Terms** listed at the beginning of each chapter appear in boldface type on first introduction and are defined the first time they appear in the chapter. All terms are defined in the comprehensive glossary that appears at the back of the book.

Key Terms

accessory sinuses
cardiopulmonary bypass (heart–lung machine)
direct laryngoscopy
heart–lung transplant
indirect laryngoscopy

nasopharynx (ney-zoh-far′-ingks)—the first division of the pharynx, the area of the throat joining to the nasal cavity

• **Medical terminology** with which students may be unfamiliar appear in blue font and their definitions and pronunciations are provided the first time they appear in the chapter.

• An **Introduction** for each chapter alerts the student to information that will be covered in the chapter.

INTRODUCTION

You have reached the next stop on your journey—coding procedures of the respiratory system. Remember that the respiratory system allows the body to inhale oxygen and distribute it throughout the bloodstream to cells in the body in order to sustain life. You will learn about many different types of procedures that physicians perform, including *laryngoscopy* (to visually examine the larynx with an endoscope) and *bronchoscopy* (to visually examine the bronchi with an endoscope). Remember that an endoscopy is a procedure where the physician views the inside of the patient's body using a lighted, flexible tube with an attached lens. The CPT manual includes several coding instructions for the Respiratory subsection, including guidelines for specific categories, including endoscopies, and guidelines for individual codes. As always, it is important to review and understand guidelines before assigning codes. This stop may be a little tricky at first, but you will gain self-confidence by completing the practice exercises and applying the new information presented in this chapter. So, let's get started with the respiratory system, taking time to learn about new procedures and how to code them!

■ TABLE 24-3 EXAMPLES OF PROCEDURES IN THE LUNGS AND PLEURA SUBHEADING

Category	Procedure	Description
Incision	*Thoracostomy* (thōr-ə-'käs-tə-mē)	A chest tube or intercostal catheter is inserted into the pleural space to remove a pleural effusion, **empyema** (pus in the pleural space), or pneumothorax (air or gas in the pleural space).
	Thoracotomy (thōr-ə-'kät-ə-mē)	An incision is made into the pleural space to perform procedures on the heart and lungs, including removing neoplasms and foreign bodies and performing a biopsy.
Excision	*Pleurectomy, parietal* (plu-'rek-tə-mē)	The parietal pleura is excised to treat pleural effusion, traumatic injuries, and pleural **mesothelioma** (carcinoma, typically caused by exposure to asbestos).

- **Informational tables** appear throughout the text and define and summarize pertinent information for the reader.

- Numerous **examples** are provided throughout the text to stress the correct billing and coding guidelines.

Example: Mrs. Wilkinson, a 57-year-old established patient, sees Dr. Goldstein for continued treatment and psychotherapy for severe bipolar I disorder. Dr. Goldstein also documents that the patient currently suffers from depression from her most recent episode of bipolar disorder.

Search the Index for the main term *disorder*, subterm *bipolar*, subterm *type I*, and subterm *depressed*. Note that the fifth digit is 3, for severe bipolar disorder without mention of psychotic behavior. Then cross-reference code 296.53 to the Tabular (■ FIGURE 10-3).

4th 296 **Episodic mood disorders**

Includes: episodic affective disorders
Excludes: neurotic depression (300.4)
reactive depressive psychosis (298.0)
reactive excitation (298.1)

The following fifth-digit subclassification is for use with categories 296.0-296.6:

0	unspecified
1	mild
2	moderate
3	severe, without mention of psychotic behavior
4	severe, specified as with psychotic behavior
5	in partial or unspecified remission
6	in full remission

5th 296.5 **Bipolar I disorder, most recent episode (or current) depressed**
[0-6]

Bipolar disorder, now depressed
Manic-depressive psychosis, circular type but currently depressed

Figure 10-3 ■ Index entry for bipolar I disorder with severe depression, most recent episode, with code 296.53 cross-referenced to the Tabular.

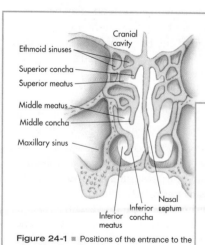

Ethmoid sinuses
Superior concha
Superior meatus
Middle meatus
Middle concha
Maxillary sinus
Cranial cavity
Nasal septum
Inferior concha
Inferior meatus

Figure 24-1 ■ Positions of the entrance to the ethmoid and maxillary sinuses.

Frontal sinus
Ethmoid sinus
Eustachian tube to middle ear
Maxillary sinus

Figure 24-2 ■ Paranasal sinuses.

- **Colored photos and anatomy diagrams** illustrate various conditions, procedures, and anatomy and physiology discussions.

TAKE A BREAK

That was a lot of informati...
review more about procedu...
practice coding.

Exercise 24.2 Incisi...
Removal of Foreign Bo...

Part 1—Theory

Instructions: Fill in the bla...

1. CPT guidelines direct you to codes _____
_____ for draining an abscess or hematoma using
an external approach.

TAKE A BREAK *continued*

appropriate. Optional: For additional p
patient's diagnosis code(s) (ICD-9-CM)

1. Jane White, a 52-year-old, presents
cal Center's ED with complaints of
and purulent (pus) discharge. Dr.
physician, assesses the patient and
and lab work. The tests reveal a nas
which *Staphylococcus aureus* caused

• **Detailed exercises** for both ICD-9-CM and
ICD-10-CM, HCPCS, and CPT-4 outline
real-world scenarios, complete with physician
names, specialties, patient names, conditions,
and the procedures that the physician
performs.

• **Workplace IQ** exercises present realistic
scenarios and ask students to problem-solve
and incorporate the higher levels of Bloom's
Taxonomy.

WORKPLACE IQ

You have worked for six months as a medical assistant for Dr. Gupta, a family care physician. You work
with Rhonda, a coding specialist, and both of you review
codes on encounter forms to ensure that they match
medical record documentation. Today, you and Rhonda
discuss the change from ICD-9-CM to ICD-10-CM.
Rhonda tells you that she is not worried about learning
ICD-10-CM code set because the implementation date
will change again. She tells you, "The implementation

date changed so many times that I couldn't even keep
track of it. I'm not in a hurry to learn ICD-10-CM
because I'm sure that the date will change again. Besides
that, insurance companies have software to change the
old codes to the new ones, and they'll take care of processing our claims. Maybe I'll learn ICD-10-CM codes
eventually."

What would you do?

DESTINATION: MEDICARE

For the Medicare exercise, you will review surgical procedures in
Medicare program transmittals from Medicare's National Coverage
Determinations Manual. Program transmittals communicate new or
changed policies and/or procedures that are incorporated into a specific program
manual. Follow these instructions to access the specific manual:

1. Go to the website http://www.cms.gov.
2. From the top banner bar, choose *Regulations & Guidance.*
3. Choose *Manuals* from the options listed under *Guidance.*
4. Choose *Internet-Only Manuals (IOMs)* listed under *Manuals.*
5. Scroll down to *Publication #*, and choose *100-03 Medicare National Coverage
Determinations (NCD) Manual.*
6. Scroll down to *Downloads*, and choose *Chapter—Coverage Determinations,
Part 2.*
7. Use the search box at the top of the screen to type in the transmittal numbers
that you need to review to answer the following questions.

Answer the following questions, using the search function (Ctrl + F) to find information that you need:

1. According to transmittal numbers 140.6, 140.7, and 140.8, under what

• **Destination: Medicare exercises** ask
students to go to Medicare's website to
research coding, billing, and reimbursement
regulations from manuals and provider guides.
Medicare is the largest payer in the United
States, and learning Medicare regulations is
imperative to successful coding.

• The **Pointers from the Pros** feature presents
interviews with healthcare professionals in a
variety of positions to offer students real-world
advice for handling many types of workplace
situations.

POINTERS FROM THE PROS: Interview with a Coding Expert

Danielle Taimuty, MA, CPC, CEMC, is
the Chief Executive Officer (CEO) of a healthcare company that offers billing, coding, and consulting services
to providers. They also develop software for patient registration, billing, coding, collections, and EHRs.

*From an information technology perspective, what do
you feel are some of the biggest challenges that providers
will face when transitioning from ICD-9-CM to ICD-
10-CM?*

*What can coders do right now to help them prepare for the
change from ICD-9-CM to ICD-10-CM?*

Buy the ICD-10-CM (draft version) and try to cross-
reference the most popular utilized codes.

*What advice can you give to new coders to help them com-
municate effectively with physicians, as physicians can sometimes be intimidating?*

Remember that their (the physician's) job is to tell the
patient news even when it is bad news. You have same

INTERESTING FACTS: What is *E. coli*, and how does it spread?

Escherichia coli (E. coli) are a large and diverse group of bacteria. Although most strains of *E. coli* are harmless, others can make you sick. Some kinds of *E. coli* cause diarrhea, urinary tract infections, respiratory illness, and pneumonia. You can become ill when you swallow *E. Coli* because when you get tiny (usually invisible) amounts of human or animal feces in your mouth, they will make you sick. Exposures that result in illness include eating contaminated food, drinking unpasteurized (raw) milk or contaminated water, swallowing lake water while swimming, touching animals in petting zoos, and eating food prepared by people who did not wash their hands well after using the toilet.

(Department of Health and Human Services, Centers for Disease Control and Prevention, www.cdc.gov/nczved/divisions/dfbmd/diseases/ecoli_o157h7/index.html, accessed 2/5/12)

• **Interesting Facts** give the student the opportunity to learn more about a given topic in each chapter.

⇨ A LOOK AHEAD TO ICD-10-CM

You learned how to assign ICD-10-CM codes in Chapter 6, and you will also have the opportunity for more practice using these codes in this chapter and future chapters. Z codes in ICD-10-CM represent the same information as V codes in ICD-9-CM. Although the coding guidelines for V codes and Z codes are generally the same, be sure to refer to ICD-10-CM Official Guidelines for Coding and Reporting for more specific information. (Directions for obtaining these guidelines are in Appendix A of this text.) In the following exercise, assign Z codes from ICD-10-CM, referencing both the Index and the Tabular.

Instructions: You already coded the following cases in this chapter using ICD-9-CM. Now assign code(s) to the same cases using ICD-10-CM, referencing both the Index and Tabular.

1. Mr. Tallent, age 65, sees Dr. Hoffman for his annual flu vaccine. Dr. Hoffman does not provide any other services. Code(s):_____

• **A Look Ahead to ICD-10-CM exercises** are found in every chapter that covers ICD-9-CM, giving students practice assigning diagnosis codes from the new code set.

CHAPTER REVIEW

Multiple Choice

Instructions: Circle one best answer to complete each statement.

1. In an outpatient setting, a primary diagnosis is also called a(n)
   a. principal diagnosis.
   b. definitive diagnosis.
   c. first-grouped diagnosis.
   d. first-listed diagnosis.

2. The main reason for a patient's encounter is typically the
   a. coexisting condition.
   b. personal history of the condition.
   c. first-listed diagnosis.

7. You should assign codes for a coexisting condition if
   a. the physician treated the patient for the condition in the past, and the patient is now cured.
   b. a specialist rendered care to the patient for the condition.
   c. the condition affects the management of the patient's main reason for the encounter.
   d. the patient was recently hospitalized for treatment of the condition.

8. When a patient has a personal history of a condition, it means that
   a. the condition is resolved and in the past, and the patient does not need further treatment for it.

• A **Chapter Review** provides students with 10 multiple choice questions to review chapter content and 10 coding exercises to further expand the coding skills they learned in the chapter.

Introduction to Medical Coding

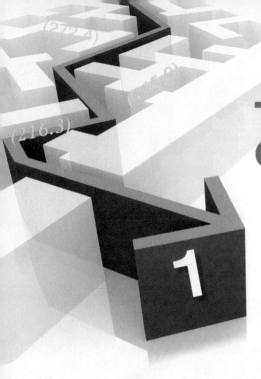

The Field of Medical Coding

Learning Objectives

After completing this chapter, you should be able to

- Spell and define the key terminology in this chapter.
- Explain common healthcare terms and processes related to medical coding.
- List the two types of insurance claim forms and explain which providers use them.
- Describe the difference between subjective and objective information in coding.
- Define a medical record and explain how to assign codes from it.
- Identify the information that is needed to establish medical necessity.
- Define insurance audit, fraud, and abuse.
- Discuss the position of a medical coder in the healthcare delivery system.
- Describe the revenue cycle and discuss how it relates to coding.
- Identify employees who work in a physician's office.
- List the steps in the revenue cycle for a new patient.
- Describe medical coding job requirements.
- List and describe medical coding job duties.
- Identify various job titles used for medical coding and explain where coding professionals work.
- Explain the relationship between billing and coding.
- Discuss the importance of national coding certifications and memberships in professional organizations.
- Define Continuing Education Units (CEUs).
- Describe other professions that are related to coding.

Key Terms

abuse
assumption coding
audit
bundled code
chart abstracting
clinician
coding
continuing education units (CEUs)
credentialed coder
diagnosis
downcoding
electronic medical record
encounter
established patient
ethical standards

False Claims Act qui tam provision
fraud
Health Insurance Portability and Accountability Act (HIPAA)
healthcare delivery system
healthcare provider
jamming
medical necessity
medical record
new patient
Office of the Inspector General (OIG) of the Department of Health and Human Services (DHHS)
revenue cycle
service
unbundling
upcoding

INTRODUCTION

Welcome to the world of medical coding! Medical **coding** is the process of assigning codes, which are made up of numbers, letters, or both, to services and procedures that patients receive and to conditions or problems that patients have. Codes are important because insurance companies require them in order to pay for patients' services and procedures. This chapter provides background information on coding, whether you want to learn coding because you would like to perform it full time or because you will perform it as part of your job. Either way, you will receive a solid foundation on which to build as you continue to expand your knowledge in subsequent chapters. You are embarking on a very interesting journey to learn a brand new subject. With the medical coding skills that you will learn, you will grow as a healthcare professional and can explore many different career options. Who knows where the road on your coding journey may lead you?

"We know what we are, but know not what we may be." —WILLIAM SHAKESPEARE

COMMON HEALTHCARE TERMS AND PROCESSES RELATED TO CODING

Coding indirectly begins when a provider renders a **service** or a procedure to a patient, which can be treatment; testing, such as a lab test; or care to prevent a disease or condition. Examples of services and procedures include performing a physical examination, removing a skin lesion, administering a flu shot, or performing surgery. A **healthcare provider** can be a place, such as a physician's office, hospital, nursing home, or clinic, or a provider can be a person, such as a physician, physician assistant, registered nurse, or physical therapist. The provider, whether a place or a person, renders healthcare to patients in the form of services and procedures. The provider bills these services or procedures to the patient's *insurance company* (also called a third-party payer, commercial insurance, or health plan). The insurance company provides medical coverage for patients to help pay for their medical care. The bills that a provider sends to insurances are called *insurance claims*, which are standardized forms that all providers are required to use to bill insurances. The claims can be on paper, or they can be in computer software, and the provider sends claims to insurances either on paper or electronically. When insurances receive providers' claims, they review them and determine whether to pay, or *reimburse*, the provider.

Insurance Claim Forms

Providers use two types of claim forms to bill insurances for a patient's services and procedures. Physicians bill insurances on the *CMS-1500 form* (■ FIGURE 1-1), which lists information about the patient, such as the name, address, insurance company name, policy number, and medical codes. Hospitals bill insurances on the *CMS-1450*, or *UB-04 form* (■ FIGURE 1-2), which also lists the patient's name, address, and insurance, along with medical codes. (Other types of providers also use the CMS-1450 form for billing). Insurances require that providers list medical codes on the claim forms that represent a patient's **diagnosis** and codes that represent a patient's procedure or service.

The patient's diagnosis is the patient's problem or condition and the reason for the patient's visit. It could be a long-term disease, short-term illness, or the diagnosis can be the reason for the visit because there is nothing wrong with the patient, such as a check-up. The coding process involves reviewing written, or narrative, documentation of the patient's diagnosis and service and determining the correct codes to assign for each.

Subjective and Objective Descriptions

You may wonder why codes exist in the first place and why providers cannot simply write a written description of a patient's diagnosis and procedure on the claim form. The reason is that written descriptions could vary from provider to provider and may not clearly describe a diagnosis, service, or procedure. One provider might describe a patient's

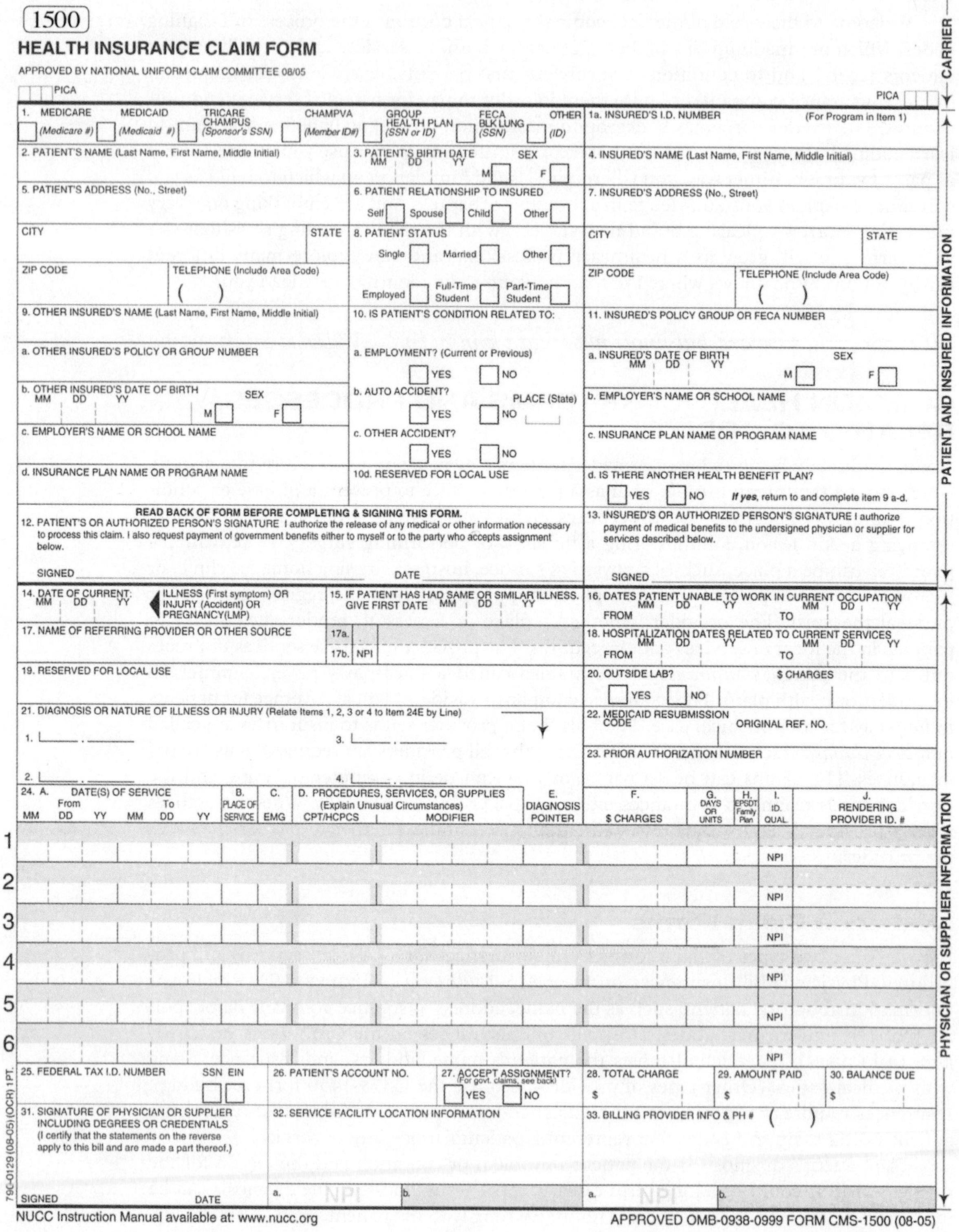
1500
HEALTH INSURANCE CLAIM FORM
APPROVED BY NATIONAL UNIFORM CLAIM COMMITTEE 08/05
PICA PICA
CARRIER
1. MEDICARE MEDICAID TRICARE CHAMPUS CHAMPVA GROUP HEALTH PLAN FECA BLK LUNG OTHER
(Medicare #) (Medicaid #) (Sponsor's SSN) (Member ID#) (SSN or ID) (SSN) (ID)
1a. INSURED'S I.D. NUMBER (For Program in Item 1)
2. PATIENT'S NAME (Last Name, First Name, Middle Initial)
3. PATIENT'S BIRTH DATE MM DD YY SEX M F
4. INSURED'S NAME (Last Name, First Name, Middle Initial)
5. PATIENT'S ADDRESS (No., Street)
6. PATIENT RELATIONSHIP TO INSURED Self Spouse Child Other
7. INSURED'S ADDRESS (No., Street)
CITY STATE
8. PATIENT STATUS Single Married Other
CITY STATE
ZIP CODE TELEPHONE (Include Area Code) ( )
Employed Full-Time Student Part-Time Student
ZIP CODE TELEPHONE (Include Area Code) ( )
9. OTHER INSURED'S NAME (Last Name, First Name, Middle Initial)
10. IS PATIENT'S CONDITION RELATED TO:
11. INSURED'S POLICY GROUP OR FECA NUMBER
a. OTHER INSURED'S POLICY OR GROUP NUMBER
a. EMPLOYMENT? (Current or Previous) YES NO
a. INSURED'S DATE OF BIRTH MM DD YY SEX M F
b. OTHER INSURED'S DATE OF BIRTH MM DD YY SEX M F
b. AUTO ACCIDENT? YES NO PLACE (State)
b. EMPLOYER'S NAME OR SCHOOL NAME
c. EMPLOYER'S NAME OR SCHOOL NAME
c. OTHER ACCIDENT? YES NO
c. INSURANCE PLAN NAME OR PROGRAM NAME
d. INSURANCE PLAN NAME OR PROGRAM NAME
10d. RESERVED FOR LOCAL USE
d. IS THERE ANOTHER HEALTH BENEFIT PLAN? YES NO *If yes,* return to and complete item 9 a-d.
READ BACK OF FORM BEFORE COMPLETING & SIGNING THIS FORM.
12. PATIENT'S OR AUTHORIZED PERSON'S SIGNATURE I authorize the release of any medical or other information necessary to process this claim. I also request payment of government benefits either to myself or to the party who accepts assignment below.
SIGNED DATE
13. INSURED'S OR AUTHORIZED PERSON'S SIGNATURE I authorize payment of medical benefits to the undersigned physician or supplier for services described below.
SIGNED
PATIENT AND INSURED INFORMATION
14. DATE OF CURRENT: MM DD YY ILLNESS (First symptom) OR INJURY (Accident) OR PREGNANCY(LMP)
15. IF PATIENT HAS HAD SAME OR SIMILAR ILLNESS. GIVE FIRST DATE MM DD YY
16. DATES PATIENT UNABLE TO WORK IN CURRENT OCCUPATION MM DD YY FROM MM DD YY TO
17. NAME OF REFERRING PROVIDER OR OTHER SOURCE
17a.
17b. NPI
18. HOSPITALIZATION DATES RELATED TO CURRENT SERVICES MM DD YY FROM MM DD YY TO
19. RESERVED FOR LOCAL USE
20. OUTSIDE LAB? YES NO $ CHARGES
21. DIAGNOSIS OR NATURE OF ILLNESS OR INJURY (Relate Items 1, 2, 3 or 4 to Item 24E by Line)
1. 2. 3. 4.
22. MEDICAID RESUBMISSION CODE ORIGINAL REF. NO.
23. PRIOR AUTHORIZATION NUMBER
24. A. DATE(S) OF SERVICE From MM DD YY To MM DD YY
B. PLACE OF SERVICE
C. EMG
D. PROCEDURES, SERVICES, OR SUPPLIES (Explain Unusual Circumstances) CPT/HCPCS MODIFIER
E. DIAGNOSIS POINTER
F. $ CHARGES
G. DAYS OR UNITS
H. EPSDT Family Plan
I. ID. QUAL.
J. RENDERING PROVIDER ID. #
1 NPI
2 NPI
3 NPI
4 NPI
5 NPI
6 NPI
25. FEDERAL TAX I.D. NUMBER SSN EIN
26. PATIENT'S ACCOUNT NO.
27. ACCEPT ASSIGNMENT? (For govt. claims, see back) YES NO
28. TOTAL CHARGE $
29. AMOUNT PAID $
30. BALANCE DUE $
31. SIGNATURE OF PHYSICIAN OR SUPPLIER INCLUDING DEGREES OR CREDENTIALS (I certify that the statements on the reverse apply to this bill and are made a part thereof.)
SIGNED DATE
32. SERVICE FACILITY LOCATION INFORMATION
a. NPI b.
33. BILLING PROVIDER INFO & PH # ( )
a. NPI b.
PHYSICIAN OR SUPPLIER INFORMATION
79O-0129 (08-05) (OCR) 1PT.
NUCC Instruction Manual available at: www.nucc.org
APPROVED OMB-0938-0999 FORM CMS-1500 (08-05)

Figure 1-1 ■ The CMS-1500 claim form.

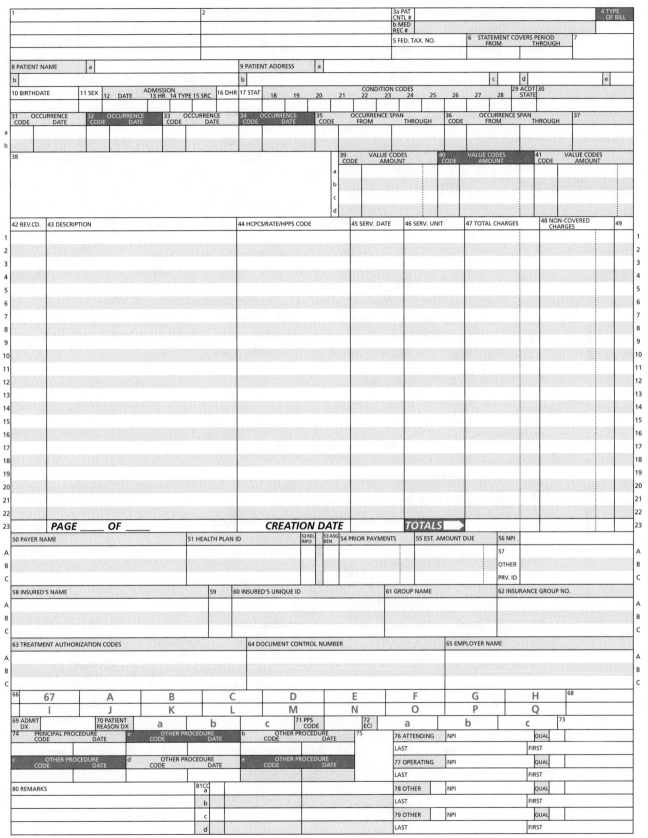

Figure 1-2 ■ The UB-04 (CMS-1450) claim form.

diagnosis as "stomach pain," whereas another might describe it as "abdominal pain," and yet another might describe it as "upper abdominal pain." If a patient has an office visit, then one provider might call it a "lengthy office visit" while another might call it an "extended exam." These descriptions illustrate *subjective information*. Subjective information is based on a person's opinion and his personal account of events that took place, as opposed to *objective information*, which is based on *facts* rather than opinion. Insurances would have a difficult time determining the exact diagnosis or procedure if providers sent written descriptions instead of codes.

Consider a group of people standing on a sidewalk and looking up at a large building. Members of the group may describe the building using subjective words like *big, large, huge, tall, massive,* or *overpowering*. The words describe their personal opinions of the building. But when they view the building objectively, they find that it is 240 feet tall. The exact measurement of 240 feet is objective information that is based on facts, not personal opinion. Everyone in the group would agree that the building is 240 feet tall because that is a fact.

Medical coding works the same way. All providers and insurances use the same set of codes that represent specific diagnoses and services, and each code represents the same objective information to everyone. Using standardized codes instead of written descriptions eliminates guesswork for providers and insurance companies. Diagnosis and procedure codes are made up of letters (alpha), or numbers (numeric), or a combination of both (alphanumeric). You will learn more about the individual coding systems for diagnoses and procedures in Chapter 2. The following are a few examples of each type of code.

Diagnosis codes:

790.29—Hyperglycemia

428.0—Congestive heart failure

V22.0—Pregnancy visit for normal first pregnancy

Procedure codes:

71010—Chest X-ray, one view

90471—Immunization administration for a vaccine

4066F—Electroconvulsive therapy (ECT) provided

G0010—Administration of hepatitis B vaccine

Medical Records

A **medical record**, also called a medical chart, contains written descriptions of what happened during a patient's service or procedure and descriptions of the patient's diagnosis. The physician or other **clinician** (person who provides hands-on patient care), such as a physician assistant, handwrites the documentation in the chart or types it into a computerized medical chart (**electronic medical record**). The clinician may also dictate (speak) the information into a recorder, and then a transcriptionist listens to the *dictation* and types the information into a document. This process is called *medical transcription*. Another method of documenting in a record is front-end speech recognition, where the computer converts speech into written text, and the transcriptionist reviews and edits the text for accuracy.

Coding Medical Records

Coding a medical record involves reading the record, interpreting the medical language in it to determine the patient's diagnosis and procedure, and then assigning the correct codes for both. Physicians and other clinicians document information in a medical record using *medical nomenclature*, a system for classifying medical terms. (Examples of medical terms include *rhinorrhea*, which is discharge from the nose, and *hypoglycemia*, a condition of low blood sugar.) Students learn medical nomenclature by studying *medical terminology*, the

■ TABLE 1-1   **MEDICAL TERMINOLOGY WORD PARTS**

hypoglycemia (hypo / glyc / emia)		
Word Part	**Definition**	**What It Means**
hypo-	prefix—beginning	under, or low
-glyc/o-	combining form—middle	sugar
-emia	suffix—end	blood condition or presence of a substance in the blood

procedure of breaking down medical words into three parts: prefix, suffix, and combining form, defining each part, and then defining the entire word. ■ TABLE 1-1 provides an example of a medical word broken down into its parts.

Read the word from back to front for its literal meaning: blood condition of under sugar. Now translate it to: a condition of low blood sugar.

A person who performs coding is called a coder. A successful coder must understand medical terminology, human anatomy and physiology, disease processes and treatments, and also understand how physicians perform specific procedures. Coding also requires excellent problem-solving, analytical, and detail-oriented skills. Think of a coder as a translator who reviews medical nomenclature, analyzes its meaning, and then translates it into diagnosis and procedure codes. This process is called **chart abstracting**.

The coder references diagnosis and procedure coding manuals to find the patient's condition and procedure and the corresponding codes. Think of the manuals as a type of dictionary or encyclopedia meant only for medical coding. Hospitals and many large physician groups have clinical coding software that replaces manuals and contains diagnosis and procedure codes so that coders can quickly locate codes. Because coding software is an additional expense, smaller providers may choose not to purchase it or cannot afford it, so they use the coding manuals instead. New coders often ask if it is possible to memorize all of the codes available, but there are thousands of codes, so it is not likely that anyone could remember all of them! Just know that you can always reference the coding manuals or coding software to ensure that you code correctly.

TAKE A BREAK

Let's take a break and then review the information with an exercise.

Exercise 1.1   Common Healthcare Terms and Processes Related to Coding

Instructions: Fill in each blank with the best answer, choosing from the list of terms.

1. A(n) _____ contains a written description of what happened during the patient's service or procedure.

2. Physicians bill insurances with the _____ form.

3. Hospitals bill insurances with the _____ form.

4. A _____ listens to dictation and types the information into a document.

5. A(n) _____ can be a person or a place.

6. A third-party payer is also called a(n) _____.

7. Medical codes can represent a(n) _____ or a(n) _____.

- Transcriptionist
- Clinician
- CMS-1450
- Healthcare provider
- Insurance company
- Procedure/service
- Medical nomenclature/chart abstracting
- Medical record
- CMS-1500
- Objective information

MEDICAL NECESSITY

Successful coding also requires knowledge of **medical necessity**, meaning that the patient's diagnosis justified the procedure that the physician performed, or the service was medically necessary. An example of a diagnosis and service meeting medical necessity is a patient who has stomach pain and the physician performs a physical examination. We can say that the stomach pain (diagnosis) justifies the reason for the examination (procedure). We can also say that the exam was medically necessary, based on the patient's diagnosis. Insurances review claims for medical necessity, and they do not pay claims with codes that do not meet medical necessity. Coders must ensure that the codes they assign meet medical necessity, but they also must assign codes that represent the documentation in the chart.

Querying the Physician

Let's say that the physician does not document medical necessity in the patient's record. The coder has to read *chart documentation* to assign codes, and if the documentation does not support medical necessity, then the codes will not either. This is where your problem-solving skills will come in handy. If you read chart documentation that shows that a patient's procedure was not medically necessary, or it is clear that the chart is missing documentation, then you always need to ask, or *query*, the physician for clarification. You will hear a saying in the field, "not documented, not done," meaning that you cannot code for procedures that the physician did not document. By talking with the physician, you will need to discuss why the documentation does not support medical necessity. It is crucial that you do not code diagnoses or procedures that the physician did not clearly document just because you believe that insurance will pay if you assign different codes.

You should also avoid making assumptions about the patient's case, called **assumption coding**. Assumption coding happens if you read chart documentation and *assume* that the patient has a specific diagnosis, even though the physician did not document it. You might read the chart and know someone who suffered symptoms similar to the patient, so you conclude that the patient has the same diagnosis as the person you know. Or you may read the chart and assume that the physician performed specific tests, even though he did not document them, just because you know someone who had the same diagnosis, and she had the tests done. Remember, it is the physician's job to diagnose and treat patients and document medical information in the patient's chart. When you code, it is your job to code directly from the physician's documentation and not add or subtract information based on your personal experience.

INSURANCE AUDITS, FRAUD, AND ABUSE

Medicare and other payers may also **audit**, or review, insurance claims, which is a process to determine whether the documentation in the record justified the procedures coded and billed on claims. Providers typically do not send copies of medical records with claims to prove why they used specific codes, so insurances have to rely on providers to code and bill appropriately. If they do not, then payers could charge providers with billing fraud or abuse.

Fraud is an intentional act of coding and billing for procedures that did not occur or coding and billing for higher level procedures than what actually occurred (**upcoding**). Some providers also commit fraud by purposely trying to gain more reimbursement by assigning multiple procedure codes for individual services that are generally represented by a single code, called a **bundled code**. If a bundled code exists, providers are required to assign it instead of separately coding for each service in the bundle. Coding for each service individually, when they should have been coded with one bundled code, is called **unbundling**. Providers may also commit fraud by **jamming**, or coding for diagnoses that do not exist so the insurance will pay for the services. Penalties for fraud can be severe, including fines and imprisonment, along with the inability to bill a specific insurance ever again or for a specified period of time. The provider also has to pay the insurance back any money it received from fraudulent claims. Anyone working for the provider who is involved with fraud could be punished.

INTERESTING FACT: Provider Bills Medicare for Equipment That Did Not Exist

A man working in California pleaded guilty to federal criminal charges of defrauding Medicare by using patients' Medicare identification numbers without their knowledge. Between August 2003 and April 2008, Melkon Gabriyelyan billed the Medicare program for more than $1,640,000 worth of fictitious equipment.

Gabriyelyan owned a durable medical equipment (DME) company in Los Angeles and admitted that he knowingly and willfully stole the identity of Medicare beneficiaries for the purpose of submitting false claims. (Department of Justice, United States Attorney's Office, Central District of California, October 16, 2008)

Reasons to Audit Claims

While fraud is intentional, **abuse** is the unintentional act of billing and coding incorrectly. It may happen because the coder was not properly trained and assigned incorrect codes. Examples of abuse are unintentionally assigning a more general code to a diagnosis when a specific one exists, unbundling codes, upcoding, or assigning a lower level code for the service than what the physician actually performed (**downcoding**). Penalties for abuse are much less severe than those for fraud and often result in the provider agreeing to develop a corrective action plan to ensure that the abuse does not continue. The plan may include new or revised procedures, training for coders, and periodic chart audits to check coding accuracy. Providers should be proactive and conduct random chart audits regularly to avoid cases of fraud or abuse.

Are you wondering why an insurance would choose to audit a provider's claims? They may want to audit claims randomly, or they may see patterns of billing and coding that do not make sense. For example, if a provider consistently billed an insurance for the highest levels of service for every patient's claim, then the insurance would question why and most likely audit the claims. It would not be common for the provider to only perform the highest level of service for every patient seen.

Insurances may also audit claims because someone contacted them to report suspected fraud. For Medicare claims, whistleblowers (people who report fraud and abuse) fall under what is called the **qui tam** (pronounced kwày tæm) **provision of the False Claims Act**. The qui tam provision states that a whistleblower can sue on behalf of the government and receive part of the money the government recovers from providers who commit fraud. Whistleblowers can be anyone, including a provider's current or past employee or a current or former patient. The *Centers for Medicare and Medicaid Services (CMS)* oversees the Medicare and Medicaid programs and works with other government agencies and law enforcement organizations to protect the Medicare program from fraud and abuse. The **Office of the Inspector General (OIG) of the Department of Health and Human Services (DHHS)** investigates cases of fraud and imposes monetary penalties on providers who are found guilty.

TAKE A BREAK

Let's take a break and then review the information with an exercise.

Exercise 1.2   Medical Necessity, Insurance Audits, Fraud, and Abuse

Instructions: Indicate whether each statement is True or False on the line preceding each statement. For statements marked False, underline the word or words that makes the statement false.

1. _____ Assigning a lower level code for a service than what the physician actually performed is called jamming.

2. _____ Abuse is intentional, and fraud is unintentional.

3. _____ Coding and billing for higher level services than what actually occurred is called upcoding.

4. _____ When one code is used to represent several individual services, it is called bundling.

5. _____ Medical necessity means that the patient's diagnosis justified the procedure performed.

6. _____ Supposition coding is when you can deduce what happened during a patient's procedure, even if the physician did not document the information.

HEALTHCARE DELIVERY AND CODING

Medical coding may be a full-time position, or coding may only be part of an individual's job duties. Coders can work for many different types of providers and other organizations, including

- physician offices or large group practices
- inpatient and outpatient hospitals
- nursing homes
- rehabilitation centers
- outpatient clinics
- urgent care clinics
- acute care hospitals
- specialty hospitals (e.g., psychiatric or rehabilitation hospitals)
- ambulatory care facilities
- mental health clinics
- laboratories
- pharmacies
- DME providers (supply items such as wheelchairs, hospital beds, and canes)
- home health agencies
- billing companies
- collection agencies
- insurance companies
- coding and auditing consulting firms
- public health departments
- post-secondary schools as educators

Wow! There are many potential employers for healthcare professionals who code. When working for a provider, coders become part of the **healthcare delivery system**, a network of people and processes working to treat patients' conditions and prevent illnesses. Coders' work is collaborative, meaning that they have to support the work of others and others have to support them. Working collaboratively also means understanding the work that others perform and why. You might say that working collaboratively is necessary whether or not you work in healthcare. That is true, but in healthcare, working together directly results in revenue: money that a provider collects for rendering services and procedures. A lot of people think that the physician is the most important person in a practice. The truth is, everyone working there is important to the provider's financial success.

Healthcare providers receive revenue primarily from two sources: insurance companies and patients. Some providers may receive money from grants that fund specific procedures or research, or individuals may donate money to larger providers, but for the most part, revenue comes only from insurance reimbursement and patient payments. The provider uses that revenue to pay expenses, including staff salaries, utilities, office supplies and equipment, monthly rent or lease for the building, the cleaning service, the answering service, and additional expenses. Think of a healthcare provider just like any other business—a grocery store, restaurant, or clothing store—it needs to earn revenue to survive and earn profits. Many physicians own their own practice, and they must earn enough money to meet their expenses. Your salary will be a direct result of the work that you and other employees perform to ensure correct insurance reimbursement and patient payments. We will discuss this work next as it applies to the revenue cycle.

The Revenue Cycle

A **revenue cycle**, also called a billing cycle, involves all of the steps that take place from the time that a patient calls a provider to schedule an appointment for a service or procedure until the patient's bill is paid in full. The revenue represents the provider's income. Each person working for a healthcare provider performs various tasks that comprise the steps in the revenue cycle, and they perform their duties while focusing on two main areas: accuracy and timeliness. Medical coding, as with many other duties involved in the revenue cycle, must be accurate and timely. To fully understand the role of medical coding in the revenue cycle, you must also understand all of the steps in the process because they all interrelate, each one affecting the other. In order to be successful at coding, you have to realize that the accuracy and timeliness of your work has a direct impact on others' work, just as their work does on yours. And most important, everyone's work has a serious impact on revenue.

Physician's Office Employees

The steps that make up the revenue cycle involve processes and people. We will discuss both as they apply to a physician's office with one location. But before we do, let's learn about the typical employees working in a physician's office and their duties so that you will have a better understanding of the revenue cycle as it applies to them (■ Figure 1-3). You may also find that many of these positions exist in other types of providers. Use this list as your reference as you read about how the employees perform the steps in the revenue cycle. The duties listed here are general ones; employees may perform more or fewer tasks, depending on the office.

* *the physician*—examines patients and performs procedures.
* *other clinicians*, such as physician assistants (PAs), certified registered nurse practitioners (CRNPs), and registered nurses (RNs), also examine patients and perform procedures but do not have the education to perform the same work as the physician. These providers are called *healthcare practitioners* or *physician extenders*.

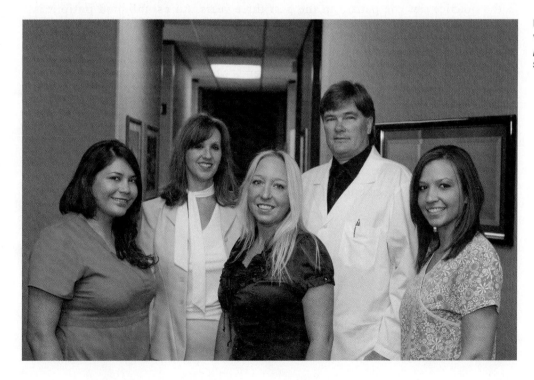

Figure 1-3 ■ Employees working in a physician's office.
Photo credit: B. Franklin / Shutterstock.

- *office manager or administrator*—oversees staff in the office, ensures that the office has enough revenue to operate, pays salaries and other expenses (called accounts payable), recruits new employees, and oversees their training.

- *medical assistant*—performs a variety of duties, including patient care, and assists with scheduling appointments, answering phones, entering patient charges, performing coding, handling insurance and patient billing and collections, and performing administrative tasks such as typing business letters.

- *billing specialist*—performs insurance billing and collections and reviews financial reports.

- *medical coder*—reads chart documentation and assigns diagnosis and procedure codes.

- *receptionist, secretary, or administrative assistant*—answers phones, schedules appointments, types business correspondence, and assists office manager as needed.

- *transcriptionist*—transcribes (types) chart documentation from the physician's dictation, which is a taped recording of the chart documentation.

- *accountant*—conducts financial analyses of all money collected and oversees banking transactions.

- *other employees or services* include the answering service to take phone calls when the office is closed, the security system to protect the practice from theft or fire, the housekeeping or cleaning company that regularly cleans the office, and the filing clerk who files medical documentation and other paperwork in patients' charts and office files.

Steps in the Revenue Cycle for a New Patient

Let's review the basic steps in the revenue cycle for a new patient in order to better understand all of the processes and people involved and how they relate to medical coding. A **new patient** is one who has never seen the physician or has not seen the physician in the past three years. In a larger group practice with physicians of different specialties, a patient is new when seeing a physician of a *different* specialty, even if another physician in the practice saw the patient in the past three years. An **established patient** is a patient who saw the same physician in the past three years. An established patient is also one visiting a large group practice to see a *different* physician who is the *same specialty* as the previous physician the patient saw. Recall that the revenue cycle begins when the patient calls to schedule an appointment and ends when the patient's bill is paid in full. You will find a list of the revenue cycle steps next, followed by the processes and people involved in each step for the case of a patient named Mr. Edward Russell. Mr. Russell will communicate with the following employees*:

- Robert R. Hoffman, M.D.—physician
- Judy—front desk receptionist
- Debbie—billing specialist
- John—coder
- Rhonda—medical assistant
- Ruth—transcriptionist
- Betsy—filing clerk

---

*Note that each employee will address the patient as "Mr. Russell" because it is customary to refer to patients as Mr., Mrs., Ms., or Dr., rather than calling them by their first name, unless they request it.

The following is a list of revenue cycle steps:

1. Preregistration
2. Insurance verification
3. Check-in and registration
4. Encounter
5. Chart documentation
6. Check-out
7. Charge entry
8. Transcription
9. Medical coding
10. Insurance claim or patient bill
11. Payment posting
12. Follow-up
13. Balance paid

   1. ***Preregistration***—*Preregistration* is the process of collecting insurance and partial demographic information, scheduling the patient's appointment, and verifying insurance coverage and benefits before the patient's appointment. It is called "pre" registration because it happens *before* the actual visit when the patient will give the provider the remaining demographic information and complete registration forms. Preregistration saves time for both the patient and the provider because part of the registration is already completed when the patient arrives at the office.

   A new patient, Edward Russell, calls to schedule an appointment for a yearly examination. The front desk receptionist, Judy, answers the call and determines the reason for the call and the length of time needed for the appointment. She schedules an appointment for Mr. Russell using the practice management software for next Monday at 3:00 p.m. and also creates an account for Mr. Russell in the software, entering his name, address, phone number, gender, and birth date. This information is called *demographic information*. It also includes the patient's social security number, employer information, and emergency contact. Judy will obtain the remaining demographic information at the time of the patient's visit. Judy asks Mr. Russell to arrive 15 minutes earlier than his appointment time to complete his registration paperwork and to also bring his driver's license or photo identification. Many providers ask for photo identification as proof of a patient's identity to ensure that the patient is not misrepresenting himself. There have been an increasing number of cases when an individual steals another's identity, takes that person's insurance card, and uses it to obtain medical services while pretending to be that person. In other cases, individuals working for healthcare providers steal another person's medical information to bill false claims to insurance and collect insurance payments. The Federal Trade Commission (FTC) and federal financial institution regulatory agencies created the Red Flags rule that ask certain providers, those who extend credit to patients and offer payment plans, to develop a Theft Prevention Program to identify and combat identity theft.

   Because the office verifies each new patient's insurance coverage and benefits before the first appointment, Judy asks Mr. Russell for his *insurance information* and adds it to his account. The insurance information includes the insurance company name, address, phone number, name of the *insured* (the person who holds the insurance policy, also called the policyholder, guarantor, or beneficiary), policy number, group number, effective date, and the insurance's website address. Insurance coverage determines whether insurance will pay for specific services; benefits are how much the insurance will pay if there is coverage. Judy asks Mr. Russell's permission to place him on hold while she asks the billing specialist, Debbie, to verify his insurance coverage and benefits on the insurance's website.

Figure 1-4 ■ Debbie verifies Mr. Russell's insurance.

Photo credit: Michal Heron/Pearson Education.

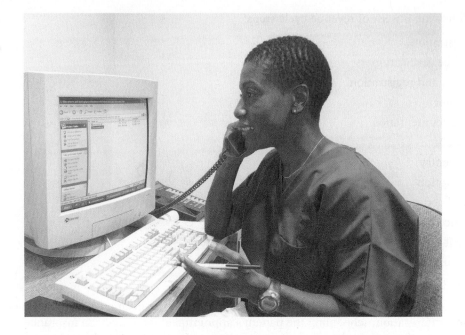

2. ***Insurance Verification***—Insurance verification is the process of determining whether a patient has insurance coverage for a service or procedure and benefits (how much the insurance will pay). Debbie works in the back office (the areas of the office that are separate from the front desk, or front office). She can verify a patient's coverage and benefits over the phone, through the insurance's website, or through a card swipe machine. She reviews the insurance information that Judy entered on Mr. Russell's account and verifies his insurance coverage and benefits through his insurance's website, documenting her findings on his account (■ FIGURE 1-4). Debbie picks up Mr. Russell's call and tells him that his insurance will cover the service; the insurance is expected to pay $100, and he is expected to pay a $20 *copayment* when he arrives for his appointment. A copayment is the amount of the patient's responsibility for the service that the insurance will *not* pay. If Mr. Russell did not have insurance, then Debbie would ask him to bring the total amount due for the service when he arrives. Debbie also asks Mr. Russell to bring his insurance card to his appointment so that the office staff can verify the information on the card and keep a copy for their records (■ FIGURE 1-5).

Insurance verification must occur before the patient's appointment for two reasons: to protect the patient from receiving a service that the insurance will not cover and to protect the provider from rendering a service that the patient's insurance or the patient may never pay.

3. ***Check-in and Registration***—On Monday at 2:45 p.m., Mr. Russell arrives for his appointment 15 minutes early to complete his registration paperwork. He *checks in* at the front desk with Judy to tell her that he has arrived for a scheduled appointment. Judy introduces herself, asks him to sign in, and also asks for his insurance card and driver's license. She copies both of them and then gives Mr. Russell registration forms, explaining that he needs to review, complete, and sign them and let her know if he has any questions (■ FIGURE 1-6).

Judy prints the *patient registration form* from the software, completed with the information that Judy obtained during Mr. Russell's call to schedule his appointment. The patient registration form contains demographic and insurance information. Mr. Russell still needs to provide his employer's information, emergency contact, marital status, and guarantor's information. You learned earlier that guarantor is another name for the policyholder or insured, or the person who holds the insurance policy. *Guarantor* is also the person who is responsible for paying the patient's bill, but the guarantor is *not* the insurance company. Providers bill insurances first and then bill any remaining balance to the guarantor. The guarantor may be a patient's spouse, parent, or legal guardian. Many times, the patient is also the guarantor.

L B GOLD HEALTH INSURANCE

Insured	EDWARD W. RUSSELL		
I.D.#	44327A87T1	**Group #**	3020822
PCP	HOFFMAN, ROBERT R. MD	**Phone**	412-555-1312
Copay	$20 PCP/$30 SPECLST/ER $150		

(Front of Insurance Card)

Member Services/Benefits	Call 1-100-555-2000/Address: 5 West Newton Parkway, East Springfield, NY 13333
Provider Questions	Call 1-100-555-6000
Copayments	Your insurance policy requires you to pay copayments at the time of service.
Nurses ASAP	Call 1-100-555-7000 for 24-hour nurse access for support and education
Emergencies	In case of an emergency, go directly to the nearest healthcare provider. You do not need prior approval. Notify your PCP within 72 hours. For emergency care out-of-state, call 1-999-555-8000 for a list of participating providers.
Mental Health/Substance Abuse	Call 1-100-555-4142 for a list of participating providers.

(Back of Insurance Card)

Figure 1-5 ■ Copy of Mr. Russell's insurance card.

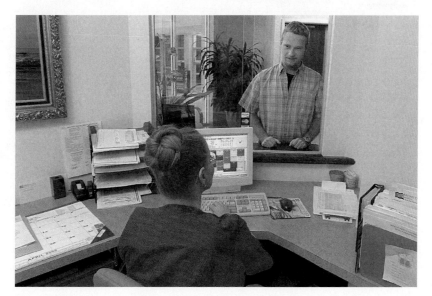

Figure 1-6 ■ Judy gives Mr. Russell his registration forms.

Photo credit: Michal Heron/Pearson Education.

Patient Registration Forms

Judy gives the patient registration form (■ FIGURE 1-7) and the additional registration forms to Mr. Russell to read, complete, and sign. He then returns the patient registration form and other forms in the packet to Judy (■ FIGURES 1-8 to 1-14):

Robert R. Hoffman, M.D.—123 Unknown BLVD, Capital City, NY 12345–2222 (412) 555–1312

Patient Information Form
Tax ID: 75–0246810
Group NPI: 1513171216

Patient Information:

Name: (Last, First) _____ ❑ Male ❑ Female Birth Date: _____

Address: _____ Phone: *(555)* _____

Social Security Number: _____ Full-Time Student: ❑ Yes ☒ No

Marital Status: ❑ Single ☒ Married ❑ Divorced ❑ Other

Employment:

Employer: _____ Phone: *(555)* _____

Address: _____

Condition Related to: ❑ Auto Accident ❑ Employment ❑ Other Accident

Date of Accident: _____ State _____

Emergency Contact: _____ **Phone: ( )** _____

Primary Insurance: _____ Phone: ( ) _____

Address: _____

Insurance Policyholder's Name: _____ ❑ M ❑ F DOB: _____

Address: _____

Phone: _____ Relationship to Insured: ☒ Self ❑ Spouse ❑ Child ❑ Other

Employer: _____ Phone: ( ) _____

Employer's Address: _____

Policy/ID No: _____ Group No: _____ Percent Covered: ____%, Copay Amt: $_____

Secondary Insurance: _____ Phone: ( ) _____

Address: _____

Insurance Policyholder's Name: _____ ❑ M ❑ F DOB: _____

Address: _____

Phone: _____ Relationship to Insured: ❑ Self ❑ Spouse ❑ Child ❑ Other

Employer: _____ Phone: ( ) _____

Employer's Address: _____

Policy/ID No: _____ Group No: _____ Percent Covered: ____%, Copay Amt: $_____

Reason for Visit: _____

Known Allergies: _____

Were you referred here? If so, by whom?: _____

Figure 1-7 ■ Sample Patient Registration form.

Figure 1-8 ■ Health History form.

ROBERT R. HOFFMAN, M.D.
HEALTH HISTORY FORM

Patient Name: _____   Date: _____

Allergies:

Are you allergic to penicillin or any other drugs?   ___Yes   ___No

If allergic to other drugs, please list: _____

Medications—Please list medications you currently take, dosage, and frequency. Please use the back of this form if you need to list more than four medications:

Medication	Dosage	How often do you take this medication?

Health History. Please check any current or past medical conditions:

Arthritis	Diabetes	Muscle pain
Cancer	Liver disorder	Asthma
Glaucoma	Kidney disorder	Paralysis
Eye problems	Hepatitis	Shortness of breath
High blood pressure	Ulcers	Lung problems
Low blood pressure	Blood in stool	Allergies
Chest pain	Thyroid disorder	Sinus problems
Irregular heart beat	Memory loss	Coughing blood
High cholesterol	Trouble balancing	Tonsillitis
Heartburn	Dizziness	Emphysema
Ankle swelling	Headaches/migraines	Chronic cough
Anemia	Neurological problems	Pneumonia
Depression	Seizures	Ear problems
Anxiety	Stroke	Hair loss
Eating disorder	Joint pain	Skin rash/itching

Please list all surgeries and dates:

Surgery	Date

Social History:

Do you smoke?	Yes	No	If yes, how many cigarettes a day?
Do you drink alcohol?	Yes	No	If yes, how much per week?
Do you consume caffeine?	Yes	No	If yes, how much per week?
Do you use recreational drugs?	Yes	No	If yes, what drug, and how much per week?

continued

Figure 1-8 ■ *continued*

Family History:

Mother: Living?	Yes		No	Age at Death:	List any diseases or illnesses:
Father: Living?	Yes		No	Age at Death:	List any diseases or illnesses:
Sister: Living?	Yes		No	Age at Death:	List any diseases or illnesses:
Sister: Living?	Yes		No	Age at Death:	List any diseases or illnesses:
Sister: Living?	Yes		No	Age at Death:	List any diseases or illnesses:
Brother: Living?	Yes		No	Age at Death:	List any diseases or illnesses:
Brother: Living?	Yes		No	Age at Death:	List any diseases or illnesses:
Brother: Living?	Yes		No	Age at Death:	List any diseases or illnesses:

I hereby certify that the information that I have provided is accurate and complete:

_____   _____

Signature of Patient or Legal Guardian   **Date**

- *Health history form*—The patient lists information about his current and past medical, family, and social history, including allergies and current medications.
- *Authorization to pay medical benefits*—The patient signs this form to authorize his insurance to pay the provider directly, instead of sending checks to him. Sometimes the wording on this form is printed at the bottom of the patient registration form.
- *Release of medical information*—The patient signs this form to authorize the office to release his medical information to his insurance, other providers, spouse, children, or anyone else he names. The wording on this form may instead be printed at the bottom of the patient registration form.
- *Billing policy*—The billing policy is a form that providers use to explain how they will bill the patient's insurance and that they will bill the patient for any balance left after insurance pays. The patient signs this form to show that he understands the policy.
- *Consent to treatment*—The consent to treatment explains any risks or side effects associated with the procedure or service for which the patient is scheduled. The patient signs the form to show that he understands the risks and side effects and still wishes to receive the procedure or service.

Figure 1-9 ■ Authorization to pay medical benefits.

ROBERT R. HOFFMAN, M.D.

AUTHORIZATION TO PAY MEDICAL BENEFITS

I authorize my insurance company to pay medical benefits directly to Robert R. Hoffman, M.D. for services and procedures that I receive at his practice:

_____   _____

Signature of Patient or Legal Guardian   **Date**

RELEASE OF MEDICAL INFORMATION

I, _____ **ACTING ON**

BEHALF OF: (Print Name of Patient or Legally Authorized Representative)

_____ **HEREBY AUTHORIZE THE RELEASE**

(Print Name of Patient) _____

OF INFORMATION AS INDICATED:

My Healthcare Information

_____ I authorize disclosure of healthcare information (related to my medical history, diagnosis, treatment, or prognosis) to all inquiries or only to the following people or entities (for example, family friends, employer, insurance companies, clergy, etc.):

List Names:

_____

_____

Limited Healthcare Information

_____ I wish to limit disclosure of only certain kinds of healthcare information (related to my medical history, diagnosis, treatment, or prognosis) to the following people or entities:

List Names   **List information that may be released**

_____   _____

_____   _____

No Information

_____ I do not authorize release of any information.

_____   _____

(Signature of Patient or Legally Authorized representative)   **(Date)**

Figure 1-10 ■ Release of medical information form.

- *Notice of HIPAA Privacy Policies and Practices*—HIPAA stands for the **Health Insurance Portability and Accountability Act**, federal laws that require providers to notify patients that they will release the patient's medical information to his insurance and other healthcare providers. The form also explains the type of information that the provider will release, to whom, and the method of delivery.

- *Acknowledgment of Receipt of the Notice of HIPAA Privacy Policies and Practices*— The patient signs this form to show that he read and understood that the provider will release his medical information as stated in the Notice of HIPAA Privacy Policies and Practices.

The forms we reviewed are the most common ones you'll find in a medical office. Providers may give patients additional registration forms or forms related to an insurance's billing requirements, depending on the situation.

Mr. Russell returns the completed registration forms to Judy, who checks them to ensure that he completed and signed all of them, and she asks if he has any questions. He does not, so she then asks him for his $20 copayment; he pays, and Judy enters his payment into the software and prints a receipt for him. Note that some providers will collect copayments, commonly called copays, *after the patient's service,* rather than before.

Judy then enters the remaining registration information into the software, using the patient registration form that Mr. Russell just completed. Judy prints a copy of Mr. Russell's completed patient registration form from the software and creates a paper medical record

Figure 1-11 ■ Billing policy.

ROBERT R. HOFFMAN, M.D.
BILLING POLICY

We're happy that you chose our office for all of your healthcare needs. It's important that you understand how we bill your insurance and you, so please review this information carefully, ask us any questions, and then sign the bottom of this form so that we know that you understand our billing policy. Thank you.

As a courtesy to you, we bill your insurance company for your services and procedures. We verify your insurance coverage and benefits before your appointment and notify you of the insurance's expected payment and your financial responsibility. We give your health insurance company up to 60 days to pay or deny, and then we turn the balance over to you. Please note, if your insurance company fails to pay or deny your services and procedures, it is your responsibility to contact your insurance directly because you have a contract with your insurance company. If your insurance company pays or denies your services, then the insurance sends an explanation of benefits to us and to you showing amount(s) paid and amount(s) denied along with denial reasons.

We will also bill your secondary insurance after your primary insurance pays. We cannot bill your secondary insurance without proof of payment from your primary insurance. Please let us know if you change or cancel your health insurance, if you move, or if you change your telephone number.

Our office participates with many different insurance companies that require patients to pay copayments. The contracts we have with insurances are legal agreements that require us to collect copayments from you AT THE TIME OF SERVICE. We are not legally permitted to allow you to receive services without paying your copayment, and then bill you after you leave the office. Therefore, we expect you to pay any copayment owed at the time of service. If you do not have your copayment, then we may reschedule your appointment.

We will bill you for any balance remaining after your primary and/or secondary insurances pay. We expect you to pay the balance due by the due date printed on the statement that we mail to you, unless you contact our office to make other arrangements. We turn unpaid balances over to a collection agency who then reports the balances to the three national credit bureaus, which can adversely affect your credit score.

We accept checks, money orders, MasterCard, VISA, and Discover. Please do not send cash payments by mail. We charge $30 for returned checks.

If you have workers' compensation or auto insurance, we are legally required to bill it instead of your health insurance. In the event that workers' compensation or auto insurance denies payment for your services, we will then bill your health insurance, or we will bill you if you don't have health insurance. If auto insurance pays your claims and then auto benefits are exhausted, we bill your health insurance. For workers' compensation or auto insurance cases in litigation, we will charge you for your services.

You can contact us Monday through Friday from 8:00 am to 5:00 pm with any billing or insurance questions at (412) 555-1312, and we will be happy to assist you.

I have read and understood the above information. The office staff has satisfactorily answered all of my questions and addressed my concerns.

_____   _____

Signature of Patient or Legal Guardian   **Date**

Figure 1-12 ■ Consent to treatment.

ROBERT R. HOFFMAN, M.D.
CONSENT TO TREATMENT

I consent to care rendered to me and understand that my care may include an examination, treatment, and diagnostic testing (lab work, x-rays). I understand that I am under Dr. Hoffman's care and supervision. I also understand that any other employees caring for me work under Dr. Hoffman's supervision.

If I am receiving a procedure, then Dr. Hoffman and other employees have explained the benefits and risks to me, and I agree to the procedure.

_____   _____

Signature of Patient or Legal Guardian   **Date**

Privacy Policy/HIPAA Form (Sample)

ROBERT R. HOFFMAN, M.D.
Notice of Privacy Policies and Practices

This Notice of Privacy and Practices (the "Notice") tells you about the ways we may use and disclose medical information about you and your rights and our obligations regarding the use and disclosure of your medical information. This Notice applies to Robert R. Hoffman, M.D. and his employees and it is effective beginning April 14, 2003.

I. OUR OBLIGATIONS.

We are required by law to:

- Make sure that the medical information we have about you is kept private, to the extent required by state and federal law;

- Give you this Notice explaining our legal duties and privacy practices with respect to medical information about you; and

- Follow the terms of the version of the Notice that is currently in effect at the time we acquire medical information about you.

II. HOW WE MAY USE AND DISCLOSE MEDICAL INFORMATION ABOUT YOU.

The following categories describe the different reasons that we typically use and disclose medical information. These categories are intended to be generic descriptions only, and not a list of every instance in which we may use or disclose medical information. Please understand that for these categories, the law generally does not require us to get your consent in order for us to release your medical information.

A. For Treatment. We may use medical information about you to provide you with medical treatment and services, and we may disclose medical information about you to doctors, nurses, technicians, medical students, or hospital personnel who are providing or involved in providing medical care to you. For example, we will provide information about the results of your test to your physicians and his or her office staff.

B. For Payment. We may use and disclose medical information about you so that we may bill and collect from you, an insurance company, or a third party for the services we provided. This may also include the disclosure of medical information to obtain prior authorization for treatment and procedures from your insurance plan. For example, we may send a claim for payment to your insurance company, and that claim may have a code on it that describes your diagnosis.

C. For Healthcare Operations. We may use and disclose medical information about you for our healthcare operations. These uses and disclosures are necessary to operate our practice appropriately and make sure all of our patients receive quality care. For example, we may need to use or disclose your medical information in order to conduct certain cost-management practices, or to provide information to our insurance carriers.

D. Quality Assurance. We may need to use or disclose your medical information for our internal processes to determine that we are providing appropriate care to our patients.

E. Utilization Review. We may need to use or disclose your medical information about you in order for us to review the credentials and actions of physicians to ensure they meet our qualifications and standards.

F. Peer Review. We may need to use or disclose your medical information about you in order for us to review the credentials and actions of physicians to ensure they meet our qualifications and standards.

G. Treatment Alternatives. We may use and disclose medical information to tell you about or recommend possible treatment options or alternatives that we believe may be of interest to you.

H. Health-Related Benefits and Services. We may use and disclose medical information to tell you about health-related benefits or services that we believe may be of interest to you.

Figure 1-13 ■ Notice of HIPAA Privacy Policies and Practices.   *continued*

I. <u>**Individuals Involved in Your Care or Payment for Your Care.**</u> We may release medical information about you to a friend or family member who is involved in your medical care, as well as to someone who helps pay for your care, but we will do so only as allowed by state or federal law, or in accordance with your prior authorization.

J. <u>**As Required by Law.**</u> We will disclose medical information about you when required to do so by federal, state, or local law.

K. <u>**To Avert a Serious Threat to Health or Safety**</u>. We may use and disclose medical information about you when necessary to prevent or decrease a serious and imminent threat to your health or safety or the health and safety of the public or another person. Such disclosure would only be to someone able to help prevent the threat, or to appropriate law enforcement officials.

L. <u>**Organ and Tissue Donation**</u>. If you are an organ donor, we may release medical information to organizations that handle organ procurement or organ, eye, or tissue transplantation or to an organ donation bank as necessary to facilitate organ or tissue donation and transplantation.

M. <u>**Research.**</u> We may use or disclose your medical information to an Institutional Review Board or other authorized research body if it has obtained your consent as required by law, or if the information we provide them is "de-identified."

N. <u>**Military and Veterans.**</u> If you are or were a member of the armed forces, we may release medical information about you as required by the appropriate military authorities.

O. <u>**Workers' Compensation.**</u> We may release medical information about you for your employer's workers' compensation or similar program. These programs provide benefits for work-related injuries. For example, if your injuries result from your employment, workers' compensation insurance or a state workers' compensation program may be responsible for payment for your care, in which case we might be required to provide information to the insurer or program.

P. <u>**Public Health Risks.**</u> We may disclose medical information about you to public health authorities for public health activities. As a general rule, we are required by law to disclose the following types of information to public health authorities, such as the Texas Department of Health. These types of information generally include the following:

- To prevent or control disease, injury, or disability (including the reporting of a particular disease or injury).

- To report births and deaths.

- To report suspected child abuse or neglect.

- To report reactions to medications or problems with medical devices and supplies.

- To notify people of recalls or products they may be using.

- To notify a person who may have been exposed to a disease or may be at risk for contracting or spreading a disease or condition.

- To notify the appropriate government authority if we believe a patient has been the victim of abuse, neglect, or domestic violence. We will only make this disclosure if you agree or when required or authorized by law.

- To provide information on certain medical devices.

- To assist in public health investigations, surveillance, or interventions.

Q. <u>**Health Oversight Activities.**</u> We may disclose medical information to a health oversight agency for activities authorized by law. These oversight activities include audits, civil, administrative, or criminal investigations and proceedings, inspections, licensure and disciplinary actions, and other activities necessary for the government to monitor the healthcare system, certain governmental benefit programs, certain entities subject to government regulation which relates to health information, and compliance with civil rights laws.

Figure 1-13 ■ Notice of HIPAA Privacy Policies and Practices. *continued*

R. <u>Lawsuits and Legal Proceedings.</u> If you are involved in a lawsuit or a legal dispute, we may disclose medical information about you in response to a court or administrative order, subpoena, discovery request, or other lawful process. In addition to lawsuits, there may be other legal proceedings for which we may be required or authorized to use or disclose your medical information, such as investigations of healthcare providers, competency hearings on individuals, or claims over the payment of fees for medical services.

S. <u>Law Enforcement.</u> We may disclose your medical information if we are asked to do so by law enforcement officials, or if we are required by law to do so. Examples of these situations are:

- In response to a court order, subpoena, warrant, summons, or similar process.

- To identify or locate a suspect, fugitive, material witness, or missing person.

- About the victim of a crime.

- About a death we believe may be the result of criminal conduct.

- About criminal conduct in our office.

- In emergency circumstances to report a crime, the location of the crime of victims, or the identity, description, or location of the person who committed the crime.

- To report certain types of wounds or physical injuries (for example, gunshot wounds).

T. <u>Coroners, Medical Examiners, and Funeral Home Directors.</u> We may disclose your medical information to a coroner or medical examiner. This may be necessary, for example, to identify a deceased person or determine the cause of death. We may also release medical information about our patients to funeral home directors as necessary to carry out their duties.

U. <u>National Security and Intelligence Activities.</u> We may disclose medical information about you to authorized federal officials for intelligence, counterintelligence, and other national security activities authorized by law.

V. <u>Inmates.</u> If you are an inmate of a correctional institution or under custody of a law enforcement official, we may disclose medical information about you to the correctional institution or the law enforcement official. This would be necessary for the institution to provide you with health care, to protect your health and safety and the health and safety of others, or for the safety and security of the correctional institution or law enforcement official.

III. <u>OTHER USES OF MEDICAL INFORMATION.</u>

There are times we may need or want to use or disclose your medical information other than for the reasons listed above, but to do so we will need your prior permission. If you provide us permission to use or disclose medical information about you for such other purposes, you may revoke that permission in writing at any time. If you revoke your permission, we will no longer use or disclose medical information about you for the reasons covered by your written authorization. You understand that we are unable to take back any disclosures we have already made with your permission, and that we are required to retain our records of the care that we provided to you.

IV. <u>YOUR RIGHTS REGARDING MEDICAL INFORMATION ABOUT YOU.</u>

Federal and state laws provide you with certain rights regarding the medical information we have about you. The following are a summary of those rights.

A. <u>Right to Inspect and Copy.</u> Under most circumstances, you have the right to inspect and/or copy your medical information that we have in our possession, which generally includes your medical and billing records. To inspect or copy your medical information, you must submit your request to do so in writing to the Robert R. Hoffman, M.D. HIPAA Officer at the address listed in Section VI below.

If you request a copy of your information, we may charge a fee for the costs of copying, mailing, or other supplies associated with your request. The fee we may charge will be the amount allowed by state law.

In certain very limited circumstances allowed by law, we may deny your request to review or copy your medical information. Under federal law, you may not inspect or copy psychotherapy notes. We will give

Figure 1-13 ▪ *continued*

you any such denial in writing. If you are denied access to medical information, you may request that the denial be reviewed. Another licensed healthcare professional chosen by the Robert R. Hoffman, M.D. will review your request and the denial. The person conducting the review will not be the person who denied your request. We will abide by the outcome of the review.

B. Right to Amend. If you feel the medical information we have about you is incorrect or incomplete, you may ask us to amend the information. You have the right to request an amendment for as long as the information is kept by Robert R. Hoffman, M.D. To request an amendment, your request must be in writing and submitted to the HIPAA Officer at the address listed in Section VI below. In your request, you must provide a reason as to why you want this amendment. If we accept your request, we will notify you of that in writing.

We may deny your request for an amendment if it is not in writing or does not include a reason to support the request. In addition, we may deny your request if you ask us to amend information that (i) was not created by us, (ii) is not part of the information kept by Robert R. Hoffman, M.D., (iii) is not part of the information which you would be permitted to inspect and copy, or (iv) is accurate and complete. If we deny your request, we will notify you of that denial in writing.

C. Right to an Accounting of Disclosures. You have the right to request an "accounting of disclosures" of your medical information. This is a list of the disclosures we have made for up to six years prior to the date of your request of your medical information, but does not include disclosures for treatment, payment, or healthcare operations (as described in Sections II A, B, and C of this Notice), or certain other disclosures. To request this list of accounting, you must submit your request in writing to the Robert R. Hoffman, M.D. HIPAA Officer at the address set forth in Section VI below. Your request must state a time period, which may not be longer than six years and may not include dates before April 14, 2003. Your request should indicate in what form you want the list (for example, on paper or electronically). The first list you request within a twelve-month period will be free. For additional lists, we may charge you a reasonable fee for the costs of providing the list. We will notify you of the cost involved and you may choose to withdraw or modify your request at that time before any costs are incurred.

D. Right to Request Restrictions. You have the right to request a restriction or limitation on the medical information we use or disclose about you in various situations. You also have the right to request a limit on the medical information we disclose about you to someone who is involved in your care or the payment for your care, like a family member or friend. We are not required to agree to your request. If we do agree, we will comply with your request unless the information is needed to provide you with emergency treatment. In addition, there are certain situations where we won't be able to agree to your request, such as when we are required by law to use or disclose your medical information. To request restrictions, you must make your request in writing to Robert R. Hoffman, M.D. HIPAA Officer at the address listed in Section VI below. In your request, you must specifically tell us what information you want to limit, whether you want us to limit our use, disclosure, or both, and to whom you want the limits to apply.

E. Right to Request Confidential Communications. You have the right to request that we communicate with you about medical matters in a certain way or at a certain location. For example, you can ask that we only contact you at home, not at work or conversely, only at work and not at home. To request such confidential communications, you must make your request in writing to Robert R. Hoffman, M.D. HIPAA Officer at the address listed in Section VI below.

We will not ask the reason for your request, and we will use our best efforts to accommodate all reasonable requests, but there are some requests with which we will not be able to comply. Your request must specify how and where you wish to be contacted.

F. Business Associates. These are some services provided in our organization through contracts with business associates. When these services are contracted, we may disclose your medical information to our business associates so that they can perform the job we have asked them to do. To protect your medical information, however, we require the business associate to appropriately safeguard your information.

G. Right to a Paper Copy of This Notice. You have the right to a paper copy of this Notice. You may ask us to give you a copy of this Notice at any time. To obtain a copy of this Notice, you must make your request in writing to Robert R. Hoffman, M.D. HIPAA Officer at the address set forth in Section VI below.

Figure 1-13 ■ Notice of HIPAA Privacy Policies and Practices. *continued*

V. CHANGES TO THIS NOTICE.

We reserve the right to change this Notice at any time, along with our privacy policies and practices. We reserve the right to make the revised or changed Notice effective for medical information we already have about you as well as any information we receive in the future. We will post a copy of the current notice, along with an announcement that changes have been made, as applicable, in our offices. When changes have been made to the Notice, you may obtain a revised copy by sending a letter to Robert R. Hoffman, M.D. HIPAA Officer at the address listed in Section VI below or by asking the office receptionist for a current copy of the Notice.

VI. COMPLAINTS.

If you believe that your privacy rights as described in this notice have been violated, you may file a complaint with Robert R. Hoffman, M.D. at the following address or phone number:

Robert R. Hoffman, M.D.

Attn: HIPAA Officer
123 Unknown Blvd.
Capital City, NY 12345-2222
(412) 555-1312

To file a complaint, you may either call or send a written letter. Robert R. Hoffman, M.D. will not retaliate against any individual who files a complaint. If you do not want to file a complaint with Robert R. Hoffman, M.D., you may file one with the Secretary of the Department of Health and Human Services.

In addition, if you have any questions about this Notice, please contact Robert R. Hoffman, M.D. HIPAA Officer at the address or phone number listed above.

I hereby certify and state that I have read, and that I fully and completely understand the HIPAA policy above.

_____   _____
Signature   (Patient)   Date

_____
Signature (Patient Representative)   (Relationship to Patient)   Witness

Figure 1-13 ▪ *continued*

for Mr. Russell that includes all of his registration forms. Note that some practice management software allows you to scan completed registration forms directly into the patient's account to eliminate using the paper chart.

Judy attaches an encounter form to the outside of his medical record so that Dr. Hoffman can complete it after Mr. Russell's service. An *encounter form* is a preprinted form, usually in two parts or copies: one copy for the office, and one copy for the patient. The encounter form includes basic patient demographic information, along with a list of commonly performed services and their procedure codes, and a list of common diagnoses and their diagnosis codes (▪ FIGURE 1-15). Providers also call an encounter form a superbill, charge slip, or charge ticket. The physician can use the encounter form to check off the patient's procedure and diagnosis because it is easier and faster than handwriting the information. At your last doctor's appointment, do you remember how the physician completed a form for you to take to the front desk after the visit? You had to give the form to the person working at the desk, who probably kept a copy and gave you a copy. The form is called an encounter form because an **encounter** is the service or procedure that the patient receives. The date of an encounter is the date of service. The encounters of patients who are hospitalized run from the date that they are admitted to the date that they are discharged—a period that is also called their episode of care.

Judy leaves Mr. Russell's chart at the front desk, and Rhonda, the medical assistant, picks it up before she goes to the waiting room to call Mr. Russell. She introduces herself to Mr. Russell and escorts him to an exam room.

ROBERT R. HOFFMAN, M.D.

ACKNOWLEDGMENT OF RECEIPT OF NOTICE OF HIPAA PRIVACY POLICIES AND PRACTICES

I understand that Robert R. Hoffman, M.D. maintains paper and electronic medical records containing information about my symptoms, past and current medical history, family medical history, and social history, as well as information that details my examinations, services, procedures, test results, treatment methods, medications, and prognoses. Robert R. Hoffman, M.D. uses this information to plan my treatment, to share my information with other healthcare professionals involved in my care and treatment, to obtain payment from my insurance company or other third party, and to assess the quality of care rendered by any healthcare professionals treating me. I understand that these activities are the normal part of healthcare medical and business operations and do not need to have my consent to take place.

I have read and understood the Notice of HIPAA Privacy Policies and Practices given to me and understand that I have the right to object to using my health information and can request that my health information be restricted. However, Robert R. Hoffman, M.D. reserves the right to refuse care to me based on those restrictions.

I want the following restrictions for using and disclosing my health information (if applicable):

____

I have read and understood the Notice of HIPAA Privacy Policies and Practices.

______________________________ ______________

Signature of Patient or Legal Guardian **Date**

Figure 1-14 ■ Acknowledgment of receipt of Notice of HIPAA Privacy Policies and Practices.

TAKE A BREAK

Let's take a break and then review registration forms with an exercise.

Exercise 1.3 Registration Forms

Instructions: Match the name of the registration form to its description, writing the letter that represents each form in the space provided.

1. _______ The patient signs this form to show that he or she agrees to a procedure and understands the risk.
2. _______ The patient completes this form with his or her demographic and insurance information.
3. _______ The patient signs this form to allow the provider to give the patient's medical information to family members.
4. _______ When the patient signs this form, he authorizes his insurance company to pay the provider directly, instead of sending payment to him.
5. _______ The patient signs this form to show that he understands what private medical and financial information the provider will release and to whom.
6. _______ When the patient signs this form, he shows that he understands how the provider will bill his insurance company and that he may owe a balance after insurance pays.
7. _______ This form is a record of information about the patient's previous surgeries and health conditions, along with information about family members' health.
8. _______ This form is for the patient to read and outlines how the provider will release his private medical and financial information and to whom.

a. Health history form
b. Authorization to pay medical benefits
c. Release of medical information
d. Billing policy
e. Notice of HIPAA Privacy Policies and Practices
f. Consent to treatment
g. Patient registration form
h. Acknowledgment of Receipt of Notice of HIPAA Privacy Policies and Practices

Robert R. Hoffman, M.D.
123 Unknown Blvd
Capital City, NY 12345
(412) 555-1312

Encounter Form

Date of Service: _____   Account Number: _____

Name (Last, First): _____

X	Code	Description	Fee	X	Code	Description	Fee	X	Code	Description	Fee
Initial				**Established**				**Special Procedures**			
	99202	Expanded Exam	60.00		99211	Minimal Exam	35.00				
	99203	Detailed Low Complexity	100.00		99212	Brief Straightforward Exam	40.00				
	99204	Comp Moderate Complexity Exam	140.00		99213	Expanded Low Complexity Exam	45.00				
	99205	Comp High Complexity Exam	160.00		99214	Detailed Moderate Complexity Exam	60.00				
					99215	Comp High Complexity Exam	90.00				
Consultations				**Laboratory**				**Prescriptions**			
	99244	Comprehensive	150.00		36415	Venipuncture	20.00				
					81000	Urinalysis	30.00				
					82948	Glucose Fingerstick	18.00				
					93000	EKG	55.00				

X	Code	Diagnosis	X	Code	Diagnosis	X	Code	Diagnosis
	466	Bronchitis. Acute		401.9	Hypertension		460	Upper Resp Tract Infection
	428.0	Congestive Heart Failure		414.9	Ischemic Heart Disease		599.0	Urinary Tract Infection
	431	CVA		724.2	Low Back Syndrome		616.10	Vaginitis
	250.00	Diabetes Mellitus		278.00	Obesity		490	Bronchitis
	625.3	Dysmenorrhea		715.9	Osteoarthritis		244.9	Acquired Hypothyroidism
	345.91	Epilepsy		462	Pharyngitis. Acule		ICD-9-CM	Other Diagnosis
	009.0	Gastroenteritis		714.0	Rheumatoid Arthritis			

Remarks/Special Instructions	New Appointment	Statement of Account	
		Old Balance	
		Today's Fee	
Referring Physician	Recall	Payment	
		New Balance	

CPT® codes, descriptions, and two-digit numeric modifiers only are copyrighted 2012 American Medical Association. All Rights Reserved.

Figure 1-15 ■ Encounter form.

4. ***Encounter***—Mr. Russell's encounter begins when Rhonda weighs him and takes his vitals: blood pressure, pulse and respiration, and temperature. She asks if he is currently taking any medications, and he replies that he is not. She documents the results in Mr. Russell's medical chart and also documents his *chief complaint*. The chief complaint is the main reason for the patient's visit and is information that the patient provides. Mr. Russell does not really have a complaint; he is there for a physical examination, but Rhonda still documents this information. She then asks Mr. Russell to wait for the physician, who is expected to arrive soon.

5. ***Chart documentation***—*Chart documentation* includes medical information that the physician and other clinicians document in the patient's record. Rhonda already documented the patient's vital signs and chief complaint in his chart. Next, Dr. Hoffman enters the exam room, introduces himself to Mr. Russell, and reads Rhonda's chart documentation. He also reviews the health history form that Mr. Russell completed. Dr. Hoffman talks with Mr. Russell about his medical history, asks him additional health-related questions, and documents more information in the record.

Dr. Hoffman then conducts Mr. Russell's physical examination and determines that he is very healthy. He tells Mr. Russell this information and asks if he has any questions. Mr. Russell does not have questions; he thanks Dr. Hoffman, and the doctor recommends that Mr. Russell return next year for another examination, unless he experiences any health problems in the meantime. Dr. Hoffman dictates the details of the exam into his recorder, being careful to include all appropriate information and not to forget any necessary details. He also completes the patient's encounter form, checking off that the patient received an office visit and that his diagnosis was an encounter for a check-up. Remember that Mr. Russell did not have any health problems, but he still needs to have a diagnosis code for his visit. There are diagnosis codes that represent reasons for a patient's visit when there is nothing wrong, this visit is called a *contact for health services*. Dr. Hoffman gives both the medical chart and encounter form to Mr. Russell, who returns them to the front desk during his check-out.

6. ***Check-out***—Patients return to the front desk after an appointment to *check-out*: schedule another appointment; arrange for additional services, such as lab or radiology tests; have office staff call their prescriptions in to pharmacies or send them electronically (electronic prescribing or e-prescribing); and pay copayments if the office collects them at check-out rather than at check-in. Upon check-out, Mr. Russell gives his encounter form to Judy, who reviews it to ensure that Dr. Hoffman did not write any additional instructions on it. Since there is no other information, and Mr. Russell already paid his copayment, Judy gives Mr. Russell the bottom copy of the encounter form. She keeps the top copy. She thanks him for coming in and tells him that the office will call to remind him of his next yearly appointment. She then places the copy of the encounter form in Debbie's mailbox so that she can enter Mr. Russell's diagnosis and procedure onto his account in the software. Then the office will be able to bill his insurance.

7. ***Charge entry***—*Charge entry*, also called charge posting, is the process of entering a patient's procedure and diagnosis onto his account in the practice management software using the encounter form. Each procedure has an associated charge that the office then bills to the patient's insurance or to the patient. Debbie performs charge entry *daily* using the information on patients' encounter forms. Before Debbie can enter charges for all patients whom Dr. Hoffman treated during the day, John, the medical coder, has to verify that the procedure and diagnosis which Dr. Hoffman checked off on each patient's encounter form matches the chart documentation. Before John can review Dr. Hoffman's documentation, Ruth, the transcriptionist, must first transcribe it.

8. ***Transcription***—Each day, Ruth listens to Dr. Hoffman's dictation and transcribes it into reports, progress notes, or letters. She has to keep up with the work because John is waiting to review the documentation to compare it to the encounter forms. When Ruth finishes transcribing, she leaves the typed documents on Dr. Hoffman's desk to review

and sign. He then leaves them in a file in his office for Betsy, the filing clerk, to file in each patient's medical record. If Dr. Hoffman reads documentation that has typing errors, then he notes the errors and returns the documentation to Ruth to correct and resubmit to him. Note that providers can also hire outside agencies to perform transcription. The transcriptionist does not have to work directly in the office.

9. ***Medical coding***—After the documentation is transcribed, reviewed, and filed in each patient's chart, John compares the documentation to the encounter form. If the chart documentation matches the encounter form, then John can give the encounter form to Debbie for charge entry. But if it does not, then John must investigate why. It could be that the documentation shows that the patient received *more* services than what the physician checked on the encounter form, less services than what the physician checked, or different diagnoses than what the physician checked. In these cases, John would need to review the discrepancies with Dr. Hoffman to correct either the chart documentation or encounter form. John finds that Mr. Russell's chart documentation matches the information on his encounter form, so he gives the encounter form to Debbie to key in the patient's charges.

10. ***Insurance claim or patient bill***—After Debbie enters charges for the day, she is ready to bill insurances. Each day, she reviews claims to bill to ensure that demographic, insurance, and coding information are accurate. Debbie then creates *electronic insurance claims* and sends them to a *claims clearinghouse*. Electronic claims are claims that providers send to insurances using the computer. A claims clearinghouse is a company that the provider pays to check claims for accuracy before forwarding them to insurances for processing. The clearinghouse has the ability to *scrub claims*, ensuring that claims have all the necessary information for insurance processing. If they are error-free, they are called *clean claims*. The clearinghouse will notify Debbie of claims with errors, called *dirty claims*, and Debbie will have to correct them before resubmitting them to the clearinghouse.

Debbie is also responsible for billing patients after their insurances pay and for billing patients who do not have insurance. Patient bills are also called *patient statements* or self-pay statements. Because Mr. Russell paid his copayment at the time of service and his insurance will pay the rest, Debbie will not need to send a patient statement to him.

11. ***Payment Posting***—Insurances pay or deny claims that Debbie bills, and they send the office an *explanation of benefits (EOB)* or a *remittance advice (RA)*, a record of how the insurance processed a claim or group of claims (■ FIGURE 1-16). The EOB or RA can be paper or electronic and provides information about each claim, including the total charge, insurance payment, denied amount (if applicable), balance owed, and additional claim information. Rhonda, the medical assistant, is in charge of *posting payments* to patients' accounts in the software, also called payment application. Posting payments involves reviewing the EOB or RA, checking claim payments for accuracy, and posting them to the patient's account, deducting them from the balance owed. Rhonda's job is to verify that insurance paid the correct amount for each claim. If they did not, she will alert Debbie, who can follow up with the insurance to determine why. Some software programs also have the capability of checking payments for accuracy.

12. ***Follow-up***—Debbie performs insurance follow-up daily, checking the status of unpaid or partially paid claims on insurance companies' websites or contacting them by telephone. After she finds out why the insurance did not pay or did not pay enough, she can perform additional follow-up, such as rebilling a claim with additional information or correcting a claim that was billed with errors. Debbie can also appeal denied claims if she believes that the insurance denied them in error. She may need to meet with John to review codes on claims if the insurance denied payment. Debbie also performs self-pay follow-up on unpaid patient bills by sending bills and collection letters and calling patients to request payments.

Medicare Remittance Advice

BENEFICIARY NAME
STREET ADDRESS
CITY, STATE ZIP CODE

CUSTOMER SERVICE INFORMATION

Your Medicare Number: 111-11-1111A

If you have questions, write or call:
Medicare (#12345)
555 Medicare Blvd., Suite 200
Medicare Building
Medicare, US XXXXX-XXXX

BE INFORMED: Beware of telemarketers offering free or discounted medicare items or services.

Call: 1-800-MEDICARE (1-800-633-4227)
Ask for Doctor Services
TTY for Hearing Impaired: 1-877-486-2048

This is a summary of claims processed from 05/10/2011 through 08/10/2011.

PART B MEDICAL INSURANCE—ASSIGNED CLAIMS

Dates of Service	Services Provided	Amount Charged	Medicare Approved	Medicare Paid Provider	You May Be Billed	See Notes Section
Claim Number: 12435-84956-84556						
Paul Jones, M.D., 123 West Street, Jacksonville, FL 33231-0024						a
Referred by: Scott Wilson, M.D.						
04/19/11	1 Influenza immunization (90724)	$5.00	$3.88	$3.88	$0.00	b
04/19/11	1 Admin. flu vac (G0008)	5.00	3.43	3.43	0.00	b
Claim Total		**$10.00**	**$7.31**	**$7.31**	**$0.00**	
Claim Number: 12435-84956-84557						
ABC Ambulance, P.O. Box 2149, Jacksonville, FL 33231						a
04/25/11	1 Ambulance, base rate (A0020)	$289.00	$249.78	$199.82	$49.96	
04/25/11	1 Ambulance, per mile (A0021)	21.00	16.96	13.57	3.39	
Claim Total		**$310.00**	**$266.74**	**$213.39**	**$53.35**	

PART B MEDICAL INSURANCE—UNASSIGNED CLAIMS

Dates of Service	Services Provided	Amount Charged	Medicare Approved	Medicare Paid You	You May Be Billed	See Notes Section
Claim Number: 12435-84956-84558						
William Newman, M.D., 362 North Street Jacksonville, FL 33231-0024						a
03/10/11	1 Office/Outpatient Visit, ES (99213)	$47.00	$33.93	$27.15	$39.02	c

THIS IS NOT A BILL—Keep this notice for your records.

Figure 1-16 ■ Sample Medicare remittance advice.

13. *Balance paid*—The ultimate goal in the revenue cycle is to ensure that insurances and patients pay in full and on time. Remember that the provider has to earn enough money to operate, including paying employees. Ideally, if everyone working in the office performs their duties correctly and on time, the accounts will be paid in full. If patients do not pay their balances after Debbie sends bills to them and calls them, then Debbie can turn their accounts over to a *collection agency*. The collection agency attempts to collect payments from patients who never paid the provider or did not pay enough. The provider has to pay the collection agency, usually a percentage of total money that the agency collects. Accounts that Debbie turns over for collection are called *bad debt accounts*, and Debbie has to *write off*, or subtract, any patient balances that she turns over for collection.

The Revenue Cycle for an Established Patient

As you read through the steps in the revenue cycle and learned about the people and processes, did you realize how much work and how many people are involved in treating patients and earning revenue? Did you notice how each person had an important role in the overall process of obtaining insurance and patient reimbursement? The processes we reviewed for a new patient are very similar to those for an established patient. For an established patient, the provider would not need to obtain registration forms but would need to verify whether any demographic or insurance information changed since the last visit and then update the information on the patient's account in the software.

TAKE A BREAK

That was a lot of information to absorb! Let's take a break and then review the information with an exercise.

| Exercise 1.4 | Healthcare Delivery and Coding |

Instructions: Complete each blank field with the best answer, referring to the steps outlined in the revenue cycle.

1. Who was the employee in charge of coding, and how often did he or she perform coding?

_____

2. What do you think would happen if the coder did not perform coding on time?

_____

3. On whom did the coder rely to do their jobs first before coding could take place?

_____

MEDICAL CODING JOB REQUIREMENTS

When Mr. Russell called to schedule his appointment, Debbie verified his insurance coverage and benefits *before his appointment* to determine the amount that his insurance would pay and the amount of money Mr. Russell would have to bring with him. It was important for Debbie to verify insurance coverage and benefits before Mr. Russell's visit in order to protect the office from billing an insurance company that might not pay for the visit and protect Mr. Russell from being told when he arrived for his appointment that his insurance would not cover his service. Debbie's role was very important to the revenue cycle because it was one of the first steps a provider takes to ensure payment.

Judy also had an important role because she had to register Mr. Russell as a new patient in the software, correctly entering his demographic and insurance information. If she made any mistakes, Mr. Russell's insurance could deny his claim because his information was inaccurate. Rhonda and Dr. Hoffman both had important roles in providing hands-on patient care and correctly documenting medical information in Mr. Russell's record. Dr. Hoffman also had to dictate information for Ruth to transcribe, and he had to be sure that he completed the patient's encounter form according to the chart documentation.

Ruth's role was also significant because she had to type the dictation so that John could review it and ensure that codes on the encounter form matched chart documentation. Only then could Debbie enter Mr. Russell's service in the software and bill it to his insurance. If the insurance did not pay, then Debbie would also have to perform follow-up to find out why. Some offices may also enter charges *before* another employee verifies charges against the medical documentation.

Many variables in the revenue cycle impact insurance and patient reimbursement, and all employees must rely on one another to perform their jobs correctly and on time to ensure financial success and patient satisfaction. Having a solid understanding of the processes involved helps you to not only envision the coder's role in a physician's office but to also realize medical coding's financial impact on the office.

We discussed how important employees are to revenue cycle processes, but you also need to understand that without the patients, there are no steps in the revenue cycle and no jobs for the employees. In other words, the primary goal of every healthcare provider should be to provide excellent care and customer service to patients to ensure that they come back and that they tell people they know about their positive experiences. In healthcare, customer service is also called *patient relations*, because everyone working in the healthcare setting relates to patients. Remember that a healthcare provider is a business, just like any other business—a grocery store, clothing store, or hardware store—and it needs revenue to survive. Customers provide that revenue, and without them, there is no business. Keep in mind that when you work for a provider, the *patients* are your customers. Treat them well, and they will return; treat them poorly, and they will go elsewhere. To lose a patient to poor service hurts everyone: the patient, the employees, and the provider's business. Treat each patient like he is the *most important* patient. Only then will you ensure that the patient is satisfied with the services, you are satisfied that you've done a great job, and all the employees are satisfied that the office will continue to generate revenue.

Recall that not everyone working in a physician's office codes on a full-time basis. Medical assistants may be responsible for coding as part of their job duties; billing specialists may also code on a part-time basis, and other office employees may spend part of their jobs coding medical records. Whether coding is all or only part of your job, there are specific traits and skills that you should possess in order to perform coding successfully:

- Knowledge of medical terminology, human anatomy and physiology, pharmacology, and disease processes, along with methods to diagnose and treat them
- Knowledge of how physicians perform specific procedures and render services
- Investigative, research, analytical, and problem-solving skills
- Ability to prioritize work effectively, handle multiple duties on a daily basis, and meet strict deadlines
- Proficiency in practice management software programs or healthcare computer systems
- Ability to follow established rules without deviating but readiness to question information that appears illogical
- Follow-up skills necessary to perform work timely and accurately
- Ability to work positively with others
- Excellent documentation and organizational skills
- Ability to follow directions well and work with minimal supervision
- Flexibility with scheduling changes
- Professionalism skills, including delivering effective and efficient services to patients

- Excellent work ethic
- Excellent oral and written communication skills
- Ability to work alone as well as with a group

MEDICAL CODING JOB DUTIES

Full- or part-time medical coders working for different provider types perform many of the same job duties; however, their duties differ depending on the coder's area of specialization. For example, coders may specialize in coding for a general practice (primary care), obstetrics and gynecology, internal medicine, or any of several other specialties. Coders can also work in hospitals, specializing in coding outpatient or inpatient services, sometimes both. The job description shown next will give you a better idea of the tasks that coders perform, whether they work in a physician office or hospital:

- Review medical record documentation in detail and perform accurate coding of diseases, conditions, procedures, and services using manuals and/or software.
- Apply knowledge of medical terminology, anatomy and physiology, pharmacology, disease processes, treatment, procedures, and services.
- Apply **ethical standards** (standards that are morally right, correct, and legal) when coding, adhering to established principles, to avoid fraudulent or abusive coding.
- Query physicians and other clinicians to clarify information in a patient's medical record, including questions on medical necessity.
- Follow coding requirements for insurance billing, including knowledge of claims forms (CMS-1500, UB-04).
- Know basics of healthcare delivery systems and revenue cycle processes, and understand how coding relates to other functions and other employees' job duties.
- Maintain confidentiality of patients' medical and financial information.
- Research, read, and interpret state, federal, and local coding and billing regulations, and apply them to coding.
- Train others in the office, including the physician, other clinicians, and the billing specialist, on coding rules, regulations, charging, and documentation requirements.
- Communicate with billing staff on claim denials, appeals, and resubmissions.
- Review services and procedures built into the *charge description master (CDM)*, a list of all services and procedures, their charges, and applicable procedure codes, in practice management software, to ensure accuracy of descriptions, procedure codes, and fees. Revise, create, or delete information as needed.

CODING JOB TITLES, OPPORTUNITIES, AND PROFESSIONAL DEVELOPMENT

Throughout the healthcare industry, providers use different job titles for coders, including:

- Medical Records Coder
- Medical Coder
- Medical Records and Health Information Technician
- Medical Records Chart Auditor
- Coder/Abstractor
- Coding Specialist
- Coder Analyst
- Coding Auditor
- Coding Consultant

Coders can work for physician offices, hospitals, other providers, insurances, and consulting firms and may be part of a team in a medical records department or health information management division. The future job growth for the medical coding field is very promising. Coders have many opportunities to advance within organizations, including to supervisory and managerial positions. Employment for coders and coding-related occupations is projected to increase 14%–20% during the 2006–2016 decade, much faster than average for all occupations because of the country's aging population (U.S. Department of Labor, Bureau of Labor Statistics, 2008–2009 Occupational Outlook Handbook). As people continue to age, they will need more healthcare services, and this increases the demand for medical coders.

Coders who work for large physician groups, hospital systems, or insurance or consulting firms have more opportunities to advance and earn higher salaries. Coders working in rural areas typically earn less than those working in suburban or urban areas. Refer to ■ Figures 1-17 through 1-19 for more information on coders' salaries by experience and workplace from the American Academy of Professional Coders (AAPC) 2011 Salary Survey.

The Relationship between Billing and Coding

Medical coding is not the same as medical billing, although people often group the two professions together as though they were the same. In smaller physician offices, or for smaller providers, the billing specialist may also perform medical coding. However, in larger physician groups with many physicians and locations, and in hospitals, there are full-time billing specialists and full-time medical coders. For larger providers, full-time billing specialists and full-time coders work very closely together to provide information, clarify issues, and ask questions. Each must understand the other's job requirements. Remember that coding must be accurate and timely in order for billing to also be correct and on time. If an insurance company denies a claim due to incorrect coding or lack of medical necessity, the billing specialist will ask for the coder's assistance to review the medical record. The coder

Figure 1-17 ■ AAPC 2011 Salary Survey: Average annual salary based on all respondents. Reprinted with permission from the American Academy of Professional Coders.

Chart C: Average annual salary based on all respondents.

Answer Options	Response
Less than $20,000	1%
$20,000-$25,000	4%
$25,001-$30,000	8%
$30,001-$35,000	15%
$35,001-$40,000	19%
$40,001-$45,000	14%
$45,001-$50,000	11%
$50,001-$55,000	8%
$55,001-$60,000	5%
$60,001-$65,000	4%
$65,001-$70,000	3%
$70,001-$75,000	2%
$75,001-$80,000	1%
$80,001-$85,000	1%
$85,001-$90,000	1%
$90,001-$100,000	1%
$100,001-$151,000+	2%

Average Salaries by Region

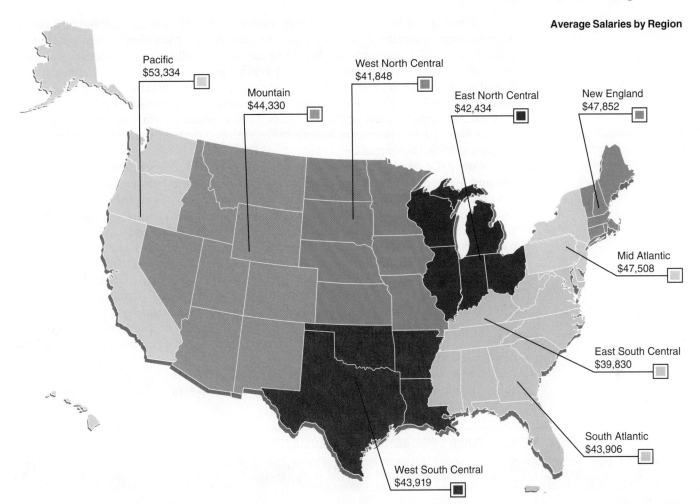

Figure 1-18 ■ AAPC 2011 Salary Survey: Average salaries by region. Reprinted with permission from the American Academy of Professional Coders.

will determine if the original codes were correct, make corrections if possible, and advise the billing specialist whether to appeal the denial and rebill the claim. Insurances have specific guidelines and regulations for both billing and coding, so both billing specialists and coders have to understand and apply all of the information to the work that they perform. Billing and coding employees share and discuss insurance regulatory information on an ongoing basis because regulations and guidelines constantly change.

Coding Certification and Membership in Professional Organizations

Salaries for certified coders are generally higher than salaries for noncertified coders. Coding certification means that a coder takes a national certification examination that

Chart E: Average wage of respondents shows disparity among group size.

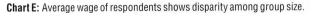

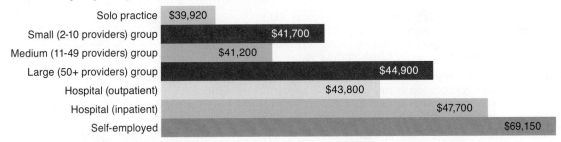

Figure 1-19 ■ AAPC 2011 Salary Survey: Average wage of respondents shows disparity among group size. Reprinted with permission from the American Academy of Professional Coders.

tests knowledge of medical terminology, anatomy and physiology, disease processes, pharmacology, procedures, and chart abstracting. A coder who has passed a national coding certification exam has exhibited mastery in the coding field and is called a **credentialed coder**. If you are interested in pursuing medical coding as a full-time career, then it is well worth your effort to pass a certification exam to earn a higher salary and become more marketable to employers. Many employers require job applicants to have national coding credentials, or the employers will not consider hiring them; other employers will hire coders without credentials but often require them to become credentialed within a specific time period.

Many different organizations offer coding examinations, courses, seminars, skills testing, and membership. Be cautious before you purchase services or pay for a professional membership from any organization without first ensuring that it is reputable and trustworthy. The majority of coding professionals choose one or both of the two most popular national medical coding organizations for professional membership and to take one or more national coding certification exams: the American Academy of Professional Coders (AAPC) and the American Health Information Management Association (AHIMA). Professional membership allows a coder to join local chapters, attend regular meetings, and participate in coding training to learn current industry trends and regulations. Members network and share ideas, suggestions, and job opportunities; they also can attend regional and national coding conferences. Becoming a member of a national coding organization enables you to take a national certification exam at a reduced rate and access members-only information, newsletters, and publications.

Here is additional information about the AAPC and AHIMA, along with information about their certifications. Refer to ■ TABLES 1-2 and 1-3 for background information

■ TABLE 1-2 **NATIONAL MEDICAL CODING ORGANIZATIONS AND CREDENTIALS OFFERED**

	American Academy of Professional Coders (AAPC)	American Health Information Management Association (AHIMA)
Year Established	1988	1928
Total Members	93,000	57,000
Membership Required for Coding Exams	Yes	No, but exam fee is higher for nonmembers
Student Membership Available	Yes	Yes
Coding Credentials Offered	• Certified Professional Coder (CPC) for physician coding • Certified Professional Coder-Apprentice (CPC-A) for physician coding without required experience • Certified Professional Coder-Hospital (CPC-H) for outpatient/facility hospital coding • Certified Professional Coder-Hospital-Apprentice (CPC-H-A) for outpatient/facility hospital coding without required experience	• Certified Coding Specialist-Physician-based (CCS-P) for physician coding • Certified Coding Specialist (CCS) for hospital coding • Certified Coding Associate (CCA) for coding without required experience, for both physician and hospital coding
Coding Credentials Nationally Recognized	Yes	Yes
Education/Experience Required for Certification Exams	Recommended: a high school diploma, coding education, associate's degree and two years of industry experience before taking certification exams	Recommended: a high school diploma, coding education, and three years of industry experience before taking certification exams
Apprentice Credentials Available	Yes: Allows coders without required experience to take certification exams and receive apprentice credentials. After coders have the necessary work experience, the AAPC removes the apprentice designation. No retesting is required.	Yes: Allows coders without required experience to take an apprentice certification exam. After coders have the necessary work experience, they take the standard exam to receive new credentials.

■ TABLE 1-3 ADDITIONAL CREDENTIALS OFFERED

AAPC	AHIMA
Certified Interventional Radiology Cardiovascular Coder (CIRCC)	Certified Health Data Analyst (CHDA)
Certified Professional Coder-Payer (CPC-P)	Certified in Healthcare Privacy and Security (CHPS)
Certified Professional Medical Auditor (CPMA)	Registered Health Information Administrator (RHIA)
AAPC certifications in coding, compliance, and reimbursement for specialty areas of medicine:	Registered Health Information Technician (RHIT)
Ambulatory Surgical Center (CASCC)	
Anesthesia and Pain Management (CANPC)	
Cardiology (CCC)	
Cardiovascular and Thoracic Surgery (CCVTC)	
Dermatology (CPCD)	
Emergency Department (CEDC)	
Evaluation and Management (CEMC)	
Family Practice (CFPC)	
Gastroenterology (CGIC)	
General Surgery (CGSC)	
Hematology and Oncology (CHONC)	
Internal Medicine (CIMC)	
Obstetrics Gynecology (COBGC)	
Orthopaedic Surgery (COSC)	
Otolaryngology (CENTC)	
Pediatrics (CPEDC)	
Plastics and Reconstructive Surgery (CPRC)	
Rheumatology (CRHC)	
Urology (CUC)	

about each organization and the coding credentials that each offer (obtained in 2010). Check both organizations' websites for more information about newly developed certifications and exam requirements.

Continuing Education

Both the AAPC and AHIMA require credentialed coders to enhance their existing skills and learn about new coding regulations, rules, and guidelines to keep current with industry trends. They must complete a specific number of **continuing education units (CEUs)** each year in order to maintain their credentials. Coders can earn CEUs by attending local chapter meetings, seminars, teleconferences, and web conferences; completing coursework; and teaching. Many employers pay a coder's membership cost because it benefits the employer when the coder develops additional coding skills and remains current in the industry. Some schools also cover the cost of a coding student's membership in a professional organization.

TAKE A BREAK

Let's take a break and then review information about coding careers with an exercise.

Exercise 1.5   Coding Job Titles, Opportunities, and Professional Development

Instructions: Fill in each blank with the best answer.

1. An individual could perform both coding and billing only when working for a _____ physician office or provider.

2. One job duty of every coder is to maintain _____ of a patient's medical and financial information.

3. A coder needs to train _____ on coding regulations, rules, and documentation and charging issues.

4. Skills required for medical coding include knowledge of medical terminology and knowledge of human _____ and _____.

5. The need for coding jobs is expected to increase _____ % to _____ % through 2016.

6. One benefit of professional _____ in a national coding organization is the ability to network with other coders and share ideas and suggestions.

7. Passing a national coding certification exam means that you are then called a _____ coder.

8. The two national coding organizations that most coders join are the _____ and _____.

9. _____ coders pass a national coding certification exam without the required work experience.

10. Coders who pass a national coding certification exam are required to maintain a specific number of _____ each year.

OTHER PROFESSIONS RELATED TO CODING

Do you remember when we discussed that coding may only be part of the job duties of some positions? You may want to work in one of these positions, and the section that follows will help you to become more familiar with them. It includes information about national membership in professional organizations and available certifications. As you move forward in your career, you might also wish to pursue supervisory or managerial positions and to obtain the relevant industry professional membership and certifications. Review ■ TABLE 1-4 for more information on positions that involve coding, their job duties, and professional organizations and certifications.

TAKE A BREAK

That was a lot of information to remember! Let's take a break and then review the information with an exercise.

Exercise 1.6   Other Professions Related to Coding

Instructions: Match the job duty to the position, writing the letter representing each position in the space provided.

1. _____ Performs administrative duties, such as coding

2. _____ Audits medical records to ensure that coding is accurate and appropriate

3. _____ Reviews providers' claims to check codes for medical necessity

4. _____ Reviews the accuracy of coding, billing, and regulatory compliance

5. _____ Checks insurance claims and codes for accuracy before billing insurance

6. _____ Registers patients' demographic and insurance information into practice management or hospital-based software

a. Registration specialist
b. Medical assistant
c. Consultant
d. Insurance claims examiner/processor
e. Billing specialist
f. Medical records auditor

TABLE 1-4 PROFESSIONS RELATED TO CODING

Position Name	Other Titles	Work Location	Common Job Duties	Professional Organization	Certification
Registration Specialist	Registration Clerk, Patient Access Specialist, Admissions Representative	Physician's office, clinic, hospital, other providers	Register patients' demographic and insurance information using practice management or hospital-based software, verify insurance coverage and benefits, code patients' diagnoses and procedures to determine medical necessity for Medicare and other payers, collect copayments and past due self-pay balances at the time of service.	National Association of Healthcare Access Management (NAHAM)	Certified Healthcare Access Associate (CHAA)
Billing Specialist	Biller, Insurance Biller, Medical Biller, Insurance Specialist, Patient Financial Services Representative, Patient Accounting Representative	Physician's office, clinic, hospital, other providers	Verify insurance coverage and benefits for patients, check insurance claims and codes for accuracy before billing insurances, bill insurances and patients, perform follow-up on unpaid claims and patient bills, communicate with patients on billing and collections issues.	American Association of Healthcare Administrative Management (AAHAM)	Certified Patient Account Technician (CPAT), Certified Clinic Account Technician (CCAT)
				American Medical Billing Association (AMBA)	Certified Medical Reimbursement Specialist (CMRS)
Medical Assistant	N/A	Physician's office, clinic, other providers	Take patients' vital signs, prepare exam rooms for patients, note chief complaint and additional documentation in patient's chart, assist physician and other clinicians with various procedures. Perform administrative duties, such as coding, scheduling, registration, billing, payment posting, and collections.	American Association of Medical Assistants (AAMA)	Certified Medical Assistant (CMA)
Insurance Claims Examiner/ Processor	Claims Examiner, Claims Processor	Insurance company or other agency that assists insurances with processing claims	Review providers' claims to check codes for medical necessity, verify insured's policy benefits to determine payment. *Note:* This position is not the same as a billing specialist who works for a healthcare provider and *sends* claims to insurance.	American Institute for Chartered Property Casualty Underwriter and Insurance Institute of America (AICPCU)	Associate in Claims (AIC)
				International Claim Association (ICU)	Associate, Life and Health Claims (ALHC) Program Fellow, Life and Health Claims (FLHC)
Consultant	Healthcare Consultant, Coding Consultant, Reimbursement Consultant, Coding Compliance Specialist	Healthcare consulting firm	Review accuracy of coding, billing, and regulatory compliance for physicians, hospitals, and other providers. May also code charts or specialize in CDM reviews, ensuring that charges built into the provider's software have correct codes and fees. Train others on coding, billing, reimbursement, and regulatory issues. Consulting positions typically require at least three years' coding experience and a coding credential. Many consulting positions are home-based and may involve national travel.	Healthcare Compliance Association (HCCA)	Certified in Healthcare Compliance (CHC), Certified in Healthcare Compliance Fellowship (CHC-F). A consultant may also have other certifications from the AAPC and AHIMA
Medical Records Auditor	Auditor, Chart Auditor	Provider, healthcare consulting firm	Audit medical records to ensure coding is accurate and appropriate; educate employees on coding, documentation, and regulatory issues.	AAPC, AHIMA	May have one or more certifications from either or both organizations

CHAPTER REVIEW

Multiple Choice

Instructions: Circle one best answer to complete each statement.

1. All providers and insurances use the same sets of codes to represent specific diagnoses and services, and each code represents the same _____ information to everyone.
   a. relevant
   b. standard
   c. objective
   d. important

2. The process in which a physician dictates into a recorder and someone else listens to the dictation and types the information into a document is called
   a. medical interpretation.
   b. medical documentation.
   c. medical dictation.
   d. medical transcription.

3. Coding a medical record involves reading the record and interpreting the medical language in it to determine the patient's
   a. charge for the visit.
   b. diagnosis and procedure.
   c. next appointment date.
   d. insurance coverage and benefits.

4. Medical _____ is defined as breaking down medical words into three parts: prefix, suffix, and combining form; defining each part; and then defining the entire word.
   a. record keeping
   b. pharmacology
   c. terminology
   d. physiology

5. All _____ and all _____ are required to use diagnosis and procedure codes.
   a. providers; insurances
   b. providers; physicians
   c. insurances; payers
   d. providers; hospitals

6. Providers need to establish medical _____ for patients, or their insurances will deny payment.
   a. terminology
   b. necessity
   c. objectivity
   d. subjectivity

7. The _____ works with other government agencies and law enforcement organizations to protect the Medicare program from fraud and abuse.
   a. Center for Medicaid Services (CMS)
   b. Center for Medicare Submissions (CMS)
   c. Centers for Medicare and Medicaid Submissions (CMS)
   d. Centers for Medicare and Medicaid Services (CMS)

8. A new patient is someone whom the physician has never seen or has not seen in the past
   a. six months.
   b. four years.
   c. two years.
   d. three years.

9. An established patient is someone whom the physician has seen within the past
   a. six months.
   b. eight months.
   c. two years.
   d. three years.

10. Whistleblowers, people who report fraud and abuse, fall under what is called the qui tam provision of the _____ Act.
    a. False Charges
    b. False Claims
    c. Fraudulent Charges
    d. Fraudulent Claims

11. _____ is the process of collecting insurance and partial demographic information, scheduling the patient's appointment, and verifying insurance coverage and benefits before the patient's appointment.
    a. Insurance verification
    b. Charge entry
    c. Preregistration
    d. Chart documentation

12. _____ must occur before the patient's appointment for two reasons: to protect the patient from receiving a service the insurance will not cover, and to protect the provider from rendering a service that the patient's insurance or the patient may never pay.
    a. Insurance verification
    b. Charge entry
    c. Preregistration
    d. Chart documentation

13. The _____ contains demographic and insurance information about the patient, including name, address, gender, birth date, and employer information.
    a. encounter form
    b. patient registration form
    c. health history form
    d. billing policy

14. The _____ is also known as the policyholder, the insured, the person who holds the insurance policy, or the person who is responsible for paying the patient's bill.
    a. patient
    b. transcriptionist
    c. patient's nearest relative
    d. guarantor

15. Another name for the date of a procedure or visit is the _____. For hospital inpatients, it is the period from the date of admission to the date of discharge, also called the episode of care.
    a. encounter
    b. counter
    c. preregistration
    d. consent

16. _____ is the name of the process when a patient returns to the front desk after an appointment to schedule another appointment, arrange for lab and radiology tests, arrange to order prescriptions, and pay copayments.
    a. Registration
    b. Preregistration
    c. Check-out
    d. Check-in

17. _____ is the process of entering a patient's procedure and diagnosis onto his account in the practice management software using information on the encounter form.
    a. Bill entry
    b. Charge entry
    c. Patient entry
    d. Copay entry

18. The _____ or _____ gives additional information about claims, including the total charge, insurance payment, and balance owed, along with other claim information.
    a. patient registration form; encounter form
    b. CMS-1500 form; CMS-1450 form
    c. explanation of benefits; remittance advice
    d. patient registration form; billing policy

19. Medical coding is not the same as _____, although people often group the two professions together as though they were the same.
    a. medical billing
    b. charge entry
    c. medical terminology
    d. patient registration

20. Salaries for _____ are generally higher than salaries for _____
    a. consultants; medical record auditors.
    b. physician coders; nonphysician coders.
    c. transcriptionists; medical assistants.
    d. certified coders; noncertified coders.

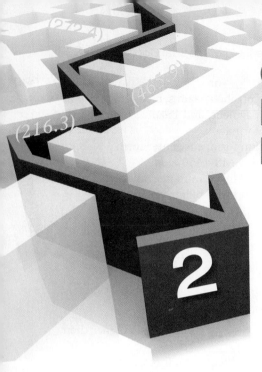

Coding Systems, Medical Records, and HIPAA Privacy and Security Rules

Learning Objectives

After completing this chapter, you should be able to

- Spell and define the key terminology in this chapter.
- Discuss the information that the ICD-9-CM and ICD-10-CM code sets classify, who created the codes, their effective dates, and their structure.
- Describe the ICD-9-CM code set for inpatient procedures, including their structure.
- Discuss the information that Level I CPT codes classify, who created them, and their structure.
- Describe the information that Level II HCPCS codes classify, who created them, and their structure.
- Identify the purpose of the National Drug Codes (NDCs) and explain their structure.
- Discuss how the healthcare industry uses diagnosis and procedure codes for statistics and tracking.
- List the types of coding references that can help coders perform diagnosis and procedure coding.
- Explain why it is important to know Medicare's coding regulations, and describe the four types of Medicare coverage.
- Describe types of medical records, including guidelines for documentation, and explain the subjective, objective, assessment, and plan (SOAP) format.
- Discuss the electronic health record (EHR) as it applies to the Health Information Technology for Economic and Clinical Health (HITECH) Act, including meaningful use and provider incentives to implement the EHR.
- Discuss the Privacy and Security Rules of the Health Insurance Portability and Accountability Act (HIPAA), confidentiality guidelines, the National Provider Identifier (NPI), and the Notice of Privacy Practices.

Key Terms

Acknowledgment of Receipt of Privacy Practices
alphabetical filing
breach of confidentiality
combination record
confidentiality
Current Procedural Terminology, Fourth Edition (CPT-4) code set
electronic health record (EHR)
electronic medical record (EMR)
Health Information Technology for Economic and Clinical Health (HITECH) Act

Healthcare Common Procedure Coding System (HCPCS)
inpatient
International Classification of Diseases, Ninth Revision, Clinical Modification (ICD-9-CM) code set
International Classification of Diseases, Tenth Revision, Clinical Modification (ICD-10-CM) code set
International Classification of Diseases, Tenth Revision, Procedure Coding System (ICD-10-PCS)
manual medical record
Medicaid
Medicare

CPT-4 codes in this chapter are from the CPT-4 2012 code set. CPT is a registered trademark of the American Medical Association.

ICD-9-CM codes in this chapter are from the ICD-9-CM 2012 code set from the Department of Health and Human Services, Centers for Disease Control and Prevention.

ICD-10-CM codes in this chapter are from the ICD-10-CM 2011 Draft code set from the Department of Health and Human Services, Centers for Disease Control and Prevention.

HCPCS Level II codes in this chapter are from the HCPCS Level II 2012 code set from the Centers for Medicare and Medicaid Services.

INTRODUCTION

During this stop on your coding journey, you'll learn about the coding systems that both healthcare providers and insurances use to code diagnoses, procedures, and services and to track and report information about patients' conditions and treatments. You'll study the coding systems in more detail and code diagnoses and procedures in later chapters. Think of this stop as a firm foundation on which to build your coding skills. You will have many opportunities to employ the skills that you learn to exercises in this chapter and continue to grow within the field of coding, utilizing your skills in the healthcare industry.

"The great thing in the world is not so much where we stand, as in what direction we are moving."—OLIVER WENDELL HOLMES

CODING SYSTEMS

■ TABLE 2-1 outlines all of the coding systems, also called code sets, for both inpatient and outpatient diagnoses and procedures. An **inpatient** is typically a patient who is hospitalized for more than 24 hours, but the inpatient stay can be less than 24 hours, depending on the physician's order. An **outpatient** is a patient who returns home or goes to another facility the same day after receiving a service or procedure at a hospital or another provider. The organizations that created each coding system add, delete, and revise codes at least once a year, and providers should always reference updated codes to avoid insurance claim denials. Refer to Table 2-1 as you read more about each coding system in further detail within this chapter.

■ TABLE 2-1   **CODING SYSTEMS**

Information that Codes Classify	Name of Code Set/Coding System	Date Created	Frequency of Additions, Deletions, and Revisions
Diagnoses—for patients of inpatient or outpatient providers	**The International Classification of Diseases, Ninth Revision, Clinical Modification (ICD-9-CM) diagnosis code set**	1979 For current use Will eventually be replaced by ICD-10-CM codes.	Twice a year, in April and October
Diagnoses—for patients of inpatient or outpatient providers	**The International Classification of Diseases, Tenth Revision, Clinical Modification (ICD-10-CM) diagnosis code set** Replaces ICD-9-CM diagnosis codes	2007 For future use Will eventually replace ICD-9-CM codes, Volumes 1 and 2.	Codes not in use yet
Procedures—for inpatients	**The International Classification of Diseases, Ninth Revision, Clinical Modification (ICD-9-CM) inpatient procedure coding system**	1979 For current use Will eventually be replaced by ICD-10-PCS codes.	Twice a year, in April and October

continued

■ TABLE 2-1 *continued*

Information that Codes Classify	Name of Code Set/Coding System	Date Created	Frequency of Additions, Deletions, and Revisions
Procedures—for inpatients	**The International Classification of Diseases, Tenth Revision, Procedure Coding System (ICD-10-PCS)** Replaces ICD-9-CM inpatient procedure codes *Healthcare Common Procedure Coding System (HCPCS)—two levels of codes:*	1998 For future use Will eventually replace ICD-9-CM codes, Volume 3.	Codes not in use yet
Procedures and services—for physicians and other providers	**HCPCS Level I: Current Procedural Terminology, Fourth Edition (CPT-4) code set**	1966 For current use	Yearly, in late summer or early fall for implementation on January 1; some CPT-4 codes are updated on January 1 and July 1 for use six months later
Procedures, services, supplies, drugs, and equipment—for Medicare patients★	**HCPCS Level II: National** Healthcare Common Procedure Coding System (HCPCS)	1980s For current use	Yearly updates, but other updates can occur throughout the year, as needed
Drug products that pharmacies typically dispense	**National Drug Codes (NDCs)**	1972 For current use	Twice a month

★Medicare requires HCPCS Level II codes, but many other insurances also mandate their use.

THE INTERNATIONAL CLASSIFICATION OF DISEASES, NINTH REVISION, CLINICAL MODIFICATION (ICD-9-CM) DIAGNOSIS CODES

Since 1948, the World Health Organization (WHO) has worked with countries worldwide to eliminate, provide statistics for, and track trends related to various diseases and conditions. Many members of WHO also belong to the United Nations, and together in 1979, these organizations created the International Classification of Diseases (ICD-9) coding system. The U.S. created its own version, which was based on WHO's ICD-9 system. This version is the **International Classification of Diseases, Ninth Revision, Clinical Modification (ICD-9-CM)**, which providers and insurances use. Two agencies within the U.S. federal government's Department of Health and Human Services (DHHS), along with the National Center for Health Statistics (NCHS) and the Centers for Medicare and Medicaid Services (CMS), are responsible for overseeing all changes and modifications to ICD-9-CM.

There are two types of ICD-9-CM codes: *diagnosis codes* for classifying inpatient and outpatient diagnoses, conditions, and reasons for encounters, which all providers and insurances use, and *inpatient procedure codes* for classifying inpatient procedures, which inpatient hospitals and insurances use. ICD-9-CM diagnosis codes classify *morbidity*—the presence of an illness, disease, or injury. It may interest you to know that the ICD-9 codes that WHO created are used to classify *mortality*—the condition that caused a patient's death. ICD-9-CM codes for diagnoses and inpatient procedures are valid until the tenth version of new and revised codes will replace them (ICD-10-CM). At press time, the DHHS and CMS announced its intent to delay the ICD-10-CM implementation date. Please refer to www.CMS.gov/ICD10 for current requirements.

Structure of ICD-9-CM Diagnosis Codes

ICD-9-CM diagnosis codes, also called I-9 codes, are three to five digits long (numeric) or can be a letter followed by up to four digits (alphanumeric). Here are some examples of codes and the conditions they represent:

- 390—Rheumatic fever without mention of heart involvement
- 428.0—Congestive heart failure, unspecified
- 808.49—Fracture of the pelvis, pelvic rim
- V72.0—Examination of eyes and vision
- E916—Struck accidentally by a falling object

THE INTERNATIONAL CLASSIFICATION OF DISEASES, TENTH REVISION, CLINICAL MODIFICATION (ICD-10-CM) DIAGNOSIS CODES

WHO updated ICD-9 codes several years ago to create the International Classification of Diseases, Tenth Revision (ICD-10), because they needed to create more classifications that better described and tracked diseases and conditions. Currently, 138 countries use ICD-10 codes to classify mortality, and 99 countries use ICD-10 codes to classify morbidity. Some countries developed their own version of diagnosis coding, based on the ICD-10 system, such as Germany's ICD-10-GM (German Modification). CMS and NCHS updated ICD-9-CM codes to create a new version, the **International Classification of Diseases, Tenth Revision, Clinical Modification (ICD-10-CM)**, structuring these codes from the ICD-10 system. ICD-10-CM codes are more specific than ICD-9-CM codes and allow detailed classifications of patients' conditions, injuries, and diseases. ICD-9-CM has 13,000 diagnosis codes, while ICD-10-CM has 120,000. The U.S. is the only country that will implement the ICD-10-CM version of codes. DHHS requires that all providers and insurances prepare for the new ICD-10-CM code set implementation before they become effective.

Structure of ICD-10-CM Diagnosis Codes

ICD-10-CM diagnosis codes, also called I-10 codes, are three to seven digits or characters long. The first character is a letter, and the second to seventh characters are letters or numbers. Here are some examples of ICD-10-CM codes and conditions they represent:

- J44.9—Bronchitis with airway obstruction
- L89.201—Pressure ulcer of hip, stage I
- O09.01—Supervision of pregnancy with history of infertility, first trimester

INTERESTING FACT: Early Diagnosis Classifications Are Over 300 Years Old

The system to classify diseases actually dates back to the 1600s in England where John Graunt, a British demographer (a person who studies population statistics), created the system. During Graunt's lifetime, no one kept records to show anyone's age when they died. Gaunt tracked many diseases that caused death in children and estimated that 36% of children would die from one of these diseases before age six. He also wrote a book, *Natural and Political Observations Made upon the Bills of Mortality,* which tracked deaths in London and helped to later determine statistics on the city's population. Other demographers and researchers found that Graunt's research and statistics were logical and valid, and his work became the foundation of diagnosis coding that we use today.

THE INTERNATIONAL CLASSIFICATION OF DISEASES, NINTH REVISION, CLINICAL MODIFICATION (ICD-9-CM) FOR INPATIENT PROCEDURE CODES

ICD-9-CM inpatient procedure codes classify procedures performed in inpatient hospitals. Insurances require inpatient hospitals to use ICD-9-CM procedure codes, along with ICD-9-CM diagnosis codes, on every inpatient claim. DHHS created ICD-9-CM inpatient procedure codes in the 1970s and implemented them in 1979 for all providers and insurances to use. DHHS oversees proposed revisions to the codes. ICD-9-CM procedure codes are valid until the tenth version of new codes will replace them.

Structure of ICD-9-CM Inpatient Procedure Codes

ICD-9-CM inpatient procedure codes can be up to four digits long. Here are some examples of codes and procedures:

- 62.0—Incision of testis
- 85.12—Open biopsy of the breast
- 31.61—Suture of laceration of larynx

THE INTERNATIONAL CLASSIFICATION OF DISEASES, TENTH REVISION, PROCEDURE CODING SYSTEM (ICD-10-PCS) FOR INPATIENT PROCEDURE CODES

The U.S. will implement a new version of the inpatient procedure codes, which CMS maintains. Several years ago, 3M Health Information Systems developed the **International Classification of Diseases, Tenth Revision, Procedure Coding System (ICD-10-PCS)** codes for CMS because the ICD-9-CM procedure coding system was old and outdated. ICD-10-PCS includes thousands of new codes to reflect advances in medicine over the past few decades and provides more specific information to describe procedures. ICD-9-CM has fewer than 4,000 procedure codes, while ICD-10-CM has almost 200,000 codes with room to add more.

Structure of ICD-10-PCS Codes

ICD-10-PCS codes, also called PCS codes, are up to seven alphanumeric characters. Here are some examples of codes and procedures:

- 02703ZZ—Dilation, coronary artery, one site, percutaneous approach
- 0UJH8ZZ—Vaginoscopy
- BW30ZZZ—Magnetic Resonance Imaging (MRI) of the abdomen

HEALTHCARE COMMON PROCEDURAL CODING SYSTEM

The Healthcare Common Procedural Coding System (HCPCS) has two divisions, or levels, of codes:

- Level I—Current Procedural Terminology, Fourth Edition (CPT-4) Codes
- Level II—National Healthcare Common Procedure Coding System Codes (pronounced "hick-picks")

Level I: Current Procedural Terminology, Fourth Edition (CPT-4) Codes

The American Medical Association (AMA) created CPT-4 codes in 1966 to classify physicians' procedures and services (performed in inpatient or outpatient settings), and other medical, surgical, and diagnostic services and procedures. Physicians, clinicians, and other providers use CPT-4 codes. The AMA maintains CPT-4 codes, including implementing yearly revisions, additions, and deletions.

Structure of CPT-4 Codes

Level I CPT-4 codes represent outpatient services and procedures and can be either five digits or four digits long, followed by the letter F or T, as shown here:

- 71010—Chest X-ray, one view
- 3470F—Rheumatoid arthritis (RA) disease activity, low (RA)[5]
- 0142T—Pancreatic islet cell transplantation through portal vein, open

Level II: National Healthcare Common Procedure Coding System Codes

CMS wanted a classification system for various services that were *not included* in CPT-4, as well as for physician and nonphysician services, medical supplies, equipment, and medications. In the 1980s, the AMA worked with CMS to develop a new set of codes, Level II **Healthcare Common Procedure Coding System (HCPCS)** codes. Examples of services, supplies, and items with HCPCS codes include ambulance services, medical and surgical supplies, drugs, nutrition therapy, durable medical equipment, orthotic and prosthetic procedures, hearing and vision services, and many other types of services that are excluded from CPT-4. Initially, providers had to assign HCPCS codes for Medicare patients; however, many other insurances found HCPCS codes to be very useful and began to require providers to use them. It is best to check individual insurance coding requirements to ensure that you report HCPCS codes on claims when applicable. CMS is in charge of maintaining Level II HCPCS codes including yearly revisions, additions, and deletions.

Structure of Level II HCPCS Codes

HCPCS codes are made up of a letter followed by four numbers and are grouped by similar items. For example, HCPCS codes beginning with the letter J, called J codes, represent drugs, and some codes beginning with the letter A represent ambulance services and medical and surgical supplies. Here are some examples of codes and what they represent:

- J2270—Injection, morphine sulfate, up to 10 mg
- V2756—Eye glass case
- A4206—Syringe with needle, sterile, 1 cc or less each
- E0130—Walker, rigid (pickup), adjustable or fixed height

The American Dental Association (ADA) created HCPCS dental service codes, called *Current Dental Terminology (CDT)* codes, or D codes, because these codes begin with the letter D. The ADA now holds the copyright to the codes.

NATIONAL DRUG CODES AND STRUCTURE

National Drug Codes (NDCs) are 11-digit codes that represent drug products. The digits identify the drug labeler (the company that manufactures the drug), the product name, and the package size. The Food and Drug Administration maintains a computer database of all NDC numbers called the NDC Directory. Insurances require pharmacies to report NDCs for all drugs they dispense and bill to insurances and patients. Here are some examples of NDCs and their corresponding drugs:

- 54868-1284-*2—Compazine tablets 5 mg
- 54569-5182-*0—amoxicillin tablets 500 mg
- 55154-7706-*0—Coumadin 7.5 mg

DIAGNOSIS AND PROCEDURE CODES FOR STATISTICS AND TRACKING

You already know that providers are required to assign diagnosis and procedure codes to patients' records to bill insurances. The codes also help various providers, organizations, and agencies to track patterns of diseases, such as how many patients the disease affected, where those patients lived, and whether or not the patients had other conditions at the same time as the disease. Do you remember hearing news about the swine flu (H1N1) virus, and how many people it affected, where they lived, and how many others were expected to contract H1N1? You may have also heard about the number of deaths that H1N1 caused. When you hear these statistics, the information often comes from DHHS, the Centers for Disease Control and Prevention, and WHO, all of which obtain part of the information they report from diagnosis codes that providers assign. WHO reported that within a year, 18,156 people died from H1N1 worldwide.

Coders enter ICD-9-CM codes into computer software, and Providers can also use the codes to analyze statistics on all patients with the same condition to determine how and why patients developed the condition. Providers can report the total number of patients treated, the time of year they were treated, their geographic locations, and how many patients died from the condition.

Like diagnosis codes, procedure codes also provide statistics for the types of services and procedures rendered to patients, how often they are provided, and in which geographic locations. Statistics help CMS, AMA, WHO, providers, and payers to track trends and predict future healthcare needs. For example, when you hear on the news that a certain number of patients in a particular city received influenza vaccines over the past week, the information comes from vaccine procedure codes that providers report.

REFERENCES FOR DIAGNOSIS AND PROCEDURE CODING

When you are coding for diagnoses and procedures in an inpatient or outpatient setting, you will want to become familiar with the coding references outlined in ■ TABLE 2-2 to help you to better understand coding guidelines and principles. Some coding reference publications are free, while others are not, so check with each publishing organization for more information.

■ TABLE 2-2 CODING REFERENCES

Name of Coding Reference	Description
ICD-9-CM Official Guidelines for Coding and Reporting	The ICD-9-CM manual contains these guidelines to help you understand the rules for assigning correct codes.
ICD-10-CM Official Guidelines for Coding and Reporting (**draft version**)	The ICD-10-CM manual contains these guidelines to help you understand the rules for assigning correct codes.
CPT® Assistant	The AMA publishes the *CPT® Assistant*, a monthly newsletter with updates on coding and billing regulations and guidance on how to assign specific codes. The CPT-4 manual contains coding references to specific issues of the *CPT® Assistant* that coders can review for additional information.
Coding guidelines in the CPT-4 manual	The CPT-4 manual contains many guidelines for coding specialty areas of medicine and specific services and procedures.
Centers for Medicare and Medicaid (CMS) manuals, local coverage determinations (LCDs), and program transmittals for Medicare coding, billing, and reimbursement	CMS publishes these documents, and providers can access the versions on the CMS website intended for their specific provider types. CMS publishes national regulations for providers across the country. There are also local regulations that apply to hospitals and other providers in certain geographic areas.
Federal Register	The federal government produces this daily publication, which coders can access to review coding rules and proposed rules before they are implemented.
National Correct Coding Initiatives (NCCI) edits	CMS publishes lists of procedure codes that providers cannot report on the same claim. Providers typically use software that reviews claims before sending them to insurance in order to find invalid codes that the provider needs to correct.
AHA (American Hospital Association) *Coding Clinic for ICD-9-CM* and *AHA Coding Clinic for HCPCS*	The AHA publishes both of these quarterly newsletters to help hospitals code diagnoses with ICD-9-CM codes and code services and supplies with HCPCS codes.
Fraud prevention and detection guidelines	The Office of Inspector General (OIG) of the DHHS publishes numerous documents outlining regulations for correct coding to prevent coding and billing fraud.
American Academy of Professional Coders (AAPC) and the American Health Information Management Association (AHIMA) articles and references	Both national coding organizations publish numerous articles on coding guidelines, as well as advice for accurate coding.

TAKE A BREAK

Let's take a break and then review more about coding systems with an exercise.

Exercise 2.1   Coding Systems

Instructions: Fill in each blank with the best answer, choosing from the list of terms. Write the letter representing each term in the space provided.

1. _____ is the presence of an illness, and _____ is the condition that caused a patient's death.

2. ICD-9-CM codes classify _____ and _____.

3. _____ codes will replace ICD-9-CM codes for diagnoses, conditions, and reasons for encounters.

4. Coding _____ help providers to accurately code inpatient and outpatient diagnoses and procedures.

5. All retail pharmacies are required to report _____ codes.

6. The AMA created _____ codes for physicians' services, and other providers also use them.

7. CMS created _____ codes for supplies and equipment.

8. The Healthcare Common Procedural Coding System includes two levels of codes: Level I _____ codes and Level II _____ codes.

a. ICD-9-CM

b. CPT-4

c. morbidity, mortality

d. mortality, morbidity

e. ICD-10-PCS

f. diagnoses, reasons for encounters

g. procedures, supplies

h. ICD-10-CM

i. references

j. NDC

k. transactions

l. HCPCS

MEDICARE REGULATIONS FOR CODING

When you perform medical coding, you not only have to learn the various coding rules and guidelines for specific code sets, or coding systems, but you also have to learn coding regulations from Medicare, along with other payers, because coding applies to billing and reimbursement. Notice that the list of coding references includes CMS publications because patients with Medicare represent a significant number of many providers' total patient populations, and coders have to follow Medicare's coding rules to ensure payment. **Medicare** is a federal government-sponsored health insurance created in 1965 for people who are age 65 or older, who are under age 65 and have certain disabilities, and who are of any age and have *end-stage renal disease (ESRD)*. Patients with ESRD have lost 95% or more of their normal kidney function and will not survive without dialysis (treatment for lost kidney function) or a kidney transplant. ESRD is also known as *chronic kidney disease (CKD) stage 5*, the most serious of CKD's five stages.

You will learn much more about Medicare coding regulations throughout this text. First, you need to know the structure of Medicare coverage composed of four parts, each of which covers a different type of service:

- *Part A Hospital Insurance*—Medicare Part A (hospital insurance) helps cover inpatient care in hospitals. It also helps cover *hospice care* (care for terminally ill patients) and some *home health care* (care patients receive in their homes). Most people do not pay an *insurance premium* (out-of-pocket amount for insurance coverage) for Part A because they or a spouse already paid for it through their payroll taxes while working.

- *Part B Medical Insurance*—Medicare Part B (medical insurance) helps cover physicians' services, outpatient care, and other medical services that Part A does not cover, such as physical and occupational therapy, and some home health care. Most people pay a monthly premium for Part B.
- *Part C Medicare Health Plan*—Insurances offer Medicare beneficiaries (insured) the option of having health insurance that replaces Medicare coverage. The coverage is designed to have similar benefits to Medicare, and only Medicare beneficiaries can qualify for it. The amount of the premium that the insured pays depends on the specific insurance plan he chooses.
- *Part D Prescription Drug Coverage*—Private companies provide this coverage, and beneficiaries may have to pay a penalty if they decide *not* to enroll when they are eligible. Most people pay a monthly premium for this coverage.

MEDICAL RECORDS

Now that you have learned about the types of coding systems you will use to code diagnoses, services, and procedures from medical records, we will discuss information found in a patient's medical record and different types of records. Another very important area we will also focus on are federal laws that you have to follow to keep information in a medical record private so that others who are not permitted to have the information will not be able to obtain it. Let's review the following areas to help you understand more about medical records:

1. Information Contained in a Medical Record
2. Structure and Organization of a Medical Record
3. Types of Medical Records
4. Conversion of Manual to Electronic Health Records
5. Medical Record Confidentiality

Information Contained in a Medical Record

Recall the steps in the revenue cycle in Chapter 1 when Judy, the front desk receptionist, created a medical record for Mr. Russell. Do you remember what types of information she included in the record? If you said demographic, insurance, and medical information, then you are correct! The patient's medical record is tied to an account number, or medical record number, usually a number that the practice management software assigns when a staff member registers a patient in the software.

Medical information in the record consists of any information related to the patient's encounter, including information on the health history form, information that the physician and other clinicians document in the patient's record for a service or procedure, lab test results, reports of radiology services (X-rays, scans), and medical records from other providers who saw the patient.

Providers also use information in medical records for *coordination of care* with other providers who also treat the patient. Coordination of care means that providers work together to ensure that the patient receives the best care and that providers in different locations are not duplicating care. One of the goals of coordinating a patient's care is to ensure *continuity of care*, which means that all providers work toward the same treatment goal for the patient.

Providers who document medical information in a patient's chart include the physician, also called a clinician, and other clinicians: physician assistant or physician associate (PA); certified registered nurse practitioner (CRNP); registered nurse (RN); physical, occupational, and speech therapist (PT, OT, ST); medical assistant (MA); psychologist; or social worker. Providers must date and sign their documentation, whether it is handwritten, transcribed, or computer-generated. Not all providers document the same type of information for a patient, and documentation depends on the provider's scope of practice (area of expertise).

Guidelines for Documenting Medical Information   Medical records are legal documents and belong to the healthcare provider, although the *information* that the patient gives to the provider belongs to the patient. Providers can use information in medical records not only to treat patients, but also to assess the quality of care that they provide, review trends and statistics for treating specific conditions, utilize the information for medical research, and provide additional information to payers. Physicians, other clinicians, and other healthcare employees have to follow rules for documenting in the medical record:

- Write legibly.

- Document timely to ensure coordination and continuity of care.

- Sign and date the documentation.

- Physicians/clinicians who supervise others must read the employee's documentation, co-sign, and date it.

- Correct errors by drawing a line through the error so that the error still shows, write the word "error" above the mistake, initial and date beside the word "error," then write the correct entry. Using liquid paper or markers to completely remove a mistake is not allowed because it makes it appear that the person documenting is trying to hide information.

- When a provider receives documentation about a patient, such as a test result or report from another physician, the provider treating the patient should review the documentation, and initial and date it before an employee files it in the patient's record.

Structure and Organization of a Medical Record

There are two basic structures for medical records:

- source-oriented medical record
- problem-oriented medical record

The **source-oriented medical record (SOMR)** is a filing system in a paper medical record where information is organized by its type or source. Providers file each source of information in a different section of the record: lab test results, radiology reports, physician documentation, and documentation from other clinicians. Information in an SOMR is not tied together and does not correlate to a specific condition; each source of information exists independently from the others. The SOMR is unstructured in its format, which makes it difficult for providers to locate information relating to a patient's specific condition or illness.

The **problem-oriented medical record (POMR)** is more organized because it groups information in the record according to the patient's specific problem or condition. The POMR contains the patient's chief complaint, health history information, specific problem(s), examination details, and the plan for treatment. Providers document patient encounters in a POMR using a **SOAP format**, which stands for subjective, objective, assessment, and plan. The SOAP format is very organized, and all of the information in a SOAP note, including the chief complaint, examination details, and test results, pertains to a specific condition. Some providers use a combination of the POMR and SOMR structures by including *both* information related to the patient's specific condition and information filed according to its source.

Information Included in the SOAP Format   The SOAP format makes it easier for the physician, and any other employee reading the patient's chart, to review documentation in a logical sequence. As a coder, you need to understand the SOAP structure so that you know where to find specific information for a patient's encounter, because it will help you to assign the correct codes. Review the following example of a patient's office visit to determine how to identify each of the four sections of the SOAP note for the visit:

- *Subjective*—Information that a *patient gives* the physician about the problem, providing details of the location of the problem, severity level, and when it occurs. Do you remember in Chapter 1 when we reviewed the definition of subjective? Subjective information is based on a person's opinion. In medical documentation, subjective information is based on the patient's opinion, *not* on the facts that the physician finds.

Examples of subjective information are when the patient tells the physician: "I've had stomach pains for the past two days. They are worse at night, about an hour after eating dinner. I've been drinking a glass of beer each night with dinner, and the past three nights I've had pork and sauerkraut." Subjective information helps the physician to better understand the patient's problem, know what follow-up questions to ask, and know where to focus the examination, procedure, or service.

- *Objective*—Information that the *physician gathers* during a patient examination and/or test results that a physician interprets. Do you remember what objective means? Objective information is based on facts, not based on a person's opinion. Objective information in a medical record is based on facts that the physician finds during the encounter.

  Examples of objective information are when the physician examines the patient and finds that he has abdominal swelling, and the patient groans in pain during the physician's hands-on exam. Other facts that the physician discovers are that the patient's skin feels moist and cold.

- *Assessment*—The assessment occurs when the physician *renders a diagnosis* of the patient's condition based on the patient's *subjective* information and the physician's *objective* information. In this encounter, the physician diagnoses the patient with abdominal pain caused by drinking alcohol and eating acidic food.

- *Plan*—The plan is *what happens next* based on the physician's assessment. A patient's plan could include a medication prescription, a follow-up appointment in two weeks, education for the patient on his condition, or lab or radiology tests, blood test, X-ray, or stress test, depending on the patient's diagnosis and need for further evaluation and treatment. In the plan for this encounter, the physician tells the patient to avoid beer and sauerkraut for a week to determine if the problem disappears and to call in a week if there is no improvement.

Transcribed Office Visit SOAP Note Review the following transcribed SOAP note for an office visit to see how the physician documented the patient's encounter using the SOAP format. The medical assistant documented the patient's chief complaint and vital signs (weight, blood pressure, temperature, and respiratory rate). You will also find definitions for abbreviations and medical terms included within the documentation.

Patient Name:	Cheryl Raines
Date of Birth:	7/15/55
Date of Service:	6/12/12
Chief Complaint:	chest congestion, cough, runny nose × 4 days
S:	55-year-old white female here today with cough and chest congestion, runny nose for the past four days. She states that her cough is productive with green mucus. She also reports that she is very tired, and her left eye has watered and been itchy since yesterday morning. Denies chills, fever, chest pain, headache, SOB (shortness of breath), and GI (gastrointestinal) disturbance. Patient states that all other systems are negative. She states that her husband experienced the same symptoms last week and is still not feeling like himself.
O:	Weight 142#, Blood pressure 120/80, Temp 98.6°, respiratory rate 17. Rhinorrhea (discharge from the nose). HEENT (head, eyes, ears, nose, and throat) otherwise negative. Chest is clear except for rhonchi (whistling or snoring sound the physician hears in the patient's chest).
A:	Acute upper respiratory infection.
P:	1. Treat with Z-Pak (an antibiotic to treat infection).
	2. Recheck if not improving or worsening.
	Robert R. Hoffman, MD

Did you notice that all of the information in the *subjective* part of the note came directly from Ms. Raines and was *her opinion*? Did you also notice that the *objective* information was from Dr. Hoffman's examination, *based on facts*? The patient's subjective information provided Dr. Hoffman with background details that told him where to focus his attention when examining Ms. Raines. In the *assessment*, Dr. Hoffman diagnosed Ms. Raines with an acute upper respiratory infection, a diagnosis that he based on both her subjective information and his objective information. For the *plan*, Dr. Hoffman wanted Ms. Raines to take Z-Pak, an antibiotic to treat her infection, and advised her to call for another appointment if she didn't improve ("Recheck if not improving or worsening.").

When you perform chart abstracting using the SOAP format, you will need to review all of the documentation, identify any diagnoses or procedures, and then assign diagnosis and procedure codes. In the previous example, the assessment part of the note listed the definitive diagnosis, an acute upper respiratory infection. The objective part of the note described the service that the physician performed, the examination, or the office visit. If the physician performed other services along with the office visit and also documented them, then you would also assign codes for them. In addition, if the visit did not result in a definitive diagnosis, then you would have to assign codes for the patient's symptoms, since the symptoms would be the only reason why Dr. Hoffman saw the patient.

TAKE A BREAK

Let's take a break and then review more about medical records with an exercise.

Exercise 2.2 Medicare Regulations for Coding Medical Records

Instructions: Indicate whether each statement is True or False on the line preceding each statement. For statements marked False, underline the word or words that make(s) the statement false.

1. _____ Coders need to follow Medicare's regulations for coding because Medicare patients represent a high proportion of many providers' total patient populations.

2. _____ Medical information in a record includes any information related to the patient's encounter, including health history and physician examinations.

3. _____ When all providers work toward the same treatment goal for a patient, it is called regularity of care.

4. _____ One guideline to follow for documenting in a medical record includes correcting errors by using a black marker to completely cover the error.

5. _____ A POMR is unstructured and makes it difficult for providers to locate information related to a patient's specific condition.

6. _____ The subjective part of a SOAP note includes information that the physician finds during the patient's examination.

7. _____ The plan part of a SOAP note is the next step for the patient's treatment, including tests, prescriptions, and follow-up visits.

TYPES OF MEDICAL RECORDS

You have learned that you can organize information in a medical record by using the SOMR structure, the POMR structure, or a combination of both. The POMR is the most common structure that providers use to organize medical records. The medical record may be in a manual (paper) format, an electronic (also called automated or computer-based) format, or a combination of manual and electronic. Patients may also keep their own personal health record (PHR), which contains all of their medical information from the different providers they have seen. Next, we will review these four types of medical records in more detail.

Manual Medical Records

Manual medical records (also called paper records) are made of a file folder that contains various file dividers with labels for specific information, such as progress notes, health history, and lab or radiology test results. Providers file information in a manual record chronologically (by date), placing papers under each labeled divider, with the most recent information at the top and the least recent information underneath in date order. Anyone reviewing the record can easily find the most current information by going to the top of the filed information underneath each divider.

Providers file manual records alphabetically by the patient's last name, first name, and middle initial, or numerically using the terminal digit system, where each record is assigned a series of three pairs of numbers and filed numerically from right to left. Refer to the examples showing records filed in the correct order using each filing system:

Alphabetical Filing—File records by the patient's last name, first name, and middle initial:

Arthur, Carrie R.

Fields, Betty J.

Johnson, Randolph A.

Neely, Jennifer B.

Neely, Jennifer T.

Paul, Mary S.

Yost, Jeffrey N.

Numeric Filing—File records from right to left in ascending order, starting with the lowest number in the last group of two on the right, then the lowest in the middle group of two, then the lowest in the first group of two on the left. If two charts have the same numbers in the last group, then file the numbers in the middle group next in ascending order. If two charts have the same numbers in both the last and middle groups, then file the numbers in the first group in ascending order. Review the following records filed in the correct order:

23-55-32

24-55-36

25-55-36

37-55-38

37-68-58

62-44-73

62-44-76

Advantages of using manual records are that information is located in one place and dividers help to classify various types of information. Disadvantages are that only one person can review the record at a time, records can become bulky as more information is added to them, and providers need to have enough room to store them or have the equipment and time to scan their images into another format.

Storing Manual Medical Records   Whether providers file manual records alphabetically or numerically, because of the confidential (private) information in medical records, providers should lock them in a filing cabinet or in a filing room and not leave records unattended where anyone can see them. Only certain employees should be allowed to access locked records. Providers may also store manual records in a separate area at the provider's location, in another location if the provider has multiple sites, or at an outside storage facility. Providers should lock stored records and restrict access to only those who need to retrieve records. Storage facilities must maintain the same safeguards to ensure that no one can access records without permission and that any records disposed of are completely destroyed and leave no paper trail.

Providers may also store manual records using less space by scanning all of the paperwork in a record and transferring each paper's image from the record to microfilm (one record per microfilm), microfiche (multiple records on a sheet of microfilm), or optical disk (one record per disk). Providers who scan manual records destroy them after scanning is complete. Providers organize and file microfilm, microfiche, or optical disk images by the patient's medical record or account number. State laws govern how long providers must keep medical records for patients no longer seen, discharged, or deceased; up to seven years is the *minimum* amount of time required throughout the U.S.

Electronic Medical Records/Electronic Health Records

Providers may also use a computer-based, or automated, medical record, called an **electronic medical record (EMR)** or **electronic health record (EHR)**. Providers store EMRs and EHRs in medical record software or through web-based technology, where providers access records using secure Internet sites. An EMR is an individual electronic record for one patient that includes all of the patient's information pertaining to *one provider*. An EHR is a comprehensive electronic record containing information about one patient that *many providers* access. The EHR is common in a health system with multiple locations of physician offices, clinics, and hospitals where different providers treat the same patient. Providers can enter information in an EMR or EHR by typing it into the record, scanning manual documents into the record, or using a device to speak information into the record so that speech translates into text (speech recognition).

Providers can locate a patient's EMR or EHR electronically using different criteria, including entering the patient's account number, medical record number, or name into a search field in the computer.

Keeping electronic records secure means that the person accessing a record should not read it in an area that is open to others walking by or working, as they could read confidential information. In addition, if you read a patient's record and have to leave your computer, then it is best to lock the computer so that no one else can review confidential patient information using your computer account. Providers must also implement technological safeguards for securing information in software and via the Internet.

One advantage of both EMRs and EHRs is that they help to streamline processes, allowing multiple providers to coordinate patient care, review patient treatments from all providers, and analyze statistical reports on the quality of care the patient received. Other advantages of EMRs and EHRs are that providers can simultaneously access the same patient's record and scan registration forms and other documents instead of keeping paper copies. Disadvantages include technical problems with software functioning properly and power outages that cause computers to go down or crash. Despite security measures implemented to protect patient records, there is always the possibility with computer software and websites that someone could access a record without permission.

Combination Records

Still other providers use a **combination record**, which combines elements of both a manual record and an EMR/EHR, with medical documentation stored in the EMR, and the patient's hardcopy forms and test results filed in a manual record. With a combination record, providers have the advantages of saving time and storage space when using the electronic record, but they face the same disadvantages associated with using a manual record.

Format of Medical Records   You also need to know that whether a medical record is on paper, electronic, or a combination of both, the healthcare provider can document different formats of reports for patients' encounters. These include the SOAP format as well as other formats for operative reports (surgeries), or hospital discharge summaries, which physicians create when discharging a patient from the hospital.

Personal Health Record

Patients may also choose to create their own **personal health record (PHR)** in order to share medical information with others, including caregivers, family members, and providers. They often create the PHR in an electronic format. A PHR is different from a provider's medical record for the patient, which the provider owns and controls. A patient owns his PHR, and it is a comprehensive record of the patient's care, regardless of where he received it. The patient adds medical information to the PHR and shares it with providers of his choice. Both providers and insurances may allow a patient to create a PHR using the provider's computer software or web-based technology giving the patient an individual user ID and password to create, revise, and access the PHR.

TAKE A BREAK

Let's take a break and then review more about medical records with an exercise.

Exercise 2.3   Types of Medical Records

Instructions: Match the term in the list to its description, writing the letter representing the term in the space provided.

1. _____ An individual electronic record for one patient including all of the patient's information pertaining to one provider.

2. _____ A record that contains dividers with labels for specific information.

3. _____ Filing according to the patient's last name, first name, and middle initial.

4. _____ The process of transferring images from a paper record to microfiche, microfilm, or optical disk.

5. _____ This record is also called a paper record.

6. _____ A comprehensive electronic record containing information about one patient that many providers access.

7. _____ An outside location where providers store medical records.

8. _____ Filing with the terminal digit system.

a. alphabetical filing
b. storage facility
c. grouping
d. personal health record (PHR)
e. chronological filing
f. electronic medical record (EMR)
g. manual medical record
h. numeric filing
i. personal health resource (PHR)
j. electronic health record (EHR)
k. scanning
l. filing cabinet
m. name filing

CONVERSION OF MANUAL TO ELECTRONIC HEALTH RECORDS

Because there are numerous advantages to using electronic medical records, many providers are converting from manual or combination records to an electronic record. Unfortunately, software or web-based technology for electronic records can be very expensive. Through 2015, the federal government will pay providers who participate with Medicare and Medicaid to transition from manual records to EHRs because it will help improve overall patient care and streamline healthcare processes. But what exactly does it mean to participate with Medicare and Medicaid?

A **participating provider** (also called a par provider) signs a contract with insurance, and the contract states how much the insurance will pay for specific services that are rendered to patients. Insurances typically pay participating providers *less* than their total charges for services. You may wonder why providers agree to participate with an insurance if the insurance will not pay the provider's total charges. A provider who participates with an insurance increases its chances of attracting patients with that insurance because patients would rather go to a participating provider than to a nonparticipating (also called nonpar) provider. When a patient visits a participating provider, his out-of-pocket expenses (the amount the patient pays) are less than if he chose a nonparticipating provider.

A provider can participate with various insurances, including Medicare and Medicaid, to ensure that patients with those insurances will choose the provider for services. Like Medicare, **Medicaid** is also a government-sponsored health insurance. It is for low-income people, although not everyone with low income qualifies for it. In the U.S., there are approximately 41 million Medicare beneficiaries and 42 million people with Medicaid. Providers participate with Medicare and Medicaid because of the high number of patients who have either or both of these insurances. A provider who does not participate with Medicare and/or Medicaid may experience severe financial distress because those patients will go elsewhere.

Health Information Technology for Economic and Clinical Health Act

The federal government will pay Medicare and Medicaid participating providers to implement EHRs because it will help improve coordination and continuity of patient care throughout the U.S. On February 17, 2009, President Obama signed into law the $787 billion *American Recovery and Reinvestment Act of 2009* (called the Recovery Act) to stimulate the economy. Part of the Recovery Act is Title IV, the **Health Information Technology for Economic and Clinical Health (HITECH) Act,** which established payment incentives to physicians and hospitals who participate with Medicare and Medicaid to implement EHRs as part of a nationwide EHR infrastructure (also referred to as a system or database). The DHHS Office of the National Coordinator for Health Information Technology (ONCHIT) is responsible for creating a nationwide health information technology infrastructure, improving healthcare quality and care coordination, and creating national standards to allow for secure electronic exchange and use of health information.

HITECH's goal is to develop a nationwide system for EHRs so that providers and insurances anywhere in the U.S. can access a patient's EHR, regardless of where the patient was last seen or the patient's type of insurance. The intent of a nationwide infrastructure for EHRs is also to enable providers and insurances to track healthcare services and trends more easily and report medical and financial information to state and government agencies.

Meaningful Use

CMS is in charge of paying incentives to providers who demonstrate what is called meaningful use of an EHR. *Meaningful use* means that providers have to prove that they will use the EHR according to the standards established in the HITECH Act for tracking patient information. These standards require them to record patients' demographic information, changes in their vital signs, and current medications; ePrescribe (send prescriptions electronically to pharmacies); and share additional patient information with pharmacies, such as medication allergies.

Through 2015, CMS will pay providers to transition from their manual records or existing EMRs or EHRs to a *nationwide* EHR. It pays Medicare-participating physicians up to $44,000 and Medicaid-participating physicians up to $63,750. CMS could pay hospitals as much as $2 million. After 2015, CMS will reduce Medicare and Medicaid payments to physicians and hospitals who fail to adopt the nationwide EHR.

Your Role in the Transition to a Nationwide EHR

Many people working in healthcare, not just information technology professionals, will assist with learning and implementing the nationwide EHR, including ensuring that providers meet HITECH requirements. Because you will need to learn how to access and use the EHR, you may also train other staff members to use it and help transition from either a manual chart or another version of EMR or EHR to the nationwide EHR. You will likely share your knowledge with physicians, clinicians, and other employees. These skills will make you more marketable to an employer.

TAKE A BREAK

Let's take a break and review more about EHRs.

| Exercise 2.4 | Conversion of Manual to Electronic Health Records, HITECH Act

Instructions: Complete each blank field with the best answer.

1. The Health Information Technology for Economic and Clinical Health (HITECH) Act established payment incentives to _____ and _____ participating physicians and hospitals to implement EHRs as part of a nationwide EHR infrastructure.

2. _____ is a government-sponsored health insurance for low-income individuals, although not everyone with low income qualifies for it.

3. _____ means that providers have to prove that they will use the EHR according to the standards established in the HITECH Act.

4. You may train other staff members and help transition from either a manual chart or another version of _____ or _____ to the nationwide EHR.

5. Having a nationwide _____ for EHRs would save providers time and resources because patients would not need an individual medical record for each provider they see.

6. A _____ is one who signs a contract with insurance, and the contract states how much the insurance will pay for specific services rendered to patients with that insurance.

MEDICAL RECORD CONFIDENTIALITY

We have reviewed the types of medical records, the information contained in them, and how providers structure that information. Whether you perform coding full-time or part time, you must follow federal laws that protect information in a patient's medical record. This means that you have to protect medical record **confidentiality** by keeping the patient's demographic, insurance, and medical information confidential, or private. Not only must you be sure not to read patient information that you are not permitted to see, but you also cannot release a patient's information to someone else who is not entitled to have it because it is illegal to do so.

As a medical coder you will be privy to sensitive patient information, including records for patients with drug addictions, sexually transmitted diseases, cancer, and many other conditions. You arc only permitted to review the aspects of records that relate to your job duties. If your job is to code a patient's diagnosis and procedure for an encounter, then you will be expected to only review the patient's medical information pertaining to that encounter, not to scan the patient's record searching for interesting information.

For years, providers tried to protect patient confidentiality and not release a patient's medical, financial, or insurance information to anyone who was not authorized to have it. Providers typically ask new employees to sign confidentiality agreements in which they agree to keep patient information confidential. Providers can terminate, or fire, employees who commit a **breach of confidentiality**, also called breaking confidentiality, which means that they release confidential information without permission. These breaches are also illegal. You will learn more about breaches in the next section.

Laws That Protect Patient Information

Federal laws include severe penalties for anyone who does not protect confidential patient information, called protected health information (PHI). The Health Insurance Portability and Accountability Act of 1996 (HIPAA) established both a **Privacy Rule** (December 2000) and a **Security Rule** (February 2003) to protect patients' health information. *Covered entities*—healthcare providers, health insurances, and claims clearinghouses—must follow the Privacy and Security Rules.

A major goal of the Privacy Rule is to ensure that providers protect individuals' information but still permit the flow of health information that is needed to provide and promote high-quality health care. The Privacy Rule permits important uses of information and still protects the patient's privacy. It also gives patients rights over their health information, including rights to examine and obtain a copy of their health records and to request corrections. The Privacy Rule requires covered entities to apply appropriate administrative, technical, and physical safeguards to protect the privacy of medical records and other PHI for whatever period the covered entity maintains the information. Providers must also apply safeguards to dispose of health information from old records discreetly and legally.

HIPAA also included *Administrative Simplification rules* through the Security Rule that established national standards to protect individuals' *electronic* PHI that a provider, insurance, or clearinghouse creates, receives, uses, or maintains. The Security Rule protects any patient's identifiable information exchanged electronically through software and/or the Internet and requires covered entities to implement administrative, physical, and technical safeguards to ensure the confidentiality, integrity, and security of electronic PHI.

Prior to the passage of HIPAA, both federal and state laws protected patient health information, but there was no single set of laws that everyone had to follow. A covered entity could release a patient's health information to others without notifying the patient. For example, a provider could release the patient's financial information to a patient's employer, who could then make employment decisions about the patient based on the information received.

HIPAA regulations require covered entities to appoint a *privacy officer*, a person who oversees processes for keeping patient information confidential. If a breach of confidentiality occurs that could harm a patient financially or otherwise, the privacy officer is in charge of notifying all involved parties. These parties include the patient, anyone who receives the patient's information, and the DHHS Office for Civil Rights (OCR). The DHHS OCR has specific requirements regarding methods and time frames for reporting and tracking breaches. You can find more information at the DHHS website at www.hhs.gov.

Privacy and Security Rule Violations   The OCR administers and enforces both the Privacy and Security Rules. Violating medical record confidentiality does not just mean that you will lose your job; it could also make you subject to fines and imprisonment. The Recovery Act established penalties for HIPAA Privacy and Security Rule violations, which can be either a *felony* (serious crime with severe punishment) or a *misdemeanor* (less serious than a felony but still punishable). Depending on the severity of the violations, penalties range from $50,000 to $250,000 and possible imprisonment.

When you are working with medical records in an electronic format, it is very easy for someone else (such as your manager) to find out whether you accessed a record without reason or permission. You need to have a computer sign-on ID and password to access electronic information. Someone else can use your ID to trace your whereabouts in the computer at any time. You leave a trail of your ID on every record you access, and time when you access it, so be very careful that you do not access records unless you need to do so in order to perform your job duties.

Anyone can report breaches of confidentiality, including your manager, the physician, a current or former patient or employee, and anyone else who suspects that his or her information, or someone else's information, was accessed or released without permission.

Guidelines for Maintaining Confidentiality

Follow these guidelines of dos and don'ts to ensure that you keep patient information confidential:

- Do not discuss a patient's demographic, medical, insurance, or financial information with another employee who is not working with the record and does not need to have the information.

- Do not repeat confidential patient information in public places within the provider's location (elevator, waiting room, front desk, hallway).

- Do not discuss patients with other employees where anyone else can hear your conversation. Go to a private place to hold the discussion.

- Do not talk with friends, family, or neighbors about a patient, no matter how interesting the patient's case may be and how tempting it could be to share it.

- Do not share your computer sign-on ID and password with anyone.
- Do refuse to answer questions about patients from people who do not need to know.
- Do report other employees to your manager or a physician if you witness them breaching patient confidentiality.
- Do lock or log off your computer when you walk away from it so that no one else can access patient information using your user ID and password.
- Do ensure that if you access patient information from outside the office, that the information is secure, whether it is in manual files or on a flash drive, laptop computer, cell phone, or personal computer linked to the Internet. An information technology professional working for your provider can help you to maintain security of electronic data transmissions.
- Do ensure that when anyone asks you for confidential patient information, do not release it without a signed authorization from the patient.

TAKE A BREAK

Let's take a break and then review workplace scenarios for maintaining confidentiality.

Exercise 2.5 Guidelines for Maintaining Confidentiality

Instructions: Read each scenario, and then explain how you would handle it in the space provided.

1. Candy, your neighbor across the street, stops you while you are cutting your grass in your front yard. She tells you that she knows that another neighbor, Alice Kline, has been coming to your office to see the physician. She asks you if Alice is all right. What should you say?

2. While you are working in the office and typing on the computer, a patient in the waiting room stands behind you and looks over your shoulder, watching what you are typing. You turn around and see her reading the information on your computer screen! What should you do?

3. You are riding on the elevator with two of your coworkers. They mention John Robbins, a patient in the office, and say that John is now receiving chemotherapy to treat his lung cancer. There are three other people in the elevator who can hear your coworkers' conversation. What should you do or say?

National Provider Identifier Standard, Transactions, and Code Sets

CMS administers and enforces other HIPAA Administrative Simplification rules through the Security Rule, which mandates the use of the *National Provider Identifier (NPI)*, a 10-digit number that is unique to each provider for electronic transmissions. All providers have an NPI and must report it on claims billed to insurances. The Administrative Simplification rules also include standards for electronic transactions and code sets. Transaction standards mean that when providers, insurances, and clearinghouses share or send electronic information through transmissions, called *electronic data interchange (EDI)*, they must use specific formats that a computer system will recognize.

Transactions include electronic communications between providers, providers and insurances, providers and claims clearinghouses, and insurances and claims clearinghouses. Examples of transactions include when a physician or hospital electronically verifies a patient's insurance eligibility and benefits, or bills insurances directly or through a claims clearinghouse. The Administrative Simplification rules require that for all electronic transmissions, all covered entities use the same codes for diagnoses (ICD-9-CM, ICD-10-CM, and ICD-10-PCS) and procedures (CPT-4 and HCPCS), as well as CDT and NDC codes.

Transactions are made up of code sets, which are the way that computers send and receive electronic information. A *code set* is written in computer language and is used to send and receive electronic transmissions, a process called encoding. Although you will hear and read about the transaction code sets, the actual work of programming computers to use the correct electronic code sets typically falls to individuals working in the field of information technology, not to a medical coder. However, you may have to review coding and claim information in practice management software to ensure that it complies with the required transaction standards. The Accredited Standards Committee (ASC) developed the standard transactions and code sets X12 version 5010 that covered entities must use for electronic transactions.

Notice of Privacy Practices and Acknowledgment of Receipt of Privacy Practices

HIPAA regulations require providers to notify patients of how they will share patients' demographic, insurance, and medical information with a **Notice of Privacy Practices**. Patients need to sign an **Acknowledgment of Receipt of Privacy Practices** to show that they have read the Notice of Privacy Practices and understand how, when, and to whom the provider will release their PHI.

The Acknowledgment of Receipt of Privacy Practices is *not* the patient's authorization to release PHI. HIPAA regulations permit providers to release PHI *without* the patient's permission for the following reasons: patient treatment and coordination of care with other providers, insurance coverage verification, insurance billing, and other health care operations, including activities that support covered entities' normal business functions.

Providers may not release patients' PHI for any other reason without the patient's permission. Patients must authorize the provider to give medical information to a patient's spouse or to leave messages on the patient's home answering machine or voice mail.

Providers can give patients copies of the Notice of Privacy Practices or post it in the waiting area for them to read. Recall from Chapter 1 that Judy gave Mr. Russell a copy of the Notice of Privacy Practices, and he had to sign an Acknowledgment stating that he had read the Notice and understood its meaning.

TAKE A BREAK

Let's take a break and then review more about confidentiality with an exercise.

Exercise 2.6   **Medical Record Confidentiality, HIPAA Privacy Rule, and Security Rule**

Instructions: Complete each blank field with the best answer.

1. A major goal of the _____ is to ensure that individuals' health information is properly protected, while allowing the flow of health information needed to provide and promote high-quality health care and to protect the public's health and well-being.

2. Your computer _____ allows someone else to trace your whereabouts in the computer at any time.

3. When you protect medical record _____, you keep the patient's demographic, insurance, and medical information private.

4. Under HIPAA, healthcare providers, health insurances, and claims clearinghouses are referred to as _____.

5. A _____ is a serious crime with severe punishment, and a _____ is a less serious (but still punishable) crime.

6. HIPAA regulations permit providers to release _____ without the patient's permission for specific reasons.

7. One way to protect private patient information is not to share your computer _____ and _____ with anyone.

8. The _____ is a 10-digit number that is unique to each provider and is used for electronic transmissions.

9. The Administrative Simplification rules require that for all electronic transmissions, providers, insurances, and claims clearinghouses must use the same codes for _____ and the same codes for _____.

10. HIPAA's Administrative Simplification rules through the _____ established national standards to protect individuals' *electronic* PHI that a provider, insurance, or clearinghouse creates, receives, uses, or maintains.

CHAPTER REVIEW

Multiple Choice

Instructions: Circle one best answer to complete each statement.

1. The code set that is currently used to classify diagnoses is
   a. ICD-10-CM.
   b. ICD-9-CM.
   c. ICD-10-PCS.
   d. CPT-4.

2. The code set that the AMA created to classify physicians' services is
   a. NDC.
   b. ICD-10-PCS.
   c. CPT-4.
   d. HCPCS Level II.

3. The new code set to classify diagnoses is
   a. ICD-10-CM.
   b. CPT-4.
   c. ICD-10-PCS.
   d. HCPCS Level II.

4. The code set that is currently used to classify inpatient procedures is
   a. ICD-10-CM.
   b. ICD-9-CM.
   c. ICD-10-PCS.
   d. HCPCS Level II.

5. The code set that CMS created to classify outpatient procedures, equipment, and supplies is
   a. NDC.
   b. ICD-10-PCS.
   c. CPT-4.
   d. HCPCS Level II.

6. The new code set for inpatient procedures that will replace ICD-9-CM, Volume 3 codes is
   a. ICD-10-CM.
   b. NDC.
   c. ICD-10-PCS.
   d. HCPCS Level II.

7. The code set that is used to classify drugs is
   a. ICD-10-PCS.
   b. NDC.
   c. CPT-4
   d. HCPCS Level II.

8. The code set that is used to classify dental services and procedures is
   a. CDT.
   b. NDC.
   c. CPT-4.
   d. HCPCS Level II.

9. Medicare Part _____ covers physicians' services and other outpatient care.
   a. A
   b. B
   c. C
   d. D

10. Medicare Part _____ covers inpatient care in hospitals.
    a. A
    b. B
    c. C
    d. D

11. When providers work together to ensure that patients receive the best care and that they do not duplicate care, it is called
    a. maintenance of care.
    b. group care.
    c. coordination of care.
    d. documentation of care.

12. The two basic structures of medical records are the
    a. MORS and MORP.
    b. SMOR and PMOR.
    c. SORM and PORM.
    d. SOMR and POMR.

13. The four sections of SOAP documentation are
    a. subjective, objective, advancement, plan.
    b. subjective, objective, assessment, plan.
    c. summary, objective, assessment, plan.
    d. subjective, objective, assessment, problem.

14. The comprehensive medical record for one patient that includes all of the patient's information that many providers can access and share is called a(n)
    a. manual medical record.
    b. personal health record.
    c. electronic medical record.
    d. electronic health record.

15. Part of the HITECH Act includes payment incentives to Medicare and Medicaid participating physicians and hospitals to
    a. implement electronic health records.
    b. implement electronic medical records.
    c. implement practice management software.
    d. implement manual medical records.

16. Meaningful use means that providers have to prove that they will
    a. bill Medicare and Medicaid claims electronically.
    b. include diagnosis and procedure codes on electronic claims.

c. use the electronic health record according to the HITECH Act's standards.

d. use the manual medical record according to the HITECH Act's standards.

17. HIPAA includes the Privacy and Security Rules to ensure that
a. patients create and control their personal health records.
b. providers protect patients' confidential information, including electronic information.
c. providers can share confidential patient information as needed.
d. providers implement electronic medical records.

18. _____ include electronic communication between providers, providers and insurances, providers and claims clearinghouses, and insurances and claims clearinghouses.
a. Connections
b. Practices
c. Authorizations
d. Transactions

19. A computer sends and receives electronic transmissions in the form of
a. code groupings.
b. electronic sets.
c. transmission sets.
d. code sets.

20. Providers notify patients of how they will share patients' demographic, insurance, and medical information with the
a. Notice of Privacy Standards.
b. Notice of Privacy Practices.
c. Notice of Security Practices.
d. Notice of HIPAA Standards.

SECTION TWO

Introduction to ICD-9-CM and ICD-10-CM Coding

(465.9)

(216.3)

(272.4)

(296.2)

(787.91)

(789.07)

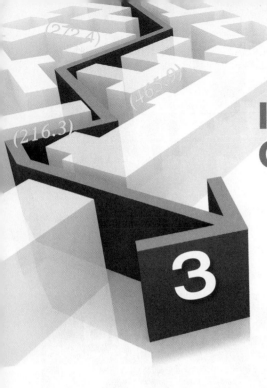

Introduction to ICD-9-CM Coding

Learning Objectives

After completing this chapter, you should be able to

- Spell and define the key terminology in this chapter.
- Define ethical standards and explain how they apply to coding.
- Discuss key points to remember when coding.
- Describe the three volumes of the ICD-9-CM manual and name the Appendices.
- Discuss the two sections of ICD-9-CM Volume 1, Tabular List.
- Explain the structure of the 17 chapters of the Classification of Diseases and Injuries, and discuss the meaning of coding to the highest level of specificity.
- List guidelines for coding to the highest level of specificity.
- Describe the structure and purpose of each of the ICD-9-CM Appendices.
- Describe the three sections of Volume 2, the Alphabetic Index.
- Define main term, subterm, and carryover line in the Alphabetic Index.
- Explain how to locate main terms and subterms and understand their structure.
- Discuss the two tables located in the Alphabetic Index and the information that they contain.

Key Terms

Alphabetic Index, Volume 2
Appendix A
Appendix B
Appendix C
Appendix D
Appendix E
carryover line
category
chapters
eponym
ethical standards
highest level of specificity
Hypertension Table
ICD-9-CM Official Guidelines for Coding and Reporting
Index to External Causes of Injury (E code)

main term
Neoplasm Table
nonessential modifier
section
subcategory
subclassification
subterm
Supplementary Classification of External Causes of Injury and Poisoning (E code)
Table of Drugs and Chemicals
Tabular List, Volume 1
Tabular List and Alphabetic Index, Volume 3
V codes—Supplementary Classification of Factors Influencing Health Status and Contact with Health Services

INTRODUCTION

During this stop on your journey, you will review the diagnosis coding manual and become familiar with its various sections. You will also learn more detail about diagnosis codes, including different types of codes and how to assign them. When you know how to use the coding manual, you will be on your way to learning more detailed information in additional chapters where you will code many different types of conditions. Do not forget

ICD-9-CM codes in this chapter are from the ICD-9-CM 2012 code set from the Department of Health and Human Services, Centers for Disease Control and Prevention.

to consult your medical references, and use them often if you do not understand a condition or want to learn more about it. The more you learn, and the more you practice what you have learned, the more successful you will be in the healthcare field!

"Learning is not attained by chance. It must be sought for with ardor and attended to with diligence."—ABIGAIL ADAMS

INTERNATIONAL CLASSIFICATION OF DISEASES, NINTH REVISION, CLINICAL MODIFICATION CODES

Recall from Chapter 2 that the diagnosis code set that providers and payers currently use is the International Classification of Diseases, Ninth Revision, Clinical Modification (ICD-9-CM). There are two types of ICD-9-CM codes:

- *Diagnosis codes*—for classifying inpatient and outpatient diagnoses, conditions, and reasons for encounters, which all providers and insurances use
- *Inpatient procedure codes*—for classifying inpatient procedures, which inpatient hospitals and insurances use

ICD-9-CM diagnosis codes classify *morbidity*, the presence of an illness, disease, or injury. The National Center for Health Statistics (NCHS) and the Centers for Medicare and Medicaid Services (CMS) oversee all changes and modifications to the ICD-9-CM. ICD-9-CM codes for diagnoses and inpatient procedures are valid until the tenth version of new and revised codes will replace them: the International Classification of Diseases, Tenth Revision, Clinical Modification (ICD-10-CM) for diagnoses, and the International Classification of Diseases, Tenth Revision, Procedure Coding System (ICD-10-PCS) for inpatient procedures. (We'll review more about ICD-10-CM codes in Chapter 6 and ICD-10-PCS codes in Chapter 16.)

Remember that ICD-9-CM diagnosis codes, or I-9 codes, are three to five digits long (numeric) or can start with the letter V or E, followed by up to four digits (alphanumeric). The first three characters are followed by a decimal point. Here are some examples of diagnosis codes and their descriptions:

- 301.7—Antisocial personality disorder
- 790.21—Impaired fasting glucose
- V26.34—Testing of male for genetic disease carrier status
- E906.1—Rat bite

ICD-9-CM inpatient procedure codes can be two to four digits long, with a decimal point after the first two digits. Here are some examples of codes and corresponding procedures:

- 06.2—Unilateral thyroid lobectomy
- 01.26—Insertion of catheter(s) into cranial cavity or tissue
- 47.01—Laparoscopic appendectomy

Providers can reference the ICD-9-CM code set for diagnoses and inpatient procedures using different formats, including a paper manual, CD-ROM, or a web-based (Internet) edition. Different publishers produce the manual in its various formats, and providers purchase the format that works best for them, but the code set is the same regardless of the format. The Centers for Disease Control (CDC) website contains the ICD-9-CM codes free of charge. The ICD-9-CM code set is divided into three volumes. In this chapter, you will learn how the volumes are structured and where to find specific information. In Chapters 4 and 5, you will also learn rules and conventions (symbols and terms) to use when coding diagnoses, as outlined in the **ICD-9-CM Official Guidelines for Coding and Reporting**. There are four organizations that review and approve the ICD-9-CM Official Guidelines, called the *Cooperating Parties*: CMS, NCHS, the American Hospital Association (AHA), and the American Health Information Management Association (AHIMA).

As you use the ICD-9-CM coding manual, you will apply various rules and conventions from the ICD-9-CM Official Guidelines (see Appendix A of this text for instructions on accessing the guidelines) and adhere to ethical coding principles. Think of the coding manual and coding rules as similar to rules for driving a car. The coding manual is like the car, and the coding rules are just like the rules of the road. Before you can operate a car, you need to learn where all of the controls are located, such as the headlights, windshield wipers, gear shift, and so on. But even if you know where to find the controls and how to use them, you still need to know the *rules* of the road to follow when driving your car. Coding works the same way; you will learn how to operate the coding manual, and you will also learn the coding rules to follow as you travel along on your coding journey and practice what you've learned!

ETHICAL CODING

You already learned that a job requirement for coding is the ability to apply **ethical standards** when coding. Ethical coding involves adhering to established principles to avoid fraudulent or abusive coding. Remember that ethical standards are standards that are morally right, correct, and legal. Both major national coding organizations, the American Academy of Professional Coders (AAPC) and the American Health Information Management Association (AHIMA) have established their own set of ethical standards, also called a code of ethics, that members of their organizations should follow when coding (■ FIGURE 3-1). Providers also develop their own ethical standards for coding. Although they might choose different wording for the standards, the basic meaning in any provider's code of ethics is the same as the information you will read from AHIMA.

Figure 3-1 ■ AHIMA Standards of Ethical Coding.

Source: Used by permission of AHIMA.

Coding professionals should:

1. Apply accurate, complete, and consistent coding practices for the production of high-quality healthcare data.

2. Report all healthcare data elements (e.g. diagnosis and procedure codes, present on admission indicator, discharge status) required for external reporting purposes (e.g. reimbursement and other administrative uses, population health, quality and patient safety measurement, and research) completely and accurately, in accordance with regulatory and documentation standards and requirements and applicable official coding conventions, rules, and guidelines.

3. Assign and report only the codes and data that are clearly and consistently supported by health record documentation in accordance with applicable code set and abstraction conventions, rules, and guidelines.

4. Query provider (physician or other qualified healthcare practitioner) for clarification and additional documentation prior to code assignment when there is conflicting, incomplete, or ambiguous information in the health record regarding a significant reportable condition or procedure or other reportable data element dependent on health record documentation (e.g. present on admission indicator).

5. Refuse to change reported codes or the narratives of codes so that meanings are misrepresented.

6. Refuse to participate in or support coding or documentation practices intended to inappropriately increase payment, qualify for insurance policy coverage, or skew data by means that do not comply with federal and state statutes, regulations and official rules and guidelines.

7. Facilitate interdisciplinary collaboration in situations supporting proper coding practices.

8. Advance coding knowledge and practice through continuing education.

9. Refuse to participate in or conceal unethical coding or abstraction practices or procedures.

10. Protect the confidentiality of the health record at all times and refuse to access protected health information not required for coding-related activities (examples of coding-related activities include completion of code assignment, other health record data abstraction, coding audits, and educational purposes).

11. Demonstrate behavior that reflects integrity, shows a commitment to ethical and legal coding practices, and fosters trust in professional activities.

Reviewed and approved by the House of Delegates 09/08.

KEY POINTS TO REMEMBER WHEN CODING

It is important to understand that you will not become an expert at coding in a short period of time. To become good at coding, you will have to invest the time and energy to practice and fine-tune your skills. In general, coding is not an activity that is simple or easy, and it is beneficial to keep this in mind as you learn coding so you do not become frustrated. Learning how to code well is a skill, just like any other skill that you have to practice.

When you code, remember that you have to read medical documentation, interpret the language in it, and determine the patient's diagnosis and procedure or service. Reading documentation in a medical record is not like reading the newspaper, a magazine, or the latest headlines on an Internet website, where you can quickly scan the information and find the general points of a story. Coding often involves reading analytically, which means reading documentation and coding manuals word for word, not skimming over the information. You may think that you understood all of the information after a quick read-through, but odds are, you probably did not. Reading documentation involves not only concentrating on the meaning of the words that you read but also applying coding rules to the documentation. Only then can you ensure that you have coded a diagnosis and procedure correctly.

Before you complete the practice exercises in this book, you should be at your best, not tired, sleepy, distracted, or hurried. If you try to retain information and code accurately when you are listening to loud music or the television, chatting with others, feeling rushed or distracted, or simply not feeling your best, you may not perform well. Wait until you are ready to learn, have the time to dedicate to it, and are free from all distractions before proceeding. Unfortunately, students often find that their answers to coding exercises are incorrect because they did not fully dedicate their time to coding. They will say that they had no idea how they found their answers because when reviewing them a second time, they do not seem to make sense. Then they realize that they coded the exercises when they were tired or rushed. Their coding answers were incorrect not because they did not understand the material, but because at the time, they were not fully devoted to it and did not concentrate hard enough.

It is also important to keep reference materials handy while you code using the ICD-9-CM manual, including a medical dictionary and books or guides on medical terminology, anatomy and physiology, and disease processes. You will also find Internet searches to be a quick, useful way to find many medical definitions. It takes extra time to look up the meaning of words and terms that you do not know, but you must take the time to find definitions. Not knowing definitions affects your ability to completely understand a patient's medical record and affects your final code assignment.

Coding can sometimes be tedious because it involves such a high level of concentration, investigation, and analytical skills, but it can also be very rewarding when you realize that you have successfully coded a particularly difficult case or learned how to apply a coding rule or payer regulation. Remember that the coding rules and payer regulations you will learn are the same whether you want to pursue a full-time coding career or just need to learn coding as part of your job. You may like coding, love coding, or only tolerate it, but no matter how you feel about it, you have to be good at it in order to perform your job successfully and to ensure that the provider for whom you work can rely on you to code accurately for correct reimbursement and avoid coding fraud and abuse.

VOLUMES AND APPENDICES OF THE ICD-9-CM MANUAL

The ICD-9-CM manual is divided into three volumes. The first two only apply to diagnosis coding; the third volume applies to inpatient procedure coding. There are also Appendices that provide you with additional coding information, as outlined below:

Diagnosis Coding:

- **Volume 1, Tabular List**—for diagnoses, contains all ICD-9-CM diagnosis codes arranged in numeric order, followed by their descriptions.
- **Volume 2, Alphabetic Index**—for diagnoses, contains the names and additional descriptions for all diagnoses, conditions, diseases, and reasons for encounters, arranged in alphabetical order. The Alphabetic Index is also called the *Index*.

Appendices:

The Appendices follow Volume 1 and provide additional information regarding patients' conditions and help to track health information:

- **Appendix A**—Morphology of Neoplasms
- **Appendix B**—Glossary of Mental Disorders (deleted October 1, 2004)
- **Appendix C**—Classification of Drugs by American Hospital Formulary Service List Number and Their ICD-9-CM Equivalents
- **Appendix D**—Classification of Industrial Accidents According to Agency
- **Appendix E**—List of Three-Digit Categories

Inpatient Procedure Coding:

- **Volume 3, Tabular List and Alphabetic Index used for Inpatient Procedures**—The Tabular List contains inpatient procedure codes in numeric order, followed by their descriptions, and the Alphabetic Index contains the names of inpatient procedures, arranged in alphabetical order.

Coding diagnoses in Volumes 1 and 2 is a two-part process:

Step 1   Look up the name of the condition in the Alphabetic Index (Volume 2), just the way you would look up a word in a dictionary. This is called looking for the **main term**, the word or words that best describe a condition or reason for an encounter. Main terms are capitalized and arranged in alphabetical order. When you find the main term, it may be in bold print, depending on the ICD-9-CM manual you use. The main term is followed by a diagnosis code. Many main terms also have **subterms**, words that are indented under the main term to provide more information about the main term. Subterms are also arranged alphabetically and also list diagnosis codes.

Step 2   Search for the diagnosis code(s) that you found in the Alphabetic Index in the Tabular List (Volume 1) to ensure that it is definitely the code that you want to assign. This is a process called *cross-referencing*. The Tabular List provides additional information, clarification, and coding instructions, so you will always need to cross-reference the code you find in the Alphabetic Index to the Tabular List to ensure that your code is correct. In addition, many times the description of a code in the Alphabetic Index does not exactly match the description of the same code in the Tabular List. The Tabular List may contain a more general description for a group of disorders, all classified under the same code. This is why it is important for you to *always cross-reference the code from the Alphabetic Index to the Tabular List* to ensure accuracy.

Coding inpatient procedure codes is also a two-step process, using Volume 3, which is divided into its own Alphabetic Index and Tabular List, created exclusively for inpatient procedures. Look up the name of the inpatient procedure in the Alphabetic Index, find the inpatient procedure code, and then cross-reference it to the Tabular List for additional clarification and final code assignment. *Never code inpatient procedures directly from the Alphabetic Index without cross-referencing the codes to the Tabular List because you risk assigning an incomplete and incorrect code.* We will review more about Volume 3 and coding inpatient procedures in Chapter 16.

TAKE A BREAK

Let's take a break and review the information you learned with an exercise.

| Exercise 3.1 | Ethical Coding, Key Points, Volumes, and Appendices in ICD-9-CM

Instructions: Match the term in the list to its description.

1. _____ should assign and report only the codes and data that are clearly and consistently supported by health record documentation.

2. It is important to keep _____ handy while you code using the ICD-9-CM coding manual.

- Volume 1, Tabular List
- Appendix C
- coding

TAKE A BREAK *continued*

3. _____ contains all ICD-9-CM diagnosis codes arranged in numeric order, followed by their descriptions.

4. The appendix that contains the List of Three-Digit Categories is _____.

5. _____ are morally right, correct, and legal.

6. The appendix for the Classification of Drugs by American Hospital Formulary Service List Number and Their ICD-9-CM Equivalents is _____.

7. _____ contains the names and additional descriptions for all diagnoses, conditions, diseases, and reasons for encounters, arranged in alphabetical order.

8. The appendix for the Morphology of Neoplasms is _____.

9. An appendix that was deleted October 1, 2004, is _____.

10. _____ involves reading analytically, which is reading documentation and the coding manuals word for word.

11. _____ contains inpatient procedure codes in numeric order, followed by their descriptions, and an Index that contains the names of inpatient procedures, arranged in alphabetical order.

12. The Appendix of Classification of Industrial Accidents According to Agency is _____.

13. A word or words that best describe a condition or reason for an encounter is called a(n) _____.

14. _____ is the process of searching for a diagnosis code in an alphabetical list of conditions and then double checking the code in the numeric list of codes.

15. Words that are indented under the main term to provide more information about the main term are called _____.

- coding professionals
- ethical standards
- reference materials
- Appendix B
- Volume 3, Alphabetic Index and Tabular List
- main term
- Appendix A
- Volume 2, Alphabetic Index
- cross-referencing
- Appendix D
- subterms
- Appendix E

ICD-9-CM VOLUME 1, TABULAR LIST

Volume 1 of the Tabular List is divided into two sections, the Classification of Diseases and Injuries and Supplementary Classifications. The *Classification of Diseases and Injuries* (Tabular List) contains 17 **chapters** that group diagnosis codes in numeric order by the body system affected or the type of disease, complication, or problem. Turn to Volume 1 in your ICD-9-CM manual, and you will find codes in the 17 chapters ranging from categories 001 to 999, as outlined in ■ FIGURE 3-2.

V Codes

V Codes, Supplementary Classification of Factors Influencing Health Status and Contact with Health Services represent reasons for encounters, other than a disease, condition, or injury, with some exceptions. You already know that insurances require providers to report diagnosis codes on claims. But what if the patient received a service but there was nothing wrong with the patient? That is where V codes are important because you assign them to show *why* the patient had a service. Examples are a patient's annual exam, visit for an oral contraceptive (birth control), fitting and adjustment of a hearing aid, or immunization for protection against a disease.

V codes can also provide additional information about a patient, even if the patient has an established diagnosis. These are the exceptions, such as personal history of cancer or family history of hypertension. In other cases, V codes can show the main reason for the

Figure 3-2 ■ ICD-9-CM Classification of Diseases and Injuries.

Chapter No.	Chapter Title	Category Range
1.	Infectious and Parasitic Diseases	001–139
2.	Neoplasms	140–239
3.	Endocrine, Nutritional, and Metabolic Diseases and Immunity Disorders	240–279
4.	Diseases of the Blood and Blood-Forming Organs	280–289
5.	Mental Disorders	290–319
6.	Diseases of the Nervous System and Sense Organs	320–389
7.	Diseases of the Circulatory System	390–459
8.	Diseases of the Respiratory System	460–519
9.	Diseases of the Digestive System	520–579
10.	Diseases of the Genitourinary System	580–629
11.	Complications of Pregnancy, Childbirth, and the Puerperium	630–679
12.	Diseases of the Skin and Subcutaneous Tissue	680–709
13.	Diseases of the Musculoskeletal System and Connective Tissue	710–739
14.	Congenital Anomalies	740–759
15.	Certain Conditions Originating in the Perinatal Period	760–779
16.	Symptoms, Signs, and Ill-Defined Conditions	780–799
17.	Injury and Poisoning	800–999

patient's encounter for therapeutic services, such as chemotherapy or radiation to treat cancer, or physical or occupational therapy. Depending on the situation, you can assign a V code as the only code, the first code, or the secondary code. You can search for V codes in Volume 2, Alphabetic Index, and cross-reference codes to categories V01–V89. In the Tabular List, V codes are not part of the 17 chapters. They are arranged in a separate section in numeric order from categories V01–V89, and you should review them to become more familiar with the type of information that they represent. Examples of V codes in the Tabular List are shown in ■ FIGURE 3-3.

E Codes

E Codes, Supplementary Classification of External Causes of Injury and Poisoning, represent an *external cause* that created the patient's condition, such as a fall from a building,

Figure 3-3 ■ Examples of V Codes from ICD-9-CM.

V24	Postpartum care and examination	
	V24.0	**Immediately after delivery**
		Care and observation in uncomplicated cases
	V24.1	**Lactating mother**
		Supervision of lactation
	V24.2	**Routine postpartum follow-up**

Activity (involving) E030

walking (on level or elevated terrain) E001.0
  an animal E019.0
walking an animal E019.0
wall climbing E004.0
warm up and cool down exercises E009.1

Figure 3-4 ■ Index to External Causes examples of E codes.

E001   Activities involving walking and running

  Excludes: walking an animal (E019.0)
               walking or running on a treadmill (E009.0)

E001.0 Walking, marching and hiking

  Walking, marching and hiking on level or elevated terrain
  Excludes: mountain climbing (E004.0)

E001.1 Running

Figure 3-5 ■ Tabular List examples of E codes.

automobile accident, or accidental overdose on a prescribed medication. E codes represent causes of injuries and/or poisonings, and you should assign them *in addition* to the diagnosis for the patient's condition. E codes are *never* the first listed diagnosis code.

For example, one of Dr. Hoffman's patients, Mr. Reynolds, was standing on a ladder to paint his house. He fell off and suffered a femur (thigh bone) fracture. The femur fracture is the diagnosis, and the external cause of the femur fracture is the fall from the ladder, represented by an E code. Mr. Reynolds' first listed diagnosis code is 821.00 for the femur fracture, and the second code is an E code of E881.0 to show how the fracture happened, a fall from a ladder. The E code provides *additional information* about the patient's diagnosis but does not represent the patient's actual condition. In Mr. Reynolds' case, the E code shows more information about his fracture: the fact that the fall caused it.

E codes actually have their own alphabetic index, called the Index to External Causes of Injury (Section 3 of Volume 2, Alphabetic Index), with external causes arranged in alphabetical order, along with their corresponding codes. E codes are listed in numeric order in a separate section of the Tabular List, categories E000–E999. You can review E codes in both the Alphabetic Index for E codes and in the Tabular List to become familiar with the types of external causes of injuries that they represent. Always cross-reference E codes from the E code Alphabetic Index to categories E000–E999. Examples of E codes in the Index to External Causes of Injury are shown in ■ FIGURE 3-4, and examples of E codes from the Tabular List are shown in ■ FIGURE 3-5. Examples include an Index entry for an injury while walking (Activity, walking) and cross-reference to code E001.0 for this injury. You will learn more about coding with V codes and E codes in Chapters 7 and 8.

STRUCTURE OF THE CLASSIFICATION OF DISEASES AND INJURIES AND CODING TO THE HIGHEST LEVEL OF SPECIFICITY

In order to code correctly, you have to understand the structure of codes in the Tabular List. Recall that the Tabular List has 17 chapters of the Classification of Diseases and Injuries. Each chapter groups diagnosis codes by the body system affected or by the type of disease, complication, or problem. Review some of the codes in the Tabular List for a better idea of how the codes appear and the conditions and diseases that they represent. You will find codes on various illnesses, diseases, and conditions. Within each of the 17 chapters, there are sections, categories, subcategories, and subclassifications of codes that start out broad and move to very specific. Let's review them and then discuss how to apply them to coding:

- **section**—a group of three-digit categories within a chapter representing related conditions or a single condition
- **category**—a three-digit code representing a single condition; some categories are further subdivided into subcategories

- **subcategory**—a four-digit code providing further specification for a category, including site of the body that the condition affects, etiology (cause of the condition), and manifestation (additional problems that occurred because of the condition). Some subcategories are further subdivided into subclassifications.

- **subclassification**—a five-digit code that includes even further specification of the subcategory, including body site affected, type of disease, and additional information to describe the condition

You already learned that an ICD-9-CM code is a minimum of three digits and a maximum of five. Think of three-digit codes as a broad category of codes that can be subdivided into four-digit subcategory codes to add more specific information. Four-digit subcategory codes can also be further subdivided into five-digit subclassification codes to add even more specific information.

When you want to find the correct code, you begin at the category level (three digits), then move to the subcategory level (four digits) if one exists, and then to the subclassification level (five digits) if one exists, to assign the most specific code available. This process is called coding to the **highest level of specificity** (pronounced spe-sə-'fi-sə-tē), meaning that you need to assign the *highest level* of a code that exists.

The process is like searching for a person's telephone number in a phone directory: You begin with a broad search of the person's last name, and you find a group of the same last name further subdivided into groups of first names, and then subdivided again into groups with middle names or middle initials. If you searched for a person's phone number, then you would not just look for his last name and begin calling each person with the same last name. You would also need to find his first name, as well as his middle name or initial before you knew that you found the correct person and phone number. You would have to be as specific as possible to know that you found the correct number for the person whom you wanted to call.

Many ICD-9-CM coding manuals will alert you when you need to assign a fourth digit to a category code or a fifth digit to a subcategory code. You will see a symbol next to a code, or a notation of 4 or 5, or 4th or 5th, to remind you that you need to code further to the fourth or fifth digit.

In the example in ■ FIGURE 3-6, you will see the breakdown of a chapter, section, category, subcategories, and subclassifications in the Tabular List. You will also see notations to tell you to code to the fourth or fifth digits. Descriptions of category, subcategory, and subclassification codes are called *code titles* or *code descriptors*. The chapter referred to in Figure 3-6 is Chapter 6 of the Tabular List, *Diseases of the Nervous System and Sense Organs*. The section (3-digit categories from 360–379) is *Disorders of the Eye and **Adnexa*** meaning parts of the eye, like the muscles behind the eyeball. You will then see the breakdown of category (3-digit), subcategory (4-digit), and subclassification (5-digit) codes with their code descriptors in bold print.

Notice the boxes with the notation "4th" and "5th," telling you that the code to the right is not specific enough to assign. In each of these cases you need to code further to a fourth or fifth digit. Review category 367 which represents *Disorders of refraction and accommodation*, but category 367 is not specific enough to assign as a code. It does not describe the *type* of refractive or accommodation eye disorder that a patient has. If you reported 367 as a patient's diagnosis on an insurance claim, then the insurance would not know what disorder the patient had because there are *many different types* of refraction and accommodation eye disorders. You then need to review the subcategory codes, as well as any further subdivisions into subclassification codes, in order to find a more specific code.

In this example, you would have to read the patient's medical documentation to determine the patient's *specific type* of refractive or accommodation eye disorder. Then you would code further by reviewing the subcategory code options for category 367 to determine if you could assign any of them (367.0, 367.1, 367.2). Notice that code 367.2 is further subdivided, meaning that you could never assign 367.2. You always have to code further.

adnexa (ad-nek′-sə)

CHAPTER

6. DISEASES OF THE NERVOUS SYSTEM AND SENSE ORGANS (320–389)

SECTION

DISORDERS OF THE EYE AND ADNEXA (360–379)

4th	**367 Disorders of refraction and accommodation**		◄*CATEGORY CODE - 3 digits*
	367.0	**Hypermetropia** Far-sightedness Hyperopia	◄*SUBCATEGORY CODE - 4 digits*
	367.1	**Myopia** Near-sightedness	◄*SUBCATEGORY CODE - 4 digits*
5th	**367.2**	**Astigmatism**	◄*SUBCATEGORY CODE - 4 digits*
		367.20 Astigmatism, unspecified	◄*SUBCLASSIFICATION CODE - 5 digits*
		367.21 Regular astigmatism	◄*SUBCLASSIFICATION CODE - 5 digits*
		367.22 Irregular astigmatism	◄*SUBCLASSIFICATION CODE - 5 digits*

Figure 3-6 ■ Chapter 6 of the Tabular List: Category 367 with its subdivisions.

Some categories in the Tabular List appropriately describe a condition and do not need to be further subdivided into subcategory or subclassification codes. Other categories are further subdivided and it is your job to keep coding higher when a subcategory and/or subclassification code is available until you are unable to code any further.

If you assign a very general code (367) to a patient's encounter when a *more specific one is available*, then you are not coding to the highest level of specificity and are, in fact, assigning an incorrect code. The insurance will question why you assigned a general code when a specific one was available and will deny payment of the patient's insurance claim.

Read Complete Code Titles

An important point to remember is that when you read many of the subcategory titles in ICD-9-CM, you must also incorporate the code title of the category above it in order to obtain the complete meaning of the code. In addition, when reading many subclassification code titles, you must incorporate the code title of the subcategory and category to understand the meaning of the subclassification code. For example, when you read the code title for subclassification code 482.82 in the Tabular List, the meaning is unclear because the title simply states, "*Escherichia coli* [*E. coli*]" (■ FIGURE 3-7).

482.82 Escherichia coli [E. coli]

Figure 3-7 ■ Code 482.82. The code title for 482.82 in the Tabular List is unclear.

A code title with only *E. coli* does not have any meaning because it does not define the patient's condition. The only way to know the complete meaning of 482.82 is to read both the subcategory (482.8) and category (482) associated with the code (■ FIGURE 3-8). Only then will you understand that 482.82 represents *other bacterial pneumonia* (category title) and *pneumonia due to other specified bacteria* (subcategory title), and that the bacteria are *E. coli* (subclassification title). You must read the category and subcategory in addition to the subclassification to understand what information code 482.82 represents.

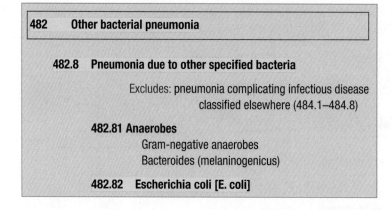

482	Other bacterial pneumonia

482.8   Pneumonia due to other specified bacteria

Excludes: pneumonia complicating infectious disease classified elsewhere (484.1–484.8)

482.81 Anaerobes
Gram-negative anaerobes
Bacteroides (melaninogenicus)

482.82   Escherichia coli [E. coli]

GUIDELINES FOR CODING TO THE HIGHEST LEVEL OF SPECIFICITY IN THE TABULAR LIST

Follow these steps to help you code diagnoses to the highest level of specificity:

1. When you review a category and you see subcategory options indented below the category, you will need to review the subcategories. Determine if the subcategories are further divided into subclassifications; which you will also need to review. In other words, do not stop coding at the category level if there is a subcategory. Do not stop coding at the subcategory level if there is a subclassification. Coding to the highest level of specificity is *mandatory*, not optional.

2. When you review a subcategory code and you need to assign a subclassification code, you will *either* see the subclassification code indented and listed below the subcategory code (■ FIGURE 3-9) or you will see a list of choices under the category for fifth-digit subclassifications (■ FIGURE 3-10).

3. If your coding manual contains symbols, review them and apply them in the Tabular List, whether you are referencing the code set in a manual, electronic, or web-based version. Review the symbols to identify whether a fourth-digit subcategory or a fifth-digit subclassification code is available, as shown in ■ FIGURES 3-11 and 3-12.

   Notice in ■ FIGURE 3-12 that the choices for the fifth digits are listed under category 789. Notice also that code 789.0 has [0-7,9] listed below it. This means that you are required to assign a fifth digit and will need to choose a fifth digit of 0-7 or 9.

4. Sometimes, you will not be able to assign the highest level code to a patient's diagnosis for two reasons: the medical record documentation does not specifically describe a diagnosis, or there is not a specific code in ICD-9-CM for the diagnosis. In these instances, you will assign a subcategory code with the words *other* or *unspecified* in its description.

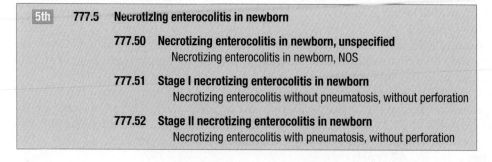

5th	777.5	Necrotizing enterocolitis in newborn

777.50   Necrotizing enterocolitis in newborn, unspecified
Necrotizing enterocolitis in newborn, NOS

777.51   Stage I necrotizing enterocolitis in newborn
Necrotizing enterocolitis without pneumatosis, without perforation

777.52   Stage II necrotizing enterocolitis in newborn
Necrotizing enterocolitis with pneumatosis, without perforation

Figure 3-10 ■ Subclassification code choices listed below the category code.

4th | **730 Osteomyelitis, periostitis, and other infections involving bone**

Excludes: jaw (526.4–526.5)
petrous bone (383.2)
Use additional code to identify organism, such as Staphylococcus (041.1)

The following fifth-digit subclassification is for use with category 730; valid digits are in [brackets] under each code. See list at beginning of chapter for definitions:

0 site unspecified
1 shoulder region   ◄**SUBCLASSIFICATION CHOICES FOR**
2 upper arm   **THE 5TH DIGIT FOR 730**
3 forearm
4 hand
5 pelvic region and thigh
6 lower leg
7 ankle and foot
8 other specified sites
9 multiple sites

These subcategory codes are called *residual subcategory codes* for you to use when there is not a more specific code in the Tabular List. Codes with *other* in their descriptions end with the number 8, and codes with *unspecified* in their descriptions end with the number 9. Refer to ■ FIGURE 3-13, which shows examples of other and unspecified codes.

In Figure 3-13, category 776 represents *Hematological disorders of newborn* (blood disorders). Subcategory choices under the category include the *specific types* of disorders. But what if the newborn had a specific hematological disorder and none of the subcategory choices identified the patient's diagnosis? Then you would assign code 776.8, *Other specified transient hematological disorders. Other specified* means that the patient's documentation specified the type of disorder, but ICD-9-CM *does not* have a code for it. You still have to assign a code for every patient's encounter, so *other specified* is as close as you can get to the diagnosis. This is a good example of why ICD-10-CM will replace ICD-9-CM codes: in order to provide greater specificity to identify many types of conditions, rather than calling them *other specified*.

But what if the newborn had a hematological disorder and the patient's documentation *did not specify* the *type* of disorder? Then you would assign code 776.9 *Unspecified hematological disorder specific to newborn. Unspecified* means that the physician did not specify the disorder in the documentation. *Unspecified* is your only choice, and you should only assign an unspecified code as a last resort. This is a good example of when you would need to query the physician to ask if there is a more definitive diagnosis for the patient. If there is, the physician can add it to the documentation and you can then assign a more specific code.

Figure 3-11 ■ Category 792 with symbol showing required fourth digit subcategory code.

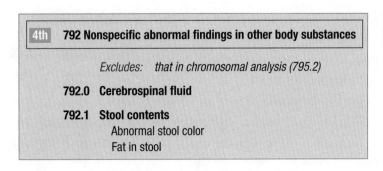

4th | **792 Nonspecific abnormal findings in other body substances**

Excludes: that in chromosomal analysis (795.2)

792.0 Cerebrospinal fluid

792.1 Stool contents
Abnormal stool color
Fat in stool

Figure 3-12 ■ Category 789 with subcategories and symbols for required fourth and fifth digits.

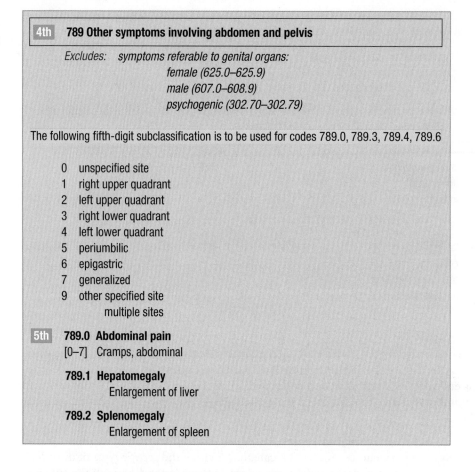

| 4th | **789 Other symptoms involving abdomen and pelvis** |

Excludes: symptoms referable to genital organs:
female (625.0–625.9)
male (607.0–608.9)
psychogenic (302.70–302.79)

The following fifth-digit subclassification is to be used for codes 789.0, 789.3, 789.4, 789.6

0   unspecified site
1   right upper quadrant
2   left upper quadrant
3   right lower quadrant
4   left lower quadrant
5   periumbilic
6   epigastric
7   generalized
9   other specified site
    multiple sites

| 5th | **789.0 Abdominal pain** |
[0–7]   Cramps, abdominal

789.1 Hepatomegaly
Enlargement of liver

789.2 Splenomegaly
Enlargement of spleen

Figure 3-13 ■ Examples of "other" and "unspecified" codes under category 776.

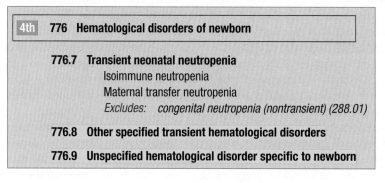

| 4th | **776   Hematological disorders of newborn** |

776.7   Transient neonatal neutropenia
Isoimmune neutropenia
Maternal transfer neutropenia
Excludes: congenital neutropenia (nontransient) (288.01)

776.8   Other specified transient hematological disorders

776.9   Unspecified hematological disorder specific to newborn

TAKE A BREAK

Wow! That was a lot to remember! Let's take a break and then review all of this new information with an exercise.

Exercise 3.2   **ICD-9-CM Volume 1 Tabular List, Structure of Classification of Diseases and Injuries, and Guidelines for Coding to the Highest Level of Specificity**

Instructions: Indicate whether each statement is True or False on the line preceding each statement. For statements marked False, underline the word(s) that make(s) the statement false.

1. _____ The Classification of Diseases and Injuries in the Tabular List contains 17 chapters that group diagnosis codes in numeric order by the body system affected or by the type of disease, complication, or problem.

2. _____ A subclassification is a group of three-digit categories within a chapter representing related conditions or a single condition.

TAKE A BREAK *continued*

3. _____ V codes represent reasons for encounters, other than a disease, condition, or injury, with a few exceptions.

4. _____ E codes represent an *external cause* that created the patient's condition, such as a fall from a building, automobile accident, or accidental overdose on a prescribed medication.

5. _____ Some subcategories are further divided into subclassifications.

6. _____ A category is a five-digit code that includes even further specification of the subcategory, including body site affected, type of disease, and additional information to describe the condition.

7. _____ A subcategory is a three-digit code representing a single condition.

8. _____ A section is a four-digit code providing further specification for a category, including site of the body that the condition affects, etiology (cause of the condition), and manifestation (additional problems that occurred because of the condition).

9. _____ The process of coding to the highest level of specificity means that you need to assign the highest level of a code that exists.

10. _____ V codes are never the first listed diagnosis code.

ICD-9-CM APPENDICES

ICD-9-CM Appendices are located after Volume 1 and provide additional information about a patient's condition, disease, or injury. Coders may not need to reference every appendix, but it is still important to understand their structure and why they exist. A list of appendices follows, and then we will review each Appendix in more detail:

- *Appendix A*—Morphology of Neoplasms
- *Appendix B*—Glossary of Mental Disorders (deleted October 1, 2004)
- *Appendix C*—Classification of Drugs by American Hospital Formulary Service List Number and Their ICD-9-CM Equivalents
- *Appendix D*—Classification of Industrial Accidents According to Agency
- *Appendix E*—List of Three-Digit Categories

Appendix A—Morphology of Neoplasms

A *neoplasm* is an abnormal new growth, such as a cancerous growth. **Morphology** is the study of structure and form of cells, organisms, and organs. When a physician diagnoses a patient with a neoplasm, like cancer, you search in the Alphabetic Index for the main term for the type of cancer, such as leukemia. You can also search the Index for the main term *neoplasm*, then search subterms showing the body site, and cross-reference the code to the Tabular List. (Neoplasm codes are listed in Chapter 2 of the Tabular List.)

morphology (mòr-fäl′-ə-jē)

You can also assign an additional *morphology code* for the neoplasm to show the *type* of cancer that a patient has, such as lymphoma, carcinoma, or glioblastoma, along with its behavior (*malignant,* life threatening; or *benign,* not life threatening). Appendix A contains morphology codes that specify types of neoplasms and their behaviors. Providers can use *morphology codes* to track the number and types of neoplasms patients have, along with types of treatment. Providers can also report morphology codes to a *cancer registry,* an organization that gathers and analyzes information and statistics about cancer. Information from cancer registries is critical for developing effective cancer prevention and control programs for specific geographic areas or populations.

The World Health Organization published an adaptation of the *International Classification of Diseases for Oncology (ICD-O)*. It contains a coded nomenclature (naming system) for the morphology of neoplasms. The morphology codes begin with the letter M, followed by four numbers that identify the histological (structure of tissues) type of neoplasm, a slash (/), and then the fifth digit, which indicates the neoplasm's behavior.

Figure 3-14 ■ Morphology codes in Appendix A of ICD-9-CM.

M912–M916	**Blood vessel tumors**
M9120/0	Hemangioma NOS
M9120/3	Hemangiosarcoma
M9121/0	Cavernous hemangioma
M9122/0	Venous hemangioma
M9123/0	Racemose hemangioma

Review examples of morphology codes with this structure in ■ FIGURE 3-14, which come from Appendix A of ICD-9-CM. Also review the descriptions and meanings of their fifth-digit behaviors in ■ TABLE 3-1. You can also find these at the beginning of Appendix A.

Appendix B—Glossary of Mental Disorders

Appendix B was deleted in 2004 because the American Psychiatric Association created the Diagnostic and Statistical Manual-IV, Text Revision (DSM-IV-TR) to classify mental disorders and help diagnosis and research various mental conditions.

Appendix C—Classification of Drugs by American Hospital Formulary Service List Number and Their ICD-9-CM Equivalents

The Classification of Drugs by American Hospital Formulary Service (AHFS) List Number, published under the direction of the American Society of Hospital Pharmacists, is a system that pharmacists use to categorize drugs. Pharmacists also review additional information about drugs that is tied to each drug's AHFS list number. In Appendix C, the list number of each drug also shows its corresponding ICD-9-CM

■ TABLE 3-1   **DESCRIPTIONS OF FIFTH-DIGIT BEHAVIORS FOR MORPHOLOGY CODES IN APPENDIX A OF THE ICD-9-CM**

Fifth Digit	Description	Meaning
/0	Benign	Neoplasm that is not life threatening
/1	Uncertain whether benign or malignant Borderline malignancy	It is not clear if the neoplasm is life threatening
/2	Carcinoma in situ (pronounced ĭn sītoo) Intraepithelial Noninfiltrating Noninvasive	Cancer (neoplasm) that is confined to one site and has not spread anywhere else in the body
/3	Malignant, primary site	Life-threatening neoplasm in the site where it was first found, and now it has spread
/6	Malignant, metastatic (spread to) site Secondary site	Life-threatening neoplasm in a site to which it has spread, although it actually started somewhere else
/9	Malignant, uncertain whether primary or metastatic site	Life-threatening neoplasm; it is not clear whether it is in a primary or secondary site

INTERESTING FACT: Prostate Cancer and Lung Cancer Are the Most Common

The graphs in ■ Figure 3-15 show that in 2006, prostate cancer was the most common cancer in men, followed by lung and bronchus cancer, then cancer of the colon and rectum. In women, lung and bronchus cancer were the most common, followed by breast cancer, then colon and rectal cancer.

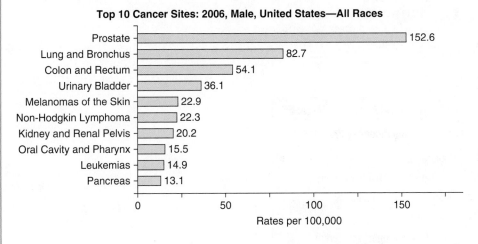

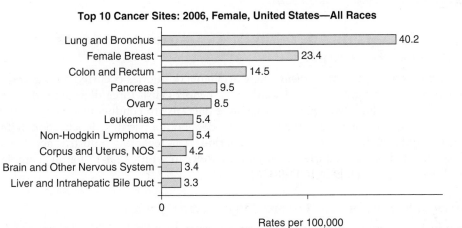

Figure 3-15 ■ Top 10 cancer sites in 2006, male and female.

Source: U.S. Cancer Statistics Working Group, U.S. Department of Health and Human Services, Centers for Disease Control and Prevention and National Cancer Institute.

code, which is the same code that you will find in the Table of Drugs and Chemicals. We will review the Table of Drugs and Chemicals later in this chapter. Refer to ■ Figure 3-16 for examples of AHFS list numbers and corresponding ICD-9-CM codes from Appendix C in ICD-9-CM.

AHFS List		ICD-9-CM Diagnosis Code
4:00	ANTIHISTAMINE DRUGS	963.0
8:00	ANTI-INFECTIVE AGENTS	
8:04	Amebacides	961.5
	hydroxyquinoline derivatives	961.3
	arsenical anti-infectives	961.1
	quinoline derivatives	961.3

Figure 3-16 ■ Appendix C—AHFS list number and corresponding ICD-9-CM code.

Figure 3-17 ■ Appendix D— Classification of Industrial Accidents According to Agency.

1	MACHINES	
11		Prime-Movers, except Electrical Motors
	111	Steam engines
	112	Internal combustion engines
	119	Others
12		Transmission Machinery
	121	Transmission shafts
	122	Transmission belts, cables, pulleys, pinions, chains, gears
	129	Others
13		Metalworking Machines
	131	Power presses
	132	Lathes

Figure 3-17 ■ Appendix D— Classification of Industrial Accidents According to Agency.

Figure 3-18 ■ Appendix E— List of three-digit categories in Chapter 1 of the Tabular List.

1. INFECTIOUS AND PARASITIC DISEASES

Intestinal infectious diseases (001–009)

001	Cholera
002	Typhoid and paratyphoid fevers
003	Other salmonella infections
004	Shigellosis
005	Other food poisoning (bacterial)

Appendix D—Classification of Industrial Accidents According to Agency

Appendix D is a list of *work locations* where accidents or injuries occurred, or a *description of the type of equipment* involved in an accident. Appendix D lists three-digit codes that labor statisticians (individuals who gather and analyze data) use to conduct further research for preventing workplace accidents and injuries. Coders do not use this classification system. The CDC and state health departments use various data regarding industrial accidents to help identify and prevent injuries to employees. Refer to ■ Figure 3-17 for an example of codes listed in Appendix D in ICD-9-CM.

Appendix E—List of Three-Digit Categories

Appendix E contains every category, in numeric order, from each of the 17 chapters in the Tabular List. Coders sometimes refer to Appendix E (■ Figure 3-18) to quickly locate a specific category and cross-reference it to the Tabular List to find the final code assignment for a patient's diagnosis.

TAKE A BREAK

Let's take a break and then review the Appendices with an exercise.

Exercise 3.3 ICD-9-CM Appendices

Instructions: Match the term in the list to its description, writing its corresponding letter in the space provided.

1. _____ The study of the science of the form, structure, and behavior of cells, organisms, and organs.

2. _____ A term describing a condition that is not life threatening.

a. malignant

b. Appendix B

TAKE A BREAK *continued*

3. _____ A list of work locations where accidents or injuries occurred, or of descriptions of the type of equipment involved in accidents.

4. _____ A term describing an abnormal new growth, such as a cancerous growth.

5. _____ Contains every category, in numeric order, from each of the 17 chapters in the Tabular List.

6. _____ Contains morphology codes, which specify types of neoplasms and their behaviors.

7. _____ An organization that gathers and analyzes information and statistics about cancer.

8. _____ Assigned to a neoplasm to show the *type* of cancer that a patient has, like lymphoma, carcinoma, and glioblastoma, along with its behavior.

9. _____ A list of disorders deleted in 2004.

10. _____ Contains a coded nomenclature for the morphology of neoplasms.

11. _____ A term describing a condition that is life threatening.

12. _____ The Classification of Drugs by American Hospital Formulary Service (AHFS) List Number that pharmacists use to categorize drugs.

c. cancer registry

d. neoplasm

e. Appendix D

f. benign

g. morphology

h. Appendix A

i. morphology code

j. International Classification of Diseases for Oncology (ICD-O)

k. Appendix C

l. Appendix E

VOLUME 2, ALPHABETIC INDEX

The Alphabetic Index has three sections: Index to Diseases and Injuries, Table of Drugs and Chemicals, and Index to External Causes of Injury (E codes).

Section 1

Index to Diseases and Injuries—contains the names and descriptions for all diagnoses, conditions, diseases, and reasons for encounters, arranged in alphabetical order as shown in ■ FIGURE 3-19. It is a good idea to place tabs in your ICD-9-CM manual to identify these sections, along with other areas that you will reference frequently.

Notice that the main terms are listed in bold, and subterms are indented under the main terms. After you review the patient's medical documentation and find the diagnosis, you'll look for it in the Index, searching for the main term and related subterms. When you find the diagnosis code, you will need to cross-reference it to the Tabular List for additional clarification and final code assignment. Turn to the Alphabetic Index in your ICD-9-CM manual to review main terms and subterms for various conditions.

Figure 3-19 ■ Alphabetic Index, Section 1—Index to Diseases and Injuries.

INDEX TO DISEASES AND INJURIES
A

AAT (alpha-1 antitrypsin) deficiency 273.4

AAV (disease) (illness) (infection) - see Human immunodeficiency virus (disease) (illness) (infection)

Abactio - see Abortion, induced

Abactus venter - see Abortion, induced

Abarognosis 781.99

Abasia (-astasia) 307.9

    atactica 781.3

    choreic 781.3

    hysterical 300.11

Substance	Poisoning	Accident	Therapeutic Use	Suicide Attempt	Assault	Undetermined
Antidepressants	969.00	E854.0	E939.0	E950.3	E962.0	E980.3
monoamine oxidase inhibitors (MAOI)	969.01	E854.0	E939.0	E950.3	E962.0	E980.3
specified type NEC	969.09	E854.0	E939.0	E950.3	E962.0	E980.3
SSNRI (selective serotonin and norepinephrine reuptake inhibitors)	969.02	E854.0	E939.0	E950.3	E962.0	E980.3
SSRI (selective serotonin reuptake inhibitors)	969.03	E854.0	E939.0	E950.3	E962.0	E980.3
tetracyclic	969.04	E854.0	E939.0	E950.3	E962.0	E980.3
tricyclic	969.05	E854.0	E939.0	E950.3	E962.0	E980.3
Antidiabetic agents	962.3	E858.0	E932.3	E950.4	E962.0	E980.4

Figure 3-20 ■ Alphabetic Index, Section 2—Table of Drugs and Chemicals.

Section 2

Table of Drugs and Chemicals—contains an alphabetical list of names of drugs and chemicals, along with their corresponding codes (■ FIGURE 3-20). The Table of Drugs and Chemicals directly follows the Index to Diseases and Injuries.

Refer to the Table of Drugs and Chemicals when a drug or chemical causes a patient to experience an adverse effect, like a poisoning. When you are coding for these cases from the Table of Drugs and Chemicals, you will assign both a code to identify *the substance that caused the adverse effect* (found in the column labeled Poisoning) and a code to identify the *external cause* of or reason for the poisoning (E codes found within the second through sixth columns of the table). You will learn more about assigning codes for poisonings later in this book.

Turn to the Table of Drugs and Chemicals in your coding manual. Review columns two through six, and you will see the reasons that poisonings occur (E codes) from the column headings. Definitions of the headings are listed next:

Accident (E850–E869)—injury or poisoning caused by a drug overdose, wrong substance given or taken, drug taken inadvertently, or drugs given to patients during medical and surgical procedures.

Therapeutic Use (E930–E949)—injury or poisoning caused by a correct substance properly administered in therapeutic or prophylactic dosage. For example, the patient had an adverse reaction to a medication that his physician prescribed.

Suicide Attempt (E950–E952)—injury or poisoning that was self-inflicted.

Assault (E961–E962)—injury or poisoning inflicted by another person with the intent to injure or kill.

Undetermined (E980–E982)—It is impossible to determine if the poisoning or injury was intentional or accidental.

Section 3

Index to External Causes of Injury (E code)—contains an alphabetical list of external causes of accidents and injuries, along with their corresponding E codes (■ FIGURE 3-21).

Turn to the Index to External Causes of Injury in your ICD-9-CM manual, which follows the Table of Drugs and Chemicals, and review the many causes of injuries. When you want to assign an E code, check this Index, and look for the external cause

Activity (involving) E030
    aerobic and step exercise (class) E009.2
    alpine skiing E003.2
    animal care NEC E019.9
    arts and handcrafts NEC E012.9
    athletics NEC E008.9
        played
            as a team or group NEC E007.9
            individually NEC E006.9
    baking E015.2
    ballet E005.0
    barbells E010.2
    BASE (Building, Antenna, Span, Earth) jumping E004.2
    baseball E007.3
    basketball E007.6

Figure 3-21 ■ Alphabetic Index, Section 3—Index to External Causes of Injury (E code).

of the patient's condition. You will then cross-reference the E code to the section of E codes in the ICD-9-CM manual. We will cover more information about E codes in Chapter 8.

MAIN TERMS, SUBTERMS, AND CARRYOVER LINES IN THE ALPHABETIC INDEX

Now that we have reviewed the three sections of the Index, let's discuss how to use Section 1: Index to Diseases and Injuries, also called the Index. This is the first step of learning how to assign diagnosis codes. When you use the Index, you have to find the patient's diagnosis in the list of diagnoses, which is arranged in alphabetical order in columns. This sounds simple enough, but in reality, there are so many different descriptions and choices for various conditions, and countless columns of information, so you have to be very careful to read all the information completely. Do you remember learning earlier in the chapter that coding involves reading information word for word? Part of reading coding information in detail involves knowing the structure of the Index so that you do not misinterpret information that you read or skip over important points that could affect your code assignment.

The Index is structured by main terms, indented subterms, and indented carryover lines. Recall from earlier in this chapter that a main term describes the patient's condition. You obtain the main term after reading the patient's medical documentation and finding the diagnosis that the physician or other clinician documented. A main term is generally one word, like *pain* or *fracture*. Main terms may also appear as phrases, such as *diaper rash*. A main term is *not* a body site. Body sites are listed as subterms under main terms.

Turn to the Index in your ICD-9-CM manual to review main terms. In the Index, main terms are capitalized and may also be printed in bold. They are followed by a corresponding code and any subterms with their corresponding codes. Notice that subterms are indented under main terms and are generally not capitalized. The main term is your starting point to find the correct code. Learning how to locate a main term is the first step to ensure that you do not waste your efforts aimlessly wandering the Index searching for the correct code to cross-reference to the Tabular List.

Subterms are listed in alphabetical order. They provide *additional information* about the main term, such as the *body site* the condition affects, the *cause* of the condition, *complications* of the condition, and whether the condition is *acute* (happened suddenly) or is *chronic* (long term). A subterm is followed by its corresponding code. A subterm is also called an *essential modifier*, a word or term that is *necessary for you to read* before you choose a code from the Index.

Figure 3-22 ■ Main term from the Index with related subterms and carryover lines.

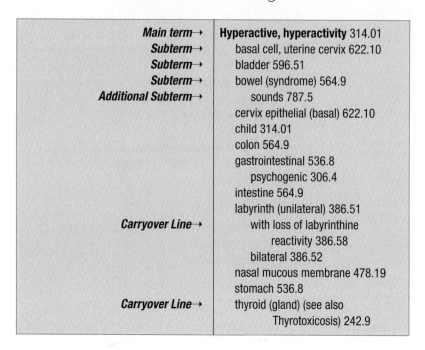

Main term→	**Hyperactive, hyperactivity** 314.01
Subterm→	basal cell, uterine cervix 622.10
Subterm→	bladder 596.51
Subterm→	bowel (syndrome) 564.9
Additional Subterm→	sounds 787.5
	cervix epithelial (basal) 622.10
	child 314.01
	colon 564.9
	gastrointestinal 536.8
	psychogenic 306.4
	intestine 564.9
	labyrinth (unilateral) 386.51
Carryover Line→	with loss of labyrinthine
	reactivity 386.58
	bilateral 386.52
	nasal mucous membrane 478.19
	stomach 536.8
Carryover Line→	thyroid (gland) (see also
	Thyrotoxicosis) 242.9

A **carryover line** is simply a line of text that continues onto a second line due to lack of space in a column. Refer to ■ FIGURE 3-22, which shows the main terms of *Hyperactive, Hyperactivity* and related subterms indented underneath them, as well as carryover lines.

In Figure 3-22, notice that the main term is *Hyperactive* or *hyperactivity*. If the physician documented that the patient suffered from hyperactivity, then you would look up the main term *hyperactivity*, find the code of 314.01, and cross-reference it to the Tabular List. You would have no reason to search further by reading subterms indented under hyperactivity because the medical documentation shows no other information.

However, if the physician documented that the patient had a hyperactive *bladder*, then you would still look up the main term of *hyperactive*, but you would also search for a subterm of *bladder*, which would take you to code 596.51 to cross-reference. Remember that main terms are *never* body sites, so it would be incorrect to search for *bladder* as the main term. If you did, then you would find the term bladder in the Index, but there would be a note to *see condition*. You would then need to search for the condition, which is *hyperactive*.

The Index may direct you to *see condition,* which means that you will need to look for the actual condition the patient has, rather than looking for the body site where the condition is located. Refer to ■ FIGURE 3-23 which shows the *see condition* instruction you'll find when you look for body sites in the Index.

You would find the same instruction of *see condition* if you searched for a word *describing* a condition, rather than the condition itself. For example, if a patient had a malignant neoplasm, and you searched for the word *malignant* as the main term, the Index would instruct you to *see condition. Malignant* is not the patient's condition; it only *describes* the condition. You would instead need to search for *neoplasm* as the main term. Words or phrases that describe conditions are often listed as subterms for the condition.

The Index could also direct you to *see also,* meaning that you may need to look for a diagnosis in an additional place in the Index. We will review more about the *see* and *see also* instructions in Chapter 4 of this text.

Keep in mind that there can be multiple ways to find a specific diagnosis code in the Index (see ■ FIGURE 3-24), but the best and quickest method is to identify the main term and then look for it in the Index, along with any related subterms. *When you find the code you need, always cross-reference it to the Tabular List to review additional information before assigning the final code.*

Leg - *see* condition

Stomach - *see* condition

Finger - *see* condition

Figure 3-23 ■ See condition instruction from the Index.

Main term - Alzheimer's→
Subterm - dementia→
 	
OR
	Alzheimer's
	dementia (senile)
	   with behavioral disturbance 331.0
	     [294.11]
	   without behavioral disturbance 331.0
	     [294.10]
	disease or sclerosis 331.0
	   with dementia - see Alzheimer's, dementia

Main term - dementia→
 	
Subterm - Alzheimer's→
	Dementia 294.8
	alcohol-induced persisting (see also
	   Psychosis, alcoholic) 291.2
	Alzheimer's - see Alzheimer's, dementia
	arteriosclerotic (simple type) (uncomplicated)
	   290.40
	with
	   acute confusional state 290.41
	   delirium 290.41
	   delusions 290.42
	   depressed mood 290.43

Figure 3-24 ■ Examples of different ways to search the Index for Alzheimer's disease, senile dementia.

Locating and Understanding the Structure of Main Terms and Subterms

Follow these guidelines for assistance with locating and understanding main terms and subterms:

1. Main terms can describe the patient's symptom(s) if there is no definitive (definite) diagnosis established that caused the symptoms. Symptoms can include pain, nausea, and itching.

2. Main terms can also be an **eponym**, a disease or condition named after a person, often the physician who discovered the disease or a famous person who suffered from it, like Lou Gehrig's Disease. You can search for the name itself as the main term, or you can search under the main term of *disease* or *syndrome*, with the name of the condition listed as a subterm.

3. A main term is *not* a body site, so if a patient's diagnosis describes the problem and the body site affected, then you will need to look first for the problem (main term), and then look further for the body site (subterm).

4. A **nonessential modifier** is a supplementary word or phrase in parentheses ( ) following a main term or subterm. It provides additional information but does not need to be present in the diagnosis. Refer to ■ FIGURE 3-25 to see an example of a nonessential modifier for **lymphadenopathy** (enlarged, diseased lymph nodes).

   In Figure 3-25, *lymphadenopathy* is followed by the nonessential modifier, *general*, shown in parentheses, with code 785.6. This means that if the patient's diagnosis is general lymphadenopathy, the code to cross-reference to the Tabular List is 785.6. If the patient's diagnosis is lymphadenopathy without mention of general, you would cross-reference the same code, 785.6. You can ignore the nonessential modifier in this case because it does not have to be part of the patient's diagnosis in order for you to assign code 785.6.

   Another example, is if the patient's diagnosis is *acquired* lymphadenopathy due to toxoplasmosis. The code to cross-reference is 130.7, and the subterm includes the

lymphadenopathy
(lĭm-făd'n-ŏp'ə-thē)

Lymphadenopathy (general) 785.6
   due to toxoplasmosis (acquired) 130.7
   congenital (active) 771.2

Figure 3-25 ■ Main term lymphadenopathy with nonessential modifier.

nonessential modifier of *acquired*. But if the patient's diagnosis is lymphadenopathy due to toxoplasmosis without any mention of acquired, then you could ignore the nonessential modifier of *acquired* and still assign the code 130.7.

The nonessential modifier is an optional word or term that you apply when it is part of the diagnosis documented in the patient's record. The fact that the nonessential modifier is in parentheses means that it is optional; use it when it is appropriate. The nonessential modifier does not have to be part of the patient's diagnosis.

5. Subterms modify, or further describe, a main term. Subterms are also called *essential modifiers,* meaning that it is necessary for you to review them to ensure that you choose the correct code. In other words, it is *not an option* to ignore subterms.

6. Not all main terms have subterms.

7. A subterm can have its own indented subterm(s) that further describe it, so you have to follow the indentations carefully to ensure that you apply the correct subterm to either the main term or another subterm.

8. Lists of subterms can continue throughout several columns, and when they do, you have to carefully follow the indentations to know which subterms modify a main term and which modify other subterms that appeared in previous columns.

TAKE A BREAK

Let's take a break and then review information about Volume 2 with an exercise.

Exercise 3.4   Volume 2, Alphabetic Index—Main Terms, Subterms, Carryover Lines

Instructions: Complete each blank field with the best answer.

1. A(n) _____ is an injury or poisoning that is self-inflicted.

2. _____ contains an alphabetical list of the names of drugs and chemicals, along with their corresponding codes.

3. A(n) _____ is an injury or poisoning caused by taking an overdose of a drug, taking the wrong substance, taking a drug inadvertently, or taking a drug given during a medical or surgical procedure.

4. A subterm is also called a(n) _____, a word or term that you must read before choosing a code from the Index.

5. _____ is an injury or poisoning that resulted from taking a correct substance properly administered in therapeutic or prophylactic dosage (for example, a patient had an adverse reaction to a medication that his physician prescribed).

6. _____ contains the names and descriptions for all diagnoses, conditions, diseases, and reasons for encounters, arranged in alphabetical order.

7. A(n) _____ is a disease or condition named after a person.

8. A(n) _____ is a supplementary word or phrase in parentheses ( ) following a main term or subterm that provides additional information but that doesn't need to be present in the diagnosis.

TABLES IN THE ALPHABETIC INDEX

There are many different variations of two diagnoses, *hypertension* (elevated, or high, blood pressure) and neoplasms. Because each diagnosis has multiple choices of codes, there is a table in the Alphabetic Index for each condition that groups all of the choices together to make it easier for you to find the correct codes. To locate the hypertension table in the Index, look for the main term, *hypertension*. To find the neoplasm table, look under the word *neoplasm*. Now we will review more about both of these tables.

In the **Hypertension Table** (■ FIGURE 3-26), look at the main term *hypertension*. Notice that there are various types of hypertension, shown with nonessential modifiers and subterms. Did you also notice that there are columns labeled *malignant, benign,* and *unspecified*? In order to code hypertension correctly, you not only have to know the type of hypertension the patient has, but you also have to know whether the hypertension is *malignant*

Hypertension Table..	Malignant	Benign	Unspecified
Hypertension, hypertensive (arterial) (arteriolar) (crisis) (degeneration) (disease) (essential) (fluctuating) (idiopathic) (intermittent) (labile) (low renin) (orthostatic) (paroxysmal) (primary) (systemic) (uncontrolled) (vascular)...	401.0	401.1	401.9
with			
chronic kidney disease			
stage I through stage IV, or unspecified	403.00	403.10	403.90
stage V or end stage renal disease	403.01	403.11	403.91

Figure 3-26 ■ Hypertension Table in the Alphabetic Index.

hypertension (abrupt onset), *benign hypertension* (can be stable over many years), or *unspecified hypertension* (no documentation in the medical record whether it is malignant or benign).

In the **Neoplasm Table** (■ FIGURE 3-27), you will see the main term *neoplasm* followed by many subterms for body sites where the neoplasm is located. When you are coding neoplasms, you need to know the *location* of the neoplasm, as well as whether the neoplasm is malignant, benign, displays uncertain behavior, or is unspecified. Notice that there are columns for these choices.

Notice in Figure 3-27 that there are six columns in the neoplasm table for choosing the neoplasm behavior. The behaviors in the neoplasm table match neoplasm behaviors

Figure 3-27 ■ Neoplasm Table in the Alphabetic Index.

	Malignant Primary	Malignant Secondary	Malignant Ca in situ	Benign	Uncertain Behavior	unspecified
Neoplasm, neoplastic	199.1	199.1	234.9	229.9	238.9	239.9

Notes - 1. The list below gives the code numbers for neoplasms by anatomical site. For each site there are six possible code numbers according to whether the neoplasm in question is malignant, benign, in situ, of uncertain behavior, or of unspecified nature. The description of the neoplasm will often indicate which of the six columns is appropriate; e.g., malignant melanoma of skin, benign fibroadenoma of breast, carcinoma in situ of cervix uteri.

Where such descriptors are not present, the remainder of the Index should be consulted where guidance is given to the appropriate column for each morphological (histological) variety listed; e.g., Mesonephroma-see Neoplasm, malignant; Embryoma-see also Neoplasm, uncertain behavior; Disease, Bowen's-see Neoplasm, skin, in situ. However, the guidance in the Index can be overridden if one of the descriptors mentioned above is present; e.g., malignant adenoma of colon is coded to 153.9 and not to 211.3 as the adjective "malignant" overrides the Index entry "Adenoma-see also Neoplasm, benign."

2. Sites marked with the sign * (e.g., face NEC*) should be classified to malignant neoplasm of skin of these sites if the variety of neoplasm is a squamous cell carcinoma or an epidermoid carcinoma and to benign neoplasm of skin of these sites if the variety of neoplasm is a papilloma (any type).

abdomen, abdominal	195.2	198.89	234.8	229.8	238.8	239.89
cavity	195.2	198.89	234.8	229.8	238.8	239.89
organ	195.2	198.89	234.8	229.8	238.8	239.89
viscera	195.2	198.89	234.8	229.8	238.8	239.89
wall	173.5	198.2	232.5	216.5	238.2	239.2
connective tissue	171.5	198.89	-	215.5	238.1	239.2
abdominopelvic	195.8	198.89	234.8	229.8	238.8	239.89
accessory sinus-see Neoplasm, sinus						
acoustic nerve	192.0	198.4	-	225.1	237.9	239.7

outlined in Appendix A – Morphology of Neoplasms. Remember that Appendix A categorizes neoplasms by types of cancer, while the Neoplasm Table categorizes neoplasms by body site. Both Appendix A and the Neoplasm Table also categorize neoplasms by their behaviors. Here are the neoplasm behaviors in the Neoplasm Table:

- *Malignant primary*—life-threatening neoplasm in the site where it was first found, and it has since spread.
- *Malignant secondary*—life-threatening neoplasm in the new site to which it has spread, although it started in a different location.
- *Malignant Ca in situ*—life-threatening cancer that is confined to one site and has not spread anywhere else.
- *Benign*—neoplasm that is not life threatening.
- *Uncertain behavior*—It is unclear whether the neoplasm is benign or malignant.
- *Unspecified (whether malignant or benign)*—The medical record does not specify the type of neoplasm.

You will practice coding from both the Hypertension and Neoplasm Tables in later chapters in this book. Refer to your ICD-9-CM coding manual to see both tables in their entirety to become more familiar with them.

TAKE A BREAK

Let's take a break and then review the Tables with an exercise.

| Exercise 3.5 | Tables in the Alphabetic Index |

Instructions: Complete each blank field with the best answer.

1. _____ is a life-threatening neoplasm in a new site to which it has spread, after starting somewhere else.

2. Hypertension with an abrupt onset is called _____ hypertension.

3. _____ hypertension can be stable over many years.

4. The _____ shows various types of hypertension, along with choices for malignant, benign, and unspecified.

5. The term for elevated, or high blood pressure, is _____.

6. _____ is a life-threatening neoplasm in the site where it was first found, and it has since spread to other locations.

7. The _____ shows various choices for body sites where a neoplasm is located.

8. _____ is a life-threatening cancer that is confined to one site and has not spread anywhere else in the body.

CHAPTER REVIEW

Multiple Choice

Instructions: Circle one best answer to complete each statement.

1. The types of ICD-9-CM codes are
   a. diagnosis codes, inpatient procedure codes, and outpatient procedure codes.
   b. inpatient procedure codes and outpatient procedure codes.
   c. diagnosis codes and inpatient procedure codes.
   d. diagnosis codes and outpatient procedure codes.

2. The four organizations that review and approve the ICD-9-CM Official Guidelines are called the
   a. cooperating parties.
   b. negotiating parties.
   c. coding parties.
   d. guideline parties.

3. The ICD-9-CM manual is divided into _____ volumes.
   a. two   b. three
   c. four   d. five

4. The Classification of Diseases and Injuries contains _____ chapters that group diagnosis codes in numeric order.
   a. 13
   b. 15
   c. 17
   d. 21

5. Assign a(n) _____ for cases in which the patient has nothing wrong, but you still need to provide a reason for the service.
   a. inpatient procedure code
   b. V code
   c. E code
   d. outpatient procedure code

6. Each chapter of the Classification of Diseases and Injuries includes a
   a. section, category, and subcategory.
   b. section, category, subcategory, and subclassification.
   c. section, subcategory, subclassification, and tables.
   d. section, category, subcategory, subclassification, and tables.

7. Subclassification codes are
   a. either indented under the subcategory code or listed below the category.
   b. either indented under the chapter or listed below the category.
   c. only indented under the subcategory code.
   d. only listed below the category.

8. Various formats of the ICD-9-CM code set provide you with _____ that are printed next to codes so that you can determine if you need to code to the fourth or fifth digit.
   a. colored pages
   b. regulatory guidelines
   c. symbols
   d. lists

9. You should use a residual subcategory code when
   a. there isn't a more specific code in the Alphabetic Index.
   b. you are coding from the neoplasm or hypertension tables.
   c. you are coding with E codes.
   d. there isn't a more specific code in the Tabular List.

10. Residual category codes contain the words _____ and _____ in their descriptions.
    a. none, unspecified
    b. other, unspecified
    c. unlisted, other
    d. unlisted, unspecified

11. The _____ located after Volume 1 Tabular List provide additional information about a patient's condition, disease, or injury.
    a. listings
    b. tables
    c. glossaries
    d. appendices

12. _____ codes identify types of cancer.
    a. Morphology
    b. V codes
    c. E codes
    d. Hypertension

13. Coders will sometimes refer to the _____ to quickly locate a specific category and cross-reference it to the Tabular List.
    a. List of Three-Digit Chapters
    b. List of Three-Digit Sections
    c. List of Three-Digit Categories
    d. List of Three-Digit Subcategories

14. Volume 1 Alphabetic Index contains _____ sections.
    a. two
    b. three
    c. four
    d. five

15. The Index is structured by _____, _____, and _____.
    a. chapters, main terms, subterms
    b. chapters, subterms, carryover lines
    c. main terms, subterms, carryover lines
    d. sections, main terms, subterms

16. Two instructions in the Index that direct you to search somewhere else for a condition are
    a. see, see also.
    b. refer, refer also.
    c. look, look also.
    d. review, review also.

17. Main terms can describe the patient's _____ if there is no definitive diagnosis established.
    a. body site
    b. left or right side
    c. body temperature
    d. symptoms

18. The _____ gives code choices to describe patients with elevated, or high, blood pressure.
    a. Hyperactive Table
    b. Hypertension Table
    c. Hypotension Table
    d. Distention Table

19. The _____ gives code choices to describe patients with abnormal growths.
    a. Neoplasm Table
    b. Carcinoma Table
    c. Protoplasm Table
    d. Growth Table

20. When the medical record does not state whether the behavior of a patient's abnormal growth is malignant or benign, you code it as _____.
    a. unremarkable behavior
    b. unclear behavior
    c. unknown behavior
    d. unspecified behavior

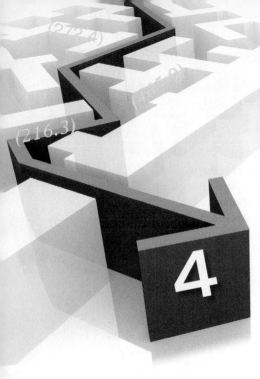

ICD-9-CM Coding Conventions and General Coding Guidelines

4

Learning Objectives

After completing this chapter, you should be able to

- Spell and define the key terminology in this chapter.
- List the Coding Conventions for ICD-9-CM.
- Define includes notes, excludes notes, and inclusion terms in the Tabular List.
- Explain the purpose of ICD-9-CM General Coding Guidelines.
- Describe the meaning of coding to the highest level of specificity.
- Explain when it is appropriate to code signs and symptoms.
- Describe when it is appropriate to assign multiple codes and combination codes.
- Define a late effect and explain how to code it.
- Explain the meaning of an impending or threatened condition and describe how to code for it.
- Discuss the purpose of ICD-9-CM's chapter-specific coding guidelines.
- List the steps to follow to perform correct coding.
- Name additional points to remember when coding.

Key Terms

coding conventions
coding to the highest level of specificity
combination code
etiology

General Coding Guidelines
manifestation
multiple coding
sign
symptom

INTRODUCTION

Remember that you had to learn the format of the ICD-9-CM coding manual and where to locate specific information before you could learn the rules that apply to coding. Just like learning the operating controls of a car, you learned the "controls," or structure, of the coding manual. The only way that you can successfully code diagnoses is to understand how to apply specific rules for assigning codes. There are many rules to follow, which we will review in this chapter. Use the information in this chapter as a reference tool after you have moved on to other chapters where you will combine these rules with chapter-specific coding guidelines. Your goal is to always continue learning so that you will be successful in the healthcare field.

"Seeing much, suffering much, and studying much are the three pillars of learning."—BENJAMIN DISRAELI

ICD-9-CM codes in this chapter are from the ICD-9-CM 2012 code set from the Department of Health and Human Services, Centers for Disease Control and Prevention.

SECTIONS OF ICD-9-CM OFFICIAL GUIDELINES FOR CODING AND REPORTING

Diagnosis coding rules are called the ICD-9-CM Official Guidelines for Coding and Reporting. The Centers for Medicare and Medicaid Services (CMS) and the National Center for Health Statistics (NCHS) created the Guidelines for all three volumes of ICD-9-CM so that providers will know how to use the coding manual and follow the same guidelines for coding diagnoses. In fact, the Health Insurance Portability and Accountability Act (HIPAA) requires you to follow ICD-9-CM Official Guidelines for Coding and Reporting when coding. No matter what form of the manual you use to code (paper, CD-ROM, or web-based), you will find ICD-9-CM guidelines in it, typically located at the very beginning.

There are four sections of rules in ICD-9-CM Official Guidelines for Coding and Reporting, outlined in ■ TABLE 4-1. (You can also find the guidelines on the CDC website; see Appendix A of this text.)

Our main focus of this book is on coding diagnoses and procedures in outpatient settings, so for the next several chapters, you will learn how to code diagnoses for outpatients. However, we will also cover how to assign diagnosis and procedure codes for inpatient settings in Chapters 15 and 16.

In this chapter, we will review the Conventions and General Coding Guidelines found in Section I of ICD-9-CM Official Guidelines for Coding and Reporting. (Section I applies to coding diagnoses in both outpatient and inpatient settings.) You can also find the Guidelines in your coding manual. We will review more about coding for outpatient diagnoses in Chapter 5.

Section I of the Guidelines contains coding conventions, which are terms, abbreviations, symbols, and punctuation that direct you to find the correct code. Section I also contains **General Coding Guidelines**, written rules that you should follow when you are coding. When you review conventions and guidelines, note the following points to help you to better understand them:

- The term *encounter* includes all types of patient visits and services, including hospital admissions.

- The term *provider* includes a physician or any other qualified health care practitioner, such as a physician assistant (PA), certified registered nurse practitioner (CRNP),

■ **TABLE 4-1   FOUR SECTIONS OF ICD-9-CM OFFICIAL GUIDELINES FOR CODING AND REPORTING**

Section I	Section II	Section III	Section IV
Conventions, General Coding Guidelines, Chapter-Specific Coding Guidelines	Selection of Principal Diagnosis (inpatient settings)	Reporting Additional Diagnoses (inpatient settings)	Diagnostic Coding and Reporting Guidelines for Outpatient Services
Section I has three divisions: **A—Conventions for ICD-9-CM** *(Section I A is covered in this chapter.)* **B—General Coding Guidelines** *(Section I B is covered in this chapter.)* **C—Chapter-Specific Coding Guidelines (corresponding to each of the 17 chapters of the Tabular List)** *(Chapter-specific guidelines are covered in other chapters in this book.)*	Section II includes guidelines for selection of the principal diagnosis (the reason for the episode of care) for inpatient settings. *(Section II is covered in Chapter 15.)*	Section III includes guidelines for reporting additional diagnoses in inpatient settings. *(Section III is covered in Chapter 15.)*	Section IV includes guidelines for reporting diagnoses for outpatient services. *(Section IV is covered in Chapter 5.)*

physical therapist (PT), or other medical professional who is legally accountable for establishing a patient's diagnosis.

- The Alphabetic Index is also referred to as the *Index*.
- The Tabular List is also referred to as the *Tabular*.
- When you see examples from the Alphabetic Index and the Tabular List, you may also see the symbols 4th or 5th, which alert you to assign a fourth or fifth digit to the code.

SECTION I A—CONVENTIONS FOR ICD-9-CM

Coding conventions are terms, abbreviations, symbols, and punctuation that are incorporated into both the Alphabetic Index and Tabular List for Volumes 1, 2, and 3. Think of the conventions as road signs that direct you to go another possible direction, continue on your current path, or stop and turn around. The important point to remember is that ICD-9-CM manual will guide you and help you, but you have to pay attention to its messages and explanations, many of which are in the form of conventions.

Refer to ■ TABLE 4-2 for a list of coding conventions and their meanings as you learn about each convention in more detail. Different companies publish the ICD-9-CM code set, along with the CDC, so depending on the version that you use, you may find special symbols and notes in addition to the standard coding conventions. We will discuss what

■ TABLE 4-2   **CONVENTIONS FOR ICD-9-CM**

1. Format	
ICD-9-CM uses an indented format for ease in reference. The Alphabetic Index contains main terms and subterms in alphabetical order. Cross-reference codes in the Index to the Tabular List.	
2. Abbreviations	
a. *Alphabetic Index* abbreviations	
NEC—Not elsewhere classifiable	Medical documentation specifies the diagnosis, but there is no specific code in ICD-9-CM.
b. *Tabular List* abbreviations	
NEC—Not elsewhere classifiable	Medical documentation specifies the diagnosis, but there is no specific code in ICD-9-CM.
NOS—Not otherwise specified	Medical documentation is insufficient to allow for a more accurate code assignment.
3. Punctuation—Alphabetic Index or Tabular List	
Brackets [ ]	Used in Tabular List to enclose synonyms, alternative wording, or explanatory phrases.
Italicized Brackets *[ ]*	May be used in the Index of some coding manuals to identify manifestation codes that you should sequence second.
Parentheses ( )	Used in the Tabular List and the Index to enclose words or terms that may or may not be present in the diagnostic statement (called nonessential modifiers).
Colon :	Used in the Tabular List after an incomplete term to list more information after the colon.
Brace }	May be used in some coding manuals in the Tabular List to connect words written to the left of it to words written to the right.
4. Includes Notes, Excludes Notes, Inclusion Terms, Note—Tabular List	
Includes	Appears after a three-digit code title to further define a category.
Excludes	Appears under a code and lists terms excluded from the code.
Inclusion Terms	Lists terms included under four-digit and five-digit codes.
Note	Gives additional information about conditions and how to code them.
5. Other and Unspecified Codes—Tabular List	
a. "Other" or "Other specified" codes	

- Medical documentation specifies the diagnosis, but there is no specific code in ICD-9-CM.
- Codes with "other" or "other specified" in their titles usually have a fourth digit of 8 and a fifth digit of 9.

continued

■ TABLE 4-2 *continued*

b. "Unspecified" codes

- Medical documentation is insufficient to allow for a more accurate code assignment.
- Codes with "unspecified" in the title usually have a fourth digit of 9 and a fifth digit of 0.

6. Etiology/manifestation convention—Tabular List
"Code first," "use additional code," and "in diseases classified elsewhere" notes

- Certain conditions have both an etiology (cause) and multiple body system manifestations (conditions due to the underlying etiology).
- Assign two codes: The first code is the etiology, the second is the manifestation.

7. "And"—Tabular List

When the word "and" appears in a code title, it can mean either "and," but it can also mean "or."

8. "With"—Alphabetic Index

- In the Index, refer to the word "with" immediately following a main term.
- Do not sequence (list) "with" in alphabetical order.

9. "See," "See Also," and "See Category"—Alphabetic Index or Tabular List

- The word "see" in the Tabular List or after a main term or subterm in the Index means to look elsewhere.
- The phrase "see also" after a main term or subterm in the Index means to also reference another main term/subterm.
- The phrase "see category" appears in the Tabular List or after a main term in the Index. It means to look for information under a specific category in the Tabular List.

---

each convention means and review examples of conventions. You can review information about each convention and work with your own coding manual to compare your findings with the examples shown in this chapter.

You will also have the opportunity to practice what you learn by completing coding exercises. Remember that there is more than one way to search for a main term in the Index, so the examples do not show every option. It will be helpful for you to begin using your own manual. If you are working with a paper manual, then you may want to label various sections of it with tabs to make it easier to find information quickly.

1. FORMAT

The first coding convention is *format*, and ICD-9-CM uses an *indented* format in the Index and Tabular List. Remember that in the Index, main terms are listed in alphabetical order, and many main terms have indented subterms (essential modifiers), also listed in alphabetical order. Subterms help further describe main terms. Subterms can also have additional indented subterms (in alphabetical order) that help to modify them. Indented subterms are also listed in alphabetical order. Refer to ■ FIGURE 4-1 to see a main term with indented subterms in the Index.

In the Tabular List, code titles, or descriptors, for categories (three-digit), subcategories (four-digit), and subclassifications (five-digit) may be printed in bold, depending on ICD-9-CM manual. In the examples in this book, you will see main terms in bold. Main terms can also have indented words and terms under the code title that provide you with important notes or supplementary information to consider before you assign the code. ■ FIGURE 4-2 shows indented information under the code title for 244.3, which gives more information about the condition.

Hypothyroidism (acquired) 244.9
complicating pregnancy, childbirth, or puerperium 648.1
congenital 243
due to
   ablation 244.1
      radioactive iodine 244.1
      surgical 244.0

Figure 4-1 ■ Index—main term and subterms.

Figure 4-2 ■ Code 244.3 from the Tabular List.

244.3	**Other iatrogenic hypothyroidism**
	Hypothyroidism resulting from:
	P-aminosalicylic acid [PAS]
	Phenylbutazone
	Resorcinol
	Iatrogenic hypothyroidism NOS
	Use additional E to identify drug

Information indented under code titles may be in *italicized* type, which alerts you to apply specific coding guidelines. We will review these guidelines later in this chapter. Whether you are referencing the Index or Tabular List, be sure to pay attention to indented information because it can affect your final code assignment.

Main Terms

Main terms describe the patient's condition, illness, injury, or reason for an encounter in a single word or a phrase. Main terms can also describe symptom(s), such as nausea or fever, if there is no definitive (definite) diagnosis that caused the symptoms. Remember that main terms can also be eponyms and that a main term is *not* a body site.

Before moving forward, it will be helpful for you to practice identifying main terms in a diagnostic statement in Exercise 4.1 so that you can follow along with the coding examples provided in this chapter and perform the exercises.

TAKE A BREAK

Exercise 4.1 **Format**

Instructions: Underline or circle the main term in each diagnostic statement. Keep your medical dictionary handy in case you need to define terms.

1. Leg pain
2. Acute cystitis
3. Cerebral angiospasm
4. Curschmann's disease
5. Hemorrhagic telangiectasia
6. Rectal sphincter relaxation
7. Pneumococcal myocarditis
8. Otitis media

2. ABBREVIATIONS

The next coding conventions are the abbreviations *NEC* (not elsewhere classifiable), that you will find in both the Index and the Tabular List, and *NOS* (not otherwise specified), that you will only find in the Tabular List. Let's discuss these in more detail.

A. Index Abbreviation—NEC "Not Elsewhere Classifiable"

The abbreviation NEC, not elsewhere classifiable, means that the physician documented a specific diagnosis for a patient, but ICD-9-CM does not have a specific code for it. A code described with NEC is often a more general code, but you have to use it because you do not have another choice, as shown in Example 1.

> **Example 1:** Dr. Hoffman documents that Mr. Wales has anterior lower cervical syndrome.
>
> 1. To find the code for the patient's diagnosis, look in the Index for the main term, remembering that the main term is not a body site.
>
> 2. Search for the word *syndrome*. When you find it, look for the body site as a subterm, which is *cervical*.

> **Syndrome**–see also **Disease**
>   cervical (root) (spine) NEC 723.8
>   disc 722.71
>   posterior, sympathetic 723.2
>   rib 353.0
>   sympathetic paralysis 337.09
>   traumatic (acute) NEC 847.0

Figure 4-3 ■ Index entry showing Syndrome, cervical.

3. In ■ FIGURE 4-3, you can see that syndrome is the main term, and cervical is a subterm.
4. Now search for *anterior* and *lower* as further subterms, and you will find that they do not exist. There are no options for you to code any further by choosing *anterior* or *lower* as subterms under cervical. This means that the condition is not classified elsewhere, or "not elsewhere classifiable."

Notice in Figure 4-3 that the abbreviation NEC follows the subterm *cervical* and its nonessential modifiers (words in parentheses that are optional). NEC means that the physician documented the patient's diagnosis as *anterior lower cervical syndrome*, but there is no equivalent code for it in ICD-9-CM. The closest that you will come to finding a code for *anterior lower cervical syndrome* is *cervical syndrome NEC*, which has a code of 723.8. You cannot code any further because the code set does not classify the diagnosis any further.

B. Tabular List Abbreviation—NEC "Not Elsewhere Classifiable"

Just as in the Index, the abbreviation NEC in the Tabular List means that the physician documented a specific diagnosis for a patient, but ICD-9-CM does not have a code for it.

Titles for these types of codes can include the words *other* or *other specified* and may also include the abbreviation NEC. The phrase *other* or *other specified* in the Tabular List means that the physician specified the patient's condition in the documentation, but there is no ICD-9-CM code for it. In Example 1, we found code 723.8 in the Index for Mr. Wales' diagnosis of *anterior lower cervical syndrome*. Let's cross-reference 723.8 to the Tabular List to see the code title, which includes the word *other*. The indented information below it contains the abbreviation NEC (■ FIGURE 4-4).

Notice that the code title for 723.8 is *Other syndromes affecting cervical region*. Indented under the code is the phrase *cervical syndrome NEC*, which is included in code 723.8. Notice that there are also separate conditions classified as *other*, such as Klippel's disease. This means that there are no ICD-9-CM codes for these conditions; they are simply *Other syndromes affecting cervical region*.

Keep in mind that when you see NEC describing a code in either the Index or Tabular List, it should be a red flag to you to only assign it after ensuring that there is not a more specific code describing the condition. Review all of the possible subterms in the Index and indented information in the Tabular List, including coding notes, *before assigning an NEC code*.

> **723.8   Other syndromes affecting cervical region**
>   Cervical syndrome NEC
>   Klippel's disease
>   Occipital neuralgia

Figure 4-4 ■ Tabular List NEC.

C. Tabular List Abbreviation—NOS "Not Otherwise Specified"

The abbreviation NOS, not otherwise specified, is different from NEC, and in fact, it means just the opposite. Whereas NEC means that the physician documented the patient's diagnosis, but it is not in ICD-9-CM, NOS means that the physician *did not document the diagnosis specifically* enough for you to assign an exact code. NOS appears in the Tabular List and means that the diagnosis is *unspecified*. The Tabular List may include the word *unspecified* with the code title.

Are you wondering why the physician would not completely document a patient's diagnosis? Some reasons are that the physician did not have any additional information to support a more definitive diagnosis, did not completely finish documenting, was waiting for the patient's lab or radiology test results before rendering a diagnosis, or was waiting for records from another physician in order to review additional information before assigning a specific diagnosis. Do you remember learning that if you do not code to the highest level of specificity, you risk the insurance not paying for the patient's service or paying too little? That is why it is important for you to query, or ask, the physician to clarify the patient's diagnosis. You can explain to the physician that you need to assign the most specific code so that you do not jeopardize reimbursement. Only assign a code with NOS in its description as a *last resort*. Refer to Example 2 to better understand when to use an NOS code.

Example 2: Dr. Hoffman documents that Mrs. Williams has a headache, but he did not specify what type of headache.

1. Search the Index for the main term, *headache*, as shown in ■ FIGURE 4-5.
2. Notice that you have several choices for the type of headache indented under the main term, *headache*. But Dr. Hoffman did not document the *type of headache* the patient has, so you have to choose code 784.0 to cross-reference to the Tabular List (■ FIGURE 4-6).

```
Headache 784.0
    allergic 339.00
    associated with sexual activity 339.82
    cluster 339.00
        chronic 339.02
        episodic 339.01
    daily
    chronic 784.0
    new persistent (NPDH) 339.42
```

Figure 4-5 ■ Index entry for headache.

```
784.0   Headache
            Facial pain
            Pain in head NOS
        Excludes:   atypical face pain (350.2)
                    migraine (346.0–346.9)
                    tension headache (307.81)
```

Figure 4-6 ■ Tabular list showing NOS.

Code 784.0 represents *headache*, and *pain in the head NOS* is indented underneath, meaning that the patient's diagnosis is an unspecified headache, or *not otherwise specified*.

There is nothing more to code because there is no more specific information in the documentation. In this case, you would query Dr. Hoffman to obtain more information about Mrs. Williams' *type of headache* to avoid assigning an NOS code. But if Dr. Hoffman cannot provide any more information, then you would have to assign code 784.0 as the last resort.

The abbreviations NEC and NOS are often confusing and sometimes are mistakenly used interchangeably, even though they have different meanings. In summary, the abbreviation NEC, not elsewhere classifiable, means that the physician documented a specific diagnosis for a patient, but ICD-9-CM doesn't have a specific code for it. The abbreviation NOS, not otherwise specified, means that the physician *did not* document a more specific diagnosis, so you cannot assign a specific code.

3. PUNCTUATION

Various types of punctuation appear throughout the Tabular List and Index to provide additional information to help you code accurately. Refer to ■ TABLE 4-3 for a list of each type of punctuation as you review the types in more detail.

A. Brackets [ ]—Tabular List

In the Tabular List, *brackets* enclose synonyms (different words that have the same meaning), alternative wording, explanatory phrases, and abbreviations. Refer to ■ FIGURE 4-7 to see two examples of abbreviations enclosed in brackets in the Tabular List.

B. Italicized Brackets *[ ]* —Index

Italicized brackets are not part of the standard conventions from ICD-9-CM's Official Guidelines. However, your coding manual may show *italicized brackets* in the Index to enclose codes for manifestations. A **manifestation** is a problem that develops from an underlying condition or disease, called an **etiology**. The etiology *causes* the manifestation. (The etiology/manifestation coding convention is also covered later in this chapter.) Refer

■ TABLE 4-3   **PUNCTUATION CONVENTIONS**

Punctuation	Location	Meaning
Brackets [ ]	Tabular List	Enclose synonyms, alternative wording, or explanatory phrases.
Italicized Brackets *[ ]*	Index	Enclose manifestation codes that you should sequence second: may be used in some coding manuals.
Parentheses ( )	Tabular List and Index	Enclose words or terms that may or may not be present in the diagnostic statement (called nonessential modifiers).
Colon :	Tabular List	Used after an incomplete term to list more information.
Brace }	Tabular List	Connects words written on the left of the brace to words written on the right: may be used in some coding manuals.

Figure 4-7 ■ Brackets in the Tabular List.

> **5th** 491.2 Obstructive chronic bronchitis
>
> 491.21 With (acute) exacerbation
> Acute exacerbation of chronic obstructive pulmonary disease [COPD]
>
> 616.10 Vaginitis and vulvovaginitis, unspecified
> Vaginitis:
> NOS
> postirradiation
> Vulvitis NOS
> Vulvovaginitis NOS
> Use additional code to identify organism,
> such as Escherichia coli [E. coli] (041.4),

to Example 3 for more information on italicized brackets associated with etiology/manifestation coding:

diabetes mellitus
(mel′-ət-əs)

Example 3: Mrs. Gold has **diabetes mellitus,** a condition in which the pancreas does not produce enough insulin (insulin regulates glucose, also called sugar), resulting in too much sugar in the patient's blood. During her office visit, Dr. Hoffman documents diabetes and also diagnoses her with gangrene of the foot (tissue death from a lack of blood supply). It is a complication of diabetes.

Gangrene and diabetes have an etiology/manifestation relationship. The etiology, or underlying cause of the gangrene, is diabetes. The manifestation, or result of the etiology, is gangrene. The patient would not have had gangrene of her foot if she had not first had diabetes. Coding a manifestation and an etiology involves assigning two codes: one for the etiology (which you should assign first) and the other for the manifestation (which you should assign second). It is mandatory to assign two codes when there is an established etiology/manifestation relationship, which is called *mandatory multiple coding.*

Are you wondering how you will know if gangrene and diabetes have an etiology/manifestation relationship? The wonderful part about coding in ICD-9-CM is that your book tells you how to code; you just need to pay attention and "hear" what the book says. We already know two important facts about Mrs. Gold's encounter: She has diabetes mellitus and gangrene of the foot. Let's find the two codes for this case, beginning with *gangrene.*

1. Search the Index for the main term *gangrene* (■ FIGURE 4-8).

2. When you search for *gangrene* in the Index, you will find code 785.4, but if you just stop there, then you are not coding the patient's complete diagnosis because she also has diabetes.

3. Look a little further, and find the connecting word *with,* then find *diabetes (mellitus)* as a subterm indented under *with.* You will see two codes: 250.7, listed

> Gangrene, gangrenous (anemia) (artery) (cellulitis) (dermatitis) (dry) (infective) (moist)
> (pemphigus) (septic) (skin) (stasis) (ulcer) 785.4
> with
> arteriosclerosis (native artery) 440.24
> bypass graft 440.30
> autologous vein 440.31
> nonautologous biological 440.32
> diabetes (mellitus) 250.7 *[785.4]*
> due to secondary diabetes 249.7 *[785.4]*

Figure 4-8 ■ Index entry for gangrene.

785.4	**Gangrene**
	Gangrene:
	NOS
	spreading cutaneous
	Gangrenous cellulitis
	Phagedena
	Code first any associated underlying condition

Figure 4-9 ■ Tabular List entry for gangrene.

first, and 785.4, listed second in italicized brackets. In the Index, codes in italicized brackets are *manifestation* codes, and you always assign them as *secondary* to an etiology code. The Index shows the etiology code 250.7 immediately before the manifestation code.

4. You have to cross-reference both the etiology and the manifestation code before final code assignment, and you can cross-reference in any order. Let's start by cross-referencing the manifestation code 785.4 to the Tabular List (■ FIGURE 4-9).

5. Refer to the note under 785.4 instructing you to *Code first any associated underlying condition*, meaning that you should assign the code for the underlying condition (etiology) first. The patient's underlying condition (etiology) is diabetes, so report the code for diabetes first and the code for gangrene second (manifestation). Remember that ICD-9-CM will direct you to the correct codes, but you have to pay attention to its messages. You now know that you will assign code 785.4 second, and you also have to search for diabetes in the Index to find the diabetes code. You will learn more about etiology/manifestation coding later in this chapter.

For this example, when you find *gangrene with diabetes* in the Index, the code in italicized brackets *[785.4]* immediately alerts you that it is a manifestation code and that you should assign it second. If you ignore the fact that the code is in italicized brackets, then when you cross-reference 785.4 to the Tabular List, the Tabular List will remind you again that it is a manifestation code with the instruction to *Code first any associated underlying condition*. ICD-9-CM provides you with messages in both the Index and the Tabular List to help you code the etiology first and the manifestation second.

C. Parentheses ( )—Tabular List and Index

You have already learned that *parentheses* enclose supplementary words, called *nonessential modifiers*, that may be present or absent in the diagnosis without affecting the code that is assigned. Parentheses can also enclose additional information that will help you code correctly.

Recall from Chapter 3 that in the Index, a nonessential modifier follows main terms, and it can also follow subterms. It provides additional information about the main term or subterm but does not need to be present in the diagnosis.

In the Tabular List, nonessential modifiers follow code titles and also do not need to be part of the diagnosis. Refer to ■ FIGURES 4-10 and 4-11 for examples of information contained in parentheses in the Index and the Tabular List.

Eruption
creeping 126.9
drug - see Dermatitis, due to, drug
Hutchinson, summer 692.72
Kaposi's varicelliform 054.0
napkin (psoriasiform) 691.0
polymorphous
light (sun) 692.72

Figure 4-10 ■ Parentheses in the Index.

732.3 Juvenile osteochondrosis of upper extremity
Osteochondrosis (juvenile) of:
capitulum of humerus (of Panner)
carpal lunate (of Kienbock)
hand NOS

Figure 4-11 ■ Parentheses in the Tabular List.

294.1 Dementia in conditions classified elsewhere
Dementia of the Alzheimer's type
Code first any underlying physical condition as:
dementia in:
Alzheimer's disease (331.0)
cerebral lipidoses (330.1)
dementia with Lewy bodies (331.82)
dementia with Parkinsonism (331.82)
epilepsy (345.0–345.9)

Figure 4-12 ■ Colons in the Tabular List.

D. Colon :—Tabular List

You will find *colons* in the Tabular List after incomplete terms that need one or more modifiers to further specify a condition. A colon typically precedes a list of information, or choices, as shown in ■ FIGURE 4-12. When you see a list of information following a colon, it means that any one of the items in the list could apply to the code that you review.

Figure 4-12 shows code 294.1, *Dementia in conditions classified elsewhere*. Notice the instruction *Code first any underlying physical condition as:* followed by *dementia in:*. This instruction is followed by a list of underlying conditions that are present with dementia. If the patient has one of those conditions with dementia, then you should assign the underlying condition code first and dementia second. In this case, the colon precedes a list of conditions to code first.

E. Brace }—Tabular List, Used in Some Versions of ICD-9-CM

The last punctuation convention is the *brace*, which connects words written to the left of it to words written to the right, as shown in ■ FIGURE 4-13. The brace is not part of the standard conventions in the Official Guidelines, but you may see it in your coding manual.

In Figure 4-13, read the information to the left of the brace and add the information to the right: "compression, brain (stem)," or "herniation, brain (stem)." The patient does not need to have *both* compression and herniation of the brain stem in order for you to assign code 348.4. Either can apply; a patient could have compression *or* herniation of the brain stem to assign code 348.4. The information that appears to the right of the brace applies to more than one term on the left, so the information to the right was only written once to save space.

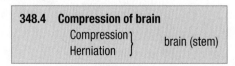

348.4 **Compression of brain**
Compression ⎫
Herniation ⎬ brain (stem)

Figure 4-13 ■ Brace in the Tabular List.

TAKE A BREAK

Let's take a break and then review abbreviations and punctuation with an exercise.

Exercise 4.2 **Abbreviations and Punctuation**

Instructions: Match the term in the list to its description, writing the letter of the term on the line preceding each description.

1. _____ The physician didn't document the diagnosis specifically enough for you to assign a more exact code.

2. _____ Enclose nonessential modifiers that may be present in or absent from the diagnosis without affecting the code number assigned.

3. _____ The physician documented a specific diagnosis for a patient, but ICD-9-CM doesn't have a code for it.

4. _____ Connects words written to the left of it to words written to the right.

5. _____ In the Index, these enclose codes for manifestations.

6. _____ This is listed after incomplete terms that need one or more modifiers to make the term assignable to a given category.

7. _____ In the Tabular List, these enclose synonyms, alternative wording, explanatory phrases, and abbreviations.

a. colon
b. brace
c. italicized brackets
d. NEC
e. parentheses
f. NOS
g. brackets

4. INCLUDES NOTES, EXCLUDES NOTES, INCLUSION TERMS, AND NOTE IN THE TABULAR LIST

Includes notes and excludes notes appear under a chapter or section and under category, subcategory, and subclassification codes. *Includes notes* further define, or provide examples of, content for a chapter, section, or code title. *Excludes notes* indicate that the terms listed as excluded should be coded elsewhere.

A. Includes and Excludes Notes

Includes and Excludes notes in the Tabular List provide you with key clues and convey important information for assigning your final code. Many new coders are often eager to assign the first code that they cross-reference from the Index to the Tabular List, and they overlook includes or excludes notes that would have changed the final code assignment. When you cross-reference a *code* to the Tabular List and read its description or title, be sure to check for includes or excludes notes. Also check for includes and excludes notes outlined for the *category* of the code that you cross-reference and for the *section* and the *chapter* that contain the code. Sometimes includes and excludes notes apply to an entire chapter, section, or category.

■ FIGURE 4-14 shows excludes notes that apply to Chapter 3 of the Tabular List. It is best to review these notes when searching for any codes in Chapter 3 to ensure that you are not searching for a condition excluded from the chapter (codes 775.0–775.9). Notice that just

---

3. ENDOCRINE, NUTRITIONAL AND METABOLIC DISEASES, AND IMMUNITY DISORDERS (240–279)

Excludes: **endocrine and metabolic disturbances specific to the fetus and newborn (775.0–775.9)**

Note: All neoplasms, whether functionally active or not, are classified in Chapter 2. Codes in Chapter 3 (i.e., 242.8, 246.0, 251–253, 255–259) may be used to identify such functional activity associated with any neoplasm, or by ectopic endocrine tissue.

Figure 4-14 ■ Chapter 3 excludes notes.

Figure 4-15 ■ Includes and excludes for category 249.

5th **249 Secondary diabetes mellitus**
Includes: diabetes mellitus (due to) (in) (secondary) (with): drug-induced or chemical induced infection
Excludes: gestational diabetes (648.8) hyperglycemia NOS (790.29) neonatal diabetes mellitus (775.1) nonclinical diabetes (790.29) Type I diabetes - see category 250 Type II diabetes - see category 250

under the excludes notes is a **Note** that contains additional information for you to review when you are searching for codes in Chapter 3. You will read more about the note later in this chapter.

Excludes notes basically mean to go somewhere else if you are looking for a condition in the excludes list. Excludes notes make your job easier because they not only list the conditions that are excluded, but they also provide you with the codes to reference if you need to search for one of the excluded conditions.

■ FIGURE 4-15 shows both includes and excludes notes pertaining to category 249. If you are attempting to code one of the conditions listed under Includes, then you are in the right place. But if you are attempting to code one of the conditions listed under Excludes, then you are in the wrong place and instead need to go to the code or category listed for the excluded condition.

Both includes and excludes notes can also apply to a subcategory or subclassification, as shown in ■ FIGURES 4-16 and 4-17.

Excludes notes also apply to *congenital* conditions (present at birth) and *acquired* conditions (developed after birth). When you cross-reference a code for either type of condition, you will see Excludes notes for the other condition because you cannot report both an acquired condition and a congenital condition together.

B. Inclusion Terms—Tabular List

Inclusion terms are types of conditions that are indented under a subcategory or subclassification code title (■ FIGURE 4-18).

Figure 4-16 ■ Excludes notes for a subcategory code.

5th **250.3** **Diabetes with other coma**
[0-3] Diabetic coma (with ketoacidosis) Diabetic hypoglycemic coma Insulin coma NOS
Excludes: diabetes with hyperosmolar coma (250.2)

Figure 4-17 ■ Excludes notes for a subclassification code.

277.85 **Disorders of fatty acid oxidation**
Carnitine palmitoyltransferase deficiencies (CPT1, CPT2) Glutaric aciduria type II (type IIA, IIB, IIC) Long chain 3-hydroxyacyl CoA dehydrogenase deficiency (LCHAD) Long chain/very long chain acyl CoA dehydrogenase deficiency (LCAD, VLCAD) Medium chain acyl CoA dehydrogenase deficiency (MCAD) Short chain acyl CoA dehydrogenase deficiency (SCAD)
Excludes: primary carnitine deficiency (277.81)

Figure 4-18 ■ Inclusion terms.

571.8 **Other chronic nonalcoholic liver disease**
Chronic yellow atrophy (liver) Fatty liver, without mention of alcohol

709.2   Scar conditions and fibrosis of skin
Adherent scar (skin)
Cicatrix
Disfigurement (due to scar)
Fibrosis, skin NOS
Scar NOS

Painful - see also Pain
scar NEC 709.2

Figure 4-19 ■ Index entry for painful scar.

Figure 4-20 ■ Tabular List showing code 709.2.

Notice that inclusion terms indented under code 571.8 are *Chronic yellow atrophy (liver)* and *Fatty liver, without mention of alcohol*. A patient does not have to have *both* conditions in order to assign code 571.8; the patient could have either condition. Or the patient could have another type of disease that falls under the code title of *Other chronic nonalcoholic liver disease* and that is not one of the conditions listed in either of the inclusion terms. Conditions listed within inclusion terms simply mean that they are possible options for code assignment. Inclusion terms can also list synonyms for a specific condition. You may not find an inclusion term under every code title.

Cross-Referencing Codes

When you are cross-referencing a code from the Index to the Tabular List, the wording in the Index may not exactly match the code title or inclusion terms in the Tabular List. ICD-9-CM is structured this way in order to save space in the Tabular List. When you are in doubt, always go back to the Index to verify the description of your code selection, and trust the Index for the *wording* of your final code assignment. Refer to ■ Figure 4-19 which shows the Index entry for "painful scar." The Index lists code 709.2 for *painful scar NEC*, but when you cross-reference 709.2 in the Tabular List, *painful scar NEC* is nowhere to be found (■ Figure 4-20).

What happened to *painful scar* in the Tabular List? The exact wording of *painful scar* does not exist in the Tabular. However, you can still assign code 709.2 because painful scar is a *scar condition*, and code 709.2 represents *scar conditions*. The Tabular List does not include every single word that describes a scar, so that is why you do not see the word *painful* listed for 709.2. If you are in doubt, then go back to the Index, look for the main term *painful*, subterm *scar*, and the Index will again lead you to code 709.2. Trust the information that you find in the Index.

C. Note

Sometimes, you will also find a Note in the Tabular List directing you how to assign codes. ■ Figure 4-21 is an example of a Note for Chapter 1 of the Tabular List. It is very important to pay attention to any Notes to ensure that you assign the correct codes.

CLASSIFICATION OF DISEASES AND INJURIES

1. INFECTIOUS AND PARASITIC DISEASES (001–139)

Note: Categories for "late effects" of infectious and parasitic diseases are to be found at 137–139.

Figure 4-21 ■ Tabular List showing a Note.

5. OTHER, OTHER SPECIFIED, AND UNSPECIFIED CODES—TABULAR LIST

We reviewed codes in the Tabular List with "other," "other specified," and "unspecified" in their titles when we discussed the abbreviations NEC and NOS. "Other" and "other specified" in code titles in the Tabular List correlate to a code's Index entry with the abbreviation NEC.

A. Other or Other Specified Codes

Assign codes titled *other* or *other specified* (usually a diagnosis code with a fourth digit of 8 or a fifth digit of 9) in the Tabular List when the physician documented a specific diagnosis for a patient but ICD-9-CM does not have a code for it. Index entries with NEC designate codes that are described as other or other specified in the Tabular List. Code titles in the Tabular List can include the words *other* or *other specified* and may also include the abbreviation NEC.

B. Unspecified Codes

Assign codes titled *unspecified* (usually a diagnosis code with a fourth digit of 9 or a fifth digit of 0) when the physician did not document the diagnosis specifically enough for you to assign a more exact code. Recall that you may also find the abbreviation NOS in the Tabular List with the code title, which means that the diagnosis is *unspecified*. The word *unspecified* may also be included in the code title instead of the abbreviation NOS.

TAKE A BREAK

That was a lot of information to cover! Let's take a break and then review more with an exercise.

Exercise 4.3 Includes Notes, Excludes Notes, Inclusion Terms, Other, Other Specified, and Unspecified Codes

Instructions: Refer to the Tabular List to answer the following questions.

1. Can you code acute cerebrovascular insufficiency with transient focal neurological signs and symptoms from category 435? yes no

   Why or why not? _____

2. Can you code for an enlarged prostate from category 600? yes no

   Why or why not? _____

3. Review inclusion terms under subcategory 704.2. Does the patient need to have all of the conditions listed as inclusion terms in order for you to assign code 704.2? yes no

   Why or why not? _____

4. What condition(s) are included in the section Organic Psychotic Conditions (290–294) in Chapter 5—Mental Disorders? _____

5. If you assigned code 377.9 to a patient's encounter, then did the physician document the type of optic nerve and visual pathway disorder? yes no

   How do you know? _____

6. Is cavitary prostatitis part of code 601.8 or 601.9? ___
   _____

   How do you know? _____

7. Refer to category 680 and its subcategories to answer the following questions:

   a. Is a boil included as a condition with category 680? yes no

   b. A patient has a boil on the top of his head. What code should you assign? _____

   c. A female patient has a boil on her external genitalia. What code should you assign? _____

   d. What code should you assign for a boil on the buttocks? _____

6. ETIOLOGY/MANIFESTATION CONVENTION—TABULAR LIST

Do you remember earlier in the chapter when we discussed how in the Index, italicized brackets contain manifestation codes? We discussed that certain conditions have both an underlying etiology (cause) and manifestation (result of the etiology). ICD-9-CM requires you to code the underlying condition first and code the manifestation second. Recall that in the Index, the etiology code is listed first, and the manifestation code appears second in italicized brackets. The italicized brackets are your clue to assign the code in italicized brackets second. ICD-9-CM provides additional hints, or notes, in the Tabular List to help you code the etiology and manifestation in the correct order, including the following notes:

A. **Code First**

B. **Use Additional Code**

C. **In Diseases Classified Elsewhere**

A. Code First

Code first is a note in the Tabular List that indicates how to sequence, or list, etiology and manifestation codes. When you find a manifestation code contained in italicized brackets in the Index and cross-reference it to the Tabular List, you will see a note to *code first* the underlying disease or etiology.

For instance, ▪ FIGURE 4-22 shows the Index entry for diabetic **retinopathy** (a disease/disorder of the innermost part of the eye). Diabetic retinopathy is a manifestation of diabetes, which is the etiology.

retinopathy
(re-tə-ˈnä-pə-thē)

The Index tells you that these two conditions have an etiology/manifestation relationship because when you search for the main term, retinopathy, and the subterm, diabetic, you will see diabetes as the first code listed (250.5) and a second code for retinopathy (362.01) listed in italicized brackets. Code 250.5 is the etiology, and 362.01 is the manifestation. You have already learned that any time you find a code contained in italicized brackets, it is a manifestation code that you assign secondary to the etiology code. When you cross-reference the manifestation code 362.01 to the Tabular List, you find a *Code first* note with subcategory 362.0, as shown in ▪ FIGURE 4-23.

If you overlook the fact that a manifestation code is in slanted brackets in the Index and you have to assign it second, then ICD-9-CM reminds you again when you cross-reference the code to the Tabular List. It directs you to *Code first* the condition that is the etiology (diabetes). It is important to remember that the *Code first* note can also apply to certain codes that are not part of an etiology/manifestation relationship.

B. Use Additional Code

Use additional code is another note in the Tabular List to help you sequence etiology and manifestation codes in the correct order. In Figure 4-23, you saw the instruction to *Code first diabetes* under the manifestation code of 362.0 for diabetic retinopathy. The choices

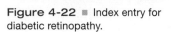

Retinopathy (background) 362.10
  arteriosclerotic 440.8 *[362.13]*
  atherosclerotic 440.8 *[362.13]*
  central serous 362.41
  circinate 362.10
  Coat's 362.12
  diabetic 250.5 *[362.01]*

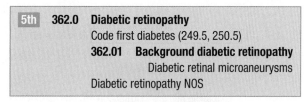

5th	**362.0**	**Diabetic retinopathy**
		Code first diabetes (249.5, 250.5)
	362.01	**Background diabetic retinopathy**
		Diabetic retinal microaneurysms
		Diabetic retinopathy NOS

Figure 4-22 ▪ Index entry for diabetic retinopathy.

Figure 4-23 ▪ Tabular List with Code first note.

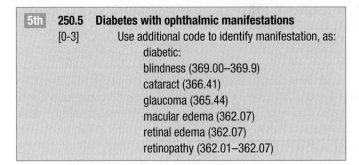

5th	250.5	**Diabetes with ophthalmic manifestations**
[0-3]		Use additional code to identify manifestation, as:
		diabetic:
		blindness (369.00–369.9)
		cataract (366.41)
		glaucoma (365.44)
		macular edema (362.07)
		retinal edema (362.07)
		retinopathy (362.01–362.07)

Figure 4-24 ▪ Tabular List with Use additional code note.

for diabetes codes were 249.5 and 250.5. Do you think that when you cross-reference the diabetes (etiology) codes to the Tabular List that you will see an instruction to code the manifestation second? If you said yes, then you are correct! The *Use additional code* note appears with an etiology code to alert you to assign a secondary code for the manifestation. Once again, ICD-9-CM tells you exactly what to do; you just have to pay attention to its instructions. Look at ▪ FIGURE 4-24 to see diabetes code 250.5 cross-referenced to the Tabular List and the instruction to *Use additional code* to assign the manifestation second (retinopathy).

In Figure 4-24, the instruction *Use additional code to identify manifestation, as:* means that you should assign a code *in addition to*, or *after*, another code. When you check the list of conditions under the *Use additional code* instruction, you find diabetic retinopathy, meaning that you assign the code for it *after the etiology* code for diabetes. If a patient has more than one manifestation of diabetes, then you can assign more than one code from category 250. You may assign as many manifestation codes as you need to fully describe the patient's complete condition. Sequence category 250 diabetes codes first, followed by the manifestation codes.

When a patient has both an etiology and a manifestation, the Tabular List provides instructions for the order in which to sequence both codes. The Tabular lists a *Code first* instruction with the manifestation code and a *Use additional code* instruction with the etiology code. Keep in mind that just like the *Code first* note, the note to *Use additional code* may apply to certain codes that are not part of the etiology/manifestation relationship.

C. In Diseases Classified Elsewhere

The Tabular List also includes a note called *in diseases classified elsewhere* as part of the code title for a manifestation, as shown in ▪ FIGURE 4-25. This note means that the condition is part of another disease. In Figure 4-25, cerebellar ataxia is classified in other diseases, which you should code first, including alcoholism, myxedema, and neoplastic disease.

Not every manifestation code has *in diseases classified elsewhere* in the title, but you will see a *use additional code* note to remind you of the order of sequencing the etiology and manifestation codes.

334.4	**Cerebellar ataxia in diseases classified elsewhere**
	Code first underlying disease, as:
	alcoholism (303.0–303.9)
	myxedema (244.0–244.9)
	neoplastic disease (140.0–239.9)

Figure 4-25 ▪ Tabular List with in diseases classified elsewhere note.

TAKE A BREAK

Let's take a break and then assign codes for etiologies and manifestations.

Exercise 4.4   **Etiology/Manifestation Convention and Notes**

Instructions: Assign codes to the following conditions using both the Index and Tabular List. Each answer will have two codes, and you will need to list codes in the correct order. Main terms are underlined for you.

1. <u>Diabetic</u> cataract.

   1st code:_____   2nd code:_____

2. <u>Tuberculous</u> abscess of the hip from tuberculosis osteomyelitis.

   1st code:_____   2nd code:_____

3. Female <u>infertility</u> due to anterior pituitary disorder.

   1st code:_____   2nd code:_____

7. AND—TABULAR LIST

In the Tabular List, when you see the word *and* in a code title, you can interpret it to mean and/or. In ■ FIGURE 4-26, category 342 represents *hemiplegia and hemipareseis*, but it can also mean hemiplegia *or* hemiparesis. Category 342 captures both conditions together or each condition separately. Just because you see the word *and* in the code title, it does not mean that the patient has to have both conditions in order for you to assign the code.

8. WITH—ALPHABETIC INDEX

Many times in the Index, the word *with* follows a main term. *With* is not an alphabetized subterm for a main term but instead is a word that *connects* main term to subterms. Notice that in ■ FIGURE 4-27 the word *with* follows the main term *rhinitis*, connecting *rhinitis* to subterms indented under *with*.

Here are some other words and phrases immediately following a main term that connect it to subterms:

- and
- associated with
- complicated (by)
- due to
- during
- following
- for
- in
- involving
- of
- secondary to
- with mention of
- without

342	**Hemiplegia and hemiparesis**

Figure 4-26 ■ Tabular List category 342 with the word *and*.

Figure 4-27 ■ Index entry showing with.

> **Rhinitis** (atrophic) (catarrhal) (chronic) (croupous) (fibrinous) (hyperplastic) (hypertrophic) (membranous) (purulent) (suppurative) (ulcerative) 472.0
> with
>   hay fever (see also Fever, hay) 477.9
>   with asthma (bronchial) 493.0
>
>   sore throat - see Nasopharyngitis

9. SEE, SEE ALSO, SEE CATEGORY—ALPHABETIC INDEX

The Index contains three different instructions containing the word *see*:

A. *see*—Look elsewhere.

B. *see also*—Look in an additional place.

C. *see category*—Go to a specific category in the Tabular List.

A. See

The instruction *see* in the Tabular List or following a main term/subterm in the Index tells you to go elsewhere to find a code. It means that you are looking in the wrong place. ■ FIGURE 4-28 includes an example of "see" in the Index, and ■ FIGURE 4-29 includes "see" in the Tabular List.

    Both instructions tell you to look elsewhere for the code(s) to assign.

B. See Also

The *see also* instruction following a main term/subterm in the Index tells you that there is *another* main term/subterm that you can reference to find the code you need (■ FIGURE 4-30). However, you do not need to follow the *see also* instruction if the original main term that you searched provides the necessary code.

C. See Category

The *see category* instruction in the Tabular List or after a main term in the Index tells you to go to a specific category in the Tabular List when you are searching for a condition. You would go directly to the Tabular List to find the category and review the code choices.

    For an example of the *see category* instruction, imagine that you are searching for the condition of *late effect of syringomyelitis* in the Index, with a main term of *syringomyelitis* and subterm of *late effect*. (**Syringomyelitis** is inflammation of the spinal cord, associated with the formation of cavities or openings.) A *late effect* is a problem that develops after the initial

syringomyelitis
(si-ringo'-mī-ə-lītis)

Figure 4-28 ■ Index entry with see instruction.

> **Rhythm**
>   heart, abnormal 427.9
>   fetus or newborn - see Abnormal, heart rate

Figure 4-29 ■ Tabular List with see instruction.

> **010   Primary tuberculous infection**
>
> Requires fifth digit. See beginning of section 010–018 for codes and definitions.

Figure 4-30 ■ Index entry with see also instruction.

> **Rhinopharyngitis** (acute) (subacute) (see also Nasopharyngitis) 460

> **Syringomyelitis 323.9**
>
> late effect - see category 326

Figure 4-31 ■ Index entry with see category, cross-referenced to the Tabular List.

> **572.2 Hepatic encephalopathy**
>   Hepatic coma
>   Hepatocerebral intoxication
>   Portal-systemic encephalopathy
> Excludes: hepatic coma associated with viral hepatitis - see category 070

Figure 4-32 ■ See category in the Tabular List.

condition (syringomyelitis) has passed. ■ FIGURE 4-31 shows that there is a note to *see category 326* beside the subterm *late effect*. This means that you do not have a choice; if you want to find the correct code, you should go directly to category 326 in the Tabular List, also shown in Figure 4-31. ■ FIGURE 4-32 shows an example of "see category" in the Tabular List.

TAKE A BREAK

Let's take a break and then review the information with an exercise.

Exercise 4.5   **And, With, See, See Also, See Category**

Instructions: Assign codes to the following conditions using both the Index and Tabular List. Main terms are underlined for you. Each coding problem has one answer.

1. <u>Abnormal</u> Papanicolaou smear with atypical squamous cells, significance undetermined.

   Code: _____

2. <u>Abortion</u> with complications of excessive hemorrhage.

   Code: _____

3. Chronic <u>abscess</u> of the accessory sinus, sphenoidal, with sinus infection.

   Code: _____

SECTION I B—GENERAL CODING GUIDELINES

Congratulations! You have learned the Coding Conventions outlined in Section I A of ICD-9-CM Official Guidelines for Coding and Reporting. Next, we will review Section I B, General Coding Guidelines. You will be glad to know that you are already familiar with some of the information outlined in the General Coding Guidelines. As with the Coding Conventions, it will be helpful for you to work through examples shown here using your own coding manual. You will also have many opportunities to practice what you learned by completing coding exercises.

There are 17 General Coding Guidelines, the titles of which are outlined in ■ TABLE 4-4. The General Coding Guidelines apply when you are coding *all conditions*. We will discuss each guideline in detail. In addition, there are guidelines that apply only to specific chapters of the Tabular List, and you will learn those guidelines in later chapters in this book. You will also learn guidelines that apply to inpatient procedure codes in Chapter 16 of this text.

1. Use Both the Alphabetic Index and Tabular List When Coding

Use both the Alphabetic Index and the Tabular List when you are locating and assigning a code. Do not rely only on the Alphabetic Index or the Tabular List because that can lead to errors in code assignments and less specificity in code selection, which can also cause insurance billing errors.

■ TABLE 4-4   **GENERAL CODING GUIDELINES FOR ICD-9-CM**

SECTION I B   General Coding Guidelines for ICD-9-CM
1. Use Both the Alphabetic Index and Tabular List when Coding
2. Locate Each Term in the Alphabetic Index
3. Level of Detail in Coding
4. Code(s) 001.0 through V91.99
5. Selection of Codes 001.0 through 999.9
6. Signs and Symptoms
7. Conditions that Are an Integral Part of a Disease Process
8. Conditions that Are *not* an Integral Part of a Disease Process
9. Multiple Coding for a Single Condition
10. Acute and Chronic Conditions
11. Combination Code
12. Late Effects
13. Impending or Threatened Condition
14. Reporting Same Diagnosis Code More than Once
15. Admissions/Encounters for Rehabilitation
16. Documentation for Body Mass Index (BMI) and Pressure Ulcer Stages
17. Syndromes

2. Locate Each Term in the Alphabetic Index

Locate each main term in the Alphabetic Index, then verify the code selected in the Tabular List. Read and follow the coding instructions that appear in both the Alphabetic Index and the Tabular List.

3. Level of Detail in Coding

Code diagnosis codes to their highest number of digits available, a practice called **coding to the highest level of specificity**. You already know that ICD-9-CM diagnosis codes have three digits (categories), four digits (subcategories), or five digits (subclassifications). Coding to the highest level of specificity means assigning a subcategory if one exists and assigning a subclassification code if one exists.

For example, in ■ FIGURE 4-33, you will see part of the Tabular List entry for code 410, *Acute myocardial infarction*. Code 410 has fourth digits that describe the location of the infarction (e.g., 410.0, Of anterolateral wall) and fifth digits that identify the episode of care. It would be incorrect to report a code in category 410 without a fourth and fifth digit.

4. Code(s) 001.0 through V91.99

and

5. Selection of Codes 001.0 through 999.9

Both guidelines 4 and 5 mean that code ranges in the Tabular List are 001.0 to V91.99, and you must assign codes within this range to identify diagnoses, symptoms, conditions, problems, complaints, or other reason(s) for the encounter, visit, or hospital admission.

6. Signs and Symptoms

Codes that describe symptoms and signs, as opposed to diagnoses, are acceptable for reporting purposes when the provider has not established a related definitive diagnosis. A **sign** is objective evidence of disease that the physician discovers, commonly through an examination. A **symptom** is subjective evidence of disease that the patient reports to

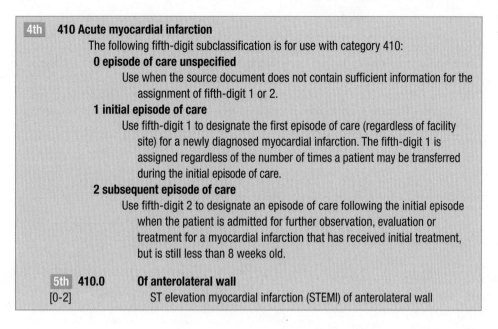

Figure 4-33 ■ Code 410 in the Tabular List.

the physician. In the physician's medical documentation of a patient's encounter, she will document signs and symptoms, along with a definitive diagnosis if one exists. The definitive diagnosis is the patient's final diagnosis that the physician reports, after examining the patient and reviewing test results. Sometimes, there is no diagnosis, only a sign or a symptom, because the physician does not or cannot establish a definitive diagnosis.

For example, during her office visit Mrs. Harper tells Dr. Hoffman that she is nauseated (symptom). Dr. Hoffman examines her but cannot discover a reason for her nausea. There is no definitive diagnosis, only the symptom of nausea. You would code nausea because there is no other reason for the patient's encounter.

Likewise, during a physical examination of Mr. Walton, Dr. Hoffman observes that the patient has memory loss (sign), but he cannot determine why. There is no definitive diagnosis, only the sign of memory loss. You would code memory loss because there is no other reason for the patient's encounter.

Chapter 16 of the Tabular List (780.0–799.9) contains many, but not all, codes for symptoms and signs. You will code these conditions in Chapter 13 of this book.

7. Conditions That Are an Integral Part of the Disease Process

Do not assign codes for signs and symptoms that are integral to (associated routinely with) a disease process, unless you are instructed to do so by the classification in ICD-9-CM. When you are coding a patient's condition, it is not necessary for you to code signs or symptoms of a specific condition along with the definitive diagnosis. It is *assumed* that if a patient has a specific diagnosis, then the patient *also has* the signs and symptoms associated with it, so you do not need to report them. If you are not sure whether the signs and symptoms documented in the patient's chart are part of the specific diagnosis, then you should query the physician for clarification. You can also review your medical references for more information.

For example, heartburn, arm pain, and shortness of breath are all symptoms of a myocardial infarction (heart attack). A patient with a definitive diagnosis of myocardial infarction would not need to have additional codes assigned for heartburn, arm pain, and shortness of breath because it is assumed that these are common symptoms of the definitive diagnosis. However, if a patient had heartburn, but the physician found no evidence of a myocardial infarction or any other condition, then you *would* code heartburn because there is no other reason for the patient's encounter.

8. Conditions That Are Not an Integral Part of the Disease Process

Code additional signs and symptoms that are not routinely associated with a disease process. This means that if a patient has other signs or symptoms that are *unrelated* to the definitive diagnosis, then you should code those signs and symptoms separately. Again, if you are not sure whether signs and symptoms are related to a disease, you should query the physician.

TAKE A BREAK

Let's take a break and then review coding guidelines 1–8 with an exercise.

| Exercise 4.6 | General Coding Guidelines 1–8 |

Instructions: Underline the main term for each diagnosis, and assign codes using both the Index and Tabular List. Determine whether to assign more than one code. Refer to your medical dictionary or conduct web searches to define medical terms and to determine if conditions listed are symptoms of another diagnosis.

1. Gastroenteritis and nausea due to *Salmonella*.
   Code(s): _____

2. Generalized abdominal pain.
   Code(s): _____

3. Respiratory infection with cough.
   Code(s): _____

4. Flatulence and bloating.
   Code(s): _____

9. Multiple Coding for a Single Condition

In addition to the etiology/manifestation convention that requires two codes to fully describe a single condition affecting multiple body systems, there are other single conditions that also require more than one code, called **multiple coding**. (You may also assign multiple codes for multiple conditions.) Notes in the Tabular List that apply to assigning multiple codes for a single condition are *Use additional code, Code first,* and *Code, if applicable, any causal condition first.* You are already familiar with two of these notes from our review of etiology/manifestation coding, and you have reviewed examples of them. Definitions of the notes follow:

- *Use additional code*—The *Use additional code* note alerts you to add a secondary code to a condition. It can apply to an etiology/manifestation relationship or other conditions that need to be described using more than one code.

- *Code first*—A *Code first* note alerts you to assign a code for an underlying condition (etiology) first, before reporting the manifestation code.

- *Code, if applicable, any causal condition first*—This note instructs you to assign a code for the cause of a condition (causal condition) if the cause is present *before* assigning a code for the condition itself. ■ FIGURE 4-34 shows code 707.1 *Ulcer of lower limbs, except pressure ulcer.* The *Code, if applicable, any causal condition first* note precedes a list of conditions that are all *causes* of an ulcer of the lower limbs. If one of these conditions caused the ulcer, then you would assign the code for the causal condition first and assign code 707.1 for the ulcer second.

Figure 4-34 ■ Code, if applicable, any causal condition first note.

707.1	Ulcer of lower limbs, except pressure ulcer
	Ulcer, chronic, of lower limb:
	neurogenic } of lower limb
	trophic
	Code, if applicable, any causal condition first:
	atherosclerosis of the extremities with ulceration (440.23)
	chronic venous hypertension with ulcer (459.31)
	chronic venous hypertension with ulcer and inflammation (459.33)

You may also need to assign multiple codes to more fully describe conditions for late effects (problems that develop from an illness that has passed), complication codes, infections, and obstetric codes (pregnancy, childbirth, and time following delivery). Please see the specific ICD-9-CM coding guidelines for further instructions for coding these conditions. The instructions are also outlined throughout this book.

TAKE A BREAK

Let's take a break and then practice assigning multiple codes.

Exercise 4.7   **General Coding Guideline 9—Multiple Coding for a Single Condition**

Instructions: Underline the main term and assign codes to the following conditions using both the Index and Tabular List. Determine whether to assign more than one code, and follow any notes listed in ICD-9-CM. Refer to your medical dictionary or conduct web searches to define medical terms.

1. Meningitis due to listeriosis.

   Code(s): _____

2. Vernal conjunctivitis with limbar and corneal involvement.

   Code(s): _____

3. Acute pyelonephritis due to *E. coli* with necrotic renal medullary lesion.

   Code(s): _____

10. Acute and Chronic Conditions

Assign two codes for a condition that is described as both acute (subacute) and chronic unless there is a combination code that describes both conditions. An *acute* condition starts quickly [has a rapid onset (start)]; a *subacute* condition exists at a level that is between acute and chronic, and a *chronic* condition typically lasts three months or more. If you need to assign separate codes for the acute and chronic conditions, then sequence the acute condition *first* and the chronic condition *second*.

For example, a patient suffers from acute and chronic nasopharyngitis. When you search the Index for the main term, nasopharyngitis (■ Figure 4-35), you see that *acute* is a nonessential modifier and the code is 460. *Chronic* is a subterm of nasopharyngitis with code 472.2. You need to cross-reference both codes to the Tabular List before final code assignment.

In ■ Figure 4-36 when you are cross-referencing acute nasopharyngitis to the Tabular List, notice that the code title for 460 includes the word *acute*. Also notice that the *Excludes* note shows that nasopharyngitis, chronic (472.2) is excluded from code 460. You have to code chronic nasopharyngitis separately and sequence it second.

In ■ Figure 4-37, when you are cross-referencing chronic nasopharyngitis to the Tabular List, notice that the code title for 472.2 includes the word chronic. Also notice that the

Nasopharyngitis (acute) (infective) (subacute) 460
     chronic 472.2

Figure 4-35 ■ Index entry for acute and chronic condition.

460   Acute nasopharyngitis [common cold]
        Coryza (acute)
        Nasal catarrh, acute
        Nasopharyngitis:
           NOS
           acute
           infective NOS
        Rhinitis:
           acute
           infective
        Excludes: nasopharyngitis, chronic (472.2)

Figure 4-36 ■ Tabular List of acute condition.

Figure 4-37 ■ Tabular List of chronic condition.

472.2	**Chronic nasopharyngitis**
	Excludes: acute or unspecified nasopharyngitis (460)

Figure 4-38 ■ Combination code in the Tabular List.

518.84	**Acute and chronic respiratory failure**
	Acute on chronic respiratory failure

Excludes note shows that nasopharyngitis, acute (460) is excluded from code 472.2. You have to code the acute condition separately and sequence it first. The final code assignment is 460 (acute nasopharyngitis) and 472.2 (chronic nasopharyngitis).

Do you remember reading that the ICD-9-CM manual will instruct you to code correctly? The rule for coding acute and chronic conditions is another example of how the manual tells you what to code. The coding rule from the General Coding Guidelines goes a step further by telling you that you need to sequence the acute condition first and the chronic condition second. If there were one code for a condition that included both acute and chronic conditions, then you would only assign that code, and you would not need two separate codes for acute and chronic. One code that represents two conditions is covered next under Combination Code.

11. Combination Code

A **combination code** is a single code used to classify

- Two diagnoses,
- A diagnosis with an associated secondary process (manifestation), or
- A diagnosis with an associated complication.

You can identify combination codes by referring to subterm entries in the Index and by reading the inclusion and exclusion notes in the Tabular List. ■ FIGURE 4-38 shows a condition that is both acute and chronic and a combination code represents both conditions.

Only assign the combination code when it fully identifies the condition(s) or when the Index directs you to assign it. Do not assign multiple codes when the classification provides a combination code that clearly identifies all of the elements documented in the diagnosis. When the combination code lacks necessary specificity in describing the manifestation or complication, assign an additional code to describe it.

TAKE A BREAK

Let's take a break and then review acute and chronic conditions and combination codes with an exercise.

Exercise 4.8 General Coding Guidelines 10 and 11—Acute and Chronic Conditions and Combination Codes

Instructions: Underline the main term and assign codes to the following conditions using both the Index and Tabular List. Determine whether to assign more than one code. Refer to your medical dictionary or conduct web searches to define medical terms.

1. Illegally induced abortion complicated by damage to pelvic organs.

   Code(s): _____

2. Open wound of auditory canal (external ear) with complication.

   Code(s): _____

3. Acute and chronic areola abscess.

   Code(s): _____

4. Acute and chronic adenitis of mesenteric lymph node.

   Code(s): _____

12. Late Effects

A *late effect* is the residual effect (condition that is produced) after the acute phase of an illness or injury has passed, or terminated. Even though the acute phase of an illness is over, the illness has caused another problem. There is no time limit for assigning codes for late effects. The late effect may be apparent early, such as in cerebrovascular accident (CVA - stroke) cases, or it may occur months or years later, such as a condition that develops due to a previous, prior, or old injury. Here are some examples of late effects:

- Arthritis (residual, or late effect) that the patient developed 15 years after suffering a pelvic (hip) fracture (acute illness that has now passed)

- Shin splints (pain in the lower leg- residual, or late effect) that the patient developed a few months after suffering a tibial (lower leg) fracture (acute illness that has now passed)

- Stiffness of the hand (residual, or late effect) that the patient developed six months after suffering a burn to the hand (acute illness that has now passed)

- Back pain (residual, or late effect) that the patient developed several years after suffering a back injury (acute illness that has now passed)

- Dysphagia (difficulty swallowing- residual, or late effect) that the patient developed shortly after suffering a stroke (acute illness that has now passed). (A stroke happens when a ruptured artery, ruptured blood vessel, or blood clot impairs blood flow to the brain, which can cause brain damage and death.)

When you are coding a late effect caused by another condition, assign two codes. First assign the code for the patient's current condition (the residual effect), then assign a second code to describe the condition that caused the problem (the previous illness or injury that has now passed). The exception to this rule is conditions that are late effects of strokes, which you typically report using one code. You can find these codes by searching the Index for the main term: late, subterm: effect(s) (of), subterm: name of the residual condition.

When you read the medical documentation, key phrases and words alert you that the patient's condition is the late effect of another condition that has now passed, such as old, past, previous, due to, and caused by.

Let's review how to assign the residual and late effect codes using the example of a patient with scarring on his neck caused by burns he sustained four months ago. The scars are constricting his airway, and he needs surgery to remove them.

The patient's current condition (residual) is scarring. The burns caused the scars, but if you only code for the scars and ignore the fact that the patient has them because of a *previous* injury (burns), then you are not coding the complete diagnosis. You would be leaving out important information showing *why* the patient has scars. The first code that you will assign is for the patient's current condition, the residual condition of scars. Look for the main term *scar* in the Index (■ FIGURE 4-39).

Now, cross-reference code 709.2 to the Tabular List for final code assignment (■ FIGURE 4-40).

The second code that you will assign is for a *late effect* of a burn. You must code the fact that the scar is a *late effect of a burn* to tell the entire story about the patient's condition. A patient could have a scar for a number of reasons, and it is your job to show *why* the patient has the scar. When you are coding a late effect, look under the main term *late,*

709.2	Scar conditions and fibrosis of skin
	Adherent scar (skin)
	Cicatrix
	Disfigurement (due to scar)
	Fibrosis, skin NOS
	Scar NOS

Scar, scarring - see also Cicatrix 709.2

Figure 4-39 ■ Index entry for scar.

Figure 4-40 ■ Scar in the Tabular List.

Figure 4-41 ■ Index entry for late effect of a burn.

Late - see also condition
    effect(s) (of) - see also condition
        burn (injury classifiable to 948–949) 906.9
            extremities NEC (injury classifiable to 943 or 945) 906.7
                hand or wrist (injury classifiable to 944) 906.6
            eye (injury classifiable to 940) 906.5
            face, head, and neck (injury classifiable to 941) 906.5
            specified site NEC (injury classifiable to 942 and 946–947) 906.8

Figure 4-42 ■ Late effect of burn injury in the Tabular List.

4th   906   Late effects of injuries to skin and subcutaneous tissues

    906.5   Late effect of burn of eye, face, head, and neck
        Late effect of injury classifiable to 940–941

then look for the subterm, *effect(s) (of)*, then look for the subterm showing the disease or injury that the patient *previously* had. In this case, look for *late, effect(s) (of), burn*. You will see *face, head, and neck* as a subterm (■ FIGURE 4-41).

Now, cross-reference code 906.5 for late effect of burn injury of the neck to the Tabular List for the final code assignment (■ FIGURE 4-42). The two codes that you'll assign are 709.2 for scar and 906.5 for the *late effect* of a burn.

Do you know why you did not assign a code for the acute phase of the illness, the burn? It is because the burn is in the *past*. It no longer exists. However, it caused a *new* problem for the patient, the scar. You always code a condition that no longer exists as a *late effect* if it created a new problem for the patient. If you code burn, it would mean that the patient is currently being treated for a burn, which is untrue.

A patient can also have more than one residual condition caused by the acute illness that has passed. Be very careful when you are coding late effects to ensure that you only code the patient's current residual condition, along with the reason for it (late effect of the previous condition that has now passed). *Never* assign a code for the acute phase of an illness or injury with a code for the late effect of that same illness/injury. We will cover more about coding late effects in Chapter 8 of this text.

INTERESTING FACT: Strokes Responsible for Most Long-Term Disabilities

Each year in the United States, there are more than 780,000 strokes. Stroke is the third leading cause of death in the country and causes more serious long-term disabilities than any other disease. Nearly three-quarters of all strokes occur in people over the age of 65, and the risk of having a stroke more than doubles each decade after the age of 55. A stroke occurs when the blood supply to part of the brain is suddenly interrupted or when a blood vessel in the brain bursts. The National Institutes of Health, through the National Institute of Neurological Disorders and Stroke, developed the "Know Stroke, Know the Signs, Act in Time" campaign to help educate the public about the symptoms of stroke and the importance of getting to the hospital quickly. The symptoms include

✔ Sudden **NUMBNESS** or weakness of face, arm, or leg, especially on one side of the body
✔ Sudden **CONFUSION**, evident through trouble speaking or understanding speech
✔ Sudden **TROUBLE SEEING** in one or both eyes
✔ Sudden **TROUBLE WALKING**, dizziness, loss of balance or coordination
✔ Sudden **SEVERE HEADACHE** with no known cause

(National Institute of Neurological Disorders and Stroke, National Institutes of Health, stroke.nih.gov/materials/actintime.htm, accessed 11/20/11)

TAKE A BREAK

Let's take a break and then review and code residuals and associated causes.

| Exercise 4.9 | **General Coding Guideline 12—Late Effects** |

Part 1

Instructions: Identify the residual condition and cause for the following conditions.

1. Contracture of scar of the throat from previous burn.

   Residual condition: _____

   Cause: _____

2. Dysphagia from previous stroke.

   Residual condition: _____

   Cause: _____

3. Osteoarthritis of the elbow due to old fracture.

   Residual condition: _____

   Cause: _____

4. Left side facial droop from prior stroke.

   Residual condition: _____

   Cause: _____

5. Knee arthritis from old sports injury.

   Residual condition: _____

   Cause: _____

6. Emotional lability from prior stroke.

   Residual condition: _____

   Cause: _____

Part 2: General Coding Guideline 12—Late Effects

Instructions: Code the following residual conditions, along with their causes. Sequence the residual first. Remember to search under "late effect" to find causes, and remember that the coding rules are different for late effects of a stroke. (Do not code previous conditions as current conditions.) Use both the Index and Tabular List. Refer to your medical dictionary or conduct web searches to define medical terms.

1. Contracture of scar of the leg muscles from previous burn.

   Code for residual condition (late effect): _____

   Code for cause: _____

2. Left side facial drooping from prior stroke.

   Code for residual condition (late effect): _____

   Code for cause: _____

3. Emotional lability from prior stroke.

   Code for residual condition (late effect): _____

   Code for cause: _____

13. Impending or Threatened Condition

Certain conditions are described as "impending" or "threatened." *Impending* means that a condition is about to occur; *threatened* means that a condition might occur.

Examples of impending conditions:

- cerebrovascular accident (stroke)
- coronary syndrome (narrow coronary artery, causing a reduction in oxygen to the heart)
- delirium tremens (mental confusion from excessive drinking or alcohol withdrawal)
- myocardial infarction (heart attack)

Examples of threatened conditions:

- abortion
- labor
- miscarriage
- premature delivery or labor

Code any condition that is described at the time of discharge as "impending" or "threatened" as follows:

- If the condition occurred, then code it as a confirmed diagnosis, *not* as impending or threatened.

Threatened

abortion or miscarriage 640.0 `5th`
  with subsequent abortion (see also
    Abortion, spontaneous) 634.9 `5th`
  affecting fetus 762.1
labor 644.1 `5th`
  affecting fetus or newborn 761.8
  premature 644.0 `5th`

Figure 4-43 ■ Index entry for threatened premature labor.

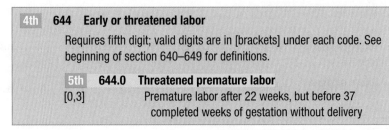

`4th` **644 Early or threatened labor**
  Requires fifth digit; valid digits are in [brackets] under each code. See beginning of section 640–649 for definitions.

`5th` **644.0 Threatened premature labor**
[0,3]   Premature labor after 22 weeks, but before 37 completed weeks of gestation without delivery

Figure 4-44 ■ Threatened premature labor in Tabular List.

- If the condition did *not* occur, then code it as an impending or threatened condition. Look for the condition as the main term in the Index, then determine whether the condition has a subterm available for "impending" or "threatened." You can also search for main terms "impending" and "threatened," with the condition listed as a subterm.

- If subterms "impending" or "threatened" are *not* listed for the condition, or if the condition is *not* listed as a subterm under "impending" or "threatened," then code the underlying condition(s), not the condition that is described as impending or threatened.

For example, if a patient's documentation showed "threatened premature labor," then you would search for the main term, *threatened*, subterm *labor*, subterm *premature* (■ FIGURE 4-43).

You would find code 644.0 to cross-reference to the Tabular List, which requires a fifth digit, depending on the patient's condition (■ FIGURE 4-44).

You also need to choose a fifth digit of 0 or 3 (choices listed in brackets under code 644.0). A list of choices appears in ■ FIGURE 4-45. The fifth digit of 0 is correct because the episode of care is unspecified, and your final code assignment is 644.00.

Figure 4-45 ■ Fifth digits available for 644.0.

The following fifth-digit subclassification is for use with categories 640–649 to denote the current episode of care:

0 unspecified as to episode of care or not applicable
1 delivered, with or without mention of antepartum condition
  Antepartum condition with delivery
  Delivery NOS (with mention of antepartum complication during current episode of care)
  Intrapartum
    obstetric condition (with mention of antepartum complication during current episode of care)
  Pregnancy, delivered (with mention of antepartum complication during current episode of care)
2 delivered, with mention of postpartum complication
  Delivery with mention of puerperal complication during current episode of care
3 antepartum condition or complication
  Antepartum obstetric condition, not delivered during the current episode of care
4 postpartum condition or complication
  Postpartum or puerperal obstetric condition or complication following delivery that occurred:
    during previous episode of care
    outside hospital, with subsequent admission for observation or care

TAKE A BREAK

Let's take a break and then code impending and threatened conditions.

Exercise 4.10   General Coding Guideline 13—
Impending or Threatened Condition

Instructions: Code the following conditions using both the Index and Tabular List. Refer to your medical dictionary or conduct web searches to define medical terms.

1. Impending stroke.

   Code: _____

2. Threatened miscarriage affecting fetus.

   Code: _____

3. Impending delirium tremens.

   Code: _____

4. Threatened premature labor at 19 weeks gestation (antepartum), pregnancy not terminated.

   Code: _____

14. Reporting Same Diagnosis Code More Than Once

Do not report the same ICD-9-CM diagnosis code more than once for a patient's encounter because it is unnecessary. This rule applies to bilateral conditions (those that affect both sides) or two different conditions that are classified using the same ICD-9-CM diagnosis code.

15. Admissions/Encounters for Rehabilitation

Rehabilitation is a branch of medicine that focuses on key areas: physical therapy (PT), occupational therapy (OT), and speech therapy (ST). (This type of rehabilitation is not related to drug rehabilitation, in which physicians and clinicians help patients with drug and alcohol addictions.) Patients receive therapeutic rehabilitation services in both inpatient and outpatient settings, as well as at home. Here is some additional information that will help you to better understand rehabilitation services:

- *Physical therapy*—helps patients recover lost physical abilities after illness or injury by treating problems they have with their joints, bones, and muscles. Physical therapists use exercise, massage, water, light, heat, ice, and electric stimulation as components of treatment modalities (methods).

  Hand therapy is another type of physical rehabilitation. Hand therapists focus their work solely on hand functioning, working with patients to regain muscle strength and ability after an illness or injury.

- *Occupational therapy*—helps patients recover lost cognitive (thinking) abilities and motor (movement) skills after an illness or injury by teaching patients how to read, write, and perform job duties again so that they can return to work. Occupational therapists also work with patients to regain abilities to perform activities of daily living, (ADLs) like grocery shopping, using the telephone, operating a computer, reading, cooking, and cleaning.

- *Speech therapy*—helps patients recover lost verbal communication abilities after an illness or injury by teaching them how to communicate through language, swallowing, and movement exercises.

Physical, hand, occupational, and speech therapists can also work with patients who have congenital conditions (present at birth). For all types of therapy, a physician must write an order for the therapy and specify the frequency of treatment before therapists can work with a patient.

When the purpose of the admission or encounter is for rehabilitation services, you will assign the first diagnosis code from category *V57 Care involving use of rehabilitation procedures*. Code the patient's actual condition as an *additional* diagnosis.

You only need to assign one code from category V57. However, you should assign code *V57.89 Other specified rehabilitation procedures*, if the patient receives more than one type of rehabilitation during a single encounter. Let's look at Example 4 to understand how to correctly assign codes for an encounter for rehabilitation:

Example 4: Mrs. Rumey suffered a neck sprain in a motor vehicle accident and has an encounter at an outpatient rehabilitation center for physical therapy for exercise and heat application.

1. Because the main reason for her encounter is for rehabilitation, you will assign a code from category V57 first, and a code for the neck sprain second.

2. For the first code, look for the main term, *admission*, with the connecting word *for* indented underneath. Then look for the subterm, *rehabilitation*, subterm, *physical* (■ FIGURE 4-46). This will lead you to code V57.1.

3. Now, cross-reference code V57.1 to the Tabular List for final code assignment (■ FIGURE 4-47).

4. Assign code V57.1 as the first code for Mrs. Rumey's encounter.

5. Did you notice the *Use additional code* note in Figure 4-47? It reminds you to assign an additional code for the patient's diagnosis. Do you know the main term that you will search for in the Index for neck sprain? If you said sprain, then you are correct. The subterm, *neck*, will be indented under the main term, *sprain* (■ FIGURE 4-48), and you will need to search through several subterms before reaching *neck*. This will lead you to code 847.0.

6. Now, cross-reference 847.0 to the Tabular List for final code assignment (■ FIGURE 4-49).

Code 847.0 is the correct code to assign for the neck sprain. Final codes for Mrs. Rumey's encounter are V57.1 (encounter for physical rehabilitation) and 847.0 (neck sprain). You will learn more about assigning V codes in Chapter 7.

Admission (encounter)
    as organ donor - see Donor
    by mistake V68.9
    for
        rehabilitation V57.9
            multiple types V57.89
            occupational V57.21
            orthoptic V57.4
            orthotic V57.81
            physical NEC V57.1
            specified type NEC V57.89
            speech(-language) V57.3
            vocational V57.22

Figure 4-46 ■ Index entry for admission for rehabilitation.

4th   **V57** **Care involving use of rehabilitation procedures**
    Use additional code to identify underlying condition
    V57.0 Breathing exercises
    V57.1 Other physical therapy
        Therapeutic and remedial exercises, except breathing

Figure 4-47 ■ Encounter for physical rehabilitation in the Tabular List.

> **Sprain, strain** (joint) (ligament) (muscle) (tendon) 848.9
>
> neck 847.0

Figure 4-48 ■ Index entry for neck strain.

> **4th   847   Sprains and strains of other and unspecified parts of back**
>
> Excludes: lumbosacral (846.0)
>
> 847.0 Neck
>
> Anterior longitudinal (ligament), cervical
>
> Atlanto-axial (joints)
>
> Atlanto-occipital (joints)
>
> Whiplash injury

Figure 4-49 ■ Neck sprain in the Tabular List.

16. Documentation for Body Mass Index and Pressure Ulcer Stages

Before we review guidelines for coding body mass index (BMI) and pressure ulcers, it is important to understand what both terms means *BMI* is a measurement for determining whether an individual is underweight, normal weight, overweight, or obese. BMI is a calculation of a person's body weight divided by the square of his height.

A *pressure ulcer,* also called a bedsore, pressure sore, or **decubitus** ulcer, develops due to lack of blood supply to a specific area of the body. It is most common on the buttocks of patients who are bedridden or in a wheelchair and happen because of lack of movement. These patients cannot move much on their own and may have no one to help them move, so pressure ulcers develop. Pressure ulcers are classified into four stages with each stage becoming progressively worse:

decubitus (di′kyoo-bi-tus)

* Stage I—skin redness, hardness, and warmth, with itching and/or pain (■ FIGURE 4-50)
* Stage II—skin loss of the first or second layer of the skin (epidermis and dermis); appears as a blister or an abrasion (■ FIGURE 4-51)
* Stage III—skin loss of both layers of the skin, along with loss of deeper subcutaneous tissue (under the skin); appears as a crater in the skin (■ FIGURE 4-52)
* Stage IV—most destructive stage with skin loss of epidermis, dermis, and subcutaneous tissue; damage to the muscles, bones, and additional body structures; could cause necrosis (death of tissue) (■ FIGURE 4-53)

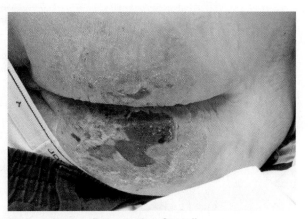

Figure 4-50 ■ Pressure ulcer Stage I.

Source: Pearson Education/PH College.

Figure 4-51 ■ Pressure ulcer Stage II.

Photo credit: Custom Medical Stock/Slaven.

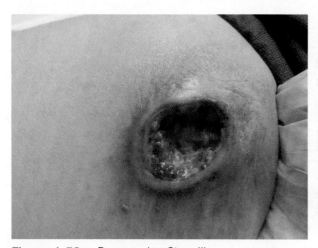

Figure 4-52 ■ Pressure ulcer Stage III.
Photo credit: Custom Medical Stock.

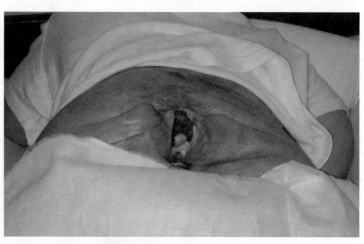

Figure 4-53 ■ Pressure ulcer Stage IV.
Photo credit: Prentice Hall Health.

Clinicians other than the physicians directly involved in the patient's care typically document BMI and pressure ulcer stages; a dietitian often documents the BMI, and nurses often document pressure ulcer stages. However, the patient's own physician/clinician or attending physician/clinician must document the *associated diagnosis* (such as overweight, obesity, or pressure ulcer). If there is conflicting medical record documentation, either from the same clinician or different clinicians, then you should query the patient's physician/clinician for clarification.

Report the BMI and pressure ulcer *stages* as *secondary* diagnoses and report the patient's condition (overweight, pressure ulcer) as the *primary* diagnosis. As with all other secondary diagnosis codes, only assign the BMI and pressure ulcer stage codes when they meet the definition of a reportable additional diagnosis. (See Section III of the Official Guidelines, Reporting Additional Diagnoses covered in Chapter 15 of this text.) Example 5 shows how to determine code assignment for a pressure ulcer and its stage.

Example 5: Dr. Hoffman saw Mr. Tate today for an examination. He diagnosed Mr. Tate with a pressure ulcer on his lower back, Stage I.

1. You need to assign two codes for Mr. Tate's encounter, the first code is for the pressure ulcer and the second code is for the *stage* of the ulcer (stage I).

2. Look in the Index for the main term, *ulcer*, subterm, *pressure*, subterm, *back*, subterm, *lower* (■ FIGURE 4-54). You will then see code 707.03 to cross-reference to the Tabular List for final code assignment (■ FIGURE 4-55).

Notice the *Use additional code* note under subcategory 707.0, alerting you to code the pressure ulcer stage as a secondary code. It directs you to the code range 707.20–707.25.

Ulcer, ulcerated, ulcerating, ulceration, ulcerative 707.9
  pressure 707.00
    with
      abrasion, blister, partial thickness skin loss involving epidermis and/or dermis 707.22
      full thickness skin loss involving damage or necrosis of subcutaneous tissue 707.23
      gangrene 707.00 [785.4]
      necrosis of soft tissues through to underlying muscle, tendon, or bone 707.24
    ankle 707.06
    back
      lower 707.03
      upper 707.02

Figure 4-54 ■ Index entry for pressure ulcer of the lower back.

5th	707.0	**Pressure ulcer**
		Bed sore
		Decubitus ulcer
		Plaster ulcer
		Use additional code to identify pressure ulcer stage (707.20–707.25)
	707.00	**Unspecified site**
	707.01	**Elbow**
	707.02	**Upper back**
		Shoulder blades
	707.03	**Lower back**
		Coccyx
		Sacrum

Figure 4-55 ■ Code 707.03 in the Tabular List.

Ulcer, ulcerated, ulcerating, ulceration, ulcerative 707.9
  pressure 707.00
    stage
      I (healing) 707.21
      II (healing) 707.22
      III (healing) 707.23
      IV (healing) 707.24
      unspecified (healing) 707.20

Figure 4-56 ■ Index entry for Stage I pressure ulcer.

5th	707.2	**Pressure ulcer stages**
		Code first site of pressure ulcer (707.00–707.09)
	707.20	**Pressure ulcer, unspecified stage**
		Healing pressure ulcer NOS
		Healing pressure ulcer, unspecified stage
	707.21	**Pressure ulcer stage I**
		Healing pressure ulcer, stage I
		Pressure pre-ulcer skin changes limited to persistent focal erythema

Figure 4-57 ■ Code 707.21 in the Tabular List.

You can either turn to that code range to find the code, or start in the Index. We will start in the Index so that you better understand how to find the pressure ulcer stage.

3. To find the code for Stage I pressure ulcer, look in the Index for the main term, *ulcer*, subterm, *pressure*, subterm, *stage*, subterm, *I (healing)*, leading you to code 707.21 (■ FIGURE 4-56). Cross-reference code 707.21 to the Tabular List for final code assignment (■ FIGURE 4-57).

Notice the *Code first* note in the Tabular under subcategory code 707.2, alerting you to code first the *site* of the pressure ulcer, which you have already done. Your final code assignment for Mr. Tate's encounter is 707.03 (pressure ulcer of the lower back), and 707.21 (Stage I pressure ulcer).

Next, review Example 6 to determine code assignment for an overweight patient, and you will code for both overweight and the BMI.

Example 6: Mrs. Reid, a 35-year-old patient, came into the office today for an examination. Dr. Hoffman diagnosed her as overweight with a BMI of 27 (the BMI range for overweight is 25–29.9).

1. You need to assign two codes for Ms. Reid's encounter, the first code for overweight and the second code for the BMI. Look in the Index for the main term, *overweight* (■ FIGURE 4-58).

Figure 4-58 ■ Index entry for overweight.

Figure 4-59 ■ Code 278.02 in the Tabular List.

Overweight (see also Obesity) 278.02

> **4th** **278** **Overweight, obesity and other hyperalimentation**
> Excludes: hyperalimentation NOS (783.6)
> poisoning by vitamins NOS (963.5)
> polyphagia (783.6)
> **5th** **278.0 Overweight and obesity**
> Excludes: adiposogenital dystrophy (253.8)
> obesity of endocrine origin NOS (259.9)
> Use additional code to identify Body Mass Index (BMI) if known (V85.0–V85.54)
> **278.00 Obesity, unspecified**
> Obesity NOS
> **278.01 Morbid obesity**
> Severe obesity
> **278.02 Overweight**

2. Notice in Figure 4-58 that there is a note to "see also Obesity." For this patient's encounter, you do not need to reference obesity because Dr. Hoffman did not document that the patient is obese, only that she is overweight. The Index leads you to code 278.02, which you need to cross-reference to the Tabular for final code assignment (■ Figure 4-59).

Notice in Figure 4-59 that there is a *Use additional code* note under subcategory 278.0 directing you to assign the patient's BMI as a secondary code. Once again, you may either turn to the code range given or start your search in the Index, which we will do next. Search the Index for the main term, *BMI (body mass index)*, subterm, *adult*, subterm, *27.0–27.9* (■ Figure 4-60). You will then see code V85.23 to cross-reference to the Tabular for final code assignment (■ Figure 4-61).

Your final code assignment for Mrs. Reid's encounter is 278.02 for overweight and V85.23 for a BMI of 27. You can calculate your own BMI through the CDC's website at http://www.cdc.gov.

Figure 4-60 ■ Index entry for BMI of 27.

BMI (body mass index)
  adult
    25.0–25.9 V85.21
    26.0–26.9 V85.22
    27.0–27.9 V85.23
    28.0–28.9 V85.24
    29.0–29.9 V85.25
    30.0–30.9 V85.30
    31.0–31.9 V85.31
    32.0–32.9 V85.32

Figure 4-61 ■ Tabular List for BMI of 27.

> **4th** **V85** **Body mass index (BMI)**
> Kilograms per meters squared
> Note: BMI adult codes are for use for persons over 20 years old
> **V85.0 Body Mass Index less than 19, adult**
> **V85.1 Body Mass Index between 19–24, adult**
> **5th** **V85.2** **Body Mass Index between 25–29, adult**
> **V85.21 Body Mass Index 25.0–25.9, adult**
> **V85.22 Body Mass Index 26.0–26.9, adult**
> **V85.23 Body Mass Index 27.0–27.9, adult**
> **V85.24 Body Mass Index 28.0–28.9, adult**
> **V85.25 Body Mass Index 29.0–29.9, adult**

Figure 4-62 ■ Index entry for syndrome.

> **Syndrome** - see also Disease
>   5q minus 238.74
>   abdominal
>   acute 789.0
>   migraine 346.2
>   muscle deficiency 756.79
>   Abercrombie's (amyloid degeneration) 277.39
>   abnormal innervation 374.43
>   abstinence
>   alcohol 291.81
>   drug 292.0
>   neonatal 779.5
>   Abt-Letterer-Siwe (acute histiocytosis X) (M9722/3) 202.5
>   Achard-Thiers (adrenogenital) 255.2

17. Syndromes

Follow the Alphabetic Index guidance when coding a *syndrome,* which is another term for disease. When you search for a syndrome, look under the main term *syndrome,* then under the subterm for the type of syndrome (■ FIGURE 4-62). If there is no entry in the Index, then assign codes for the documented *manifestations* of the syndrome.

TAKE A BREAK

Let's take a break and then code conditions from coding guidelines 14–17.

Exercise 4.11   **General Coding Guidelines 14–17**

Instructions: Code the following conditions using both the Index and Tabular List. Refer to your medical dictionary or conduct web searches to define medical terms.

1. Patient has an encounter for physical therapy with range of motion exercises. Patient is suffering from an ankle sprain.

   Code(s): _____

2. Patient has an encounter for speech therapy. Patient is suffering from a brain injury without loss of consciousness.

   Code(s): _____

3. Patient has a pressure ulcer of the coccyx, stage II.

   Code(s): _____

4. Physician diagnoses an adult patient as obese with a BMI of 35.2.

   Code(s): _____

5. Patient is underweight with a BMI of 18.7.

   Code(s): _____

6. Patient has Gilbert's syndrome.

   Code(s): _____

STEPS TO FOLLOW FOR CORRECT CODING

The steps that follow summarize the information we have covered regarding coding conventions and General Coding Guidelines in this chapter. You can apply these steps as you code all types of diagnoses:

1. Read the patient's medical documentation and determine the diagnosis(es). Then determine the main term(s) for which you need to search in the Index.

2. Look up the main term in the Index. The main term is capitalized and may be in bold print. It is followed by a diagnosis code.

3. Many main terms also have subterms (essential modifiers) arranged alphabetically. Subterms are indented under the main term to provide more information about the main term. Follow the indented format and review applicable subterms to ensure that you have reviewed all necessary information before you choose a code.

4. Review nonessential modifiers, which are words in parentheses that follow a main term. Follow coding conventions in both the Index and Tabular, including NEC and NOS.

5. When you read information in the Index, understand that the word "and" can mean both "and" as well as "or." The word "with" is a connector between the main term and subterms.

6. Follow instructions for "see," "see also," and "see category."

7. Cross-reference the diagnosis code that you find to the Tabular List for final code assignment.

8. Review information describing conditions as "other," "other specified," and "unspecified." Assign an unspecified code only as a last resort.

9. Pay attention to instructions for coding an etiology/manifestation relationship: "code first," "use additional code," "in diseases classified elsewhere," and "code, if applicable, any causal condition first."

10. Code from the Tabular List to the highest level of specificity, assigning the highest level code available for a given category. Code to the subcategory (fourth digit) if one exists, and code to the subclassification (fifth digit) if one exists.

11. Ensure that you code the complete diagnostic statement, assigning multiple codes if applicable.

12. Query the physician/clinician if you have questions about diagnoses documented in the patient's record.

CHAPTER REVIEW

Multiple Choice

Instructions: Circle one best answer to complete each statement.

1. Terms, abbreviations, symbols, and punctuation that direct you in both the Alphabetic Index and Tabular List are called coding
   a. sections.   b. conventions.
   c. guidelines.   d. acronyms.

2. Written rules to follow when you are coding are called coding
   a. sections.   b. conventions.
   c. guidelines.   d. acronyms.

3. How many sections make up ICD-9-CM's Official Guidelines for Coding and Reporting?
   a. three   b. four
   c. five   d. six

4. The convention that means there is medical documentation that specifies the diagnosis, but there is no specific code in ICD-9-CM, is
   a. code first.   b. NOS.
   c. etiology/manifestation. d. NEC.

5. The underlying cause of another condition is called a(n)
   a. syndrome.   b. etiology.
   c. sign.   d. manifestation.

6. Code signs and symptoms when
   a. there is no definitive diagnosis.
   b. they are integral to the disease process.
   c. the patient has discussed them with the physician.
   d. the physician documents them.

7. A(n) _____ is a single code used to classify two diagnoses, a diagnosis with an associated secondary process, or a diagnosis with an associated complication.
   a. multiple code   b. unspecified code
   c. combination code   d. late-effect code

8. A condition lasting three months or more is called a(n) _____ condition.
   a. impending   b. threatened
   c. acute   d. chronic

9. When the reason for the patient's encounter is for _____, assign a code from category V57 as the first code and assign a code for the patient's diagnosis as a secondary code.
   a. BMI measurement
   b. a pressure ulcer dressing change
   c. rehabilitation services
   d. treatment of chronic conditions

10. The residual condition after the acute phase of an illness or injury has passed is called a(n)
    a. manifestation.   b. late effect.
    c. etiology.   d. acute condition.

11. Assigning more than one code for a single condition or more than one condition is called
    a. combination coding.   b. advanced coding.
    c. extra coding.   d. multiple coding.

12. _____ enclose manifestation codes that you should sequence second.
    a. Parentheses   b. Brackets
    c. Italicized brackets   d. Braces

13. _____ is a note in the Tabular List indicating how to sequence etiology and manifestation codes.
    a. Assign first   b. Code first
    c. Sequence first   d. See also

14. _____ follows a main term in the Index and is a word that connects main terms to subterms.
    a. And   b. Also
    c. With   d. See

15. The _____ instruction following a main term in the Index tells you that there is *another* main term that you can reference to find the code that you need.
    a. see also   b. see
    c. see category   d. see main term

16. There are _____ stages of pressure ulcers, ranging from the least severe to the most severe.
    a. three   b. four
    c. five   d. six

17. A condition that is about to occur is called a(n) _____ condition.
    a. acute   b. impending
    c. chronic   d. threatened

18. The type of rehabilitation that helps patients to recover cognitive abilities and motor skills is called
    a. physical therapy.   b. occupational therapy.
    c. speech therapy.   d. hand therapy.

19. When coding pressure ulcers,
    a. only assign the code for the pressure ulcer stage because it is understood that the patient already has a diagnosis that caused the pressure ulcer.
    b. assign the patient's diagnosis as the second code, and assign the pressure ulcer stage as the first code.
    c. only assign the code for the patient's diagnosis; no code is needed for the pressure ulcer stage.
    d. assign the patient's diagnosis as the first code, and assign the pressure ulcer stage as the second code.

20. A measurement for determining whether an individual is underweight, normal weight, overweight, or obese is
    a. Weight Body Mass (WBM).
    b. Body Mass Measurement (BMM).
    c. Physical Mass Index (PMI).
    d. Body Mass Index (BMI).

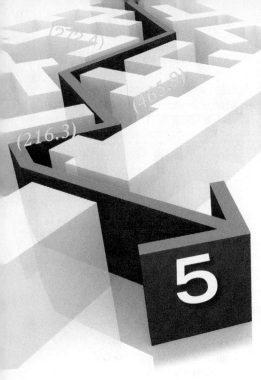

Diagnostic Coding and Reporting Guidelines for Outpatient Services

Learning Objectives

After completing this chapter, you should be able to

- Spell and define the key terminology in this chapter.
- List the differences between inpatient and outpatient coding guidelines.
- Explain how to select the first-listed condition.
- Explain how to code for outpatient surgery and observation stays.
- Describe how to use codes 001.0 through V89.
- Explain how to report ICD-9-CM diagnosis codes accurately.
- Discuss how to select codes 001.0 through 999.9.
- State the guidelines for coding symptoms and signs.
- Demonstrate how to code encounters for circumstances other than a disease or injury.
- Discuss the level of detail in coding.
- Apply ICD-9-CM codes for the diagnosis, condition, problem, or other reason for encounter/visit.
- Identify and explain how to code uncertain diagnoses and chronic diseases.
- Describe how to code all documented conditions that coexist, including personal and family history.
- Discuss how to code for patients receiving diagnostic services only.
- Demonstrate how to code for patients receiving therapeutic services only.
- Know how to code for patients receiving preoperative evaluations only.
- Identify and describe coding for ambulatory surgery and routine outpatient prenatal visits.
- Explain how to use the Index and Tabular List for outpatient encounters.

Key Terms

ambulatory surgery
causal relationship
contraindication
first-listed diagnosis
observation
outpatient provider

preoperative evaluation
principal diagnosis
probable/suspected
questionable
rule out
surgical clearance
working diagnosis

INTRODUCTION

You probably realize by now that your coding journey can take many twists and turns and will also direct you down the paths of outpatient coding, as well as inpatient coding! In Chapter 4, you learned the Conventions and General Coding Guidelines from Section I of ICD-9-CM's Official Guidelines for Coding and Reporting, which apply to outpatient and inpatient encounters. You also practiced using the Conventions and Guidelines to code various conditions. You had your first road trip, operating ICD-9-CM manual while following the rules of the road. In this chapter, you will learn rules of the road strictly for

ICD-9-CM codes in this chapter are from the ICD-9-CM 2012 code set from the Department of Health and Human Services, Centers for Disease Control and Prevention.

■ TABLE 5-1   FOUR SECTIONS OF ICD-9-CM OFFICIAL GUIDELINES FOR CODING AND REPORTING

Section I	Section II	Section III	Section IV
Conventions, General Coding Guidelines, Chapter-Specific Coding Guidelines	Selection of Principal Diagnosis (inpatient settings)	Reporting Additional Diagnoses (inpatient settings)	Diagnostic Coding and Reporting Guidelines for Outpatient Services
Section I has three divisions: **A—Conventions for ICD-9-CM** *(Section I A is covered in Chapter 4.)* **B—General Coding Guidelines** *(Section I B is covered in Chapter 4.)* **C—Chapter-Specific Coding Guidelines—correspond to each of the 17 chapters of the Tabular List** *(Chapter-specific guidelines are covered in other chapters in this book.)*	Section II includes guidelines for selection of principal diagnosis (reason for the episode of care) for inpatient settings. *(Section II is covered in Chapter 15.)*	Section III includes guidelines for reporting additional diagnoses in inpatient settings. *(Section III is covered in Chapter 15.)*	Section IV includes guidelines for reporting diagnoses for outpatient services. *(Section IV is covered in this chapter.)*

outpatient encounters. Recall from Chapter 4 that there are four sections of the Guidelines (**■** TABLE 5-1). You already learned about Section I of the Guidelines in Chapter 4. We will cover sections II and III in Chapter 15.

This chapter covers Section IV of the Guidelines, Diagnostic Coding and Reporting Guidelines for Outpatient Services. Section IV applies to **outpatient providers**, including emergency departments, outpatient hospitals, ambulatory surgery centers (ASCs), outpatient clinics, and outpatient urgent care centers. Be aware that although an emergency department is located within an acute care hospital and some patients are admitted to the hospital directly from the emergency department, the services provided in the emergency department itself are considered to be outpatient services. Within the Guidelines, you will see the terms *encounter*, *admission*, and *visit* used interchangeably to describe outpatient services.

You will continuously refer to these guidelines as you code diagnoses in future chapters because they contain a lot of important rules that you need to follow. As you work through the examples and exercises in this chapter, you will notice many medical terms and procedures. You can find their pronunciations in the side margins of the page, as well as their definitions if the terms are not defined for you in the chapter itself. You should practice pronouncing words and learning their definitions, not only because it will affect how well you code, but also because it will make you a much more qualified and marketable employee when you are working in the healthcare field. You will need to be able to effectively communicate with others, including the physician, your manager, other employees, and patients, and knowing the proper pronunciations and definitions of words will help make your communications successful. There is much information to cover, but with time, patience, and practice, you can do it!

"If you grit your teeth and show real determination, you always have a chance."—CHARLIE BROWN (CHARLES SCHULZ)

OUTPATIENT AND INPATIENT CODING GUIDELINES

In Section I, you learned that Conventions (road signs) and General Guidelines (rules of the road) apply to both outpatient and inpatient services. However, coding for outpatient services differs from inpatient services in specific ways.

■ **TABLE 5-2   DIAGNOSTIC CODING AND REPORTING GUIDELINES FOR OUTPATIENT SERVICES**

SECTION IV

A. Selection of first-listed condition

   1. Outpatient surgery

   2. Observation stay

B. Codes from 001.0 through V91.99

C. Accurate reporting of ICD-9-CM diagnosis codes

D. Selection of codes 001.0 through 999.9

E. Codes that describe symptoms and signs

F. Encounters for circumstances other than a disease or injury

G. Level of detail in coding

   1. ICD-9-CM codes with 3, 4, or 5 digits

   2. Use of full number of digits required for a code

H. ICD-9-CM code for the diagnosis, condition, problem, or other reason for encounter/visit

I. Uncertain diagnosis

J. Chronic diseases

K. Code all documented conditions that coexist

L. Patients receiving diagnostic services only

M. Patients receiving therapeutic services only

N. Patients receiving preoperative evaluations only

O. Ambulatory surgery

P. Routine outpatient prenatal visits

One of these differences is that inpatient providers (including acute care, short- and long-term care, and psychiatric hospitals) refer to the first diagnosis for a patient as the **principal diagnosis**. The Uniform Hospital Discharge Data Set (UHDDS) definition of a principal diagnosis is "the condition established after study (tests, exams) to be *chiefly responsible* for occasioning the admission of the patient to the hospital." Outpatient providers (physician offices, outpatient surgery centers, urgent care clinics) refer to the first diagnosis as the primary diagnosis, or **first-listed diagnosis**, the reason for the patient's encounter.

There are also inpatient coding guidelines for coding inconclusive (not definitive) diagnoses, such as a condition that the physician believes may be probable or suspects may be present, or situations when the physician orders testing to rule out a specific condition. Guidelines for inconclusive diagnoses only apply to *inpatient* settings. You'll learn the inpatient diagnosis coding guidelines (Sections II and III) in Chapter 15 of this text.

■ TABLE 5-2 summarizes guidelines contained in Section IV—Reporting Diagnoses for Outpatient Services. You can use Table 5-2 as a reference as you review each guideline in more detail, work through the coding examples using your own manual, and practice the coding exercises. The Guidelines are explained to you throughout this chapter, but you can also find instructions for accessing them in Appendix A in this text. Throughout this book, the Alphabetic Index is also called the Index, and the Tabular List is also called the Tabular.

SECTION IV—DIAGNOSTIC CODING AND REPORTING GUIDELINES FOR OUTPATIENT SERVICES

Let's review each of the following guidelines and examples so that you can better understand how to apply the guidelines when you are coding various types of diagnoses and conditions.

A. Selection of the First-Listed Condition

When you are determining the first-listed, or primary, diagnosis, follow ICD-9-CM's Coding Conventions, General Coding Guidelines, and Chapter-Specific Coding Guidelines. If you are not able to determine the first-listed diagnosis using the Conventions and Guidelines, then refer to rules outlined in Section IV—Diagnostic Coding and Reporting Guidelines for Outpatient Services. We will discuss those rules next.

It is important to understand that many times, patients will not have a definitive diagnosis during the initial encounter or visit, and the physician will provide a definitive diagnosis during a subsequent (follow-up) visit. You still have to code both the initial and subsequent visits, but each will have a different diagnosis.

For example, during an initial visit for an annual check-up, the physician may order a lab test to determine if the patient has a specific condition, although the patient has no symptoms. The physician does not yet know if the patient has the condition, so you cannot code it. Instead, you will assign a *V code* as the first-listed diagnosis to show the *reason* for the visit, the annual check-up. Remember that you can assign V codes to show why a patient had an encounter when the patient has nothing wrong.

Then the physician will either send a sample (e.g., blood, urine) obtained in the office to an outside lab for testing or send the patient to a nearby lab (such as a hospital lab department) to provide the sample. The lab will send the test results to the physician. He can then review the test results and ask the patient to return for a follow-up visit. The physician will discuss the results with the patient and provide a *definitive* diagnosis at that time. During the second visit, you can code the *definitive diagnosis* as the first-listed diagnosis. Follow these steps to determine the first-listed diagnosis:

1. The first-listed diagnosis is the *main reason* for the encounter such as a flu shot or annual check-up. Ask yourself these questions: "What was the main reason for the patient's visit?" and "What was the physician's final diagnosis for the patient?" If the physician provided a final diagnosis, then it becomes the *main reason* for the patient's visit.

2. If the reason for the visit was a symptom (patient reported) or sign (physician observed), but another condition *caused* the symptom, then do not code the symptom. Instead, code the *condition* that caused it. Remember that you should not code symptoms and signs that are an integral part of the disease process. *Only code a symptom or sign when there is no definitive diagnosis.* You may be wondering how you will know if a condition is a symptom or sign of another condition. In this book, you will learn how to determine this from various coding examples and exercises. Also, if you are unsure if a condition is a symptom or sign of another condition, then you should check medical reference materials or conduct an Internet search to find out more about a condition's symptoms and signs. You can also query the physician.

3. Patients can have more than one diagnosis for an encounter. It is your job to determine the order in which to sequence the diagnoses, assigning the first-listed diagnosis as the *main reason* for the visit and/or the physician's definitive diagnosis. Code additional conditions secondary to the first-listed diagnosis. The order in which you code additional diagnoses will depend on the medical documentation and if there are conventions or guidelines in ICD-9-CM telling you the order in which to assign the diagnoses.

Refer to the following examples of patient encounters in order to choose the first-listed diagnosis. The encounters are with Dr. Hoffman, a general practitioner, also called a family practice or primary care physician. A general practitioner sees patients for many different conditions and can refer patients to specialists for additional treatment. Patients often refer to their general practitioner as the "family doctor."

Examples of the First-Listed Diagnosis for Encounters

1. Mr. Lorde, a 45-year-old new patient, has an encounter because of cough, congestion, and runny nose for the past four days. After examination and further lab testing, Dr. Hoffman diagnoses the patient with an acute upper respiratory infection and prescribes an antibiotic.

   First-listed diagnosis: acute upper respiratory infection (465.9)

   Cough, congestion, and runny nose are all symptoms of the infection, and you should not code them.

2. Mrs. Simon, a 72-year-old established patient, sees Dr. Hoffman for removal of a benign mole from her cheek. Mrs. Simon tells Dr. Hoffman that she also needs a prescription refill for Crestor®, a medication to treat **hyperlipidemia**. Dr. Hoffman checks previous notes in the record regarding the diagnosis and asks the patient questions about the condition and side effects of the medication that she may have experienced. He writes the prescription refill.

   First-listed diagnosis: benign mole of the cheek (216.3)

   Second diagnosis: hyperlipidemia (272.4); this condition is a secondary diagnosis because it was not the main reason for the patient's visit, but the physician reviewed information and questioned the patient about the condition. He also wrote a prescription refill for a drug to treat it.

3. Mr. Hemmfield, a 70-year-old established patient, sees Dr. Hoffman for a general medical exam. During the visit, the patient tells Dr. Hoffman that he has experienced depression for the past three months since his wife died. Dr. Hoffman counsels the patient on managing his depression and also refers Mr. Hemmfield to a psychologist for regular counseling sessions. He diagnoses the patient with moderate acute depression.

   First-listed diagnosis: general exam (V70.9)

   Second diagnosis: moderate acute depression (296.22)

4. Miss Wright, a 21-year-old established patient, is a college student who works part-time as a nurse's aide in a skilled nursing facility (SNF). She sees Dr. Hoffman with complaints of watery diarrhea multiple times a day and abdominal cramps. The medical assistant who took Miss Wright's vital signs found that her oral temperature was elevated to 102°. Dr. Hoffman suspects that Miss Wright may have contracted the *Clostridium difficile (C. diff.)* toxin from a nursing home patient. He obtains a stool sample to send to the lab immediately. He tells Miss Wright that someone from the office will call her the following day to discuss the test results.

   First-listed diagnosis: diarrhea (787.91)

   Second diagnosis: generalized abdominal cramps (789.07)

   Third diagnosis: fever (780.60)

   Note that you can only code symptoms for this encounter and cannot code C. diff. because the lab test has not confirmed it. List the diagnoses in the order in which the physician documents them, unless there are guidelines or conventions in ICD-9-CM for the order in which to assign the diagnoses.

5. Miss Wright returns the following day (and still has the same symptoms), and Dr. Hoffman confirms that her stool test was positive for the *C. difficile* toxin. He diagnoses her with **enteritis** caused by *C. diff.*, prescribes Flagyl®, an antibiotic, advises the patient to drink plenty of fluids, and asks her to follow up with him within a week for an exam and further testing.

   First-listed diagnosis: enteritis, Clostridium difficile (008.45)

   Diarrhea, abdominal cramps, and fever are all symptoms of the C. diff. infection (the definitive diagnosis), and you should not code them.

Margin glossary:

hyperlipidemia (hī′pĕr-lipi-dē-mē-ă)—condition of elevated lipids, or fats, in the blood

Clostridium difficile (C. diff.) (klo-strid′-ee-um dif′-uh-seel)—bacteria that cause diarrhea and more serious intestinal conditions, like colitis

enteritis (ent-ə-rīt′-əs)—inflammation of the intestines

TAKE A BREAK

Let's take a break and then code first-listed diagnoses.

Exercise 5.1	Selection of the First-Listed Condition

Instructions: Review each patient's encounter with Dr. Hoffman. Determine which condition is the first-listed diagnosis, and determine if there is another condition that should be listed as a secondary diagnosis. Using both the Index and Tabular, assign codes for both the first-listed and any secondary diagnoses. With some encounters, it takes two visits before the diagnosis is confirmed.

1. Mr. Homer, a 58-year-old established patient, sees Dr. Hoffman for a swollen ankle and ankle pain. Mr. Homer also has essential **hypertension**, which is controlled with medication. Dr. Hoffman diagnoses Mr. Homer with an ankle sprain, writes a prescription for pain medicine, and provides pain management instructions. Dr. Hoffman also writes a prescription refill for Mr. Homer's hypertension medication and answers the patient's questions about the medication.

    First-listed diagnosis: _____

    Code: _____

    Is there a secondary diagnosis? yes no If yes, please

    list: _____ Code: _____

2. Mrs. Leeds, a 35-year-old new patient, visits Dr. Hoffman for a check-up because she does not feel well. During the exam, the patient complains that she has "low energy levels." Dr. Hoffman diagnoses her as obese, calculating a BMI of 36.3. He discusses weight control measures and good eating habits.

    First-listed diagnosis: _____

    Code: _____

    Is there a secondary diagnosis? yes no If yes, please

    list: _____ Code: _____

3. Mr. North is a 40-year-old established patient who returns for a follow-up visit to discuss the results of his cholesterol test, which reveal that he has hyperlipidemia. Dr. Hoffman counsels him on reducing his weight, exercising more, eating a low-fat/low-cholesterol diet, and taking vitamins. He also prescribes Lipitor® for hyperlipidemia.

    First-listed diagnosis: _____

    Code: _____

    Is there a secondary diagnosis? yes no If yes, please

    list: _____ Code: _____

4. Miss Smith, a 19-year-old established patient, visits Dr. Hoffman for a gynecological exam. She tells Dr. Hoffman that she felt small lumps around her anus. Dr. Hoffman conducts a breast and pelvic exam and obtains a Papanicolaou (Pap) smear to send to an outside lab. During the exam, he discovers that Miss Smith has a sexually transmitted disease, genital warts, called **human papillomavirus (HPV)**. He prescribes Condylox® Gel for the warts. He also counsels the patient on protected sex and asks her to return in three weeks for a follow-up visit.

    First-listed diagnosis: _____

    Code: _____

    Is there a secondary diagnosis? yes no If yes, please

    list: _____ Code: _____

5. Miss Smith returns three weeks later for a follow-up exam. Dr. Hoffman tells her that her Pap smear test results were normal. He conducts an exam and determines that the genital warts are gone. He advises Miss Smith to call for another appointment if she experiences further problems.

    First-listed diagnosis: _____

    Code: _____

    Is there a secondary diagnosis? yes no If yes, please

    list: _____ Code: _____

Physician Services and Procedures Performed Outside the Office   As you are determining the first-listed diagnosis, it is also important to understand that when you are working for a physician's office or clinic, you may code and bill services and procedures that the physician performs in the office or clinic, as well as services and procedures that he performs at other locations. For example, physicians may work part time in the office and part time performing surgeries at a hospital or an ASC. Physicians may conduct bedside exams for hospitalized patients and also examine patients who reside in SNFs. When physicians provide services and procedures outside the office, they typically complete an encounter form for the patient that shows the patient's diagnosis and procedure. Then they return the encounter form to the office for review, coding verification, and insurance and patient billing. You should always follow ICD-9-CM guidelines for coding diagnoses.

hypertension (hī-pər-ten′-chən)—high blood pressure

human papillomavirus (HPV) (pāp′ə-lō-mə-vī′rəs)—virus causing warts in the genital area, feet, and hands

osteoarthritis (ăs-tē-ō-är-thrīt′-əs)—arthritis causing a breakdown of tissues and cartilage (connective tissue) surrounding a joint

atrial fibrillation (ā′-trē-əl fi-brə-lā′-shən)—irregular contractions of heart muscles

abdominal hysterectomy (ab-dah′-mih-nul his-tə-rek′-tə-mē)—removal of the uterus through an incision in the lower abdomen

intramural uterine fibroids (in-tră-myū′-răl yoo′-teh-rin fī′-broyds)—fibroid tumors located inside the wall of the uterus, made up of connective tissue and muscle

cardiac catheterization (kär′-dē-ak kath-ĕ-ter-ĭ-za′-shun)—catheter (flexible tube) insertion into the patient's blood vessel to view blood flow to the heart; also called a heart catheterization or heart "cath"

coronary artery disease—also called ischemic heart disease; condition in which the coronary arteries cannot maintain blood flow to the heart

Outpatient Surgery When a physician performs outpatient surgery, code the reason for the surgery as the first-listed diagnosis (reason for the encounter). Assign additional codes if the patient has other diagnoses that affect the surgery or management of the patient's condition. Sometimes, a patient is scheduled for surgery but has a **contraindication** (problem that affects another condition) that would make starting or continuing surgery unwise. The physician then cancels the surgery. *Even when surgery is cancelled due to a contraindication, code the reason for the surgery as the first-listed diagnosis. Report the contraindication(s) as secondary diagnoses.*

Here are some examples of scheduled surgeries with contraindications:

- A patient is scheduled for hip replacement surgery due to localized **osteoarthritis** of the hip, but after receiving anesthesia before the surgery, the patient experiences **atrial fibrillation**. The surgery is postponed until the patient's condition is stabilized.

First-listed diagnosis: localized osteoarthritis of the hip (reason for surgery)

Additional diagnosis: atrial fibrillation

- A patient is scheduled for an **abdominal hysterectomy** because of **intramural uterine fibroids** and has an anxiety attack before surgery because she is afraid. The surgery is rescheduled.

First-listed diagnosis: intramural uterine fibroids (reason for surgery)

Additional diagnosis: anxiety, or panic, attack

- A patient is scheduled for a **cardiac catheterization** due to **coronary artery disease** (also called ischemic heart disease), but his blood pressure is too high, and surgery would be dangerous, so it is cancelled.

First-listed diagnosis: coronary artery disease (reason for surgery)

Additional diagnosis: hypertension

TAKE A BREAK

Let's take a break and then code the first-listed diagnosis for outpatient surgeries.

Exercise 5.2 **Outpatient Surgery**

Instructions: Determine the first-listed diagnosis for the following patients' surgeries. Ask yourself, "What was the reason for the surgery?" Then write the answer as the first-listed diagnosis, and assign the code after referencing the Index and cross-referencing the Tabular.

1. Mr. Jansen, age 78, is admitted to the hospital for outpatient surgery to remove a **mature senile cataract** from the lens of his left eye and undergo an intraocular lens replacement. The patient has been suffering from blurred vision and sees colored halos around lights. Dr. Mons performs the surgery, and it is successful.

   First-listed diagnosis (reason for the surgery): _____

   _____

   Code: _____

2. Mr. Stein, a 54-year-old, has chronic constipation and nausea. He is admitted to the hospital for outpatient surgery to repair a *recurrent* (returning) *unilateral* (one side) **femoral hernia with obstruction**. Dr. Niles performs the surgery and there are no complications.

   First-listed diagnosis (reason for the surgery): _____

   _____

   Code: _____

3. Mrs. Winter, a 61-year-old, suffers from depression and is admitted to the hospital as an outpatient for a diagnostic colonoscopy due to **melena** (bloody stool). Dr. Rice performs the procedure and finds no abnormalities.

   First-listed diagnosis (reason for the surgery): _____

   _____

   Code: _____

4. Ms. Pierce, a 48-year-old, is admitted to the hospital for an outpatient **laparascopic cholecystectomy** (gallbladder removal with a laparascope) to treat **cholelithiasis** (gall stones). Because of her excessive weight and the amount of fat in her abdomen, her abdominal wall is too thick to complete the procedure, so Dr. Moon discontinues it.

   First-listed diagnosis (reason for the surgery): _____

   _____

   Code: _____

INTERESTING FACT: Laparoscopy, Surgery with a Camera

A **laparoscopy** is a method of performing surgery in which a physician inserts a thin, rigid tube through a small incision (about 1 cm long) in the patient's abdomen (■ FIGURE 5-1). The laparoscope has a light and a camera on the end so that the physician can see the patient's internal pelvic organs. Physicians can then insert surgical instruments into the abdomen to perform the surgical procedure. Laparoscopy replaces traditional surgical procedures requiring larger incisions, and it is common for hysterectomies and cholecystectomies.

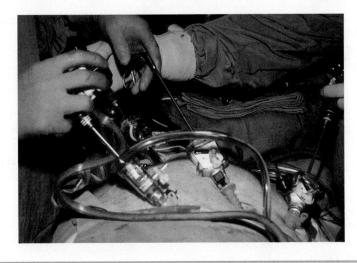

Figure 5-1 ■ A surgeon performs a cholecystectomy using laparoscopy.

Photo credit: Glenn Vanstrum, M.D./Custom Medical Stock Photo.

Observation Stay   Before you can apply coding guidelines related to **observation**, you first need to understand what observation services are. Patients under observation care typically begin as patients in a hospital's emergency department, but their diagnoses are unclear. The physician overseeing the patient's care does not have enough information about the patient's condition to either admit the patient to the hospital as an inpatient or discharge the patient to home or another facility (such as a SNF).

When a patient's diagnosis is unclear, the physician admits the patient for observation to watch the patient's *progression* (movement forward) or *regression* (movement backward), placing the patient in a separate area of the hospital or within the emergency department. The physician and other clinicians, such as nurses, then monitor the patient, administer and/or order tests, provide treatment, and continue to assess the patient's status. Remember that a patient under observation is considered an *outpatient*.

Within 24–48 hours, the physician can usually determine if there is a definitive diagnosis after reviewing the patient's status and test results. The physician then either admits or discharges the patient. On rare occasions, it may take up to 72 hours to determine a patient's definitive diagnosis. There are two coding guidelines related to observation:

1. When a patient is admitted for observation for a medical condition, assign a code for the medical condition as the *first-listed* diagnosis. Refer to the following example.

Example: Ms. Johns, a 40-year-old patient, presents to the hospital emergency department experiencing shortness of breath (SOB), and **diaphoresis**. Since these are symptoms of a **myocardial infarction (MI)**, the emergency physician, Dr. Quinn, orders a series of tests to determine if Ms. Johns is having an MI. Test results reveal no evidence of an MI. *The first-listed diagnosis is shortness of breath (786.05), and the second diagnosis is diaphoresis (780.8).*

2. When a patient presents for outpatient surgery and then develops complications requiring admission to observation, code the reason for the surgery as the first-listed diagnosis. Assign code(s) for the complication(s) as secondary diagnoses.

mature senile cataract (kat′-uh-rakt)—condition in which the lens of the eye becomes opaque (cloudy, white) due to age, trauma, or disease

femoral hernia with obstruction (fe′-mə-rəl)—condition in which a portion of the intestine protrudes through the abdominal wall, creating a bulge near the inside of the thigh (femur), and blood cannot flow properly to the intestine

melena (mə-lē′-nə)—black stool containing blood

laparascopic cholecystectomy (lap-uh-ruh-skawp′-ik kō-lī-sĭ-stĕk′-′tə-mē)

cholelithiasis (kō-lə-li-thī′-ə-səs)

laparoscopy (lap-uh-ros′-kuh-pee)

diaphoresis (dī-ə-fə-rē′-səs)—excessive sweating

myocardial infarction (MI) (mī-ō-kär′dē-əl in-fahrk′-shuhn)—heart attack; in this situation blood cannot flow properly to the heart, causing death of heart tissue

TAKE A BREAK

Let's take a break and then code the first-listed diagnosis for observation encounters.

Exercise 5.3   Observation Stay

Instructions: Using both the Index and the Tabular List, determine the first-listed diagnosis and any secondary diagnoses for the following patients admitted for observation.

1. Candace Linn, a 10-year-old, is admitted for observation because of diarrhea, nausea, and vomiting.

   First-listed diagnosis (reason for observation): _____

   _____

   Code: _____

   Secondary diagnosis (additional reason for observation): _____

   Code(s): _____

2. David Guy, a 12-year-old, is admitted for observation because of constipation, lack of appetite, and generalized abdominal pain. His mother reveals that David has taken over-the-counter cough medicine for the past several days for a cold. Dr. Quinn believes that the cough medicine caused the constipation. He administers an enema to relieve the constipation and continues to monitor the patient.

   First-listed diagnosis (reason for observation): _____

   _____

   Code: _____

   Secondary diagnosis (additional reason(s) for observation): _____

   Code(s): _____

3. Mrs. Henry, a 75-year-old, has same-day (outpatient) surgery for cataract removal on her right eye with an intraocular lens (IOL) replacement. She develops **pyrexia postoperatively** and is admitted for observation.

   First-listed diagnosis (reason for surgery): _____

   _____

   Code: _____

   Secondary diagnosis (complication): _____

   _____

   Code: _____

4. Mrs. Simon, a 63-year-old, is admitted for outpatient upper eyelid **blepharoplasty** surgery because of **ptosis** of the upper eyelids and she wants to look younger. Postoperatively, she vomits excessively and is admitted for observation.

   First-listed diagnosis (reason for surgery): _____

   _____

   Code: _____

   Secondary diagnosis (complication): _____

   _____

   Code: _____

5. Mr. Moore, a 72-year-old, develops **arrhythmia** after an outpatient **polypectomy** due to colon polyps. He is admitted for observation.

   First-listed diagnosis (reason for surgery): _____

   _____

   Code: _____

   Secondary diagnosis (complication): _____

   _____

   Code: _____

---

pyrexia (pī-rek′-sē-ə)—fever

postoperatively—after surgery

blepharoplasty (blef′ă-ro-plast-tē)—upper or lower eyelid surgery to remove fat and excess skin and tissue for cosmetic or medical reasons

ptosis (toh′-sis - the p is silent)—drooping

arrhythmia (ā-rith′-mē-ə)—abnormal heart rhythm

B. Codes 001.0 through V91.99

Both guidelines B (codes 001.0–V91.99) and D (001.0–999.9) show code ranges in the Tabular List, and you must assign codes within these ranges to identify diagnoses, symptoms, conditions, problems, complaints or other reason(s) for the encounter/visit or hospital admission, including assigning V codes when appropriate. These guidelines are the same as ICD-9-CM's General Coding Guidelines, Section I B 4 and 5.

C. Accurate Reporting of ICD-9-CM Diagnosis Codes

In order for you to determine the correct ICD-9-CM diagnosis codes, the documentation should describe the patient's condition, using terminology which includes specific diagnoses, as well as symptoms, problems, or reasons for the encounter. There are ICD-9-CM codes to describe all of these diagnoses and reasons.

This guideline means that the physician or other clinician should clearly document a patient's diagnosis and any symptoms in the medical record. The guideline also means that you have to assign codes based on the documentation. If you are unsure of information in the medical record, always query the physician or other clinician for clarification.

polypectomy (poli-pek′-tŏ-mē)—surgical excision of a polyp (growth)

D. Selection of Codes 001.0 through 999.9

Select codes 001.0 through 999.9 to describe the reason for the encounter. These codes appear in the section of ICD-9-CM for the classification of diseases and injuries (e.g., infectious and parasitic diseases; neoplasms; symptoms, signs, and ill-defined conditions; etc.). Again, just as with guideline B, this guideline means that you must assign diagnosis codes within the range of 001.00 to 999.9 unless the reason for the encounter applies to a V code description. In that case you would assign codes from V01.0–V91.99.

E. Codes that Describe Symptoms and Signs

As you learned in Chapter 4, the guideline in Section I B 6 states that codes describing symptoms and signs, as opposed to diagnoses, are acceptable for reporting purposes when the provider has not established (confirmed) a related definitive diagnosis. Remember that a sign is objective evidence of a disease that the physician discovers, commonly through an examination. A symptom is subjective evidence of disease that the patient reports to the physician. In the physician's medical documentation of a patient's encounter, he documents signs and symptoms, along with a definitive diagnosis, if one exists. The definitive diagnosis is the first-listed diagnosis that the physician reports, after reviewing subjective information, conducting an examination, and reviewing test results.

Sometimes, there is no definitive diagnosis, only a sign or a symptom. In the Tabular List, Chapter 16—Symptoms, Signs, and Ill-defined Conditions (codes 780.0–799.9), contains codes for symptoms. You will learn more about signs and symptoms and will code them later in this chapter under Guideline I—Uncertain Diagnosis, and also code them in Chapter 13 of this book.

F. Encounters for Circumstances Other than a Disease or Injury

Recall that V codes are from the Supplementary Classification of Factors Influencing Health Status and Contact with Health Services (V01.0–V91.99). They represent reasons for outpatient encounters other than a disease, condition, or injury. Examples are a patient's annual exam, a visit to obtain a prescription for an oral contraceptive (birth control), fitting and adjustment of a hearing aid, or immunization for protection against a disease.

V codes can also provide additional information about a patient, even if the patient has an established diagnosis. Examples are personal history of cancer (malignant neoplasm) (Index entries: history, personal) or family history of hypertension (Index entries: history, family). In a handful of exceptions, V codes can show the main reason for the patient's encounter when the patient already has a health problem, like an encounter for chemotherapy or radiation to treat cancer or an encounter for physical therapy (rehabilitation). You can assign a V code as the only code, first code, or secondary code.

Locate V codes in the Index by searching for the main term and then cross-referencing to the V code section in the Tabular. You can look at V codes in the Tabular by turning to the code range V01.0–V91.99 located immediately after code 999.9. There are ICD-9-CM chapter-specific guidelines for V codes, and you will learn how to assign V codes later in this chapter, as well as in Chapter 7.

G. Level of Detail in Coding

Remember to always assign codes to the highest level of specificity, checking for both subcategory and subclassification codes for every category. Let's review more about the level of detail when coding diagnoses.

ICD-9-CM Codes with Three, Four, or Five Digits You already learned that the ICD-9-CM is composed of codes with three, four, or five digits. Codes with three digits are included in ICD-9-CM as the heading of a category of codes that may be further subdivided by fourth (subcategory) and/or fifth (subclassification) digits, which provide greater specificity.

Use of Full Number of Digits Required for a Code Assign a three-digit code only if it is not further subdivided into a subcategory and subclassification. If a fourth-digit subcategory and/or a fifth-digit subclassification exist, then you must assign them. A code is invalid if you have not coded it to the full number of digits required for that code.

Recall from Chapter 4 that you should always code diagnosis codes to their highest number of digits available, a practice that is called coding to the highest level of specificity. Coding to the highest level of specificity means assigning a subcategory if one exists and assigning a subclassification code if one exists.

H. ICD-9-CM Code for the Diagnosis, Condition, Problem, or Other Reason for Encounter/Visit

Many times, you will find that a patient's medical documentation for a service or procedure includes more than one diagnosis. One of the most difficult tasks when coding is determining whether to code all of the diagnoses that a physician documents and deciding on the order in which to assign multiple codes. Always code the reason for the encounter as the first-listed diagnosis. You practiced assigning codes as first-listed diagnoses earlier in this chapter. When you want to find the reason for the encounter/visit, follow these steps:

1. Read the documentation for a patient's service or procedure, and determine the *main reason* for the encounter. First assign the code for the diagnosis, condition, problem, or other reason for encounter/visit shown in the medical record to be chiefly responsible for the services provided. The physician may treat a patient for multiple conditions, but typically only *one* of the conditions is the *main reason* for the encounter. Assign the code for the main reason first. If the physician treated two conditions equally, then you can assign codes in any order.

2. List additional codes that describe any coexisting conditions (diagnoses that exist at the same time) only if the physician treated the patient for the conditions, or if the conditions affect the management of the patient's main reason for the encounter.

    For example, if a physician treated a patient for **chronic kidney disease (CKD)**, and the patient also had hypertension, you would code both conditions, assigning the code for CKD first because the treatment focused on the CKD. Even though the physician only treated the CKD, hypertension is a condition that is directly related to CKD and could affect the management of the patient's CKD. In fact, hypertension and CKD have a **causal relationship**, a relationship in which one condition can cause the other. When you are not sure whether two conditions are related, query the physician for clarification. As you practice the coding exercises in this book, use reference materials to review more about coexisting conditions.

3. In some cases, the first-listed diagnosis may be a symptom when the physician has not established (confirmed) a diagnosis. Code symptoms and signs as the first diagnosis when there is not a definitive diagnosis. You have also coded these types of encounters earlier in this chapter.

chronic kidney disease (CKD)—condition in which the kidneys can no longer remove toxins from the blood

I. Uncertain Diagnosis

Physicians do not always know a patient's definitive diagnosis. They may order radiology or laboratory tests to find the source of the patient's symptoms. Physicians document in the patient's record that a diagnosis is **probable** or **suspected** (likely to be present), or **questionable** (may or may not be present), meaning that they are not sure of the diagnosis yet. They may also document that they are ordering specific tests to "**rule out**" (eliminate the possibility of) a particular diagnosis. They may also say that a diagnosis is a "**working diagnosis**," meaning that it is not yet definitive, or proven, but seems probable.

When you see documentation of a patient's encounter that describes a diagnosis as "probable," "suspected," "questionable," "rule out," or "working diagnosis," it means that the physician is not sure of the patient's definitive diagnosis. You cannot code a diagnosis that is not definitive. Instead, code the main reason for the encounter, including symptoms, signs, abnormal test results, or other reasons. Please note that not all providers follow this coding rule. In acute care (inpatient) settings, long-term or short-term care settings, and psychiatric hospitals, you can code a diagnosis as though it is established even if the physician documents it as probable, suspected, questionable, rule out, or working. Review the following examples of uncertain diagnoses, and then code the encounters in Exercise 5.4.

Examples of uncertain diagnoses

- Mr. Williams, a 58-year-old established patient, sees Dr. Hoffman because of severe low back pain and **dysuria** that he has experienced over the past few weeks. Dr. Hoffman orders a **prostate-specific antigen (PSA) blood test** to *rule out* prostate cancer. Mr. Williams will go to the local hospital's lab department for the test.

  For this encounter, you can only code symptoms because Dr. Hoffman has to wait for the results of the PSA test and cannot yet confirm that the patient has prostate cancer. Symptoms and corresponding codes are

  > low back pain—724.2, dysuria—788.1

dysuria (dis-yr′-ē-ə)—painful urination

prostate-specific antigen (PSA) blood test—screening test for prostate cancer to determine the number of PSAs in the blood; prostate cells produce PSAs

- Mrs. Miller, a 46-year-old established patient, sees Dr. Hoffman because of vomiting, diarrhea, chills, and fatigue that she has had for three days. The medical assistant takes the patient's temperature, and it is 102°. Dr. Hoffman *suspects* that Mrs. Miller may have the H1N1 swine flu, so he sends her to a nearby hospital lab for a nasal swab H1N1 swine flu test.

  For this encounter, you can only code the patient's symptoms, because Dr. Hoffman has not confirmed that she has the H1N1 swine flu. Symptoms and corresponding codes are

  > vomiting—787.03, diarrhea—787.91, chills with fever—780.60, and fatigue—780.79

- Mr. Thomas, a 62-year-old established patient, sees Dr. Hoffman because of intense headaches that will not stop, even with over-the-counter pain medicine. The patient reports that the headaches have occurred over the past month, and he also reports he had recent short-term memory loss. Dr. Hoffman feels that a **glioblastoma** may be *probable*. He orders a **magnetic resonance imaging (MRI)** scan of the brain. (An MRI is a radiology test that will show if there is a brain tumor.) Mr. Thomas will have the scan in the local hospital's radiology department.

  For this encounter, you can only code the patient's symptoms, since Dr. Hoffman has not confirmed that Mr. Thomas has a glioblastoma. Symptoms and corresponding codes are

  > headache—784.0, memory loss—780.93

glioblastoma (glē -ō-bla-stō′-mə)—malignant brain tumor that grows rapidly with poor prognosis (outcome)

magnetic resonance imaging (MRI) (rez′-ə-nəns)—radiology test using magnetic fields to view body structures

TAKE A BREAK

Let's take a break and then review coding uncertain diagnoses with an exercise.

Exercise 5.4   Uncertain Diagnosis

Instructions: Determine the conditions to code for the following patients' encounters with Dr. Hoffman. Use both the Index and the Tabular before final code assignment.

1. Julie Lewis, age 21, is an established patient who sees Dr. Hoffman for a sore throat and fatigue. The medical assistant documents that Ms. Lewis has a fever. During the exam, Dr. Hoffman notes that Julie has swollen lymph nodes in her neck. He sends her to a nearby hospital's lab for a blood test because he believes that mononucleosis is *probable*.

   Condition(s): _____

   Code(s): _____

2. Edward Johnson, a 13-year-old established patient, sees Dr. Hoffman because of a persistent cough with mucus. Upon exam, Dr. Hoffman hears wheezing sounds in the patient's lungs. He obtains a sputum culture to send to the lab and orders a chest X-ray because of *suspected* bronchitis. The patient will visit a nearby hospital for the chest X-ray.

   Condition(s): _____

   Code(s): _____

3. Joe Adams, a 16-year-old established patient, sees Dr. Hoffman because of a painful boil on his leg. Dr. Hoffman evacuates the pus from the boil and obtains a culture from the boil drainage to send to the lab for a wound culture test. Because the patient is a high-school wrestler, Dr. Hoffman *suspects* that he

continued

TAKE A BREAK *continued*

may have a **methicillin-resistant *Staphylococcus aureus* (MRSA) infection** (■ FIGURE 5-2), called community-associated (CA)-MRSA. CA-MRSA is spread by contact with an infected person's skin and starts as a painful boil.

Condition(s): _____

Code(s): _____

4. Nancy Mitchell, age 58, is an established patient who sees Dr. Hoffman for a severe throat and fever. Dr. Hoffman obtains a throat culture to send to the lab to *rule out* strep throat. The lab test will identify if Group A streptococci (strep) bacteria are present.

Condition(s): _____

Code(s): _____

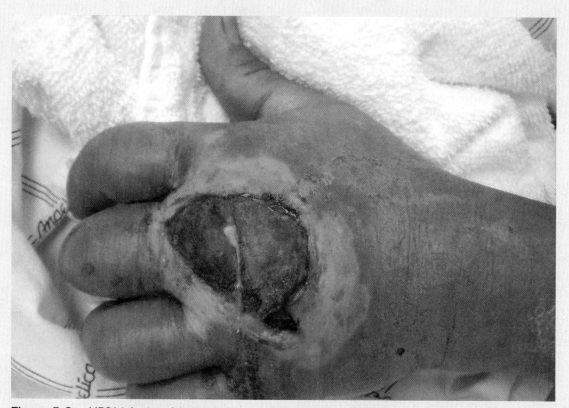

Figure 5-2 ■ MRSA infection of the hand. *Photo credit:* Gregory Moran, M.D./CDC.

J. Chronic Diseases

methicillin-resistant *Staphylococcus aureus* (MRSA) infection (meth-ə-sil'-ən stăf'ə-lō-kŏk-əs aw'-ree-əs)—skin infection that is resistant to methicillin (antibiotic); infection is spread by skin-to-skin contact, skin abrasions, contaminated surfaces, and poor hygiene

Physicians treat chronic diseases on an ongoing basis, and you can code and report them as many times as the patient receives treatment and care for the condition(s). Remember that a chronic condition is one that typically lasts three or more months.

For example, during a new patient's exam, the physician determines that the patient has diabetes, a chronic condition. You can code diabetes, along with any other diagnoses the physician documents. When the patient returns for a follow-up visit for diabetes management, you would again assign a code for diabetes. Just because you reported a code for diabetes for the first encounter does not mean that you do not ever have to code it again. Keep in mind that when you code an outpatient encounter, you need to review the medical documentation for that encounter only and then code accordingly. You should not incorporate past documentation or previous diagnoses from other encounters for the patient. Code each outpatient encounter individually.

TAKE A BREAK

Let's take a break and then code chronic diseases.

| Exercise 5.5 | **Chronic Diseases** |

Instructions: Code chronic conditions for the following patients' encounters. Use both the Index and the Tabular before assigning the final code.

1. Mark Moore, age 16, sees Dr. Wilson, his dermatologist, for management of **acne vulgaris**.

   Code(s): _____

2. Ralph Anderson, a 60-year-old established patient, sees Dr. King, his oncologist, for **palliative** treatment of prostate cancer (primary site) which has **metastasized** to the bone (secondary site).

   Code(s): _____

3. Debbie Nelson, a 48-year-old established patient, sees Dr. Hoffman for management of diabetes and hypertension.

   Code(s): _____

4. Dr. Gonzalez, a neurologist, sees Mr. Morris, age 72, an established patient, for management of **Parkinson's disease**.

   Code(s): _____

5. Dr. Hoffman sees Mrs. Cook, an 82-year-old established patient, for an **A1C test** for diabetes management.

   Code(s): _____

K. Code All Documented Conditions that Coexist

You have already learned in Guideline H how to determine the reason for an encounter. You also learned that you should list additional codes that describe any coexisting conditions (diagnoses that exist at the same time) only if

- the physician treated the patient for the condition(s), or
- the condition(s) affect the management of the patient's main reason for the encounter.

Do you remember in Chapter 1 when we discussed how the patient's diagnosis has to support the procedure or service? We said that a service or procedure has to be medically necessary. The insurance company decides if a service is medically necessary by ensuring that the diagnosis code justifies the service. When you try to determine whether to code a coexisting condition, think about whether the diagnosis for the condition will support medical necessity for the service or procedure. Review the following examples of encounters involving coexisting conditions and decide whether you should code them:

> **Example:** Mr. Collins, a 48-year-old established patient, sees Dr. Hoffman for an office visit to manage hyperlipidemia, and Dr. Hoffman prescribes a medication refill for the condition. During the visit, Mr. Collins says that he was recently promoted at work and has experienced job stress from the additional responsibilities. However, he states that he has started an exercise regimen and has been more relaxed lately. He said that he feels he will be successful in his new role.
>
> For Mr. Collins' encounter, code only hyperlipidemia because it is the reason for the encounter and establishes the medical necessity that is needed to bill the patient's insurance for the encounter. Mr. Collins said he suffered from stress, but he told Dr. Hoffman that he successfully manages it. Dr. Hoffman did not treat the patient for stress, and it did not affect the management of his hyperlipidemia, so you do not need to code it as a coexisting condition.

> **Example:** Mrs. Sanchez is a 32-year-old established patient who sees Dr. Hoffman for a check-up for asthma and prescription refill for asthma medication. During the visit, Mrs. Sanchez asks Dr. Hoffman to look at her right great toe (big toe) because it "feels hard." She tells him that she thinks it's an ingrown toenail and that she soaked it in warm water the previous day. Dr. Hoffman examines the toenail and tells

acne vulgaris (vŭl-gā′ris)—ordinary acne

palliative (pal′-lee-uh-tiv)—care to relieve symptoms

metastasized (meh-tas′-tuh-sized)—spread from one location to another

Parkinson's disease—disorder of the central nervous system; symptoms, which worsen as the disease progresses, include tremors, loss of balance and motor skills, and difficulty speaking

A1C test—glucose blood test that diabetic patients receive about every three months

the patient that it does not appear to be infected. Upon further examination with a magnifier, he finds that there is a large piece of fuzz stuck under her nail, which he removes.

For Mrs. Sanchez's encounter, only code asthma because it is the reason for the encounter and establishes the medical necessity needed to bill the patient's insurance for the visit. Dr. Hoffman examined the patient's great toe but did not treat her for any condition; he only removed fuzz, so do not code a "hard" toe as a coexisting condition.

Example: Mrs. Ward, a 68-year-old established patient, sees Dr. Hoffman for management of hypertension and diabetes. During the visit, Dr. Hoffman determines that Mrs. Ward's hypertension medication is ineffective, so he prescribes a new one.

For Mrs. Ward's encounter, code both hypertension and diabetes, as the patient saw Dr. Hoffman for both conditions. The coexisting conditions will both support medical necessity needed for the visit. You can sequence the codes in any order, unless ICD-9-CM guidelines or conventions direct you to code in a specific order.

TAKE A BREAK

Let's take a break and then practice coding coexisting conditions.

Exercise 5.6   Code All Documented Conditions That Coexist

Instructions: Determine whether to code coexisting conditions for the following patients' encounters with Dr. Hoffman. Remember to code conditions that affect the management of the patient, that the physician treated, and/or that support medical necessity. Use both the Index and the Tabular before assigning the final code.

1. Mrs. Bailey, age 42, is an established patient who sees Dr. Hoffman for removal of several skin tags from her neck. The patient has been taking an anti-emetic for nausea during her menstrual cycle and has three refills left, so Dr. Hoffman does not need to write a new prescription.

   What condition(s) should you code? _____

   _____

   What code(s) should you assign? _____

   _____

2. Mrs. Watson, a 70-year-old established patient, sees Dr. Hoffman for management of malignant hypertensive CKD. The CKD is Stage III.

   What condition(s) should you code? _____

   _____

   What code(s) should you assign? _____

   _____

3. Ms. Price, a 26-year-old established patient, sees Dr. Hoffman for management of anxiety. Dr. Hoffman writes a prescription refill for Ms. Price's anti-anxiety medication. During the visit, Ms. Price says that she has a mole on her back that she'd like Dr. Hoffman to examine. Dr. Hoffman looks at the mole and determines that it's benign, requiring no intervention.

   What condition(s) should you code? _____

   _____

   What code(s) should you assign? _____

   _____

Personal or Family History as a Coexisting Condition   When determining whether to code coexisting conditions, you also need to remember these additional rules:

1. Do not code conditions that the physician previously treated and that no longer exist *unless* a past condition affects current care or influences the patient's treatment. If a past condition affects current care or influences treatment, then assign a V code as a *secondary* code for *personal* history of the past condition (V10–V15). V codes for personal history of a condition help to clarify why a patient may have a *current* condition. When you are coding a personal history, search the Index for the main term, *history (personal) of.*

When a condition is classified as personal history, it means that the patient had the condition at one time, and it is now gone. It is history, in the past, no longer a condition for which the patient needs treatment. However, many times historical conditions affect current conditions and their treatment.

For example, the physician sees a patient for management of lung cancer. The patient has a personal history of breast cancer and had a left breast total **mastectomy**. Even though the patient's breast was removed, the cancer had eventually spread to the lung. In order to code the full details of the patient's case, you need to assign a code for malignant neoplasm of the lung (secondary site—197.0), and then assign a code for personal history of breast cancer (V10.3). The personal history of breast cancer explains why the patient currently has lung cancer.

2. Assign a V code as a *secondary* code if the patient has a *family* history of a condition that affects current care or influences treatment (V16—V19). Just like personal history, family history V codes are necessary to tell the entire story of a patient's current condition. When coding a family history, search the Index for the main term, *history (personal) of*, subterm, *family*.

For example, a patient sees the physician for a physical examination. During the exam, the physician determines that the patient is overweight, a condition that can make a patient prone to developing diabetes. Her BMI is 28. The patient also has a family history of **diabetes mellitus**. Even though the physician determines that the patient does not have diabetes, he counsels her on better eating habits to lose weight. Because the patient also has a family history of diabetes, the physician tells her that she is more likely to become diabetic than someone without a family history of diabetes. He provides her with additional literature on diabetes that includes suggestions to better manage her health. For this encounter, you would code

1. overweight (278.02)

2. BMI of 28 (V85.24)

3. V code for family history of diabetes mellitus (V18.0)

You assign a V code because the family history influences the patient's treatment and explains why the physician provided additional counseling. Notice that V code for family history is not the secondary code because you need to report the BMI secondary to the diagnosis of overweight.

You can locate codes in the Index for personal history by searching *history, personal* and family history by searching *history, family*.

mastectomy (ma-stek′-tə-mē)—surgical removal of part or all of the breast, which may include removal of muscles and lymph nodes

diabetes mellitus—high glucose (sugar) levels that result when the pancreas does not produce the correct amount of insulin (hormone) or the body's cells do not utilize insulin properly

appendectomy (a-pən-dek′-tə-mē)—surgical removal of the appendix

hysterectomy (his-tə-rek′-tə-mē)—surgical removal of the uterus

TAKE A BREAK

Let's take a break and then code encounters for patients with personal or family histories.

Exercise 5.7   Personal or Family History as a Coexisting Condition

Instructions: Determine whether to code a personal or family history as a coexisting condition for the following patients' encounters with Dr. Hoffman. Remember to only code personal or family histories if they affect current care or influence the patient's treatment. Use both the Index and the Tabular before assigning the final code. (Hint: When coding histories, search the Index for the main term, *history (personal) of.*)

1. Mrs. Clark, age 28, has an initial visit with Dr. Hoffman for chills and body aches. On her health history questionnaire, Mrs. Clark notes her past history of surgeries, an **appendectomy** due to appendicitis and a **hysterectomy** due to uterine fibroid tumors. Dr. Hoffman diagnoses Mrs. Clark with influenza.

What condition(s) should you code? _____

_____

What code(s) should you assign? _____

_____

continued

TAKE A BREAK *continued*

2. Nathan Hill, a 12-year-old established patient, saw Dr. Hoffman yesterday because of a severe cough with mucus. Upon exam, Dr. Hoffman heard wheezing sounds in the patient's lungs. He obtained a sputum culture to send to the lab and ordered a chest X-ray because of suspected bronchitis. Today, the patient returns, and Dr. Hoffman explains that the sputum culture and the chest X-ray were positive for bronchitis. Nathan has a personal history of allergy to **penicillin**, so Dr. Hoffman prescribes a different antibiotic to treat the patient's bronchitis.

   What condition(s) should you code? _____

   _____

   What code(s) should you assign? _____

   _____

3. Mr. Young is a 35-year-old new patient who sees Dr. Hoffman for a check-up. (*Hint: Index entry: admission for general exam.*) Mr. Young notes on his health history questionnaire that he has a past history of pelvic fractures following a motor vehicle accident 10 years

ago. Dr. Hoffman determines that Mr. Young is healthy and asks him to return in a year for his annual exam.

   What condition(s) should you code? _____

   _____

   What code(s) should you assign? _____

   _____

4. Mrs. Peterson is a 62-year-old new patient who sees Dr. Hoffman for a persistent smoker's cough and **dyspnea**. Mrs. Peterson notes on her health history questionnaire that she has a past history of tobacco use and was a chronic cigarette smoker. Dr. Hoffman *suspects* that the patient may have emphysema brought on by her past smoking. He orders several different tests and tells Mrs. Peterson to visit the local hospital to have the tests performed.

   What condition(s) should you code? _____

   _____

   What code(s) should you assign? _____

   _____

penicillin—antibiotic drug used to treat infections

dyspnea (dis(p)'-nē-ə)— difficulty breathing

L. Patients Receiving Diagnostic Services Only

Diagnostic services include laboratory or radiology tests or procedures to help diagnose a condition. They are performed when a patient experiences certain symptoms and the physician suspects a specific diagnosis but needs more testing to substantiate it.

Patients can receive diagnostic tests at hospitals, *outside labs* (outside the physician's office), outpatient clinics, and ASCs, facilities where physicians perform outpatient surgeries. Sometimes physicians perform their own diagnostic tests *on-site* (at the provider's location), like lab or radiology tests, which allows them to review test results before the patient leaves the office.

Examples of laboratory services include tests to determine if specific substances are present in a patient's body, such as a prescription medication or recreational drug, and tests to measure how well the patient's body or a particular organ functions. Examples of radiology services include X-rays, ultrasounds, MRIs (■ FIGURE 5-3), computed tomography (CT) scans (■ FIGURE 5-4), positron emission tomography (PET) scans, and many others that allow clinicians to view various areas of the body for abnormalities. Scans are often called "imaging studies."

The physician interprets, or reviews, the test result to determine the patient's diagnosis and then documents it in the medical record.

When you assign diagnosis codes for patients receiving diagnostic tests, it is important to remember that you will not know the definitive diagnosis until the physician interprets the patient's test result. You may code encounters in which a physician *orders* a diagnostic test, but the patient has not had the test yet. In that case, you can only code the *reason* that the physician ordered the test, such as a sign or symptom.

Follow these rules when coding encounters that are *only* for diagnostic services. The examples relate to coding for both the physician's services and other outpatient facilities:

1. Sequence first the diagnosis, condition, problem, or other reason for the diagnostic encounter/visit. The physician will document in the medical record the chief reason for providing diagnostic services.

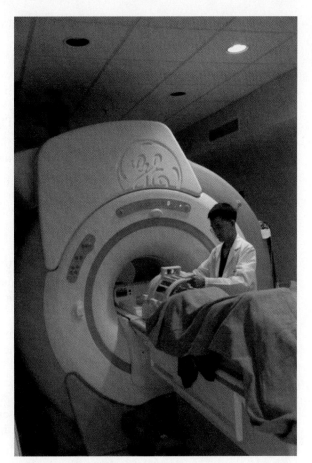

Figure 5-3 ▪ Patient in an MRI scanner.

Photo credit: Journal of NIH Research.

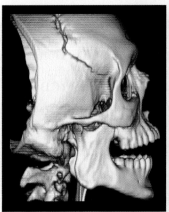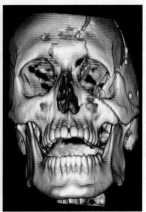

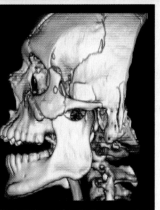

Figure 5-4 ▪ 3-D CT scan reconstruction showing fractures of the left side of the face and skull of a 24-year-old man.

Photo credit: Kallista Images/ Custom Medical Stock Photo.

2. Sequence any other codes for diagnoses (e.g., chronic conditions) as additional diagnoses.

> **Example:** Dr. Hoffman sees Mr. Lee, a 58-year-old established patient, for shortness of breath and chronic cough. The patient has a personal history of smoking but quit six months ago. Dr. Hoffman orders a chest X-ray, along with other diagnostic tests, to determine if Mr. Lee has emphysema. The patient will receive the tests at the local hospital.
>
> *Diagnoses: shortness of breath (786.05), chronic cough (786.2), personal history of smoking (V15.82).*
>
> *Mr. Lee has not had any diagnostic tests yet, so there is no definitive diagnosis, only symptoms and a personal history of smoking, which could be related to the symptoms.*

3. When the patient receives a routine diagnostic service but does not have an associated diagnosis, sign, or symptom, assign code V72.5 (radiology exam—Index entry: examination, radiological—Index entry: examination, laboratory) and/or a code from subcategory V72.6 (lab exam for blood or urine testing).

> **Example:** Mr. Green, age 34, has no symptoms, but needs to have a general health lab *panel test* (a series of tests performed together from one specimen).
>
> *Diagnosis: lab exam for blood testing (V72.62)*

4. When the patient receives a *routine* diagnostic service and also receives a nonroutine diagnostic test to evaluate a sign, symptom, or diagnosis during the *same encounter*,

   • Assign V72.5 (radiology exam) and/or a code from subcategory V72.6 (lab exam for blood or urine testing) for the *routine* diagnostic service and

   • Assign a code describing the reason for the *nonroutine* diagnostic service.

complete blood count (CBC)—lab tests on blood cells to determine cell counts

> **Example:** Dr. Hoffman sees Mrs. Carter, a 38-year-old new patient, for a physical exam. She provides a blood specimen for a routine lab test to check cholesterol. During the exam, Mrs. Carter tells Dr. Hoffman that she has felt fatigued and weak during the past couple of weeks. Dr. Hoffman decides to write an order for the lab to also perform a **complete blood count (CBC)**.
>
> *Diagnosis: encounter for routine lab test (cholesterol) (V72.6), fatigue and weakness (780.79)*
>
> *Fatigue and weakness are symptoms related to a nonroutine CBC test. The lab test for cholesterol is the routine lab test.*

5. Code the definitive diagnosis for outpatient encounters documented for diagnostic tests when the physician reviewed and interpreted the test report, and the final report is available at the time of coding. Do not code related signs and symptoms as additional diagnoses.*

> **Example:** Mrs. Ross visits Williton's radiology clinic for a screening mammogram. Dr. Snyder, the radiologist at the clinic, reviews and interprets the mammogram and determines that there are no abnormalities.
>
> *Diagnosis: encounter for screening mammogram (V76.12)*
>
> Dr. Snyder did not find any abnormalities in the patient's mammogram. His interpretation of the test was available at the time of coding.

*Please note: This outpatient coding rule differs from the coding practice in the hospital inpatient setting regarding abnormal findings on test results. Please refer to Chapter 15 of this book.

TAKE A BREAK

Let's take a break and then code encounters for patients receiving diagnostic services.

Exercise 5.8 Patients Receiving Diagnostic Services Only

Instructions: Assign codes for the following encounters involving diagnostic services, referring to the guidelines outlined in this section. Use both the Index and the Tabular before assigning the final code.

1. Mrs. Davis is a 61-year-old patient who presents to the local hospital's radiology department for a **diagnostic mammogram** that Dr. Hoffman ordered because Mrs. Davis has a lump in her right breast.

   What condition(s) should you code? _____

   _____

   What code(s) should you assign? _____

   _____

2. Mr. Martinez, a 46-year-old patient, sees Dr. Hoffman for a general medical exam. During the exam, Mr. Martinez tells Dr. Hoffman that he has felt very tired lately but cannot determine why. Dr. Hoffman orders a lab panel test to determine Mr. Martinez's

overall health. The patient will visit the local hospital's lab department for the test.

   What condition(s) should you code? _____

   _____

   What code(s) should you assign? _____

   _____

3. Mrs. Harris, a 29-year-old patient, visits the local hospital's lab department to have blood drawn for tests to determine her medication levels.

   What condition(s) should you code? _____

   _____

   What code(s) should you assign? _____

   _____

4. Miss Baker, a 28-year-old patient, sees Dr. Hoffman because of constant nausea. He orders a blood test to check for pregnancy.

   What condition(s) should you code? _____

   _____

   What code(s) should you assign? _____

   _____

M. Patients Receiving Therapeutic Services Only

Therapeutic means to heal, or to cure. Therapeutic services are services that help a patient to manage a disease or eliminate it. Examples of therapeutic services are chemotherapy or radiation to treat cancer, rehabilitation or physical therapy to treat a fracture, occupational or speech therapy to treat a stroke, respiratory therapy to treat breathing problems, medications to treat diseases, dialysis to treat kidney failure, and various other services or procedures to treat illnesses and diseases.

To code an encounter for a patient who receives only therapeutic services, sequence first the diagnosis, condition, problem, or other reason for the encounter for therapeutic services. Sequence second any additional codes for other diagnoses, including chronic conditions.

Example: Mr. Stewart, a 73-year-old patient, sees the respiratory therapist at an outpatient hospital. The patient has **chronic obstructive pulmonary disease (COPD),** and the therapist provided oxygen treatments and instructions for at-home use. The patient also suffers from congestive heart failure.

First-listed diagnosis: COPD (496)

Second diagnosis: congestive heart failure (428.0)

The only exception to this rule is that when the primary reason for the admission or encounter is chemotherapy, radiation therapy, immunotherapy, or rehabilitation. The V code for **dialysis** and dialysis catheter care also includes a note to "use additional code to identify the associated condition." This means that when you are coding an encounter for dialysis or dialysis catheter care, you should *assign a V code first* and assign the code for the

diagnostic mammogram (dahy-uhg-nos′-tik mam′-ə-gram)—X-ray of soft tissue of the breast that provides more definitive information about a neoplasm

chronic obstructive pulmonary disease (COPD)—lung disease characterized by inflammation of bronchi (airways), called bronchitis, or by destruction of the air sacs (alveoli) of the lungs

dialysis (dī-al′-ə-səs)—procedure to cleanse the body of toxins (poisons) when the kidneys can no longer remove toxins from the blood

asthma (az'-mə)—condition in which the airways are obstructed so that breathing is difficult

diagnosis of the condition second. Recall that V codes can also provide additional information about a patient, even if the patient has an established diagnosis. When the reason for the patient's encounter is for chemotherapy, radiation therapy, immunotherapy, rehabilitation, dialysis, or dialysis catheter care, you will assign two codes:

- 1st code—Assign a V code to show that the encounter is for chemotherapy, radiation therapy, rehabilitation, dialysis, or dialysis catheter care. (Index entry: admission for)
- 2nd code—Assign a code for the diagnosis or problem that required the service.

> **Example:** Mrs. Jenkins, a 24-year-old patient, sees a physical therapist at an outpatient rehabilitation center. Mrs. Jenkins suffered an open fracture of her femur shaft in a motor vehicle accident and needs gait training.
>
> *Diagnoses: Encounter for physical rehabilitation (V57.1), open fracture of shaft of the femur (821.11)*

asthma with status asthmaticus (stat'-əs az-mat'-i-kəs)—serious asthma attack that threatens life

TAKE A BREAK

Let's take a break and then code encounters for patients receiving therapeutic services.

Exercise 5.9   Patients Receiving Therapeutic Services Only

Instructions: Assign codes for the following encounters involving therapeutic services. Use both the Index and the Tabular before assigning the final code.

1. Mr. Sanders, a 59-year-old patient, has an encounter at an outpatient rehabilitation clinic. He sees the speech therapist for treatment of dysphagia.

   Code(s): _____

2. Mr. Wood, a 47-year-old patient, has an encounter at an outpatient clinic to manage acute kidney failure.

While he is there, the physician decides to begin peritoneal dialysis treatment in the clinic and also counsels the patient on the procedure.

   Code(s): _____

3. Ms. Bennett, age 26, has an encounter at an outpatient hospital for chemotherapy to treat a malignant neoplasm of the breast (Ca in situ).

   Code(s): _____

4. Mr. Washington, a 43-year-old patient, has an encounter at an outpatient hospital for respiratory therapy to treat **asthma with status asthmaticus**.

   Code(s): _____

N. Patients Receiving Preoperative Evaluations Only

lumbar spinal fusion surgery—joining one or more lumbar vertebrae to stop pain

lumbar degenerative disc disease (dǐ-jěn'-ər-ə-tǐv)—low back pain caused by a breakdown in the lumbar disc and structures around the lumbar spine

obstructive sleep apnea (OSA) (ap'-nē-ə)—condition that interrupts a patient's breathing during sleep; throat muscles block the patient's airway

A **preoperative evaluation** (one that occurs before a surgery or procedure) is an examination and testing to ensure that a patient is healthy enough for surgery. When a patient is scheduled for surgery, it is imperative that the patient be in good health not only to survive the surgery, but also to endure anesthesia and its after effects. If the surgeon feels that the patient may be at risk during the surgery, he will request that another physician, such as a general practitioner, conduct a preoperative evaluation to assess the patient's overall health and determine if the patient has **surgical**, or medical, "**clearance**" for surgery. Clearance means that a physician has determined that the patient's medical condition is stable enough for surgery. The general practitioner may order specific diagnostic tests in addition to performing an exam and may determine that the patient cannot have surgery because of one or more health problems.

Patients with lung or heart conditions may not be good candidates for surgery because they cannot endure the anesthesia they will need during the procedure. Patients who are overweight or obese are also at risk during surgery because their increased weight makes them more likely to develop infections, and they may also have hypertension or dyspnea, which makes surgery risky. Elderly patients and infants may also be at risk during surgery because they are too weak to withstand surgical procedures.

For patients receiving preoperative evaluations only, follow these steps:

- 1st code—Sequence first a code from category V72 *(Special investigations and examinations)* to describe the pre-op evaluations (Index entries: examination, preoperative or preprocedural).

- 2nd code—Assign a code for the condition to describe the reason for the surgery as an additional diagnosis.

- Additional codes—Code any findings related to the pre-op evaluation.

> **Example:** Mrs. Long, a 39-year-old established patient, sees Dr. Hoffman for surgical clearance for an abdominal hysterectomy due to chronic pelvic pain. The patient also has benign hypertension. Dr. Hoffman conducts a general exam and approves the surgery.
>
> 1. *Preoperative examination (V72.83)*
> 2. *Chronic pelvic pain (625.9)*
> 3. *Benign hypertension (401.1)*

vestibular neurectomy (ve-stib′-yə-lər nū-rek′-tŏ-mē)—surgery that cuts part of the cochleovestibular cranial nerve to correct vertigo (dizziness); *cochleovestibular* refers to the location of the cochlea inside the inner ear, and *vestibular* pertains to the auditory nerve of the inner ear

Meniere's disease (men′-yərz)—disorder of the labyrinth of the ear, causing dizziness, tinnitus (ringing in the ears), nausea, and hearing loss; also called Meniere's syndrome

mitral valve replacement surgery (mī′-trăl)—replacement of the mitral valve with a metal or animal tissue valve

TAKE A BREAK

Let's take a break and then code encounters for patients receiving preoperative evaluations.

Exercise 5.10 **Patients Receiving Preoperative Evaluations Only**

Instructions: Assign codes for the following encounters involving preoperative evaluations. Use both the Index and the Tabular before assigning the final code.

1. Mrs. Johnson, a 33-year-old established patient, sees Dr. Hoffman for surgical clearance for a **lumbar spinal fusion surgery** to treat **lumbar degenerative disc disease**. The patient also has **obstructive sleep apnea (OSA)**. Dr. Hoffman approves the surgery.

   Diagnosis to code first: _____

   Code: _____

   Diagnosis to code second: _____

   Code: _____

   Additional diagnosis to code: _____

   _____

   Code(s): _____

2. Dr. James sends Mr. Winden, a 42-year-old established patient, to Dr. Hoffman for a surgical clearance consult. Mr. Winden needs to have a **vestibular neurectomy** for unilateral **Meniere's disease**. Dr. Hoffman approves the surgery.

   Diagnosis to code first: _____

   Code: _____

   Diagnosis to code second: _____

   Code: _____

3. Mr. Stipp, a 61-year-old established patient, sees Dr. Frazier for surgical clearance for **mitral valve replacement surgery** needed for coronary artery disease. The patient has a history of a **coronary artery bypass graft (CABG)** to treat **angina**. Dr. Frazier approves the surgery.

   Diagnosis to code first: _____

   Code: _____

   Diagnosis to code second: _____

   Code: _____

   Additional diagnosis to code: _____

   Code(s): _____

O. Ambulatory Surgery

For **ambulatory surgery** (outpatient surgery after which the patient leaves the same day), code the diagnosis for which the surgery was performed. If the postoperative (after surgery) diagnosis is different from the preoperative (before surgery) diagnosis, then *code the postoperative diagnosis*, since it is the most definitive.

coronary artery bypass graft (CABG)—creation of a new blood vessel (graft) from an artery or vein to make a new passage for blood to flow to the heart, when coronary arteries are blocked; CABG is pronounced "cabbage"

angina (an-jī′-nə)—chest pain

palmar (pahl′-mahr)—pertaining to the palm of the hand

ganglion (gan′-glē-ən)—either a group of nerve cells or a cyst (sac containing fluid) that forms on a tendon

carpal tunnel decompression (kär′-pal)—procedure to treat carpal tunnel syndrome

carpal tunnel syndrome (CTS)—a condition in which the tendons of the wrist pinch the median nerve, causing pain and discomfort

cystoscopy (sis-tos′- kŏ-pē)—procedure to view the urinary bladder with a flexible tube inserted into the urethra

transitional cell carcinoma—cancer occurring in the urinary system, including the urinary bladder and kidneys

esophagogastroduodenoscopy (EGD) (ĕ-sofă-gō-gas-trō-dūō-den-os′-kŏ-pē)—use of an endoscope to examine the interior of a patient's esophagus (esophago-), stomach (gastro-), and duodenum (duodeno-)

Example: Mrs. Gonzales, a 33-year-old, presents to ambulatory surgery to excise a ganglion cyst on her left ring finger. Her preoperative diagnosis is left **palmar** mass, and her postoperative diagnosis is **ganglion** of left ring finger tendon sheath (■ FIGURE 5-5).

Condition to code: ganglion of left ring finger tendon sheath (727.42)

Code the postoperative diagnosis because the surgeon determined that the mass was a ganglion, which he removed. Ganglion is more specific than "mass."

Figure 5-5 ■ Patient with recurrent ganglion of the thumb.
Photo credit: Science Photo Library/Custom Medical Stock Photo.

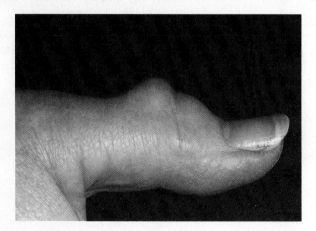

It is especially important to remember this coding rule if you are abstracting a chart because the physician documents *both* a pre-op and a post-op diagnosis. Many times, these diagnoses are the same. But you have to carefully review the documentation to choose the post-op diagnosis if the diagnoses are different.

TAKE A BREAK

Let's take a break and then code ambulatory surgery encounters.

Exercise 5.11 Ambulatory Surgery

Instructions: Assign codes for the following encounters involving ambulatory surgeries. Use both the Index and the Tabular before assigning the final code.

1. Mrs. Russell, a 48-year-old patient, presents to ambulatory surgery for left **carpal tunnel decompression**. Her pre-op diagnosis is left **carpal tunnel syndrome (CTS)**, and her post-op diagnosis is the same.

   Condition to code: _____

   Code: _____

2. Mr. Ford, an 88-year-old patient, presents to ambulatory surgery for a **cystoscopy** to check for neoplasms.

He has a personal history of **transitional cell carcinoma** of the bladder. The physician does not find any evidence of recurrence.

Condition to code: _____

Code: _____

3. Mr. Graham, a 53-year-old patient, presents to ambulatory surgery for an **esophagogastroduodenoscopy (EGD)** with biopsy and a **colonoscopy**. The physician also performs a polypectomy. His pre-op diagnosis is abdominal pain. Post-op diagnoses are colon polyps, **pancolonic diverticulosis**, and **antral gastritis**.

Conditions to code: _____

Codes: _____

colonoscopy (kō-län-ə′-skäp-ee)—use of an endoscope (fiberoptic tube) to view the inside of the colon

P. Routine Outpatient Prenatal Visits

Prenatal means before birth. A routine prenatal visit is when a pregnant patient visits the physician for a status check of her pregnancy, and there are no complications. Ultrasound is a typical diagnostic test that physicians perform on pregnant patients (■ FIGURE 5-6). Ultrasound bounces sound waves off body tissues and converts the echoes of the sound waves into pictures called sonograms.

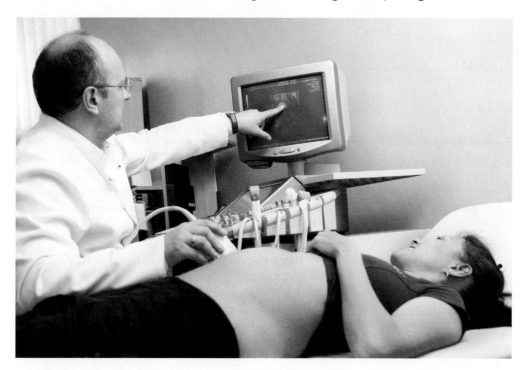

Figure 5-6 ■ An obstetrician performs ultrasound during a prenatal visit.

Photo credit: Dmitry Kalinovsky / Shutterstock.com.

For routine outpatient prenatal visits in which no complications are present, assign one of the following codes:

* V22.0—Supervision of normal *first* pregnancy
* V22.1—Supervision of *other* normal pregnancy (not the first pregnancy)
  Index entries are *pregnancy, supervision of.*

If the pregnant patient has a prenatal visit and the physician finds a complication, do not assign a V code. *Instead, assign the code for the complication.* Chapter 11 of the Tabular List contains all pregnancy complication codes. You will practice coding pregnancy complications in Chapter 14 of this book.

> **Example:** Mrs. West, a 28-year-old established patient, has an encounter for **prenatal** visit. She is pregnant with her second child. She sees Dr. Owens, her **obstetrician**. Dr. Owens finds no complications.
>
> *Code: V22.1—Supervision of other normal pregnancy*

pancolonic diverticulosis (pan-kō-lon′-ic dī-vur-tik-yoo-loh′-sis)—condition characterized by bulging pouches (diverticula) within the colon or intestine

antral gastritis (an′-trəl ga-strī′-təs)—bacterial infection in the lower part of the stomach (antrum)

prenatal (prē-nā′təl)—before birth

obstetrician (ob-stĕ-trish′-ŭn)—a physician who specializes in care of patients during pregnancy, childbirth, and the period that follows childbirth

TAKE A BREAK

Let's take a break and then code routine outpatient prenatal visits.

Exercise 5.12 **Routine Outpatient Prenatal Visits**

Instructions: Assign codes for the following encounters involving routine outpatient prenatal visits. Use both the Index and the Tabular before assigning the final code.

1. Mrs. Gibson, a 25-year-old new patient, is pregnant with her first child. She sees Dr. Owens for a prenatal visit, and there are no complications.

   Code: _____

2. Mrs. Gomez, a 34-year-old established patient, has an encounter with Dr. Owens for a prenatal visit. She is pregnant with her third child and is doing well.

   Code: _____

3. Mrs. Henry, a 31-year-old established patient, is pregnant with her second child. She sees Dr. Owens for a prenatal visit without complications.

   Code: _____

CHAPTER REVIEW

Multiple Choice

Instructions: Circle one best answer to complete each statement.

1. In an outpatient setting, a primary diagnosis is also called a(n)
   a. principal diagnosis.
   b. definitive diagnosis.
   c. first-grouped diagnosis.
   d. first-listed diagnosis.

2. The main reason for a patient's encounter is typically the
   a. coexisting condition.
   b. personal history of the condition.
   c. first-listed diagnosis.
   d. secondary diagnosis.

3. Coding for a physician can involve
   a. coding only services that the physician provides at the office.
   b. coding only services that the physician provides at a hospital.
   c. coding services that the physician provides at the office and in the hospital.
   d. coding only services that the physician provides at a hospital and SNF.

4. If the reason for a patient's visit was a symptom, but another condition caused the symptom, you should
   a. code the symptom.
   b. code the condition that caused the symptom.
   c. sequence the symptom code first and the condition code second.
   d. sequence the condition code first and the symptom code second.

5. When a patient presents to hospital outpatient surgery and develops complications requiring admission to observation, you should
   a. code the complication.
   b. code the reason for the surgery.
   c. sequence the complication code first and the reason for surgery code second.
   d. sequence the reason for surgery code first and the complication code second.

6. You should report codes for patients with chronic diseases
   a. as many times as the patients receive treatment and care for the condition(s).
   b. on the first visit only; you do not report chronic disease codes for subsequent visits.
   c. by assigning a V code to show that the patient's encounter involved a chronic disease.
   d. only if the physician treated the patient for the chronic disease within the past six months.

7. You should assign codes for a coexisting condition if
   a. the physician treated the patient for the condition in the past, and the patient is now cured.
   b. a specialist rendered care to the patient for the condition.
   c. the condition affects the management of the patient's main reason for the encounter.
   d. the patient was recently hospitalized for treatment of the condition.

8. When a patient has a personal history of a condition, it means that
   a. the condition is resolved and in the past, and the patient does not need further treatment for it.
   b. the condition was diagnosed in the past, and the patient is receiving current treatment.
   c. one or more of the patient's family members suffered from the condition in the past.
   d. the patient is receiving medications to treat the condition.

9. Chemotherapy, radiation therapy, immunotherapy, and rehabilitation services are all classified as _____ services
   a. observation
   b. diagnostic
   c. preoperative
   d. therapeutic

10. There are _____ V codes available to code for routine outpatient prenatal visits without complications.
    a. two   b. three
    c. four   d. five

Coding Assignments

Instructions: Assign code(s) for the following cases, using both the Index and Tabular. Some cases will have more than one code. Refer to the guidelines outlined in this chapter for assistance.

1. Mrs. Hall, a 62-year-old established patient, has an encounter at the outpatient rehabilitation facility for gait training with a physical therapist, due to a closed tibial fracture.

   Code(s): _____

2. Mr. Hernandez, a 46-year-old established patient, sees Dr. Wright, a dermatologist, for a follow-up for treatment of atopic dermatitis (eczema). Mr. Hernandez developed a *Staphylococcus aureus* infection of the skin. He also has a personal history of allergy to penicillin.

   Code(s): _____

3. Mrs. Evans, a 24-year-old patient, sees Dr. Hoffman for coughing, body aches, and chills. Her temperature at the office is 102°. Dr. Hoffman diagnoses Mrs. Evans with influenza.

    Code(s): _____

4. Dr. Hoffman sees Mr. Murphy, age 35, for a check-up. Dr. Hoffman diagnoses the patient with benign hypertension and writes a prescription for medication to treat it. On Mr. Murphy's health history form, he wrote that he sustained a clavicle fracture in a motor vehicle accident four years ago.

    Code(s): _____

5. Mrs. Cooper, a 72-year-old patient, is admitted to the hospital's observation unit postoperatively. She underwent an appendectomy to treat acute appendicitis. After surgery, she developed severe nausea and vomiting.

    Code(s): _____

6. Kelly Torres, a 16-year-old established patient, sees Dr. Hoffman for a sore throat and neck, along with left ear pain, all of which have lasted for a week. Dr. Hoffman diagnoses Ms. Torres with otitis media and writes a medication prescription.

    Code(s): _____

7. Mr. Gray, age 54, is an established patient who sees Dr. Hoffman for essential hypertension. Dr. Hoffman writes a prescription refill.

    Code(s): _____

8. Mrs. Long, a 39-year-old established patient, sees Dr. Hansen for surgical clearance for a transurethral resection of the prostate due to benign prostatic hypertrophy (BPH). The patient also has benign hypertension. Dr. Hansen approves the surgery.

    Code(s): _____

9. Ms. Henderson, age 30, is an established patient who sees Dr. Hoffman for pain and swelling of her right ankle. He diagnoses her with ankle sprain, advises her to use crutches and an ankle splint, take an over-the-counter (OTC) pain medication, and elevate her ankle with an ice pack.

    Code(s): _____

10. Mr. Hughes, a 48-year-old patient, is admitted to the hospital's observation unit for shortness of breath and excessive sweating. Dr. Sullivan orders tests to rule out an MI.

    Code(s): _____

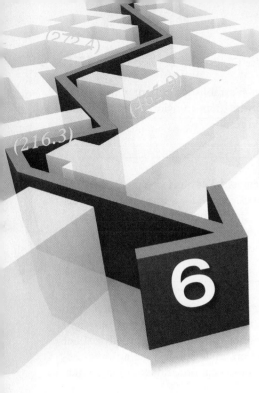

Introduction to ICD-10-CM Coding

Learning Objectives

After completing this chapter, you should be able to

- Spell and define the key terminology in this chapter.
- Describe the purpose of the change to ICD-10-CM.
- Identify the reason to accept the change to ICD-10-CM.
- Identify the elements in ICD-10-CM that are the same as in ICD-9-CM and the elements that are different.
- Describe ICD-10-CM changes that apply to coding all diagnoses.
- Describe your role in the transition to ICD-10-CM.
- Define General Equivalence Mappings (GEMs).

Key Terms

Code also note
crosswalk
default code
Excludes1 note

Excludes2 note
General Equivalence Mappings (GEMs)
placeholder "x"
seventh character
use of codes for reporting purposes

INTRODUCTION

Now that you have learned ICD-9-CM coding conventions and coding guidelines and have coded many types of diagnoses, it is time to embark on a new road along your coding journey. It involves applying what you have already learned about the ICD-9-CM code set to a brand new code set, ICD-10-CM, which will eventually replace ICD-9-CM. Along this road, we will make several stops to investigate different destinations, learning more about ICD-10-CM and the differences between ICD-9-CM and ICD-10-CM.

It may surprise you to learn that there are many similarities between ICD-9-CM and ICD-10-CM. You will take small steps as we cover new information to give you time to grasp the changes and then practice coding with ICD-10-CM codes. You can also apply your knowledge of ICD-10-CM in Chapters 7–14 because you will have the opportunity to code diagnoses using both the ICD-9-CM and ICD-10-CM code sets.

You will make two new stops in this chapter and in subsequent chapters called Pointers from the Pros, which are interviews with healthcare professionals who provide you with real-world advice as you embark on your healthcare career. You also will complete an

ICD-9-CM codes in this chapter are from the ICD-9-CM 2012 code set from the Department of Health and Human Services, Centers for Disease Control and Prevention.

ICD-10-CM codes in this chapter are from ICD-10-CM 2012 Draft code set from the Department of Health and Human Services, Centers for Disease Control and Prevention.

activity called Workplace IQ, real-world scenarios to help you learn how to handle workplace situations. Let's begin learning about ICD-10-CM.

"Change is the law of life. And those who look only to the past or present are certain to miss the future."—JOHN F. KENNEDY

THE CHANGE TO ICD-10-CM

The WHO updated ICD-9 codes several years ago with the International Classification of Diseases, Tenth Revision (ICD-10), because they needed to create more classifications that better described and tracked diseases and conditions. Currently, 138 countries use ICD-10 to classify mortality, and 99 countries use ICD-10 to classify morbidity. Some countries developed their own version of diagnosis coding that is based on the ICD-10 system, such as Germany creating the ICD-10-GM (German Modification). The CMS and the NCHS updated ICD-9-CM codes with ICD-10-CM, structuring them from WHO's ICD-10 system. CMS and NCHS also will oversee all changes and modifications to the ICD-10-CM code set.

ICD-10-CM, or I-10, codes are more specific than ICD-9-CM codes and allow for detailed classifications of patients' conditions, injuries, and diseases. ICD-9-CM has approximately 13,000 diagnosis codes, while ICD-10-CM has approximately 120,000. The U.S. is the only country that will implement ICD-10-CM codes. The change means that outpatient providers have to use the new code set for outpatient services (ICD-10-CM). Remember that inpatient providers will implement the ICD-10-PCS code set. ICD-10-CM diagnosis codes were created in 2007 and consist of three to seven alphanumeric characters. Although there have been many changes to ICD-10-CM codes since they were first developed, there is not a set schedule yet for regular additions, deletions, and revisions because the codes have not yet been implemented.

The DHHS requires all outpatient and inpatient providers, insurances, claims clearinghouses, and billing and collection agencies to ensure that they are prepared for the new ICD-10-CM code set implementation. At press time, DHHS and CMS announced its to delay the ICD-10-CM implementation date. Please refer to www.CMS.gov/ICD10 for current requirements.

The CDC is part of DHHS, and you can find more information about ICD-10-CM on the CDC's website at www.cdc.gov. You can also find the ICD-10-CM manual on the site for free, if you do not have access to an ICD-10-CM manual to reference.

New Codes Provide Greater Specificity

When you think of the changeover from ICD-9-CM to ICD-10-CM code sets, remember that ICD-9-CM codes were created in 1979, over 30 years ago. Many ICD-9-CM codes are outdated, and the code set did not allow enough room to expand and include many different types of conditions. ICD-10-CM codes capture countless diagnoses that either did not exist in 1979 or did not have codes representing them. ICD-10-CM codes also provide more details about a patient's encounter, such as whether the provider sees the patient for the first time or for a follow-up visit, the type of blood a patient has, or the nature of a patient's injury.

Just think of the ICD-10-CM code set as a larger dictionary to search for codes with greater specificity. It does not mean that you have to memorize every code (you couldn't!); it just means that you will be able to obtain a better, more specific definition for a patient's condition or reason for encounter.

Because the new code set has greater specificity, providers and payers can use ICD-10-CM codes to track many types of information about patients' conditions and the types and number of treatments that patients receive. They can gather coding information using computer system reports and analyze the information to

- Measure the quality, safety, and effectiveness of patient care, and report this information to patients.

epidemic (ĕp i-dĕm′ ik)—widespread occurrence within a population, community, or region, of an infectious disease, spread by a pathological organism that is transmitted through humans, animals, or insects

pandemic (pan-dem′-ik)—disease occurring over a wide geographic area and affecting a large population

- Conduct medical research and *clinical trials* (treatment provided to a group of patients to test if a medication, procedure, or medical device is safe and effective).
- Determine the health status of specific populations, understand their risk factors for developing certain conditions, and study conditions to determine whether they reach an **epidemic** level or **pandemic** level.
- Improve and monitor providers' performance treating patients, and review the costs of providing care to specific populations.
- Investigate and prevent healthcare coding and billing fraud and abuse, and study healthcare policies for treating patients.

Accepting the Change to ICD-10-CM

It is sometimes difficult to accept change because it can often be uncomfortable and intimidating. However, many changes mean improved processes and easier methods, so even though it may be awkward and time consuming to learn new things, investing the time and effort to learn pays off in the long run by ultimately saving time. Changing from ICD-9-CM to ICD-10-CM will improve many different areas of healthcare. The ICD-10-CM code set has many changes that can sometimes be difficult to learn. One important point to remember is that when you work in healthcare, there is *constant change* because healthcare regulations and rules constantly change. Many people are afraid to learn the ICD-10-CM code set and are intimidated by it; in fact, some are transitioning out of the coding profession in order to avoid learning ICD-10-CM! But it is necessary to learn the new code set in order to code successfully. Remaining in 1979 when ICD-9-CM was created and holding onto the old ways of doing things results in having a lot of outdated information and being unable to track patient care appropriately.

Why Learn Both ICD-9-CM and ICD-10-CM?

Are you wondering why you have to know ICD-9-CM coding in the first place when ICD-10-CM is just going to replace it anyway? ICD-10-CM codes will not be effective for at least two years, so providers, insurances, and claims clearinghouses will still have to use the ICD-9-CM codes until then. Even after ICD-10-CM codes become effective, providers and claims clearinghouses may still have outstanding claims with service dates *before* ICD-10-CM's implementation date, including claims that need to be billed, rebilled, or appealed. There will be a transition time when providers and claims clearinghouses will use both code sets to bill insurances, and insurances will use both code sets to process claims. The fact that you will know how to assign codes from both code sets will make you more marketable to potential employers.

COMPARISON OF ICD-9-CM AND ICD-10-CM

You will have a much better understanding of ICD-10-CM codes once you learn the similarities and differences between ICD-9-CM and ICD-10-CM. Let's review more about the code structures, Tabular List, and coding conventions.

Code Structures

■ TABLE 6-1 compares ICD-9-CM with ICD-10-CM code structures. You already know that ICD-9-CM diagnosis codes, also called I-9 codes, are three to five characters long. The first character can be a number or letter, and the remaining characters are numbers.

The first character of an ICD-10-CM code is a letter, the second and third characters are numbers, and the fourth to seventh characters can be letters or numbers. Here are some examples of ICD-10-CM codes and conditions they represent:

- J44.9—Bronchitis with airway obstruction
- L89.201—Pressure ulcer of hip, stage I
- O09.01—Supervision of pregnancy with history of infertility, first trimester

Refer to Table 6-1 to compare structures of the two code sets.

■ TABLE 6-1 **CODE STRUCTURES IN ICD-9-CM AND ICD-10-CM**

Character Detail	ICD-9-CM Example: 790.21	ICD-10-CM Example: L89.201
Character 1	Numeric or Alpha (V or E)	Alpha (Capital letter A–Z, except U, which is not used)
Character 2	Numeric	Numeric
Character 3	Numeric	Numeric
Character 4	Numeric	Numeric or Alpha
Character 5	Numeric	Numeric or Alpha
Character 6	N/A	Numeric or Alpha
Character 7	N/A	Numeric or Alpha
		Character 7 is only used in specific chapters related to pregnancy, musculoskeletal, injuries, and external causes of morbidity.
Minimum number of characters	3	3
Maximum number of characters	5	7
Decimal placement after characters	Use decimal after first three characters	Use decimal after first three characters
Alpha characters	Alpha characters (V or E) are reported as capital letters.	Alpha characters can be reported as capital or lowercase letters.
Placeholder character	N/A	ICD-10-CM uses an "x" to hold the place of missing characters when it is necessary to assign a 7th character.

Tabular List

The ICD-10-CM code set created thousands of new codes, and the expansion of the code set also required creating additional chapters. While ICD-9-CM has 17 chapters and two supplementary classifications (V codes and E codes), ICD-10-CM has 21 chapters without supplementary classifications. Refer to ■ TABLE 6-2 to review chapter numbers, titles, and category ranges for each code set.

■ TABLE 6-2 **COMPARISON OF TABULAR LIST CHAPTERS BETWEEN ICD-9-CM AND ICD-10-CM**

ICD-9-CM Chapter Number	Chapter Title	Category Range	ICD-10-CM Chapter Number	Chapter Title	Category Range
1	Infectious and Parasitic Diseases	001–139	1	Certain Infectious and Parasitic Diseases	A00–B99
2	Neoplasms	140–239	2	Neoplasms	C00–D49
3	Endocrine, Nutritional, and Metabolic Diseases and Immunity Disorders	240–279	3	Disease of the Blood and Blood-forming Organs and Certain Disorders Involving the Immune Mechanism	D50–D89
4	Diseases of the Blood and Blood-Forming Organs	280–289	4	Endocrine, Nutritional, and Metabolic Diseases	E00–E89
5	Mental Disorders	290–319	5	Mental and Behavioral Disorders	F01–F99
6	Diseases of the Nervous System and Sense Organs	320–389	6	Diseases of the Nervous System	G00–G99
7	Diseases of the Circulatory System	390–459	7	Diseases of the Eye and Adnexa	H00–H59
8	Diseases of the Respiratory System	460–519	8	Diseases of the Ear and Mastoid Process	H60–H95

continued

■ TABLE 6-2 *continued*

ICD-9-CM			ICD-10-CM		
Chapter Number	Chapter Title	Category Range	Chapter Number	Chapter Title	Category Range
9	Diseases of the Digestive System	520–579	9	Diseases of the Circulatory System	I00–I99
10	Diseases of the Genitourinary System	580–629	10	Diseases of the Respiratory System	J00–J99
11	Complications of Pregnancy, Childbirth, and the Puerperium	630–679	11	Diseases of the Digestive System	K00–K94
12	Diseases of the Skin and Subcutaneous Tissue	680–709	12	Diseases of the Skin and Subcutaneous Tissue	L00–L99
13	Diseases of the Musculoskeletal System and Connective Tissue	710–739	13	Diseases of the Musculoskeletal System and Connective Tissue	M00–M99
14	Congenital Anomalies	740–759	14	Diseases of the Genitourinary System	N00–N99
15	Certain Conditions Originating in the Perinatal Period	760–779	15	Pregnancy, Childbirth, and the Puerperium	O00–O9A
16	Symptoms, Signs, and Ill-Defined Conditions	780–799	16	Certain Conditions Originating in the Perinatal Period	P00–P96
17	Injury and Poisoning	800–999	17	Congenital Malformations, Deformations, and Chromosomal Abnormalities	Q00–Q99
Supplementary Classification	V codes—Supplementary Classification of Factors Influencing Health Status and Contact with Health Services	V01–V91	18	Symptoms, Signs, and Abnormal Clinical and Laboratory Findings, Not Elsewhere Classified	R00–R99
Supplementary Classification	E codes—Supplementary Classification of External Causes of Injury and Poisoning	E000–E999.1	19	Injury, Poisoning, and Certain Other Consequences of External Causes	S00–T88
			20	External Causes of Morbidity	V01–Y99
			21	Factors Influencing Health Status and Contact with Health Services	Z00–Z99

adnexa (ad-nek′-sə)—joined, or associated anatomic parts

mastoid process (măs′ toyd prō′ ses)—bone behind the ear that is well developed in adults but inconspicuous in children

Notice that ICD-9-CM's Chapter 6 Diseases of the Nervous System and Sense Organs (eye and ear) was separated into three chapters in ICD-10-CM: Chapter 6, Diseases of the Nervous System; Chapter 7, Diseases of the Eye and **Adnexa**; and Chapter 8, Diseases of the Ear and **Mastoid Process**. Two additional chapters include Chapter 20, External Causes of Morbidity, which replaces the supplementary classification of E codes in ICD-9-CM, and Chapter 21, Factors Influencing Health Status and Contact with Health Services, which replaces the supplementary classification of V codes in ICD-9-CM.

Coding Conventions

You learned in Chapter 4 the coding conventions that are part of ICD-9-CM's Official Guidelines. You will be glad to know that many of the coding conventions remain unchanged in ICD-10-CM, so you can still apply the same conventions when assigning ICD-10-CM codes.

The coding conventions that are *new* are as follows:

- Use of codes for reporting purposes
- Placeholder "x"
- Use of seventh character
- Excludes Notes-two types
- Code also note
- Default codes
- Syndromes

We will review more about these changes when we discuss major differences between both code sets, covered in the next section. Refer to ■ TABLE 6-3 to review coding conventions that remain the same in ICD-10-CM. Refer to Appendix A of this text for directions on locating the coding conventions in ICD-10-CM Official Guidelines for Coding and Reporting. We will not review details on each coding convention again because you already learned them in Chapter 4.

■ **TABLE 6-3 CODING CONVENTIONS THAT REMAIN THE SAME IN ICD-10-CM**

1. Format

The code set uses an indented format for ease in reference. The Alphabetic Index contains main terms and subterms in alphabetical order. Cross-reference codes in the Index to the Tabular List.

2. Abbreviations

a. Alphabetic Index abbreviations

NEC—Not elsewhere classifiable	Medical documentation specifies the diagnosis, but there is no specific code in the code set.

b. Tabular List abbreviations

NEC—Not elsewhere classifiable	Medical documentation specifies the diagnosis, but there is no specific code in the code set.
NOS—Not Otherwise specified	Medical documentation is insufficient to allow a more accurate code assignment.

3. Punctuation—Alphabetic Index or Tabular List

Brackets [ ]	Used in Tabular List to enclose synonyms, alternative wording, or explanatory phrases.
	Used in the Index to identify manifestation codes that you should sequence second.
Parentheses ( )	Used in the Tabular List and the Index to enclose words or terms that may or may not be present in the diagnostic statement (called nonessential modifiers).
Colon :	Used in the Tabular List after an incomplete term to list more information after the colon.

4. Includes notes, Inclusion Terms, and Note—Tabular List

Includes	Appears after a three-digit code title to further define a category.
Inclusion Terms	Lists terms that are included under certain codes to show conditions that are included with a specific code.
Note	Gives additional information about conditions and how to code them.

5. Other and unspecified codes—Tabular List

a. "Other" or "Other specified" codes

- Medical documentation specifies the diagnosis, but there is no specific code in the code set.
- In ICD-9-CM, codes with "other" or "other specified" in their titles usually have a fourth digit of 8 and a fifth digit of 9.

b. "Unspecified" codes

- Medical documentation is insufficient to allow a more accurate code assignment.
- In ICD-9-CM, codes with "unspecified" in the title usually have a fourth digit of 9 and a fifth digit of 0.

continued

■ **TABLE 6-3** *continued*

6. Etiology/manifestation convention—Tabular List

"Code first," "Use additional code," and "In diseases classified elsewhere" notes

- Certain conditions have both an etiology (cause) and multiple body system manifestations (conditions that are due to the underlying etiology).
- Assign two codes: the first code is the etiology, the second is the manifestation.
- Assign one code for both the etiology and manifestation, if applicable.

7. "And"—Tabular List

When the word "and" appears in a code title, it can mean "and," but it can also mean "or."

8. "With"—Alphabetic Index

- In the Index, refer to the word "with" immediately following a main term.
- "With" is not a subterm and is not listed in alphabetical order with other subterms.

9. "See," "See also," "See category"—Alphabetic Index or Tabular List

- The word "see" in the Tabular List or after a main term/subterm in the Index means to look elsewhere.
- The phrase "see also" after a main term/subterm in the Index means to also reference another main term/subterm.
- The phrase "see category" appears in the Tabular List or after a main term in the Index. It means to look for information under a specific category in the Tabular List.

TAKE A BREAK

Let's take a break and then review similarities and differences between code structures, Tabular List, and coding conventions in ICD-9-CM and ICD-10-CM.

Exercise 6.1 **The Change to ICD-10-CM, Comparison of ICD-9-CM to ICD-10-CM**

Instructions: Refer to Tables 6-1, 6-2, and 6-3 to answer the following questions, writing your answers in the spaces provided.

1. ICD-9-CM codes have a minimum of _____ characters and a maximum of _____ characters. ICD-10-CM codes have a minimum of _____ characters and a maximum of _____ characters.

2. Which character in ICD-10-CM is only used in specific chapters? _____

3. ICD-10-CM added _____ chapters and eliminated two _____ classifications.

4. ICD-10-CM uses a(n) _____ to hold the place of missing characters when you need to assign a seventh character, and it is called a(n) _____ .

5. In ICD-10-CM, the letters _____ and _____ are used to begin codes in more than one chapter.

6. The Tabular List abbreviations _____ and _____ remain the same in ICD-10-CM.

7. In ICD-10-CM, Diseases of the Genitourinary System are located in chapter _____ and cover codes _____ to _____ .

8. The notes "Code first," "Use additional code," and "In diseases classified elsewhere" are used in the _____ / _____ convention.

9. In ICD-9-CM, "unspecified" codes are used when _____ is insufficient to allow a more accurate code assignment, and they usually have a fourth digit of _____ and a fifth digit of _____ .

Code Set Similarities

Although there are major differences between the code sets, which you will soon review, there are many similarities between ICD-9-CM and ICD-10-CM Alphabetic Index, Tabular List, Official Guidelines for Coding and Reporting, and requirements related to the HIPAA. After reviewing the similarities in ■ TABLE 6-4, you may feel more comfortable learning the new ICD-10-CM code set.

■ **TABLE 6-4   SIMILARITIES BETWEEN ICD-9-CM AND ICD-10-CM CODE SETS**

ALPHABETIC INDEX SIMILARITIES	

Index Structure	The Alphabetic Index of ICD-10-CM has the same structure as ICD-9-CM. It contains
	• An Alphabetic Index of Diseases and Injuries
	• Two tables listed at the end of the Index of Diseases and Injuries:
	  - Table of Neoplasms
	  - Table of Drugs and Chemicals
	  ★ *The Hypertension Table does not exist in ICD-10-CM.*
	• An Alphabetic Index of External Causes
	Follow the same steps for locating codes in the Index for ICD-10-CM as you would for ICD-9-CM.

Main Terms and Subterms (essential modifiers)	The Alphabetic Index in both code sets lists main terms in bold and in alphabetical order; subterms are listed alphabetically and indented underneath main terms.
Carryover Lines	Carryover lines appear in the Alphabetic Index of both ICD-9-CM and ICD-10-CM.
Nonessential Modifiers	In both the ICD-9-CM and ICD-10-CM Alphabetic Index, nonessential modifiers are listed in parentheses after main terms.

TABULAR LIST SIMILARITIES	
Chapter Structure	Chapters in the Tabular List of both code sets have similar structures, with minor exceptions. The Tabular List is divided into chapters based on body system, condition, etiology, signs and symptoms, injuries and poisonings, factors influencing health status, and external causes of morbidity.
Code Order	Codes in the Tabular List of ICD-9-CM and ICD-10-CM are listed in numeric order or alphanumeric order.
Codes in Bold	Codes in the Tabular List of ICD-9-CM and ICD-10-CM are listed in bold.
Specificity in Coding	When using the ICD-9-CM or ICD-10-CM Tabular List, coders must assign codes to the highest level of specificity.
Notes	Notes in the ICD-9-CM and ICD-10-CM Tabular List appear at the beginning of chapters or at the beginning of subdivisions within the chapters.

OFFICIAL GUIDELINES FOR CODING AND REPORTING SIMILARITIES	
Official Guidelines for Coding and Reporting	Coders must follow the Official Guidelines for Coding and Reporting for ICD-10-CM codes, and follow coding conventions and the General Coding Guidelines, just as they followed the Official Guidelines for ICD-9-CM. Guidelines are still separated into four sections. The General Coding Guidelines in ICD-10-CM are similar to the Guidelines in ICD-9-CM. Many coding conventions in ICD-10-CM still have the same meaning as conventions in ICD-9-CM, such as abbreviations, punctuation, symbols, and notes. Refer to Table 6-3 to review coding conventions that are the same in ICD-9-CM and ICD-10-CM.

SIMILARITIES IN HIPAA REQUIREMENTS	
HIPAA Requirements	HIPAA requires providers to follow the Official Guidelines for each code set.

WORKPLACE IQ

You have worked for six months as a medical assistant for Dr. Gupta, a family care physician. You work with Rhonda, a coding specialist, and both of you review codes on encounter forms to ensure that they match medical record documentation. Today, you and Rhonda discuss the change from ICD-9-CM to ICD-10-CM. Rhonda tells you that she is not worried about learning ICD-10-CM code set because the implementation date will change again. She tells you, "The implementation date changed so many times that I couldn't even keep track of it. I'm not in a hurry to learn ICD-10-CM because I'm sure that the date will change again. Besides that, insurance companies have software to change the old codes to the new ones, and they'll take care of processing our claims. Maybe I'll learn ICD-10-CM codes eventually."

What would you do?

bilateral (bī-lăt′ ĕr-ăl)—both the right and left sides of the body, or the right and left members of paired organs

pathophysiology (path-oh -fiz-ē- ăl′-ə-jē)—changes in body functions that accompany a syndrome or disease

puerperium (pyūr-pir′-ē-əm)—period between childbirth and the return of the uterus to its normal size, about six weeks

sequela (si-kwe′-lə)—abnormal condition resulting from a previous disease

congenital (kän-jen′-ə-tel)—existing at or dating from birth

acquired (ă-kwīrd′)—developed after birth

do not resuscitate (DNR) (ri-suhs′-i-teyt)—a direction from a patient or family to medical staff not to employ life-saving measures

Code Set Differences

There are almost 60,000 more ICD-10-CM codes than ICD-9-CM codes, which means that many of the new codes represent diseases and conditions that did not exist in ICD-9-CM. The codes are also more detailed, allowing you to assign a higher level of specificity than what was previously possible. The greater detail represents more information about a patient's condition, including when the physician treated the patient, such as for an *initial encounter* (first visit/treatment) or *subsequent encounter* (any visit/treatment after the first encounter). Detailed codes in ICD-10-CM also provide the stage of a pregnancy, such as the first, second, or third *trimester* (a period of three months).

It is important to understand that because ICD-10-CM codes are much more specific than ICD-9-CM codes, you will be required to be well versed in human anatomy, physiology, pharmacology, disease processes, diagnostic methods, and treatment. Without having advanced knowledge of these areas, you will not be able to assign codes accurately. This does not mean that you did not have to know the same information when you were assigning ICD-9-CM codes. It means that you will have to know *more than ever* before to interpret medical documentation, locate errors to query the physician or other clinician, and assign the correct codes.

Be sure to keep your reference materials handy when you are working through the coding exercises in this chapter and subsequent chapters because you will need to refer to them often. References can include a medical dictionary and textbooks on anatomy, physiology, pharmacology, and disease processes, diagnoses, and treatment. Remember that you can also find additional information through website searches, but be sure that you only rely on reputable websites, such as websites from national organizations and companies, rather than blogs or personal accounts from individuals.

■ TABLE 6-5 is an overview of the differences between ICD-9-CM and ICD-10-CM to help you better understand the overall picture of where and/or why changes occurred. You will then review some of the differences in more detail later in this chapter. Refer to Table 6-5 as you work through the coding examples and exercises. Table 6-5 is also located in Appendix B of this text and will help you review how individual changes apply to specific chapters in the Tabular. Note that the 2010 draft version of ICD-10-CM codes is used in this book; however, ICD-10-CM codes will most likely be updated again before they are implemented. ICD-10-CM was designed to leave additional room to expand and add even more codes.

■ TABLE 6-5 OVERVIEW OF DIFFERENCES BETWEEN ICD-9-CM AND ICD-10-CM

TABULAR LIST CHANGES	ICD-9-CM	ICD-10-CM
Total Number of Codes	Approximately 14,000	Approximately 70,000
Total Number of Tabular Chapters	17, plus two supplementary classifications (V codes and E codes)	21, with no supplementary classifications Four new chapters were created: • Diseases of the Eye and Adnexa • Diseases of the Ear and Mastoid Process • External Causes of Morbidity • Factors Influencing Health Status and Contact with Health Services
	Chapters are divided into: Sections, groups of categories (3 characters).	*Chapters are divided into:* *Subchapters*, also called *blocks*. Subchapters are divided into groups of categories (3 characters).
	Each chapter *does not* provide a summary of sections within the chapter.	Each chapter begins with a summary of blocks within the chapter.
	Sections are divided into: Categories (3 characters).	*Subchapters are divided into:* Categories (3 characters).

■ **TABLE 6-5** *continued*

TABULAR LIST CHANGES	ICD-9-CM	ICD-10-CM
		If a category has no further subdivision, it is called a **code**.
	A category can represent one disease or a group of related diseases or conditions.	A category can represent one disease or a group of related diseases or conditions.
	Category codes (3 characters) are valid codes if they are not further subdivided into 4- or 5-character codes.	Category codes (3 characters) are valid as codes if they are not further subdivided into 4-, 5-, or 6-character codes. If they are further subdivided, then you must code them to the highest level of specificity.
	Categories are divided into:	*Categories are divided into:*
	Subcategories (4 characters)	Subcategories (4, 5, or 6 characters)
		Each level of a subdivision after a category is called a subcategory.
	Subcategories are divided into:	*Subcategories are divided into:*
	Subclassifications (5 characters).	Codes (4, 5, 6, or 7 characters)
		Codes are the *final level* that cannot be further subdivided. Remember that a code can also be 3 characters.
		Codes that are 7 characters are always called codes because 7 is the maximum number of characters in any code.
Code Ranges	001.0–999.9 (Tabular chapters)	A00.0–Z99.89 (Tabular chapters)
	V01.0–V91.99	Supplementary classifications were removed.
	(V code supplementary classification)	
	E000.0–E999.1	
	(E code supplementary classification)	
Code Titles	Code titles can be incomplete.	Code titles are more complete.
	The coder needs to add information from a category title when reading a subcategory or subclassification title.	In many cases, the coder does not need to add information from a category title when reading a subcategory or code title.

CODE STRUCTURE CHANGES	ICD-9-CM	ICD-10-CM
Code Length	Up to 5 alphanumeric characters.	Up to 7 alphanumeric characters.
Use of Letters in Codes	The first character of an ICD-9-CM code is a number or the letter V or E.	The first character of an ICD-10-CM code is always a capital letter and can be any letter except U. The letter U is reserved for additional code expansion and does not currently exist in the ICD-10-CM code set.
		The first character applies to a specific chapter because all codes in the chapter will start with the same letter. However, letters D and H are each used in two chapters.
	The second, third, fourth, and fifth characters are numbers. There is no sixth or seventh character.	The second and third characters are numbers. The fourth, fifth, sixth, and seventh characters can be numbers or any letter except U.
Highest Level of Codes	The highest code level is 5 characters.	The highest code level is 7 characters.
Codes with Five or Six Characters	Many categories show a list of choices for the fifth digit that applies to subcategory codes.	The list of choices for the fifth digit has been eliminated. Codes with five and six characters have code titles that include information that applies to the fifth or sixth character. There is no longer any need to reference a category to find choices for the fifth character.

continued

■ TABLE 6-5 *continued*

CHANGES TO LEVEL OF CODE DETAIL	ICD-9-CM	ICD-10-CM
Laterality	Not used	Laterality has been added to codes to identify whether the patient's condition affects the left or right side, if it is **bilateral**, or if the side is unspecified.
Advances in Medicine	Codes reflect limited advances in medicine.	Codes reflect numerous advances in medicine and include conditions that were not previously identified. Codes are more specific regarding anatomy, physiology, **pathophysiology**, treatments, and updated medical terminology.
Additional Detail	Codes are limited to the amount of detail they provide.	Codes were expanded to further define many disorders and provide more detail about the following conditions: diabetes, postoperative complications, injuries, substance abuse, alcohol abuse, ambulatory and managed care encounters.
Patient Risk Factors	Limited codes exist for patient risk factors.	Specific codes identify patients' *risk factors*. Risk factors are problems that patients experience which could lead to health issues. Examples include tobacco use, lack of exercise, inappropriate diet and eating habits, gambling, and high-risk sexual behavior. All of these risk factors could cause health problems if the patient does not change his behavior and lifestyle.
Codes for Pregnancy, Childbirth, and the Puerperium	Codes include a fifth digit to identify the patient's **episode of care**, the time period when the physician or other clinician treats the patient for a specific condition. Episodes of care include treating the patient's condition before, during, or after delivery. Codes do not identify if a pregnancy condition is present in a specific trimester.	Fifth digits identifying the patient's episode of care were eliminated. Instead, individual code titles identify this information. Codes identify whether a pregnancy condition is present in the first, second, or third trimester.

CHANGES TO CODING CONVENTIONS	ICD-9-CM	ICD-10-CM
Use of Codes for Reporting Purposes	This rule does not exist in ICD-9-CM coding conventions. However, it means to report codes to their highest level of specificity, including categories, subcategories, and subclassifications, which has always been a rule for ICD-9-CM coding.	The coding rule "**Use of codes for reporting purposes**" was added to ICD-10-CM coding conventions. It means to always code to the highest level of specificity when reporting codes to insurances, claims clearinghouses, billing and collection agencies, or any other organizations. In ICD-10-CM, a code that cannot be further subdivided is called a "code." Always report codes, rather than categories or subcategories that can be further subdivided. Also be sure to report applicable seventh characters.
Use Placeholder "x" to fill in a Missing Character	Not used.	Some codes require a seventh character but do not have an applicable fourth, fifth, or sixth character. You are still required to assign the seventh character, even though the characters before the seventh may be missing. For example, some codes are five characters long, don't have an applicable sixth character, but require a seventh character to identify encounter information. It is mandatory to fill in the space of the missing sixth character with a **placeholder "x"** so that the seventh character is in the correct place. The code is invalid if you do not add the "x" to hold the place of the sixth character before adding the seventh. ICD-10-CM placeholder "x" was created to allow additional code expansion in case the placeholder "x" is someday replaced by an actual character with a specific meaning.

■ TABLE 6-5   *continued*

CHANGES TO CODING CONVENTIONS	ICD-9-CM	ICD-10-CM
The Seventh Character Provides Episode of Care and Additional Information	Not used.	The **seventh character** provides more information about a patient's encounter, including the patient's episode of care, the time period when the physician or other clinician treats the patient. Examples of a seventh character for injuries and external causes of injuries are • A—Initial encounter • D—Subsequent encounter • S—**Sequela** Seventh characters can also provide additional information about fractures and other types of encounters.
Not elsewhere classifiable (NEC) and not otherwise specified (NOS)	One code can represent both NEC and NOS.	NEC codes and NOS codes are listed separately. There are no codes that combine NEC and NOS. The meanings of NEC and NOS remain the same as in ICD-9-CM.
Brace }	Used in the Tabular in some coding manuals to connect words written to left of it to words written to the right.	Not used.
Excludes Notes in the Tabular List	There is one type of Excludes Notes which means that the terms listed as excluded should be coded elsewhere.	Excludes Notes were revised to include: • Excludes1 • Excludes2 There are two types of Excludes Notes. The **Excludes1 note** means "NOT CODED HERE!" An Excludes1 note appears under codes in the Tabular. It lists conditions and their corresponding codes that are excluded from the code that you cross-reference. It is similar to the Excludes note in ICD-9-CM. The Excludes1 note is a warning that two conditions cannot ever occur together. For example, if you cross-reference a **congenital** condition, an Excludes1 note would show the **acquired** form of the same condition. You could not code both conditions together. The **Excludes2 note** means "not included here." When you cross-reference a code to the Tabular, and it has an Excludes2 note, it means that the condition listed in the note is not typically part of the code that you cross-referenced. The Excludes2 note is a warning that two conditions are not likely to occur together, but they could. For example, a chronic condition typically is not also an acute condition, but it could be. When an Excludes2 note appears under a code, it is acceptable to assign both the code and the Excludes2 code together if the patient has both conditions.
Code Also Note	Not used.	A **"code also" note** is a new convention that you may need to assign two codes to fully describe a condition. The note does not provide you with the order in which to sequence the codes.
Default Codes	Codes are listed next to main terms in the Index, but they are not called default codes.	A **default code** is a new convention. It is the code listed next to a main term in the Index. The default code represents the condition that is most commonly associated with the main term, or it is the unspecified code for the condition. When a physician documents a condition in the medical record but does not provide enough specific information, assign the default code of "unspecified." Always query the physician about the documentation before assigning a code that is unspecified.

continued

■ **TABLE 6-5** *continued*

CHANGES TO CODING CONVENTIONS	ICD-9-CM	ICD-10-CM
Syndromes	Instructions for coding syndromes appear in the Official Guidelines under the General Coding Guidelines.	Instructions for coding syndromes have not changed but were moved from ICD-9-CM General Coding Guidelines to coding conventions in ICD-10-CM. When you search for a syndrome, look under the main term *syndrome* and look for the subterm that describes the type of syndrome. In the absence of Index guidance, assign codes for the documented *manifestations* of the syndrome.

CHANGES TO SUPPLEMENTARY CLASSIFICATIONS	ICD-9-CM	ICD-10-CM
V codes— Supplementary Classification of Factors Influencing Health Status and Contact with Health Service	V codes are included in their own Supplementary Classification, rather than within a chapter in the Tabular.	There is no separate Supplementary Classification of V codes. Any conditions previously represented by V codes are now included in Chapter 21—Factors Influencing Health Status and Contact with Health Services. Chapter 21 includes codes for many conditions that are not in ICD-9-CM. It includes codes for lifestyle problems, such as high-risk behaviors, lack of exercise, and inappropriate diet. Also included are codes for blood types and **do not resuscitate (DNR)** status.
E codes— Supplementary Classification of External Causes of Injury and Poisoning	E codes are included in their own Supplementary Classification, rather than within a chapter in the Tabular.	There is no separate Supplementary Classification of E codes. Any conditions previously represented by E codes are now included in Chapter 20—External Causes of Morbidity.

ADDITIONAL CHANGES	ICD-9-CM	ICD-10-CM
Multiple Codes and Combination Codes	Assign multiple codes for an etiology/manifestation relationship, external cause of poisoning and substance that caused the poisoning, symptoms and related conditions, and when the patient has more than one diagnosis that cannot be represented by a combination code.	In many cases, assign only one combination code that represents both the etiology and manifestation, both the external cause of poisoning and poison substance, and both symptoms and their related conditions. In other cases, there can be multiple ICD-10-CM codes that are represented by a single ICD-9-CM code.
Morphology Codes	Morphology codes, codes beginning with the letter M, are listed in the Index and cross-referenced to Appendix A— Morphology of Neoplasms.	Codes for morphology of neoplasms are listed in the Index and cross-referenced to the Tabular. They no longer appear in a separate Appendix.
Hypertension Table	Located in the Index. The Hypertension Table separates hypertension into malignant, benign, and unspecified.	The Hypertension Table has been removed. Under the main term *hypertension* in the Index, malignant and benign have been added as nonessential modifiers.
Appendices	There are four Appendices—A, C, D, and E.	Not used.
Hyphen (Dash)	Not used.	A hyphen (dash) can appear after a code in the Index or Tabular to show that you need to add more characters to the code to make it valid. Examples are as follows: I87.0— I83.— Both of these codes need an additional character in order to be considered valid codes.

TAKE A BREAK

Let's take a break and then review ICD-9-CM and ICD-10-CM code set similarities and differences.

Exercise 6.2   Code Set Similarities and Differences

Instructions: Refer to information covered under code set similarities and differences, as well as to Tables 6-4 and 6-5, to answer the following questions. Write your answers in the spaces provided.

1. In both the ICD-9-CM and ICD-10-CM Alphabetic Index, _____ _____ are listed in parentheses after main terms.

2. ICD-10-CM chapters are divided into _____, which are also called _____. These are further divided into _____, each of which consists of three characters. The next level of subdivision is called a _____, which has four, five, or six characters. _____ are the final level that cannot be further subdivided.

3. In ICD-10-CM, the list of choices for the _____ digit has been eliminated. Codes with five and six characters have _____ _____ that include information which applies to the fifth or sixth character. There is no longer any need to reference a _____ to find choices for the fifth character.

4. In ICD-10-CM, laterality has been added to codes to identify if the patient's condition affects the _____ or _____ side, if it is _____, or whether the side is _____.

5. Under Pregnancy, Childbirth, and the Puerperium, ICD-10-CM eliminated fifth digits identifying the patient's _____ of care. Codes identify whether a pregnancy condition is present in the first, second, or third _____.

6. When you cross-reference a code to the Tabular and it has a(n) _____ note, it means that the condition listed in the note should never be sequenced with the code that you cross-referenced. Do not report both codes.

7. When a(n) _____ note appears under a code, it is acceptable to assign both codes together if the patient has both conditions.

ICD-10-CM CHANGES THAT AFFECT ALL CONDITIONS

Now that we reviewed several tables that describe the changes in ICD-10-CM, we will specifically review 10 changes to teach you how to assign I-10 codes. In subsequent ICD-9-CM chapters in this book, you will have the chance to practice additional ICD-10-CM coding at the end of each chapter. You will also learn about specific ICD-10-CM coding guideline changes. As we review the 10 changes, it will be helpful to follow along in your own coding manual. Here are the changes:

1. Chapter structures in the Tabular List
2. Code titles
3. Code structure and use of letters
4. Codes with five and six characters
5. Laterality added to codes
6. Use of placeholder "x" and seventh character extension
7. Excludes1 and Excludes2 notes
8. Code also note
9. Multiple codes and combination codes
10. Hyphen, or dash

1. Chapter Structures in the Tabular List

You already know that there are 21 chapters in the Tabular List, including four new chapters that did not exist in ICD-9-CM, and that the supplementary classifications for V codes and E codes have been removed. Codes in the Tabular are arranged in alphabetical order from categories and codes A00–Z99. Each chapter is divided into subchapters, also called blocks, which represent groups of three-character categories. Each chapter begins with a summary of blocks contained in the chapter (■ FIGURE 6-1). Notice in Figure 6-1

Certain infectious and parasitic diseases (A00-B99)

Includes: diseases generally recognized as communicable or transmissible
Use additional code for any associated drug resistance (Z16)
Excludes1:   carrier or suspected carrier of infectious disease (Z22.-)
                 certain localized infections—see body system-related chapters
                 infectious and parasitic diseases complicating pregnancy, childbirth and the
                      puerperium (O98.-)
                 influenza and other acute respiratory infections (J00-J22)
Excludes2:   infectious and parasitic diseases specific to the perinatal period (P35-P39)

This chapter contains the following blocks:

A00-A09	Intestinal infectious diseases
A15-A19	Tuberculosis
A20-A28	Certain zoonotic bacterial diseases
A30-A49	Other bacterial diseases
A50-A64	Infections with a predominantly sexual mode of transmission
A65-A69	Other spirochetal diseases
A70-A74	Other diseases caused by chlamydiae
A75-A79	Rickettsioses
A80-A89	Viral infections of the central nervous system

that blocks are ranges of three-character categories that can represent one disease or a group of related diseases or conditions.

Each block within a chapter contains categories, and many categories are subdivided into subcategories. Category codes (three characters long) are valid to assign as codes if they are *not* further subdivided into subcategories of additional characters. When a category has subdivisions, you need to assign the subdivisions until you have coded to the highest level of specificity. Each level of a subdivision after a category is called a subcategory.

An interesting point about assigning I-10 codes is that a category is only referred to as a category when it *can* be subdivided into subcategories. If it cannot be subdivided into subcategories, it is called a *code* because you cannot code it any higher. The same is true for subcategories: When they have subdivisions, or additional subcategories, they are still called subcategories. If they do not have additional subdivisions, they are called codes because you cannot code them any higher.

A final code assignment is always called a code. Any category or subcategory that still has subdivisions can *never* be a code because it has not been coded to the highest level of specificity. In ■ FIGURE 6-2, notice that code A09 in the Tabular List is three characters long. It has no subcategories and cannot be coded any higher, so A09 is a code (not a category). It would only remain a category if it had additional subcategories.

Notice also in ■ FIGURE 6-3 that the four-character subcategory A01.0 is further subdivided into five-character codes, not additional subcategories. The five-character codes are called *codes* because they cannot be further subdivided and represent a final code assignment at the highest level of specificity. Category A01 is also further subdivided into four-character codes: A01.1, A01.2, A01.3, and A01.4. They are codes because they do not have subcategories and cannot be coded any higher.

In ICD-10-CM, codes can be three to seven characters long. In ICD-9-CM, codes can be three to five characters long. ICD-10-CM codes with seven characters are always called codes because seven is the maximum number of characters in any code and the

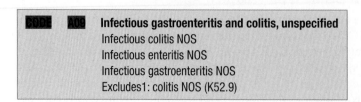

CODE   A09   **Infectious gastroenteritis and colitis, unspecified**
             Infectious colitis NOS
             Infectious enteritis NOS
             Infectious gastroenteritis NOS
             Excludes1: colitis NOS (K52.9)

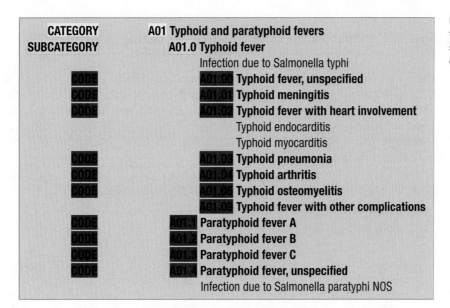

Figure 6-3 ■ Category A01 in the Tabular List is further subdivided, so it remains a category, not a code.

highest level of a code. The seventh character is called an extension; we will review examples of extensions later in this chapter.

2. Code Titles

Code titles for ICD-10-CM codes in the Tabular List are more complete than code titles in ICD-9-CM. Recall that when you read many of the subcategory titles in ICD-9-CM, you must also incorporate the code title of the category above it to obtain the complete meaning of the code. In addition, when you read many subclassification code titles, you must incorporate the code title of the subcategory and category to understand the meaning of the subclassification code. In comparison, ICD-10-CM code titles are complete. Review ■ FIGURE 6-4, which shows an example of an incomplete code title in ICD-9-CM. Then compare it with ■ FIGURE 6-5, which shows a complete code title in ICD-10-CM.

3. Code Structure and Use of Letters

While ICD-9-CM codes can be up to five characters long, ICD-10-CM codes can be up to seven characters, which allows for greater code specificity. The first character of an ICD-9-CM code can be a number or the letter V or E (supplementary classifications); characters two through five are numbers. ICD-10-CM codes begin with a capital letter (except U). Specific letters correspond to certain chapters, except for letters D and H, each of that is found in two chapters. The second and third characters of ICD-10-CM codes are numbers, while characters 4–7 can be a number or any letter except U. In the following examples, you will compare the same diagnosis in ICD-9-CM to ICD-10-CM to better understand the changes to the ICD-10-CM code structure and see how codes appear using both letters and numbers. You will notice that ICD-10-CM provides more code choices for conditions that were grouped under one code in ICD-9-CM. Let's get started by reviewing the first example!

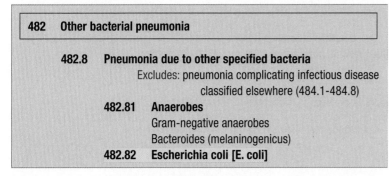

482	Other bacterial pneumonia

	482.8	Pneumonia due to other specified bacteria
		Excludes: pneumonia complicating infectious disease classified elsewhere (484.1-484.8)
	482.81	**Anaerobes**
		Gram-negative anaerobes
		Bacteroides (melaninogenicus)
	482.82	**Escherichia coli [E. coli]**

Figure 6-4 ■ Incomplete code title for 482.82 in ICD-9-CM.

J15	**Bacterial pneumonia, not elsewhere classified**

J15.5	**Pneumonia due to Escherichia coli**

Figure 6-5 ■ Complete code title for J15.5 in ICD-10-CM.

INTERESTING FACTS: What is *E. coli*, and how does it spread?

Escherichia coli (E. coli) are a large and diverse group of bacteria. Although most strains of *E. coli* are harmless, others can make you sick. Some kinds of *E. coli* cause diarrhea, urinary tract infections, respiratory illness, and pneumonia. You can become ill when you swallow *E. Coli* because when you get tiny (usually invisible) amounts of human or animal feces in your mouth, they will make you sick. Exposures that result in illness include eating contaminated food, drinking unpasteurized (raw) milk or contaminated water, swallowing lake water while swimming, touching animals in petting zoos, and eating food prepared by people who did not wash their hands well after using the toilet.

(Department of Health and Human Services, Centers for Disease Control and Prevention, www.cdc.gov/nczved/divisions/dfbmd/diseases/ecoli_o157h7/index.html, accessed 2/5/12)

Escherichia coli (E. coli)
(esh-ə-rik′ ē-ə kō′-lī)—
bacteria that form acid and gas on many carbohydrates, normally present in the human intestine

hydrocephalus (hī drō-sĕf′ ă -lŭs)—abnormal increase in the amount of cerebrospinal fluid within the cranial cavity

Example 1—Congenital hydrocephalus in ICD-9-CM and ICD-10-CM
Several conditions are listed in ICD-9-CM under the code title **congenital hydrocephalus**, meaning that one or more of them are included in code 742.3 (■ FIGURE 6-6). Now review ■ FIGURE 6-7, and notice how many of the conditions that were previously grouped together under one code for *congenital hydrocephalus* now have their own code in ICD-10-CM.

> **742.3   Congenital hydrocephalus**
>   Aqueduct of Sylvius:
>   anomaly
>   obstruction, congenital
>   stenosis
>   Atresia of foramina of Magendie and Luschka
>   Hydrocephalus in newborn
>
>   Excludes: hydrocephalus:
>   acquired (331.3-331.4)
>   due to congenital toxoplasmosis (771.2)
>   with any condition classifiable to 741.9 (741.0)

Figure 6-6 ■ Congenital hydrocephalus in the Tabular List in ICD-9-CM.

> **Q03   Congenital hydrocephalus**
>
>   Includes: hydrocephalus in newborn
>   Excludes1: Arnold-Chiari syndrome, type II (Q07.0-)
>   acquired hydrocephalus (G91.-)
>   hydrocephalus due to congenital toxoplasmosis (P37.1)
>   hydrocephalus with spina bifida (Q05.0-Q05.4)
>   **Q03.0 Malformations of aqueduct of Sylvius**
>   Anomaly of aqueduct of Sylvius
>   Obstruction of aqueduct of Sylvius, congenital
>   Stenosis of aqueduct of Sylvius
>   **Q03.1 Atresia of foramina of Magendie and Luschka**
>   Dandy-Walker syndrome
>   **Q03.8 Other congenital hydrocephalus**
>   **Q03.9 Congenital hydrocephalus, unspecified**

Figure 6-7 ■ Congenital hydrocephalus in the Tabular List in ICD-10-CM.

By providing a separate code for many of the conditions that previously were grouped together, ICD-10-CM gives a greater level of specificity to the conditions.

Example 2—Visual field defects in ICD-9-CM and ICD-10-CM Review
■ FIGURE 6-8 for the various types of **visual field defects** that are listed as subclassification codes under subcategory 368.4 in ICD-9-CM.

Now review ■ FIGURE 6-9, and notice how many more choices you have for coding various types of visual field defects using ICD-10-CM codes.

visual field defects (vĭzh′ ū-ăl)—inadequate vision

368.4	**Visual field defects**
368.40	**Visual field defect, unspecified**
368.41	**Scotoma involving central area** Scotoma: central centrocecal paracentral

Figure 6-8 ■ Visual field defects in the Tabular List in ICD-9-CM.

H53.4 Visual field defects
H53.40 Unspecified visual field defects
H53.41 Scotoma involving central area
Central scotoma
H53.411 Scotoma involving central area, right eye
H53.412 Scotoma involving central area, left eye
H53.413 Scotoma involving central area, bilateral
H53.419 Scotoma involving central area, unspecified eye

Figure 6-9 ■ Visual field defects in the Tabular List in ICD-10-CM.

Did you notice how much more specific ICD-10-CM codes are in their description of various visual field defects? ICD-10-CM codes specify whether the left or right eye has the condition, whether both eyes have it, or if the information is not specified.

4. Codes with Five and Six Characters

Because many codes in ICD-9-CM need a fifth digit, you have to go to the category and reference a list of common fifth digit choices. In ■ FIGURE 6-10, notice the fifth digit choices for categories 010–018. Codes 013.0 and 013.1 require you to choose a fifth digit.

In ICD-10-CM, codes with both five and six characters have code titles that include information that applies to the fifth or sixth character. Notice that the five-character codes in ■ FIGURE 6-11 have complete meanings, and you are not required to go to a category in order to find a list of choices for the fifth character. This makes coding more efficient.

5. Laterality Added to Codes

ICD-9-CM codes have no choices for *laterality*, the side of the body that the condition affects, such as right or left, or bilateral sides. In ICD-10-CM, there are code choices for left, right, and bilateral. For bilateral sites, the final character of the code indicates laterality. An unspecified side code is also provided if the physician does not identify the side in the medical record. If a condition is bilateral but there is no code for it, assign separate

Figure 6-10 ■ Fifth digit choices for codes 013.0 and 013.1 in ICD-9-CM.

TUBERCULOSIS (010-018)

Includes: infection by Mycobacterium tuberculosis (human) (bovine)
Excludes: congenital tuberculosis (771.2)
           late effects of tuberculosis (137.0-137.4)

The following fifth-digit subclassification is for use with categories 010-018:

0 unspecified
1 bacteriological or histological examination not done
2 bacteriological or histological examination unknown (at present)
3 tubercle bacilli found (in sputum) by microscopy
4 tubercle bacilli not found (in sputum) by microscopy, but found by bacterial culture
5 tubercle bacilli not found by bacteriological examination, but tuberculosis confirmed histologically
6 tubercle bacilli not found by bacteriological or histological examination, but tuberculosis confirmed by other methods [inoculation of animals]

013	Tuberculosis of meninges and central nervous system

Requires fifth digit. See beginning of section 010-018 for codes and definitions.

013.0 Tuberculous meningitis
[0-6]

    Tuberculosis of meninges (cerebral) (spinal)
Tuberculous:
  leptomeningitis
  meningoencephalitis
Excludes: tuberculoma of meninges (013.1)

013.1 Tuberculoma of meninges
[0-6]

Figure 6-11 ■ Fifth digit choices for codes 013.0 and 013.1 in ICD-10-CM.

A17 **Tuberculosis of nervous system**
    A17.0   **Tuberculous meningitis**
        Tuberculosis of meninges (cerebral)(spinal)
        Tuberculous leptomeningitis
        Excludes1: tuberculous meningoencephalitis (A17.82)
    A17.1   **Meningeal tuberculoma**
        Tuberculoma of meninges (cerebral) (spinal)
        Excludes2: tuberculoma of brain and spinal cord (A17.81)
    A17.8   **Other tuberculosis of nervous system**
        A17.81 Tuberculoma of brain and spinal cord
            Tuberculous abscess of brain and spinal cord
        A17.82 Tuberculous meningoencephalitis
            Tuberculous myelitis
        A17.83 Tuberculous neuritis
            Tuberculous mononeuropathy
        A17.89 Other tuberculosis of nervous system
            Tuberculous polyneuropathy
    A17.9   **Tuberculosis of nervous system, unspecified**

> **H93 Other disorders of ear, not elsewhere classified**
> **H93.0 Degenerative and vascular disorders of ear**
> Excludes1: presbycusis (H91.1)
> **H93.01 Transient ischemic deafness**
> **H93.011 Transient ischemic deafness, right ear**
> **H93.012 Transient ischemic deafness, left ear**
> **H93.013 Transient ischemic deafness, bilateral**
> **H93.019 Transient ischemic deafness, unspecified ear**
> **H93.09 Unspecified degenerative and vascular disorders of ear**
> **H93.091 Unspecified degenerative and vascular disorders of right ear**

Figure 6-12 ■ ICD-10-CM has code options for laterality.

codes for both the left and right side. Refer to ■ FIGURE 6-12 for examples of laterality in code descriptors. Specifying laterality helps to better establish medical necessity and increases the probability that the insurance will pay claims accurately.

TAKE A BREAK

Let's take a break and then review ICD-10-CM code changes.

Exercise 6.3 **ICD-10-CM Changes 1–5**

Instructions: Complete the following statements using the list of terms provided.

1. Each chapter in ICD-10-CM is divided into subchapters, also called _____.

2. _____ codes are valid to assign as codes if they are *not* further subdivided into subcategories of 4-, 5-, or 6-characters.

3. Any category or subcategory that still has _____ can never be a code because it has not been coded to the highest level of specificity.

4. The seventh character is called a(n) _____.

5. In ICD-10-CM, codes with both five and six characters have code _____ that include information that applies to the fifth or sixth character.

6. By providing a separate _____ for many of the conditions that were previously grouped together, ICD-10-CM gives a greater level of _____ to the conditions.

blocks
category
code(s)
condition(s)
diagnosis
extension(s)
laterality
letter(s)
number(s)
specificity
subchapter(s)
subdivision(s)
titles

6. Use of Placeholder "x" and Seventh Character Extension

ICD-9-CM has very limited code choices for providing information about a patient's encounter. The seventh character of an ICD-10-CM code provides additional information, such as whether an encounter is initial or subsequent. Seventh characters also provide information about fracture care, including the type of encounter for the fracture.

Some codes require a seventh character to show information about an encounter, but the codes do not have an applicable fourth, fifth, or sixth character. They have already been coded to their highest level of specificity, except for the seventh character. You are still required to assign the seventh character, even though characters before the seventh may be missing.

- The seventh character must be in the seventh position of the code, so you must place an "x" in place of the missing characters to ensure that the code is complete and has a total of seven characters.

Figure 6-13 ■ ICD-10-CM requires seventh characters for category T18.

> **T18 Foreign body in alimentary tract**
> Excludes2: foreign body in pharynx (T17.2-)
> The appropriate 7th character is to be added to each code from category T18
> > A initial encounter
> > D subsequent encounter
> > S sequela
>
> **T18.0 Foreign body in mouth**
> **T18.1 Foreign body in esophagus**
> Excludes2: foreign body in respiratory tract (T17.-)
> > **T18.10 Unspecified foreign body in esophagus**
> > **T18.100 Unspecified foreign body in esophagus causing compression of trachea**

- Add the placeholder "x" when a code contains fewer than six characters but requires a seventh character.
- The ICD-10-CM placeholder "x" was created to allow for additional code expansion in case the placeholder "x" is someday replaced by an actual character with a specific meaning.

Refer to ■ FIGURE 6-13 to review examples of codes that need the placeholder "x."

Notice in Figure 6-13 the instruction under category T18 that tells you to add a seventh character to all codes beginning with category T18. Seventh character choices are

- A—Initial encounter
- D—Subsequent encounter
- S—Sequela

Refer to Figure 6-13 to review the following example of a code from category T18 that uses the placeholder "x:"

> **Example:** A patient's diagnosis is *foreign body in mouth*, represented by subcategory T18.0. It is the patient's *initial* encounter. You must add letter A as the *seventh* character since it represents an initial encounter. The instruction under category T18 is to add a seventh character to any codes beginning with T18. But subcategory T18.0 is only *four* characters. What do you do?
>
> You need to add the placeholder "x" to code T18.0 *in the spaces where there are missing characters* until you reach the seventh character. The code to assign is T18.0xxA. Because there is no fifth or sixth character in T18.0, you have to place an "x" in the space of the missing fifth and sixth characters in order to extend the code to the seventh position. You can then add the seventh character. When ICD-10-CM requires seven characters, your final code assignment must be seven characters long.

closed—covered by unbroken skin

open—a fracture in which the patient's skin is broken

routine—customary or regular

delayed—impeded or slow progress

nonunion (non-yün′-yən)— failure of the fragments of a broken bone to heal together

Now that you reviewed how to add the placeholder "x," you will review more examples of seventh character extensions. As you saw in Figure 6-13, seventh character extension options include initial encounter, subsequent encounter, and sequela. There are also seventh character extensions that identify types of encounters to treat specific fractures (■ FIGURE 6-14).

Notice that for fractures classified under category S22, you need to add a seventh character to identify whether the encounter was initial or subsequent, as well as the type of fracture the physician treats, including (**closed, open, routine** healing, **delayed** healing, or **nonunion**). Refer to ■ FIGURE 6-15 for an example of seventh character extensions for single and multiple fetuses in pregnancy. Remember that when you have to add a seventh character, and you do not already have six characters, add the placeholder "x" where there are missing characters.

For some codes in ICD-10-CM, the placeholder "x" is already present in the fifth position (■ FIGURE 6-16).

S22 Fracture of rib(s), sternum and thoracic spine

> The appropriate 7th character is to be added to each code from category S22
> A fracture not identified as open or closed should be coded to closed
>> A initial encounter for closed fracture
>> B initial encounter for open fracture
>> D subsequent encounter for fracture with routine healing
>> G subsequent encounter for fracture with delayed healing
>> K subsequent encounter for fracture with nonunion
>> S sequela

S22.0 Fracture of thoracic vertebra

> **S22.00 Fracture of unspecified thoracic vertebra**
>> **S22.000 Wedge compression fracture of unspecified thoracic vertebra**
>> **S22.001 Stable burst fracture of unspecified thoracic vertebra**
>> **S22.002 Unstable burst fracture of unspecified thoracic vertebra**
>> **S22.008 Other fracture of unspecified thoracic vertebra**
>> **S22.009 Unspecified fracture of unspecified thoracic vertebra**

Figure 6-14 ■ ICD-10-CM requires seventh characters in order to describe encounters for fractures.

One of the following 7th characters is to be assigned to code O33.6. 7th character 0 is for single gestations and multiple gestations where the fetus is unspecified. 7th characters 1 through 9 are for cases of multiple gestations to identify the fetus for which the code applies. The appropriate code from category O30, Multiple gestation, must also be assigned when assigning code O33.6 with a 7th character of 1 through 9.

> 0 not applicable or unspecified
> 1 fetus 1
> 2 fetus 2
> 3 fetus 3
> 4 fetus 4
> 5 fetus 5
> 9 other fetus

O33.6 Maternal care for disproportion due to hydrocephalic fetus

Figure 6-15 ■ ICD-10-CM requires seventh characters for O33.6.

T36.6 Poisoning by, adverse effect of an underdosing of rifampicins

> **T36.6x Poisoning by, adverse effect of and underdosing of rifampicins**
>> **T36.6x1 Poisoning by rifampicins, accidental (unintentional)**
>> Poisoning by rifampicins NOS
>> **T36.6x2 Poisoning by rifampicins, intentional self-harm**

Figure 6-16 ■ Placeholder "x" in the fifth position of a code.

> **S61.0 Open wound of thumb without damage to nail**
>   Excludes1: open wound of thumb with damage to nail (S61.1-)

Figure 6-17 ■ Excludes1 note under a code in ICD-10-CM.

7. Excludes1 and Excludes2 Notes

Excludes notes in the Tabular List of ICD-9-CM indicate that the terms listed as excluded should be coded elsewhere. Excludes notes appear under a chapter, a section, or category, subcategory, or subclassification codes.

In ICD-10-CM, Excludes notes were eliminated and replaced by Excludes1 and Excludes2 notes, which can appear under a chapter, subchapter (block), category, subcategory, or code. The Excludes1 note means "NOT CODED HERE!" When you cross-reference a code to the Tabular and it has an Excludes1 note, it means that the condition listed in the note should never be sequenced with the code that you cross-referenced. In other words, do not report both codes together (■ FIGURE 6-17).

In Figure 6-17, code S61.0 is for an *open wound of thumb without damage to nail*. The Excludes1 note shows that you cannot report a code for an *open wound of thumb with damage to nail (S61.1-)* and report code S61.0. It does not make sense to assign both codes together because a patient could not have an open wound *without* nail damage and an open wound *with* nail damage. The Excludes1 note warns you of codes that you should not report with another code.

The Excludes2 note means "not included here." When you cross-reference a code to the Tabular and it has an Excludes2 note, it means that the condition listed in the note is not *typically* part of the code that you cross-referenced. The Excludes2 note is an alert that two conditions *most likely* will not occur together, but they could.

For example, a chronic condition can have an Excludes2 note listing the same condition, only in the acute form. A chronic condition typically is not also an acute condition, but it could be. When an Excludes2 note appears under a code, it is acceptable to assign both the code and the Excludes2 code together if the patient has both conditions (■ FIGURE 6-18).

Notice in Figure 6-18 that code C43.5 represents *malignant* **melanoma** *of trunk*. The Excludes2 note lists *malignant neoplasm of anus* and *malignant neoplasm of scrotum* as conditions *not typically* found with a malignant neoplasm of the trunk. However, a patient can have either or both of those conditions in the Excludes2 note, along with a malignant melanoma of the trunk. Therefore, although the Excludes2 note alerts you that a specific condition does not typically occur with another condition, they could occur together, and you could code both of them.

Review ■ FIGURE 6-19 for an example of a category with both Excludes1 and Excludes2 notes.

melanoma (mĕl ă-nō′ mă)—cancerous black mole or tumor that develops in the pigment cells of the skin

> **C43.5 Malignant melanoma of trunk**
>   Excludes2: malignant neoplasm of anus NOS (C21.0)
>   malignant neoplasm of scrotum (C63.2)

Figure 6-18 ■ Excludes2 note under a code in ICD-10-CM.

> **S37 Injury of urinary and pelvic organs**
>   Code also any associated open wound (S31.-)
>   Excludes1: obstetric trauma to pelvic organs (O71-)
>   Excludes2: injury of peritoneum (S36.81)
>   injury of retroperitoneum (S36.89-)

Figure 6-19 ■ Category with both Excludes1 and Excludes2 notes in ICD-10-CM.

TAKE A BREAK

Let's take a break and then review the placeholder "x," seventh characters, and Excludes notes in ICD-10-CM codes.

Exercise 6.4   ICD-10-CM Changes 6 and 7

Instructions: Answer the following questions using the ICD-10-CM Tabular.

1. Refer to code M48.42 for a fatigue fracture. If the patient's encounter was initial, what code would you assign? _____

2. Refer to code O60.14 for *Preterm labor third trimester with preterm delivery third trimester*. If this is a single-gestation pregnancy, what code would you assign? _____

3. Refer to code S22.22 for *Fracture of body of sternum*. If this is a subsequent encounter for fracture with delayed healing, what code would you assign? _____

4. Review the Excludes1 note for category range M50–M54. What condition is excluded from the categories? _____

5. Review the Excludes2 note for category C7a. What conditions are excluded from this category but can be coded together if they are documented in the medical record? _____

6. Review the Excludes1 and Excludes2 codes for category F32 for *Major depressive disorder, single episode*. What condition(s) should never be coded with codes from this category? _____

8. Code Also Note

A code also note is a new convention that alerts you that you may need to assign two codes in order to fully describe a condition. The *code also* note does not provide you with the order in which to sequence the codes. It appears under a category, subcategory, or code. Refer to examples of *code also* notes under codes shown in ■ FIGURE 6-20.

ICD-9-CM does not contain *code also* notes. Other notes instructing you to assign more than one code, that are in both ICD-9-CM and ICD-10-CM, are *use additional code, code first,* and *in diseases classified elsewhere.*

9. Multiple Codes and Combination Codes

In ICD-9-CM, assign either multiple codes or a combination code for an etiology/manifestation relationship, external cause of poisoning and substance that caused the poisoning, and symptoms and related conditions. In ICD-10-CM, there are many more combination codes that are represented by *multiple* codes in ICD-9-CM.

For example, if a patient has diabetic retinopathy with type II diabetes, you would have to code it in ICD-9-CM using multiple codes to show an etiology/manifestation relationship: diabetes is the etiology, and diabetic retinopathy is the manifestation. Refer to ■ FIGURE 6-21 to review multiple codes in the Index when you are searching for the main term retinopathy, subterm diabetic.

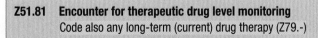

Z51.81	**Encounter for therapeutic drug level monitoring**
	Code also any long-term (current) drug therapy (Z79.-)
F51.05	**Insomnia due to other mental disorder**
	Code also associated mental disorder
F80.4	**Speech and language development delay due to hearing loss**
	Code also type of hearing loss (H90.-, H91.-)

Figure 6-20 ■ Code also notes appearing under codes in ICD-10-CM.

Retinopathy (background) 362.10
  arteriosclerotic 440.8 [362.13]
  atherosclerotic 440.8 [362.13]
  central serous 362.41
  circinate 362.10
  Coat's 362.12
  diabetic 250.5 [362.01]

Figure 6-21 ■ Diabetic retinopathy in the ICD-9-CM Index, looking under the main term retinopathy.

Diabetes, diabetic (mellitus) (sugar) E11.9
- with
- - retinopathy E11.319

Figure 6-22 ■ Diabetic retinopathy in the ICD-10-CM Index under the main term diabetes.

ICD-10-CM eliminates the need to assign *two codes* to many etiology/manifestation relationships. Refer to ■ FIGURE 6-22 to review diabetic retinopathy in the ICD-10-CM Index, and notice that there is *only one code* to cross-reference to the Tabular List. Then cross-reference E11.319 to the Tabular in order to assign the code (■ FIGURE 6-23).

In ICD-10-CM, you only need to assign one code, E11.319, for the condition of diabetic retinopathy. Do you see how ICD-10-CM combination codes will save time because you do not have to cross-reference multiple codes? ICD-10-CM coding makes your job much easier and more efficient.

When ICD-10-CM requires two codes for an etiology/manifestation, you will see the etiology code listed first in the Index, followed by the manifestation code in brackets, just as in ICD-9-CM. You will also see sequencing notes in the Tabular for etiology/manifestation codes: a "use additional code" note with the etiology code, and a "code first" note with the manifestation code. In most cases the manifestation codes also have in the code title, "in diseases classified elsewhere." Codes with this title are a component of the etiology/manifestation convention.

10. Hyphen (Dash)

In the ICD-10-CM Index and Tabular, you will find a hyphen (dash) at the end of a category or subcategory to show that you need to add more characters in order to make a valid code. Many times in the Tabular, you will find codes with the hyphen appearing within notes and coding instructions, such as *Excludes1, Excludes2,* and *use additional code.*

ICD-9-CM does not use hyphens after codes, but some versions of the ICD-9-CM code set use symbols with codes, such as a checkmark or box, to alert you to add a fourth or fifth digit. You already reviewed examples of codes with these symbols in previous chapters. ■ FIGURE 6-24 shows examples of the hyphen in the Index, and ■ FIGURE 6-25 shows examples of the hyphen in the Tabular.

Figure 6-23 ■ Diabetic retinopathy cross-referenced to the ICD-10-CM Tabular.

E11.3 Type 2 diabetes mellitus with ophthalmic complications
  E11.31 Type 2 diabetes mellitus with unspecified diabetic retinopathy
    E11.311 Type 2 diabetes mellitus with unspecified diabetic retinopathy with macular edema
    E11.319 Type 2 diabetes mellitus with unspecified diabetic retinopathy without macular edema

Figure 6-24 ■ Examples of the hyphen in the ICD-10-CM Index.

Lobster-claw hand Q71.6-

Masculinovoblastoma D27.-

Mastoiditis (coalescent) (hemorrhagic) (suppurative) H70.9-
- acute, subacute H70.00-
- - complicated NEC H70.09-

H72 **Perforation of tympanic membrane**
Includes: persistent post-traumatic perforation of ear drum
postinflammatory perforation of ear drum
Code first any associated otitis media (H65.-, H66.1-, H66.2-, H66.3-, H66.4-, H66.9-, H67.-)
Excludes1: acute suppurative otitis media with rupture of the tympanic membrane (H66.01-)
traumatic rupture of ear drum (S09.2-)

Figure 6-25 ■ Examples of the hyphen in the ICD-10-CM Tabular.

You have now learned about the major changes in ICD-10-CM that apply to coding all diagnoses. We will review changes to the coding guidelines for specific conditions in subsequent chapters in this book.

diabetic osteomyelitis (dī-a-bet′-ik os-tee-oh -mī-ə-līt′-əs) infectious and painful inflammatory bone disease caused by diabetes

TAKE A BREAK

Let's take a break and then review the code also note, multiple and combination codes, and the hyphen.

Exercise 6.5   **ICD-10-CM Changes 8–10**

Instructions: Assign multiple codes to the following diagnoses in ICD-9-CM and a combination code or multiple codes for the same conditions in ICD-10-CM. Use both the Index and the Tabular.

1. **Diabetic osteomyelitis**

   ICD-9-CM multiple codes _____

   ICD-10-CM multiple codes: _____

2. **Gangrene** of the toe due to diabetes

   ICD-9-CM multiple codes _____

   ICD-10-CM combination code: _____

3. **Pick's disease** with behavioral disturbance

   ICD-9-CM multiple codes _____

   ICD-10-CM multiple codes: _____

4. **Insomnia** due to **depression**

   ICD-9-CM multiple codes _____

   ICD-10-CM multiple codes: _____

5. Nutritional and metabolic **cardiomyopathy**

   ICD-9-CM multiple codes _____

   ICD-10-CM multiple codes: _____

6. **Premenstrual tension syndrome with menstrual migraine**

   ICD-9-CM multiple codes _____

   ICD-10-CM multiple codes: _____

Instructions: For questions 7–9, assign ICD-10-CM codes to the following diagnoses, paying close attention to the hyphens in the index to ensure that you code to the highest level of specificity. Use both the Index and the Tabular.

7. **Di Guglielmo's disease**

   ICD-10-CM code(s) _____

8. **Diastasis** of ankle muscle

   ICD-10-CM code(s) _____

9. Primary acute **iridocyclitis**

   ICD-10-CM code(s) _____

YOUR ROLE IN THE TRANSITION TO ICD-10-CM

You already know that the change to ICD-10-CM means that you will have to use ICD-10-CM codes to replace ICD-9-CM codes. Recall also that ICD-10-PCS will replace ICD-9-CM Volume 3 inpatient procedure codes. When you think about the transition to ICD-10-CM and ICD-10-PCS, keep in mind that it will not be simple or fast. Think about the steps of the revenue cycle that you learned in Chapter 1. Do you remember all of the different areas that coding affected in Dr. Hoffman's office? ICD-10-CM will affect all of these areas and ultimately affect the way that you perform your job duties.

gangrene (găng′ grēn)—death of tissue or bone due to loss of blood supply

Pick's disease (pix)—rare and fatal degenerative disease of the nervous system

insomnia (ĭn-sŏm′ nē-ah)—prolonged inability to sleep

depression (dē-prĕsh′ ŭn)—altered mood disorder, a symptom of which is loss of interest in things that are usually pleasurable

cardiomyopathy (kärd-ē-ō-mī-ăp′-ə-thē)—structural or functional disease of heart muscle, enlargement of the heart, or rigidity and loss of flexibility of the heart walls

premenstrual tension syndrome (prē-men′-struhl ten′-shun sin′-drōm)—emotional instability, insomnia, fatigue, anxiety, and depression prior to menstruation

menstrual migraine (men′-strul mī′-grān)—recurrent and often one-sided severe headache that occurs during menstruation

Di Guglielmo's disease (dē-gū-lyē-el′mōs)—a syndrome in which large numbers of nucleated red cells appear in the bone marrow and blood, also known as erythemic myelosis

diastasis (dī-as′-t ə-səs)—abnormal separation of parts that normally are joined together

All providers, insurances, claims clearinghouses, and billing and collection agencies throughout the U.S. will need to take all steps necessary to ensure that their computer software is updated to receive and send electronic healthcare transactions, including claims, using ICD-10-CM codes. They also have to make sure that all staff members involved with ICD-10-CM coding receive proper training on how to use the new code set. There is much work to do to prepare!

You may also be required to assist with practice management software changes and may have to work with a claims clearinghouse, billing, or collection agency. You may also help to create statistical reports using the new code set. And you may have to train other employees on using ICD-10-CM codes, including training the physician. The more information you know about ICD-10-CM, the more successful you will be in your job, and your employer will be glad to have your help because transitioning to ICD-10-CM is a huge undertaking. Let's review the changes that Dr. Hoffman and his office staff will need to make to prepare for the transition to ICD-10-CM.

Preparing Encounter Forms

Recall from Chapter 1 that Dr. Hoffman completed an encounter form (also called a super-bill) for Mr. Russell. Encounter forms have common diagnoses and corresponding codes already printed on them because it makes it easier for the physician to just check a box on the form indicating the patient's diagnosis. Because Dr. Hoffman's encounter forms have ICD-9-CM codes printed on them, new forms will need to be created, and Dr. Hoffman will have to become familiar with them before ICD-10-CM codes are implemented.

Implementing Information Technology Changes

Recall also that Debbie, the billing specialist, entered Mr. Russell's charge for his visit into the practice management software, along with his diagnosis code, so that she could bill his insurance. This means that the software Debbie uses will have to accept ICD-10-CM codes. The practice management software is currently set to accept a five-character ICD-9-CM code, not a seven-character ICD-10-CM code. Debbie will need to contact the information technology staff who work for her *software vendor*, a company that sells and services software, to ask them to change the software to accept the 7-character ICD-10-CM codes. She also will need to ensure that the software vendor includes ICD-10-CM codes on all of her electronic claims billed to the claims clearinghouse.

POINTERS FROM THE PROS: Interview with a Coding Expert

Danielle Taimuty, MA, CPC, CEMC, is the Chief Executive Officer (CEO) of a healthcare company that offers billing, coding, and consulting services to providers. They also develop software for patient registration, billing, coding, collections, and EHRs.

From an information technology perspective, what do you feel are some of the biggest challenges that providers will face when transitioning from ICD-9-CM to ICD-10-CM?

Contacting the vendors for software updates, implementing updates, testing of claims with clearinghouse, maintaining a larger database (to store information) because of the need for two datasets (ICD-9-CM and ICD-10-CM), speed issues based on maintaining two coding datasets, larger backups (to save information) and employee training.

What can coders do right now to help them prepare for the change from ICD-9-CM to ICD-10-CM?

Buy the ICD-10-CM (draft version) and try to cross-reference the most popular utilized codes.

What advice can you give to new coders to help them communicate effectively with physicians, as physicians can sometimes be intimidating?

Remember that their (the physician's) job is to tell the patient news even when it is bad news. You have same job, but yours is to tell the physicians what they need to hear to protect themselves. Always have written backup ready for the advice you are providing. It is not always easy, but if you can remember that you are helping them and guiding them much like they do with their patients, it becomes a little easier.

(Used by permission of Danielle Taimuty.)

Also recall that Debbie sends any unpaid patient bills to a collection agency for follow-up. She will need to work with both her software vendor and the collection agency to ensure that the collection agency is able to accept ICD-10-CM codes if Debbie sends the collection agency patients' claims to rebill to insurances. In addition, Debbie creates statistical reports for Dr. Hoffman, reporting on patients' diagnoses and treatment. Diagnosis codes are also in each patient's EHR, so Debbie will need to ensure that the EHR can accommodate ICD-10-CM codes.

iridocyclitis (ĭr ĭd-ō-sĭ-klī'tĭs)—inflammation of the iris and ciliary body

Participating in Additional Training

John, Dr. Hoffman's coder, will have to learn the new ICD-10-CM code set so that he can assign accurate codes to patients' records. Because ICD-10-CM codes are much more specific than ICD-9-CM codes, John will need to be sure that he is well versed in updated medical terminology and advanced anatomy, physiology, disease processes, and treatment. Debbie will have to learn ICD-10-CM, too, because she has to understand information on the claims that she sends to insurances. The office manager and medical assistant will learn more about ICD-10-CM codes because they both occasionally assist with coding and billing duties. Dr. Hoffman will need to ensure that he understands the basics of the new code set and documents completely in patients' records so that John and anyone else who codes can code accurately.

Dr. Hoffman's office manager will need to find a school or professional organization that offers ICD-10-CM training in a classroom, online, or through webinars. It is important to understand that providers have to plan for the transition to ICD-10-CM and not wait until the last minute; otherwise, they may not be able to accomplish all of their goals on time.

GENERAL EQUIVALENCE MAPPINGS

CMS and the CDC created **General Equivalence Mappings (GEMs)** that electronically convert ICD-9-CM codes to ICD-10-CM codes. GEMs also can convert ICD-9-CM Volume 3 inpatient procedure codes to ICD-10-PCS codes. GEMs are not intended to be a substitute for actual coding because GEMs map ICD-9-CM codes to ICD-10-CM codes without taking the patient's medical record into account. GEMs are a way to compare two different sets of information, not a coding tool. CMS refers to GEMs as a **crosswalk**, which means that many ICD-9-CM codes have an equivalent ICD-10-CM code. However, it is important to note that not all ICD-9-CM codes have an ICD-10-CM code equivalent.

Providers, insurances, claims clearinghouses, billing and collection agencies, and state and federal health organizations can also use GEMs for healthcare statistics and research reporting. For example, insurances keep records of patients' diagnoses from claims received and reimbursement for those claims. After ICD-10-CM codes become effective, the only record of patients' diagnoses that insurances will have are from ICD-9-CM codes, unless they use GEMs to convert the old code set to the new one.

FINAL NOTES ON ICD-10-CM

Keep in mind that the ICD-10-CM code set is considered to be a draft version until it is finalized. Refer to Appendix A in this text for directions on accessing the code set and the Official Guidelines for Coding and Reporting. Also remember that Current Procedural Terminology (CPT) and Healthcare Common Procedure Coding System (HCPCS) code sets will not change.

The CMS-1500 form (Figure 1-1) was revised and will accommodate ICD-10-CM codes. The form includes the addition of eight fields for diagnosis codes and letters that represent the fields, rather than numbers, which were used previously. The National Uniform Claim Committee (NUCC) revised the CMS-1500 form, and CMS and the Office of Management and Budget (OMB) both need to approve the draft version (■ FIGURE 6-26) before it is finalized, and providers can use it to bill insurances.

1500

DRAFT - NOT FOR OFFICIAL USE

CARRIER

HEALTH INSURANCE CLAIM FORM

APPROVED BY NATIONAL UNIFORM CLAIM COMMITTEE (NUCC) 02/12

☐☐☐ PICA | PICA ☐☐☐

1. MEDICARE ☐ (Medicare #) MEDICAID ☐ (Medicaid #) TRICARE ☐ (ID#/DoD#) CHAMPVA ☐ (Member ID#) GROUP HEALTH PLAN ☐ (ID#) FECA BLK LUNG ☐ (ID#) OTHER ☐ (ID#)

1a. INSURED'S I.D. NUMBER (For Program in Item 1)

2. PATIENT'S NAME (Last Name, First Name, Middle Initial)

3. PATIENT'S BIRTH DATE MM | DD | YY SEX M☐ F☐

4. INSURED'S NAME (Last Name, First Name, Middle Initial)

5. PATIENT'S ADDRESS (No. Street)

6. PATIENT RELATIONSHIP TO INSURED Self☐ Spouse☐ Child☐ Other☐

7. INSURED'S ADDRESS (No. Street)

CITY STATE

8. RESERVED FOR NUCC USE

CITY STATE

ZIP CODE TELEPHONE (Include Area Code) ( )

ZIP CODE TELEPHONE (Include Area Code) ( )

9. OTHER INSURED'S NAME (Last Name, First Name, Middle Initial)

10. IS PATIENT'S CONDITION RELATED TO:

11. INSURED'S POLICY GROUP OR FECA NUMBER

a. OTHER INSURED'S POLICY OR GROUP NUMBER

a. EMPLOYMENT? (Current or Previous) ☐YES ☐NO

a. INSURED'S DATE OF BIRTH MM | DD | YY SEX M☐ F☐

b. RESERVED FOR NUCC USE

b. AUTO ACCIDENT? PLACE (State) ☐YES ☐NO

b. OTHER CLAIM ID (Designated by NUCC)

c. RESERVED FOR NUCC USE

c. OTHER ACCIDENT? ☐YES ☐NO

c. INSURANCE PLAN NAME OR PROGRAM NAME

d. INSURANCE PLAN NAME OR PROGRAM NAME

10d. CLAIM CODES (Designated by NUCC)

d. IS THERE ANOTHER HEALTH BENEFIT PLAN? ☐YES ☐NO *If yes,* complete item 9, 9a and 9d.

READ BACK OF FORM BEFORE COMPLETING & SIGNING THIS FORM.

12. PATIENT'S OR AUTHORIZED PERSON'S SIGNATURE I authorize the release of any medical or other information necessary to process this claim. I also request payment of government benefits either to myself or to the party who accepts assignment below.

SIGNED ______ DATE ______

13. INSURED'S OR AUTHORIZED PERSON'S SIGNATURE I authorize payment of medical benefits to the undersigned physician or supplier for services described below.

SIGNED ______

PATIENT AND INSURED INFORMATION

14. DATE OF CURRENT ILLNESS, INJURY, or PREGNANCY (LMP) MM | DD | YY QUAL.

15. OTHER DATE QUAL. MM | DD | YY

16. DATES PATIENT UNABLE TO WORK IN CURRENT OCCUPATION FROM MM | DD | YY TO MM | DD | YY

17. NAME OF REFERRING PROVIDER OR OTHER SOURCE

17a.

17b. NPI

18. HOSPITALIZATION DATES RELATED TO CURRENT SERVICES FROM MM | DD | YY TO MM | DD | YY

19. ADDITIONAL CLAIM INFORMATION (Designated by NUCC)

20. OUTSIDE LAB? ☐YES ☐NO $ CHARGES

21. DIAGNOSIS OR NATURE OF ILLNESS OR INJURY Relate A-L to service line below (24E) ICD Ind.

A. ____ B. ____ C. ____ D. ____
E. ____ F. ____ G. ____ H. ____
I. ____ J. ____ K. ____ L. ____

22. RESUBMISSION CODE ORIGINAL REF. NO.

23. PRIOR AUTHORIZATION NUMBER

24. A. DATE(S) OF SERVICE From MM DD YY To MM DD YY	B. PLACE OF SERVICE	C. EMG	D. PROCEDURES, SERVICES, OR SUPPLIES (Explain Unusual Circumstances) CPT/HCPCS MODIFIER	E. DIAGNOSIS POINTER	F. $ CHARGES	G. DAYS OR UNITS	H. EPSDT Family Plan	I. ID. QUAL.	J. RENDERING PROVIDER ID. #
1								NPI	
2								NPI	
3								NPI	
4								NPI	
5								NPI	
6								NPI	

25. FEDERAL TAX I.D. NUMBER SSN EIN ☐☐

26. PATIENT'S ACCOUNT NO.

27. ACCEPT ASSIGNMENT? (For govt. claims, see back) ☐YES ☐NO

28. TOTAL CHARGE $

29. AMOUNT PAID $

30. Rsvd for NUCC Use $

31. SIGNATURE OF PHYSICIAN OR SUPPLIER INCLUDING DEGREES OR CREDENTIALS (I certify that the statements on the reverse apply to this bill and are made a part thereof.)

SIGNED DATE

32. SERVICE FACILITY LOCATION INFORMATION

a. NPI b.

33. BILLING PROVIDER INFO & PH. # ( )

a. NPI b.

PHYSICIAN OR SUPPLIER INFORMATION

NUCC Instruction Manual available at: www.nucc.org *PLEASE PRINT OR TYPE* OMB APPROVAL PENDING

Figure 6-26 ■ Draft of the revised CMS-1500 form. *Source:* http://www.nucc.org/.

CHAPTER REVIEW

Multiple Choice

Instructions: Circle one best answer to complete each statement.

1. ICD-10-CM codes can be up to _____ characters long.
   a. five
   b. six
   c. seven
   d. eight

2. Categories in the Tabular List are arranged in alphabetical order from
   a. 100–999.
   b. A–Z.
   c. A00–Z99.
   d. A001–Z999.

3. A final code assignment is always called a
   a. code.
   b. category.
   c. subcategory.
   d. block.

4. You may be asked to _____ other healthcare employees on the ICD-10-CM code set or on using the codes in practice management software.
   a. schedule
   b. hire
   c. train
   d. bill claims with

5. The side(s) of the body that a condition affects, such as the right or left eye or bilateral sides, is called
   a. bilateral.
   b. unilateral.
   c. ICD-10-CM.
   d. laterality.

6. When you are required to assign the seventh character, even though characters before the seventh are missing, use the placeholder
   a. -.
   b. x.
   c. 0.
   d. z.

7. When you cross-reference a code to the Tabular List, what note means that you should never sequence the condition listed in the note with the code that you cross-referenced?
   a. Excludes1
   b. Excludes2
   c. Code also
   d. Use additional code

8. In the ICD-10-CM Index and Tabular, what mark at the end of a category or subcategory shows that you need to add more characters to make it a valid code?
   a. x
   b. dot
   c. arrow
   d. hyphen

9. Which of the following is not a likely role that you will have in the transition to ICD-10-CM?
   a. Changing encounter forms to show ICD-10-CM codes
   b. Testing how the software will work using ICD-10-CM codes
   c. Becoming well-versed in updated medical terminology and advanced anatomy, physiology, disease processes, and treatment
   d. Explaining ICD-10-CM codes to patients

10. GEMs electronically convert ICD-9-CM codes to ICD-10-CM codes
    a. for statistics and tracking purposes.
    b. to substitute the correct code in patients' medical records.
    c. to eliminate the need for coder training in ICD-10-CM.
    d. to allow insurance companies to recode claims that were submitted with ICD-9-CM codes.

Coding Assignments

Instructions: You already reviewed the following cases in Chapter 5 using ICD-9-CM. Now, you will assign codes to the same cases using ICD-10-CM, referencing both the Index and Tabular. Write the condition(s) to code on the line provided, then assign ICD-10-CM codes.

1. Mrs. Peterson is a 62-year-old new patient who sees Dr. Hoffman for a persistent smoker's cough and dyspnea. Mrs. Peterson notes on her health history questionnaire that she has a past history of tobacco use and was a chronic cigarette smoker. Dr. Hoffman *suspects* that the patient may have emphysema brought on by her past smoking. He orders several different tests, and Mrs. Peterson will visit the local hospital to have the tests performed.

   What condition(s) should you code? _____
   _____

   What code(s) should you assign? _____
   _____

2. Mrs. Bailey, a 42-year-old established patient, sees Dr. Hoffman for removal of several skin tags from her neck. The patient is taking an anti-emetic for nausea during her menstrual cycle and has three refills left, so Dr. Hoffman doesn't need to write a new prescription.

   What condition(s) should you code? _____

   _____

   What codes should you assign? _____

   _____

3. Mark Moore, a 16-year-old established patient, sees Dr. Wilson, his dermatologist, for management of acne vulgaris.

   What condition(s) should you code? _____

   _____

   What code(s) should you assign? _____

   _____

4. Dr. Gonzalez, a neurologist, sees Mr. Morris, an established patient, for management of Parkinson's disease.

   What condition(s) should you code? _____

   _____

   What code(s) should you assign? _____

   _____

5. Mrs. Russell, a 48-year-old patient, presents to ambulatory surgery for left carpal tunnel decompression. Her pre-op diagnosis is left carpal tunnel syndrome, and her post-op diagnosis is the same.

   What condition(s) should you code? _____

   _____

   What code(s) should you assign? _____

   _____

6. Mrs. West, a 28-year-old established patient, has an encounter for a prenatal visit. She is pregnant with her second child. She sees Dr. Owens, her obstetrician. Dr. Owens finds no complications.

   What condition(s) should you code? _____

   _____

   What code(s) should you assign? _____

   _____

7. Mrs. Evans, a 24-year-old patient, sees Dr. Hoffman because she is coughing and has body aches and chills. Her temperature at the office is 102°. Dr. Hoffman diagnoses Mrs. Evans with influenza.

   What condition(s) should you code? _____

   _____

   What code(s) should you assign? _____

   _____

8. Dr. Hoffman sees Mr. Murphy, age 35, for a check-up. Dr. Hoffman diagnoses the patient with benign hypertension and writes a prescription for medication to treat it. On Mr. Murphy's health history form, he wrote that he sustained a clavicle fracture in a motor vehicle accident four years ago.

   What condition(s) should you code? _____

   _____

   What code(s) should you assign? _____

   _____

9. Kelly Torres, a 16-year-old established patient, sees Dr. Hoffman for a sore throat and neck, along with left ear pain, that all have lasted for a week. Dr. Hoffman diagnoses Ms. Torres with otitis media and writes a medication prescription.

   What condition(s) should you code? _____

   _____

   What code(s) should you assign? _____

   _____

10. Ms. Henderson, age 30, is an established patient who sees Dr. Hoffman for pain and swelling of her right ankle. He diagnoses her with ankle sprain, advises her to use crutches and an ankle splint, take an over-the-counter (OTC) pain medication, and elevate her ankle with an ice pack.

    What condition(s) should you code? _____

    _____

    What code(s) should you assign? _____

    _____

SECTION THREE

ICD-9-CM and ICD-10-CM Coding

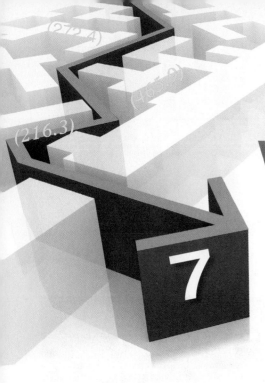

V Codes

Learning Objectives

After completing this chapter, you should be able to

- Spell and define the key terminology in this chapter.
- Describe the purpose of V codes.
- Discuss four reasons to assign V codes.
- Define and demonstrate how to code from the 15 categories of V codes.

Key Terms

counseling
diagnostic examinations or tests
follow-up care

health status V codes
preventive health care
routine and administrative examinations
screening

INTRODUCTION

One of the next stops on your coding journey is to assign different types of V codes, the Supplementary Classification of Factors Influencing Health Status and Contact with Health Services (V01–V91.99). You previously practiced assigning V codes, and you will continue to build on your coding knowledge by practicing with many more exercises, which will enable you to correctly assign diagnosis codes and understand more about coding specific conditions.

There is a new exercise in this chapter, which you will see in many other chapters, called Destination: Medicare. It includes many different types of exercises that will help you to better understand Medicare's coding, billing, and reimbursement regulations by navigating the CMS website. So let's move on now to V codes and keep learning and practicing.

"What we have to learn to do, we learn by doing." —ARISTOTLE

HEALTH STATUS AND CONTACT WITH HEALTH SERVICES (SUPPLEMENTARY CLASSIFICATION V01–V91.99)

oral contraceptive (or′-əl kon-trə-sep′tiv)—a pill, typically containing estrogen or progesterone, that prevents conception

Do you remember that V codes represent reasons for encounters, other than a disease, condition, or injury? Examples of when to assign V codes are to describe a patient's annual exam, a visit to obtain a prescription for an **oral contraceptive**, the fitting and adjustment of a hearing aid, or an immunization for protection against a disease. V codes also can provide additional information about a patient, even if the patient has an established diagnosis.

ICD-9-CM codes in this chapter are from the ICD-9-CM 2012 code set from the Department of Health and Human Services, Centers for Disease Control and Prevention.

ICD-10-CM codes in this chapter are from the ICD-10-CM 2012 Draft code set from the Department of Health and Human Services, Centers for Disease Control and Prevention.

■ **TABLE 7-1   GUIDELINES FOR ASSIGNING V CODES (SUPPLEMENTARY CLASSIFICATION V01–V91)**

Four common reasons to assign V codes are to describe an encounter for:
1. A patient who is not ill but needs a healthcare service, such as a checkup, or a patient who is not ill but has a personal or family history of an illness.
2. A patient who has a resolving disease or injury and who needs aftercare, or a patient who has a chronic long term condition and needs continuous care.
3. A patient who has circumstances or problems that influence his health status but that are not current illnesses or injuries.
4. A newborn; the V code indicates birth status on the infant's and mother's charts during the delivery encounter.
V codes can be used in any healthcare setting.
There are 15 types of V codes:
1. Contact with/exposure to communicable diseases
2. Inoculations and vaccinations
3. Status of health (disease carrier or sequelae)
4. Personal and family history of illnesses or conditions
5. Screening for disease
6. Observation
7. Aftercare for treatment recovery or healing after initial treatment
8. Follow-up care after completed treatment
9. Donors of blood or body tissue
10. Counseling
11. Obstetrics and related conditions
12. Newborn, infant, and child care
13. Routine and administrative examinations
14. Miscellaneous V codes—reasons for encounters excluded from other categories
15. Nonspecific V codes—reasons for encounters for nonspecific conditions
Providers assign specific V codes as the principal or first-listed diagnosis. (See Official Guidelines for Coding and Reporting for a list of codes.)

Examples are personal history of cancer, family history of hypertension, absence of an organ, or dependence on a wheelchair. In a handful of exceptions, V codes can show the main reason for the patient's encounter for therapeutic services, such as chemotherapy or radiation to treat cancer, or an encounter for physical or occupational therapy.

There are numerous V codes that represent many different health situations, and it is often difficult to know why and when you should assign V codes. It is also difficult to know how to find main terms for V codes. Keep in mind that there may be more than one main term that will lead you to the correct code, and not all main terms are listed in this chapter. Refer to ■ TABLE 7-1 to become familiar with V code guidelines and the 15 different categories of V codes. Then we will review more detailed information about each category, including examples of more complex coding exercises.

Four Reasons to Assign V Codes

As shown in Table 7-1, you will assign V codes (V01–V91) when the patient has an encounter for reasons other than a disease or injury (codes 001–999). You already know that insurances require ICD-9-CM codes in order to pay claims. V codes help to establish medical necessity for performing services when the patient has nothing wrong. They also help to provide additional information about the patient or the patient's personal or family medical history. In some cases, V codes provide more information about the encounter. The four main reasons to assign V codes are for

1. A patient who is not ill.

Examples: annual check-up, pre-employment physical, encounter or admission for normal pregnancy visit, contraceptive management, **genetic counseling**, organ donation, **prophylactic** care, **inoculations** or health screenings, counseling on health-related issues, or family history of a disease or condition (hypertension, diabetes).

2. A patient who has a resolving disease or injury and needs *aftercare*, or a patient who has a chronic condition and needs continuous care.

Examples of aftercare: breast reconstruction following a mastectomy; fitting and adjustment of a **prosthetic**, such as an artificial arm or leg; cast change; or removal or replacement of a **catheter**.

Examples of continuous care chemotherapy, radiation, or immunotherapy for an existing condition, such as a malignant neoplasm; or dialysis for renal disease.

3. A patient who has circumstances or problems that influence his health status but are not current illnesses or injuries.

Examples: transplanted organ (kidney, heart, lung), or artificial device (heart valve, shoulder joint, knee joint).

4. A newborn; the V code indicates birth status on the infant's and mother's charts during the delivery encounter.

Examples: single liveborn; twin, mate liveborn; twin, mate stillborn.

You can find V codes in the Alphabetic Index and then cross-reference them to the supplementary section on V codes in the Tabular List (V01–V91).

Use V Codes in Any Healthcare Setting

You can assign V codes in any healthcare setting as a first-listed code (principal diagnosis code in the inpatient setting) or as a secondary code, depending on the circumstances of the encounter. There are specific V codes that you can assign as a first-listed diagnosis, and can only assign others only as secondary codes. *(See Section I.C.18.e, V Codes that May Only Be the Principal/First-Listed Diagnosis in the Official Guidelines for Coding and Reporting.)*

TYPES OF V CODES

There are 15 different types of V codes, and it is important to become familiar with each of them in order to better understand the types of codes that are available to use in various circumstances. Always refer to the V code guidelines outlined in this chapter. (You will find directions for accessing ICD-9-CM Official Guidelines for Coding and Reporting in Appendix A of this text.) Let's review each type of V code, along with the main term(s) to search for in the Index to find the codes. You will also see several examples from the ICD-9-CM manual for assigning more complicated V codes.

1. Contact with/Exposure to Communicable Diseases

Assign a V code for a patient who was exposed to a **communicable** disease, which can occur through close personal contact with an infected person. A patient may also be exposed to a communicable disease just by being in close proximity to others who have it, which commonly occurs when the disease has reached epidemic proportions.

---

genetic counseling (jə-net′ik kown′səl-ing)—guidance that a medical professional provides to individuals with an increased risk of having children with a specific disorder because they pass on specific genes through reproduction

prophylactic (prō-fi-lăk′tĭk)—protective or preventive

inoculations (ĭ-no-ku-la′shəns)—introducing a substance into the body to produce immunity to a specific disease

aftercare (af′tər-kār)—the care, treatment, help, or supervision given to persons after they have been discharged from a healthcare institution or facility

prosthetic (prŏs′ thē-tĭc)—an artificial device used to replace a missing body part

catheter (kăth′ ĕ-tĕr)—hollow, flexible tube inserted into a body cavity, duct, or vessel to remove or inject fluids or to open a passageway

communicable (kə myu′-nĭk-ə-bəl)—transmitted from person to person

When you assign a V code for contact with or exposure to a communicable disease (V01), the patient cannot show any sign or symptom of the disease. If the patient exhibits signs or symptoms, do not assign a V code. Instead, assign a code for the sign, symptom, or definitive diagnosis.

You may assign V codes for contact with or exposure to a communicable disease as a first-listed code in order to establish medical necessity to test for the presence of the disease. More commonly, you will assign these V codes as secondary codes to show that the patient has a *potential risk* of developing a disease because she was exposed to it. There are also V codes from categories V15 and V87 for exposure to hazardous substances or body fluids.

Main Term(s): Exposure, contact with

Refer to the following example to code for contact with a disease:

Example: Mr. Brown, age 65, is an established patient who sees Dr. Hoffman, his family physician. Mr. Brown says that while he was attending a birthday party, one of the guests told several people that she was "just getting over the swine flu." He was in close proximity to this guest because the party was crowded. Dr. Hoffman sends the patient to the local hospital's lab department for a nasal swab HINI swine flu test.

To find a V code showing Mr. Brown's contact with the infected person, look in the Index under the main term *contact*, connecting word *with*, subterm *communicable disease*, and subterm *viral NEC*. Cross-reference code V01.79 to the Tabular (■ Figure 7-1).

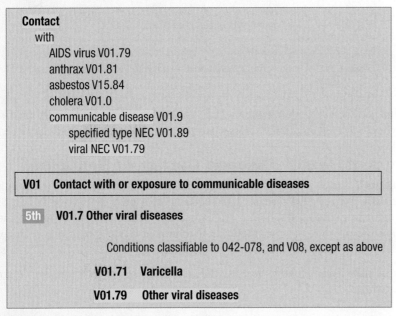

Figure 7-1 ■ Index entry for contact with communicable disease with V01.79 cross-referenced to the Tabular.

2. Inoculations and Vaccinations

Assign V codes (V03–V06) for patients who receive prophylactic inoculations or **vaccinations** against diseases. You may assign these V codes as the first-listed code if they represent the reason for the patient's encounter. Assign them as secondary codes if the patient receives the inoculation or vaccination as *part of* **preventive health care** (care that prevents illness), such as a well-baby visit. For preventive health visits, assign a separate V code for preventive care as the first-listed diagnosis, and assign an additional V code for the inoculation or vaccination.

vaccinations (vak-sĭ-naʹ shəns)—introducing a substance into the body to produce immunity to a specific disease

Main Term(s): Vaccination

Refer to the following example to code for a vaccination.

> **Example:** Kelly Walker is a 15-month-old established patient who sees Dr. Hoffman for a well-child exam and a *Hemophilus influenzae* type B (Hib) vaccine (**booster dose**). The vaccine is part of the patient's routine vaccination schedule.
>
> Assign two codes to this encounter: a V code for the preventive exam and a V code for the vaccine. For the first V code, search the Index for the main term *examination* and subterm *childcare*. Cross-reference code V20.2 to the Tabular (■ FIGURE 7-2).

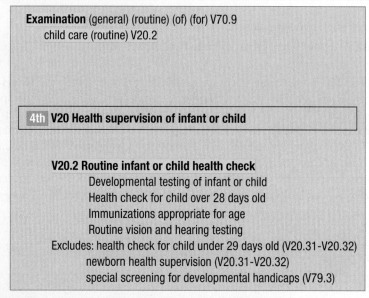

Examination (general) (routine) (of) (for) V70.9
  child care (routine) V20.2

4th V20 Health supervision of infant or child

V20.2 Routine infant or child health check
  Developmental testing of infant or child
  Health check for child over 28 days old
  Immunizations appropriate for age
  Routine vision and hearing testing
  Excludes: health check for child under 29 days old (V20.31-V20.32)
    newborn health supervision (V20.31-V20.32)
    special screening for developmental handicaps (V79.3)

Figure 7-2 ■ Index entry for well-child exam with V20.2 cross-referenced to the Tabular.

For the additional V code for the vaccine, search the Index for the main term *vaccination* and subterm *Hemophilus influenzae*. Cross-reference code V03.81 to the Tabular (■ FIGURE 7-3).

3. Status of Health (Disease Carrier or Sequelae)

Health status V codes provide additional information about a patient, including whether the patient is a carrier of a disease, has sequelae of a past disease or condition, or has another factor influencing his health status, such as a transplanted organ. Status codes also include the presence of prosthetic or mechanical devices resulting from past treatment. Refer to the following guidelines when assigning V codes to show health status.

1. A status code is informative because the status may affect the course of treatment and its outcome.

Figure 7-3 ■ Index entry for *Haemophilus influenzae* vaccination with V03.81 cross-referenced to the Tabular.

Vaccination
  Hemophilus influenzae, type B [Hib] V03.81

4th V03 Need for prophylactic vaccination and inoculation against bacterial diseases

5th V03.8 Other specified vaccinations against single bacterial diseases

V03.81 Hemophilus influenza, type B [Hib]

2. A status code is distinct from a history code. The history code indicates that the patient *no longer* has the condition.

3. Do not assign a status code with a diagnosis code from one of the body system chapters if both codes provide the same information.

   • For example, do not assign code *V42.1, Heart transplant status,* with code *996.83, Complications of transplanted heart.* Because code 996.83 already shows that the patient has a transplanted heart, it is repetitive to also assign V42.1, which shows the same information.

Review ■ TABLE 7-2 to become more familiar with the purpose and meaning of V code status categories, subcategories, and subclassifications and to learn how to find them in the Index.

Human Immunodeficiency Virus (HIV) (ĭm ū-nō-dĕ-fīsh′ ĕn-sē)—the virus that causes AIDS

constitutional (kon-stĭ-too′shən-əl)—relating to the development and growth of a person

sterilization (ster′ĭ-lĭ-za′ shən)—surgical procedure to eliminate the capacity to reproduce

■ TABLE 7-2   **STATUS CODE CATEGORIES, SUBCATEGORIES, AND SUBCLASSIFICATIONS**

Category, Subcategory, Subclassification	Title	Assign for a Patient Who	Index Main Term or Subterm
V02	Carrier or suspected carrier of infectious diseases	Carries specific disease organisms but does not have any signs or symptoms. (Carriers can still transmit the infection to others.)	Carrier
V07.5X	Use of agents affecting estrogen **receptors** and **estrogen** level	Receives a cancer-prevention drug that affects estrogen receptors and estrogen levels	Long term drug use; Use of
V08	Asymptomatic **Human Immunodeficiency Virus (HIV)** infection status	Tests positive for HIV but does not have any signs or symptoms	Infection
V09	Infection with drug-resistant microorganisms	Has an infection that is resistant to drug treatment. Sequence the infection code first.	Look under drug name, subterm resistant
V21	**Constitutional** states in development	Is obese, had short stature in childhood, had low birth weight, is experiencing puberty, or is demonstrating rapid growth	Constitutional
V22.2	Pregnant state, incidental	Is pregnant. V22.2 is a secondary code when the pregnancy does not complicate the reason for the visit.	Pregnancy
V26.5x	**Sterilization** status	Was sterilized and cannot reproduce (male or female)	Sterilization
V42	Organ or tissue replaced by transplant	Received animal or human organ or tissue transplants. Do not assign if there are complications.	Transplant(ed)
V43	Organ or tissue replaced by other means	Received artificial or mechanical devices as transplants. Do not assign if there are complications.	Replacement by artificial or mechanical device or prosthesis
V44	Artificial opening status	Has an artificial opening, such as a **tracheostomy** or **colostomy**. Do not assign if there are complications.	Artificial
V45	Other postsurgical states	Previously had a transplanted organ removed or has an implanted device, such as a pacemaker. Do not assign if there are complications.	Status
V46	Other dependence on machines	Is dependent on machines for survival, such as an oxygen tank or wheelchair. Do not assign if there are complications.	Status
V49.6	Upper limb **amputation** status	Had upper limbs amputated. Do not assign if there are complications.	Absence
V49.7	Lower limb amputation status	Had lower limbs amputated. Do not assign if there are complications.	Absence

continued

■ **TABLE 7-2** *continued*

Category, Subcategory, Subclassification	Title	Assign for a Patient Who	Index Main Term or Subterm
V49.81	Asymptomatic postmenopausal status (age-related) (natural)	Is past **menopause**	Postmenopausal
V49.82	**Dental sealant** status	Had a sealant applied to teeth to protect them	Status
V49.83	Awaiting organ transplant status	Is waiting for an organ to become available for a transplant	Awaiting organ transplant status
V49.86	Do not resuscitate status	Does not want to be resuscitated in a life-threatening situation, and this information is documented	Status
V49.87	Physical restraint status	Is placed in restraints during the encounter due to aggressive behavior that could harm others or the patient. (This code does not apply to patients who are restrained during a procedure.)	Status
V58.6x	Long-term (current) drug use	Uses a prescribed drug continuously, such as aspirin therapy, for the long-term treatment of a condition or for prophylactic use. Do not assign a code from this subcategory for patients who have drug addictions.	Status; Administration, prophylactic
V83	Genetic carrier status	Carries a gene associated with a specific disease, which they may pass to offspring who may develop that disease. The patient does not have the disease and is not at risk of developing the disease.	Carrier of
V84	Genetic susceptibility status	Carries a gene associated with a specific disease that increases the risk that the patient will develop the disease. Do not assign a code from this category as a principal or first-listed code.	Family, familial
V85	BMI	Has a BMI measurement that the physician documents. Assign codes from this category as secondary codes.	BMI
V86	Estrogen receptor status	Has a positive or negative estrogen receptor status from cancer treatment. Assign codes from this category as secondary codes.	Status
V88	Acquired absence of other organs and tissue	Is missing organs or tissue because of surgery or injury. (The patient was not born without the organs or tissue.)	Status
V90	Retained foreign body	Has a foreign body, such as metal, glass, plastic, that is retained somewhere in the body	Foreign body, retained

tracheostomy (trā kē-ŏs′ tō-mē)—surgical formation of an opening into the trachea through the neck

colostomy (kō-lŏs′ tō -mē)—surgical formation of an opening in the colon through the abdominal wall to evacuate the bowel

amputation (ăm pū-tā′ shŭn)—surgical or traumatic removal of all or part of a limb

Refer to the following example for assigning a status V code.

Example: Mr. Winner, a 60-year-old patient, sees his **cardiologist**, Dr. Bryan, for recent intermittent mild chest pain. Mr. Winner had a **pacemaker** implanted six months ago. Dr. Bryan orders several tests for the patient. Mr. Winner will visit the local hospital to have the tests performed, then follow up with Dr. Bryan in one week.

For this case, you need to assign two codes, the first for the patient's symptom of chest pain and the second for the presence of his pacemaker. It is important to code for the pacemaker because it may be related to the patient's symptoms. As you have already learned how to code symptoms, you know that in order to code the chest pain, you search the Index for the main term *pain* and subterm *chest*. Cross-reference code 786.50 to the Tabular for final code assignment.

For the pacemaker status V code, search the Index for the main term *status*, subterm *cardiac*, subterm *device*, and subterm *pacemaker*. Cross-reference code V45.01 to the Tabular. The codes to assign in this example are 786.50 and V45.01.

menopause (mĕn' ō-pawz)—when menstruation permanently ends, usually between the ages of 45 and 55

TAKE A BREAK

Let's take a break and then practice assigning V codes.

Exercise 7.1   Contact with Diseases, Inoculations or Vaccinations, Status of Health

Instructions: Assign V codes to the following patient cases, using both the Index and the Tabular. Refer to the main terms that were previously outlined for assistance locating V codes.

1. Ms. White, a 29-year-old established patient, sees Dr. Hoffman for an office visit. Ms. White recently helped a neighbor stand up out of bed. He had an **abscess** on the bottom of his foot. When he put his foot on the floor, the abscess burst, and the fluid inside hit Ms. White's glasses. She believes that some of it could have gotten into her eye. Ms. White says that her neighbor may be positive for HIV, the virus that causes **Acquired Immunodeficiency Syndrome (AIDS)**. She tells Dr. Hoffman that as a precaution she wants to be tested for HIV. Dr. Hoffman obtains a blood sample and sends it to the lab to test for HIV.

   Code(s): _____

2. Mrs. Denner brings her 8-week old son, Tyrone, to see Dr. Flynn, a pediatrician, for the child's diphtheria, tetanus, pertussis (DTaP) vaccination.

   Code(s): _____

3. Mrs. Parson brings her daughter, Ann, age 6, to see Dr. Hoffman as a precautionary measure because she feels that Ann may have been exposed to another child with measles. Since it has been more than 30 days since the suspected exposure, Dr. Hoffman administers a vaccine instead of performing a screening.

   Code(s): _____

4. Mr. Tallent, age 65, sees Dr. Hoffman for his annual flu vaccine. Dr. Hoffman does not provide any other services.

   Code(s): _____

5. Ms. Johnson, age 32, sees Dr. Noolan for genetic counseling, as she is a genetic carrier of the gene that causes cystic fibrosis.

   Code(s): _____

6. Dr. Hoffman documents that Ms. Reichard's height and weight give her a BMI of 27.5.

   Code(s): _____

4. Personal and Family History of Illnesses or Conditions

In Chapter 5, you learned about personal and family history and how to assign codes for them. You can assign applicable history codes to any medical record, regardless of the reason for the patient's visit. Code personal and family history of an illness when it affects the management of the patient and the type of treatment the physician provides. Refer to the following guidelines for coding personal and family histories.

1. Do not code conditions that the physician previously treated and no longer exist *unless* a past condition affects current care or influences the patient's treatment. If it does, assign a personal history V code as a secondary code for *personal* history of the past condition (V10–V15). V codes for personal history of a condition help to clarify why a patient may have a *current* condition.

2. Assign a family history V code as a secondary code if the patient has a *family* history of a condition that affects current care or influences treatment (V16–V19). Just like personal history, family history V codes are necessary to tell the entire story of a patient's current condition. You may assign family history codes along with screening codes to explain the need for a test or procedure.

3. Use caution when you are assigning the following category and subcategory:

   • V14—Personal history of allergy to medicinal agents

   • V15.0—Allergy, other than to medicinal agents

dental sealant (dĕn'tăl sē'lənt)—plastic material applied to teeth that have imperfections

cardiologist (kăr dĭ-ŏl'ō-jist)—a medical doctor who specializes in treating the heart

pacemaker (pās'ma-kər)—electrical device for stimulating or steadying heartbeat

abscess (ăb' sĕs)—a localized collection of pus surrounded by inflamed tissue

Acquired Immunodeficiency Syndrome (AIDS) (ă'-kwīrd ĭm ū-nō dĕ-fĭsh' ĕn-sē)—a severe disorder of the immune system caused by a virus and transmitted through sexual contact or exposure to infected blood or blood components

■ **TABLE 7-3   CATEGORIES OF HISTORY V CODES**

Category	Title
V10	Personal history of malignant neoplasm.
V12	Personal history of certain other diseases.
V13	Personal history of other diseases.
	Exception: V13.4—*Personal history of arthritis,* and V13.6—*Personal history of congenital (corrected) malformations.* These conditions are lifelong, so they are not true history codes.
V14	Personal history of allergy to medicinal agents.
V15	Other personal history presenting hazards to health.
	Exception: V15.7—*Personal history of contraception.* V15.7 does not typically present a health hazard to the patient. (Please see the Official Guidelines for additional exceptions.)
V16	Family history of malignant neoplasm.
V17	Family history of certain chronic disabling diseases.
V18	Family history of certain other specific diseases.
V19	Family history of other conditions.
V87	Other specified personal exposures and history presenting hazards to health. (Please see the Official Guidelines for a list of exceptions.)

A person who had a past allergic reaction to a substance should almost always be considered allergic to the substance. This means that you will not assign a personal history code to these cases because the patient's allergy is a current condition, not a past history condition. However, there are cases in which a patient has an allergic reaction to a substance one time and never again. In these cases, it is appropriate to assign a personal history of allergy to medicines or other substances. Be sure to read the patient's documentation thoroughly, and query the physician for clarification.

Main Term(s): History (personal) of, or History (personal) of, subterm family

Refer to ■ TABLE 7-3 to become familiar with categories of history V codes.
Refer to the following example to code for history.

Example: Ms. Smith sees Dr. Hoffman to discuss her risk for developing breast cancer, which runs in her family. (Both her mother and grandmother suffered from it.)

To find a V code showing the patient's family history of breast cancer, search the Index for the main term *history,* subterm *family,* subterm *malignant neoplasm,* and subterm *breast.* Cross-reference code V16.3 to the Tabular.

5. Screening for Disease

A **screening** is a test, like a blood test, or an exam for the presence of a disease or other conditions that may cause a disease, called disease *precursors.* For example, hypertension is a precursor for coronary artery disease, meaning that because a patient has hypertension, it increases his risk of developing coronary artery disease. Screenings are especially important because they identify problems even in **asymptomatic** patients. Early detection of a disease or precursor helps physicians to provide care and counseling to patients as quickly as possible.

Here are some common screenings that physicians recommend for groups who are more likely to develop specific conditions:

- Routine mammogram for women over age 40 to test for breast cancer (■ FIGURE 7-4)

- **Fecal occult blood test** for men and women over age 50 to test for colon cancer

- **Amniocentesis** to rule out a fetal **anomaly** for pregnant women over age 35. (The incidence of **Down's syndrome** is higher for this group.)

---

asymptomatic (a-simp-to-mat´ik)—showing no symptoms of disease

fecal occult blood test (fe´kəl ŏ-kult´)—chemical test to detect blood in the feces that cannot be seen with the naked eye

amniocentesis (ăm n ĭ -ō-sĕn-tē´ s ĭ s)—surgical puncture of the amniotic sac to obtain a sample of amniotic fluid containing fetal cells

anomaly (ə-nom´ə-le)—abnormal condition

Down's syndrome—congenital condition caused by the presence of an extra copy of chromosome 21, resulting in learning difficulties and physical differences

INTERESTING FACT: **Families Talk Turkey and Health History on Thanksgiving**

The U.S. Surgeon General has declared Thanksgiving Day to be National Family History Day and is encouraging Americans to share a meal and their family health history. This information can help your doctor recommend tests and screenings. Family members share genes, behaviors, lifestyles, and environments, all of which may affect their risk of developing health problems. Most people have a family health history of common chronic diseases (cancer, heart disease, or diabetes) and other health conditions (high blood pressure and high cholesterol). The relatives whose family health history are most relevant are your parents, brothers and sisters, and children, followed by grandparents, uncles and aunts, nieces and nephews, half-brothers, half-sisters, great uncles, great aunts, and cousins. Common questions to ask include "Do you have any chronic diseases, such as heart disease, or health conditions such as high blood pressure, cholesterol, or diabetes? Have you had any other serious diseases, such as cancer or stroke? How old were you when you developed these diseases? What diseases did your deceased relatives have? How old were they when they died, and what caused their deaths?"

(Department of Health and Human Services, Centers for Disease Control and Prevention, www.cdc.gov/Features/FamilyHealth History/, accessed 11/20/10.)

Do not confuse screenings with *diagnostic* **examinations or tests**. Physicians conduct or order diagnostic exams or tests when the patient has a *sign or symptom* of a suspected condition. In these cases, *code the sign or symptom* to justify the exam or test unless there is a definitive diagnosis.

Refer to the following guidelines for assigning V codes to screenings.

1. Assign a screening code as the first-listed code if the reason for the visit is specifically the screening test or exam.

2. Assign a screening code as an *additional* code if the provider performs the screening during an office visit for a diagnosed condition.

3. Do not assign a separate V code for screening if the screening is normally part of a procedure, such as a Pap smear (screening) taken during a routine pelvic examination. Instead, assign the appropriate V code or other diagnosis code to describe the encounter.

4. If a patient's screening reveals a specific diagnosis, code the diagnosis as *secondary* to the V code for the screening.

5. The V code indicates that a screening test or exam is planned.

Main Term(s): Screening

Categories:

- V28—**Antenatal** screening
- V73–V82—*S*pecial screening examinations

antenatal (an-te-na′təl)— before birth

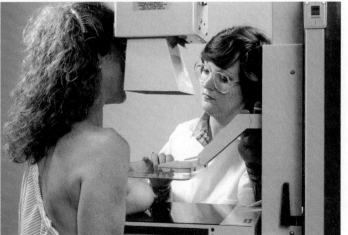

Figure 7-4 ■ Patient receiving a screening mammogram.
Photo credit: Bill Branson/National Cancer Institute.

Refer to the following example for assigning a V code for screening:

> **Example:** Mrs. Nelson, a 43-year-old patient, visits the radiology department at Washington Bryant Memorial Hospital for a screening mammogram for breast cancer.
>
> Search the Index for the main term *screening*, subterm *malignant neoplasm*, subterm *breast*, and subterm *mammogram*. Cross-reference code V76.12 to the Tabular.

6. Observation

Assign V codes for observation when a physician observes a patient for a suspected condition but does not find any evidence of it. These are the three observation V code categories, which you should only use in rare circumstances:

- V29—Observation and evaluation of newborns for suspected condition not found. (For a newborn, sequence a code from categories V30–V39—*Liveborn Infants According to the Type of Birth* first, and report a code from category V29 second.)
- V71—Observation and evaluation for suspected condition not found
- V89—Suspected maternal and fetal conditions not found

Do not assign V codes for observation if the patient has an injury, illness, or any signs or symptoms that are related to the suspected condition. Instead, assign a code for the injury, illness, sign, or symptom. (Also assign an E code to identify an external cause that is responsible for the patient's condition, sign, or symptom. You will learn how to assign E codes later in this chapter and in Chapter 8.)

You already learned how to code observation cases with signs, symptoms, and conditions in Chapter 5. Refer to the rules outlined next for additional guidance on assigning V codes for observations for conditions not found.

1. Assign an observation V code as the principal diagnosis only.
   - *Exception*: On a newborn's chart, assign the observation code second. If the infant is under *observation* with no condition found, assign an observation code from category V29—*Observation and evaluation of newborns for suspected condition not found* as a *secondary* diagnosis.
   - You may also assign additional codes using the V code for newborn observation, but only if they are unrelated to the observation of the suspected condition.
2. Assign codes from subcategory V89.0—*Suspected maternal and fetal conditions not found* in very limited cases on a maternal record when the mother's encounter is for a suspected maternal or fetal condition which the physician then rules out.
   For example, an abnormal test result may cause the physician to suspect that there is a maternal or fetal condition present. But the physician then rules out the condition because there is no evidence of it. Assign codes from subcategory V89.0 as a first-listed or additional code, depending on the case.
3. Assign additional codes with subcategory V89.0—*Suspected maternal and fetal conditions not found* only if they are unrelated to the suspected condition.
4. Do not assign codes from subcategory V89.0—*Suspected maternal and fetal conditions not found* for encounters for antenatal screening of the mother.
5. If the patient shows signs or symptoms that are related to the suspected condition, then do not assign a V code for observation; assign a code for the signs or symptoms. If the physician *confirms* a patient's suspected condition, do not assign a V code for observation. Instead, code the confirmed condition.
6. For encounters for suspected fetal conditions that are *inconclusive* (no result) following testing and evaluation, assign the appropriate code from category 655, 656, 657 or 658.

Main Term(s): Observation

Refer to the following example for coding a newborn observation:

Example: Mrs. North delivers Gabrielle North, a single liveborn, at Washington Bryant Memorial Hospital. The delivery is normal without any complications. However, Mrs. North is **Group B Streptococcus (GBS)** positive but asymptomatic. Dr. Gold, the **neonatologist**, observes the **neonate** because she is at risk for developing **sepsis** due to her mother's GBS-positive status. Gabrielle is also asymptomatic. After observation, Dr. Gold finds nothing wrong with Gabrielle and discharges her home.

During an encounter for delivery, you must assign codes to both the mother's chart and the infant's chart; you'll learn more about this in Chapter 14. In this example, assign only the V codes to the infant's chart, the first code for the outcome of delivery (single liveborn) and the second code for observation of the infant with no conditions found.

To find the first code for outcome of delivery, search the Index for the main term *newborn*, subterm *single*, and subterm *born in hospital*. Cross-reference code V30.00 to the Tabular (■ FIGURE 7-5). Next, assign the V code for observation of the neonate (newborn) with no conditions found. Search the Index for the main term *observation*, subterm *newborn*, and subterm *infectious*. Cross-reference code V29.0 to the Tabular (■ FIGURE 7-6).

Group B streptococcus (GBS) (strep-to-kok′əs)—serious bacterial infection that can be passed from mother to fetus and is a leading cause of death and disability in newborns

neonatologist (ne-o-na-tol′ə-jist)—a physician who specializes in the study and treatment of newborns

neonate (ne′o-nāt)—newborn infant, often defined as 28 days or younger

sepsis (sep′sis)—severe infection from disease-causing organisms, especially bacteria, in the blood or tissues

---

Newborn (infant) (liveborn)

single

born in hospital (without mention of cesarean delivery or section) V30.00

LIVEBORN INFANTS ACCORDING TO TYPE OF BIRTH (V30-V39)

Note: These categories are intended for the coding of liveborn infants who are consuming health care [e.g., crib or bassinet occupancy].

The following fourth-digit subdivisions are for use with categories V30-V39:

0 Born in hospital
1 Born before admission to hospital
2 Born outside hospital and not hospitalized

The following two fifths-digits are for use with the fourth-digit .0, Born in hospital:

0 delivered without mention of cesarean delivery
1 delivered by cesarean delivery

V30 Single liveborn

V31 Twin, mate liveborn

V32 Twin, mate stillborn

V33 Twin, unspecified

V34 Other multiple, mates all liveborn

V35 Other multiple, mates all stillborn

V36 Other multiple, mates live- and stillborn

V37 Other multiple, unspecified

V39 Unspecified

Figure 7-5 ■ Index entry for single liveborn, born in hospital with V30.00 cross-referenced to the Tabular.

Observation (for) V71.9

   newborn V29.9

      cardiovascular disease V29.8

      congenital anomaly V29.8

      genetic V29.3

      infectious V29.0

4th **V29 Observation and evaluation of newborns for suspected condition not found**

Note: This category is to be used for newborns, within the neonatal period (the first 28 days of life), who are suspected of having an abnormal condition resulting from exposure from the mother or the birth process, but without signs or symptoms, and which, after examination and observation, is found not to exist.

Excludes: suspected fetal conditions not found (V89.01-V89.09)

V29.0 Observation for suspected infectious condition

V29.1 Observation for suspected neurological condition

V29.2 Observation for suspected respiratory condition

Figure 7-6 ■ Index entry for newborn observation with V29.0 cross-referenced to the Tabular.

TAKE A BREAK

Let's take a break and then practice assigning more V codes.

Exercise 7.2   **Personal and Family History, Screening for Disease, and Observation**

Instructions: Assign V codes to the following patient cases, using both the Index and the Tabular. For some cases, you may also need to assign a second code. Refer to the main terms listed for each type of V code for assistance finding codes in the Index.

1. Ms. Cronin, age 32, reports to Williton Medical Center's radiology department for a mammogram. Dr. Hoffman recommended that she begin mammograms before the usual age because she has been found to be susceptible to the breast cancer. She is a carrier of an abnormal BRCA1 gene (breast cancer gene 1).

   Code(s): _____

2. Dr. Hoffman notes that for patient Kim Elstein, both Ms. Elstein's mother and grandmother had breast cancer.

   Code(s): _____

3. Mr. Newton brings his son Jason, age 5, to see Dr. Hoffman for a precautionary measles screening.

   Code(s): _____

4. Kelly Reichard, age 22, requests that Dr. Hoffman perform an HPV screening.

   Code(s): _____

5. Dr. Moon, a gastroenterologist, diagnoses Mr. Swindel, age 72, with primary colon cancer, after finding it during a routine colonoscopy. (Hint: The second code is for a malignant neoplasm.)

   Code(s): _____

6. Dr. Flynn, a pediatrician, places newborn Katie Partin under observation for a suspected respiratory problem. She was born at Washington Bryant earlier today via cesarean section. (Hint: Start with the Index entry *newborn* for the first code).

   Code(s): _____

7. Aftercare for Treatment Recovery or Healing after Initial Treatment

Aftercare involves healing or treatment. Assign aftercare visit codes for two reasons:

1. To show that the encounter is for current treatment to heal a condition which was previously treated (healing or recovery phase).

2. To describe treatment related to the long-term consequences of a disease.

Refer to ■ TABLE 7-4 for aftercare V code categories, subcategories, and subclassification code titles, main terms, and subterms.

Do not assign an aftercare V code if the patient's treatment is for a current, acute disease or injury. Instead, assign the diagnosis code for the disease or injury. Exceptions include encounters for chemotherapy, radiotherapy, and immunotherapy to treat neoplasms. For those encounters, assign the V code for chemotherapy, radiotherapy, and immunotherapy as the first-listed code:

- V58.0—Radiotherapy (also called radiation)
- V58.11—Encounter for antineoplastic chemotherapy
- V58.12—Encounter for antineoplastic immunotherapy

■ TABLE 7-4   **AFTERCARE V CODES**

Category, Subcategory, Subclassification	Title	Main Term/Subterm
V51.0	Encounter for breast reconstruction following mastectomy	Admission, for, cosmetic surgery
V52	Fitting and adjustment of prosthetic device and implant	Fitting
V53	Fitting and adjustment of other device	Fitting
V54	Other **orthopedic** aftercare	Aftercare
V55	Attention to artificial openings	Admission, for, attention to
V56	Encounter for **dialysis** and dialysis catheter care	Admission, for, dialysis
V57	Care involving the use of rehabilitation procedures	Admission, rehabilitation
V58.0	**Radiotherapy**	Admission, for, therapy
V58.11	Encounter for **antineoplastic chemotherapy**	Admission, encounter
V58.12	Encounter for antineoplastic **immunotherapy**	Admission, encounter
V58.3x	Attention to dressings and sutures	Admission
V58.41	Encounter for planned postoperative wound closure	Aftercare, following surgery, for
V58.42	Aftercare, surgery, neoplasm	Aftercare, following surgery, for
V58.43	Aftercare, surgery, trauma	Aftercare, following surgery, for
V58.44	Aftercare involving organ transplant	Aftercare, following surgery, for
V58.49	Other specified aftercare following surgery	Aftercare, following surgery, for
V58.7x	Aftercare following surgery	Aftercare, following surgery, for
V58.81	Fitting and adjustment of **vascular** catheter	Admission
V58.82	Fitting and adjustment of nonvascular catheter	Admission
V58.83	Monitoring therapeutic drug	Admission
V58.89	Other specified aftercare	Aftercare

orthopedic (or-tho-pe′dik)—relating to a deformity, disorder, or injury of the skeletal structure

dialysis (dī′al′i sis)—removing waste from the body due to loss of kidney function

radiotherapy (rā dĭ-ō-thĕr′ă-pē)—treatment of disease by X-rays and radioactive substances

antineoplastic (an-ti-ne-o-plas′tik)—inhibiting or preventing the growth and spread of malignant or cancerous cells

chemotherapy (kē mō-thĕr′ă-pē)—use of chemical agents in the treatment or control of disease, especially cancer

immunotherapy (ĭm mū-nō-thĕr′ă pē)—treatment of disease by inducing, enhancing, or suppressing an immune response

vascular (văs′- kŭ-lar)—relating to or containing blood vessels

Assign the neoplasm(s) code second. If a patient receives both radiation and chemotherapy therapy during the same encounter, then assign both codes V58.0 and V58.11, and sequence either one first.

Refer to the following guidelines for assigning aftercare codes.

1. Assign aftercare codes as first-listed codes to explain the specific reason for the encounter. Assign an aftercare code as an additional code if the patient receives aftercare in addition to other services.

2. Assign aftercare codes with other aftercare codes or other diagnosis codes to provide better detail of an aftercare encounter visit.

3. Assign aftercare codes for an encounter in any order.

4. Certain aftercare V code categories need a secondary diagnosis code to describe the resolving condition or sequelae because it is not listed in the code title.

5. Assign status V codes with aftercare V codes to indicate the nature of the aftercare.
   - For example, you may assign status code V45.81—*Aortocoronary bypass status*, with aftercare code V58.73—*Aftercare following surgery of the circulatory system, NEC*.

6. You may assign a transplant status V code to identify the organ transplanted, in addition to code V58.44—*Aftercare following organ transplant*.

7. Do not assign a status V code when the aftercare code already shows the patient's status.
   - For example, the aftercare code V55.0—*Attention to tracheostomy* already shows that the patient had a tracheostomy (status), so you would not need to assign an additional status code, V44.0—*Tracheostomy status*.

Refer to the following example for assigning an aftercare V code.

Example: Mrs. Garcia, a 48-year-old patient, has an encounter for chemotherapy at Williton Cancer Center to treat a primary malignant neoplasm of the left lower breast (■ FIGURE 7-7).

Figure 7-7 ■ A colored x-ray showing a malignant tumor (solid white mass) in the left breast. Breast cancer is the most common type of cancer in women.

Photo credit: National Cancer Institute.

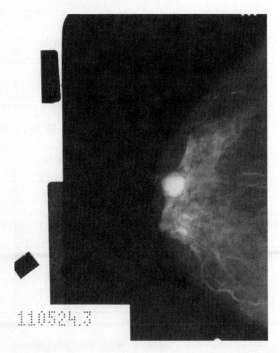

Assign a V code for chemotherapy as the first-listed code because the main reason for the encounter was to administer chemotherapy. Assign a secondary code for the malignant breast neoplasm.

Figure 7-8 ■ Index entry for admission for chemotherapy with V58.11 cross-referenced to the Tabular.

> **Admission** (encounter)
>
> > for
> >
> > > therapy
> > >
> > > > blood transfusion, without reported diagnosis V58.2
> > > > breathing exercises V57.0
> > > > chemotherapy, antineoplastic V58.11
> > > >
> > > > > prophylactic NEC V07.39
> > > > >
> > > > > > fluoride V07.31
>
> ---
>
> **4th**   **V58 Encounter for other and unspecified procedures and aftercare**
>
> Excludes: convalescence and palliative care(V66.0-V66.9)
>
> > **V58.0 Radiotherapy**
> > Encounter or admission for radiotherapy
> > Excludes: encounter for radioactive implant - code to condition
> > radioactive iodine therapy-code to condition
>
> > **5th V58.1 Encounter for chemotherapy and immunotherapy for neoplastic conditions**
> > Encounter or admission for chemotherapy
> > Excludes: chemotherapy and immunotherapy for nonneoplastic conditions-code to condition
> >
> > > **V58.11   Encounter for antineoplastic chemotherapy**
> > > **V58.12   Encounter for antineoplastic immunotherapy**

For the first code, search the Index for the main term *admission*, connecting word *for*, subterm *therapy*, and subterm *chemotherapy*. Cross-reference code V58.11 to the Tabular (■ FIGURE 7-8).

Next, assign the code for the primary malignant neoplasm of the left lower breast. Recall from Chapter 3 that a primary neoplasm is the site where the physician first found the neoplasm, and it has spread. Search the Neoplasm Table in the Index under the main term *neoplasm*, subterm *breast*, subterm *lower*, and subterm *malignant primary*. Cross-reference 174.8 in the Tabular (■ FIGURE 7-9).

8. Follow-up Care after Completed Treatment

Follow-up care occurs when the patient sees the physician for monitoring after treatment of a disease, condition, or injury is completed. When you assign a follow-up care V code to show the reason for the encounter, it means that the physician has fully treated the patient's condition, and it no longer exists. Be careful not to confuse follow-up V codes with aftercare V codes. Aftercare V codes represent encounters for *current treatment for a healing condition* or its sequelae, not follow up *after completed treatment*.

You may also assign follow-up codes with history codes to provide the full picture of the healed condition and its treatment. Sequence the follow-up code first, followed by the history code. If the physician finds a recurring condition during the follow-up visit, do not assign a V code for the follow-up. Instead, assign the diagnosis code for the recurring condition.

Main Term(s): Follow-up

Follow-up V Code Categories:

- V24—**Postpartum** care and evaluation

- V67—Follow-up examination

Refer to the following example for coding a follow-up visit.

postpartum (pōst-pahr′ təm)—six weeks after childbirth

Figure 7-9 ■ Index entry for primary malignant breast neoplasm from the Neoplasm Table with 174.8 cross-referenced to the Tabular.

	Malignant Primary	Malignant Secondary	Malignant Ca in situ	Benign	Uncertain Behavior	unspecified
Neoplasm, neoplastic	**199.1**	**199.1**	**234.9**	**229.9**	**238.9**	**239.9**
breast (connective tissue) (female) (glandular tissue) (soft parts)	174.9	198.81	233.0	217	238.3	239.3
lower	174.8	198.81	233.0	217	238.3	239.3

> **4th** 174 Malignant neoplasm of female breast

Includes: breast (female)
        connective tissue
        soft parts
      Paget's disease of:
        breast
        nipple
Use additional code to identify estrogen receptor status (V86.0, V86.1)
Excludes: skin of breast (172.5, 173.5)

    174.8 Other specified sites of female breast
        Ectopic sites
        Inner breast
        Lower breast

Final code assignments for this example are V58.11 and 174.8.

Example: Mrs. Scott, a 35-year-old patient, sees Dr. Jules, her obstetrician, for a follow-up visit two weeks after the birth of her first child.

Search the Index for the main term *follow-up*, subterm *postpartum*, and subterm *routine*. Cross-reference code V24.2 to the Tabular.

9. Donors of Blood or Body Tissue

cadaveric (kə-dav′ər-ik)—relating to a dead body

Assign V codes to encounters for donors of blood or body tissue (V59), including organs, bone, and skin. These codes are only for living individuals who are donating to others, not donating to themselves. These codes do not identify **cadaveric** donations.

WORKPLACE IQ: What Would You Do?

You are working as a medical assistant for Dr. Gupta, a family care physician. Part of your job involves verifying that codes on the patient's encounter form match medical record documentation. Today, Kelly, the billing specialist, tells you that she just finished reviewing insurance claims for accuracy before billing insurance. She believes that one of the claims has the codes in the wrong order and tells you, "Take a look at this claim for Emma Patterson for her chemotherapy encounter. You assigned a V code first and the neoplasm code second. I thought you had to code the neoplasm first because that is her diagnosis, and I don't want to bill the insurance until we correct the codes."

What would you do?

Main Term(s): Donor

Refer to the following example for assigning a V code for an organ donor.

> **Example:** Deena Parker, a 36-year-old organ donor, has an encounter at Washington Bryant to donate a kidney to her mother, Ruth Parker. Ruth Parker suffers from end-stage renal disease (ESRD) and needs a kidney transplant to survive.
>
> Assign the V code for Deena Parker's encounter by searching the Index for the main term *donor* and subterm *kidney*. Cross-reference code V59.4 to the Tabular.

TAKE A BREAK

Let's take a break and then practice assigning V codes for after-care, follow-up, and donors of blood and body tissue.

> **Exercise 7.3**   **Aftercare, Follow-Up, and Donors**

Instructions: Assign V codes to the following patient cases, using both the Index and the Tabular. Refer to the main terms listed for each type of V code for assistance finding codes in the Index.

1. Mr. Swindel has an outpatient encounter for chemotherapy that is directed at his primary colon cancer.

   Code(s): _____

2. Mr. Risner, age 26, sees Dr. Grisham, orthopedist, for removal of a cast from his arm.

   Code(s): _____

3. Eva Russel, age 42, is admitted to Valley Hospital to donate bone marrow for her sister, Clare Russell.

   Code(s): _____

4. Mr. Wicks, age 73, sees his cardiologist, Dr. Bergin, to get his cardiac pacemaker reprogrammed.

   Code(s): _____

5. Mrs. Silva presents to Williton Medical Center's physical therapy department for physical therapy after a below-the-knee amputation of the right leg.

   Code(s): _____

6. Mrs. Day receives a fitting for a breast prosthesis following her mastectomy.

   Code(s): _____

10. Counseling

Assign **counseling** V codes when a patient or family member receives assistance in the aftermath of an illness or injury or when they need support to cope with family or social problems. Do not assign V codes for counseling when the patient has an established diagnosis and the encounter is for a service when counseling is *integral* to (part of) standard treatment.

Main Term(s): Counseling

The counseling V code categories and subcategories are listed in ■ TABLE 7-5.

■ TABLE 7-5   CATEGORIES OF COUNSELING V CODES

V25.0	General counseling and advice for contraceptive management
V26.3	Genetic counseling
V26.4	General counseling and advice for procreative management
V61.X	Other family circumstances
V65.1	Person consulted on behalf of another person
V65.3	Dietary surveillance and counseling
V65.4	Other counseling, not elsewhere classified

Refer to the following example to assign a V code for counseling.

> **Example:** Mr. Edwards, a 44-year-old established patient, sees Dr. Hoffman because he and his wife are not getting along. He reports that his wife is working two jobs and is under constant stress. He adds that she is emotional all the time, and he is upset and does not know how to handle the situation. Dr. Hoffman counsels the patient on stress management techniques and refers him to a marital counselor for regular counseling sessions.
>
> To find a code for counseling, search the Index for the main term *counseling* and subterm *marital*. Cross-reference code V61.10 to the Tabular.

11. Obstetrics and Related Conditions

obstetrics (ob-stet′riks)— branch of medicine that deals with the care of women during pregnancy, childbirth, and the recuperative period following delivery

You learned about V codes for pregnancy (prenatal) visits in Chapter 5. There are two types of codes for pregnancies: V codes for pregnancy visits when there are no pregnancy complications, and diagnosis codes for pregnancy visits when there *are* pregnancy complications. When there is a complication, assign codes from the **obstetrics** chapter in the Tabular List (Chapter 11—Complications of Pregnancy, Childbirth, and the Puerperium). (You will learn how to assign codes from Chapter 11 in a later chapter in this book.) There are two V code choices for a normal pregnancy encounter without complications, which you should always assign as the first-listed code.

- V22.0—Supervision of normal first pregnancy
- V22.1—Supervision of other normal pregnancy (not the first pregnancy)

During a *delivery encounter* (an encounter when the physician delivers a newborn), you must assign a code from category V27 indicating the outcome of delivery on the mother's chart, such as a single liveborn or the mate of a twin. For the mother's chart, always assign a code from category V27 as a secondary code.

Also assign a code for the outcome of delivery as the first-listed code (V30–V39) to the infant's chart. The first-listed code will show whether the delivery was normal or complicated (C-section). We will also cover this information in the next section.

If the physician or other clinician provides family planning services (contraceptive or procreative management) either during a pregnancy visit or during a postpartum (after delivery) visit, assign the appropriate V code for family planning. (See Section I.C.11., the Obstetrics Guidelines, for further instruction on the use of these codes.)

Review ■ TABLE 7-6 to become more familiar with V code categories for obstetrics and related conditions. Main terms are also listed in the table.

Refer to the following example to assign a V code to a prenatal encounter:

> **Example:** Mrs. West, a 28-year-old established patient, has an encounter for a prenatal visit with her obstetrician, Dr. Owens. She is pregnant with her second child. Dr. Owens finds no complications.
>
> To assign a code for this visit, search the Index for the main term *pregnancy*, subterm *supervision*, and subterm *normal*. Cross-reference code V22.1 to the Tabular.

12. Newborn, Infant, and Child Care

Newborn, infant, and child care falls into one of the three following categories:

1. Category V20—*Health supervision of infant or child* (includes visits for immunizations and exams)
2. Category V29—*Observation and evaluation of newborns and infants for suspected condition not found*
   You already learned how to assign codes from category V29 earlier in this chapter (Figure 7-6).

■ TABLE 7-6 CATEGORIES OF V CODES FOR OBSTETRICS AND RELATED CONDITIONS

Category, Subcategory, Subclassification	Title	Main Term or Subterm
V22	Normal pregnancy	Pregnancy, supervision
V23	Supervision of high-risk pregnancy	Pregnancy, supervision
	Exception: V23.2—*Pregnancy with history of abortion.* Code 646.3—Recurrent pregnancy loss, from the Obstetrics chapter, is required to indicate a history of abortion during a pregnancy.	
V24	Postpartum care and evaluation	Postpartum, observation
V25	Encounter for contraceptive management	Admission, for
	Exception: V25.0x—*General counseling and advice*	
V26	Procreative management	Management
	Exception: V26.5x—*Sterilization status,* V26.3—*Genetic counseling and testing,* V26.4—*General counseling and advice*	
V27	Outcome of delivery	Outcome of delivery
V28	Antenatal screening	Screening
V91	Multiple gestation placenta status	Gestation

3. Categories V30–V39 represent *birth status* (type of birth). Assign a code from V30–V39 as the first-listed code on the infant's chart to show the type of birth during the delivery encounter (single liveborn; liveborn with mate) (Figure 7-5). Assign additional codes for any other conditions. After the delivery encounter, you will not assign V30 again (birth only happens one time to the patient). Note that if the newborn is transferred from the hospital where birth took place to another hospital, the receiving hospital does not assign a code from V30–V39 because the first hospital already coded the birth.

Main term(s): Admission, observation, newborn

Refer to the following example to assign a V code for health supervision of a child:

Example: Mrs. Mendoza brings her two-year-old, Vincent, to Dr. Hoffman to receive immunizations. Vincent has no current health issues.

To assign a V code to Vincent's encounter, search the Index for the main term *admission,* connecting word *for,* subterm *examination,* subterm *health supervision,* and subterm *child.* Cross-reference code V20.2 to the Tabular.

TAKE A BREAK

Let's take a break and then practice assigning V codes for counseling, obstetrics, and child care.

Exercise 7.4 V Codes—Counseling, Obstetrics and Related Conditions, and Newborn, Infant, and Child Care

Instructions: Assign V codes to the following patient cases, using both the Index and the Tabular. Refer to the main terms listed for each type of V code for assistance with finding codes in the Index.

1. Miss Kurth, age 20, sees Dr. Hoffman to obtain a prescription refill for oral contraceptives.

   Code(s):_____

2. Ms. Asbury is six weeks pregnant with her first child and will turn 35 years old next month, so her pregnancy is considered an elderly pregnancy. She sees her obstetrician, Dr. Gerard, for her first prenatal visit.

   Code(s):_____

continued

TAKE A BREAK *continued*

3. Thirty-one weeks later, Ms. Asbury gives birth to a healthy baby girl, Marie, via normal vaginal delivery. Assign the V code for Ms. Asbury's delivery encounter.

Code(s):_____

4. Baby Marie Asbury was born today in the hospital via vaginal delivery. Code Marie's record.

Code(s):_____

5. Two weeks after giving birth, Ms. Asbury sees Dr Gerard for a routine postpartum follow-up examination. Everything is normal.

Code(s):_____

6. Mrs. Asbury takes Marie to Dr. Flynn, a pediatrician, for a 14-day health check.

Code(s):_____

13. Routine and Administrative Examinations

V codes for **routine and administrative examinations** describe encounters such as a general check-up or a pre-employment physical. Administrative exams refer to exams that patients need for reasons other than illnesses, such as exams for a life insurance policy, driver's license, marriage license, or admission to a camp or school. Do not assign these codes if the patient's exam is for signs or symptoms of a suspected condition or to treat a specific condition. Instead, code the signs, symptoms, or diagnosis. Follow the guidelines listed next for additional assistance assigning V codes for routine and administrative exams:

1. If the physician finds a condition during a routine exam, assign the condition code *secondary to* the V code for the routine exam.

2. Assign history codes and codes for pre-existing and chronic conditions as additional codes for a routine exam, as long as the examination is for administrative purposes and not focused on any particular condition.

preprocedural (pro-se′jər ăl)—the time shortly before a surgical operation

3. Assign pre-operative examination and **preprocedural** laboratory examination V codes only when a physician sees the patient for surgery clearance and does not render any treatment. You learned about surgical clearance encounters in Chapter 5.

Main Term(s): Admission, examination, test

Categories:

- V20.2—Routine infant or child health check
- V70—General medical examination
- V72—Special investigations and examinations
  - Assign codes V72.5—*Radiological examination not elsewhere classified* and/or V72.62—*Laboratory examination ordered as part of a routine general medical examination* if the patient encounter is for routine laboratory or radiology testing in the absence of any signs, symptoms, or associated diagnosis. If the provider performs routine testing during the same encounter as a nonroutine test to evaluate a sign, symptom, or diagnosis, it is appropriate to assign *both* the V code and the code describing the reason for the nonroutine test. You already learned about assigning codes for routine tests in Chapter 5.

Refer to the following example to assign a V code for an administrative exam:

Example: Mr. Howard, a 47-year-old established patient, sees Dr. Hoffman for an examination that the patient's insurance company requires before they can offer him a life insurance policy. Dr. Hoffman finds Mr. Howard to be in excellent health.

To assign a V code to Mr. Howard's encounter, search the Index for the main term *admission*, connecting word *for*, subterm *examination*, and subterm *insurance certification*. Cross-reference code V70.3 to the Tabular.

14. Miscellaneous V Codes—Reasons for Encounters Excluded from Other Categories

The miscellaneous V codes capture a number of other health care encounters that do not fall into any of the other V code categories. Certain codes identify the reason for the encounter; others are additional codes that provide useful information which may affect a patient's care and treatment.

Miscellaneous V codes can describe encounters for prophylactic removal of breasts, ovaries, or another organ because the patient is **genetically** predisposed to cancer or has a family history of cancer. For these encounters, assign V50.4—*Prophylactic organ removal* as the principal or first-listed code. Assign additional codes for genetic susceptibility to cancer and any applicable family history code.

genetically—relating to heredity and variation of organisms

If the patient has a malignancy at one site and has prophylactic removal at another site to prevent either a new primary malignancy or metastatic (spreading) disease, then assign a code from V50.4—*Prophylactic organ removal* as the first-listed code, and assign an additional code for the malignancy. For example, you would use this code if a female patient had a malignant neoplasm of the left breast and had a healthy right breast removed to prevent another malignant neoplasm. Do not assign V50.4 if the patient has organ removal *to treat* a malignancy, such as the removal of the testes to *treat* prostate cancer. Refer to ■ TABLE 7-7 for a list of miscellaneous V code categories, subcategories, subclassifications, main terms, and subterms.

Refer to the following example to assign a miscellaneous V code.

Example: Mrs. Coleman, a 73-year-old established patient, sees Dr. Hoffman because of sleeping issues. She explains that since she retired, she has no trouble initially falling asleep but wakes up six to seven times a night and falls back to sleep again each time, waking up in the morning extremely tired. Dr. Hoffman recommends an **over-the-counter (OTC)** sleep aid and also recommends that Mrs. Coleman find new activities to keep herself occupied. They discuss possible options for activities.

over-the-counter (OTC)—medications that are sold lawfully without a prescription

To code Mrs. Coleman's encounter, search the Index for the main term *problem* and subterm *sleep, lack of*. Cross-reference code V69.4 to the Tabular.

■ TABLE 7-7   MISCELLANEOUS V CODES

Category, Subcategory	Title	Main Term or Subterm
V07	Need for isolation and other prophylactic or treatment measures	Prophylactic
	Exception: V07.5X—*Use of agents affecting estrogen receptors and estrogen levels*	
V40.31	Wandering in diseases classified elsewhere	Wandering
	Example: A patient with Alzheimer's disease frequently wanders away from home. Code first the underlying condition that caused the wandering.	
V50	Elective surgery for purposes other than remedying health states	Surgery, admission
V58.5	Orthodontics	Orthodontics
V60	Housing, household, and economic circumstances	Person, living (in)
V62	Other psychosocial circumstances	Problem (with)
V63	Unavailability of other medical facilities for care	Unavailability of medical facilities
V64	Persons encountering health services for specific procedures, not carried out	Procedure
V66	Convalescence and Palliative Care	Admission
V68	Encounters for administrative purposes	Admission, issue of
V69	Problems related to lifestyle	Problem (with)

POINTERS FROM THE PROS: Interview with an Office Manager

For several years, Christine Ringer has worked as the office manager for a family care physician and a physician assistant. She ensures that her staff provides excellent customer service and patient care. She also oversees all registration, charge entry, coding, billing, and collections processes.

Describe the qualities that a good coder should have.

A good coder must be detail-oriented and thorough. It also helps if you enjoy investigative work.

Discuss why a medical assistant should have coding training.

Medical assistants are required to include ICD-9-CM codes on all test orders. They also need to understand the importance of documenting every service they provide (i.e., immunizations, phlebotomy, urinalysis, etc.). If they understand how their duties impact the bottom line (insurance and patient reimbursement), they are more likely to (document thoroughly). I also think it makes them feel that their job is important and encourages them to do it well.

Why do you feel that coders make mistakes when coding?

They are impatient or simply don't have the time to properly investigate a service.

(Used by permission of Christine Ringer.)

15. Nonspecific V Codes—Reasons for Encounters for Nonspecific Conditions

Nonspecific V codes represent very general information about a patient's encounter. Use these codes with caution because they are repetitive when they are used with other V codes that have the same general meaning but provide more specific information. There is almost no reason to assign nonspecific V codes in an inpatient setting. *Assign nonspecific V codes as a last resort* in the outpatient setting *only when* the physician's documentation is too general to allow you to assign more precise codes. As always, you should query the physician for clarification before assigning a nonspecific V code. Refer to ■ TABLE 7-8 for a list of nonspecific V code categories, subcategories, main terms, and subterms.

Refer to the following example to assign a nonspecific V code:

Example: Ms. Carlson visits Dr. Fowler, an obstetrician/gynecologist, for a pregnancy check-up. Ms. Carlson is considered a high-risk patient because she had an abortion of her first pregnancy.

To code Ms. Carlson's encounter, search the Index for the main term *pregnancy*, subterm *supervision*, subterm *previous*, and subterm *abortion*. Cross-reference code V23.2 to the Tabular.

■ TABLE 7-8 **NONSPECIFIC V CODES**

Category, Subcategory	Title	Main Term or Subterm
V11	Personal history of mental disorder	History
V13.4	Personal history of arthritis	History
V13.6	Personal history of congenital malformations	History
V15.7	Personal history of contraception	History
V23.2	Pregnancy with history of abortion	Pregnancy
V40	Mental and behavioral problems	Problem
	Exception: V40.31—*Wandering in diseases classified elsewhere*	
V41	Problems with special senses and other special functions	Problem
V47	Other problems with internal organs	Problem
V48	Problems with head, neck, and trunk	Problem
V49	Problems with limbs and other problems	Problem
	Excludes limb amputations. (See the Official Guidelines for Coding and Reporting for additional exceptions.)	

TAKE A BREAK

Let's take a break and then practice assigning V codes for routine exams, miscellaneous situations, and nonspecific V codes.

Exercise 7.5 Routine and Administrative Examinations, Miscellaneous V Codes, Nonspecific V Codes

Instructions: Assign V codes to the following patient cases, using both the Index and the Tabular. Refer to the main terms listed for each type of V code for assistance with finding codes in the Index.

1. Mr. Brewer, age 45, sees Dr. Hoffman for his annual exam and asks if he should have a colonoscopy because his brother recently passed away from colon cancer.

   Code(s):_____

2. Ms. Koons brings her 12-year-old daughter, Maggie, to Dr. Hoffman for a physical for summer camp.

   Code(s):_____

3. Mr. Rucker, age 50, sees Dr. Dunford, a general surgeon, for a pre-operative examination prior to a planned cholecystectomy (gall bladder removal).

   Code(s):_____

4. Later that day, Mr. Rucker presents to Washington Bryant's laboratory for pre-operative blood work.

   Code(s):_____

5. Ms. Fleming, age 32, elects to have a prophylactic mastectomy because she is susceptible to breast cancer. She is a carrier of an abnormal BRCA1 gene (breast cancer gene 1). Her mother, grandmother, and sister have also had breast cancer.

   Code(s):_____

6. Dr. Milburn, a plastic surgeon, performs a face lift on Mrs. Byrne for cosmetic reasons.

   Code(s):_____

DESTINATION: MEDICARE

The CMS website contains the *Medicare Learning Network (MLN)*, which provides training and education on Medicare regulations and issues. In this exercise, your Medicare destination is one of MLN's computer-based training modules called the *World of Medicare*. The *World of Medicare* covers basic information about the Medicare program and is a good place to start learning more about Medicare before you begin researching Medicare regulations in future chapters. Follow the instructions listed next to access the *World of Medicare*.

1. Go to the website http://cms.gov.

2. At the top of the screen on the yellow banner bar, choose *Outreach & Education*.

3. Scroll down to *Medicare Learning Network*, and choose *MLN Products*.

4. Choose *Web-Based Training (WBT)*.

5. Scroll down and under *Related Links*, and click on *Web-Based Training (WBT) Courses*.

6. You will then see a list of web-based training courses. Click on *World of Medicare—Developed January 2010, Revised January 2011*.

7. If you never accessed the MLN's computer-based training, then you will have to register as a new user. Registration is free and takes a few minutes. After you have registered, you will only need your login and password each time you access the computer-based MLN. After registering, click *Web-Based Training Courses*, and click the *World of Medicare* again.

8. On the next screen, click the radio button for *No credits* or *Continuing Education Units (CEU)*. (CMS grants 1 CEU to coders who are certified through the American Academy of Professional Coders (AAPC) for scoring 70% or higher on the posttest for a computer-based training module.) Then click *Take Course*. You will take both a pretest and posttest so that you can monitor how well you learned the material.

⇨ A LOOK AHEAD TO ICD-10-CM

You learned how to assign ICD-10-CM codes in Chapter 6, and you will also have the opportunity for more practice using these codes in this chapter and future chapters. Z codes in ICD-10-CM represent the same information as V codes in ICD-9-CM. Although the coding guidelines for V codes and Z codes are generally the same, be sure to refer to ICD-10-CM Official Guidelines for Coding and Reporting for more specific information. (Directions for obtaining these guidelines are in Appendix A of this text.) In the following exercise, assign Z codes from ICD-10-CM, referencing both the Index and the Tabular.

Instructions: You already coded the following cases in this chapter using ICD-9-CM. Now assign code(s) to the same cases using ICD-10-CM, referencing both the Index and Tabular.

1. Mr. Tallent, age 65, sees Dr. Hoffman for his annual flu vaccine. Dr. Hoffman does not provide any other services. Code(s):_____

2. Ms. Cronin, age 32, reports to Williton Medical Center's radiology department for a mammogram. Dr. Hoffman recommended that she begin mammograms before the usual age because she has been found to be susceptible to the breast cancer. She is a carrier of an abnormal BRCA1 gene (breast cancer gene 1). Code(s):_____

3. Mr. Swindel has an outpatient encounter for chemotherapy directed at his primary colon cancer. Code(s):_____

4. Ms. Asbury gives birth to a healthy baby girl, Marie, via normal vaginal delivery. Assign the Z code for Ms. Asbury's delivery encounter (mother's record). Code(s):_____

5. Mr. Rucker, age 50, sees Dr. Dunford, a general surgeon, for a pre-operative examination prior to a planned cholecystectomy (gall bladder removal). Code(s):_____

6. Dr. Flynn, a pediatrician, places newborn Katie Partin under observation for a suspected respiratory problem. She was born at Washington Bryant earlier today via cesarean section. No current conditions were found. Code(s):_____

CHAPTER REVIEW

Multiple Choice

Instructions: Circle one best answer to complete each statement.

1. Which of the following is *not* a reason to assign V codes?
   a. A patient who is not ill
   b. A patient who has a resolving disease or injury and who receives aftercare
   c. A patient who is receiving healthcare because of problems or circumstances that influence his or her health status
   d. A pregnant woman who is experiencing serious complications

2. In order to assign a V code for exposure to a communicable disease, the patient
   a. must exhibit signs and symptoms.
   b. must identify how she was exposed to the disease.
   c. cannot show any sign or symptom of the disease.
   d. cannot have had an inoculation or vaccination against the disease.

3. Which of the following is *not* a health status V code?
   a. AIDS-related diseases
   b. Carrier or suspected carrier of infectious diseases
   c. Asymptomatic HIV infection status
   d. Do not resuscitate status

4. Personal and family history codes are used
   a. to document a patient's family members' past surgeries.
   b. for conditions that the physician previously treated, that no longer exist and no longer affect current care.
   c. only for the patient's initial visit.
   d. when the history of an illness affects the management of the patient and the type of treatment the physician provides.

5. Screenings are especially important because they identify problems even if the patient is
   a. contagious.
   b. asymptomatic.
   c. terminal.
   d. recovering.

6. Assign V codes for observation in all the following encounters *except*
   a. when the patient shows signs or symptoms that are related to the suspected condition.
   b. when the mother's encounter is for a suspected maternal or fetal condition, which the physician then rules out.
   c. for observation and evaluation of newborns for suspected condition not found.
   d. when a physician observes a patient for a suspected condition but does not find any evidence of it.

7. Assign aftercare visit codes
   a. if the patient's treatment is for a current, acute disease or injury.
   b. to show that the encounter is for current treatment for a healing condition.
   c. when the physician finds a recurring condition.
   d. when the patient sees the physician for a surgical complication.

8. Assign follow-up visit codes
   a. if the physician finds a recurring condition.
   b. to show that the encounter is for a surgical complication.
   c. for treatment of the sequelae of a healed condition.
   d. when the patient sees the physician for monitoring after treatment of a disease, condition, or injury is completed.

9. Assign counseling V codes when
   a. a mental health condition exists.
   b. the patient has an established diagnosis, and the encounter is for a service in which counseling is integral to standard treatment.
   c. a patient or family member receives assistance in the aftermath of an illness or injury.
   d. the patient seeks a second opinion on his condition.

10. Obstetric and newborn-related V codes are *not* used to describe
    a. the outcome of delivery on the mother's chart during a delivery encounter.
    b. the outcome of delivery code on the infant's chart during a delivery encounter.
    c. complications of pregnancy.
    d. routine prenatal visits.

Coding Assignments

Instructions: Assign ICD-9-CM code(s) to the following cases, referencing both the Index and Tabular.

1. Janice Deaver, a 30-year-old pregnant patient, arrives at the Emergency Department at Washington Bryant Memorial Hospital with a Colles fracture. After examination, the ED physician, Dr. Smyther, states that the fracture does not affect her pregnancy in any way. He treats her and discharges her.

   Code(s):_____

2. Mrs. Harbaugh, an 82-year-old, sees Dr. Lightner, a pulmonologist, for a periodic check-up. She has end-stage chronic obstructive pulmonary disease (COPD) and also has a tracheostomy tube to aid in her breathing.

   Code(s):_____

3. Mrs. Buss, a 28-year-old, sees Dr. Gerard, obstetrician/gynecologist (OB/GYN), for a routine prenatal visit. She became pregnant via *in vitro* fertilization technology. Everything is going fine so far in this pregnancy.

   Code(s):_____

4. Karen Jensen goes into labor and dilates quickly. She and her husband Danny, are on route to Washington Bryant, which is about 20 minutes away. They soon realize that she is going to deliver before they get to the hospital, so they stop in a parking lot and call 911. The operator gives Danny instructions on caring for his wife until the paramedics arrive. The paramedics deliver a healthy boy, Scott. An ambulance then transports Karen and Scott to the hospital, and they are both admitted. Code for the outcome of delivery on Scott's record after his hospital admission.

   Code(s):_____

5. Baby Scott Jensen is circumcised the next day.

   Code(s):_____

6. Mr. Cheng, a 62-year-old, presents to Washington Bryant's outpatient radiology department for radiotherapy directed at his bladder cancer.

   Code(s):_____

7. Amanda Dykes, age 64, receives a screening for osteoporosis due to a family history of the condition. The test is negative.

   Code(s):_____

8. Robert Curtin, a 35-year-old, has agreed to donate a kidney for his brother, Clarence, who suffers from ESRD and is on dialysis. Mr. Curtin is admitted to Williton Medical Center for a left nephrectomy.

   Code(s):_____

9. Mr. Larrabee, age 47, sees his optometrist, Dr. Byrd, for a routine vision examination.

   Code(s):_____

10. Mrs. Pearson, age 32, visits her gynecologist, Dr. Gerard, for insertion of an intrauterine contraceptive device (IUD).

    Code(s):_____

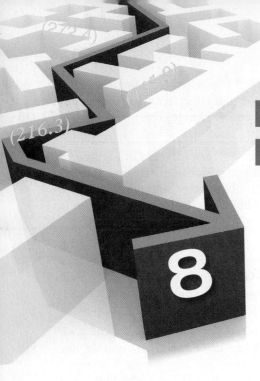

E Codes, Injuries, Burns

8

Learning Objectives

After completing this chapter, you should be able to

- Spell and define the key terminology in this chapter.
- Explain the purpose of E codes and guidelines for assigning E codes.
- Identify different types of injuries and applicable coding guidelines.

Key Terms

activity code
adverse effect
burn
dislocation
external cause status
fracture
medical misadventure

open wound
poisoning
rule of nines
sprain
strain
superficial injury
terrorism
total body surface area (TBSA)
toxic effect

INTRODUCTION

During this stop on your coding journey, you will learn how to assign E codes, the Supplementary Classification of External Causes of Injury and Poisoning. You learned in Chapter 3 that E codes represent an *external cause* that created a patient's condition, such as a fall from a building, automobile accident, or accidental overdose of a prescribed medication.

You will also learn how to assign codes for poisonings, injuries, and adverse, toxic, and late effects. All the coding guidelines are from the ICD-9-CM Official Guidelines for Coding and Reporting, and you can review additional information in the Guidelines. Let's continue on your journey by learning about assigning E codes!

"It is good to have an end to journey towards, but it is the journey that matters in the end."—Ursula K. LeGuin

ICD-9-CM codes in this chapter are from the ICD-9-CM 2012 code set from the Department of Health and Human Services, Centers for Disease Control and Prevention.

ICD-10-CM codes in this chapter are from the ICD-10-CM 2012 Draft code set from the Department of Health and Human Services, Centers for Disease Control and Prevention.

SUPPLEMENTAL CLASSIFICATION OF EXTERNAL CAUSES OF INJURY AND POISONING (E-CODES, E000, E800–E999)

E codes represent *external causes* that created the patient's condition—injury, poisoning, adverse effect, toxic effect, or late effect—such as an automobile accident, an accidental overdose of a prescribed medication, or a fall from a building. You will assign E codes *in addition* to the diagnosis for the patient's condition. *E codes are never the first-listed diagnosis code.*

> **Example:** One of Dr. Hoffman's patients, Mr. Reynolds, was standing on a ladder to paint his house. He fell off and suffered a femur (thigh bone) fracture.
>
> The femur fracture is the diagnosis, and the *external cause* of the femur fracture is the fall from the ladder, represented by an E code. Mr. Reynolds' first-listed diagnosis code is 821.00 (femur fracture), and the second code is E881.0 (fall from a ladder). The E code provides *additional information* about the patient's diagnosis but does not represent the patient's *actual condition.*

E codes actually have their own Alphabetic Index, called the Index to External Causes of Injury (Section 3 of Volume 2—Alphabetic Index), in which external causes are arranged in alphabetical order, along with their corresponding codes. The Tabular List groups E codes in numeric order from categories E000 to E999. To become familiar with the types of external causes and injuries that E codes represent, review E codes in both the Index to External Causes of Injury and the Tabular List. Place tabs in your coding manual so that you can easily find the Index for E codes and the supplementary classification of E codes. Examples of E codes in the Index to External Causes of Injury and in the Tabular List are shown in ■ FIGURE 8-1.

It is a provider's decision to assign E codes. E codes help providers, payers, and other organizations review injury statistics to develop methods for injury prevention. E codes capture the following information:

- How the injury, poisoning, or adverse effect happened (cause), such as accidental medication overdose, motor vehicle accident, fall down a flight of stairs, or boating accident
- The intent behind the injury, poisoning, or adverse effect, including unintentional, accidental, or intentional, such as suicide or assault

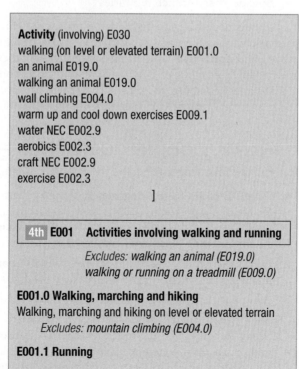

Figure 8-1 ■ Alphabetic Index for E codes and in the Tabular List (Supplementary Classification of External Causes of Injury and Poisoning.

■ **TABLE 8-1** **GUIDELINES FOR ASSIGNING E CODES**

Supplemental Classification of External Causes of Injury and Poisoning (E000, E800–E999)

Guidelines for Specific Situations Involving E Codes:

1. Place of Occurrence
2. Adverse Effects, Poisonings, and Toxic Effects
3. Child and Adult Abuse
4. Unknown or Suspected Intent, Undetermined Cause
5. Late Effects of External Cause
6. Misadventures and Complications of Care
7. Terrorism
8. Activity Codes
9. External Cause Status

- The patient's status (i.e., whether the patient is in the military or a civilian)
- The associated activity and place where the event occurred. Specific E codes represent injuries that occur during activities such as running, climbing, sports, housework, exercise, and dancing, among others.

Major categories of E codes include

- Transport accidents (accidents involving transportation, such as trains, boats, automobiles)
- Poisoning and adverse effects of drugs, medicinal substances, and **biologicals**
- Accidental falls
- Accidents caused by fire and flames
- Accidents due to natural and environmental factors
- Late effects of accidents, assaults, or self-injuries
- Assaults or purposely inflicted injuries
- Suicide or self-inflicted injuries

biologicals (bī-o-loj′ĭ-kəls)—relating to life or living organisms

Guidelines for assigning E codes apply to various providers, including hospitals, outpatient clinics, emergency departments (EDs), other ambulatory care settings, providers' offices, and **nonacute** care settings, except when other specific guidelines apply. There are several different types of guidelines relating to E codes from the Official Guidelines for Coding and Reporting (■ TABLE 8-1). We will first review general coding guidelines for E codes and then review each guideline for specific situations.

nonacute (non-ə-kūt′)—not having a sudden onset, sharp rise, or short course

GENERAL CODING GUIDELINES FOR E CODES

Refer to the following guidelines when you are assigning E codes to patients' records.

1. Assign E codes from categories E800–E999 with any code in the range of 001–V91 for an injury, poisoning, or adverse effect from an external cause. You may also assign an activity E code (categories E001–E030) with any code from 001–V91 to represent situations when an activity caused or contributed to a condition.

2. Only assign an E code to the patient's *initial* encounter, not to subsequent encounters involving treatment for the same injury or illness.

3. Assign as many E codes as necessary to fully explain each cause of illness or injury, including an E code for the place of occurrence.

4. Select E codes from the Index to External Causes, located after the Alphabetic Index to diseases. Cross-reference E codes to their supplementary classification in the Tabular List, and be sure to follow any Includes and Excludes notes in the Tabular List.

5. Do not assign an E code as a principal (first-listed) diagnosis.

6. Do not assign E code(s) with **systemic inflammatory response syndrome (SIRS)** (995.9).

7. When a patient has multiple external causes of injuries, assign an E code for each external cause of injury. Refer to the Official Guidelines (Section I. C. 19.) for the order in which to assign multiple external causes of injuries involving abuse, terrorism, catastrophic events, and transport accidents, beginning with the most serious injury as the first-listed E code.

8. If the provider's practice management software allows only one E code to be reported, report the E code for the cause or intent that is most related to the first-listed diagnosis. Now, let's now review guidelines for assigning E codes to specific situations.

1. Place of Occurrence

The *place of occurrence* describes the place *where* the event occurred, *not* the patient's activity at the time of the event. Code from category E849 to describe the place of occurrence *in addition* to the E code for the cause of the injury or illness. Examples of places of occurrence include home, farm, cinema, beach, market, office, parking lot, and many others. Refer to category E849 in the Tabular to review options for place of occurrence.

Main Term(s): Accident, subterm *occurring*

Refer to the following example to assign E codes for an accident and the place where it occurred.

> **Example:** Emma Patterson, an 88-year-old, arrives at Williton Medical Center's ED because she fell out of bed in her hotel room. Her husband called the ambulance to transport her because she was in pain and unable to walk. Dr. Mills, the emergency physician, diagnoses Mrs. Patterson with a **closed fracture** of the **pubis** and contacts an orthopedic surgeon to discuss further **orthopedic** treatment.
>
> For Mrs. Patterson's encounter, assign the code for the pubic fracture as the first-listed code, then assign two E codes: the type of fall and the place of occurrence.
>
> For the first-listed code, search the Index for the main term *fracture* and subterm *pubis*, and cross-reference code 808.2 to the Tabular. When you are coding fractures, always assume that the fracture is closed (skin not broken) unless the documentation states that it is open (breaks the skin). Next, assign the E code for the type of fall by searching the Index to External Causes for the main term *fall*, connecting word *from*, and subterm *bed*, and cross-reference code E884.4 to the Tabular (■ FIGURE 8-2).
>
> The last code that you will need to assign is for the *place of occurrence*, which was a hotel. Search the Index to External Causes for the main term *accident*, subterm *occurring*, and subterm *hotel*, and cross-reference code E849.6 to the Tabular (■ FIGURE 8-3).
>
> Final code assignment for this case is 808.2 (fracture), E884.4 (fall from bed), and E849.6 (accident in a hotel).

2. Adverse Effects, Poisonings, and Toxic Effects

Recall that the Table of Drugs and Chemicals is part of the Alphabetic Index, listed in Section 2 (■ FIGURE 8-4). Turn to the Table to become more familiar with the information shown. Use the Table of Drugs and Chemicals to find codes for poisonings, adverse effects of drugs, medicinal and biological substances, and toxic effects. The Table of Drugs and Chemicals contains an alphabetical list of names of drugs and chemicals, along with their corresponding codes.

Do not code directly from the Table of Drugs and Chemicals. Always cross-reference codes to the Tabular List. Did you notice that the Table of Drugs and Chemicals also

---

Sidebar definitions:

systemic inflammatory response syndrome (SIRS) (sis-tem′ik in-flam′-ə-tōr-ē)—also called sepsis; severe illness in which bacteria invade the bloodstream

closed fracture (frak′chər)—break in a bone that does not puncture the skin

pubis (pu′bis)—one of the three sections of the hip bone

orthopedic (ôr-thu pě′dik)—pertaining to treatment of skeletal disorders

Figure 8-2 ■ Index to External Causes entry for fall from bed with E884.4 cross-referenced to the Tabular.

Fall, falling (accidental) E888.9
  from, off
      aircraft (at landing, take-off) (in-transit) (while alighting, boarding) E843
          resulting from accident to aircraft - see categories E840-E842
      animal (in sport or transport) E828
      animal-drawn vehicle E827
      balcony E882
      bed E884.4

4th **E884**	**Other fall from one level to another**

E884.0 Fall from playground equipment
Excludes: recreational machinery (E919.8)

E884.1 Fall from cliff

E884.2 Fall from chair

E884.3 Fall from wheelchair
    Fall from motorized mobility scooter
    Fall from motorized wheelchair

E884.4 Fall from bed

Figure 8-3 ■ Index entry for hotel as the place of occurrence with E849.6 cross-referenced to the Tabular.

Accident (to) E928.9

  occurring (at) (in)

    hotel E849.6

PLACE OF OCCURRENCE (E849)

Note: The following category is for use to denote the place where the injury or poisoning occurred.

E849.6 Public building
      Building (including adjacent grounds) used by the general public or by a
          particular group of the public, such as:
          airport
          bank
          cafe
          casino
          church
          cinema
          clubhouse
          courthouse
          dance hall
          garage building (for car storage)
          hotel

ICD-9-CM Table of Drugs and Chemicals (FY10)

Substance	Poisoning	Accident	Therapeutic Use	Suicide Attempt	Assault	Undetermined
Antidepressants	969.00	E854.0	E939.0	E950.3	E962.0	E980.3
monoamine oxidase inhibitors (MAOI)	969.01	E854.0	E939.0	E950.3	E962.0	E980.3
specified type NEC	969.09	E854.0	E939.0	E950.3	E962.0	E980.3
SSNRI (selective serotonin and norepinephrine reuptake inhibitors)	969.02	E854.0	E939.0	E950.3	E962.0	E980.3
SSRI (selective serotonin reuptake inhibitors)	969.03	E854.0	E939.0	E950.3	E962.0	E980.3
tetracyclic	969.04	E854.0	E939.0	E950.3	E962.0	E980.3
tricyclic	969.05	E854.0	E939.0	E950.3	E962.0	E980.3
Antidiabetic agents	962.3	E858.0	E932.3	E950.4	E962.0	E980.4
Antidiarrheal agents	973.5	E858.4	E943.5	E950.4	E962.0	E980.4
Antidiuretic hormone	962.5	E858.0	E932.5	E950.4	E962.0	E980.4

Figure 8-4 ■ Table of Drugs and Chemicals from the Index.

contains E codes showing reasons for adverse effects, poisonings, and toxic effects? Here are the categories of E codes from the Table of Drugs and Chemicals:

- *Accidental poisoning (E850–E869)*—injury or poisoning caused by an accidental drug overdose, wrong substance given or taken, drug taken inadvertently, or drugs given to patients during medical and surgical procedures
- *Therapeutic use (E930–E949)*—injury or poisoning caused by a substance correctly prescribed and properly administered in therapeutic or prophylactic dosage (example: a patient having an adverse reaction to a medication that his physician prescribed)
- *Suicide attempt (E950–E952)*—injury or poisoning that is self-inflicted
- *Assault (E961–E962)*—injury or poisoning inflicted by another person with the intent to injure or kill
- *Undetermined (E980–E982)*—unknown whether the poisoning or injury was intentional or accidental (rarely assigned)

The properties of certain drugs, medicinal and biological substances, or combinations of substances may cause toxic reactions. ICD-9-CM classifies drug toxicity into three categories that we will review next: adverse effects, poisonings, and toxic effects.

Adverse Effects (E930–E949)

An **adverse effect**, also called an adverse reaction or side effect, occurs when a patient's drug or medicinal and biological substance is correctly prescribed and properly administered, but the patient has an adverse reaction to it. Some adverse reactions occur **systemically** or only in a certain body site or system. Adverse effects can occur when a patient

- has a disease that affects the way the patient's body absorbs a drug.
- takes more than one prescribed drug simultaneously, which can cause a specific reaction.
- is allergic to a drug.
- has any other factors that change the way the body **metabolizes** a drug.

To code for adverse effects of a drug:

1. Code first the reaction to the drug, such as respiratory failure or nausea and vomiting.

systemically (sis-tem′ik lē)—affecting the entire body or organism

metabolizes (mě tab′ō līzs)—chemical processes by which cells produce the substances and energy needed to sustain life

2. Assign an *additional E code* (E930–E949) to identify the substance that caused the patient's condition and the reason for it (therapeutic use). You can find the these E codes in the Table of Drugs and Chemicals under the Therapeutic Use column.

If the patient has other conditions that affect the encounter, then assign additional codes for them. Remember to always assign the E code last. Refer to the following example for coding an adverse effect of a drug.

> **Example:** Mr. Morgan, a 43-year-old established patient, sees Dr. Hoffman because of the problems he is having when he takes prochlorperazine, a medication to treat his anxiety. Mr. Morgan developed nausea after taking the prescribed amount of the medicine, and after discussing the situation with him, Dr. Hoffman writes a prescription for a different drug.
>
> Codes to assign for this encounter are 787.02 (nausea—reaction to the drug), 300.00 (anxiety—the reason the patient took the drug), and E939.1 (therapeutic use of prochlorperazine).
>
> To find the E code, locate *prochlorperazine* in the Table of Drugs and Chemicals. Then go to the column for Therapeutic Use and cross-reference code E939.1 to the Tabular (■ FIGURE 8-5).

ICD-9-CM Table of Drugs and Chemicals (FY10)

Substance	Poisoning	Accident	Therapeutic Use	Suicide Attempt	Assault	Undetermined
Prochlorperazine	969.1	E853.0	E939.1	E950.3	E962.0	E980.3

4th E939   Psychotropic agents

E939.0 Antidepressants
Amitriptyline
Imipramine
Monoamine oxidase [MAO] inhibitors

E939.1 Phenothiazine-based tranquilizers
Chlorpromazine
Fluphenazine
Phenothiazine
Prochlorperazine
Promazine

Figure 8-5 ■ Therapeutic Use of Prochlorperazine in the Table of Drugs and Chemicals with E839.1 cross-referenced to the Tabular.

Poisonings   A **poisoning** occurs when a drug, medicinal substance, or biological substance that is not properly prescribed or correctly administered causes the patient to experience a reaction. Poisonings can occur for many reasons:

- taking the incorrect dose of a prescribed drug, sometimes because a provider gave the incorrect dose
- taking a nonprescription medication with a prescribed medication
- taking an illegal drug
- using a prescribed medication with alcohol
- intentionally overdosing on a drug

Poisonings (960–979) indicate that the dose, patient, substance, or route of administration was incorrect, while adverse effects indicate that the dose, patient, substance, or route of administration was correct (therapeutic use) but the patient had a bad reaction to the drug. To code poisonings, you still need to reference the Table of Drugs and Chemicals, but you will use it differently than when you code for adverse effects. Assign poisoning codes in the following order:

1. First, code the drug poisoning. (Use the Poisoning column in the Table of Drugs and Chemicals.)
2. Assign an additional code for the patient's condition that the poisoning caused.
3. Last, assign an E code for the reason that caused the poisoning. You should never assign an E code from the Therapeutic Use column for a poisoning, as these codes are reserved for adverse effects. It is important to note that not all providers assign an E code for poisonings.

Refer to the following example for coding a poisoning.

Example: Natalie Richardson, a 28-year-old, presents to Washington Bryant's ED because of confusion and nausea she experienced after taking her antidepressant medication. Her husband accompanies her. Dr. Quinn, the ED physician, determines after discussion with the patient's husband that Mrs. Richardson had incorrectly taken double doses of the drug, which caused her reactions. Mrs. Richardson undergoes **gastric lavage** and receives **intravenous (IV)** fluids and continuous monitoring.

Codes for this encounter include: 969.00 (antidepressant poisoning), 298.9 (confusion), 787.02 (nausea), and E854.0 (accidental poisoning). Refer to ■ FIGURE 8-6 to review both the poisoning code and the E code from the Table of Drugs and Chemicals to cross-reference to the Tabular.

gastric lavage (gas′trik lah-vahzh′)—procedure that empties stomach contents

intravenous (IV) (in-trə-ve′nəs)—administered into a vein

ICD-9-CM Table of Drugs and Chemicals (FY10)

Substance	Poisoning	Accident	Therapeutic Use	Suicide Attempt	Assault	Undetermined
Antidepressants	969.00	E854.0	E939.0	E950.3	E962.0	E980.3

Figure 8-6 ■ Antidepressant poisoning and E code in the Table of Drugs and Chemicals.

Toxic Effects   A **toxic effect** occurs when a patient ingests or is exposed to a harmful substance, such as alcohol, gasoline, acid, lead, carbon monoxide, pesticides, or detergents. ICD-9-CM classifies toxic effect codes to categories 980–989, and you can find codes for toxic effects in the Table of Drugs and Chemicals. When a patient experiences a toxic effect from a substance, assign codes in the following order:

1. First, code the toxic substance. (Use the Poisoning column in the Table of Drugs and Chemicals.)
2. Assign a secondary code for the patient's condition that the toxic substance caused.
3. Last, assign an additional E code that shows the intent of the toxic effect.

Example: A grandmother brings her 2-year-old grandson to the local hospital's ED because he accidentally ingested isopropyl (rubbing) alcohol. The child is experiencing abdominal pain and lethargy (tiredness). The physician and other clinical staff assess and treat the patient.

Codes for this encounter are 980.2 (toxic substance), 789.00 (abdominal pain—condition resulting from the toxic effect), 780.79 (lethargy—condition resulting from the toxic effect), and E860.3 (intent—accidental). You can find both the code for the isopropyl alcohol (toxic substance) and the E code for intent in the Table of Drugs and Chemicals (■ FIGURE 8-7).

ICD-9-CM Table of Drugs and Chemicals (FY11)

Substance	Poisoning	Accident	Therapeutic Use	Suicide Attempt	Assault	Undetermined
Alcohol	980.9	E860.9		E950.9	E962.1	E980.9
absolute	980.0	E860.1		E950.9	E962.1	E980.9
beverage	980.0	E860.0	E947.8	E950.9	E962.1	E980.9
amyl	980.3	E860.4		E950.9	E962.1	E980.9
antifreeze	980.1	E860.2		E950.9	E962.1	E980.9
butyl	980.3	E860.4	—	E950.9	E962.1	E980.9
dehydrated	980.0	E860.1	—	E950.9	E862.1	E980.9
beverage	980.0	E860.0	E947.8	E950.9	E962.1	E980.9
denatured	980.0	E860.1		E950.9	E962.1	E980.9
deterrents	977.3	E858.8	E947.3	E950.4	E962.0	E980.4
diagnostic (gastric function)	977.8	E858.8	E947.8	E950.4	E962.0	E980.4
ethyl	980.0	E860.1		E950.9	E962.1	E980.9
beverage	980.0	E860.0	E947.8	E950.9	E962.1	E980.9
grain	980.0	E860.1		E950.9	E962.1	E980.9
beverage	980.0	E860.0	E947.8	E950.9	E962.1	E980.9
industrial	980.9	E860.9		E950.9	E962.1	E980.9
isopropyl	980.2	E860.3		E950.9	E962.1	E980.9

4th **980** **Toxic effect of alcohol**

980.0 Ethyl alcohol
　　Denatured alcohol
　　Ethanol
　　Grain alcohol

Use additional code to identify any associated:
　acute alcohol intoxication (305.0)
　　in alcoholism (303.0)
　drunkenness (simple) (305.0)
　pathological (291.4)

980.1 Methyl alcohol
　　Methanol
　　Wood alcohol

980.2 Isopropyl alcohol
　　Dimethyl carbinol
　　Isopropanol
　　Rubbing alcohol

Figure 8-7 ■ Toxic effect and E code from the Table of Drugs and Chemicals, cross-referenced to the Tabular.

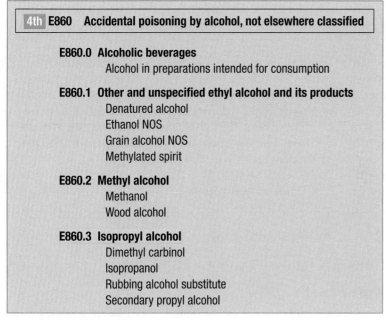

4th	**E860**	**Accidental poisoning by alcohol, not elsewhere classified**

E860.0 Alcoholic beverages
Alcohol in preparations intended for consumption

E860.1 Other and unspecified ethyl alcohol and its products
Denatured alcohol
Ethanol NOS
Grain alcohol NOS
Methylated spirit

E860.2 Methyl alcohol
Methanol
Wood alcohol

E860.3 Isopropyl alcohol
Dimethyl carbinol
Isopropanol
Rubbing alcohol substitute
Secondary propyl alcohol

Figure 8-7 ■ *continued*

TAKE A BREAK

Let's take a break and then practice assigning codes using the Table of Drugs and Chemicals.

Exercise 8.1   **Place of Occurrence, Adverse Effects, Poisonings, and Toxic Effects**

Instructions: Assign diagnosis codes, including poisoning codes and E codes, to the following patient cases, using the Index, the Tabular, and the Table of Drugs and Chemicals.

1. Dr. Hoffman treats new patient Wayne Virgil for a skin rash that he developed after he took an initial dose of penicillin, an antibiotic that was correctly prescribed to him.

   Code(s): _____

2. Dr. Mills treats Carlos Kern in Williton Medical Center's ED for intoxication with delirium from digitalis glycosides (a medication to regulate heartbeat), which the patient took as prescribed.

   Code(s): _____

3. Ralph Vargas drives himself to the Williton Medical Center ED for sudden onset of shortness of breath. Dr. Mills diagnoses him with an allergic reaction to penicillin. His physician prescribed the penicillin in error because he overlooked the note in the chart about Mr. Virgil's penicillin allergy.

   Code(s): _____

4. Leah Farwell's sister finds her unconscious in her home. She calls 911 for an ambulance, which transports her to Williton's ED. Ms. Farwell took a number of heroin shots and is experiencing atrial fibrillation (irregular, rapid heartbeat). Dr. Mills documents that the patient accidentally overdosed on heroin.

   Code(s): _____

5. A coworker finds Rodney Huss, a mechanic, unconscious but alive in the garage where he works. Mr. Huss left a suicide note on the garage floor. An ambulance transports him to Williton. Dr. Mills diagnoses the patient with carbon monoxide poisoning and administers treatment.

   Code(s): _____

6. On her day off, Sue Burrus, age 28, is at home stripping wood furniture inside on a rainy day. She gets a severe headache and begins vomiting after breathing in the fumes of the chemical she was using to strip the furniture. She calls her neighbor, who takes her to Williton's ED. Dr. Mills diagnoses her with acetone toxicity from chemical fumes.

   Code(s): _____

WORKPLACE IQ

You are working as a medical assistant for Dr. Gupta, a family care physician. Part of your job involves comparing medical documentation in the patient's record to the information on the patient's encounter form. You also check patients in at the front desk. Mrs. Arnold arrives for an appointment today with her husband. While he is taking out his insurance card for you to copy, Mr. Arnold tells you that his wife hurt her ankle when she fell down the basement stairs at their house.

Later, when you are reviewing the chart documentation, you notice that Dr. Gupta stated that Mrs. Arnold suffered an ankle sprain from a fall, but he did not document any other information about the fall. You know how and where the fall occurred, because Mr. Arnold told you, and you could easily find E codes for the type of accident and place of occurrence.

What would you do?

3. Child and Adult Abuse

Child and adult abuse can be either intentional or accidental. First, assign a code for the patient's condition. When the cause of an injury or neglect is *intentional*, next assign an E code from E960–E968—*Homicide and injury purposely inflicted by other persons* as the first-listed E code (main term *assault* or *neglect*). Assign an additional code to identify the perpetrator of abuse from category E967— *Child and adult battering and other maltreatment* (main term *abuse*).

In cases of *accidental* neglect, assign E904.0—*Abandonment or neglect of infant and helpless person* as the first-listed E code (main term *abandonment*).

4. Unknown or Suspected Intent, Undetermined Cause

If the *intent* (accident, suicide attempt, assault) of the cause of an injury or poisoning is *unknown, unspecified, questionable, probable, or suspected*, then code the intent as *undetermined* E980–E989. You should assign these codes only as a last resort when the physician did not document the intent in the patient's record.

When you know the intent of an injury or poisoning but do not know the *cause*, assign one of the following codes:

- E928.9—Unspecified accident
- E958.9—Suicide and self-inflicted injury by unspecified means
- E968.9—Assault by unspecified means

You should only assign these codes in rare instances because providers should document the cause in the patient's record.

Remember to first assign a code(s) for the patient's condition before assigning an E code.

5. Late Effects of External Cause

In Chapter 4, you learned that a late effect is a residual condition that remains after the acute phase of an illness has passed, such as facial paralysis after a stroke. We also reviewed how to code late effects. There are also late effects that appear after an injury or poisoning occurred. ICD-9-CM does not set a time limit for coding late effects of external causes. If the patient's late effect is due to a previous injury or poisoning, then assign a code for the patient's condition first, and assign an E code for the late effect second. (There are no late-effect E codes for adverse effects.) To find an E code for a late effect, search the Index to External Causes under the main term *late effect of* (■ FIGURE 8-8).

Figure 8-8 ■ Late effects in the Index to External Causes.

Late effect of
  accident NEC (accident classifiable to E928.9) E929.9
    specified NEC (accident classifiable to E910-E928.8) E929.8
  assault E969
  fall, accidental (accident classifiable to E880-E888) E929.3
  fire, accident caused by (accident classifiable to E890-E899) E929.4
  homicide, attempt (any means) E969
  injury due to terrorism E999.1

Do not assign a late-effect E code if the patient's encounter is for a *current* injury or poisoning. You can also assign a late-effect E code for subsequent visits when the physician treats a late effect of the initial injury or poisoning.

TAKE A BREAK

Let's take a break and then practice assigning more E codes.

Exercise 8.2   Child and Adult Abuse, Unknown or Suspected Intent, Undetermined Cause, and Late Effects of External Cause

Instructions: Assign diagnosis codes, including E codes and poisoning codes, to the following patient cases, using both the Index and the Tabular. Each coding problem requires multiple codes. Refer to the main terms previously outlined for assistance locating codes.

1. Four-year-old Megan Salvador's grandmother brings her to Williton's ED for evaluation after her mother severely beat her. Dr. Mills diagnoses Megan with severe contusions to the face, back, and arms. He also reports the abuse to local police.

   Code(s): _____

2. A neighbor takes Alan Lemke, age 89, to Williton's ED for treatment of a left broken arm. His adult daughter became frustrated while caring for him and hit him with his cane. Dr. Mills reviews the patient's X-rays, which show that the shaft of the right radius has a greenstick fracture. He contacts local police to file a report of elder abuse against the patient's daughter.

   Code(s): _____

3. Mrs. Miles brings Laurie Miles, age 5, to Williton's ED for a gunshot wound to the leg after her 9-year-old brother shot her with their father's police revolver. It is unclear whether the shooting was intentional or accidental.

   Code(s): _____

4. Leah Farwell sees her cardiologist, Dr. Woods, for treatment of arrhythmia. Dr. Woods documents that the arrhythmia is a late effect of the patient's accidental heroin overdose.

   Code(s): _____

5. Dr. Grisham, an orthopedist, treats established patient, Steve Earnest, age 28, for low back pain, which is a late effect of an auto accident that happened three years ago.

   Code(s): _____

6. Mrs. Silvers brings her son Johnny, age 18 months, to Williton's emergency department after she found him unconscious. She also found an open whiskey bottle next to him.

   Code(s): _____

6. Misadventures and Complications of Care

Misadventure means mistake. A **medical misadventure** can be any problem that a patient develops that a physician or other clinician caused, either directly (through hands-on care) or indirectly (through failure to react to a patient's concerns or symptoms). Refer to the examples that follow for a better understanding of medical misadventures.

Example 1: A patient had abdominal surgery, and the physician and operating room staff failed to realize that a surgical instrument remained in the patient's body. The physician sutured the patient's wound closed. Later, the patient suffered from internal punctures and ruptured blood vessels.

psychiatrist (sə-kī′-ə-trəst)—a physician specializing in the diagnosis and treatment of mental disorders

Example 2: A patient visits a **psychiatrist** to treat her depression and anxiety. The physician prescribes medication for the patient to take twice a day and asks her to follow up with him in two months. Several days later, the patient calls the physician to report breathing problems. He tells her not to worry and says that he will see her at her next appointment. Later, the patient's breathing becomes so difficult that she is near death and spends several days in the hospital recovering.

Example 3: A patient needs cataract surgery on his left eye. He is prepped for surgery, and the physician mistakenly performs the surgery on the opposite eye.

The E code range of E870–E876 is for misadventures that the provider *documents as misadventures* in the patient's record. In other words, you cannot assume that a misadventure occurred simply by reading the circumstances of the patient's encounter. The physician or other clinician must specifically document that the patient's condition resulted from the provider's lack of or improper care. To code misadventures, search under the main term *misadventure(s)*.

Assign a code from category E878 or E879 if the provider documents the patient's abnormal reaction to or complication from a surgical or medical procedure but does not mention misadventure as the cause. Turn to these categories of codes in your ICD-9-CM manual to become more familiar with them.

7. Terrorism

When the Federal Bureau of Investigation (FBI) identifies the cause of an injury as **terrorism** (not suspected terrorism), the first-listed E code should be a code from category E979—*Terrorism* (main term *terrorism*). You can find the FBI's definition of terrorism in the note under category E979 (■ FIGURE 8-9). When you assign a code from E979, do not assign additional E codes from assault categories.

Assign code E979.9—*Terrorism, secondary effects* when the patient's condition develops after a terrorist event, not during the event.

8. Activity Codes

Assign an **activity code** from category E001–E030 to describe the activity that caused or contributed to the injury or other health condition, such as walking, running, sports, building and construction, and food preparation. Activity codes are not applicable to poisonings, adverse effects, misadventures, or late effects. Assign activity codes as *secondary E codes* to provide additional information, unless there are no other E codes applicable to the patient's situation. Search for the main term *activity* in the E code Index to see a list of activity choices.

E979	Terrorism
	Injuries resulting from the unlawful use of force or violence against persons or property to intimidate or coerce a Government, the civilian population, or any segment thereof, in furtherance of political or social objective

Figure 8-9 ■ The definition of terrorism under category E979.

9. External Cause Status

Category E000 is for **external cause status**, which represents the *work status* or *recreational status* of the patient at the time the injury occurred. Assign a code from category E000 *External cause status* in *addition to* any other E code that you assign for an encounter, including E codes for activities, transport accidents, and falls. Do not assign a code from category E000 along with an E code for poisonings, adverse effects, misadventures, or late effects. Codes from category E000 cannot stand alone, so you should only assign them when you are assigning another E code that represents the cause of the patient's injury. Turn to your ICD-9-CM manual and locate external cause status codes under the main term *external cause status*.

Now you have finished learning guidelines for assigning E codes. Next you will learn how to code different types of injuries.

TAKE A BREAK

Let's take a break and then practice assigning more E codes.

Exercise 8.3 **Misadventures and Complications of Care, Terrorism, Activity Codes, and External Cause Status**

Instructions: Assign diagnosis codes, including E codes, to the following patient cases, using both the Index and the Tabular. Refer to the main terms previously outlined for assistance locating codes.

1. Nathan Dowdell, age 16, sees Dr. Grisham, an orthopedic surgeon, for a new shoulder injury. Dr. Grisham diagnoses a full-thickness tear of the left rotator cuff capsule, which happened while Nathan was pitching a baseball.

   Code(s): _____

2. Jose Whittaker, age 72, reports to outpatient surgery for removal of a senile cortical cataract on his left eye. Clinicians prep him for surgery, but his physician mistakenly performs the surgery on the opposite eye.

   Code(s): _____

3. In 2001, Dr. Hoffman treated Gerald Fitts, age 27, for anthrax exposure during the domestic terrorism scares. What codes would you have assigned for his encounter?

   Code(s): _____

4. Dr. Grisham treats Bryan Woody, an established patient, for adhesive capsulitis (inflammation of tissue surrounding the shoulder joint). The condition is a late effect of a gradual onset rotator cuff (muscles and tendons connecting the arm to the shoulder joint) tear from an injury he sustained while in the military.

   Code(s): _____

5. Assign only the external cause status and activity codes for the following case that you already coded earlier in the chapter: On her day off, Sue Burrus, age 28, is at home stripping wood furniture inside on a rainy day. She gets a severe headache and begins vomiting after breathing in the fumes of the chemical she was using on the furniture. She calls her neighbor who takes her to Williton's ED. Dr. Mills diagnoses her with acetone toxicity from chemical fumes.

   Code(s): _____

6. Dr. Hoffman treats an established patient, Dennis Doss, age 79, for monoplegia (paralysis of a single limb) of his left leg (his dominant side), which is a late effect of a previous surgery when the physician mistakenly punctured the patient's leg. This information is documented in the patient's record.

   Code(s): _____

GUIDELINES FOR CODING INJURIES

You already learned how to assign E codes for external causes of injuries. Now let's discuss how to assign codes for the specific injuries, which may or may not involve assigning additional E codes. Patients can have many different kinds of injuries, including injuries that cause temporary or permanent damage to organs, tissues, arteries, veins, or bones. Injuries can be the result of accidents (external causes), but they do not have to be. Because there are numerous injury types, you will not learn how to code all of them in this chapter, but you will learn how to assign codes for the most common injuries, including fractures, dislocations, sprains and strains, open wounds, superficial injuries, and burns. For these injuries, assign codes from Chapter 17—Injury and Poisoning (800–999) of the Tabular List, and assign any applicable E codes. Referring to Chapter 17 will help you become more familiar with injury types. You can also review guidelines for coding injuries not covered in this chapter in the Official Guidelines for Coding and Reporting.

Fractures (800–829)

Fractures, also called traumatic fractures, are broken bones that can occur for many different reasons: trauma, such as a fall or an auto accident; an underlying disease or condition, such as osteoporosis; or repeated stress to a bone, such as through gymnastics exercises. It is important to know the differences among *traumatic* (related to an injury or wound), *pathologic* (caused by disease) and *stress* fractures (due to continued stress on a bone) because the codes are different for each type of fracture.

Patients with fractures experience pain, swelling, numbness, bleeding, and paralysis, which can vary according to the type of fracture. Depending on how the bone is broken, fractures can be **displaced, nondisplaced, transverse,** or **oblique.** Physicians diagnose fractures from exams, X-rays, and other radiology tests. Physicians repair fractures using various methods, depending on the severity of the fracture, including **casts, splints, straps,** *open reduction* (a repair when skin is broken) and *closed reduction* (a repair when skin is closed). You will learn more about these procedures in Chapter 17 when you assign procedure codes for these services.

Traumatic fractures are included in categories 800–829. When you are coding for fractures, search the Index for the main term *fracture* and then search subterms for the *body site* where the fracture occurred. You can find the fracture site in the physician's documentation and/or radiology test results documented in the record. Always query the physician if you need clarification.

To code the fracture, you also need to determine if the patient has an *open fracture,* also called a compound fracture (when the fractured bone breaks through the skin) (■ FIGURE 8-10), or a *closed fracture,* also called a simple fracture (when the fractured bone does not break through the skin).

There are several different types of both open and closed fractures. The physician may specifically state in the patient's medical documentation that a fracture is open or closed. Or the physician may only list the *type* of fracture, and you will need to know which type is open or closed (■ TABLE 8-2).

---

displaced (dis plās′d)—moved from the usual or proper place

nondisplaced—in the normal location and alignment

transverse (trans-vərs′)—lying across the long axis of the body or of a part

oblique (o-blēk′)—situated in a slanting position

casts (kasts)—rigid casings used to prevent movement of diseased or broken body parts

splints (splĭnts)—rigid devices used to prevent motion of a fractured joint

straps (străpz)—strips or pieces of overlapping adhesive plaster

---

Figure 8-10 ■ Compound fracture.

Photo credit: © Robert Malota / Dreamstime.com.

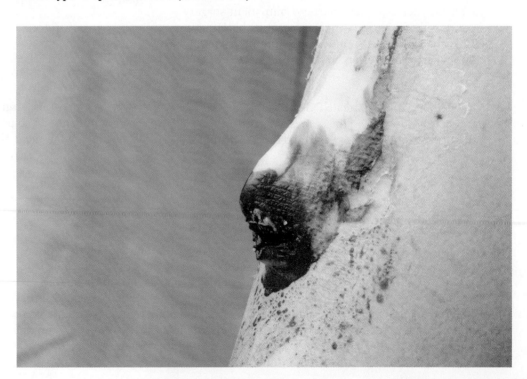

■ TABLE 8-2   **FRACTURE TYPES AND DEFINITIONS**

Closed Fracture Types	Definition
comminuted (■ Figure 8-11)	splinters or crushes the bone into numerous pieces
depressed	forms an indentation that is sunk below the surrounding area
elevated	rises above the surrounding area
fissured	extends partially through a bone, with no displacement of the bony fragments
greenstick (■ Figure 8-12)	bends the bone for an incomplete fracture
impacted	drives one fragment into another portion of the same bone or into an adjacent bone
linear	runs in a line
simple	does not break through the skin, also called closed
slipped **epiphysis**	shows slippage of the end of a long bone
spiral	runs around the axis of the bone

Open Fracture Types	Definition
compound	breaks through the skin, also called open
infected	has been invaded by disease-causing microorganisms
missile	was caused by a projectile, such as a bullet or a piece of shrapnel
puncture	pierces the skin
with foreign body	contains an external object

comminuted (kom′ĭ-noot′əd)

fissured (fish′ərd)

epiphysis (ə-pif′ə-sis)

You should assume that a fracture is closed if the physician *does not* document the type of fracture or specify whether the fracture is open or closed. Refer to the example listed next for coding a fracture.

Example: Jason Bell, a 12-year-old, presents to Williton Medical Center's ED for a tibial shaft fracture. His mother accompanies him. The ED physician examines Jason and orders an X-ray before starting treatment.

Because there is no documentation stating whether the fracture is open or closed, code it as closed. ■ FIGURE 8-13 shows the Index entry for tibial shaft fracture, with code 823.20 cross-referenced to the Tabular.

Multiple Fractures   When a patient has multiple fractures, assign a code for each fracture. Sequence multiple fractures in the order of their severity, assigning a code for the most severe fracture first, based on medical documentation. Code each fracture separately unless the ICD-9-CM guidelines provide different instructions, or you can assign a combination code for multiple fractures (main term *fracture*, subterm *multiple*). Assign combination codes when

- There is insufficient documentation in the medical record detailing each fracture and its location.
- The provider's computer software for reporting coding statistics does not have room to list multiple codes, so you must assign a combination code.
- ICD-9-CM does not provide enough specificity at the fourth-digit or fifth-digit level, so you must choose a combination code.

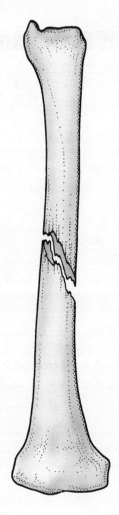

Figure 8-11 ■ Comminuted fracture.

Source: Doring Kindersley.

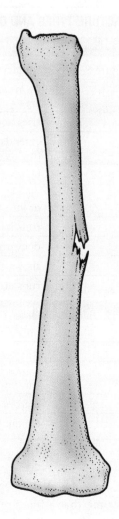

Figure 8-12 ■ Greenstick fracture.

Source: Doring Kindersley.

Figure 8-13 ■ Index entry for tibial shaft fracture with 823.20 cross-referenced to the Tabular.

Fracture (abduction) (adduction) (avulsion) (compression) (crush) (dislocation) (oblique) (separation) (closed) 829.0

tibia (closed) 823.80

shaft 823.20
with fibula 823.22
open 823.32

4th	823	Fracture of tibia and fibula

The following fifth-digit subclassification is for use with category 823:
0 tibia alone
1 fibula alone
2 fibula with tibia

5th **823.2 Shaft, closed**
[0-2]

POINTERS FROM THE PROS: Interview with a Referral Specialist

Patrick Gaudio works as a primary care check-in referral specialist for a large physician group. He registers patients and coordinates the insurance referral process, following insurances' procedures for referring patients to other providers for lab and radiology tests. Mr. Gaudio assigns diagnosis codes to test orders, ensuring that diagnoses meet the conditions of medical necessity before the test is performed.

What interests you the most about the job that you perform?

Patient interaction. I try to give every patient at least one minute worth of personal time so as to make them feel important.

What are the most challenging aspects of your job?

Multitasking and being able to handle a very large patient turnover at a quick rate.

What advice can you give to coding students to help them to prepare to work successfully in the healthcare field?

Be willing to meet the subject matter with an open mind. What appears to be little more than a jumble of numbers is, indeed, a very important element of the healthcare industry.

(Used by permission of Patrick L. Gaudio.)

Turn to the Official Guidelines for additional instructions for coding multiple bilateral or unilateral fractures of the same limb or bone (Section I C 17b).

Fracture Aftercare and Complications Be sure not to confuse a patient's current fracture treatment with fracture *aftercare*. Examples of *current* treatment are surgery, emergency department encounter, and when a new physician evaluates and treats the patient. Code fractures using the *aftercare* codes (subcategories V54.0, V54.1, V54.8, or V54.9) for encounters when the patient already completed active treatment and now needs routine fracture care during the healing or recovery phase (main term *aftercare*). Examples of fracture aftercare are cast change or removal, removal of **external** or **internal fixation device**, medication adjustment, and follow up visit.

Assign separate codes when the patient has fracture complications, such as **malunion** and **nonunion**, during healing or recovery. Do not assign separate codes for superficial injuries (abrasions) if they are part of the fracture injury.

external fixation device (ek-stur′nəl fik-sa′shən də-vīs′)—device that stabilizes a body part, usually to keep fractured bones in alignment by attaching bones together with pins, rods, plates, or screws, which are attached to another device placed on the outside of the body, and adjusted to maintain position during and after healing

internal fixation device (in tərn′əl)—device inserted surgically to stabilize a body part, usually to keep fractured bones in alignment, attaching bones together with pins, rods, plates, or screws, which are not visible on the outside of the body.

TAKE A BREAK

Let's take a break and then review types of fractures and practice assigning codes for them.

Exercise 8.4   Coding Injuries: Fractures

Part 1—Theory

Instructions: Refer to Table 8-2 and complete each statement.

1. A closed fracture, which does not break the skin is also called a(n) _____ fracture.

2. A fracture that has been invaded by disease-causing organisms is called a(n) _____ fracture.

3. An incomplete fracture that bends the bone is called a(n) _____ fracture.

4. A bullet can cause a(n) _____ fracture.

5. A fracture that rises above the surrounding area is called a(n) _____ fracture.

6. A(n) _____ fracture contains a splintered bone.

Part 2—Coding

Instructions: Assign diagnosis codes, including E codes, to the following patient cases, using both the Index and the Tabular. Refer to Table 8-2 for fracture types.

1. Jessica Neill sees Dr. Hoffman for removal of a case, which Dr. Mills previously applied in Williton's emergency department.

   Code(s): _____

continued

TAKE A BREAK *continued*

2. Dr. Mills treats Vince Chenoweth, age 15, for a fractured right heel. Vince fell from the high bar while practicing gymnastics.

   Code(s): _____

3. Keith Cruz, a 27-year-old, arrives in Williton's ED with severe left leg pain. Dr. Mills diagnoses him with a compound fracture of the shaft of his left tibia.

   Code(s): _____

4. At Williton's ED, Dr. Mills diagnoses Delores Corder, a 34-year-old, with a Colles' fracture (radius fracture above the wrist) of her right wrist.

   Code(s): _____

5. Dr. Mills treats Ryan Loftis, age 45, in Williton's ED for an open fracture of the base of his skull with a subarachnoid (small cavity on the surface of the brain) hemorrhage. The patient was unconscious for 90 minutes after his injury, but then regained consciousness.

   Code(s): _____

6. Mrs. McCleary brings her mother, age 86, to Valley's Urgent Care Center for right hip pain and difficulty walking. Dr. Foster diagnoses the patient with a right hip fracture which osteoporosis caused.

   Code(s): _____

---

malunion (mal-ūn′yon)—incomplete or faulty joining of bones or tissues after a fracture or wound

nonunion failure of a fracture to heal

rheumatoid arthritis (roo′mə-toid ahr-thri′tis)—joint disease that causes pain, swelling, stiffness, and loss of joint functions

Dislocations (830–839)

A **dislocation** occurs when a bone or joint moves from its usual location. Dislocations cause pain, swelling, and the inability to move a joint. Falls, transport accidents, **rheumatoid arthritis**, joint disorders, and sports accidents can all cause dislocations. You may be familiar with a specific type of elbow dislocation that often occurs in early childhood, called Nursemaid's Elbow. It is a ligament tear that dislocates the upper end of the **radius**. It happens when someone pulls too hard on someone else's arm, causing pain and the inability to move the arm or elbow. Physicians treat Nursemaid's Elbow by returning the radius and ligament to their correct positions and applying a sling and ice. As the injury heals, pain decreases, and the elbow starts to function properly again.

Like fractures, dislocations can also be open or closed (■ Figure 8-14).

Figure 8-14 ■ Closed ankle dislocation.

Photo credit: BATES, M.D. / Custom Medical Stock Photo.

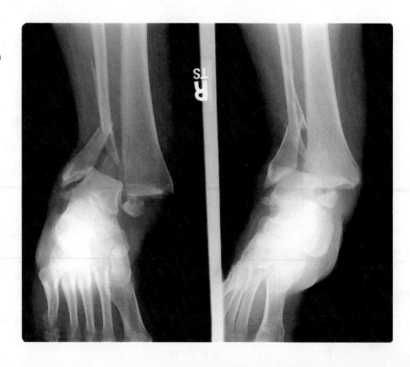

If the physician does not document whether the dislocation is open or closed, assume that it is closed. Physicians diagnose dislocations by performing exams and X-rays or other radiology tests. They treat dislocations with **manipulation**, splints, casts, or surgery. When you are assigning codes for dislocations, search the Index for the main term *dislocation*, then search subterms for the *body site* of the dislocation. You may need to further specify information about the body site, including whether the injury is **anterior, posterior, medial,** or **lateral.** Refer to the following example for coding a dislocation.

Example: Mary Richardson, a 35-year-old, arrives at Williton Medical Center's ED by ambulance. She is suffering from rib pain. The ED physician examines Ms. Richardson, reviews her X-ray, and determines that she has a dislocated rib.

Since the documentation does not specify whether the dislocation is open or closed, code it as closed. ■ FIGURE 8-15 shows the Index entry for dislocated rib, followed by the cross-reference of code 839.69 to the Tabular.

radius (ra′de-əs)—the bone on the thumb side of the human forearm

manipulation (mə-nip′u-la′shən)—process of moving or adjusting with the hands

anterior (an-tĕr′e-ər)—relating to the front surface of the body

posterior (pos-tĕr′e-ər)—situated at or toward the back side of the body

medial (me′de-əl)—lying or extending in the middle

lateral (lat′ər-əl)—relating to the side

Dislocation (articulation) (closed) (displacement) (simple) (subluxation) 839.8

Note "Closed" includes simple, complete, partial, uncomplicated, and unspecified dislocation.

"Open" includes dislocation specified as infected or compound and dislocation with foreign body.

"Chronic," "habitual," "old," or "recurrent" dislocations should be coded as indicated under the entry "Dislocation, recurrent"; and "pathological" as indicated under the entry "Dislocation, pathological."

For late effect of dislocation see Late, effect, dislocation.

    rib (cartilage) (closed) 839.69
        congenital 756.3
        open 839.79

| 4th | 839 | Other, multiple, and ill-defined dislocations |

| 5th | 839.6 | Other location, closed |

        839.61   Sternum
                  Sternoclavicular joint

        839.69   Other
                  Pelvis

Figure 8-15 ■ Index entry for rib dislocation with 839.69 cross-referenced to the Tabular.

Review the note listed under the main term *dislocation* for additional information about coding dislocations.

Sprains and Strains (840–848)

When you are coding for sprains and strains, it is important to remember that the terms are not interchangeable. A **sprain** is more serious than a strain. It is a sudden or violent twist or wrench of a joint, causing the stretching or tearing of connective tissue and often rupturing of blood vessels. Sprains to the wrist, knee, and ankle are the most

edema (ə-de′mə)—swelling or abnormal excess accumulation of fluid in cells, connective tissue, or body cavity

braces (brās-es)—appliances that support a movable body part in the correct position while allowing motion of the part

spasms (spaz′əms)—sudden involuntary contractions of a muscle or group of muscles

common. You may have heard of a sprained ankle, which can occur while playing sports or from a fall on ice, on stairs, or when walking on an irregular surface. The individual loses his balance, and his foot turns inward, stretching the ligaments. Patients with sprains experience **edema**, pain, bruising, and lack of movement. Physicians diagnose sprains by performing exams and radiology tests, and they treat them with ice, elevation, strapping, **braces**, splints, and pain medication. When coding sprains, locate the main term *sprain, strain* in the Index, and then search for the subterm of the *body site* affected.

A **strain** can occur to a person who is playing sports, exercising, or doing any activity. It involves bodily injury from excessive tension, effort, or use of muscles and tendons. You may have heard someone say that he "pulled a muscle," which refers to a strain, not a sprain. Common strains happen in the calves, thighs, shoulders, and lower back. Symptoms of strains include pain, soreness, weakness, **spasms**, and inability to have complete *range of motion* (movement at various angles) in the affected area. Physicians diagnose strains by conducting exams and sometimes by performing radiology tests. Treatment for strains includes rest, ice, elevation, pain medications, and compression by bandaging. To code a strain, search the Index for the main term *sprain, strain*, and then search subterms for the *body site* affected.

Open Wounds (870–897)

Open wounds, which involve broken skin, can encompass one or more layers of skin or go deeper into muscles, nerves, and organs. Once a patient's skin is broken, there is a greater chance of developing infection because the skin protects the body from many types of bacteria and disease.

Patients experience different symptoms from open wounds, including pain, swelling, bleeding, and infection. Wounds can occur from trauma, insect bites, stepping on a nail or other sharp object, or working with equipment and tools. Pressure ulcers, which you learned about in a previous chapter, also can lead to open wounds. Physicians treat open wounds in various ways, depending on the type and severity of the wound, including **debridement**, **sutures**, and **grafts**.

debridement (di-brēd′-mənt)—removal of damaged or contaminated tissue

sutures (soo′chərs)—surgical methods used to close a wound or join tissues with fine thread

grafts—to implant living tissue surgically

When you are coding open wounds, search the Index for the main term *wound, open*, and then search subterms for the *body site* affected. You can also locate open wounds by searching for the *type of wound* in the Index. Refer to ■ TABLE 8-3 for types of open wounds and their definitions.

ICD-9-CM also classifies wounds as complicated or without complications. A complicated wound has delayed healing or treatment, contains a foreign body, or is infected. If the patient suffers from an infection, be sure to assign a code for the infection, in addition to the code for the open wound.

■ TABLE 8-3   TYPES OF OPEN WOUNDS

Type of Open Wound	Definition
abrasion	rubbing or scraping of the surface layer of cells or tissue
amputation	surgical removal of all or part of a limb
avulsion (■ FIGURE 8-16)	tearing away of a body part
cut	opening or wound made by a sharp edge
incision	cut or wound of body tissue, especially in surgery
laceration	jagged wound or cut
penetrating	passing or piercing into or through the skin
perforating	making a hole through the skin
puncture	piercing the skin

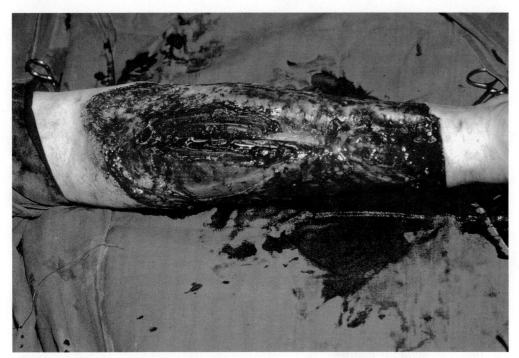

Figure 8-16 ■ Avulsion of a forearm draped for surgery. *Photo credit:* © SHOUT / Alamy.

TAKE A BREAK

Let's take a break and then practice assigning more codes for more injuries.

Exercise 8.5   Dislocations, Sprains and Strains, and Open Wounds

Instructions: Assign diagnosis codes, including E codes, to the following patient cases, using both the Index and the Tabular. Refer to the main terms previously outlined for assistance locating codes.

1. Dr. Burns, an emergency physician at Williton Medical Center, treats new patient Patrick Banks, a high school football player, age 16 for a tear of the left lateral meniscus (knee cartilage) in the anterior horn (front of the meniscus). Patrick sustained the tear when another football player tackled him during practice.

    Code(s): _____

2. Dr. Grisham, an orthopedic surgeon, treats established patient, Mrs. Yanez, age 31, for a subsequent encounter for an infection in her dislocated right elbow.

    Code(s): _____

3. Mrs. Smythe, age 72, arrives at Williton because of severe right leg pain. Dr. Burns examines her and finds that her left leg is strained.

    Code(s): _____

4. Rudy Arwood, a 45-year-old new patient, sees Dr. Hoffman for a lumbar strain from playing golf.

    Code(s): _____

5. Dr. Burns treats Shawn Herrmann, age 38, in Williton's ED for a laceration that penetrated the bone on her right index finger. It happened when she was preparing dinner, and she cut herself with a butcher knife.

    Code(s): _____

6. An ambulance transports Rachel Slade, age 27, to Williton's ED. Dr. Burns removes shrapnel from a puncture wound on her left calf.

    Code(s): _____

Superficial Injuries (910–919)

Superficial, or **surface**, **injuries** include abrasions, blisters, nonvenomous insect bites, splinters, and scratches. ICD-9-CM classifies superficial injuries under categories 910–919. When you are assigning codes for superficial injuries, search the Index for the main term *injury*, subterm *superficial*.

When the patient has both a superficial injury, such as an abrasion or contusion, and a more serious injury of the same body site, assign a code for the more serious injury. Do not code the superficial injury. Refer to the following example to code a superficial injury.

> **Example:** Mrs. Cole, a 57-year-old established patient, sees Dr. Hoffman because she has itchy red skin on her face and neck. Dr. Hoffman determines that the condition is from bed bug bites. Dr. Hoffman prescribes antibiotic cream and discusses methods of eliminating bed bugs from her home.
> ■ FIGURE 8-17 shows the Index entry for nonvenomous insect bite, with code 910.4 cross-referenced to the Tabular.

Additional Notes on Injuries

When you are coding injuries, follow these guidelines:

1. Assign separate codes for each type of injury, unless there is a combination code that describes all of the injuries.
2. Sequence the code for the most serious injury first.
3. Do not assign injury codes for normal, healing surgical wounds or for surgical wound complications.
4. When a primary injury results in minor damage to **peripheral nerves** or blood vessels, assign at least two codes. Sequence first the code for the primary injury, assign additional code(s) from 950–957—*Injury to nerves and spinal cord* and/or 900–904—*Injury to blood vessels*.

peripheral nerves (pə-rif′ər-əl nərvz)—nerves outside the brain and spinal cord

Burns (940–949)

A **burn** is a bodily injury resulting from exposure to heat, caustics, electricity, or some radiations. Burns can damage the skin, underlying tissues, muscles, and organs. Causes of burns include fire; hot liquids; sun; steam; hot objects, such as a pot, pan, or iron (thermal burns); and friction (rope and rug burns). Burns occur under many different circumstances, including fires in a building or in an auto accident, children playing on or around a hot stove or iron, and people playing with matches or explosives, such as firecrackers. Patients can also experience airway burns from inhaling steam, smoke, or chemical fumes.

Burn symptoms include pain; blisters; red, white, charred, or peeling skin; edema; and fever. Patients with severe burns may also experience shock and have blue lips and fingernails, clammy and pale skin, and feel faint and disoriented. Patients with airway burns have burns on the face, neck, head, and mouth, as well as coughing, wheezing, and breathing problems.

ICD-9-CM classifies burns in categories 940–949 according to the depth and extent of the burn, as well as by the cause of the burn (E code). Burns are classified as first, second, or third degree, as follows:

epidermis (ep-ĭ-dur′mis)—outer protective layer of the skin

erythema (er-ə-thē′mə)—abnormal skin redness from dilation (widening) and congestion of capillaries

dermis (dur′mis)—sensitive connective tissue layer of the skin located below the outer layer of skin, the epidermis

blistering (blis′tər-ing)—having a local swelling of the skin that contains watery fluid

partial-thickness—affecting both the outer (epidermis) and underlying (dermis) layer of skin

full-thickness—including the muscles and blood supply

- First degree— injury to the **epidermis**, with **erythema** and edema (superficial)
- Second degree—injury to the epidermis and possibly the **dermis**, with erythema, edema, and **blistering** (**partial-thickness**)
- Third degree—the most critical type of burn with injury to the epidermis, dermis, and subcutaneous tissue and can also include muscles and bones (**full-thickness**)

■ FIGURE 8-18 shows types of burns.

Physicians diagnose burns by examining the patient, and they treat burns in the office or at a hospital, depending on the severity of the patient's condition. Burn treatment includes providing pain relief, preventing infection, using bandages, performing debridement (clean-

Injury 959.9

> Note For abrasion, insect bite (nonvenomous), blister, or scratch, see Injury, superficial.
>
> For laceration, traumatic rupture, tear, or penetrating wound of internal organs, such as heart, lung, liver, kidney, pelvic organs, whether or not accompanied by open wound in the same region, see Injury, internal.
>
> For nerve injury, see Injury, nerve.
>
> For late effect of injuries classifiable to 850-854, 860-869, 900-919, 950-959, see Late, effect, injury, by type.

    superficial 919

> Note Use the following fourth-digit subdivisions with categories 910-919:
>
> .0   abrasion or friction burn without mention of infection
>
> .1   abrasion or friction burn, infected
>
> .2   blister without mention of infection
>
> .3   blister, infected
>
> .4   insect bite, nonvenomous, without mention of infection
>
> .5   insect bite, nonvenomous, infected
>
> .6   superficial foreign body (splinter) without major open wound and without mention of infection
>
> .7   superficial foreign body (splinter) without major open wound, infected
>
> .8   other and unspecified superficial injury without mention of infection
>
> .9   other and unspecified superficial injury, infected
>
> For late effects of superficial injury, see category 906.2.

    face (any part(s), except eye) (and neck or scalp) 910

4th 910   Superficial injury of face, neck, and scalp except eye

Includes: cheek
            ear
            gum
            lip
            nose
            throat
Excludes: eye and adnexa (918.0-918.9)

    910.0 Abrasion or friction burn without mention of infection

    910.1 Abrasion or friction burn, infected

    910.2 Blister without mention of infection

    910.3 Blister, infected

    910.4 Insect bite, nonvenomous, without mention of infection

Figure 8-17 ■ Index entry for nonvenomous inset bite with 910.4 cross-referenced to the Tabular.

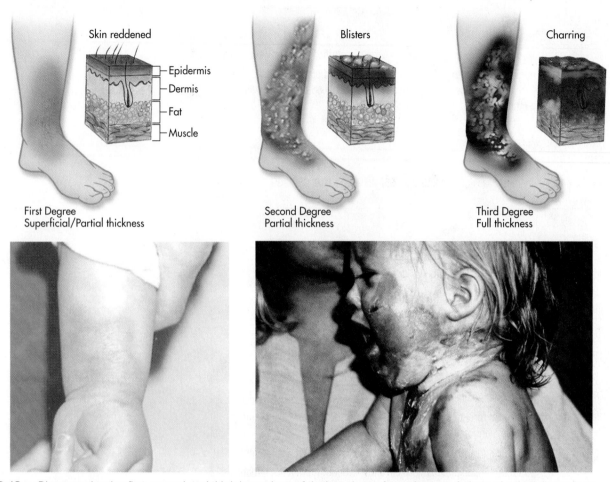

Figure 8-18 ■ Diagrams showing first, second, and third degree burn of the leg; photo of a sunburn, and photo of a third degree burn.

Diagrams source: Anatomy and Physiology for Health Professions, Colbert, Ankney, Lee, Pearson Prentice-Hall (2007) p. 178.

Photo credits: Michal Heron/Pearson Education.

skin grafts—replacements of damaged skin with skin from another part of the body or from a donor

ing), and ensuring that the patient has adequate fluids and calories to help the body to heal. Physicians can also perform **skin grafts** to replace burned skin and tissues (■ FIGURE 8-19), taking the graft from the patient or from a human or animal donor, such as a pig.

Severely burned patients may be critically ill and require acute care to save their lives. Physicians may recommend a *hyperbaric oxygen (HBO) chamber* for patients, an enclosed area with pure oxygen to aid the burn healing process.

Guidelines for Coding Burns   It is important to understand the coding guidelines for burns, especially when a patient has multiple burns or has other conditions in addition to a burn. Coding for burns can be complex and you should read through this section carefully. Follow along in your ICD-9-CM manual as you read the example. Let's review several coding guidelines for burns and then discuss how to correctly assign codes:

1. In the Index, locate the main term *burn*, search subterms for the *body site* where the burn occurred, then search subterms for the *degree* of burn.

2. When a patient has multiple burns, sequence first the code for the highest degree of burn out of all of the burns the patient sustained (third, second, first).

3. When a patient has both internal and external burns, review medical documentation for the reason for the patient's admission to determine which code to assign as the principal or first-listed diagnosis.

4. When a provider admits a patient to the hospital for burn injuries and *other related conditions*, such as smoke inhalation and/or respiratory failure, review medical documentation for the reason for the patient's admission to determine the code to assign as the principal or first-listed diagnosis.

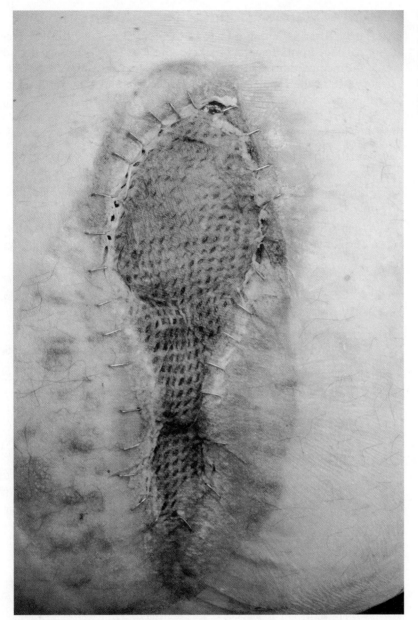

Figure 8-19 ■ Split thickness skin graft covering an open abdominal wound. Physicians perform skin grafting when the wound cannot be sutured or will not heal on its own.

Photo credit: Slaven / Custom Medical Stock Photo.

5. Code a nonhealing burn the same way that you would code an acute burn. Code **necrosis** of burned skin as a nonhealing burn.

6. If a burn site is infected, assign code 958.3—*Posttraumatic wound infection, not elsewhere classified* as an additional code.

7. Assign separate codes for each burn site. Do not use category 946—*Burns of multiple specified sites* unless the physician does not document burn sites. Avoid category 949— *Burn, unspecified* because it is extremely vague. Instead, query the physician for additional information.

8. If a patient has multiple burns of the *same* body site, but the burns are different degrees, then assign *one code with the subcategory for the highest degree* of burn (940–947).

9. Code encounters for the treatment of the late effects of burns (i.e., scars or joint contractures) for the residual condition (sequelae) followed by the appropriate late effect of external cause code (906.5–906.9).

10. When both a current burn and sequelae of an old burn exist, assign both a sequelae with a late-effect code and a current burn code.

11. Assign E codes representing the causes of a burns, if it is appropriate.

necrosis (nə-krō′sis)—death of cells or tissues through injury or disease

Assign Additional Code(s) for Percentage of Body Surface Burned

After assigning a code for a first, second, or third degree burn, assign an additional code from category 948 that represents the percentage of body surface burned, even if the medical documentation does not specify the burn site (■ FIGURE 8-20). Turn to category 948 in the Tabular List to review code choices and fifth-digit options for third-degree burns.

Burn units often gather statistical information using codes from category 948. Note the following information when you are assigning a code from category 948:

- Fourth digits identify the percentage of total body surface burned (burns of all degrees added together).
- Fifth digits identify the percentage of body surface involved in a *third-degree* burn only, if the patient had a third-degree burn.
- Assign a fifth digit of zero (0) when less than 10% of the body surface is affected by a burn of any degree, or no body surface is involved in a third-degree burn.

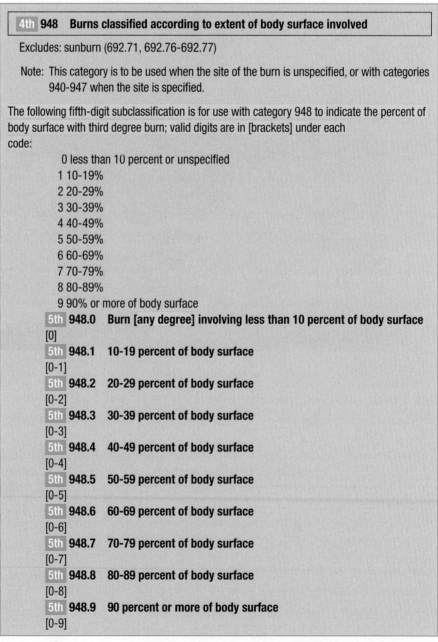

4th **948**	**Burns classified according to extent of body surface involved**	

Excludes: sunburn (692.71, 692.76-692.77)

Note: This category is to be used when the site of the burn is unspecified, or with categories 940-947 when the site is specified.

The following fifth-digit subclassification is for use with category 948 to indicate the percent of body surface with third degree burn; valid digits are in [brackets] under each code:

      0 less than 10 percent or unspecified
      1 10-19%
      2 20-29%
      3 30-39%
      4 40-49%
      5 50-59%
      6 60-69%
      7 70-79%
      8 80-89%
      9 90% or more of body surface

5th **948.0** **Burn [any degree] involving less than 10 percent of body surface**
[0]

5th **948.1** **10-19 percent of body surface**
[0-1]

5th **948.2** **20-29 percent of body surface**
[0-2]

5th **948.3** **30-39 percent of body surface**
[0-3]

5th **948.4** **40-49 percent of body surface**
[0-4]

5th **948.5** **50-59 percent of body surface**
[0-5]

5th **948.6** **60-69 percent of body surface**
[0-6]

5th **948.7** **70-79 percent of body surface**
[0-7]

5th **948.8** **80-89 percent of body surface**
[0-8]

5th **948.9** **90 percent or more of body surface**
[0-9]

Figure 8-20 ■ Category 948 in the Tabular.

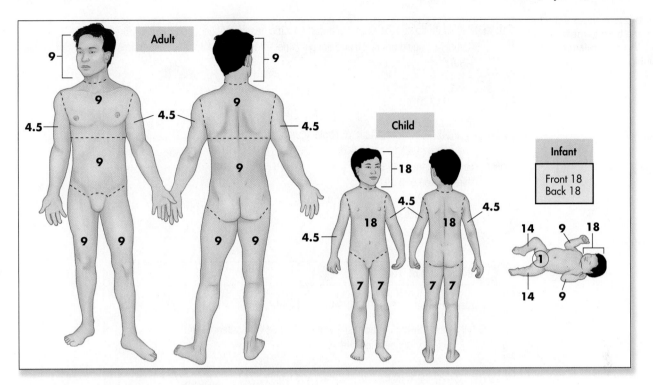

Figure 8-21 ■ The rule of nines for an adult, child, and infant.

Source: Anatomy and Physiology for Health Professions, Colbert, Ankney, Lee, Pearson Prentice-Hall (2007) p. 178.

ICD-9-CM bases category 948 on the **"rule of nines"** for adults to estimate the percentage of **total body surface area (TBSA)** burned, the percentage burned out of the total area of the entire body. The rule of nines divides the body into several sections and each section represents a percentage of TBSA and is divisible by 9, as illustrated in ■ FIGURE 8-21.

Physicians document percentages of body surfaces burned and/or use body diagrams of the rule of nines to show percentages. Physicians may also deviate from the rule of nines when necessary to accommodate infants and children, who have proportionately larger heads than adults, and for patients who have large buttocks, thighs, breasts, or abdomens. They also may use a Lund-Browder chart to estimate percentage of burns for infants and children. Let's review the following example to code two different degrees of burns, then assign a third code for the TBSA burned:

Example: Blanche McDonald, a 69-year-old, is admitted to Williton Medical Center's burn unit through the ED to treat a second-degree burn covering the upper left arm (4.5% TBSA) and third-degree burns to the breasts (9% TBSA).

1. Sequence first the highest degree of burn, the third-degree burns to the breasts.

2. Assign a second code for the second-degree burn of the upper left arm.

3. Assign a third code from category 948 representing the percentage of TBSA burned (all burns added together), adding a fifth digit to show the percentage of *third-degree burn* only.

For the third-degree burn, search the Index for the main term *burn*, subterm *breast(s)*, and subterm *third-degree*, and then cross-reference code 942.31 to the Tabular (■ FIGURE 8-22).

For the second-degree burn of the upper left arm, search the Index for the main term *burn*, subterm *arm*, subterm *upper*, and subterm *second-degree*. Then cross-reference code 943.23 to the Tabular (■ FIGURE 8-23).

For the third code, refer to category 948 to find the code that represents the total TBSA burned, which is 13.5% (code 948.1). Then locate the fifth digit representing the percentage of *third-degree burn* only, which is 9% (fifth digit 0) (■ FIGURE 8-24).

Figure 8-22 ■ Index entry for third-degree burn to the breasts with 942.31 cross-referenced to the Tabular.

Burn (acid) (cathode ray) (caustic) (chemical) (electric heating appliance) (electricity) (fire) (flame) (hot liquid or object) (irradiation) (lime) (radiation) (steam) (thermal) (x-ray) 949.0

    breast(s) 942.01
        with
            trunk - see Burn, trunk, multiple sites
        first degree 942.11
        second degree 942.21
        third degree 942.31
            deep 942.41
                with loss of body part 942.51

4th **942** **Burn of trunk**

Excludes: scapular region (943.0-943.5 with fifth-digit 6)

The following fifth-digit subclassification is for use with category 942:
        0 trunk, unspecified site
        1 breast
        2 chest wall, excluding breast and nipple
        3 abdominal wall
            Flank
            Groin
        4 back [any part]
            Buttock
            Interscapular region
        5 genitalia
            Labium (majus) (minus)
            Penis
             Perineum
            Scrotum
            Testis
            Vulva
        9 other and multiple sites of trunk

    5th **942.0** **Unspecified degree**
    [0-5,9]

    5th **942.1** **Erythema [first degree]**
    [0-5,9]

    5th **942.2** **Blisters, epidermal loss [second degree]**
    [0-5,9]

    5th **942.3** **Full-thickness skin loss [third degree NOS]**
    [0-5,9]

If you do not remember that category 948 shows codes for percentages of TBSA burned, you can also find code choices in the Index by searching for the main term *burn*, subterm, *extent*.

For this example, assign the following codes:

1. 942.31—third-degree burn to the breasts
2. 943.23—second-degree burn to the upper left arm
3. 948.10—13.5% TBSA burned, with 9% representing a third-degree burn

Burn (acid) (cathode ray) (caustic) (chemical) (electric heating appliance) (electricity) (fire) (flame) (hot liquid or object) (irradiation) (lime) (radiation) (steam) (thermal) (x-ray) 949.0

arm(s) 943.00
    first degree 943.10
    second degree 943.20
    third degree 943.30
        deep 943.40
            with loss of body part 943.50
    lower - see Burn, forearm(s)
    multiple sites, except hand(s) or wrist(s) 943.09
        first degree 943.19
        second degree 943.29
        third degree 943.39
            deep 943.49
                with loss of body part 943.59
    upper 943.03
        first degree 943.13
        second degree 943.23
        third degree 943.33
            deep 943.43
                with loss of body part 943.53

4th 943 Burn of upper limb, except wrist and hand

The following fifth-digit subclassification is for use with category 943:
    0 upper limb, unspecified site
    1 forearm
    2 elbow
    3 upper arm
    4 axilla
    5 shoulder
    6 scapular region
    9 multiple sites of upper limb, except wrist and hand

5th 943.0 Unspecified degree
[0-6,9]

5th 943.1 Erythema [first degree]
[0-6,9]

5th 943.2 Blisters, epidermal loss [second degree]
[0-6,9]

Figure 8-23 ■ Index entry for second-degree burn to the upper arm with 943.23 cross-referenced to the Tabular.

Figure 8-24 ■ Percentage of TBSA burned and percentage of third-degree burn, shown by code 948.10 in the Tabular.

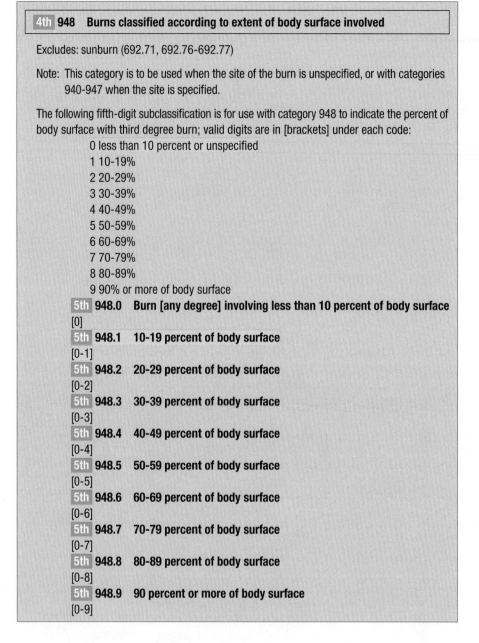

| **4th** | **948** | **Burns classified according to extent of body surface involved** |

Excludes: sunburn (692.71, 692.76-692.77)

Note: This category is to be used when the site of the burn is unspecified, or with categories 940-947 when the site is specified.

The following fifth-digit subclassification is for use with category 948 to indicate the percent of body surface with third degree burn; valid digits are in [brackets] under each code:

0 less than 10 percent or unspecified
1 10-19%
2 20-29%
3 30-39%
4 40-49%
5 50-59%
6 60-69%
7 70-79%
8 80-89%
9 90% or more of body surface

5th 948.0 Burn [any degree] involving less than 10 percent of body surface
[0]

5th 948.1 10-19 percent of body surface
[0-1]

5th 948.2 20-29 percent of body surface
[0-2]

5th 948.3 30-39 percent of body surface
[0-3]

5th 948.4 40-49 percent of body surface
[0-4]

5th 948.5 50-59 percent of body surface
[0-5]

5th 948.6 60-69 percent of body surface
[0-6]

5th 948.7 70-79 percent of body surface
[0-7]

5th 948.8 80-89 percent of body surface
[0-8]

5th 948.9 90 percent or more of body surface
[0-9]

INTERESTING FACTS: Statistics on Fires, Burn Injuries, and Burn Infections

✔ On average in the U.S. in 2004, someone died in a fire every 135 minutes, and someone was injured every 30 minutes.

✔ Each year in the U.S., 1.1 million burn injuries require medical attention.

✔ Approximately 50,000 burn injuries require hospitalization each year.

✔ Approximately 20,000 of these injuries are major burns involving at least 25% of the total body surface, and approximately 4,500 of these people die.

✔ Up to 10,000 people in the U.S. die every year of burn-related infections.

✔ Only 60% of Americans have an escape plan in the event of a fire, and of those, only 25% have practiced it.

✔ Smoke alarms cut your chances of dying in a fire in half.

(Department of Health and Human Services, Centers for Disease Control and Prevention, emergency.cdc.gov/masscasualties/burns. asp, accessed 11/19/10.)

TAKE A BREAK

Let's take a break and then practice assigning codes for superficial injuries and burns.

Exercise 8.6   **Superficial Injuries, Additional Guidelines for Superficial and Primary Injuries, and Burns**

Instructions: Assign diagnosis codes, including E codes, to the following patient cases, using both the Index and the Tabular. Refer to the main terms previously outlined, as well as to steps for coding burns, for assistance with locating codes.

1. Dr. Hoffman treats Mr. Pooler, a 28-year-old established patient, for a blister on his right heel.

   Code(s): _____

2. Mr. Sterling drives his wife, Paula, to Williton's ED after she fell off a ladder. Dr. Burns, the ED physician, treats the bruises on her left leg and a left wrist sprain.

   Code(s): _____

3. Mrs. Bateman brings her daughter, Pearl, age 4, to Williton's ED. Dr. Mills, an emergency physician, treats a first-degree burn on Pearl's left cheek (less than 10% TBSA), which she sustained while playing with her mother's cigarette lighter.

   Code(s): _____

4. Luis Will, age 15, is rearranging wood in the family's fireplace when his clothes catch on fire. His father transports him to Williton's ED. Dr. Mills treats Luis for first-degree burns and documents the following: foot (1% TBSA), lower left leg (8% TBSA) and buttocks (8% TBSA).

   Code(s): _____

5. A house fire injures Beverly Chacon, a 50-year-old. An ambulance transports her to Williton's ED. Dr. Mills treats third-degree burns to her left arm, second-degree burns to her right arm, and first-degree burns to both hands. He uses a diagram with the rule of nines to show the following: left arm (8% TBSA), right arm (8% TBSA), each hand (1% TBSA).

   Code(s): _____

6. Bessie Raines, age 62, arrives at Williton's ED by ambulance. Dr. Mills treats her for multiple burns and documents the following on the rule of nines diagram: third-degree burns to the face (9% TBSA), deep third-degree burns to both forearms and hands (total of 11% TBSA), and second-degree burns to the back (18% TBSA). He admits her to Williton's Burn Unit for further treatment.

   Code(s): _____

DESTINATION: MEDICARE

In Chapter 7, you learned about the *World of Medicare* through the Medicare Learning Network (MLN). Healthcare providers access Medicare billing, coding, coverage, and reimbursement information through the CMS website. It is important to understand that CMS's regulations, and other payers regulations, change frequently. You always have to search for the most recent documentation on the CMS website to ensure that you review updated regulations for coding, billing, and reimbursement.

CMS publishes *National Coverage Determinations (NCDs),* regulations that apply to all providers across the U.S., and *Local Coverage Determinations (LCDs),* regulations that apply to providers in specific geographic areas, which can supersede NCDs. In order to become familiar with CMS regulations, you must review and interpret information in NCDs and LCDs, as well as information in many other bulletins and guidelines that CMS releases. In this exercise, you will access CMS's manual of NCDs to practice finding specific reimbursement information. Access the NCD manual by following these steps:

1. Go to the website http://www.cms.gov.

2. At the top of the screen on the yellow banner bar, choose *Regulations & Guidance.*

3. Under *Guidance,* choose *Manuals.*

continued

4. On the left side of the screen, choose *Internet-Only Manuals (IOMs)*.

5. Scroll through the pages listing *Publication #* and choose *100-03 Medicare National Coverage Determinations (NCD) Manual*.

6. Scroll down to *Downloads,* and choose ncd103c1_Part1 [PDF, 479KB], which will take you to the Medicare National Coverage Determinations Manual Chapter 1, Part 1 (Sections 10 – 80.12) Coverage Determinations.

   Chapter 1—Coverage Determinations, Part 1 Sections 10–80.12.

To find specific information in the manual, you can hit the *Ctrl* key and the *F* key to go to the search field and type in what you are looking for, or click directly in the search field at the top of the document. Then answer the following questions about Medicare reimbursement for HBO therapy:

1. Does Medicare cover HBO therapy for crush injuries and suturing of severed limbs? _____

2. How many days have to pass without measurable signs of healing with standard wound care before Medicare will pay for HBO therapy? _____

3. How often do providers have to evaluate patients' wounds during HBO therapy? _____

⤷ A LOOK AHEAD TO ICD-10-CM

Recall that E codes do not exist in ICD-10-CM; V codes replaced them in Chapter 20 of ICD-10-CM (V00–V99). Injuries, poisonings, and other consequences of external causes are in Chapter 19 of ICD-10-CM (S00–T88). Late effects in the I-10 Index are listed under *sequelae*, not under *late*, as they were listed in I-9. Burn codes in I-10 differentiate between the left and right sides of the body. Refer to instructions for accessing the ICD-10-CM guidelines in Appendix A of this text to review the guidelines for these conditions.

Instructions: Assign codes from ICD-10-CM to cases that you previously coded in this chapter using ICD-9-CM. Reference both the Index and the Tabular.

1. Dr. Hoffman treats a new patient, Wayne Virgil, for a skin rash that he developed after taking an initial dose of penicillin, an antibiotic that was correctly prescribed to him. Code(s): _____

2. Nathan Dowdell, age 16, sees Dr. Grisham, an orthopedic surgeon, for a new shoulder injury. Dr. Grisham diagnoses a full-thickness tear of the left rotator cuff capsule, which happened while Nathan was pitching a baseball. Code(s): _____

3. Jose Whittaker, age 72, reports to outpatient surgery for removal of a senile cortical cataract on his left eye. Clinicians prep him for surgery, but his physician mistakenly performs the surgery on the opposite eye. Code(s): _____

4. Dr. Grisham treats established patient, Mrs. Yanez, age 31, for a subsequent encounter for an infection in her dislocated right elbow. Code(s): _____

5. Keith Cruz, a 27-year-old, arrives in Williton's ED with severe left leg pain. Dr. Mills diagnoses him with a compound fracture of the shaft of his left tibia. Code(s): _____

6. Bessie Raines, age 62, arrives at Williton's ED by ambulance. Dr. Mills treats her for multiple burns and documents the following on the rule of nines diagram: third-degree burns to the face (9%), deep third-degree burns to both forearms and hands (total of 11%), and second-degree burns to the back (18%). He admits her to Williton's Burn Unit for further treatment. Code(s):_____

CHAPTER REVIEW

Multiple Choice

Instructions: Circle one best answer to complete each statement.

1. Which of the following is *not* a category in the Table of Drugs and Chemicals?
   a. Therapeutic use
   b. Suicide attempt
   c. Assault
   d. Terrorism

2. If the patient's late effect is due to a previous injury or poisoning, then how should you assign codes?
   a. Assign an E code for the late effect only.
   b. Assign a code for the late effect first, and assign an E code for the patient's condition second.
   c. Assign a code for the patient's condition first, and assign an E code for the late effect second.
   d. Assign an E code for the patient's condition first, and assign a late effect code second.

3. Which of the following E codes would you *not* typically assign in addition to another E code?
   a. External status (E000)
   b. Activity (E001–E030)
   c. Place of occurrence (E849)
   d. Accidental falls (E880–E888)

4. The time limit for assigning codes for a late effect of an external cause is
   a. three months.
   b. one year.
   c. five years.
   d. not applicable; there is no time limit.

5. Which of the following types of fractures is open?
   a. Infected
   b. Comminuted
   c. Impacted
   d. Spiral

6. If the physician does not document the *type* of fracture, or document whether the fracture is open or closed, then code the fracture as
   a. open.
   b. closed.
   c. comminuted.
   d. unspecified.

7. Patients with sprains may experience
   a. edema, pain, bruising, and lack of movement.
   b. fractures or dislocations.
   c. bleeding and paralysis.
   d. residual hemiplegia.

8. Which of the following is *not* used to locate the main term for an open wound?
   a. The entry "Wound, open"
   b. Body site
   c. Type of wound
   d. Index

9. A _____-degree burn involves injury to the epidermis and possibly the dermis, with erythema, edema, and blistering.
   a. first
   b. second
   c. third
   d. fourth

10. When a provider admits a patient to the hospital for burn injuries and other related conditions, such as smoke inhalation and/or respiratory failure, how do you select the principal, or first-listed, diagnosis?
    a. The highest degree of burn is the principal diagnosis.
    b. First-degree burns are the first-listed diagnosis.
    c. The nonburn injury is the principal diagnosis.
    d. The circumstances of admission govern the selection.

Coding Assignments

Instructions: Assign ICD-9-CM code(s) to the following cases, referencing both the Index and Tabular. Also assign E codes where appropriate.

1. Dr. Burns treats Edward Toon, age 19, in the Williton Medical Center's ED for stab wounds to the chest and arms after a gang fight on the street.

   Code(s): _____

2. Gloria Cushman, a 48-year-old, is walking in the street after dark on a rainy night, when a man hits her with his car. It was dark, and he did not see her. At Williton's ED, Dr. Burns treats Ms. Cushman for a concussion. X-rays show that the lower ends of her right ulna and radius are fractured.

   Code(s): _____

3. Shelley Pyle, age 67, walks through her living room when her cat darts in front of her, causing her to stumble. She loses her balance, falls over an ottoman, sprains her wrist, and suffers contusions to her calf. She waits until the next day to see how she is feeling, then comes in to see Dr. Hoffman to make sure nothing is broken. Dr. Hoffman says that the extensive hematoma (collection of blood from a broken blood vessel) on the calf is

due to her long-term Coumadin® therapy. X-rays show no fractures. The wrist sprain is at the radiocarpal joint, the joint between the distal (farthest) end of the radius and the carpal bones.

Code(s): _____

4. Justin Busby, a 79-year-old, has pharyngeal (pertaining to the pharynx, or throat) dysphagia (difficulty swallowing), which Dr. Hoffman determines is a late effect of a medication reaction suffered earlier this year from accidental poisoning.

Code(s): _____

5. Danielle Burchett, a city bus driver, assists a disabled passenger out of his wheelchair. She has difficulty holding him steady, and they both fall to the ground. Fortunately, the passenger only has minor abrasions and requires no medical attention, but Miss Burchett travels to Williton's ED, where Dr. Mills diagnoses her with a dislocated right shoulder, acromioclavicular joint. No bones are broken. Dr. Mills treats her and then discharges her to home.

Code(s): _____

6. Gerald Sorrell, age 22, was trapped in a barn fire. Dr. Mills treats him in Willition's ED for third-degree burns to his left forearm (4% TBSA), and second-degree burns to his left upper arm and shoulder (5% TBSA), as well as smoke inhalation. Dr. Mills admits him to Williton's Burn Unit for further treatment.

Code(s): _____

7. Irma Morris, a type 2 diabetic who regularly takes metformin, an antidiabetic medication, experiences nausea, vomiting, and tachycardia (rapid heart beat) after sharing a bottle of wine with her boyfriend, Don. She forgot that she should avoid alcohol while on metformin. Don brings her to the emergency department where Dr. Mills treats her and stabilizes her condition. He then discharges her to home.

Code(s): _____

8. Delores Corder, age 62, is in the hospital recovering from a hysterectomy (removal of the uterus) when she develops a urinary tract infection. Dr. Dunford documents that the infection happened because hospital clinicians did not follow sterile procedures when maintaining her urinary catheter. Lab tests show the infectious bacteria is *Pseudomonas aeruginosa*. Dr. Dunford begins administration of the antibiotic ciprofloxacin.

Code(s): _____

9. Opal Griffiths, a 56-year-old, presents to Williton's ED where Dr. Mills treats her for whiplash. Mrs. Griffiths was a passenger in a car that another vehicle rear-ended at a stop light.

Code(s): _____

10. Dr. Mills treats Holly Dawkins, age 19, in Williton's ED after someone sexually assaulted her. A lab urine test was positive for flunitrazepam (a strong, hypnotic sedative). Dr. Mills determines that someone gave Ms. Dawkins the drug in order to sexually assault her. He contacts local police, who arrive at the hospital to interview Ms. Dawkins.

Code(s): _____

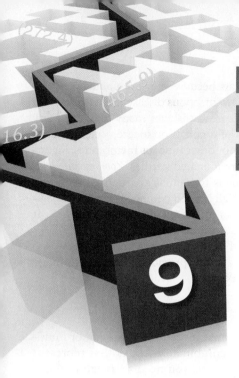

Infectious Diseases and Endocrine, Blood, and Nervous System Disorders

Learning Objectives

After completing this chapter, you should be able to

- Spell and define the key terminology in this chapter.
- Describe and apply the guidelines for coding infectious and parasitic diseases.
- Define combination and multiple codes, and discuss how to assign them.
- Interpret and utilize guidelines for coding HIV and AIDS.
- Review and apply the guidelines for coding endocrine, nutritional, and metabolic diseases and immunity disorders.
- Discuss and interpret guidelines for coding diseases of the blood and blood-forming organs.
- Interpret and review guidelines for coding diseases of the nervous system and sense organs.

Key Terms

blood
central nervous system (CNS)
endocrine system

infectious disease
nervous system
nutritional disorders
peripheral nervous system (PNS)

INTRODUCTION

The next stop on your coding journey is to learn more about disorders and conditions categorized in specific chapters of ICD-9-CM, beginning with infectious and parasitic diseases. Remember that knowing how physicians diagnose, treat, and prevent disorders is an important part of coding correctly. Taking the time to learn about the diagnoses that you code ensures that you will perform your job well. There is not time to code all disorders in every ICD-9-CM chapter, but you will learn about some of the most common conditions that you may be likely to code. You have traveled far on your journey and made great strides. There is still much to do and much to learn!

"Every day you may make progress. Every step may be fruitful. Yet there will stretch out before you an ever-lengthening, ever-ascending, ever-improving path." —WINSTON CHURCHILL

INFECTIOUS AND PARASITIC DISEASES (ICD-9-CM CHAPTER 1—001–139)

An **infectious disease** occurs when a **pathogen** enters the body, multiplies, and causes illness because the body is not strong enough to defend itself against an attack. Pathogens include **bacteria**, **viruses**, **fungi**, and **protozoa** and can invade both humans and animals. *Parasites*, which are living organisms, exist within or on their hosts, who give them nourishment and enable them to reproduce.

pathogen (path′o-jən) disease-producing agent or microorganism, such as a bacterium, fungus, protozoon, or virus

bacteria (bak-tēr′e-ə) ever-present one-celled organisms that are involved in infections and infectious diseases

viruses (vi′-rəs-es) certain types of microorganisms that grow and multiply in living cells

fungi (fun′ji) organisms that produce spores

protozoa (pro-to-zo′ə) mostly one-celled organisms

ICD-9-CM codes in this chapter are from the ICD-9-CM 2012 code set from the Department of Health and Human Services, Centers for Disease Control and Prevention.

ICD-10-CM codes in this chapter are from ICD-10-CM 2012 Draft code set from the Department of Health and Human Services, Centers for Disease Control and Prevention.

Infectious diseases often pose serious health threats because they are contagious, and people can quickly spread them to each other. This is why infectious diseases are also referred to as transmissible or communicable diseases. People spread diseases many different ways: sharing physical and sexual contact, inhaling droplets of a cough or sneeze, touching contaminated objects and then touching their eyes, mouths, or other mucous membranes, ingesting pathogens from contaminated food, and sharing contaminated needles. *Zoonotic infectious diseases* spread from animals to humans or from humans to animals, particularly rodents, cattle, and bats. According to the DHHS CDC, 60% of all human pathogens are zoonotic.

The CDC tracks, analyzes, controls, and prevents infectious diseases in the U.S. It works around the world to identify and study disease origins to try to contain diseases before they spread to the U.S. and other countries. The WHO tracks and monitors diseases on a global level, helping to stop disease threats and providing support to many countries for fighting and controlling disease outbreaks.

COMBINATION CODES AND MULTIPLE CODES

Assigning codes for infectious and parasitic diseases could involve combination or multiple codes. In Chapter 4, you learned how to assign combination codes that represent more than one diagnosis and also learned that many times, you need to assign multiple codes for multiple conditions. Do you remember how to identify when you need a combination code or multiple codes? Assign multiple codes when the patient has two diagnoses, diagnoses with an etiology/manifestation relationship, or a diagnosis and associated complication when there is no combination code available. Also follow ICD-9-CM's coding conventions, inclusion and exclusion notes, and guidelines to determine whether to assign multiple codes or a combination code. You can also identify combination codes by their titles because they describe more than one condition.

tuberculosis (tū-bĕr-kū-lō′ sĭs) infectious disease caused by the tubercle bacillus

When you are coding infectious and parasitic diseases that are excluded from Chapter 1 of the Tabular List, you may need to assign multiple codes: one code for the infectious disease (search the Index for the name of the infection or disease) and one code to identify the pathogen, or organism, that caused it (search the Index for *infection* and search subterms for the name of the organism). Generally, when you look up the infectious disease code, you will see a *Use additional code* note directing you to assign an additional code for the organism. Sequence the infectious disease code first, unless ICD-9-CM directs you to code otherwise. In other cases, you may need to assign combination codes representing *both* the infection and the pathogen.

whooping cough (hūp′ ĭng) acute contagious infection of the respiratory tract, usually seen in young children

septicemia (sĕp-tĭ-sē′ mĭ-ă) abnormal condition in that bacteria are present in the blood

candidiasis (kăn dĭ-dī′ ă -sĭs) a fungal infection of the skin or mucous membranes caused by a species of Candida yeast

Sometimes you may have difficulty determining if the condition that you are coding is an infectious disease. If you are not sure, research the condition in your medical references or on the Internet to learn more about it. Examples of infectious diseases include **tuberculosis**, **whooping cough**, **septicemia**, and **candidiasis**. Review the following example to assign *multiple codes* representing an infectious disease and the bacteria that caused it.

cellulitis (sĕl-ū-lī′ tĭs) spreading inflammation of subcutaneous or connective tissue

Example: Margaret Johnson, a 32-year-old, presents to Williton Medical Center's ED with complaints of redness, swelling, and tenderness of her right buttock. She also has fever and chills. After examination and study, Dr. Mills, the ED physician, determines that the patient has Group A streptococcal **cellulitis** (■ FIGURE 9-1). He removes dead tissue from the wound on the buttock and starts the patient on IV antibiotics.

To code this case, first look for the main term *cellulitis* in the Index, subterm *buttock*, and check to see if there is a combination code that includes *both* cellulitis and Group A streptococcus, the bacteria that caused the condition (■ FIGURE 9-2).

Since there is no combination code for both the condition and the bacteria, cross-reference code 682.5 to the Tabular for final code assignment of the cellulitis (■ FIGURE 9-3). You will need to assign a separate code for the bacteria.

Did you notice the *Use additional code* note under category 682? Find the code for Group A streptococcus by searching the Index for the main term *infection*, subterm *streptococcal*, subterm *group*, and subterm *A* and cross-referencing code 041.01 to the Tabular (■ FIGURE 9-4).

Did you also see the note under category 041 alerting you that the bacteria code is in addition to the code for the infection? For Ms. Johnson's case, sequence first code 682.5 for cellulitis, then code 041.01 for Group A streptococcus.

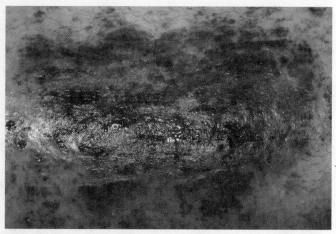

Figure 9-1 ■ Cellulitis of the buttocks.

Photo credit: DR P. MARAZZI/SCIENCE PHOTO LIBRARY / Custom Medical Stock Photo.

Cellulitis (diffuse) (with lymphangitis) (see also Abscess) 682.9
    abdominal wall 682.2
    anaerobic (see also Gas gangrene) 040.0
    ankle 682.6
    anus 566
    areola 611.0
    arm (any part, above wrist) 682.3
    auditory canal (external) 380.10
    axilla 682.3
    back (any part) 682.2
    breast 611.0
        postpartum 675.1
    broad ligament (see also Disease, pelvis, inflammatory) 614.4
        acute 614.3
    buttock 682.5

Figure 9-2 ■ Index entry for cellulitis.

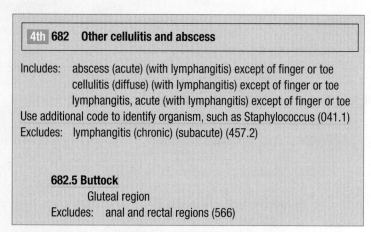

4th 682   Other cellulitis and abscess

Includes: abscess (acute) (with lymphangitis) except of finger or toe
           cellulitis (diffuse) (with lymphangitis) except of finger or toe
           lymphangitis, acute (with lymphangitis) except of finger or toe
Use additional code to identify organism, such as Staphylococcus (041.1)
Excludes: lymphangitis (chronic) (subacute) (457.2)

       682.5 Buttock
           Gluteal region
       Excludes: anal and rectal regions (566)

Figure 9-3 ■ Code 682.5 cross-referenced to the Tabular.

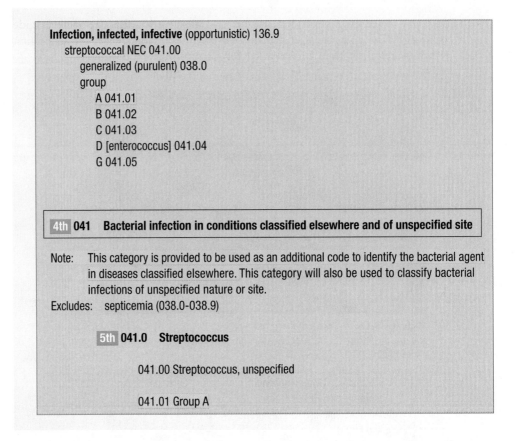

Infection, infected, infective (opportunistic) 136.9
  streptococcal NEC 041.00
    generalized (purulent) 038.0
    group
      A 041.01
      B 041.02
      C 041.03
      D [enterococcus] 041.04
      G 041.05

| 4th 041 | Bacterial infection in conditions classified elsewhere and of unspecified site |

Note: This category is provided to be used as an additional code to identify the bacterial agent in diseases classified elsewhere. This category will also be used to classify bacterial infections of unspecified nature or site.
Excludes: septicemia (038.0-038.9)

  | 5th 041.0 | Streptococcus |

    041.00 Streptococcus, unspecified

    041.01 Group A

Review the next example to assign a *combination code* for an infectious disease and the bacteria that caused it.

gastroenteritis (gas-tro-en tər-i'tis) inflammation of the membrane lining the stomach and the intestines

antiemetic (an-te-ə-met'ik) agent that prevents or stops vomiting

Example: Tracy Thompson, a 26-year-old, presents to Williton Medical Center's ED with complaints of vomiting, nausea, stomach pain, and diarrhea. After examining her, Dr. Mills determines that the patient has **gastroenteritis** due to salmonella (bacteria) food poisoning, and he starts the patient on an IV **antiemetic**.

Search the Index for the main term *gastroenteritis*, and then determine if there is a combination code representing *both* the infectious disease and the bacteria that caused it (■ FIGURE 9-5).

Gastroenteritis (acute) (catarrhal) (congestive) (hemorrhagic) (noninfectious) (see also Enteritis) 558.9

salmonella 003.0

Figure 9-5 ■ Index entry for gastroenteritis.

Code 003.0 represents *both* the condition of gastroenteritis and the Salmonella bacteria that caused it, so you do not need to assign an additional code for salmonella. ■ FIGURE 9-6 shows code 003.0 cross-referenced to the Tabular.

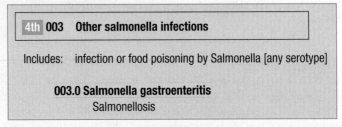

| 4th 003 | Other salmonella infections |

Includes: infection or food poisoning by Salmonella [any serotype]

  003.0 Salmonella gastroenteritis
    Salmonellosis

Figure 9-6 ■ Code 003.0 cross-referenced to the Tabular.

When coding causes of infectious diseases, search the main term *infection*, then search the following subterms:

- name of the bacteria
- name of the virus
- fungus
- parasitic
- protozoal

You may not always know the type of virus that causes an infectious disease because it is not always included in the documentation. This may be because the physician is waiting for test results or does not know specifically what caused the patient's illness, just that it is a virus. You can still assign a code for an *unspecified virus* by searching the main term *infection*, subterm *virus*, and subterm *unspecified nature or site*.

TAKE A BREAK

That was a lot of information to remember! Let's take a break and then practice assigning combination and multiple codes for infectious and parasitic diseases.

| Exercise 9.1 | Infectious and Parasitic Diseases, and Combination and Multiple Codes

Instructions: Code the following patient cases, using both the Index and the Tabular. Refer to the main terms previously outlined for assistance locating codes.

1. Daniel Blackman, a new patient, age 19, sees Dr. Hoffman for general lack of energy, fatigue, loss of appetite, fever, and chills. Dr. Hoffman suspects infectious mononucleosis, which is confirmed by a blood test.

   Code(s): _____

2. Sonya Kerr, a 27-year-old established patient, sees Dr. Hoffman because she has had bloody diarrhea and is worried that she might have cancer. She tells Dr. Hoffman that she recently ate hamburgers at a pool party, and the symptoms started a few days later. Dr. Hoffman diagnoses Ms. Kerr with hemorrhagic colitis (inflammation and bleeding of the colon) due to *E. coli*. Dr. Hoffman tells her it should clear up in about a week and instructs her to call him if it does not.

   Code(s): _____

3. Mike Pollock, age 47, is a new patient who sees Dr. Hoffman due to blisters and scabs on his face and the left side of his body. He is also having unexplained pain. Dr. Hoffman diagnoses Mr. Pollock with herpes zoster.

   Code(s): _____

4. Sharon Putnam, a 30-year-old established patient, sees Dr. Hoffman with complaints of dark urine, fever, vomiting, and yellowing skin. After conducting a physical examination, Dr. Hoffman tells her that she has viral hepatitis A. He recommends rest and tells her to avoid alcohol and fatty foods.

   Code(s): _____

5. Dr. Hoffman treats established patient, Mr. Marchand, age 60, for pneumonia due to rickettsia.

   Code(s): _____

6. Carlos Choate, a 44-year-old nursing assistant, sees Dr. Hoffman for his annual PPD test (Purified Protein Derivative, the skin test for tuberculosis). The test is positive, which explains his recent weight loss, fatigue, and coughing. A bacterial culture confirms tuberculosis, due to the *Mycobacterium tuberculosis*. An X-ray shows that the tuberculosis consists of nodules in the lung.

   Code(s): _____

HUMAN IMMUNODEFICIENCY VIRUS AND ACQUIRED IMMUNODEFICIENCY SYNDROME

It is important to understand how to assign codes for HIV and HIV-related illnesses because they are common infectious conditions. ICD-9-CM created specific guidelines to code HIV and related diagnoses. HIV destroys blood cells that provide the body with immunity to fight infections and diseases. A person with HIV has a compromised immune system and is more susceptible to various illnesses, including **Kaposi's sarcoma**, a form of cancer (■ FIGURE 9-7). An individual may be HIV positive for many years and be asymptomatic before developing AIDS. AIDS is a group of symptoms representing the diseases, infections, and disorders

Kaposi's sarcoma (kăp′ ō-sēz sär-kō′ mǎ) common AIDS-related cancer that causes violet-colored vascular lesions and diseased lymph nodes

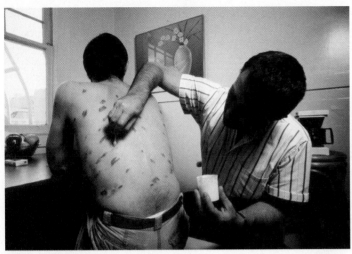

Figure 9-7 ■ A clinician applies medication to an HIV/AIDS patient with Kaposi's sarcoma lesions.

Photo credit: © Chuck Nacke/Alamy.

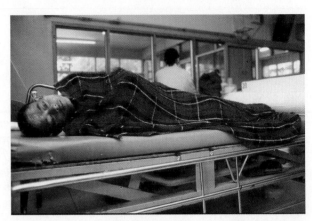

Figure 9-8 ■ An AIDS patient at a hospice facility in Thailand.

Photo credit: © Jack Picone/Alamy.

immunity (ĭ-mu′nĭ-te) protection of the body from a disease that infection causes

that a patient eventually contracts because his body does not have enough **immunity** to fight them. HIV infections first appeared in the U.S. in the 1970s. Researchers believe that the origin of HIV is zoonotic because African chimpanzees carried the illness and passed it to human hunters who were exposed to the animals' infected blood.

HIV infection is spread by many methods, including

- having unprotected vaginal, anal, or oral sex (sex without a condom) with a partner who is HIV positive or who has AIDS; having multiple sex partners or other sexually transmitted diseases (STDs) increase the risk of contracting HIV.
- sharing needles, syringes, rinse water, or other equipment used to inject drugs.
- being born to an infected mother; a mother with HIV can pass it to her child during pregnancy, birth, or breastfeeding.

Symptoms of HIV infection include rapid weight loss; cough; recurring fever; night sweats; fatigue; pneumonia; swollen lymph glands; diarrhea lasting more than a week; white spots on the tongue, in the mouth, or in the throat; red, brown, pink, or purple blotches on or under the skin or inside the mouth, nose, or eyelids; memory loss; and depression. The symptoms mean that the patient has an HIV-related condition that has developed into AIDS. Many patients with AIDS deteriorate rapidly, and their prognosis is poor because there is no cure (■ FIGURE 9-8).

Physicians diagnose HIV infection using several different types of lab tests. Treatment includes combinations of drug therapy to increase immunity and enable the patient to fight off diseases and disorders for as long as possible, sometimes many years, before developing AIDS. CDC sponsored clinical trials in other countries to test the effectiveness of a **prophylactic** (preventive) pill to prevent HIV infection. The pill is called tenofovir, brand name Viread®, and the trials showed promising results. The CDC also completed a study in 2010 for tenofovir use in the U.S.

prophylactic (prō-fə-′lak-tik)

Coding Guidelines for HIV and AIDS

Let's review guidelines for coding HIV and HIV-related illnesses because the ICD-9-CM guidelines can sometimes be confusing. Follow these ICD-9-CM guidelines when coding an HIV infection if a patient is *asymptomatic* and when coding AIDS if the patient has an HIV-related illness (symptomatic):

1. Assign code V08 for a patient with an asymptomatic HIV infection (main term *infection*, subterm *HIV*, or main term *human immunodeficiency virus*, subterm *infection*). In order for you to assign V08, the physician has to document confirmation of HIV by noting that the patient has HIV, is HIV positive, had an HIV test that was positive, or

is known to have HIV. The patient must be *asymptomatic*. Do not assign V08 if the physician documents "AIDS" or any HIV-related illness. You would instead assign code 042, which we will discuss next.

2. Assign code 042 for a patient with an HIV-related illness (AIDS). The physician must document that the patient's condition is related to HIV or is AIDS. You can find code 042 by searching the Index for the main term *AIDS* or main term *infection*, subterm *HIV*, connecting word *with*, subterm *symptoms, symptomatic*.

3. After a patient develops an HIV-related illness, he is no longer HIV *asymptomatic*, and you can *never* assign code V08 for him again. Only assign code V08 *until the patient develops symptoms*, and then assign code 042. After you have assigned code 042 to one encounter, you will *always* assign 042 to every subsequent encounter, whether or not the physician treats the patient for an HIV-related illness. Sequence code 042 based on the reason for the patient's encounter:

   • Assign 042 *first* if a patient is admitted or *seen for an HIV-related condition*. Medical documentation will most likely include wording that the patient's illness is *due to, caused by, caused from, following*, or *a result of* AIDS. If you are not sure if AIDS caused the condition, then query the physician. Assign additional diagnosis codes for all reported HIV-related conditions or any other conditions that are pertinent to the encounter.

   • Assign 042 *second* if a patient has or previously had an HIV-related condition and the *reason for the current encounter is unrelated* to HIV (such as a traumatic injury). First, sequence the code for the unrelated condition. Assign 042 as the second code. Assign additional codes for any documented HIV-related conditions.

4. Assign code 795.71—*Inconclusive serologic test for Human Immunodeficiency Virus [HIV]* for patients with an inconclusive HIV test and the physician does not provide a definitive diagnosis of HIV or document an HIV-related illness. To locate this code, search the Index for *findings (abnormal)*, subterm *serological*, subterm *human immunodeficiency virus (HIV)*, subterm *inconclusive*.

5. When a patient has an encounter for an HIV test, assign code V73.89—*Screening for other specified viral disease* (Index entries: *Screening (for), disease, viral, specified type*.) Assign code V69.8—*Other problems related to lifestyle* as a secondary code if an asymptomatic patient is in a known high-risk group for HIV (Index entries: *problem (with), lifestyle, specified NEC*). Assign code V01.79—*Exposure to HIV* if it is known that the patient was exposed to HIV (Index entry: *exposure to*).

6. If the patient receiving an HIV test shows signs, symptoms, illness, or a confirmed HIV-related diagnosis, then code the signs, symptoms, illness or diagnosis. Assign V65.44—*HIV counseling* as an additional counseling code if the physician counseled the patient during the encounter for the test (Index entries: *counseling, HIV*).

   • When a patient returns to be informed of his or her HIV test results and the test results are negative, assign code V65.44—*HIV counseling*.

   • If the results are positive, but the patient is asymptomatic, assign code V08. Assign V65.44 for counseling if appropriate.

   • If the results are positive and the patient is *symptomatic*, assign code 042 first. Sequence secondary codes for the HIV-related symptoms or diagnosis. Assign V65.44 for counseling if appropriate.

Review the following examples for coding HIV and AIDS encounters. Follow along with your ICD-9-CM manual to practice finding codes in the Index and cross-referencing them to the Tabular:

Example 1: Frank Campbell, a 55-year-old patient, returns to see his primary care physician, Dr. Turner, for the results of his HIV test. Dr. Turner tells Mr. Campbell that he is HIV positive. The patient is asymptomatic, and Dr. Turner counsels him on managing the infection.

Codes to assign for this case: V08—*asymptomatic HIV* (■ FIGURE 9-9), V65.44—*HIV counseling* (■ FIGURE 9-10).

Figure 9-9 ■ Index entry for asymptomatic HIV with code V08 cross-referenced to the Tabular.

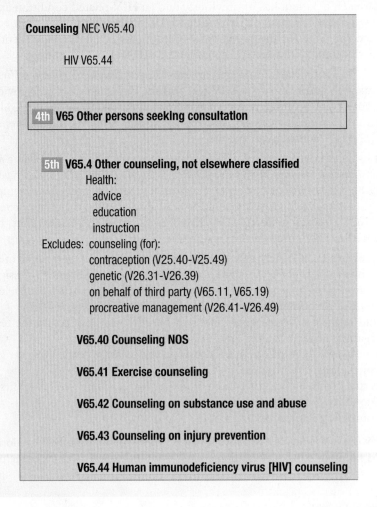

Human immunodeficiency virus (disease) (illness) 042
   infection V08
      with symptoms, symptomatic 042

V08 Asymptomatic human immunodeficiency virus [HIV] infection status

    HIV positive NOS

Note: This code is ONLY to be used when NO HIV infection symptoms or conditions are
      present. If any HIV infection symptoms or conditions are present, see code 042.
Excludes: AIDS (042)
      human immunodeficiency virus [HIV] disease (042)
      exposure to HIV (V01.79)
      nonspecific serologic evidence of HIV (795.71)
      symptomatic human immunodeficiency virus [HIV] infection (042)

Figure 9-10 ■ Index entry for HIV counseling with code V65.44 cross-referenced to the Tabular.

Counseling NEC V65.40

    HIV V65.44

4th V65 Other persons seeking consultation

    5th V65.4 Other counseling, not elsewhere classified
      Health:
        advice
        education
        instruction
Excludes: counseling (for):
      contraception (V25.40-V25.49)
      genetic (V26.31-V26.39)
      on behalf of third party (V65.11, V65.19)
      procreative management (V26.41-V26.49)

    V65.40 Counseling NOS

    V65.41 Exercise counseling

    V65.42 Counseling on substance use and abuse

    V65.43 Counseling on injury prevention

    V65.44 Human immunodeficiency virus [HIV] counseling

Example 2: Randy Morgan, a 38-year-old, presents to Williton Medical Center's ED for a right ankle fracture. Dr. Mills examines the patient, applies a splint, and prescribes a pain medication, instructing Mr. Morgan to avoid bearing weight on his right foot for five days. During the encounter, the patient provides past health history, including the fact that he has AIDS.

Codes to assign for this case: 824.8—*closed ankle fracture* (■ FIGURE 9-11), 042—
AIDS, secondary code because the encounter is not due to AIDS (■ FIGURE 9-12).

Fracture (abduction) (adduction) (avulsion) (compression) (crush) (dislocation) (oblique)
(separation) (closed) 829.0

ankle (malleolus) (closed) 824.8

4th **824 Fracture of ankle**

824.0 **Medial malleolus, closed**
Tibia involving:
ankle
malleolus

824.1 **Medial malleolus, open**

824.2 **Lateral malleolus, closed**
Fibula involving:
ankle
malleolus

824.3 **Lateral malleolus, open**

824.4 **Bimalleolar, closed**
Dupuytren's fracture, fibula
Pott's fracture

824.5 **Bimalleolar, open**

824.6 **Trimalleolar, closed**
Lateral and medial malleolus with anterior or posterior lip of tibia

824.7 **Trimalleolar, open**

824.8 **Unspecified, closed**
Ankle NOS

Figure 9-11 ■ Index entry for closed ankle fracture with code 824.8 cross-referenced to the Tabular.

AIDS 042

HUMAN IMMUNODEFICIENCY VIRUS (HIV) INFECTION (042)

042 **Human immunodeficiency virus [HIV] disease**

Acquired immune deficiency syndrome
Acquired immunodeficiency syndrome
AIDS
AIDS-like syndrome
AIDS-related complex
ARC
HIV infection, symptomatic
Use additional code(s) to identify all manifestations of HIV
Use additional code to identify HIV-2 infection (079.53)
Excludes: asymptomatic HIV infection status (V08)
exposure to HIV virus (V01.79)
nonspecific serologic evidence of HIV (795.71)

Figure 9-12 ■ Index entry for AIDS with code 042 cross-referenced to the Tabular.

Example 3: Jennifer Reed, a 42-year-old, is admitted to Williton Medical Center for pneumonia due to AIDS.

Codes to assign for this case: 042—*AIDS*, first-listed code because the encounter is due to AIDS, and 486—*pneumonia*. Try coding this case on your own using your ICD-9-CM manual by searching for these codes in the Index and cross-referencing them to the Tabular.

Review these additional guidelines for coding HIV or an HIV-related illness (AIDS):

1. When the patient's encounter is for an HIV-related illness during pregnancy, childbirth, or the puerperium (up to six weeks after childbirth), assign codes as follows:
    *   Sequence first code of 647.6X—*Other specified infectious and parasitic diseases in the mother classifiable elsewhere, but complicating the pregnancy, childbirth or the puerperium.* (Index entries: *disease, virus, complicating pregnancy, childbirth, or the puerperium*). You must always first assign codes from Chapter 11 in the Tabular (Complications of Pregnancy, Childbirth, and the Puerperium).
    *   Sequence second code 042.
    *   Assign additional code(s) for the HIV-related illness(es).

2. When an HIV-positive *asymptomatic* patient has an encounter during pregnancy, childbirth, or the puerperium, assign the codes as follows:
    *   Sequence first code 647.6X—*Other specified infectious and parasitic diseases in the mother classifiable elsewhere, but complicating the pregnancy, childbirth or the puerperium.* You will learn more about coding pregnancy encounters in Chapter 14 of this text.
    *   Sequence second code V08.

TAKE A BREAK

Let's take a break and then practice assigning codes for HIV and AIDS.

Exercise 9.2   Human Immunodeficiency Virus (HIV) and Acquired Immunodeficiency Syndrome (AIDS)

Instructions: Code the following patient cases, using both the Index and the Tabular. Refer to the main terms outlined for assistance locating codes, and refer to the coding guidelines in the previous section.

1. Dr. Hoffman diagnoses established patient, Arthur Tardif, age 42, with Kaposi's sarcoma due to AIDS. Mr. Tardif was previously diagnosed as HIV positive.

    Code(s): _____

2. Jason Moreno, age 26, is an AIDS patient with Kaposi's sarcoma, which AIDS caused. He arrives at Williton Medical Center's ED with a broken great toe on his right foot.

    Code(s): _____

3. Samantha Farber, a 32-year-old established patient, sees Dr. Hoffman for HIV testing, even though she has not had any HIV-related conditions or symptoms.

She admits to having a high-risk lifestyle with multiple sexual partners, one of whom is infected with HIV. Dr. Hoffman discusses how to make the needed lifestyle changes and refers her to a community mental health center for counseling.

Code(s): _____

4. Samantha Farber returns to see Dr. Hoffman to discuss her positive HIV test result. He counsels her on managing her diagnosis and possible future outcomes.

    Code(s): _____

5. Patsy Wallace, a 28-year-old, sees Dr. Gerard, obstetrician/gynecologist (OB/GYN), for a prenatal check-up at 12 weeks. She is HIV positive but has no other problems.

    Code(s): _____

6. Ronald Douglas, age 50, has an HIV test. He sees Dr. Hoffman today for the result, and Dr. Hoffman informs him that the result is inconclusive. He orders another HIV test, which Williton Medical Center's lab will perform.

    Code(s): _____

ENDOCRINE, NUTRITIONAL AND METABOLIC DISEASES, AND IMMUNITY DISORDERS (ICD-9-CM CHAPTER 3—240–279)

The **endocrine system** is made up of glands that secrete **hormones** into the bloodstream (■ FIGURE 9-13).

Disorders of the endocrine system occur when the body secretes too few, too many, or no hormones. Endocrine system disorders may be congenital (existing at birth) or *acquired* (happening after birth). *Endocrinology* literally means the study of (-ology) to secrete (crin/o) within (end/o), or the study of diagnosis, treatment, and prevention of endocrine system disorders. An *endocrinologist* specializes in treating disorders of the endocrine system. Some diseases of the endocrine system include diabetes mellitus, which we will review later in this section, **Cushing's syndrome**, and **premature menopause**.

Nutritional disorders occur when the body lacks nutrients for good health (e.g., Vitamin A deficiency) or receives too many nutrients. Examples of nutritional disorders are **malnutrition** and **calcium deficiency**.

Metabolic disorders happen when the body reacts abnormally to chemical processes and cannot maintain **homeostasis**. There are either too many or too few of the chemicals that

hormones (hor' mōns) chemical substances that endocrine glands secrete to regulate specific body processes

Cushing's syndrome (koosh' ings) rare condition caused by excess corticosteroid hormones in the body, characterized chiefly by obesity of the trunk and face, high blood pressure, fatigue, and loss of calcium from the bones

premature menopause (men'o-pawz) when menstruation stops before it normally should; affects a small percentage of women ages 15–45

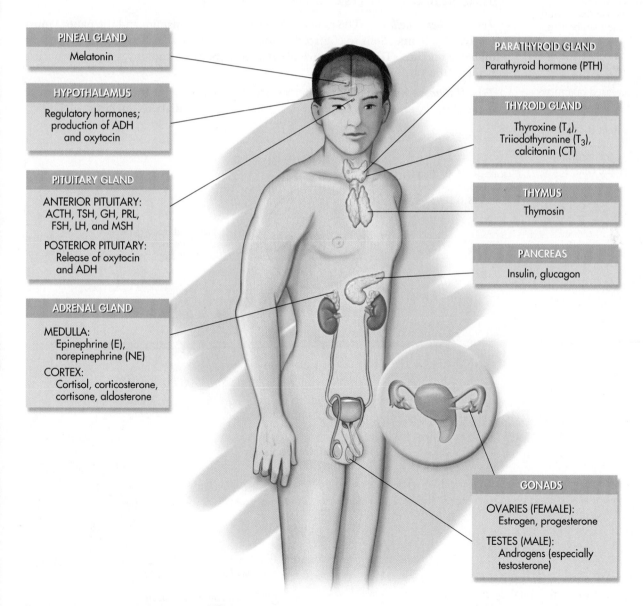

PINEAL GLAND	PARATHYROID GLAND
Melatonin	Parathyroid hormone (PTH)

HYPOTHALAMUS	THYROID GLAND
Regulatory hormones; production of ADH and oxytocin	Thyroxine (T$_4$), Triiodothyronine (T$_3$), calcitonin (CT)

PITUITARY GLAND	THYMUS
ANTERIOR PITUITARY: ACTH, TSH, GH, PRL, FSH, LH, and MSH / POSTERIOR PITUITARY: Release of oxytocin and ADH	Thymosin

ADRENAL GLAND	PANCREAS
MEDULLA: Epinephrine (E), norepinephrine (NE) / CORTEX: Cortisol, corticosterone, cortisone, aldosterone	Insulin, glucagon

GONADS

OVARIES (FEMALE): Estrogen, progesterone

TESTES (MALE): Androgens (especially testosterone)

Figure 9-13 ■ Endocrine glands and their hormones.

malnutrition (mal-noo-trish′ən) any disorder of inadequate nutrition

calcium deficiency (kal′se-əm de-fish′ən-se) less than the normal amount of calcium, the most abundant mineral in the body

homeostasis (hō-mē-ō-stā′sĭs) stability; the state of equilibrium maintained in the body's internal environment by adjusting its physiological processes

hypercalcemia (hī ñ pĕr-kăl-sē′ mĭ-ă) abnormally large amount of calcium in the blood

Wilson's disease rare, progressive disease that is due to a defect in the metabolism of copper

hypogammaglobulinemia (hi-po-gam-ə-glob-u-lĭ-ne′me-ə) decreased quantity of antibodies in the blood

graft-versus-host disease reaction in that the cells of transplanted tissue immuno-logically attack the cells of the host organism

the body requires to be healthy, which can happen because specific organs do not function properly. Examples of metabolic disorders are **hypercalcemia** and **Wilson's disease**.

Immunity disorders occur when the body's immune system cannot fight off bacteria, viruses, fungi, or protozoa, or when the patient has an autoimmune disorder when the immune system actually attacks itself (called an *overactive immune response*). Types of immunity disorders include **hypogammaglobulinemia** and **graft-versus-host disease**.

There are many endocrine, nutritional, metabolic, and immunity disorders and diseases, too many for you to code in this chapter. So, we'll review one of the most common endocrine disorders, diabetes mellitus, which you can then practice coding.

Diabetes Mellitus

The *pancreas* is an organ that produces insulin, a hormone that lowers blood sugar, to help the body's cells metabolize fats and carbohydrates (■ FIGURE 9-14). A patient with diabetes mellitus has increased levels of glucose (called high blood sugar) either because the pancreas does not properly produce insulin, or because the body's cells do not respond correctly to the insulin the pancreas produces.

There are three main types of diabetes mellitus:

- *Type I diabetes mellitus*—The pancreas does not produce insulin, and the patient must receive insulin injections to control the disease. Type I is also called insulin-dependent diabetes mellitus (IDDM) or juvenile diabetes (because the onset typically occurs before puberty).

- *Type II diabetes mellitus*—The pancreas produces insulin, but the body does not use it correctly. Type II is also called non-insulin-dependent diabetes mellitus (NIDDM)

Figure 9-14 ■ Diagram of how the body controls blood sugar levels.

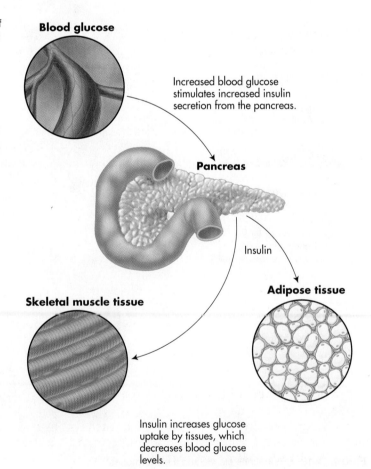

Blood glucose

Increased blood glucose stimulates increased insulin secretion from the pancreas.

Pancreas

Insulin

Adipose tissue

Skeletal muscle tissue

Insulin increases glucose uptake by tissues, which decreases blood glucose levels.

or adult-onset diabetes. Type II is more prevalent than type I. To control type II, patients can take medication and sometimes take insulin.

- *Gestational diabetes*—This type can occur during the second and third trimesters of pregnancy in women who are not diabetic prior to pregnancy. Gestational diabetes means that the body does not use insulin correctly. It may cause complications during the pregnancy. It typically resolves after pregnancy but increases the risk of developing type II diabetes later in life. Be careful not to confuse gestational diabetes with *diabetes mellitus in pregnancy*, which means that a pregnant woman *already had* diabetes before she became pregnant.

It is important to note that patients also can have congenital diabetes and drug-induced diabetes, also called *secondary diabetes*, which another condition caused. Many times, if the first condition is resolved, the secondary diabetes will also resolve.

Do not confuse *secondary diabetes* documented in a patient's record with assigning a *secondary code* for diabetes because they do not mean the same thing. Also note that secondary diabetes is not necessarily type II diabetes just because it is called "secondary." Patients can also have a *prediabetes* diagnosis, a condition in that blood glucose levels are higher than the normal range but not yet high enough for a diagnosis of diabetes mellitus. You can find normal lab values, including glucose, in Appendix C of this text.

Symptoms of diabetes include

- **polyuria**
- **polydipsia**
- **polyphagia**
- unexplained weight loss
- sudden vision changes
- fatigue
- numbness or tingling in hands or feet
- slow-healing sores

Many people have no symptoms or do not recognize them, so they do not know that they have diabetes.

Risk factors for type I diabetes are genetic, autoimmune, and environmental. Risk factors for type II diabetes include obesity, lack of physical activity, advanced age, family history of diabetes, or prior history of gestational diabetes. High-risk groups for type II are African, Hispanic, Latino, and Asian Americans.

Physicians diagnose diabetes by using one or more fasting plasma glucose blood tests. Before the test, patients must fast for at least eight hours. The normal fasting blood glucose (blood sugar) ranges from 70 to 105 mg/dL (milligrams per deciliter), and a patient with diabetes has a reading of 126 mg/dL or higher.

There is no cure for diabetes, and treatment for both type I and type II includes eating a healthy diet and exercising. Both type I and type II diabetics regularly monitor their glucose levels to control diabetes. Patients with diabetes who fail to manage their disease (called *uncontrolled diabetes*), who smoke, or who have hypertension are at risk for developing more serious conditions, such as problems with the eyes, heart, kidneys, and blood vessels. Diabetics can suffer nerve damage and poor circulation that may result in amputations of toes, feet, and legs, as well as open wounds (■ FIGURE 9-15). They also can become blind from unmanaged **glaucoma** and **diabetic retinopathy**.

Diabetic patients see many different providers, including a primary care physician who monitors their progress, an endocrinologist, an **ophthalmologist**, a **podiatrist**, and a *diabetes educator* who teaches patients how to manage their disease, including eating a healthy diet.

Coding Guidelines for Diabetes Mellitus Patients with diabetes often have complications, and there is an etiology/manifestation relationship between diabetes and any complications. In Chapter 4, you learned how to assign codes using the etiology/manifestation coding convention for a patient with diabetic retinopathy. You also assigned codes for diabetic patients' encounters in Chapter 5. Refer to the following guidelines for

polyuria (pŏl-ē-ū′ rĭ-ă) frequent urination

polydipsia (pol-e-dip′se-ə) excessive thirst and intake of fluid

polyphagia (pol-e-fa′jə) excessive eating

glaucoma (glaw-kō′ mă) disease of the eye in that pressure within the eyeball damages the optic disc, impairing vision and sometimes progressing to blindness

diabetic retinopathy (ret-ĭ-nop′ə-the) disorder of the blood vessels of the retina, occurring as a complication of poorly controlled diabetes mellitus and often leading to blindness

ophthalmologist (ŏf-thăl-mŏl′ ō-jĭst) medical doctor who specializes in the study of the eye

podiatrist (po-di′ə-trist) physician who specializes in treating disorders of the foot

Figure 9-15 ■ Wound debridement in a diabetic foot ulcer using larvae that eat the dead tissue.

Photo credit: © Scott Camazine / Alamy.

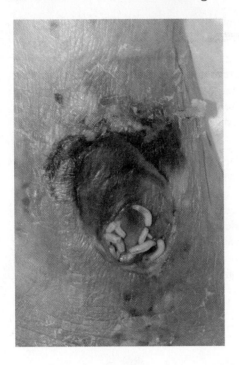

additional clarification when you are assigning codes for diabetes mellitus, secondary diabetes mellitus, and any associated manifestations. Turn to category 250 in your ICD-9-CM manual to review subcategory and subclassification choices for diabetes.

Diabetes Mellitus

1. Category 250—*Diabetes mellitus* includes diabetes with and without complications. The following are mandatory fifth digits to assign to codes from category 250:
   - 0—type II or unspecified type, not stated as uncontrolled
   - 1—type I, [juvenile type], not stated as uncontrolled
   - 2—type II or unspecified type, uncontrolled
   - 3—type I, [juvenile type], uncontrolled

2. If the physician does not document the type of diabetes mellitus, *code it as type II.*

3. All type I diabetics use insulin, and type II diabetics may also use insulin. If the physician does not document the type of diabetes but *does state that the patient uses insulin,* assign the appropriate fifth digit for type II.

4. For type II patients who routinely use insulin, assign code V58.67—*Long-term (current) use of insulin.* Do not assign V58.67 if the physician administers insulin *temporarily* to bring a type II patient's blood sugar under control during an encounter.

5. When assigning codes for diabetes and its associated conditions, sequence first a code(s) from category 250 (etiology). Sequence second the code for the condition (manifestation). Be careful not to confuse a condition that diabetes caused with a condition that is also present with diabetes.

   For example, a patient could have a diabetic cataract, which diabetes caused. Another patient could have diabetes and a senile cataract, which diabetes did not cause. Always query the physician if you are not sure about an etiology/manifestation relationship involving diabetes.

6. Assign as many codes from category 250 and as many associated manifestation codes as are necessary to identify all of a patient's associated conditions.

Secondary Diabetes Mellitus

1. Category 249—*Secondary diabetes mellitus* includes secondary diabetes with and without complications. Other conditions always cause secondary diabetes, such as **cystic fibrosis**, malignant neoplasm of pancreas, **pancreatectomy**, and an adverse

cystic fibrosis (sĭs′ tĭk fī-brō′ sĭs) hereditary disease that usually appears in early childhood, involves functional disorder of the exocrine glands, and is marked by faulty digestion and breathing difficulty

pancreatectomy (pan-kre-ə-tek′tə-me) surgical removal of all or part of the pancreas

effect of a drug or poisoning. Turn to category 249 in your ICD-9-CM manual to review subcategory code choices and the following fifth digits to assign to codes from category 249:
- 0—not stated as uncontrolled, or unspecified
- 1—uncontrolled

2. For secondary diabetes patients who routinely use insulin, assign code V58.67—*Long-term (current) use of insulin.* Do not assign V58.67 if the physician administers insulin *temporarily* to bring a patient's blood sugar under control during an encounter.

3. When you are assigning codes for secondary diabetes and its associated conditions or manifestations, sequence first a code(s) from category 249 (etiology). Sequence second the code for the condition (manifestation).

4. Assign as many codes from category 249 and any associated manifestation codes as are necessary to identify all of the patient's associated conditions. ICD-9-CM lists manifestation codes under secondary diabetes code with a specific manifestation.

5. Sequence secondary diabetes codes and the cause of secondary diabetes based on the reason for the encounter.

6. If the reason for the encounter is to treat secondary diabetes, then first assign a code from category 249. Sequence second a code for the *cause* of secondary diabetes.

7. If the reason for the encounter is to treat the condition that caused the secondary diabetes, then first assign a code for that condition. Sequence second a code for the *secondary diabetes* from category 249.

8. You can find additional coding guidelines for secondary diabetes, diabetic retinopathy, diabetic macular edema, diabetes mellitus complicating pregnancy, gestational diabetes, and insulin pump malfunction in the Official Guidelines for Coding and Reporting.

TAKE A BREAK

Let's take a break and then practice assigning codes for endocrine, nutritional, and metabolic diseases, as well as immunity disorders and diabetes mellitus.

Exercise 9.3   Endocrine, Nutritional, and Metabolic Diseases and Immunity Disorders

Instructions: Code the following patient cases, using both the Index and the Tabular. Refer to instructions outlined in the previous section for assistance.

1. Sondra Davidson, age 30, sees Dr. Herrera, an endocrinologist, at Williton's Endocrinology Clinic to discuss the results of her diagnostic tests. She currently suffers from obesity and essential hypertension, and she bruises easily. Dr. Herrera diagnoses Ms. Davidson with Cushing's syndrome and discusses treatment options with her.

   Code(s): _____

2. Mildred Hopkins, age 48, visits Williton's Endocrinology Clinic today. Dr. Herrera previously diagnosed her with Vitamin K deficiency due to prolonged antibiotic use. She meets with the clinic's dietician for nutrition counseling. (Hint: One of the codes that you will assign is a V code.)

   Code(s): _____

3. Lisa Wade, age 35, has trouble sleeping, a rapid heart rate (tachycardia), diarrhea, and bulging eyes. After examination and testing, Dr. Herrera diagnoses the patient with Graves' disease and discusses therapeutic and medicinal options with her.

   Code(s): _____

4. Dr. Hoffman sees Carol Walters, age 50, who complains of sharp pains in her great toe, along with edema and swelling. Ms. Walters is also overweight. After conducting an examination and further testing, Dr. Hoffman determines that the patient has gout due to a diet that is heavy in red meat. He discusses dietary changes with Ms. Walters and refers her to the Williton's Endocrinology Clinic for nutrition counseling.

   Code(s): _____

5. Lawrence Amick, age 51, sees Dr. Herrera for diabetes monitoring. Mr. Amick has required insulin for the past six months to control the diabetes.

   Code(s): _____

6. Dr. Hoffman diagnoses new patient Kathleen Grizzle, age 13, with type I diabetes and immediately starts her on insulin.

   Code(s): _____

continued

TAKE A BREAK *continued*

7. Dr. Herrera sees established patient, Victor Magness, a 48-year-old, for management of uncontrolled diabetes due to chronic pancreatitis.

   Code(s): _____

8. Michael Franz, an established patient, age 62, sees Dr. Hoffman for management of an ulcer on his right foot due to diabetes.

   Code(s): _____

9. An ambulance rushes Clarence Currie, a 53-year-old diabetic, to Williton's ED for weakness, shortness of breath, and severe abdominal pain with vomiting. Dr. Burns, an ED physician, diagnoses the patient with uncontrolled diabetes with ketoacidosis.

   Code(s): _____

10. Dr. Lombard, a neurologist (physician who diagnoses and treats nerve disorders), treats new patient, Sarah Benavidez, age 71, for peripheral autonomic neuropathy (various symptoms that nerve damage causes). She is also a type II diabetic.

    Code(s): _____

DISEASES OF THE BLOOD AND BLOOD-FORMING ORGANS (ICD-9-CM CHAPTER 4—280-289)

erythrocytes (ĕ-rīth′ rō-sīts)

leukocytes (′lü-kə-′sīts)

thrombocytes (thrŏm′ bō-sīts)

hematology (hē-mă-tŏl′ ō-jē)

hematologist (hēmă-tŏl′ ō-jĭst)

anemia (ă-nē′ mĭ-ă) disorder characterized by a reduction in the number of circulating red blood cells, the amount of hemoglobin, or the volume of packed red cells

coagulation defects (ko-ag-u-la′shən) disorders in the way that blood thickens or clots

purpura (pur′ pū-ra) purplish discoloration of the skin when blood discharges into the tissues

white blood cell diseases any disorders that affect colorless blood cells

inherited (in-her′-ət ed) having received a trait from one's parents by genetic transmission

aplastic anemia (a-plas′tik) form of anemia in that the capacity of the bone marrow to generate red blood cells is defective

hemolytic anemia (he-mo-lit′ik) anemia caused by excessive destruction of red blood cells

Blood has many important functions in the body to maintain homeostasis, including delivering nutrients, eliminating wastes, transporting oxygen and hormones, and fighting infections. The body performs these functions using **erythrocytes** (red blood cells—RBCs), **leukocytes** (white blood cells—WBCs), and **thrombocytes** (platelets). Blood is made up of cells, platelets, and plasma (■ FIGURE 9-16). **Hematology** literally means the study of (-ology) blood (hemat/o), or the study of the diagnosis, treatment, and prevention of blood disorders. A **hematologist** specializes in treating disorders of the blood. Examples of blood disorders are **anemia, coagulation defects, purpura**, and **white blood cell diseases**. We will focus on learning more about anemia, a very common blood disorder. According to the CDC, there are over *400 types of anemia* affecting 3.5 million people in the U.S.

Anemia

Anemia occurs when the body does not have enough RBCs to carry oxygen from the lungs throughout the body. This may happen because the body simply cannot produce enough RBCs, there is a process in the body that destroys RBCs, or there is blood loss, which is the most common cause of anemia. Surgery, digestive or urinary tract bleeding, cancer, trauma, and heavy menstrual periods can all result in excessive blood loss.

The body may not produce an adequate number of RBCs due to an **inherited** or acquired condition, such as **aplastic anemia**; lack of iron; lack of the hormone erythropoietin, which produces RBCs; having cancer or HIV; being pregnant, which can cause low levels of iron; **hemolytic anemia**; **sickle cell anemia**; and **thalassemias** (all three are inherited disorders). Other types of anemia include **iron-deficiency anemia** (■ FIGURE 9-17), **pernicious anemia**, and **Cooley's anemia**.

Symptoms of anemia vary depending on the type of anemia, but general symptoms include fatigue, pale skin, weakness, and **dyspnea**. Treatment for anemia also varies with the type but may include iron and vitamin supplements, **blood transfusions**, and methods to help stimulate RBC production. Physicians diagnose anemia through blood tests that provide RBC counts and additional information about the structure of RBCs.

Coding Guidelines for Anemia in Chronic Illness ICD-9-CM subcategory 285.2 contains subclassification codes for anemia in chronic illness, including chronic kidney disease (CKD), neoplastic disease, and other chronic illnesses. Turn to subcategory 285.2 to review subclassification choices, and refer to the following guidelines when coding from subcategory 285.2:

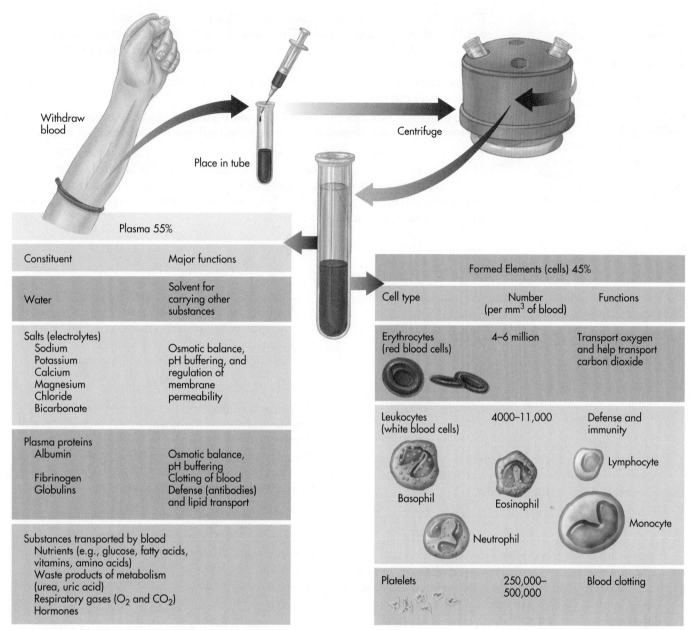

Withdraw blood

Place in tube

Centrifuge

Plasma 55%

Constituent	Major functions
Water	Solvent for carrying other substances
Salts (electrolytes) Sodium Potassium Calcium Magnesium Chloride Bicarbonate	Osmotic balance, pH buffering, and regulation of membrane permeability
Plasma proteins Albumin Fibrinogen Globulins	Osmotic balance, pH buffering Clotting of blood Defense (antibodies) and lipid transport
Substances transported by blood Nutrients (e.g., glucose, fatty acids, vitamins, amino acids) Waste products of metabolism (urea, uric acid) Respiratory gases (O_2 and CO_2) Hormones	

	Formed Elements (cells) 45%	
Cell type	Number (per mm^3 of blood)	Functions
Erythrocytes (red blood cells)	4–6 million	Transport oxygen and help transport carbon dioxide
Leukocytes (white blood cells) Basophil Eosinophil Neutrophil	4000–11,000	Defense and immunity Lymphocyte Monocyte
Platelets	250,000–500,000	Blood clotting

Figure 9-16 ■ Blood components separated by a centrifuge.

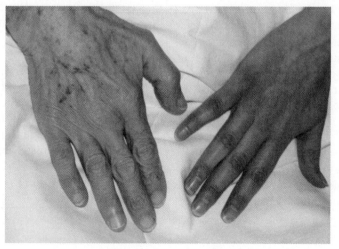

Figure 9-17 ■ Patient with iron-deficiency anemia (left); Patient with a normal hand (right).

Photo credit: Westminster Hospital / Photo Researchers, Inc.

sickle cell anemia (sik'-əl) anemia that is common in people of West African or Mediterranean descent; in affected individuals, red blood cells are abnormally shaped like a sickle (crescent-shaped), are sticky, and block blood flow

thalassemias (thăl-ă-sē' mĭ-ăs) hereditary anemia occurring in populations bordering the Mediterranean Sea and in Southeast Asia; causes reduced hemoglobin (protein that carries oxygen to red blood cells)

1. When assigning a code from subcategory 285.2, also assign a code for the chronic condition that caused the anemia (CKD, neoplastic disease, or other chronic disease):
   - Assign codes from 285.2 as the principal or first-listed code if the reason for the encounter is to treat anemia.
   - Assign codes from 285.2 as secondary codes if anemia treatment is *part of* the encounter but not the main reason for it.
2. When assigning code 285.21—*Anemia in chronic kidney disease*, also assign a code from category 585—*Chronic kidney disease*, to indicate the stage of chronic kidney disease.
3. When assigning code 285.22—*Anemia in neoplastic disease* (disease pertaining to a neoplasm), also assign a code for the neoplasm that caused the anemia. Code 285.22 represents anemia that is due to a malignancy, *not* anemia due to antineoplastic chemotherapy drugs. Assign code 285.3—*Antineoplastic chemotherapy induced anemia* when chemotherapy caused the anemia.

TAKE A BREAK

Let's take a break and then practice assigning codes for blood disorders and anemia.

Exercise 9.4 **Diseases of the Blood and Blood-Forming Organs**

Instructions: Code the following patient cases, using both the Index and the Tabular. Refer to instructions outlined in the previous section for assistance.

1. Dr. Jennings, a hematologist, sees established patient, Patty Neal, age 25, to review results of blood tests to monitor her medication to treat hemophilia A (an inherited blood clotting disorder).

   Code(s): _____

2. Mrs. Barnett brings her son, Tyler, to see Dr. Jennings for the results of his blood tests. Tyler has experienced frequent nosebleeds and bruises easily. Tyler's family history is positive for bleeding disorders. Dr. Jennings diagnoses Tyler with von Willebrand disease (a bleeding disorder) and discusses medication therapy with Mrs. Barnett.

   Code(s): _____

3. Dr. Hoffman sees Maggie Lowe, age 7, for a red, freckled skin rash on her legs and buttocks. Her mother accompanies her to the visit. Dr. Hoffman recently treated Maggie for an upper respiratory infection (URI). After an examination, he determines that Maggie has allergic purpura as a result of the URI. He states that it should resolve without further treatment and instructs Mrs. Lowe to call in a week if it does not.

   Code(s): _____

4. Dr. Hoffman admits Steve Green, age 62, to Williton Medical Center for severe anemia due to primary prostate cancer with metastasis to the bone. Clinicians give him blood transfusions and then discharge him home.

   Code(s): _____

5. Dr. Burns, Williton's ED physician, admits Thomas Slay, age 81, to Williton Medical Center for aplastic anemia and pancytopenia (shortage of all types of blood cells, including red and white blood cells and platelets). The patient receives a blood transfusion.

   Code(s): _____

6. Dr. Burns admits Victoria Coen, a 59-year-old, to Williton Medical Center for anemia due to chemotherapy (antineoplastic drugs) for metastatic lung cancer. (Hints: The secondary cancer site is not documented, but you still need to assign a code for it. This case also needs an E code from the Table of Drugs and Chemicals.)

   Code(s): _____

7. Earl Sledge, age 52, reports to Williton Medical Center's outpatient infusion center for treatment of anemia due to stage II CKD. The infusion center provides intravenous medication infusions and therapeutic injections.

   Code(s): _____

8. Gregory Lasley, a 63-year-old established patient, sees Dr. Hoffman's registered nurse for a vitamin B-12 injection for pernicious anemia. Dr. Hoffman recently diagnosed him during routine blood tests performed during his annual physical.

   Code(s): _____

9. Mrs. Rigby brings her daughter, Wanda, 7 months old, to Williton Medical Center's ED with fever, cough, and shortness of breath. After a thorough workup (an exam and testing), Dr. Mills diagnoses her with acute chest syndrome due to sickle cell anemia (with crisis). Clinicians administer oxygen and IV antibiotics in the ED, after which Dr. Mills admits her to the hospital for further treatment.

   Code(s): _____

POINTERS FROM THE PROS: Interview with a Coder

Janet Lord's job title is Coder II at a large physician group and she has worked in healthcare for 23 years. She audits anesthesia records for compliance and completeness; assigns ICD-9-CM, CPT-4, and anesthesia base units; and obtains missing medical information needed for coding.

What are the most challenging aspects of your job?

Incomplete documentation is always a challenge. It is sometimes overly time consuming to track down information that should have been included up front.

Please give an example of a time when you educated a physician(s) on processes of coding and the outcome.

I worked closely with our pain management physicians to set up a chronic pain clinic. They relied on my advice as far as proper coding and documentation. They were eager to learn, and it all turned out great.

What advice would you like to give to coding students to help them prepare to work successfully in the healthcare field?

Learn the medical terminology; learn that pronunciation and spelling are important. Read all that you can as often as you can.

(Used by permission of Janet F. Lord.)

DISEASES OF THE NERVOUS SYSTEM AND SENSE ORGANS (ICD-9-CM CHAPTER 6—320–389)

The **nervous system** is made of a framework of nerves throughout the body that process, receive, and send messages through nerve impulses that tell the body what to do and how to react. The nervous system consists of the **central nervous system (CNS)**, including the brain and spinal cord, that enables the body to see, hear, touch, taste, and smell, and the **peripheral nervous system (PNS)**, which contains nerves outside the CNS that control voluntary functions (muscle movement) and involuntary functions (cardiac, glands) (■ FIGURE 9-18). The sense organs are the eye and the ear, which work in conjunction with the nervous system.

Neurology literally means the study of (-ology) nerves (neuro), and *neurologists* are physicians who specialize in the diagnosis, treatment, and prevention of nervous system disorders. You may have heard of *neurosurgery*, which is the branch of medicine that specializes in surgically correcting nervous system disorders. Nervous system disorders can have many different causes, including trauma, neoplasms, **degenerative** diseases, or congenital conditions. Symptoms of disorders vary, depending on the patient's condition, but common symptoms include headache, muscle weakness, vision, hearing, or memory loss, weakness, seizures, and mental impairment. Common disorders of the CNS include **bacterial meningitis, Parkinson's disease**, and **epilepsy**. Common disorders of the PNS include **Bell's palsy**, carpal tunnel syndrome, and **polyneuropathy**.

Pain is also a nervous system disorder, and ICD-9-CM provides extensive guidelines for coding pain. Here are some of the guidelines:

1. Assign codes from category 338—*Pain, not elsewhere classified* with codes from other categories and chapters to provide more detail about acute or chronic pain and neoplasm-related pain.

2. For acute pain, assign a code from subcategory 338.1—*Acute pain*. For chronic pain, assign a code from subcategory 338.2—*Chronic pain*. If the physician does not specify if the pain is acute or chronic, then do not assign codes from category 338 unless it is post-**thoracotomy** pain, postoperative pain, neoplasm-related pain, or central pain syndrome.

3. Do not assign codes from subcategories 338.1 or 338.2 if the physician documents an underlying (definitive) diagnosis. The exception is if the reason for the patient's encounter is pain control or management, and *not* management of the underlying condition; in that case, assign codes from 338.1 or 338.2.

iron-deficiency anemia anemia characterized by low or absent iron in the blood

pernicious anemia (pər-nĭsh′ əs) type of anemia usually seen in older adults, caused when the patient's intestines cannot absorb vitamin B12

Cooley's anemia (koo′ lees) group of inherited forms of anemia causing a shortened life span of red blood cells; also known as thalassemia

dyspnea (dĭsp-nē′ ă) difficulty breathing

blood transfusions (transfu′zhəns) injections of blood from one person into the bloodstream of another

degenerative (dĭ′-jen-ə-rāt-ĭv) causing degeneration or deterioration

bacterial meningitis (men-in-jī′tĭs) rapidly developing inflammation of the subarachnoid space located within the layers of tissue covering the brain and spinal cord, caused by bacteria

Parkinson's disease (păr′ kĭn-sŭnz) progressive neurological disorder from degeneration of nerve cells in the part of the brain that controls movement

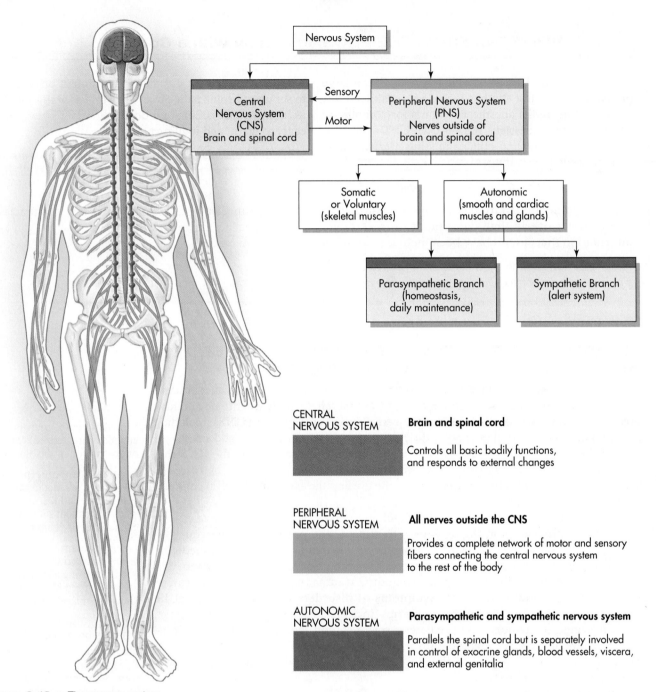

Figure 9-18 ■ The nervous system.

4. Category 338 codes are acceptable as principal diagnosis or first-listed code when
    • Pain control or pain management is the reason for the admission/encounter. Report the underlying cause of the pain as an additional diagnosis.
    • The encounter is for the insertion of a neurostimulator (stimulates nerve functions) for pain control.

5. Assign pain as a secondary diagnosis when the reason for the encounter is to treat the underlying cause of the pain.

6. Assign code 338.3—*Neoplasm related pain (acute) (chronic)* to pain that is documented as being related to, associated with, or due to cancer, a primary or secondary malignancy, or a tumor, *regardless* of whether the pain is acute or chronic.

WORKPLACE IQ

You are working as a medical assistant for Dr. Gupta, and one of your jobs is to compare diagnoses on patients' encounter forms with medical record documentation for accuracy. Over the past few weeks, you have read a lot of documentation on patients who have cancer. Three of them are terminally ill, and their health is declining rapidly. Reading all of the records is very sad and upsetting, and you do not want to continue to work on the cancer cases.

What would you do?

7. Assign 338.3 as the principal or first-listed code when the reason for the admission or encounter is pain control or management. Code the underlying neoplasm as an additional diagnosis.

8. When the reason for the admission or encounter is management of the neoplasm, and the physician also documents pain associated with the neoplasm, assign the neoplasm code first and code 338.3 second.

9. Assign subcategory 338.2 to chronic pain. There is no time frame that defines when pain becomes chronic pain. Rely on the provider's documentation to guide you, and query the physician if you are not sure. Chronic pain syndrome (CPS) and chronic pain do not mean the same thing. Patients with CPS typically do not respond well to treatment. Do not assume that you should code chronic pain when the provider specifically documents CPS. Instead, assign code 338.4—*Chronic pain syndrome.*

For more information on coding pain, refer to the Official Guidelines; and you can find directions for accessing them in Appendix A of this text.

Eye Disorders

ICD-9-CM classifies external and internal eye disorders to categories 360–379 (Disorders of the eye and **adnexa**).

Ophthalmology literally means the study of (-ology) the eye (ophthalm/o). Ophthalmologists are physicians who specialize in diagnosing and treating medical eye disorders, including performing surgery. **Optometry** literally means measurement (-metry) of the eye (opt/o). **Optometrists** are physicians who specialize in conducting eye examinations, diagnosing and treating disorders, performing procedures, and prescribing corrective lenses.

It is important to not only become familiar with the anatomy of the eye to correctly code diagnoses, but also to understand how the eye functions. Review your medical references and conduct Internet research to understand more about eye disorders and treatment.

Refer to ■ FIGURE 9-19 to review **lacrimal** eye structures and ■ FIGURE 9-20 to review internal eye structures.

There are many different types of eye disorders, and you will next learn about two of the most common disorders: *glaucoma* and *cataracts.*

Glaucoma is known as the silent killer of sight because a patient may have glaucoma for a long time and not know it until they develop serious vision problems. Physicians diagnose glaucoma when patients have high **intraocular pressure (IOP)**, causing a build-up of too much fluid in the eye, although not all patients with glaucoma have high IOP. There are different types of glaucoma and they can lead to optic nerve damage, eventually causing blindness if not properly treated or if treatment fails. Physicians measure glaucoma's severity in stages, from mild to severe. There is no cure for glaucoma, but patients can manage it with regular eye exams and medications or surgery to reduce IOP. However, any damage that occurs to the optic nerve cannot be reversed.

Symptoms of glaucoma include seeing colored halos around lights, having severe headaches, and experiencing nausea, vomiting, eye pain, and peripheral (on the side)

---

polyneuropathy (pol-e-nŏŏ-rop′ə-the) disturbance or disorder of several peripheral nerves at the same time

thoracotomy (thō-răk-ŏt′ō-mē) incision into the chest wall

adnexa (ăd-něk′ să) adjoining anatomical parts

ophthalmology (of-thul-măl′-ə-jē)

optometry (op-tom′-i-tree)

optometrists (op-tom′-i-trists)

lacrimal (lăk′ rĭm-ăl) pertaining to tears

intraocular pressure (IOP) the pressure of fluid in the eye against the membranes of the eye

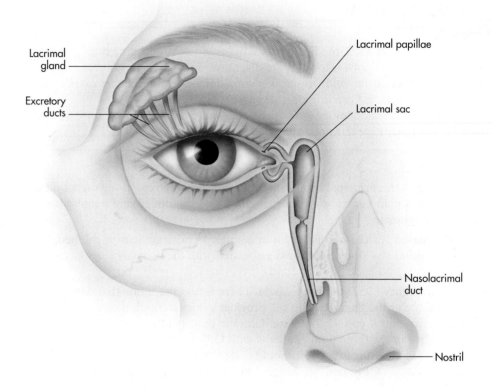

Figure 9-19 ■ Lacrimal eye structures.

Source: Anatomy and Physiology for Health Professions, Colbert, Ankney, Lee, Pearson Prentice-Hall (2007) p. 250.

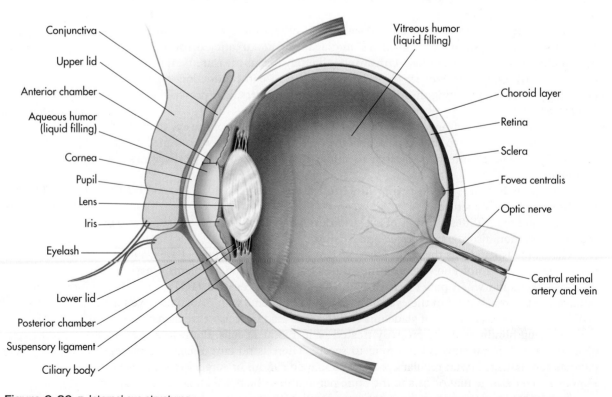

Figure 9-20 ■ Internal eye structures.

Source: Anatomy and Physiology for Health Professions, Colbert, Ankney, Lee, Pearson Prentice-Hall (2007) p. 251.

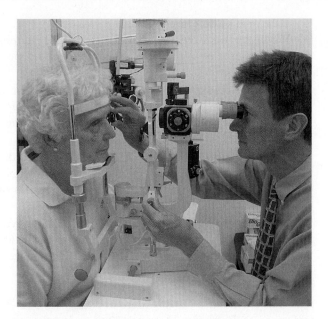

Figure 9-21 ■ A physician examines a patient's internal eye structures using a slit lamp.

Photo credit: Pearson owned, Michal Heron Image/Pharmaceutical Care Management Association.

vision loss. Risk factors for glaucoma include previous trauma to the eye, such as being hit in the eye with an object or a penetrating wound; diabetes; family history of glaucoma; severe nearsightedness or farsightedness; using steroid drops in the eye; previous eye surgeries; and being over age 60 or of African-American descent. Keep in mind that glaucoma may affect both eyes or only one eye.

The word cataract comes from the Greek word *cataractos*, meaning waterfall. When you look at a waterfall, the water appears cloudy or white, not clear. Cataracts cause cloudy or blurred vision on the lens of the eye. Physicians diagnose cataracts by conducting an examination of the lens using a **slit lamp** (■ FIGURE 9-21).

Risk factors for a cataract include eye trauma, eye surgery, smoking, diabetes, and being over age 60. Treatment for cataracts includes outpatient surgery, when the physician breaks up the cataract and suctions it out of the eye, then removes the lens and replaces it with a clear *intraocular lens (IOL)*. The patient's natural lens has small muscles called *zonules* that move the lens, enabling it to focus near or far. The IOL is set to a specific level of visual acuity. Depending on the patient's vision after surgery, an optometrist may also have to prescribe corrective lenses for the patient.

Turn to your ICD-9-CM manual to reference codes in the Tabular as you review the following ICD-9-CM guidelines for coding glaucoma:

1. Code first the type of glaucoma classified to subcategories 365.1–365.6. Assign *an additional code* from subcategory 365.7—*Glaucoma stage* to identify the glaucoma stage (unspecified, mild, moderate, severe, or indeterminate). *Never* assign codes from 365.7 as the principal or first-listed diagnosis.

   Assign code 365.74—*Indeterminate stage glaucoma* for glaucomas where the physician documents that she cannot clinically determine the stage. Do not confuse code 365.74 with code 365.70—*Glaucoma stage, unspecified,* which you should assign when there is *no documentation* regarding the stage of the glaucoma.

slit lamp lamp with a narrow flat opening that projects a beam of intense light into the eye for microscopic study

INTERESTING FACT: Early Physicians Suctioned Cataracts Using their Mouths

Centuries ago, Roman and Greek physicians pioneered cataract surgery using a thin tube which they placed on the patient's eye. The physician then physically sucked the cataract out of the eye, which required a tremendous amount of respiratory effort. Not surprisingly, there were many complications, including infections, and the lens falling into the back of the eye, causing blindness. Cataract surgery is one of the most common surgeries that physicians perform today.

2. **Bilateral glaucoma with same stage:**
   When a patient has bilateral glaucoma and the physician documents that each eye has the same type and stage, assign only one code for the *type* of glaucoma and one code for the *stage*.

3. **Bilateral glaucoma, same type with different stages:**
   When a patient has bilateral glaucoma of the same type and the physician documents that each eye has a different stage, assign one code for the *type* of glaucoma and one code for the *highest glaucoma stage*.

4. **Bilateral glaucoma with different types and different stages:**
   When a patient has bilateral glaucoma and the physician documents that each eye has a different *type* and a different *stage*, assign *a code for each type* of glaucoma and *only one code for the highest glaucoma stage*.

5. **Patient admitted with glaucoma and stage evolves during the admission:**
   If a patient is admitted with glaucoma and the stage progresses and changes during the admission, then assign a code for highest stage documented.

Ear Disorders

ICD-9-CM classifies ear disorders to categories 380–389 (Diseases of the ear and mastoid process). Refer to ■ FIGURE 9-22 to review the structure of the ear.

Otolaryngology literally means the study of (-ology) the ear (ot/o) and the larynx (laryng/o). **Otolaryngologists** are physicians who diagnose and treat ear, nose, and throat disorders. You may have heard of an ENT (ear, nose, and throat) physician. They are also called **otorhinolaryngologists**.

There are also many different types of ear disorders. You will learn about two common disorders: otitis media and tinnitus.

Bacteria or viruses cause **otitis media**, a middle ear infection that is common in children, in which the patient can have fluid build-up in the middle ear. Otitis media can also be acute or chronic. Symptoms include pain, **tinnitus** (ringing in the ears), fever, and nausea. Risk factors for otitis media include being under age five, more-than-average pacifier use, family history of the condition, allergies, and close contact with others who are ill, such as in a daycare center. Physicians diagnose otitis media by examining the ear with an **otoscope** (■ FIGURE 9-23). Treatment varies, depending on the patient's age and severity of the condition, and may include **antibiotics**, pain medications, and **analgesic** ear drops.

---

otolaryngology (oh-toh-lar-ing-ʹgol-uh-jee)

otolaryngologists (ōt-ō-lar-ən-ʹgäl-ə-jəsts)

otorhinolaryngologists (ōt-ō-rī-nō-lar-ən-gälʹ-ə-jəsts)

otitis media (ō-tīʹ tĭs mēʹ dē-ă)

tinnitus (tĭn-īʹ tŭs)

otoscope (oʹto-skōp) instrument for inspecting the ear

antibiotics (anʹti-bi-otʹiks) substances that are used chiefly in the treatment of infectious bacterial diseases, derived entirely or in part from a microorganism that destroys or stops the growth of bacteria

analgesic (ăn-ăl-jēʹ zĭk) medication to reduce or eliminate pain

---

Figure 9-22 ■ Ear structures.

Source: Anatomy and Physiology for Health Professions, Colbert, Ankney, Lee, Pearson Prentice-Hall (2007) p. 254.

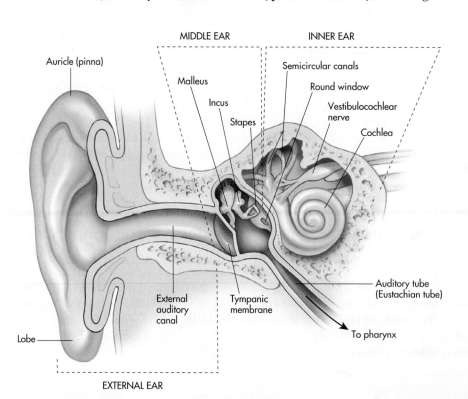

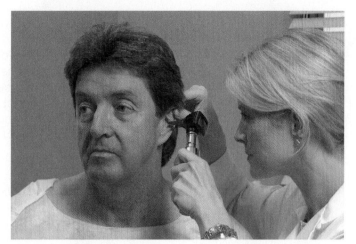

Figure 9-23 ■ A physician examines a patient's ear using an otoscope.

Photo credit: Michal Heron owned by PE/Pharmaceutical Care Management Association.

Tinnitus is commonly called *ringing in the ears*. Patients with tinnitus also complain that they hear buzzing, roaring, or clicking sounds, and they may also experience **pulsatile** tinnitus. Tinnitus can be the result of hearing loss from advanced age or be noise-induced, caused by repeatedly listening to loud music or working in a very noisy environment, like working with a jackhammer. Reactions to medications can also cause tinnitus. Physicians diagnose tinnitus by examining the neck and head and through hearing and radiology tests, such as a computed tomography (CT) scans. Treatment for tinnitus varies, depending on the cause. When patients have tinnitus from hearing loss, which is the most common cause, there is no treatment. Tinnitus generally worsens as the hearing loss worsens.

pulsatile (pul′sə-tīl) characterized by a rhythmical pulsation

TAKE A BREAK

Let's take a break and then practice assigning codes for nervous system and sense organs disorders.

Exercise 9.5   Diseases of the Nervous System and Sense Organs

Instructions: Code the following patient cases, using both the Index and the Tabular. Refer to instructions outlined in the previous sections for assistance.

1. Gwendolyn Pappas, age 39, comes to the pain management clinic at Williton Medical Center for treatment of chronic low back and hip pain, which is the late effect of automobile accident injuries from several years ago. (Hint: You will need to assign two different late effect codes for this case.)

   Code(s): _____

2. Benjamin Villareal, age 67, sees his oncologist, Dr. Valore, for pain management related to lung cancer.

   Code(s): _____

3. Chad Bumgarner, a 70-year-old, complains of acute pain in his chest following coronary artery bypass graft (CABG) surgery. Dr. Bergin, the cardiologist, determines that the pain is due to the thoracotomy (cutting the chest) required for the operation. He prescribes Vicodin®, a pain medication.

   Code(s): _____

4. Vera Dillingham, age 55, sees Dr. Fisher, an ophthalmologist, for management of acute angle-closure glaucoma, which affects both eyes. The left eye is a mild stage, and the right eye is a moderate stage.

   Code(s): _____

5. Brandon Moser, age 74, sees Dr. Fisher for his monthly retinal injections to manage age-related wet macular degeneration (breakdown of the macula, the tissue where light focuses to allow clear central vision). Mr. Moser has the condition in both eyes.

   Code(s): _____

6. Bruce Franks, a 6-year-old established patient, sees Dr. Kerr, an ENT, for a tympanoplasty (surgical repair of the middle ear) due to chronic serous (containing fluid) otitis media.

   Code(s): _____

7. Dr. Hoffman refers Betty Caldwell, age 63, to see Dr. Kerr because of complaints of ringing in her ears. After examination and testing, Dr. Kerr diagnoses Mrs. Caldwell with age-related pulsatile tinnitus.

   Code(s): _____

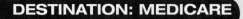

DESTINATION: MEDICARE

Medical nutrition therapy for diabetes involves educating diabetes patients on proper diet and changes to their lifestyles to help manage the disease. Medicare will reimburse providers for medical nutrition therapy services, but there are specific guidelines for the frequency and type of therapy that providers render. Access *Medicare's Medical Nutrition Therapy* National Coverage Determination (NCD) following the steps listed next, and then answer the questions that follow:

1. Go to the website http://www.cms.gov.

2. In the search field at the top right, type *medical nutrition therapy.*

3. Choose the search result *(NCD) for Medical Nutrition Therapy.* The NCD number is 180.1.

1. What diagnoses does Medicare approve in order to reimburse providers for a patient's medical nutrition therapy?

2. How can a Medicare beneficiary receive more than the approved hours of therapy treatment?

A LOOK AHEAD TO ICD-10-CM

ICD-10-CM classifies endocrine, nutritional, and metabolic diseases in Chapter 4 (E00–E90), diseases of the blood and blood-forming organs and certain disorders involving the immune mechanism in Chapter 3 (D50–D89), diseases of the nervous system in Chapter 6 (G00–G99), diseases of the eye and adnexa in Chapter 7 (H00–H59), and diseases of the ear and mastoid process in Chapter 8 (H60–H95). There are currently no ICD-10-CM coding guidelines for Chapters 3, 7, or 8. There are coding guidelines for Chapters 4 and 6, and one major addition in Chapter 6 are guidelines for assigning codes to identify conditions occurring on the patient's **dominant** or **nondominant** side.

dominant side the side that is predominant, such as right-handed or left-handed

nondominant side the side that is not predominant, either the right or left side

Instructions: Assign ICD-10-CM codes to the following cases that you previously coded in ICD-9-CM, using both the ICD-10-CM Index and the Tabular. (Refer to ICD-10-CM Official Guidelines for additional information; directions for accessing the guidelines are located in Appendix A of this text.)

1. Sharon Putnam, a 30-year-old established patient, sees Dr. Hoffman with complaints of dark urine, fever, vomiting, and yellowing skin. After conducting a physical examination, Dr. Hoffman tells her that she has viral hepatitis A. He recommends rest and tells her to avoid alcohol and fatty foods. Code(s): _____

2. Lawrence Amick, age 51, sees Dr. Herrera for diabetes monitoring. Mr. Amick required insulin for the past six months to control the diabetes. Code(s): _____

3. Michael Franz, an established patient, age 62, sees Dr. Hoffman for management of an ulcer on his right foot due to diabetes. Code(s): _____

4. Samantha Farber, a 32-year-old established patient, sees Dr. Hoffman for HIV testing, even though she has not had any HIV-related conditions or symptoms. She admits to having a high-risk lifestyle with multiple sexual partners, one of whom is infected with HIV. Dr. Hoffman discusses how to make the needed lifestyle changes and refers her to a community mental health center for counseling. Code(s): _____

5. Dr. Hoffman admits Steve Green, age 62, to Williton Medical Center for severe anemia due to primary prostate cancer with metastasis to the bone. Clinicians give him blood transfusions and then discharge him home. Code(s): _____

6. Vera Dillingham, age 55, sees Dr. Fisher, an ophthalmologist, for management of acute angle-closure glaucoma, which affects both eyes. The left eye is a mild stage, and the right eye is a moderate stage. Code(s): _____

CHAPTER REVIEW

Multiple Choice

Instructions: Circle one best answer to complete each statement.

1. When you are coding causes of infectious diseases, search for the main term
   a. bacteria.
   b. infection.
   c. protozoal.
   d. virus.

2. If a patient has an encounter for an HIV-related illness, you should
   a. assign code V08—*Asymptomatic human immunodeficiency virus (HIV) infection status* first, and assign a code for the illness second.
   b. assign a code for the illness first, and assign code V08—*Asymptomatic human immunodeficiency virus (HIV) infection status* second.
   c. assign code 042—*Human immunodeficiency virus (HIV) disease* first, and assign the code for the illness second.
   d. assign the code for the illness first, and assign code 042—*Human immunodeficiency virus (HIV) disease* second.

3. Which of the following is *not* a form of diabetes?
   a. Type I
   b. Type II
   c. Gestational
   d. Prediabetes

4. Secondary diabetes is
   a. drug or illness-induced.
   b. the same as type II diabetes.
   c. sequencing diabetes as the secondary code.
   d. prediabetes.

5. Which of the following is *not* a disorder of the endocrine system?
   a. Cushing's syndrome
   b. Wilson's disease
   c. Gestational diabetes
   d. Bell's palsy

6. Anemia occurs when the body does not have enough
   a. ABCs.
   b. CBCs.
   c. RBCs.
   d. WBCs.

7. Anemia due to antineoplastic chemotherapy drugs is coded when
   a. a malignancy caused the anemia.
   b. chemotherapy caused the anemia.
   c. CKD caused the anemia.
   d. none of the above.

8. When the reason for the admission/encounter is management of pain related to cancer, code the pain as
   a. acute.
   b. chronic.
   c. the primary diagnosis.
   d. the secondary diagnosis.

9. Pain is coded as chronic when the physician documents the pain as
   a. chronic.
   b. acute.
   c. chronic pain syndrome.
   d. lasting more than three weeks.

10. Which physician specializes in the diagnosis, treatment, and prevention of disorders of the blood?
    a. endocrinologist
    b. neurologist
    c. hematologist
    d. oncologist

Coding Assignments

Instructions: Assign ICD-9-CM code(s) to the following cases, referencing both the Index and Tabular.

1. Beth Claussen, age 21, sees Dr. Hoffman to obtain her HIV test result, which is negative.

   Code(s): _____

2. Carlos Wolff, a 44-year-old, sees Dr. Hoffman to obtain his HIV test result, which is inconclusive. Dr. Hoffman plans to schedule another HIV test for the patient.

   Code(s): _____

3. Alan Ratcliffe, age 47, sees Dr. Mayhew, his endocrinologist, for uncontrolled diabetes. He also has nephropathy due to diabetes.

   Code(s): _____

4. Grace Gonzales, a 62-year-old, had a three-hour glucose tolerance test and a complete chemistry analysis at her last office visit. Two weeks later, she sees Dr. Hoffman for a prescription to treat her iron (Fe)-deficiency anemia and for follow-up to discuss her lab tests. Dr. Hoffman tells Mrs. Gonzales that her glucose level was too high and that she has the potential to develop diabetes. He gives her a 1,500-calorie diabetic diet to follow.

   Code(s): _____

5. Olivia Wages, age 18, comes to the infusion center at Williton Medical Center for treatment of staphylococcal meningitis.

   Code(s): _____

6. Chris Medellin, age 35, comes to the pain clinic at Williton Medical Center for treatment of chronic pain syndrome.

   Code(s): _____

7. Pamela Vickery, a 37-year-old, is admitted to Williton for a lumbar spinal fusion (surgery to decrease back pain between lumbar vertebra). Dr. Kerr, an orthopedist, previous diagnosed Mrs. Vickery with spinal stenosis in her lumbar region. He told her that if she could not control the pain, then she could have corrective surgery. After unsuccessful efforts to manage the pain, she decided to have the surgery.

   Code(s): _____

8. Stanley Peach, a 67-year-old, experiences chronic pain from a herniated cervical disc (when discs that connect vertebra are displaced or move out of place). He comes to the pain management clinic at Williton Medical Center for medication injections to help eliminate the pain.

   Code(s): _____

9. Sandra Hanes, a 61-year-old, sees neurologist Dr. Lombard for ongoing migraine headaches. The migraines make her vomit and make her extremely sensitive to light, but she does not experience aura (visual problems, such as flashing lights and blurred vision). The current episode has lasted for more than 72 hours. Her diagnosis is common migraine with status migrainosus (migraine lasting more than 72 hours).

   Code(s): _____

10. Elizabeth Searles, age 60, complains of ringing and buzzing in her ears and difficulty hearing. Dr. Kerr, her ENT, examines her ears and notes a structural defect. He diagnoses her with objective tinnitus.

    Code(s): _____

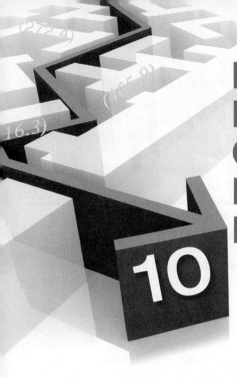

Mental Disorders; Respiratory, Digestive, Genitourinary, Skin, and Musculoskeletal System Disorders

10

Learning Objectives

After completing this chapter, you should be able to

- Spell and define the key terminology in this chapter.
- Review and apply the guidelines for coding mental disorders.
- Code respiratory diseases according to correct coding guidelines.
- Describe and code diseases of the digestive system.
- Discuss coding guidelines for diseases of the genitourinary system, and correctly assign codes.
- Demonstrate how to code disorders of the skin and connective tissue.
- Describe coding guidelines for musculoskeletal system disorders, and code these conditions.

Key Terms

digestive system
genitourinary system
integumentary system

mental disorder
musculoskeletal system
respiratory system

| INTRODUCTION

The next stop on your coding journey is to learn more about disorders and conditions categorized in specific chapters of ICD-9-CM, beginning with mental disorders. It is important to note that when you work in healthcare, you may only work in one specialty area, such as in a primary care physician's office. If so, you will most likely code the same diagnoses repeatedly because of the specific nature of the physician's practice. The benefit to learning how to code many specialties is that you will be better prepared to work in any specialty because your coding education will be well rounded. You will also be better prepared to work in a facility including multiple specialties, such as a hospital.

Coding all disorders in every specialty is beyond the scope of this chapter, but you will learn about some of the most common conditions. You will also have the chance to apply previous coding rules and conventions that you learned by completing exercises in this chapter. Keep in mind that you can keep track of specific coding rules by making notes in your code book or on the computer if you use an online ICD-9-CM code set. The notes will help you to remember how to code specific conditions. Let's continue on your journey and further expand your knowledge!

"Be curious always! For knowledge will not acquire you: you must acquire it."—SUDIE BACK

ICD-9-CM codes in this chapter are from the ICD-9-CM 2012 code set from the Department of Health and Human Services, Centers for Disease Control and Prevention.

ICD-10-CM codes in this chapter are from the ICD-10-CM 2012 Draft code set from the Department of Health and Human Services, Centers for Disease Control and Prevention.

MENTAL DISORDERS (ICD-9-CM CHAPTER 5—290–319)

Mental literally means pertaining to (-al) the mind (ment/o), and a **mental disorder** is a problem with or in the mind. Mental disorders are real conditions that patients experience, not imagined ones. They can take many forms, such as **anxiety**, depression, **schizophrenia**, **dementia**, and **behavioral disorders**.

Although the field of mental health has progressed significantly over the past century, there has been a *stigma* (negative perception) attached to mentally ill patients. In other words, many people do not consider the specialty of mental health to be valid. People still believe that the mentally ill imagine their own disorders and can cure themselves by simply "snapping out of it." They may refer to the mentally ill using derogatory terms such as "crazy," "nuts," or "psycho," or may state that mentally ill individuals simply like to complain and pretend to be ill to gain attention. They also may not believe that individuals have actual mental health disorders, insisting that they are just "weird" or "eccentric."

Before providers fully understood how to care for the mentally ill and meet their unique needs, they kept them in mental hospitals that were called *insane asylums* (an outdated term for a facility that houses the mentally ill). Families with mentally ill relatives did not understand how to care for them, so they placed them in asylums and left them there for the rest of their lives. Many caretakers neglected them and never provided the necessary treatment or nurturing; others beat or abused the patients, causing much more harm than good.

Today, this type of behavior is considered abusive and is illegal, but the mental illness stigma still exists, partly because it is not easy for people to understand mental disorders, because they cannot find physical evidence of them. You can see many other conditions, such as a deformity or a blocked artery, but many mental health conditions lack physical proof that they exist. It is important to understand that even though you cannot see a mental health problem, it is just as valid as any other health condition elsewhere in the body.

Providers who diagnose and treat mentally ill patients include psychiatrists, psychologists, and social workers. **Psychiatry** literally means treatment or specialty (-iatry) of the mind (psych/o). **Psychology** literally means the study of (-ology) the mind (psych/o). **Psychiatrists** are physicians who specialize in the field of mental health, diagnosing and treating patients, providing individual, family, and group **psychotherapy**, and prescribing medications. **Psychologists** are not physicians but are specially trained therapists with psychology degrees who also diagnose and treat mental health patients through psychotherapy but cannot prescribe medications.

Social work involves utilizing community resources to help patients. *Social workers* hold degrees in social work and may also have degrees in psychology. They provide *interdisciplinary* (involving many disciplines) care to patients, including therapy, and also help patients find outside resources to assist them. These include day care services for patients' children, domestic violence shelters for physically and verbally abused patients, and assistance applying for Medicaid for indigent patients. Social workers can also work for schools, helping students to deal with stress, depression, and anxiety, and working with students' families to help them create a positive home environment. Other healthcare providers are involved in treating mental health patients, such as registered nurses and other types of physicians, depending on each patient's situation.

Mental health services can be inpatient, if the patient is too ill to function independently, or can be in an outpatient hospital, clinic, physician's or psychologist's office, or *community-based mental health center* (outpatient clinic which individual counties operate within a state). Mental health patients also receive services in a *Partial Hospitalization Program (PHP)*, a program that patients attend during the day which provides group therapy and activities, education, and counseling. Patients in a PHP are not ill enough to be hospitalized but are not well enough for regular outpatient visits. They need more intensive treatment, which the PHP can provide. Both hospitals and community-based mental health centers have PHPs.

anxiety—involuntary bodily reaction to stress, which creates feelings of uneasiness, apprehension, or worry

schizophrenia (skĭz ō -frĕn ē- ă)—a mental disorder with psychotic symptoms such as delusions, hallucinations, and disordered thinking

dementia (dē-mĕn′ shē-ă)— a collection of symptoms marked by memory loss and loss of other cognitive functions, such as perception, thinking, reasoning, and remembering

behavioral disorders— mental health problems that lead to disruptive behavior, such as attention deficit disorder (ADD)

psychiatry (sī-kahy′-uh-tree)

psychology (sī -kol′-uh-jee)

psychiatrists (sī-kahy′-uh-trists)

psychotherapy (sī kō-thĕr′ ă-pē)—treatment of mental disorders through verbal and nonverbal communication techniques, such as counseling

psychologists (sī -kol′-uh-jists)

Many different types of mental disorders are congenital; others are acquired from disease, injury, drugs, or trauma. You will learn about some of the most common mental disorders and how to code them, including anxiety disorders, depression, and bipolar disorder. There are no specific ICD-9-CM Official Guidelines for coding mental disorders, and you will need to follow instructional notations in the code book for direction on correctly assigning codes.

Anxiety Disorders

Anxiety is a normal part of life, and everyone experiences it. Normal reactions to feelings of anxiety include coping appropriately with situations and not acting irrationally. *Anxiety disorders* occur when a person has an abnormal reaction to feelings of anxiety, which manifests itself in many different symptoms, including worry, irritability, sweating, nausea, fatigue, and diarrhea. Specific symptoms may be more or less severe, depending on the individual patient. Anxiety disorders can be debilitating, causing the sufferer to withdraw from the real or imagined situation that caused the anxiety, such as work, school, shopping, or driving. A patient may also experience anxiety or panic attacks that happen without warning, making the patient feel as though he is dying, out of control, and about to experience something very bad.

Causes of anxiety include hereditary factors, where anxiety disorders are common among members of the same family; a chemical imbalance in the brain (brain disorder) that causes the patient to have irrational fears and symptoms of anxiety; traumatic events, such as a car crash, fire, or death of a loved one; and drug-induced, where illegal drug use or a prescription medication causes the anxiety. Physicians and clinicians diagnose anxiety disorders by examining the patient and asking him questions about his family, health, and social history. They also determine if there is an underlying medical problem that is causing the anxiety, which then requires specific treatment. Anxiety disorder treatment includes psychotherapy to help patients learn and practice effective techniques for dealing with anxiety, along with prescription medication.

Here are some common anxiety disorders:

- *Generalized Anxiety Disorder*   chronic worry or anxiety without reason, with symptoms of headaches, muscle tension, trembling, and sweating.
- *Obsessive-Compulsive Disorder (OCD)*   repetitive behaviors (compulsions) and/or unwanted thoughts or obsessions, with persistent rituals, of hand washing, counting, and cleaning.
- *Post-Traumatic Stress Disorder (PTSD)*   worry or anxiety about past traumatic events, such as a car accident, natural disaster, physical attack, or military combat. Symptoms include anxiety and fear over flashbacks that relive the traumatic event.
- *Panic Disorder*   fear and anxiety so severe that it causes shortness of breath (SOB), dizziness, nausea, vomiting, chest pain, sweating, and loss of control.
- *Social Anxiety Disorder*   fear and anxiety surrounding a specific social setting, such as being watched while eating out. Symptoms include becoming overly self-conscious of one's actions, sweating, nausea, and difficulty expressing oneself.

When you are coding anxiety disorders, be sure to query the physician if the chart documentation does not include the specific type of anxiety disorder. Review the following example for coding an anxiety disorder encounter:

Example: Mrs. Wells, a 35-year-old new patient, sees Dr. Hunter, a psychiatrist, for a psychiatric evaluation. She states that she has difficulty with everyday tasks. Mrs. Wells states that she has to lock and relock the door, sometimes 10 times or more, and has to review the mail a second or third time before she feels that she can throw it away. After Dr. Hunter obtains Mrs. Wells' past family, medical, and social history, and asks her some additional questions, he diagnoses her with OCD. Dr. Hunter provides psychotherapy, prescribes medication, and then asks her to schedule a follow-up appointment.

Search the Index for the main term *disorder* and subterm *obsessive-compulsive*, and then cross-reference code 300.3 to the Tabular (■ FIGURE 10-1).

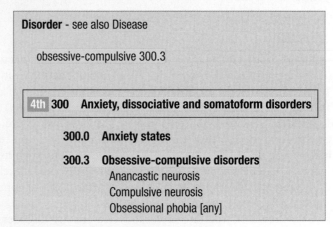

Figure 10-1 ■ Index entry for obsessive-compulsive disorder with code 300.3 cross-referenced to the Tabular.

Depression

Depression, another common mental disorder, is when the patient consistently withdraws from activities that he used to enjoy, avoids interactions with others, and has no hope for the future. Patients suffering from depression frequently feel tired, agitated, or sad and have trouble remembering, concentrating, and sleeping. They may also think that suicide is the answer to solving their problems.

Like anxiety, causes of depression include hereditary factors, brain disorder, traumatic events, taking illegal drugs or prescription medications, or drinking alcohol. Patients can suffer from depression due to the death of a loved one or pet, loss of a job, relocation to a new area, or other major life change, like a marriage, divorce, or having a physical or mental disability. Sadness is a normal reaction to loss, but depression occurs when a person's sadness does not lessen over time but becomes worse. Physicians and clinicians diagnose depression through an examination and obtaining the patient's health, family, and social history. Patients with depression benefit from prescription medication and psychotherapy.

Turn to your ICD-9-CM manual to review category 296, which includes major depressive disorder and bipolar disorders, discussed next. All subcategory codes under category 296 require a fifth digit to identify whether the patient's condition is unspecified, mild, moderate, severe, or in partial or full remission (improving or lessening).

Refer to the following example to code a patient's encounter for depression.

Example: Mr. Jones, a 28-year-old established patient, sees Dr. Goldstein, a psychiatrist, for psychotherapy. Dr. Goldstein documents that the patient suffers from recurring major depressive disorder in partial remission.

Search the Index for the main term *depression*, subterm *major*, and subterm *recurrent episode*. Then cross-reference code 296.3 to the Tabular, and assign the fifth digit (■ FIGURE 10-2).

Note that the fifth digit 5 specifies partial remission, and code 296.35 is the final code assignment. Always query the physician if you are not sure about the specific type of the patient's depression.

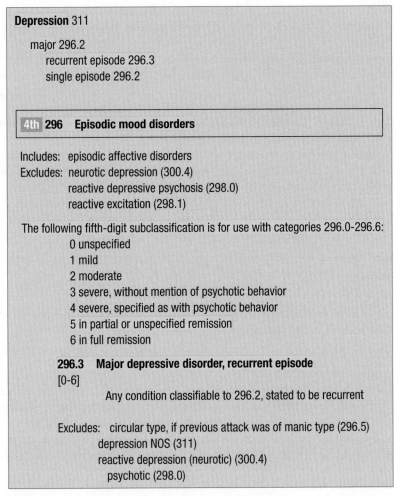

Depression 311

major 296.2
recurrent episode 296.3
single episode 296.2

| 4th | 296 | **Episodic mood disorders** |

Includes: episodic affective disorders
Excludes: neurotic depression (300.4)
reactive depressive psychosis (298.0)
reactive excitation (298.1)

The following fifth-digit subclassification is for use with categories 296.0-296.6:
0 unspecified
1 mild
2 moderate
3 severe, without mention of psychotic behavior
4 severe, specified as with psychotic behavior
5 in partial or unspecified remission
6 in full remission

296.3   Major depressive disorder, recurrent episode
[0-6]
Any condition classifiable to 296.2, stated to be recurrent

Excludes: circular type, if previous attack was of manic type (296.5)
depression NOS (311)
reactive depression (neurotic) (300.4)
psychotic (298.0)

Figure 10-2 ■ Index entry for recurrent major depressive disorder, with code 296.3 cross-referenced to the Tabular.

Bipolar Disorder

Bipolar disorder, also called manic-depressive illness, is a brain disorder where patients have severe mood changes, called *mood episodes,* ranging from very happy and overly excited (*mania,* or manic episode), to extremely sad (*depression,* or depressive episode). Some patients experience both manic and depressive symptoms during the same episode, called a *mixed state.*

Individuals with bipolar disorder can also talk fast, move from one thought or topic to another very quickly, be irritable or explosive, or act impulsively and engage in risky behaviors, such as gambling and unsafe sex. Sometimes patients also experience *psychotic* (abnormal condition of the mind) symptoms with hallucinations or delusions. During a manic episode, a patient may believe that he is wealthy, famous, or has unique powers, and during a depressive episode the patient may believe that he is a criminal, has no money, and is useless. Providers may misdiagnose patients who have psychotic symptoms as having schizophrenia, a severe mental illness with the same symptoms.

Patients with bipolar disorder often have troubled interpersonal relationships, may perform poorly at work or school, and may be suicidal. Many people have bipolar disorder and do not know it, and they may be symptomatic for several years before seeing a physician for the condition.

One risk factor for developing bipolar disorder is heredity, and children with a sibling or parent with bipolar disorder are four to six times more likely to develop the illness compared to children who do not have a family history of bipolar disorder (National Institute of Mental Health, www.nimh.nih.gov/health/publications/bipolar-disorder/what-are-the-risk-factors-for-bipolar-disorder.shtml). Mental health researchers have also found that a patient's environment may play a role in developing bipolar disorder.

Physicians diagnose bipolar disorder through a physical examination, interview with the patient, and lab test results which help to rule out any other conditions that may cause the same symptoms, such as brain tumor or stroke. Physicians will also conduct a psychiatric evaluation and treat the patient with psychotherapy and medication. There is no cure for bipolar disorder, but patients who have it can still lead positive, productive lives with appropriate treatment, which is typically lifelong.

Mental health providers reference guidelines and assign codes for bipolar disorder and other mental health conditions from the *Diagnostic and Statistical Manual of Mental Disorders, Fourth Edition (DSM-IV)*, which the American Psychiatric Association created for statistics and tracking. DSM-IV codes exist for mental disorders in adults and children, and codes also include causes of and treatment for disorders.

There are four basic types of bipolar disorders:

1. *Bipolar I Disorder*—manic or mixed episodes that last at least seven days, or severe manic symptoms that require patient hospitalization.
2. *Bipolar II Disorder*—pattern of depressive episodes.
3. *Bipolar Disorder Not Otherwise Specified (BP-NOS)*—symptoms of bipolar disorder but they do not fall under bipolar disorder I or II.
4. *Cyclothymic Disorder, or Cyclothymia*—mild form of bipolar disorder.

When coding bipolar disorder from category 296, it is very important to correctly code the *type* of bipolar disorder. Always query the physician when you do not understand information in the patient's record. ICD-9-CM classifies bipolar I disorder according to whether the patient has a single or current episode of depression, mania, or both. Fifth digits also classify specific information about the type of bipolar disorder. Turn to your ICD-9-CM manual to review the fifth-digit options for subclassification codes from category 296.

Refer to the following example to code a patient's encounter for bipolar disorder.

> **Example:** Mrs. Wilkinson, a 57-year-old established patient, sees Dr. Goldstein for continued treatment and psychotherapy for severe bipolar I disorder. Dr. Goldstein also documents that the patient currently suffers from depression from her most recent episode of bipolar disorder.
>
> Search the Index for the main term *disorder*, subterm *bipolar*, subterm *type I*, and subterm *depressed*. Note that the fifth digit is 3, for severe bipolar disorder without mention of psychotic behavior. Then cross-reference code 296.53 to the Tabular (■ FIGURE 10-3).

Many other mental disorder codes also require you to add the correct fifth digit. Be very careful to ensure that you do not guess the fifth digit and always query the physician for clarification.

Pay close attention to ICD-9-CM instructions for mental disorders to *Use additional code to identify any associated condition* or *Code first any underlying physical condition*. The patient may suffer from *a mental disorder which can cause another problem*, such as alcohol dependence (category 303), a mental disorder, which caused liver cirrhosis (571.2). ICD-9-CM requires you to code both conditions, assigning the code for alcohol dependence first and the code for liver cirrhosis second (■ FIGURE 10-4).

The patient *may also have a condition which caused the mental disorder*, such as Alzheimer's disease (331.0) that caused dementia (294.1—a mental disorder). Assign the code for Alzheimer's disease first and the code for dementia second, following the *Code first* note in the Tabular (■ FIGURE 10-5).

Disorder - see also Disease

bipolar (affective) (alternating) 296.80

Note Use the following fifth-digit subclassification with categories 296.0-296.6:

    0   unspecified
    1   mild
    2   moderate
    3   severe, without mention of psychotic behavior
    4   severe, specified as with psychotic behavior
    5   in partial or unspecified remission
    6   in full remission

atypical 296.7
specified type NEC 296.89
type I 296.7
   most recent episode (or current)
      depressed 296.5
      hypomanic 296.4
      manic 296.4
      mixed 296.6
      unspecified 296.7
   single manic episode 296.0
type II (recurrent major depressive episodes with hypomania) 296.89

4th   296   Episodic mood disorders

Includes: episodic affective disorders
Excludes: neurotic depression (300.4)
        reactive depressive psychosis (298.0)
        reactive excitation (298.1)

The following fifth-digit subclassification is for use with categories 296.0-296.6:

    0   unspecified
    1   mild
    2   moderate
    3   severe, without mention of psychotic behavior
    4   severe, specified as with psychotic behavior
    5   in partial or unspecified remission
    6   in full remission

5th   296.5   Bipolar I disorder, most recent episode (or current) depressed
[0-6]
      Bipolar disorder, now depressed
      Manic-depressive psychosis, circular type but currently depressed

Figure 10-3 ■ Index entry for bipolar I disorder with severe depression, most recent episode, with code 296.53 cross-referenced to the Tabular.

4th 303 **Alcohol dependence syndrome**

Use additional code to identify any associated condition, as:
  alcoholic psychoses (291.0-291.9)
  drug dependence (304.0-304.9)
  physical complications of alcohol, such as:
    cerebral degeneration (331.7)
    cirrhosis of liver (571.2)
    epilepsy (345.0-345.9)
    gastritis (535.3)
    hepatitis (571.1)
    liver damage NOS (571.3)

Figure 10-4 ▪ Alcohol dependence syndrome, category 303, in the Tabular with *Use additional code* note.

5th 294.1 **Dementia in conditions classified elsewhere**
Dementia of the Alzheimer's type
Code first any underlying physical condition as:
  dementia in:
    Alzheimer's disease (331.0)
    cerebral lipidoses (330.1)
    dementia with Lewy bodies (331.82)
    dementia with Parkinsonism (331.82)
    epilepsy (345.0-345.9)

Figure 10-5 ▪ Dementia subcategory code 294.1 in the Tabular with Code first note.

TAKE A BREAK

Let's take a break and then practice assigning codes for mental disorders.

Exercise 10.1 **Mental Disorders**

Instructions: Assign diagnosis codes to the following patient cases, using both the Index and Tabular. Refer to instructions outlined in the previous section for assistance.

1. George Boggs, a 23-year-old established patient, sees Dr. Goldstein, a psychiatrist, for medication management of bipolar I disorder. After questioning Mr. Boggs, Dr. Goldstein documents that the patient experienced severe manic episodes over the past several days.

   Code(s): _____

2. Jeannette Hand, a 42-year-old established patient, sees Dr. Goldstein for psychotherapy. Dr. Goldstein documents that she suffers from recurring severe major depressive disorder with psychotic behavior.

   Code(s): _____

3. Ryan Osuna, a new patient, age 41, sees Dr. Goldstein for a psychiatric evaluation because his cardiologist, Dr. Bergin, referred him. Mr. Osuna saw Dr. Bergin for shortness of breath and chest pain. Dr. Bergin ruled out cardiac-related problems and suspects a psychiatric disorder, due to Mr. Osuna's reports of extreme fear and anxiety. Dr. Goldstein diagnoses the patient with panic disorder, prescribes medication, and schedules him for psychotherapy.

   Code(s): _____

4. Eileen Cagle, age 33, sees Dr. Goldstein for ongoing management of chronic schizophrenia. He documents that the patient has not had any recent acute exacerbations.

   Code(s): _____

5. Wayne Garrido, a 56-year-old established patient, sees Dr. Hoffman for cirrhosis of the liver due to chronic alcoholism.

   Code(s): _____

6. Dr. Mills, ED physician, sees Marvin Chatman, age 27, at Williton Medical Center's ED after Mr. Chatman overdosed on LSD (an illegal hallucinogenic drug).

   Code(s): _____

DISEASES OF THE RESPIRATORY SYSTEM (ICD-9-CM CHAPTER 8—460-519)

respiratory (res′-pə-rə-tōr-ē)

cardiopulmonary (kärd-ē-ō-pul′-mə-ner-ē)

larynx (lar′inks) the voice box

pharynx (far′inks) the throat

The **respiratory system** allows the body to inhale oxygen and distribute it throughout the bloodstream to cells in the body to sustain life. The body exhales carbon dioxide, the waste product remaining after cells use oxygen. **Respiratory** literally means pertaining to or process of (-y) breathing (respirat/o). The respiratory system is also closely connected to the heart and *circulatory system* (blood flow through the heart, arteries, and veins). You may have heard the term **cardiopulmonary**, which is the system pertaining to (-ary) functions of the heart (cardi/o) and the lungs (pulmon/o) working together.

The respiratory system is divided into an upper airway (▪ FIGURE 10-6) and lower respiratory tract (▪ FIGURE 10-7). The upper airway includes the nose, **larynx**, and **pharynx**,

Figure 10-6 ■ The upper airway.

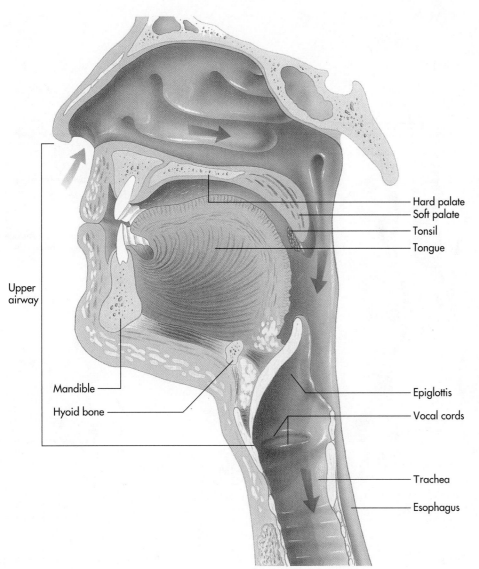

Hard palate
Soft palate
Tonsil
Tongue

Upper airway

Mandible
Hyoid bone

Epiglottis
Vocal cords

Trachea
Esophagus

and the lower respiratory tract contains the lungs; **bronchi** and **bronchioles**, branches of tubes that carry oxygen; and **alveoli**, air sacs at the ends of the bronchioles. The **diaphragm** is a muscular membrane separating the **abdominal cavity** from the **thoracic cavity**, helping the body to inhale oxygen and exhale carbon dioxide (■ FIGURE 10-8).

Respiratory disorders occur when the lungs and organs of the respiratory system do not function properly because of a congenital condition or underlying disease, such as cancer, infection, or trauma.

Pulmonology literally means the study of (-ology) the lungs (pulmon/o). A **pulmonologist** is a physician who diagnoses and treats respiratory system diseases. *Thoracic surgeons* are physicians who diagnose and treat disorders of the lungs and diaphragm. *Cardiothoracic surgeons* diagnose and treat disorders affecting both the respiratory and **cardiovascular** systems. A *respiratory therapist (RT)* is not a physician but is a trained clinician who assesses and treats patients with respiratory diseases and disorders, including delivering oxygen to patients in inpatient, outpatient, or emergency care settings.

Let's review some of the most common respiratory conditions, and then review specific ICD-9-CM guidelines for coding them, including COPD, asthma, bronchitis, and respiratory failure. We will review examples for some of the more complex cases. It is important to mention that there is a note at the beginning of the respiratory system chapter in ICD-9-CM instructing you to *Use additional code to identify infectious organism*. If an infection caused the patient's respiratory condition, then assign a code for the respiratory condition first and the infectious organism second.

bronchi (brŏng′ kī)plural of *bronchus*; the tubes that provide a passageway for air to and from the lungs

bronchioles (brong′ke-ōls)

alveoli (al-vē- ə-lī, -lē)

diaphragm (dī′ ă-frăm)

abdominal cavity—the hollow space which lies between the thorax (chest) and the pelvis

thoracic cavity (thə-ras′ik)—the body cavity containing the heart and lungs that the chest wall surrounds

pulmonology (pul-mə-nol′-ə-jē)

pulmonologist (p ul-mə-näl′-ə-jəst)

cardiovascular (kärd-ē- ō vas′-kyə-lər)—pertaining to the heart and blood vessels

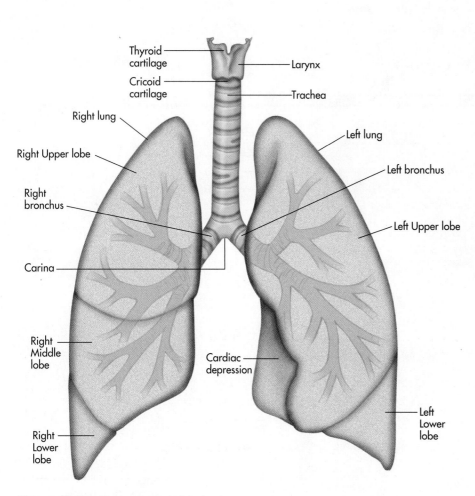

Figure 10-7 ■ The lower respiratory tract.

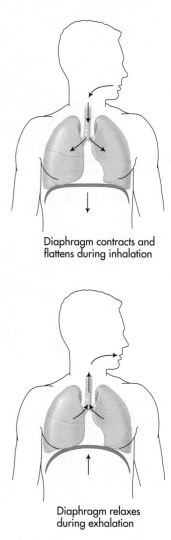

VENTILATION

Figure 10-8 ■ The diaphragm during inhalation and exhalation.

Chronic Obstructive Pulmonary Disease

COPD refers to a group of respiratory disorders that cause the patient to have breathing problems. Symptoms of COPD include shortness of breath, wheezing, cough, **sputum**, weight changes, and dizziness. The main risk factor for developing COPD is smoking, and patients can have many different types of COPD. They can develop COPD as a result of another condition, such as emphysema, cystic fibrosis, asthma, and bronchitis. Other causes include hereditary factors, exposure to air pollution, and respiratory infections.

    Physicians diagnose COPD through an examination; review of the patient's medical, family, and social history; and pulmonary function tests, including **spirometry**, which measures the speed and amount of inhaled and exhaled air using an instrument called a spirometer. Other tests assess *lung volume*, which measures whether the lungs contain too much or too little air and *diffusion capacity*, which measures how the lungs move oxygen into the bloodstream. Treatment for COPD depends on a patient's specific symptoms and other conditions present; it may include avoiding tobacco and exposure to pollutants, taking antibiotics to treat infections, and receiving oxygen therapy.

    Note that COPD is a *general* description for a group of respiratory disorders. Only assign a code for COPD when the medical documentation does not define the *type* of COPD that

sputum (spū' tŭm)—thick watery substance coughed up from the lungs

spirometry (spi-rom'ə-tre)

the physician treated, and you are unable to obtain more specific documentation. Refer to the Official Guidelines to determine when to assign a COPD code if the physician documents COPD with another condition. The guidelines for coding COPD and other respiratory conditions are outlined at the end of this section. (You can also find directions for accessing them in Appendix A of this text.) You may need to educate the physician on COPD coding guidelines to ensure that patients' medical documentation is specific enough for you to assign the correct code.

ICD-9-CM classifies COPD to category 496. However, COPD with related disorders is also included in categories 491–493. Refer to your ICD-9-CM manual to review the note under category 496 stating that you should *not* assign code 496 for COPD *along with a code from categories 491–493*, which already describe obstructive conditions.

Refer to the following example to assign a combination code for COPD with another condition.

> **Example:** Mr. Robinson, a 92-year-old new patient, sees Dr. Rutner, a pulmonologist, for shortness of breath and coughing. After examination and testing, Dr. Rutner diagnoses the patient with COPD with **emphysema** (■ FIGURE 10-9). He prescribes medication and oxygen and asks the patient to schedule a follow-up appointment.
>
> Search for the main term *disease*, subterm *lung*, subterm *obstructive*, connecting word *with*, and subterm *emphysema*. Then cross-reference code 492.8 to the Tabular (■ FIGURE 10-10).

emphysema (ĕm fĭ-sē′mă)—chronic obstructive pulmonary disease (COPD) where the alveoli (tiny air sacs in the lungs) expand, making it difficult to exhale

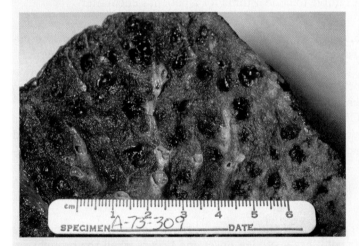
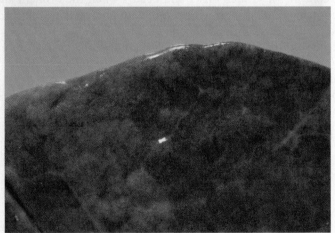

Figure 10-9 ■ Lung with emphysema (A) compared to the smooth, glistening, pink pleural surface of a healthy lung. (B)

Photo credits: (A) Dr. Edwin P. Ewing, Jr./CDC; (B): Custom Medical Stock Photo.

Disease, diseased - see also Syndrome

  lung NEC 518.89

    obstructive (chronic) (COPD) 496
      with
        acute
          bronchitis 491.22
          exacerbation NEC 491.21
        alveolitis, allergic (see also Alveolitis, allergic) 495.9
        asthma (chronic) (obstructive) 493.2
        bronchiectasis 494.0
          with acute exacerbation 494.1
        bronchitis (chronic) 491.20
          with
            acute bronchitis 491.22
            exacerbation (acute) 491.21
        decompensated 491.21
          with exacerbation 491.21
        emphysema NEC 492.8

4th **492   Emphysema**

    492.8   Other emphysema
        Emphysema (lung or pulmonary):
          NOS
          centriacinar
          centrilobular
          obstructive

Figure 10-10 ■ Index entry for COPD with emphysema with code 492.8 cross-referenced to the Tabular.

Asthma

Asthma is characterized by chronic inflammation of the bronchi, where they swell and narrow. This swelling restricts airflow and causes difficulty breathing. Symptoms include shortness of breath, coughing, chest tightness, and wheezing. The most common causes of asthma include allergic reaction to tobacco smoke, pollen, mold, dust, food, or pets, called *extrinsic asthma*, which usually begins in childhood. *Intrinsic asthma* usually appears in adulthood and is unrelated to allergies.

Physicians diagnose asthma through an examination; review of the patient's medical, family, and social history; and spirometry. Physicians treat asthma patients with **bronchodilators** and *steroids*, medications that open airways and reduce swelling. Patients can take bronchodilators orally, by injection, or through inhalers.

ICD-9-CM classifies asthma in category 493 and requires a fifth digit for the following subcategories. The following fifth-digit subclassification is for use with category 493.0–493.2 and 493.9:

0 unspecified

1 with status asthmaticus

2 with (acute) exacerbation

A fifth digit of 1 indicates that the patient's condition includes **status asthmaticus**, a medical emergency when a patient has an acute asthma attack but medication does not reduce symptoms. Status asthmaticus may lead to **cardiac arrest** and death. A fifth digit of 2 indicates that a patient's condition exacerbates (worsens).

Refer to the following example to code asthma for a patient's encounter.

> **Example:** Jamie Williams, a 12-year-old established patient, sees Dr. Rutner, a pulmonologist, for treatment of asthma. Dr. Rutner documents that Jamie is experiencing acute exacerbation of symptoms of extrinsic asthma, and the patient's medication no longer seems to work. Dr. Rutner prescribes two new medications, one oral to take daily, and the other inhaled and the other, inhaled, to take as needed.
>
> Use your ICD-9-CM manual to search the Index for the main term *asthma* and subterm *extrinsic,* and cross-reference code 493.0 to the Tabular. Note that you need to add a fifth digit, which will be 2, *with (acute) exacerbation.* Your final code assignment is 493.02.

Bronchitis

Bronchitis is inflammation of the bronchi and there are different types of bronchitis. *Acute bronchitis,* also called a chest cold, has a sudden onset and occurs when the bronchi are inflamed, swell, and produce mucus. *Chronic bronchitis* is more common in smokers and can last from a few months to over a year. *Chronic obstructive bronchitis* is a type of COPD with recurring respiratory infections. Symptoms of bronchitis include cough, shortness of breath, chest pain, fever, sputum production, sore throat, and nasal congestion. Acute bronchitis is typically infectious, which viruses from a cold or influenza can cause.

Physicians diagnose bronchitis by listening to sounds in the chest using a **stethoscope**, which is called **auscultation**. Physicians can also diagnose bronchitis with a chest X-ray, blood and sputum lab tests, and spirometry. Treatment includes medications to treat a virus or bacterial infection, nasal **decongestant**, and medications to suppress coughs and relieve pain.

Refer to the following example to code bronchitis for a patient's encounter.

> **Example:** Ms. Lopez, a 25-year-old established patient, sees Dr. Hoffman, her family physician, for a persistent cough with sputum and nasal congestion. Dr. Hoffman examines the patient and hears wheezing and crackles on auscultation of the lungs. He diagnoses the patient with acute bronchitis and prescribes an antibiotic.
>
> Use your ICD-9-CM manual to search the Index for the main term *bronchitis* and subterm *acute,* and cross-reference code 466.0 to the Tabular for final code assignment.

---

bronchodilators (brong-ko-di′la-tərs)

status asthmaticus (sta′təs az-mat'-i kəs)

cardiac arrest (kahr′de-ak)—loss of effective heart function, which results in stoppage of circulation

stethoscope (stĕth′ ō-skōp)—medical instrument used to listen to sounds of the heart, lungs, and other internal organs

auscultation (aws-kəl-ta′shən)

decongestant (de-kən-jes′tənt)—medication used for the temporary relief of nasal congestion

INTERESTING FACT: Many Jobs Are Hazardous to Lungs

Occupational disorders, or medical conditions that affect individuals working in specific jobs, can cause various respiratory symptoms, including a dry cough, shortness of breath, dizziness, fever, and weight loss. These conditions can worsen if left untreated and may even cause death. Some occupational respiratory conditions include:

✔ Pigeon fancier's disease, or pigeon fancier's lung, occurs when an individual, usually a pigeon breeder, develops a respiratory reaction to pigeon protein, found in their droppings.

✔ Cheese-washers' lung occurs when a person working in a cheese factory reacts to inhaled airborne bacteria transmitted in cheese.

✔ Farmers' lung occurs in farmers who react to inhaled dust and mold while working on a farm, typically around hay, but it can also occur in individuals who are working near tobacco, grain, and corn.

Respiratory Failure

Respiratory failure occurs when the body cannot properly inhale and distribute oxygen to the cells, or exhale and eliminate carbon dioxide. This condition leads to too little oxygen in the blood and too much carbon dioxide. *Acute respiratory failure (ARF)* is a medical emergency with a rapid onset. Many times, patients with ARF suffer from other conditions that cause ARF, such as COPD, cystic fibrosis (CF), pneumonia due to AIDS, respiratory infections, and congestive heart failure (CHF). *Chronic respiratory failure* develops over a period of days, rather than suddenly. Patients with acute or chronic respiratory failure may experience any of these symptoms: shortness of breath, chest pain, **syncope** (fainting), **cyanosis** (bluish skin due to lack of oxygen), irritability, confusion, or **tachycardia** (rapid heart rate over 100 beats per minute).

Physicians diagnose respiratory failure using various tests, including chest x-rays, CT scans, **arterial blood gases**, spirometry, and **complete blood count (CBC)** lab tests. Treatment includes oxygen therapy, bronchodilators, steroids, and antibiotics if a bacterial infection is present. Refer to the following example to code respiratory failure for a patient's encounter.

> **Example:** Mrs. Rogers, an 82-year-old, presents to Williton Medical Center's ED with shortness of breath, chest pain, and cyanosis. The ED physician administers oxygen, and after examination and study determines that Mrs. Rogers has chronic respiratory failure. He admits her for further treatment.
>
> To code this case, search the Index for the main term *failure*, subterm *respiration, respiratory*, and subterm *chronic*, and then cross-reference code 518.83 to the Tabular for final code assignment.

syncope (sĭn′ kŭ-pē)

cyanosis (sī-ă n-ō′ sĭs)

tachycardia (tăk ĭ-kăr′ dĭ-ă)

arterial blood gases (ăr-tē′ rē-ăl)—tests that measure the acidity of the blood and the levels of oxygen and carbon dioxide in the blood

complete blood count (CBC)—blood test that includes a hematocrit, hemoglobin, red and white blood cell count, and differential to diagnose blood disorders

ICD-9-CM Guidelines for Coding COPD, Asthma, Status Asthmaticus, Bronchitis, and Acute Respiratory Failure

Refer to the following guidelines for additional assistance when coding specific respiratory conditions.

1. The conditions that comprise COPD are:
   - obstructive chronic bronchitis (subcategory 491.2)
   - emphysema (category 492)

2. All asthma codes are under category 493—*Asthma*.

3. Code 496—*Chronic airway obstruction, not elsewhere classified*, is a nonspecific code. Do not assign it unless the documentation in the medical record does not specify the type of COPD that was treated. Always query the physician for specific information before assigning a nonspecific code.

4. The codes for chronic obstructive bronchitis and asthma distinguish between uncomplicated cases and those in acute exacerbation.

   - An acute exacerbation is a worsening of a chronic condition.

   - A condition is not considered to be an acute exacerbation if the patient already has a chronic condition and then develops an infection. But an infection can trigger an exacerbation.

5. Physicians may document COPD and asthma in many different ways. Assign codes based on terms that the physician documents because COPD and asthma can have the same symptoms.

   - Pay close attention to instructional notes in ICD-9-CM for coding COPD and asthma to ensure correct code assignment.

6. An acute exacerbation of asthma is an increased severity of the asthma symptoms, such as wheezing and shortness of breath. Status asthmaticus refers to a patient's failure to respond to therapy administered during an asthmatic episode. It is a life-threatening complication that requires emergency care.

7. If the provider documents status asthmaticus with any type of COPD or with acute bronchitis, sequence status asthmaticus first.

   - If a patient has asthma with status asthmaticus, assign the fifth digit 1, *with status asthmaticus* to the asthma code. Do not assign a separate code for asthma with the fifth digit 2, *with acute exacerbation*.

8. Assign code 466.0 for *Acute bronchitis due to an infectious organism*.

9. When the provider documents acute bronchitis and COPD, assign code 491.22—*Obstructive chronic bronchitis with acute bronchitis*. It is not necessary to also assign code 466.0 for acute bronchitis due to an infectious organism.

   - If a provider documents acute bronchitis and COPD with acute exacerbation, then assign code 491.22—*Obstructive chronic bronchitis with acute bronchitis*.

   - If a provider documents COPD with acute exacerbation without mention of acute bronchitis, then assign code 491.21—*Obstructive chronic bronchitis with (acute) exacerbation*.

10. Assign code 518.81—*Acute respiratory failure* as a principal diagnosis when

    - it is the condition established after study to be chiefly responsible for the admission to the hospital; and

    - the selection is supported by the Alphabetic Index and Tabular List.

    Note that chapter-specific coding guidelines (such as guidelines for obstetrics, poisoning, HIV, and newborns) may require a different sequencing order.

11. Sequence respiratory failure as a secondary diagnosis if it is present on admission or occurs after admission but does not meet the definition of principal diagnosis.

12. When a physician admits a patient to the hospital with respiratory failure and another acute condition, such as a myocardial infarction, the principal diagnosis will not be the same in every situation. This applies whether the other acute condition is a respiratory or nonrespiratory condition. Select the principal diagnosis based on circumstances of admission.

    - If both respiratory failure and the other acute condition are equally responsible for the admission to the hospital, follow the Official Guidelines for coding two or more diagnoses that equally meet the definition for principal diagnosis. Note that there may be chapter-specific sequencing rules in ICD-9-CM that you will need to follow.

    - Query the physician for clarification if the documentation does not clearly state whether acute respiratory failure and another condition are equally responsible for the admission.

WORKPLACE IQ

You are working as a coding specialist for Dr. Barnes. Today, you are coding a chart for Mrs. Foster, an 86-year-old established patient. Dr. Barnes documented that the patient's diagnosis is COPD; however, the documentation included various symptoms that are common to COPD and other respiratory disorders.

What would you do?

TAKE A BREAK

Let's take a break and then practice assigning codes for respiratory disorders.

Exercise 10.2 Diseases of the Respiratory System

Instructions: Assign diagnosis codes to the following patient cases, using both the Index and Tabular. Refer to instructions outlined in the previous section for assistance.

1. Dr. Hoffman sees Curtis Humbert, a 68-year-old established patient, for COPD.

   Code(s): _____

2. Katie Vachon, age 35, sees Dr. Hoffman because she recently experienced problems from previously diagnosed intrinsic asthma, such as shortness of breath and increased severity of wheezing. Dr. Hoffman diagnoses her with an acute exacerbation and adjusts her medication.

   Code(s): _____

3. Jerry Sweatt, a 51-year-old new patient, sees Dr. Hoffman for an expectorating cough (a cough that produces phlegm or mucus) and shortness of breath. After Mr. Sweatt has a chest X-ray and sputum culture, Dr. Hoffman diagnoses him with acute bronchitis due to *Streptococcus* bacteria, and he prescribes antibiotics.

   Code(s): _____

4. Loretta Velez, a 55-year-old established patient, sees Dr. Hoffman for management of chronic bronchitis with emphysema, which is due to her past history of tobacco use.

   Code(s): _____

5. Dr. Mills treats Gary Severance, age 72, in Williton Medical Center's ED for acute respiratory failure. After diagnostic workup, Dr. Mills diagnoses Mr. Severance with aspiration pneumonia due to gastric secretions and admits him to the hospital.

   Code(s): _____

6. Dr. Mills admits John Graf, age 36, to Williton Medical Center for sudden onset of dyspnea. After examination, Dr. Lightner, a pulmonologist, diagnoses Mr. Graf with spontaneous pneumothorax (air and gas accumulation in the chest) due to a ruptured bulla (lesion that contains fluid).

   Code(s): _____

DESTINATION: MEDICARE

Nutrition therapy is provided when a patient either cannot eat because of a medical condition or is unable to eat enough to provide the body with adequate nutrition. The patient may have had a neoplasm of the mouth or throat and may have had surgery to remove part of those structures. **Enteral** nutrition therapy, also called tube feeding, where the patient receives nutrients through a tube in the nose, stomach, or small intestine. **Parenteral** nutrition therapy is when a patient receives nutrients intravenously because of the body's inability to take in nutrients orally or by other methods. Medicare will reimburse for enteral and parenteral nutrition therapy services, but there are specific guidelines that providers must follow. Access *Medicare's National Coverage*

enteral (en′tər-əl)

parenteral (pə-ren′tər-əl)

Determinations Manual to review enteral and parenteral guidelines, then answer the questions that follow.

Medicare's National Coverage Determinations Manual:

1. Go to the website: http//:cms.gov.
2. From the top banner bar, choose *Regulations & Guidance*.
3. Choose *Manuals* from the options listed under *Guidance*.
4. Choose *Internet-Only Manuals (IOMs)* listed under *Manuals*.
5. Scroll down to *Publication #*, and choose *100-03 Medicare National Coverage Determinations (NCD) Manual*.
6. Scroll down to *Downloads*, and choose *Chapter 1—Coverage Determinations, Part 3*.
7. In the search box at the top of the screen, type in *parenteral* to locate guidelines on enteral and parenteral nutrition therapy (listed under 180.2).

Answer the following questions:

1. What type of impairment must a patient have in order for Medicare to pay for parenteral or enteral nutritional therapy?
2. How does Medicare determine whether it will pay for related supplies, equipment, and nutrients for parenteral or enteral nutritional therapy?
3. What information do providers need to include with Medicare claims in order for Medicare to pay for parenteral or enteral nutritional therapy?

DISEASES OF THE DIGESTIVE SYSTEM (ICD-9-CM CHAPTER 9—520–579)

The **digestive system** begins at the mouth, where food is ingested (taken in), and moves through digestive system organs and structures until the body excretes food waste through the anus (■ FIGURE 10-11). *Digestion* is the process of the body breaking down food when it reaches the stomach, and *absorption* is the process of the body converting food into energy. The food moves through the small intestine and large intestine and finally reaches the anus, where the body excretes unused food (waste products), a process called *defecation*.

ICD-9-CM categorizes digestive system conditions starting with disorders of the teeth, mouth, and jaw, followed by disorders of the organs and structures of the digestive tract.

There are several types of medical specialties involved in the diagnosis, treatment, and prevention of disorders of the mouth, teeth, and jaw. Review ■ TABLE 10-1 to become familiar with each specialty.

gastroenterology (gas-troh-en-tuh-rol′-uh-jee)

gastroenterologist (gas-troh-en-tuh-rol′-uh-jist)

Gastroenterology literally means the study of (-ology) the stomach (gastr/o) and small intestine (enter/o). A **gastroenterologist** is a physician who specializes in the diagnosis, treatment, and prevention of digestive system disorders. You will learn how to code common digestive system disorders, including ulcer and hernia. There are no specific ICD-9-CM Official Guidelines for digestive system disorders, and you will need to follow instructional notations and conventions for correctly assigning codes.

Ulcer

mucous membrane (mu′kəs)—thin tissue that lines body passages and cavities

An ulcer is an open sore or lesion of the eyes, skin, or **mucous membrane** (mucosa) that an infection, inflammation, trauma, or abrasion causes. In the digestive system, ulcers occur in different sites, including the esophagus and stomach. Ulcers can produce pus if they are infected and can also become necrotic. If an ulcer tears completely through the mucosa, then it is a *perforated* (torn) ulcer. Ulcers that erode through blood vessels can cause a *hemorrhage* (bleeding).

Figure 10-11 ■ The digestive system.

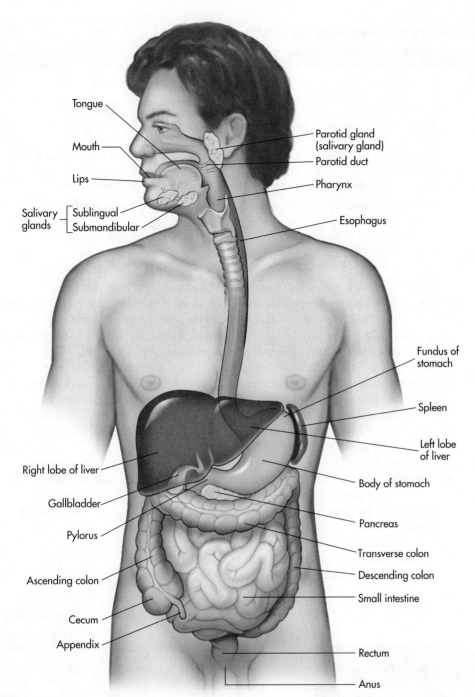

A *peptic* ulcer, also called peptic ulcer disease (PUD), is an ulcer of the esophagus, stomach (also called stomach ulcer) or duodenum (■ FIGURE 10-12).

Chronic *gastroesophageal reflux disease* (GERD), also called acid reflux, is the most common cause of esophageal peptic ulcers. It occurs when the body allows stomach acid to move backward through the digestive tract, reaching the esophagus and eroding it.

Other causes of esophageal peptic ulcers include *Helicobacter pylori* (*H. pylori*) bacterium infection, smoking or chewing tobacco, and bulimia (an eating disorder). Symptoms of esophageal peptic ulcers include heartburn; pain in the chest, neck, and throat; vomiting blood; and melena. Physicians diagnose esophageal ulcers with a barium X-ray (barium is a liquid that helps technicians see various structures on an X-ray) or endoscopy (using a camera to view inside the patient). Treatment includes prescription of antibiotics to treat infection, antacids, and proton pump inhibitors, which reduce stomach acid.

■ **TABLE 10-1   MEDICAL SPECIALTIES FOR THE MOUTH, TEETH, AND JAW**

Specialty	Definition	Physician
General Dentistry	the study, treatment, and restoration of teeth, oral cavity, and associated structures	**Dentist**
Endodontics (en-do-don'tiks)	the study and treatment of diseases and injuries affecting the dental pulp, tooth root, and periapical tissue (surrounding the tooth root)	**Endodontist**
Oral Maxillofacial Surgery (mak-sil-o-fa'shəl)	the treatment of problems with wisdom teeth, facial pain, and misaligned jaws	**Oral maxillofacial surgeon**
Orthodontics (or-tho-don'tiks)	the correction of growing or mature dental structures	**Orthodontist**
Periodontics (per-e-o-don'tiks)	the study and treatment of diseases of tissues that support the teeth	**Periodontist**
Prosthodontics (pros-tho-don'tiks)	the replacement of missing teeth and adjacent tissues with artificial substitutes, such as dentures	**Prosthodontist**

Digestive fluids, which are composed of hydrochloric acid and pepsin (an enzyme), work together to break down food. A peptic ulcer of the stomach or duodenum occurs when there is an imbalance between hydrochloric acid and pepsin, and the acid erodes the lining of the stomach or duodenum. Symptoms of stomach and duodenal ulcers include abdominal pain, heartburn, bloating, nausea, vomiting, and melena.

The most common cause of peptic ulcers of the stomach and duodenum is infection with *H. pylori* bacteria. *H. pylori* infections can spread from person to person through kissing or by ingesting infected food or water. Another cause of peptic ulcers includes using nonsteroidal anti-inflammatory drugs (NSAIDs), which are pain relievers, including ibuprofen and aspirin. NSAIDs break down the stomach's protective chemicals, which then allow stomach acid to erode the lining of the stomach. Additional factors for developing peptic ulcers include drinking alcohol and smoking, which increase stomach acid production, and stress, which itself does not cause an ulcer but does inhibit the body's ability to heal.

Physicians diagnose peptic ulcers of the stomach and duodenum with endoscopy (■ FIGURE 10-13), X-rays (■ FIGURE 10-14), and lab tests for *H. pylori* infection. Treatment includes antibiotics for infection; proton pump inhibitors; H2 receptor blockers, which reduce stomach acid; surgery to repair damage the ulcer caused; changes to dietary habits; and avoiding alcohol, smoking, and NSAIDs.

Review the following example to code a peptic ulcer for a patient's encounter.

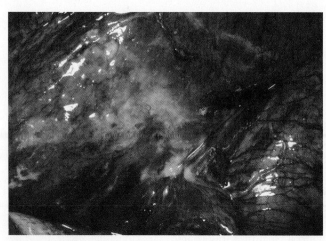

Figure 10-12 ■ Peptic ulcer in the duodenum

Photo credit: MICHAEL ENGLISH, M.D. / Custom Medical Stock Photo.

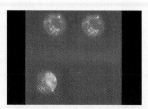

Figure 10-13 ■ Peptic ulcer of the small bowel seen through an endoscope.

Photo credit: NIH.

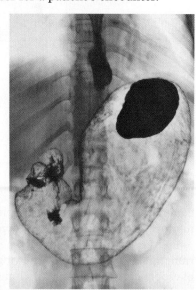

Figure 10-14 ■ Peptic ulcer of the stomach seen on x-ray (upper right, black).

Photo credit: CNRI / Photo Researchers, Inc.

Example: Mr. Phillips, a 52-year-old, presents to Williton Medical Center's ED with complaints of severe abdominal pain, heartburn, vomiting, and melena. Dr. Mills, the ED physician, examines the patient and consults with Dr. Drimond, a gastroenterologist. Dr. Drimond performs an endoscopy and determines that the patient's **pylorus** is obstructed, and the patient also has hemorrhaging. (The pylorus is the opening that allows stomach contents to empty into the small intestine (■ FIGURE 10-15). He admits the patient for a **pyloroplasty** (an enlargement of the pylorus to allow the stomach to empty faster). The patient's diagnosis is stomach ulcer with hemorrhage and obstruction.

pylorus (pī-lōr′-əs)

pyloroplasty (pī-lōr′-ə-plas-tē)

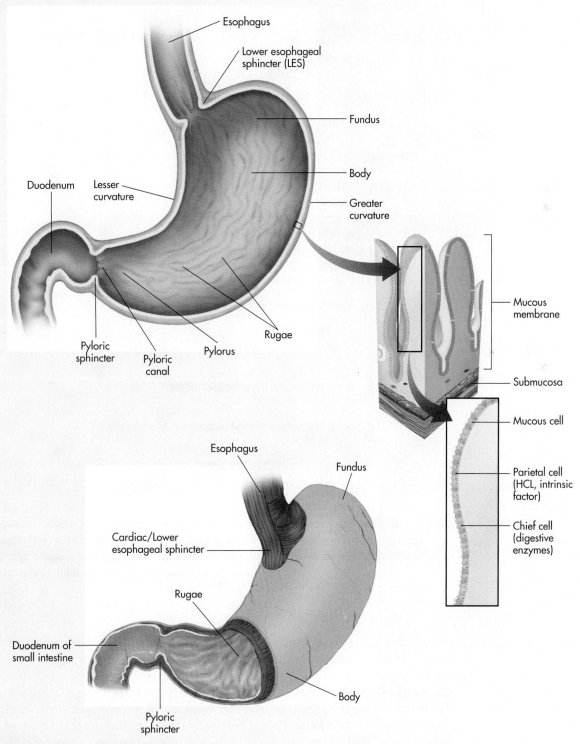

Figure 10-15 ■ The stomach and pyloris.

Figure 10-16 ■ Index entry for stomach ulcer with hemorrhage and obstruction with code 531.41 cross-referenced to the Tabular.

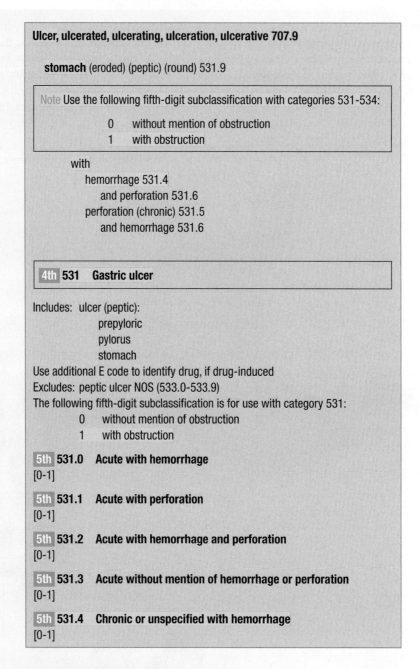

Ulcer, ulcerated, ulcerating, ulceration, ulcerative 707.9

   stomach (eroded) (peptic) (round) 531.9

> Note Use the following fifth-digit subclassification with categories 531-534:
>
>   0   without mention of obstruction
>   1   with obstruction

     with
       hemorrhage 531.4
         and perforation 531.6
       perforation (chronic) 531.5
         and hemorrhage 531.6

4th 531   Gastric ulcer

Includes: ulcer (peptic):
       prepyloric
       pylorus
       stomach
Use additional E code to identify drug, if drug-induced
Excludes: peptic ulcer NOS (533.0-533.9)
The following fifth-digit subclassification is for use with category 531:
       0   without mention of obstruction
       1   with obstruction

5th 531.0   Acute with hemorrhage
[0-1]

5th 531.1   Acute with perforation
[0-1]

5th 531.2   Acute with hemorrhage and perforation
[0-1]

5th 531.3   Acute without mention of hemorrhage or perforation
[0-1]

5th 531.4   Chronic or unspecified with hemorrhage
[0-1]

To code this case, search the Index for the main term *ulcer*, subterm *stomach*, connecting word *with*, and subterm *hemorrhage*, leading you to code 531.4 (■ FIGURE 10-16). There is also a note under the subterm *stomach* instructing you to assign a fifth digit of 0 *without mention of obstruction* or 1 *with obstruction*. Assign the fifth digit 1, and then cross-reference code 531.41 to the Tabular (Figure 10-16).

Coding hemorrhages and obstructions can be confusing. Review the information listed next for clarification when coding a hemorrhage and/or obstruction.

Coding Hemorrhage In the coding example for Mr. Phillips, there was a *combination code* for the patient's condition that included all components: stomach ulcer, with obstruction, and with hemorrhage. For many digestive disorders, ICD-9-CM *includes* hemorrhage (bleeding) as part of the code. For others, you must choose the fifth digit 0 *without mention of hemorrhage* or fifth digit 1 *with hemorrhage*. It is important to note that

| **4th** **578** | **Gastrointestinal hemorrhage** |

Excludes: that with mention of:
  angiodysplasia of stomach and duodenum (537.83)
  angiodysplasia of intestine (569.85)
  diverticulitis, intestine:
    large (562.13)
    small (562.03)
  diverticulosis, intestine:
    large (562.12)
    small (562.02)
  gastritis and duodenitis (535.0-535.6)
  ulcer:
    duodenal, gastric, gastrojejunal, or peptic (531.00-534.91)

Figure 10-17 ■ *Excludes* note from category 578 in the Tabular.

you should only assign a code for hemorrhage if the physician documents hemorrhage in the patient's chart. If you suspect that a hemorrhage may be present but the documentation is not clear, then query the physician to be sure. It is also important to remember that a physician can document the presence of a hemorrhage even if the patient *did not have active bleeding during the encounter.*

Turn to your ICD-9-CM manual to review gastrointestinal hemorrhage in the Tabular under category 578. ■ FIGURE 10-17 shows conditions that are *excluded from category 578.*

These conditions are excluded from category 578 because the hemorrhage is already part of the code for these conditions.

Assign code 578.9—*Hemorrhage of gastrointestinal tract, unspecified* when the patient has a gastrointestinal tract hemorrhage, but it is not associated with any of the conditions listed in the *Excludes* note. As you already learned, a code ending in "9," such as 578.9, is a nonspecific code that you should only assign as a *last resort,* and you should query the physician for additional information before assigning a nonspecific code.

Coding Obstruction An *obstruction,* also called an occlusion, blocks or stops organs and structures of the digestive system from performing their normal functions. The obstruction could be caused by another condition; could be the result of outside factors, such as exposure to chemicals or substances in food; or could be congenital. An obstruction can happen suddenly or develop over time.

Many codes for digestive disorders include the fifth digit 0 *without mention of obstruction* or 1 *with obstruction.* Only assign the fifth digit 1 when the documentation includes obstruction. If the physician does not document an obstruction, assign the fifth digit 0. Note that the physician does not need to specifically state "no obstruction" in order for you to assign the fifth digit 0 because it is appropriate even if there is no documentation of an obstruction.

Hernia

A *hernia* occurs when part of an organ or tissue, often a loop of intestine, protrudes outside the area that normally contains it, creating an opening and bulge. For example, a **hiatal** hernia occurs when part of the stomach protrudes through the diaphragm. There are many types of hernias, and some of the most common types are outlined in ■ TABLE 10-2. Most hernias occur in the abdominal wall when it weakens.

hiatal (hī- āt′-əl)

Symptoms of hernias vary according to the type of hernia but most include pain, heartburn, vomiting, bulging, swelling, and discomfort. Hernia causes include lung disease, lifting heavy objects, obesity, straining during a bowel movement, constipation,

■ TABLE 10-2 COMMON TYPES OF HERNIAS

Type of Hernia	Location
epigastric (ĕp ĭ-găs′ trĭc)	the region above the stomach
femoral (fĕm′ ŏr-ăl)	the space between the femoral (thigh) vein and femoral sheath
hiatal	part of the stomach protrudes through the diaphragm
incisional (in-sizh′- ən əl)	the site of a previously made incision
inguinal (ing′gwĭ-nəl)	the inguinal canal, a tubular passage through the lower layers of the abdominal wall
intervertebral disk (in-tər-vur′tə-brəl -(.)vər-′tē-)	a plate of pulp surrounded by cartilage located between each of the vertebrae in the spine
umbilical (əm-bil′ĭ-kəl)	protrusion at the navel, covered with skin

chronic coughing, previous surgery (■ Figure 10-18), pregnancy, and aging. Physicians diagnose hernias through examination by feeling the hernia and performing an X-ray in some cases. Physicians treat hernias with *manipulation* (massage) and surgery.

Hernias can be *strangulated,* which stops blood supply and causes gangrene if untreated; *incarcerated,* which causes bowel obstruction; *irreducible,* which the physician cannot correct without surgery; or *reducible,* which the physician can correct manually without surgery. Review the following example to code a hernia for a patient's encounter.

Example: Mr. Roberts, a 58-year-old patient, sees Dr. Drimond, a gastroenterologist, with complaints of groin pain, especially when lifting. Upon examination, Dr. Drimond determines that the patient has an inguinal hernia on the left side and schedules him for surgery for a hernia repair.

To code this case, search the Index for the main term *hernia* and subterm *inguinal.* Refer to the note in the Index alerting you to add a fifth digit to show whether the hernia was *unilateral* or *bilateral* and *recurrent* or *unspecified (not specified as recurrent).* Add the fifth digit 0 to show the hernia was only on the left side (unilateral) and unspecified. Then cross-reference code 550.90 to the Tabular (■ Figure 10-19).

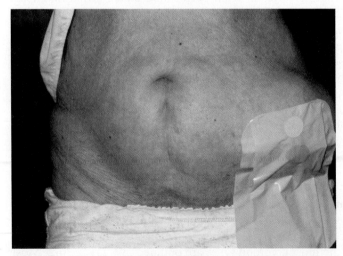

Figure 10-18 ■ View of a large swelling (incisional hernia) from the abdomen of an 85-year-old patient. The hernia was caused by a weakness in the abdominal wall after the patient underwent a colostomy. A colostomy bag is seen attached to the patient.

Photo credit: SPL/Custom Medical Stock Photo.

Hernia, hernial (acquired) (recurrent) 553.9

inguinal (direct) (double) (encysted) (external) (funicular) (indirect) (infantile) (internal) (interstitial) (oblique) (scrotal) (sliding) 550.9

Note Use the following fifth-digit subclassification with category 550:

0	unilateral or unspecified (not specified as recurrent)
1	unilateral or unspecified, recurrent
2	bilateral (not specified as recurrent)
3	bilateral, recurrent

4th 550   Inguinal hernia

Includes: bubonocele
  inguinal hernia (direct) (double) (indirect) (oblique) (sliding)
  scrotal hernia

The following fifth-digit subclassification is for use with category 550:
  0 unilateral or unspecified (not specified as recurrent)
    Unilateral NOS
  1 unilateral or unspecified, recurrent
  2 bilateral (not specified as recurrent)
    Bilateral NOS
  3 bilateral, recurrent

5th 550.9   Inguinal hernia, without mention of obstruction or gangrene
[0-3]
    Inguinal hernia NOS

Figure 10-19 ■ Index entry for unilateral inguinal hernia, unspecified, with code 550.90 cross-referenced to the Tabular.

TAKE A BREAK

Let's take a break and then practice assigning codes for digestive disorders.

Exercise 10.3   Diseases of the Digestive System

Instructions: Assign diagnosis codes to the following patient cases, using both the Index and Tabular. Refer to instructions outlined in the previous section for assistance.

1. Dr. Drimond, a gastroenterologist, sees Harold Hatchett, a 54-year-old new patient. Dr. Drimond diagnoses Mr. Hatchett with a chronic perforated peptic ulcer in his stomach that is bleeding.

   Code(s): _____

2. Dr. Drimond repairs a right inguinal hernia for Jack Covington, age 61, in Williton's outpatient surgery department.

   Code(s): _____

3. Velma Deltoro, a 67-year-old established patient, sees Dr. Drimond for a hiatal hernia, which has been bothering her more than usual. Upon examination,

Dr. Drimond finds that it is strangulated. He orders immediate surgery to prevent it from becoming gangrenous (rotting).

   Code(s): _____

4. Annette Snodgrass, a 36-year-old established patient, sees Dr. Drimond for management of GERD.

   Code(s): _____

5. Jason Rockett, age 55, comes to Williton Medical Center's outpatient surgery department for a colonoscopy. Dr. Drimond recommended the colonoscopy because he previously removed colon polyps (growths), and the patient is predisposed to developing them again. During the procedure, Dr. Drimond finds new adenomatous growths (benign neoplasms) and removes them.

   Code(s): _____

6. Brandy Audet, age 14, sees her dentist, Dr. Rye, for dental caries (decay).

   Code(s): _____

POINTERS FROM THE PROS: Interview with a Bill Review Analyst

Karen Conley, CPC-A, is a Bill Review Analyst for an organization that works with insurance companies to check providers' claims for accuracy before reimbursing them. She compares medical documentation with diagnosis and procedure codes. Ms. Conley is currently a Certified Professional Coder-Apprentice, a credential she obtained through the American Academy of Professional Coders.

What interests you the most about the job that you perform?

Most of the bills I work with involve chiropractic and physical therapy treatments, so I enjoy reviewing bills for surgeries or procedures that are a little out of the ordinary from what I usually see. Even though I'm not coding (and only reviewing codes), I feel like I'm learning more about coding as I read the operative notes and do research to ensure the coding is accurate before I release the bill (for payment).

What advice can you give to new coders to help them communicate effectively with physicians, since physicians can sometimes be intimidating?

Be willing to listen. Don't be afraid to tell the physician that you can't understand his documentation or read his handwriting. Be flexible if you can, but stand your ground if you know you are right.

What advice would you like to give to coding students to help them prepare to work successfully in the healthcare field?

Be patient! Don't expect to walk out of coding school and make $60,000 a year. Be willing to learn, because it's a continual learning process; you don't know everything when you come out of school, and you'll discover that very quickly when you start working. I also suggest that coding students sit for their (certification) exams within a year after finishing coding school. Although you'll be considered an apprentice until you have the required experience to be a full-fledged (certified coder), passing the exam is a terrific confidence builder (and doesn't hurt your resume, either!

(Used by permission of Karen Conley.)

DISEASES OF THE GENITOURINARY SYSTEM (ICD-9-CM CHAPTER 10—580–629)

genitourinary (jen-i-toh-yoor'-uh-ner-ee)

The **genitourinary system** includes the urinary system and the male and female reproductive systems, along with disorders of the breast. **Genitourinary** literally means pertaining to (-ary) the genitals (genit/o) and urine (urin/o). The urinary system, which produces and excretes urine, consists of four main organs and structures: the kidneys, ureters, urinary bladder, and urethra (■ FIGURE 10-20).

Figure 10-20 ■ The urinary system.

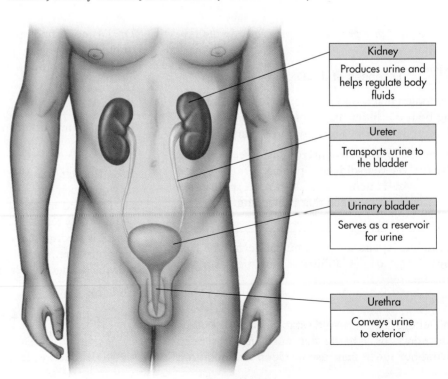

| Kidney |
| Produces urine and helps regulate body fluids |

| Ureter |
| Transports urine to the bladder |

| Urinary bladder |
| Serves as a reservoir for urine |

| Urethra |
| Conveys urine to exterior |

Figure 10-21 ■ The male reproductive system.

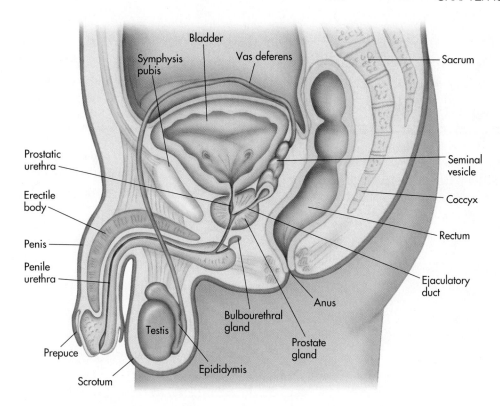

Labels:
- Symphysis pubis
- Bladder
- Vas deferens
- Sacrum
- Prostatic urethra
- Seminal vesicle
- Erectile body
- Coccyx
- Penis
- Rectum
- Penile urethra
- Ejaculatory duct
- Anus
- Prepuce
- Testis
- Bulbourethral gland
- Prostate gland
- Scrotum
- Epididymis

Urology literally means the study of (-ology) urine (ur/o). A **urologist** is a physician who specializes in the diagnosis, treatment, and prevention of male and female urinary disorders and disorders of the male reproductive system (■ FIGURE 10-21).

Nephrology literally means the study of (-ology) the kidneys (nephr/o). A **nephrologist** is a physician who specializes in the diagnosis, treatment, and prevention of kidney disorders. **Gynecology** literally means the study of (-ology) a female (gynec/o). A **gynecologist** is a physician who specializes in the diagnosis, treatment, and prevention of disorders of the female reproductive system (■ FIGURE 10-22), including the breasts, also called the *mammary glands* (■ FIGURE 10-23).

Obstetrics is the medical care of women during pregnancy, childbirth, and the puerperium. An **obstetrician** is a physician who specializes in obstetrics. You may have heard of an OB/GYN physician, which is an abbreviation for Obstetrics/Gynecology. This physician specializes in both obstetrics and gynecology. You will learn how to code obstetrical disorders in Chapter 14 of this book.

Throughout Chapter 10 in ICD-9-CM, you will see manifestation codes and *Code first* notes for underlying diseases. Follow the *Code first* notes carefully to ensure that you not only code both an etiology and a manifestation, but that you also sequence codes in the correct order. In addition, you will find *Use additional code* notes to identify infectious organisms when coding infections. Be sure to follow *Use additional code* notes carefully for correct code assignment. There are numerous genitourinary disorders in Chapter 10, and we will concentrate on learning how to code chronic kidney disease, a common disorder.

urology (yoo-rol′-uh-jee)

urologist (yoo-rol′-uh-jist)

nephrology (ni-fräl′-ə-jē)

nephrologist (ni-fräl′-ə-jist)

gynecology (gīn-ū-käl′-ū-jē)

gynecologist (gīn-ə-käl′-ə-jist)

obstetrics (əb-ste-triks)

obstetrician (äb-stə-trish′-ən)

Chronic Kidney Disease

CKD, also called renal (kidney) failure, occurs when a patient loses partial or full function of kidneys, typically over a period of time. Less severe kidney disease is called *renal insufficiency*. The job of the kidneys is to filter blood, and when kidneys do not function normally, the body cannot excrete water and waste products, which are poisonous if not removed. Kidney failure can also cause other health conditions, such as hypertension and anemia.

Symptoms of CKD include polyuria, **nocturia**, fatigue, loss of appetite, edema in the legs and under the eyes, shortness of breath, and chest pain. Causes of CKD

nocturia (nŏk-tū′ rĭ-ă)—frequent urination during the night

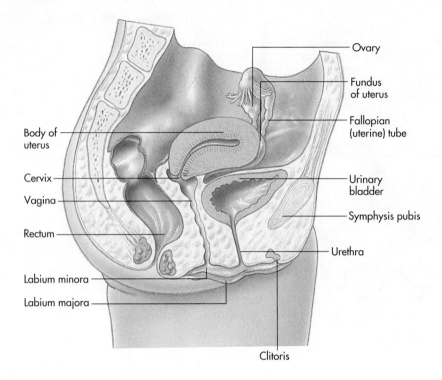

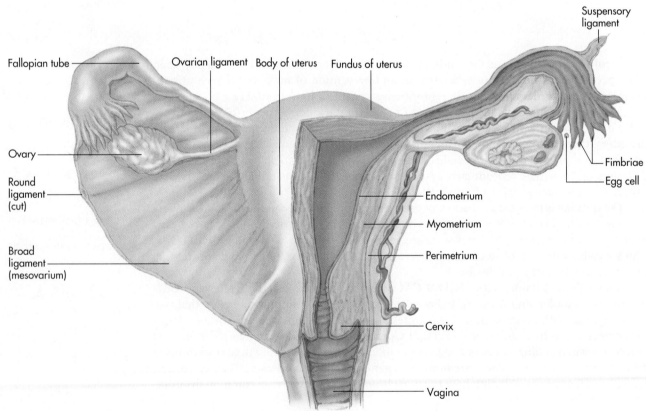

Figure 10-22 ■ The female reproductive system.

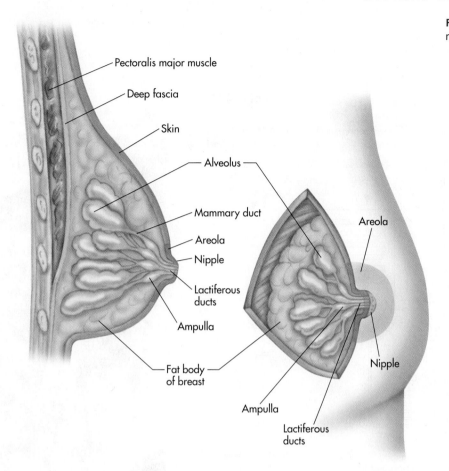

Figure 10-23 ■ The mammary glands.

- Pectoralis major muscle
- Deep fascia
- Skin
- Alveolus
- Mammary duct
- Areola
- Nipple
- Lactiferous ducts
- Ampulla
- Fat body of breast
- Ampulla
- Lactiferous ducts
- Areola
- Nipple

include diabetes mellitus, hypertension, **atherosclerosis**, **renal calculus**, NSAIDs, and aspirin.

Physicians diagnose kidney disease in stages of severity, measured by the rate at which the kidneys filter blood per minute, called glomerular filtration rate (GFR). The normal rate of GFR is 90-120 mL/min (milliliters per minute). There are five stages of kidney disease. ICD-9-CM lists CKD under category 585, with the fourth digit representing the stage of severity:

- Stage I (585.1)—slight decrease in GFR with rate over 90, kidney damage
- Stage II (585.2)—mild decrease in GFR with rate in the range of 60–89, kidney damage
- Stage III (585.3)—moderate decrease in GFR with rate in the range of 30–59, kidney damage
- Stage IV (585.4)—severe decrease in GFR with rate in the range of 15–29, kidney damage
- Stage V (585.5)—severe decrease in GFR with rate less than 15, kidney failure

Note that in ICD-9-CM there is a separate code, 585.6—*End stage renal disease* for patients with ESRD, CKD stage V, who need chronic dialysis. There are two types of dialysis, **hemodialysis** (■ FIGURE 10-24) and **peritoneal dialysis** (■ FIGURE 10-25).

Only assign code 585.9—*Chronic kidney disease, unspecified* as a *last resort* when the documentation does not include the stage of CKD.

Diagnostic tests for CKD include blood tests to measure GFR, **urinalysis** (urine lab test), and X-rays. Treatment for CKD includes dietary changes, avoiding NSAIDs and aspirin, and prescription medications. For ESRD patients, treatment also includes hemodialysis, peritoneal dialysis, and kidney transplants.

Using your ICD-9-CM manual, review the following example to code an encounter for a patient with CKD.

atherosclerosis (ăth ĕr-ō-sklĕ-rō′ sĭs)—an abnormal condition of the arteries characterized by the buildup of fatty substances and hardening of the artery walls

renal calculus (rē′ năl kal′ku-ləs)—hard deposits of mineral salts in the kidney

hemodialysis (hē mō-dī-ăl′ ĭ-sĭs)—procedure in which a catheter or tubing is connected from the fistula or graft on the patient to a dialyzer, a machine that filters the blood of toxins before returning it to the body

peritoneal dialysis (pĕr ĭ-tō-nē′ ăl dī-ăl′ ĭ-sĭs)—separation of waste from the blood by using a catheter in the peritoneum (lining of the abdominal cavity) and introducing fluid to filter waste from the blood

urinalysis (u-rĭ-nal′ ĭ-sis)

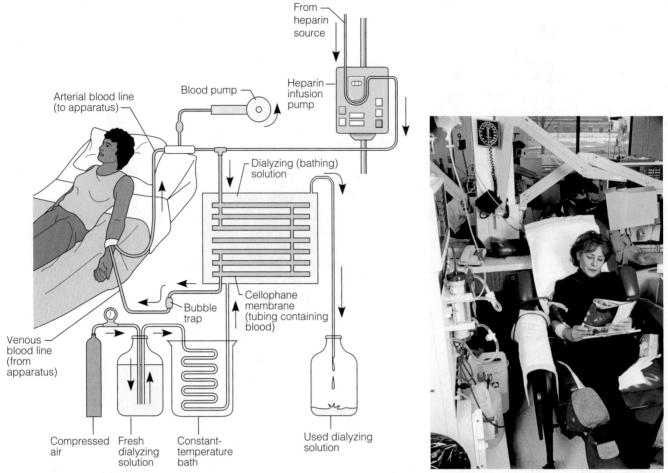

Figure 10-24 ■ A. Hemodialysis; B. A woman receiving hemodialysis at the hospital.

Photo credit: (B) Carolyn A. Mckeone/Photo Researchers, Inc.

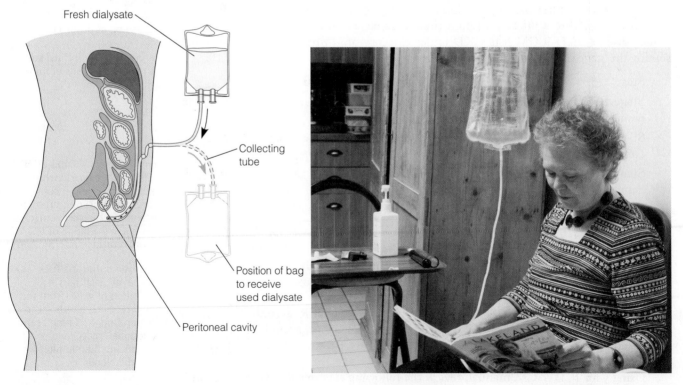

Figure 10-25 ■ A. Peritoneal dialysis; B. A woman receiving peritoneal dialysis at home.

Photo credit: (B) Life in View / Photo Researchers, Inc.

Example: Mrs. Perez, a 43-year-old established patient, has an outpatient encounter at Green Dialysis Center for one of three weekly hemodialysis treatments, due to ESRD.

Recall from Chapter 5 that when the patient's main reason for an encounter is dialysis, you need to first sequence a V code for the dialysis encounter, and then assign an additional code for the patient's condition. Search the Index for the main term *dialysis* and subterm *hemodialysis*, then cross-reference code V56.0 to the Tabular.

Next, search the Index for the main term *disease*, subterm *renal*, and subterm *end-stage*, and cross-reference code 585.6 to the Tabular. In this example, assign code V56.0 for the dialysis encounter and 585.6 for ESRD requiring chronic dialysis.

ICD-9-CM Guidelines for Coding Chronic Kidney Disease Refer to the following guidelines for additional assistance when you are coding chronic kidney disease.

1. ICD-9-CM classifies CKD on the basis of its severity using codes 585.1–585.5 Assign code 585.6 for ESRD. If the physician documents both CKD and ESRD, only assign code 585.6—*End stage renal disease*, because 585.6 already includes CKD.

2. Patients who have undergone a kidney transplant may still have some form of CKD, because the kidney transplant may not fully restore kidney function. This does not mean that a transplant complication caused the CKD. In these cases, sequence the code for the correct stage of CKD from category 585 and assign code V42.0—*Organ or tissue replaced by transplant, kidney* as an additional code. Always query the physician if the documentation does not clearly state whether a transplant complication caused the patient's CKD. Refer to the Official Guidelines for assistance when coding a transplant complication.

3. Patients with CKD may also suffer from other serious conditions, most commonly diabetes mellitus and hypertension. Refer to coding conventions in the Tabular List for assistance with sequencing CKD and any other conditions.

endometriosis (en-dō-mē-trē-ō′-sǝs)

TAKE A BREAK

Let's take a break and then practice assigning codes for genitourinary disorders.

Exercise 10.4 **Diseases of the Genitourinary System**

Instructions: Assign diagnosis codes to the following patient cases, using both the Index and Tabular. Refer to instructions outlined in the previous section for assistance.

1. Alberta Arias, age 56, has stage V chronic kidney disease and reports to Green Dialysis Center for one of her three weekly encounters for dialysis.

   Code(s): _____

2. Dennis Flint, age 80, sees his urologist, Dr. Moir, for an enlarged prostate with urinary retention, which has not significantly improved with medication. Dr. Moir adjusts Mr. Flint's medication and says that if his symptoms do not improve, he should consider surgery.

   Code(s): _____

3. Constance Portis, age 25, sees Dr. Rhodes, a nephrologist, for test results after an evaluation due to abdominal pain, urinary tract infection (due to *E. coli*), polyuria (excessive urine and frequent urination), and hematuria (blood in urine). Dr. Rhodes reviews the patient's blood tests and MRI scan results. He diagnoses her with polycystic kidney disease (cysts in the kidneys). He explains that the condition is inherited, caused by a gene that is autosomal (chromosome) recessive (inherited from both parents). Because there is no cure, Dr. Rhodes can only treat her infection and pain with medications. Dr. Rhodes states that Mrs. Portis may eventually need to have surgery for the condition.

   Code(s): _____

4. Dr. Wooten, an OB/GYN, admits established patient Jessie Grissom, age 40, to Williton Medical Center for surgery for **endometriosis** of the uterus (when cells from the lining of the womb (uterus) grow in other areas of the body).

   Code(s): _____

continued

TAKE A BREAK *continued*

5. Alicia McMurray, a 42-year-old established patient, sees Dr. Hoffman because she found lumps in both breasts and is experiencing some pain. Upon **palpation** (feeling with the hands), Dr. Hoffman diagnoses her with fibrocystic breast disease (benign breast lumps) and tells her not to worry.

Code(s): _____

6. Patsy Mattern, a 32-year-old new patient, sees Dr. Hoffman with complaints of vaginal discharge, burning, and redness in the **perineal** area (in front of the anus). He conducts a pelvic exam and takes a culture for a lab test. Two days later, he reviews the lab test results and diagnoses Ms. Mattern with bacterial vaginitis due to *Staphylococcus* and prescribes an antibiotic.

Code(s): _____

palpation (pal-pā′-shən)

perineal (per-ə-nē′-əl)

DISEASES OF THE SKIN AND SUBCUTANEOUS TISSUE (ICD-9-CM CHAPTER 12—680–709)

The **integumentary system** includes the skin, hair, hair follicles, related glands (■ FIGURE 10-26), and nails (■ FIGURE 10-27).

The skin is the largest body organ. It protects the body from harmful organisms, regulates body temperature, and produces Vitamin D, which helps bones to grow. The skin consists of three layers:

- epidermis (upper layer of skin)
- dermis (middle layer of skin)
- subcutaneous fascia (deepest layer of skin made of fatty tissue)

Figure 10-26 ■ The skin and associated glands and structures.

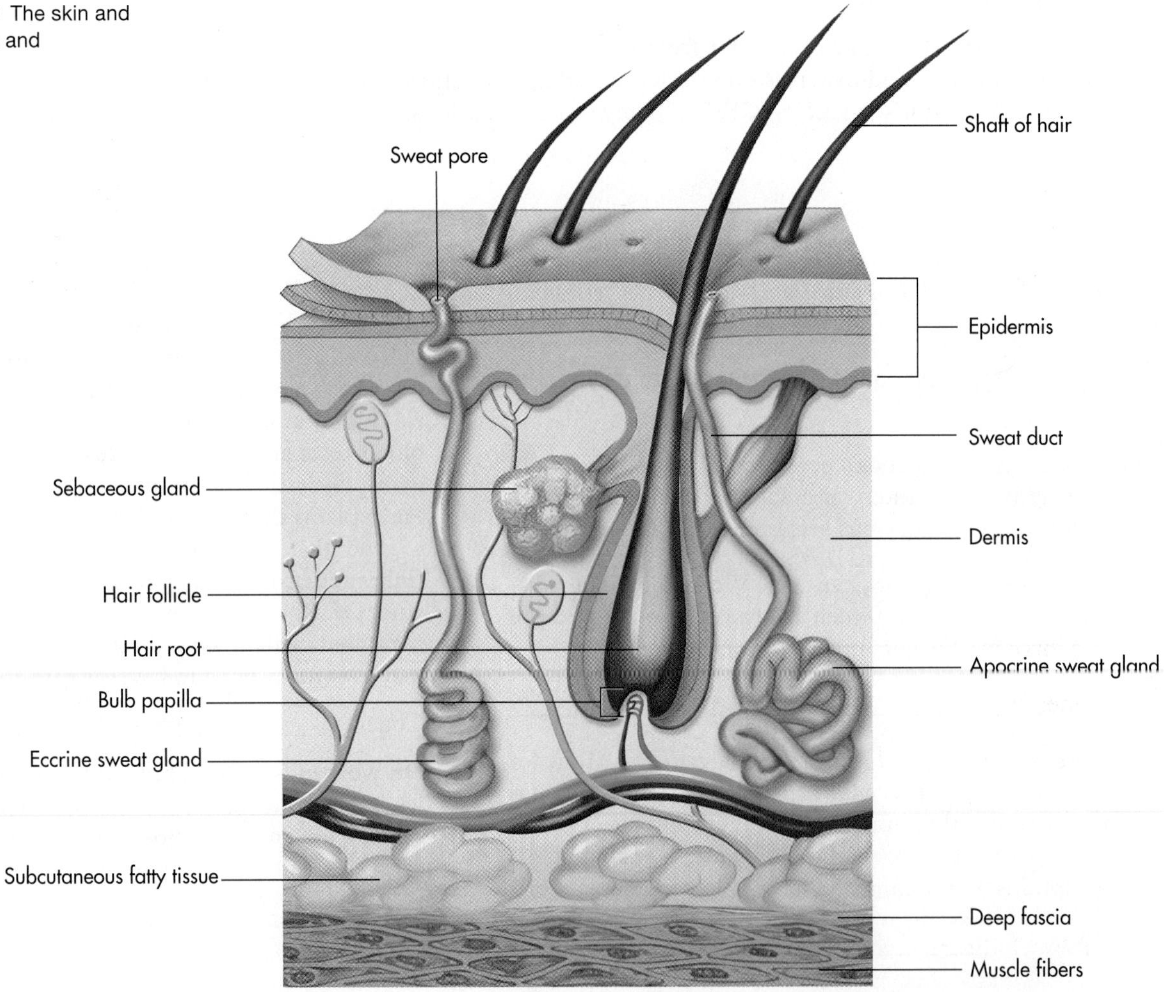

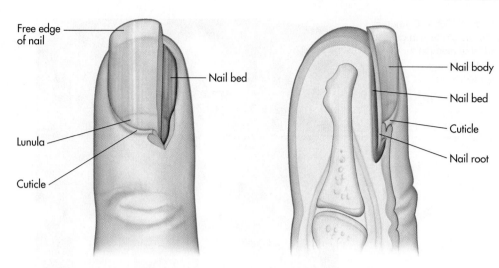

Figure 10-27 ■ Structures of a fingernail.

Free edge of nail

Nail bed

Lunula

Cuticle

Nail body

Nail bed

Cuticle

Nail root

Integumentary literally means pertaining to (-ary) a covering or skin (integument/o). **Dermatology** is the study of (-ology) the skin (dermat/o). A **dermatologist** is a physician who specializes in the diagnosis, treatment, and prevention of skin disorders. Other physicians, also treat patients for skin disorders and infections, such as a general practitioner or family physician.

Let's review coding notes for skin disorders in the Tabular and then review more about cellulitis and dermatitis. Refer to your ICD-9-CM manual as you read these notes.

integumentary (in-teg-yuh-men'-tuh-ree)

dermatology (dər-mə-täl'-ə-jē)

dermatologist (dər-mə-täl'-ə-jəst)

1. The following categories instruct you to *Use additional code* for an organism, such as *Staphylococcus* or *E. coli*, that caused the patient's condition:

    - 681—Cellulitis and abscess of finger and toe
    - 682—Other cellulitis and abscess
    - 683—Acute lymphadenitis
    - 686—Other local infections of skin and subcutaneous tissue

2. Subcategory code 695.1—**Erythema multiforme** (allergic skin disorder with lesions) (■ FIGURE 10-28) has a *Use additional code* note instructing you to

    - Assign additional codes for any manifestations of the condition, such as edema, ulcers, or infection.
    - Assign an additional E code if a drug caused erythema multiforme.
    - Assign an additional code to identify the percentage of skin exfoliation (peeling) from codes 695.50–695.59.

erythema multiforme (er-ə-the'mə məl-tə-for'-mē)

3. Subcategory code 707.0—*Pressure ulcer* has a *Use additional code* note instructing you to identify the pressure ulcer stage from codes 707.20–707.25. Remember that you already learned how to assign codes for pressure ulcers and their stages in Chapter 4 of this book. Refer to the Official Guidelines for assistance with coding *multiple* pressure ulcers and their stages.

4. Subcategory code 707.1—*Ulcer of lower limbs, except pressure ulcer* has a note to *Code, if applicable, any causal condition first* (■ FIGURE 10-29).

It is also important to note that you will *not* find *neoplasms* of the skin in Chapter 12 of ICD-9-CM. Instead, ICD-9-CM categorizes skin neoplasms in Chapter 2, along with neoplasms of other sites. You will learn more about coding neoplasms in Chapter 12 of this book.

You will next learn how to code two common skin conditions, cellulitis and dermatitis.

Cellulitis

Cellulitis is an infection of the skin and subcutaneous tissue that *Staphylococcus* and Group A *Streptococcus* bacteria most commonly cause (■ FIGURE 10-30). It often appears on the lower legs but can occur on other body sites, such as the arms or thighs.

Figure 10-28 ■ Erythema multiforme of the skin caused by an adverse reaction to antibiotics.

Photo credit: CDC.

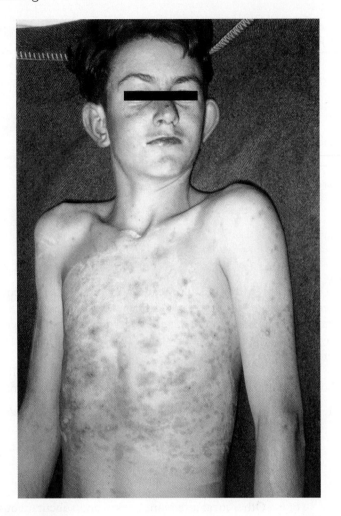

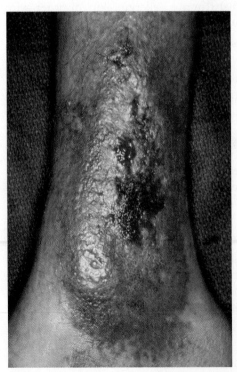

Figure 10-29 ■ Ulcer of the shin.

Photo credit: CDC.

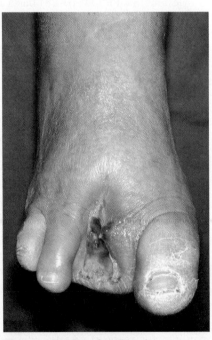

Figure 10-30 ■ Cellulitis of the toes and foot.

Photo credit: © Scott Camazine / Alamy.

Cellulitis occurs when bacteria enters the skin through an opening, such as an ulcer, laceration, abrasion, recent surgery, trauma (like an animal or insect bite), or **athlete's foot**. Patients with diabetes, HIV infection, AIDS, and CKD are at a higher risk for developing cellulitis because they have weakened immune systems that cannot properly fight off infections.

athlete's foot—ringworm (fungal) infection of the feet

Symptoms of cellulitis include erythema, edema, pain, warmth and tenderness of the affected area, fever, fatigue, and chills. Physicians diagnose cellulitis by conducting an examination of the affected area and testing for the presence of bacteria. Treatment includes antibiotics, removing any necrotic tissue, and protecting the affected area from further infection. If cellulitis is left untreated, it may become life-threatening when the bacteria spread to the bloodstream. Refer to the following example to code a patient's encounter for cellulitis.

Example: Ms. Robinson, a 36-year-old established patient, presents to Williton Medical Center's ED and sees Dr. Burns, an ED physician, with complaints of pain, redness, and swelling on her lower right leg. She states that a spider recently bit her in the affected area. After examination, Dr. Burns orders a blood test to determine if bacteria are present. The test is positive for Group A *Streptococcus*, which caused the cellulitis. Because of the severity of the infection, Dr. Burns starts the patient on IV antibiotics and admits her to the hospital.

To code this case, search the Index for the main term *cellulitis* and subterm *leg*, then cross-reference code 682.6 to the Tabular. Notice the *Use additional code* note under category 682 in the Tabular. You will need to assign an *additional code* for Group A *Streptococcus*. Search the Index for the main term *infection*, subterm *streptococcal*, subterm *group*, and subterm *A*, then cross-reference code 041.01 to the Tabular. Final code assignment for this example includes codes 682.6 and 041.01.

Dermatitis

Dermatitis is a skin inflammation, and there are different types of dermatitis, including:

- *atopic dermatitis*, also called eczema—an itchy rash
- *contact dermatitis*—an allergic rash that a chemical (such as a cleaning product) or plant (like poison ivy) causes
- **seborrheic** *dermatitis*—occurs on the face and scalp, causing dandruff

seborrheic (seb-o-re′ik)

Causes of dermatitis include allergic reactions to various substances, chemical and plant poisonings, and medical conditions. Symptoms of dermatitis include erythema, blisters, and edema. Physicians diagnose dermatitis through examination; obtaining the patient's medical, family, and social history; a **patch test**; and **skin biopsy**. Treatment includes avoiding exposure to harmful substances that cause allergic reactions or poisonings, applying wet dressings, taking NSAIDs, applying topical **corticosteroids**, and taking **antihistamines**. Refer to the following example to code a patient's encounter for dermatitis.

patch test—a skin test used primarily to diagnose allergies, in which small pieces of gauze or filter paper treated with suspected allergens are applied to the skin

skin biopsy (bi′op-se)— removal and examination of samples of skin for diagnosis

Example: Mr. Palmer, a 68-year-old established patient, sees Dr. Ferguson, a dermatologist, with complaints of redness and swelling of his hands. The patient states that he suspects the condition began when he used a new cleaning solution for his garage floor. After doing some additional questioning and examination, Dr. Ferguson determines that Mr. Palmer has contact dermatitis from the cleaning solution. He advises the patient to avoid the cleaning solution and apply a topical corticosteroid.

Use your ICD-9-CM manual to search the Index for the main term *dermatitis*, subterm *due to*, subterm *chemical*, and subterm *irritant*, then cross-reference code 692.4 to the Tabular. Notice in the Tabular under code 692.4 that the word "irritant" is not listed under *Dermatitis due to*. But the word "caustics" is listed there. *Caustics* are toxic substances that cause the patient to have a skin reaction. So code 692.4 is the final code assignment.

corticosteroids (kor-ti-ko-ster′oids)—medications used to reduce inflammation; corticosteroid is also the steroid hormone secreted by the adrenal glands (which are located above each kidney)

antihistamines (an′ti-his′tə-mēns)—agents that are used to help relieve symptoms, such as itching, in allergic responses and contact dermatitis

TAKE A BREAK

Let's take a break and then practice assigning codes for skin and subcutaneous tissue disorders.

Exercise 10.5 Diseases of the Skin and Subcutaneous Tissue

Instructions: Assign diagnosis codes to the following patient cases, using both the Index and Tabular. Refer to instructions outlined in the previous section for assistance.

1. Julie Bratcher, a 61-year-old new patient, sees Dr. Ferguson, a dermatologist, because of pain and redness on her right leg. Dr. Ferguson diagnoses Mrs. Bratcher with cellulitis, which diabetes caused. A blood test shows that *Streptococcus* is responsible for the infection. Dr. Ferguson prescribes oral antibiotics and states that if the condition does not improve within three days or if it gets worse, then he will need to admit her to the hospital to administer IV antibiotics.

   Code(s): _____

2. Mr. Delafuente brings his daughter Tara, age 12, to her pediatrician, Dr. Flynn, for blisters, redness, and itching on her arms. Dr. Flynn diagnoses the patient with contact dermatitis due to poison sumac.

   Code(s): _____

3. Jerry Rounds, age 55, sees Dr. Ferguson for a follow-up visit to check on his erythema multiforme minor (a skin infection following a herpes infection). The patient developed a herpes simplex infection after he took a sulfonamide (a medication), which another physician prescribed a month ago for inflammatory bowel disease. The herpes simplex infection shows some improvement. Dr. Ferguson estimates that 15% of Mr. Rounds' skin is exfoliated.

   Code(s): _____

4. Dr. Ferguson visits Ralph Mixon, an 84-year-old nursing home resident, for a stage II pressure ulcer on his hip.

   Code(s): _____

5. Sarah Wooden, a 47-year-old established patient, sees Dr. Ferguson for a follow-up visit to check a chronic ulcer on her right calf, which is due to postphlebitic syndrome (leg pain and edema).

   Code(s): _____

6. Louis Merkel, a 54-year-old new patient, sees Dr. Hoffman for an infected ingrown nail on his left great toe.

   Code(s): _____

DISEASES OF THE MUSCULOSKELETAL SYSTEM AND CONNECTIVE TISSUE (ICD-9-CM CHAPTER 13—710–739)

The **musculoskeletal system** includes both the skeletal and muscular systems. The skeletal system is made up of bones and joints that hold the body together and enclose and protect organs and structures (■ FIGURE 10-31). It also creates blood cells and works in conjunction with the skeletal muscles in the muscular system (■ FIGURE 10-32) to allow the body to move. Besides skeletal muscles, the body contains cardiac muscles, which form the walls of the heart, and smooth muscles, which are in all of the body's organs. Connective tissue joins structures throughout the body to provide structure and support.

orthopedic (or-thə-pēd'-ik)

Orthopedic literally means pertaining to (-ic) straight (orth/o) foot (ped/o). An *orthopedic specialist* or *orthopedic surgeon* diagnoses, treats, and prevents all musculoskeletal system disorders, not only disorders of the feet.

At the beginning of Chapter 13 in ICD-9-CM, you will see a note to *Use additional external cause code, if applicable, to identify the cause of the musculoskeletal condition* (■ FIGURE 10-33). Recall that E codes represent *external causes*, and you should sequence them last. There is also a list of fifth digits to identify the body sites involved under specific categories (Figure 10-33). Refer to the categories in your ICD-9-CM to become familiar with conditions that they represent.

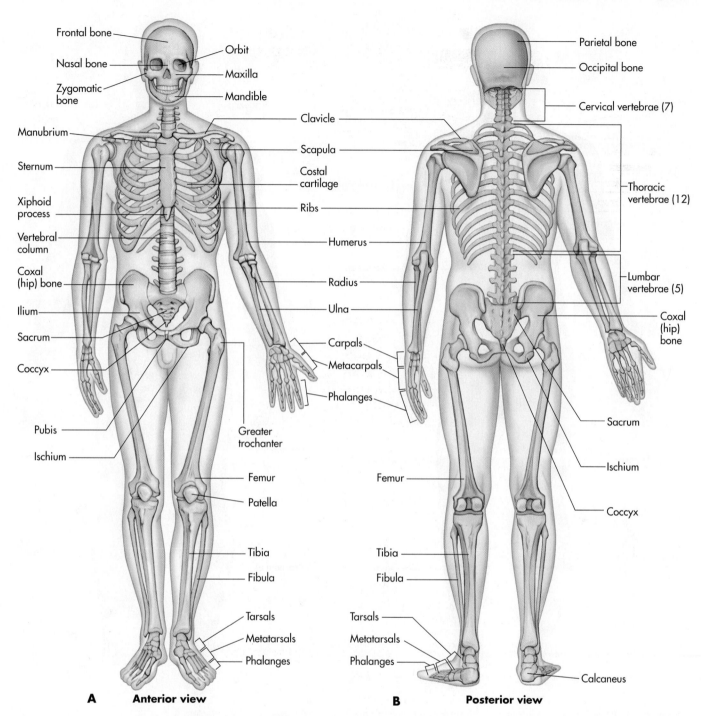

A   Anterior view

B   Posterior view

Figure 10-31 ■ The human skeleton, A. anterior (front) view and B. posterior (back) view.

Chapter 13 is divided into four sections of categories that represent the following categories:

- Categories 710–719—**arthropathy** (joint disorder) and related disorders
- Categories 720–724—**dorsopathy** (back or spine disorder)
- Categories 725–729—**rheumatism** (disorders of bones, joints, muscles, and tendons, excluding the back)
- Categories 730–739—**osteopathy** (bone disease), **chondropathy** (**cartilage** disease), and acquired musculoskeletal deformities

arthropathy (ahr-throp′ə-the)

dorsopathy (dor-sə′ path ē)

rheumatism (roo′mə-tiz-əm)

osteopathy (os te-op′ə-the)

chondropathy (kon-drop′ə-the)

cartilage (kär′ tĭ-lĭj)—fibrous connective tissue at the ends of bone, tip of the nose, and earlobes

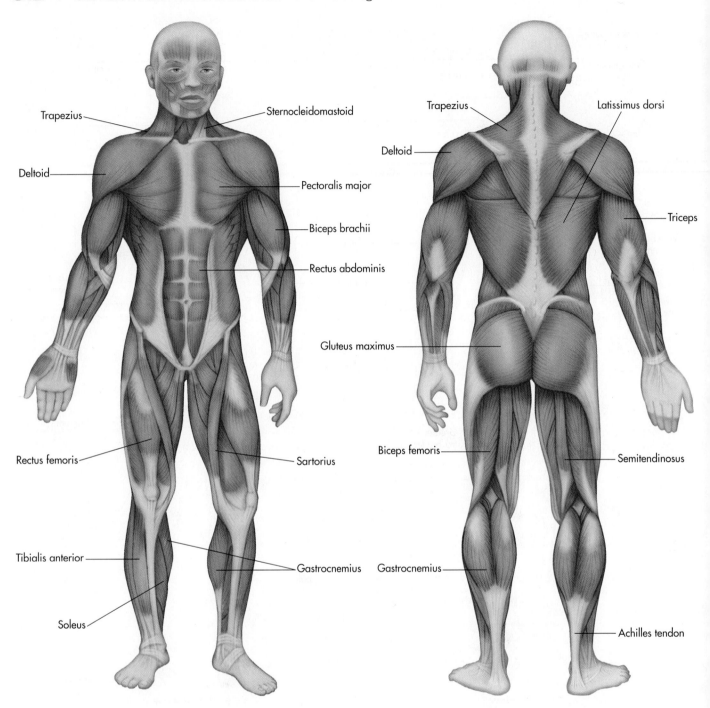

Figure 10-32 ■ The muscular system with anterior (front) and posterior (back) views of major muscles.

For many types of arthropathies, ICD-9-CM requires you to code first any underlying disease that caused the arthopathy. Be sure to follow *Code first* notes and any other conventions very carefully in order to ensure correct code assignment. For category 730, ICD-9-CM instructs you to *Use additional code to identify organism* that caused the infection. Let's review how to code pathologic fractures, a common musculoskeletal system disorder.

Pathologic Fracture

Do you remember coding fractures in Chapter 8 when you reviewed coding for injuries and poisonings? You can review the coding instructions and types of fractures as you work through this next section. ICD-9-CM classifies *pathologic* fractures, also called

> ### 13. DISEASES OF THE MUSCULOSKELETAL SYSTEM AND CONNECTIVE TISSUE (710-739)
>
> Use additional external cause code, if applicable, to identify the cause of the musculoskeletal condition
>
> The following fifth-digit subclassification is for use with categories 711-712, 715-716, 718-719, and 730:
>
>   0 site unspecified
>   1 shoulder region
>   Acromioclavicular joint(s)
>   Glenohumeral joint(s)
>   Sternoclavicular joint(s)
>   Clavicle
>   Scapula
>   2 upper arm
>   Elbow joint
>   Humerus

Figure 10-33 ■ Note to Use additional external cause code and fifth-digit choices appearing at the beginning of Chapter 13 in the Tabular.

spontaneous fractures (bone structure weakness), to Chapter 13, along with other musculoskeletal system disorders. Subcategory code 733.1 represents a pathologic fracture, and subclassification codes include pathologic fracture *sites*.

It is important to understand that the word pathologic means *caused by another condition*. Other conditions, such as neoplasms, infections, and **osteoporosis**, cause bones to be brittle and weak and make an individual prone to pathologic fractures. Osteoporosis is one of the main reasons for pathologic fractures. It is a *systemic* condition, meaning that it affects all the bones in the musculoskeletal system.

osteoporosis (ŏs tē- ō-por-ō′ sĭs)—an abnormal condition marked by decreased bone density and strength

Patients experience pathologic fractures when they perform normal activities and functions. Fractures occur during routine movements because the patient's underlying disease makes his bones weak and more likely to break. Symptoms of pathologic fractures include pain, swelling, and the inability to have normal range of motion. Physicians diagnose pathologic fractures through examinations and X-rays. They treat pathologic fractures using the same methods you learned about previously, including manipulation, cast application, and surgery.

When coding pathologic fractures, you always need to assign codes for *both* the fracture and the underlying condition that caused the fracture to occur. ICD-9-CM does not have a coding convention or note under pathologic fractures instructing you to assign two codes. If the physician only documents that the patient has a pathologic fracture but does not document the underlying cause, you should query the physician to clarify the cause.

Pathologic fractures are not the same as traumatic fractures, which result from traumatic injuries. If a minor injury causes a fracture but the patient has an underlying condition that makes him more susceptible to any type of fracture, then the fracture may not be considered traumatic. It may still be a pathologic fracture. Always query the physician for clarification if the documentation is not specific enough.

Refer to the following coding guidelines when coding pathologic fractures.

1. Assign subcategory code 733.1—*Pathologic fracture* when the fracture is newly diagnosed and the physician is actively treating the patient for the fracture. Examples of active treatment include surgery, emergency department encounter, and evaluation and treatment by a new physician.

2. Assign fracture aftercare codes (subcategories V54.0, V54.2, V54.8 or V54.9) for encounters *after* the patient completes active treatment for the fracture and receives routine care during the healing or recovery phase. Examples of fracture aftercare include cast change or removal, removal of external or internal fixation device, medication adjustment, and follow-up visits following fracture treatment.

3. Assign complication codes when there are complications of surgical treatment for fracture repairs during the healing or recovery phase.

4. Assign appropriate fracture codes for complications such as malunion and nonunion of fractures.

Refer to the following example to code a pathologic fracture.

Example: Mrs. Perkins, a 75-year-old, presents to Williton Medical Center's ED with complaints of right arm pain and swelling. Dr. Mills examines the patient, who states that she bumped her arm on a wrought-iron kitchen chair when she moved it to mop the floor. The patient's medical history reveals that she suffers from post-menopausal osteoporosis. The patient's X-ray shows a fracture of the right humerus. Dr. Mills documents a pathologic fracture of the right *humerus* (upper arm bone).

To code this case, search the Index for the main term *fracture*, subterm *pathologic*, and subterm *humerus*, then cross-reference code 733.11 to the Tabular. Now assign a code for the underlying cause of the fracture, osteoporosis, by searching the Index for the main term *osteoporosis* and subterm *postmenopausal*, then cross-reference code 733.01 to the Tabular. The final code assignment for this example is 733.11 and 733.01.

TAKE A BREAK

Let's take a break and then practice assigning codes for musculoskeletal system and connective tissue disorders.

Exercise 10.6 Diseases of the Musculoskeletal System and Connective Tissue

Instructions: Assign diagnosis codes to the following patient cases, using both the Index and Tabular. Refer to instructions outlined in the previous section for assistance.

1. Annie Norwood, an 87-year-old established patient, sees Dr. Hoffman for acute hip pain. X-rays show that she has a pathological fracture in her hip due to age-related osteoporosis.

   Code(s): _____

2. Harry Ibarra, age 78, sees Dr. Grisham, an orthopedic surgeon, for complaints of low back pain. Dr. Grisham examines the patient and orders radiological tests, which reveal collapsed vertebrae (fractured) L3 and L4 due to bone metastasis from prostate cancer.

   Code(s): _____

3. Brandon Espinosa, a 36-year-old established patient, sees Dr. Grisham for chronic knee derangement (disruption of cartilage and ligaments of the knee joint), due to an old football injury.

   Code(s): _____

4. Maureen Pearl, a 64-year-old established patient, sees Dr. Hoffman for management and monitoring of degenerative osteoarthritis, which affects her hips and knees.

   Code(s): _____

5. Dr. Grisham treats Sarah Thrasher, age 72, for chondrocalcinosis (crystal accumulation in connective tissue) of the right hand due to dicalcium phosphate crystals.

   Code(s): _____

6. Francine Broyles, a 48-year-old established patient, sees her rheumatologist, Dr. Truman, for management of fibromyalgia.

   Code(s): _____

A LOOK AHEAD TO ICD-10-CM

Refer to ■ TABLE 10-3 for a summary of the ICD-10-CM classifications and guidelines for body systems that you coded in this chapter.

Instructions: Assign ICD-10-CM codes to the following cases that you previously coded in ICD-9-CM, using both the ICD-10-CM Index and the Tabular. (Refer to ICD-10-CM Official Guidelines for additional information; directions for accessing the guidelines are located in Appendix A of this text.)

■ **TABLE 10-3 ICD-10-CM CHAPTERS AND GUIDELINES**

Chapter Title	Chapter Number	Chapter Categories	ICD-10-CM Guidelines
Mental disorders	5	F01–F99	Addition of code for pain that is psychological (in the mind)
Respiratory diseases	10	J00–J99	Revised guidelines for COPD and asthma, and COPD and bronchitis
Digestive diseases	11	K00–K94	No ICD-10-CM guidelines
Genitourinary diseases	14	N00–N99	No ICD-10-CM revisions
Skin and subcutaneous tissue disorders	12	L00-L99	New and revised guidelines for coding pressure ulcers and stages, including a combination code for an ulcer and its stage
Musculoskeletal system and connective tissue disorders	13	M00–M99	Revisions to guidelines for coding fracture sites, including addition of laterality; guidelines for osteoporosis with or without a pathologic fracture

1. George Boggs, a 23-year-old established patient, sees Dr. Goldstein, a psychiatrist, for medication management of bipolar I disorder. After questioning Mr. Boggs, Dr. Goldstein documents that the patient experienced severe manic episodes over the past several days. Code(s):_____

2. Katie Vachon, age 35, sees Dr. Hoffman because she recently experienced problems from previously diagnosed intrinsic asthma, such as shortness of breath and increased severity of wheezing. Dr. Hoffman diagnoses her with an acute exacerbation and adjusts her medication. Code(s):_____

3. Dr. Drimond repairs a right inguinal hernia for Jack Covington, age 61, in Williton's outpatient surgery department. Code(s):_____

4. Dennis Flint, age 80, sees his urologist, Dr. Moir, for an enlarged prostate with urinary retention, which has not significantly improved with medication. Dr. Moir adjusts Mr. Flint's medication and says that if his symptoms do not improve, he should consider surgery. Code(s):_____

5. Sarah Wooden, a 47-year-old established patient, sees Dr. Ferguson for a follow-up visit to check a chronic ulcer on her right calf, which is due to postphlebitic syndrome (leg pain and edema). Code(s):_____

6. Annie Norwood, an 87-year-old established patient, sees Dr. Hoffman for acute hip pain. X-rays show that she has a pathological fracture in her hip due to age-related osteoporosis. Code(s):_____

CHAPTER REVIEW

Multiple Choice

Instructions: Circle one best answer to complete each statement.

1. Which of the following is *not* a mental disorder?
   a. Schizophrenia
   b. Anxiety
   c. Dementia
   d. Erythema multiforme

2. A program that patients attend during the day which provides group therapy and activities, education, and counseling is called a(n)
   a. insane asylum.
   b. partial hospitalization program.
   c. community-based mental health center.
   d. outpatient clinic.

3. Symptoms of COPD include all of the following *except*
   a. smoking.
   b. shortness of breath.
   c. sputum.
   d. weight changes.

4. An allergic reaction to tobacco smoke, pollen, mold, dust, food, or pets is called
   a. status asthmaticus.
   b. COPD.
   c. intrinsic asthma.
   d. extrinsic asthma.

5. The digestive system includes all of the following *except*
   a. teeth.
   b. bronchus.
   c. small intestine.
   d. gallbladder.

6. A hernia that causes a bowel obstruction is called
   a. strangulated.
   b. incarcerated.
   c. irreducible.
   d. reducible.

7. The GFR is
   a. the rate at which the kidneys filter blood per minute.
   b. the rate at which a patient loses partial or full function of kidneys, typically over a period of time.
   c. a measurement of end stage renal disease.
   d. a hemodialysis measurement.

8. Which condition does *not* instruct you to use an additional code for an organism, such as *Staphylococcus* or *E. coli*, that caused the patient's condition?
   a. Cellulitis and abscess of finger and toe
   b. Acute lymphadenitis
   c. Pressure ulcer
   d. Erythema multiforme

9. Untreated cellulitis may become
   a. an HIV infection.
   b. a pressure ulcer.
   c. Group A *Streptococcus*.
   d. life-threatening.

10. Which of the following is *not* a cause of a pathologic fracture?
   a. Neoplasms
   b. Infections
   c. Falls
   d. Osteoporosis

Coding Assignments

Instructions: Assign ICD-9-CM code(s) to the following cases, referencing both the Index and Tabular.

1. Dr. Hoffman treats Kara Cutter, age 77, for pyogenic arthritis of the hip and thigh due to *Pseudomonas*.

   Code(s): _____

2. Dr. Hoffman treats Charles Claxton, age 68, for an abscessed pilonidal cyst.

   Code(s): _____

3. Dr. Moir, a urologist, treats Sarah Thrasher, a 78-year-old, for urinary urge incontinence and cystocele (the urinary bladder protrudes through the vaginal wall).

   Code(s): _____

4. Geraldine Boylan, a 36-year-old established patient, sees Dr. Rhodes, a nephrologist, for management of glomerulonephritis (inflammatory kidney disease). She has secondary diabetes from chronic pancreatitis (inflammation of the pancreas). The diabetes is causing the glomerulonephritis.

   Code(s): _____

5. Samuel Frick, age 44, sees his dentist, Dr. Abbott, for full crowns due to amelogenesis imperfecta (small, discolored teeth that wear easily).

   Code(s): _____

6. Inez Tejeda, age 24, has been unable to conceive children. Dr. Gerard, her OB/GYN, examines her and finds that she has severe pelvic adhesions, which caused infertility.

   Code(s): _____

7. Harry Stewart, age 57, has outpatient surgery at Williton Medical Center for a cholecystectomy (gall bladder removal) due to choledocholithiasis (gallstones) and chronic cholecystitis (gall bladder inflammation).

   Code(s): _____

8. Kevin Silva, age 5, was at the beach all day. Even though his mother applied sunscreen, it washed off in the water. Mrs. Silva brings him to Valley Urgent Care Center, where Dr. Foster diagnoses Kevin with a severe second-degree sunburn.

   Code(s): _____

9. Tammy Hague, a 24-year-old established patient, sees Dr. Goldstein, a psychiatrist, for a psychiatric evaluation. He diagnoses her with severe, acute, recurrent depression.

   Code(s): _____

10. Wilma Boston brings her 2-year-old son, William, to see Dr. Kerr, an ENT, because of coughing and difficulty breathing. Dr. Kerr diagnoses William with an acute exacerbation of asthmatic bronchitis.

   Code(s): _____

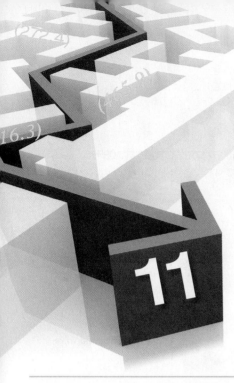

Diseases of the Circulatory System

11

Learning Objectives

After completing this chapter, you should be able to

- Spell and define the key terminology in this chapter.
- Describe and apply the guidelines for coding circulatory system disorders, including hypertension and hypertension with heart or kidney conditions.
- Describe and apply the guidelines for coding an acute myocardial infarction (AMI).

Key Terms

benign hypertension
cardiovascular disease
causal relationship
circulatory system
coronary artery bypass graft (CABG)

heart
heart disease
hypertension
hypertensive heart disease
myocardial infarction (MI)
prehypertension

INTRODUCTION

The next stop on your coding journey is to learn about coding disorders of the circulatory system, including two common diagnoses, high blood pressure and heart attack. You will learn specific information about disorders, including their causes, diagnosis, and treatment. It is beneficial for you to learn as much as you can about the conditions that you code so that you will understand when the medical documentation is incomplete or unclear. The more you know about the conditions, the more effectively you will be able to communicate with physicians and other providers. The more you know, the more you can improve your chances of advancing in your career!

"Always bear in mind that your own resolution to success is more important than any other one thing."

—ABRAHAM LINCOLN

CIRCULATORY SYSTEM (ICD-9-CM CHAPTER 7—390–459)

Before you begin coding circulatory system disorders, let's first review the anatomy of the circulatory system. As you read about the circulatory system and its functions, follow along with the diagrams to achieve a better understanding of how the heart works in conjunction with the circulation of blood throughout the body.

The **circulatory system** consists of the heart (■ FIGURE 11-1) and blood vessels—arteries and veins. Arteries transport blood away from the heart throughout the body (■ FIGURE 11-2), and veins transport blood from body tissues and lungs to the heart (■ FIGURE 11-3). Arterioles are smaller blood vessels that branch off arteries, and capillaries are the smallest blood vessels.

ICD-9-CM codes in this chapter are from the ICD-9-CM 2012 code set from the Department of Health and Human Services, Centers for Disease Control and Prevention.

ICD-10-CM codes in this chapter are from the ICD-10-CM 2012 Draft code set from the Department of Health and Human Services, Centers for Disease Control and Prevention.

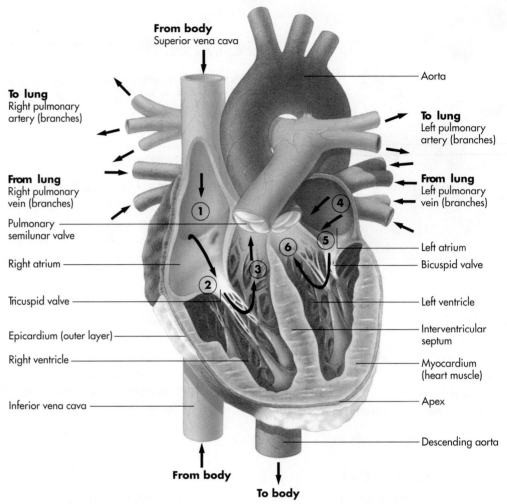

From body
Superior vena cava

To lung
Right pulmonary
artery (branches)

From lung
Right pulmonary
vein (branches)

Pulmonary
semilunar valve

Right atrium

Tricuspid valve

Epicardium (outer layer)

Right ventricle

Inferior vena cava

Aorta

To lung
Left pulmonary
artery (branches)

From lung
Left pulmonary
vein (branches)

Left atrium

Bicuspid valve

Left ventricle

Interventricular
septum

Myocardium
(heart muscle)

Apex

Descending aorta

From body

To body

RIGHT HEART PUMP

1. Deoxygenated blood returns from the upper and lower body to fill the right atrium of the heart creating a pressure against the tricuspid valve.

2. This pressure of the returning blood forces the tricuspid valve open and begins filling the ventricle. The final filling of the ventricle is achieved by the contracting of the right atrium.

3. The right ventricle contracts increasing the internal pressure. This pressure closes the tricuspid valve and forces open the pulmonary semilunar valve thus sending blood toward the lung via the pulmonary artery. This blood will become oxygenated as it travels through the capillary beds of the lung and then return to the left side of the heart.

LEFT HEART PUMP

4. Oxygenated blood returns from the lung via the pulmonary vein and fills the left atrium creating a pressure against the bicuspid valve.

5. This pressure of returning blood forces the bicuspid valve open and begins filling the left ventricle. The final filling of the left ventricle is achieved by the contracting of the left atrium.

6. The left ventricle contracts increasing internal pressure. This pressure closes the bicuspid valve and forces open the aortic valve causing oxygenated blood to flow through the aorta to deliver oxygen throughout the body.

Figure 11-1 ■ Heart valve functions and blood flow.

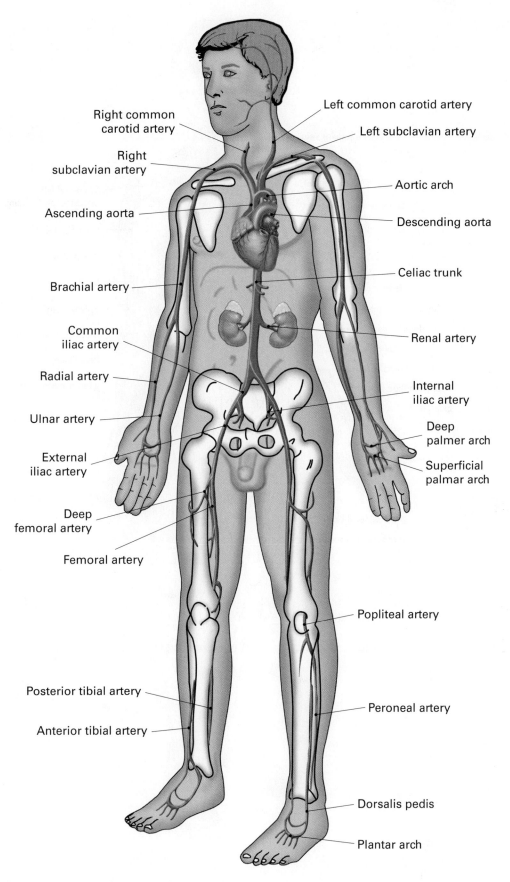

Right common
carotid artery

Right
subclavian artery

Ascending aorta

Brachial artery

Common
iliac artery

Radial artery

Ulnar artery

External
iliac artery

Deep
femoral artery

Femoral artery

Posterior tibial artery

Anterior tibial artery

Left common carotid artery

Left subclavian artery

Aortic arch

Descending aorta

Celiac trunk

Renal artery

Internal
iliac artery

Deep
palmer arch

Superficial
palmar arch

Popliteal artery

Peroneal artery

Dorsalis pedis

Plantar arch

Figure 11-2 ■ Major arteries of circulation.

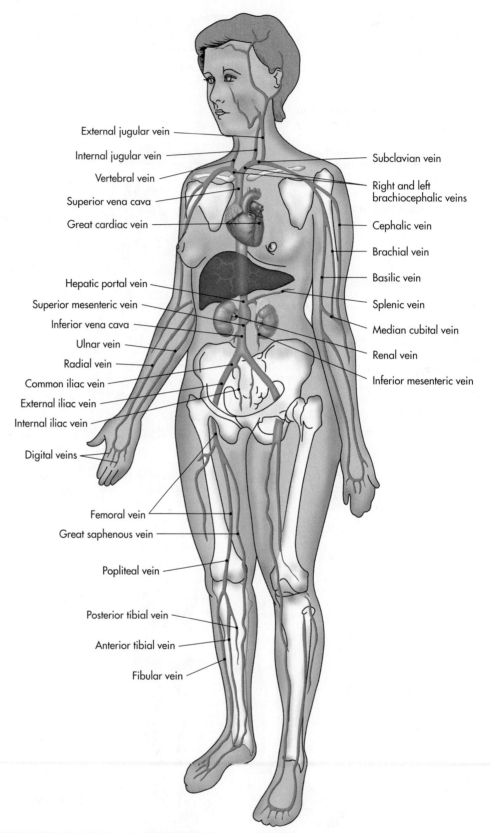

External jugular vein

Internal jugular vein

Vertebral vein

Superior vena cava

Great cardiac vein

Hepatic portal vein

Superior mesenteric vein

Inferior vena cava

Ulnar vein

Radial vein

Common iliac vein

External iliac vein

Internal iliac vein

Digital veins

Femoral vein

Great saphenous vein

Popliteal vein

Posterior tibial vein

Anterior tibial vein

Fibular vein

Subclavian vein

Right and left brachiocephalic veins

Cephalic vein

Brachial vein

Basilic vein

Splenic vein

Median cubital vein

Renal vein

Inferior mesenteric vein

Figure 11-3 ■ Major veins of circulation.

The **heart** has four chambers, two upper and two lower. The heart's upper chambers are the right and left **atria**. They receive and collect blood. The heart's lower chambers are the right and left **ventricles**. The ventricles pump blood out of the heart to other parts of the body. Some of the main blood vessels (arteries and veins) that make up the circulatory system are directly connected to the heart.

atria (ā′trēə)

ventricles (ven′-tri-kəls)

Right Side of the Heart

The superior and inferior vena cavae are the largest veins in the body. After the body's organs and tissues have used the oxygen in the blood, the vena cavae carry the oxygen-poor blood back to the right atrium of the heart. The superior vena cava carries oxygen-poor blood from the upper parts of the body, including the head, chest, arms, and neck. The inferior vena cava carries oxygen-poor blood from the lower parts of the body.

The oxygen-poor blood from the vena cavae flows into the heart's right atrium and then to the right ventricle. From the right ventricle, the blood is pumped through the pulmonary arteries to the lungs. After it has entered the lungs, the blood travels through many small, thin blood vessels called capillaries. There, the blood picks up more oxygen and transfers carbon dioxide to the lungs—a process called gas exchange. The oxygen-rich blood passes from the lungs back to the heart through the pulmonary veins.

Left Side of the Heart

The blood then enters the left atrium and is pumped into the left ventricle. From the left ventricle, the oxygen-rich blood is pumped to the rest of the body through the aorta. The *aorta* is the main artery that carries oxygen-rich blood to the body. Like all of the organs, the heart itself needs oxygen-rich blood. As blood is pumped out of the heart's left ventricle, some of it flows into the coronary arteries. The coronary arteries are located on the heart's surface at the beginning of the aorta. They carry oxygen-rich blood to all parts of the heart.

Septum

The *septum* is an internal wall of tissue that divides the right and left sides of the heart. The area of the septum that divides the atria is called the *atrial* or *interatrial* septum. The area of the septum that divides the ventricles is called the *ventricular* or *interventricular* septum.

Heart Valves

In order for the heart to work well, blood must flow in only one direction. The heart's valves ensure that it does so. Both of the heart's ventricles have an inlet valve from the atria and an outlet valve leading to the arteries. Healthy valves open and close in exact coordination with the pumping action of the heart's atria and ventricles. Each valve has a set of flaps called leaflets or cusps that seal or open the valve. This allows blood to pass through the chambers and into the arteries without backing up or flowing backward.

Each side of the heart uses an inlet valve to help move blood between the atrium and ventricle. The *tricuspid valve* performs this function between the right atrium and right ventricle. The *mitral valve* performs this function between the left atrium and left ventricle. You may have heard a heartbeat described as "lub dub." The "lub" is the sound of the tricuspid and mitral valves closing.

Each of the heart's ventricles also has an outlet valve. The right ventricle uses the *pulmonary valve* to help move blood into the pulmonary arteries. The left ventricle uses the *aortic valve* to do the same for the aorta. The "dub" is the sound of the aortic and pulmonary valves closing.

Circulation

Arterial circulation is the part of the circulatory system that involves arteries, including the aorta and pulmonary arteries. Remember, arteries are blood vessels that carry blood away from the heart. (The exception is the coronary arteries, which supply the heart muscle with oxygen-rich blood.) Healthy arteries are strong and elastic (stretchy). They become narrow in between heartbeats, and they help keep blood pressure consistent. This helps blood move through the body. Arteries and arterioles have strong, flexible walls that allow them to adjust the amount and rate of blood flowing to parts of the body.

Venous circulation is the part of the circulatory system that involves veins, including the vena cavae and pulmonary veins. Veins have thinner walls than arteries. Veins can widen as the amount of blood passing through them increases.

Capillary circulation is the part of the circulatory system where oxygen, nutrients, and waste pass between the blood and parts of the body. Capillaries are very small blood vessels. They connect the arterial and venous circulatory subsystems. Capillaries are special because they have very thin walls. Oxygen and nutrients in the blood can pass through the walls of the capillaries to the parts of the body that need them to work normally. Capillaries' thin walls also allow waste products such as carbon dioxide to pass from the body's organs and tissues into the blood, where it is taken away to the lungs.

Pulmonary circulation is the movement of blood from the heart to the lungs and back to the heart again. Pulmonary circulation includes both arterial and venous circulation. Oxygen-poor blood is pumped to the lungs from the heart (arterial circulation). Oxygen-rich blood moves from the lungs to the heart through the pulmonary veins (venous circulation). Pulmonary circulation also includes capillary circulation. Oxygen breathed in from the air passes through the lungs into the blood through the many capillaries in the lungs. Oxygen-rich blood moves through the pulmonary veins to the left side of the heart and out the aorta to the rest of the body. Capillaries in the lungs also remove carbon dioxide from the blood so that the lungs can exhale the carbon dioxide (National Institutes of Health).

CARDIOVASCULAR AND CIRCULATORY SYSTEM DISORDERS

cardiology (kärd-ē-ʹäl-ə-jē)

cardiologist (kärd-ē-ʹäl-ə-jist)

Cardiology literally means the study of (-ology) the heart (cardi/o). A **cardiologist** is a physician who specializes in the diagnosis, treatment, and prevention of disorders of the heart. A cardiovascular surgeon diagnoses and treats heart and related blood vessel disorders. *Endovascular* or *vascular surgeons* diagnose and treat disorders of arteries and veins.

coronary (kŏrʹō-nă-rē)

Heart disease is a general description for any disorder affecting the heart. You may have also heard the term **cardiovascular disease**, which is a general description for a disorder affecting the heart and related blood vessels. **Coronary** literally means pertaining to (-ary) the heart (coron/o). Sometimes people use the term heart disease to mean *coronary artery disease*, which develops when plaque (cholesterol and other substances) forms and clogs an artery, restricting blood flow. Plaque builds up in arteries from smoking, obesity, hypertension, and diabetes mellitus. Many years ago, people used to describe a heart attack or heart condition as a "coronary," which is a general term that could pertain to any number of heart disorders.

Chapter 7 of the ICD-9-CM categorizes circulatory system disorders as follows:

rheumatic (rōō-mătʹĭk)

- Categories 390–392—Acute **rheumatic** fever (joint infection that can affect the heart)

- Categories 393–398—Chronic rheumatic heart disease (heart disorder that rheumatic fever causes)

- Categories 401–405—Hypertensive disease

ischemic (is-kemʹik)

- Categories 410–414—**Ischemic** heart disease (lack of blood and oxygen to the heart)

- Categories 415–417—Diseases of pulmonary circulation

- Categories 420–429—Other forms of heart disease

cerebrovascular (ser-ə-bro-vasʹku-lər)

- Categories 430–438—**Cerebrovascular** disease (disorder of blood flow to the brain)

- Categories 440–449—Diseases of arteries, arterioles, and capillaries

lymphatics (lim-fatʹiks)

- Categories 451–459—Diseases of veins and **lymphatics** (vessels carrying lymph) and other diseases of circulatory system

Throughout Chapter 7 in the Tabular, you will find notes to *Code first underlying disease* and *Use additional code.* There are also many codes that require you to add a fifth digit to identify the presence of another disease or the episode of care. Follow coding conventions and rules closely to ensure that you assign the correct code. For example, rules for coding ischemic heart disease and cerebrovascular disease instruct you to assign an additional code to identify the presence of hypertension. As you can imagine, there are numerous circulatory system disorders and Official Guidelines and coding conventions for coding them. Because we cannot cover all of them, you will next learn how to code two of the most common disorders, hypertension and **myocardial infarction (MI)**.

TAKE A BREAK

That was a lot of information to absorb! Let's take a break and review more information about the heart and circulatory system.

Exercise 11.1   The Circulatory System and Cardiovascular and Circulatory System Disorders

Instructions: Complete the following statements using information discussed in the previous sections.

1. The heart's upper chambers are the right and left _____. They receive and collect blood. The heart's lower chambers are the right and left _____.

2. The _____ carries oxygen-poor blood from the upper parts of the body, including the head, chest, arms, and neck.

3. The _____ are located on the heart's surface at the beginning of the aorta.

4. The _____ is an internal wall of tissue that divides the right and left sides of the heart.

5. Each side of the heart uses a(n) _____ to help move blood between the atrium and ventricle.

6. Veins are blood vessels that carry blood _____ the heart.

7. Arteries are blood vessels that carry blood _____ the heart.

8. _____ is the part of the circulatory system where oxygen, nutrients, and waste pass between the blood and parts of the body.

9. Many years ago, people used to describe a heart attack or heart condition as a _____.

HYPERTENSION

Hypertension is consistently elevated blood pressure. You may wonder what it means to have elevated blood pressure. First, let's review what blood pressure is and how to measure it. Blood pressure is a *vital sign,* a measurement of body functions, along with respiratory rate, temperature, and pulse. (See Appendix C of this text for normal reference ranges of vital signs.) Blood pressure readings can provide a lot of important information about how a patient's body is functioning and whether the patient needs additional treatment for a specific condition.

Blood pressure measures the force of blood pumped through the arteries. **Systole** is the force of blood when the heart beats and contracts, and **diastole** is the force of blood when the heart relaxes and dilates (widens). In a normal blood pressure reading, such as 110/70 mm/Hg, the top number, 110, represents *systolic blood pressure*, the maximum pressure of pumping blood as the heart contracts and beats. The bottom number, 70, represents *diastolic blood pressure*, the minimum pressure of pumping blood when the heart rests in between beats.

systole (sĭs'tō-lē)
diastole (dī-ăs'tō-lē)

There are digital and manual devices to measure blood pressure. Clinicians use a stethoscope to listen to pulse sounds and a manual **sphygmomanometer**, or blood pressure cuff (■ FIGURE 11-4), to measure blood pressure in the upper arm at the **brachial artery**.

sphygmomanometer (sfĭg'mō-măn-ō mĕt-ĕr)

brachial artery (brā'ki-ăl ahr'tə-re)—artery of the upper arm

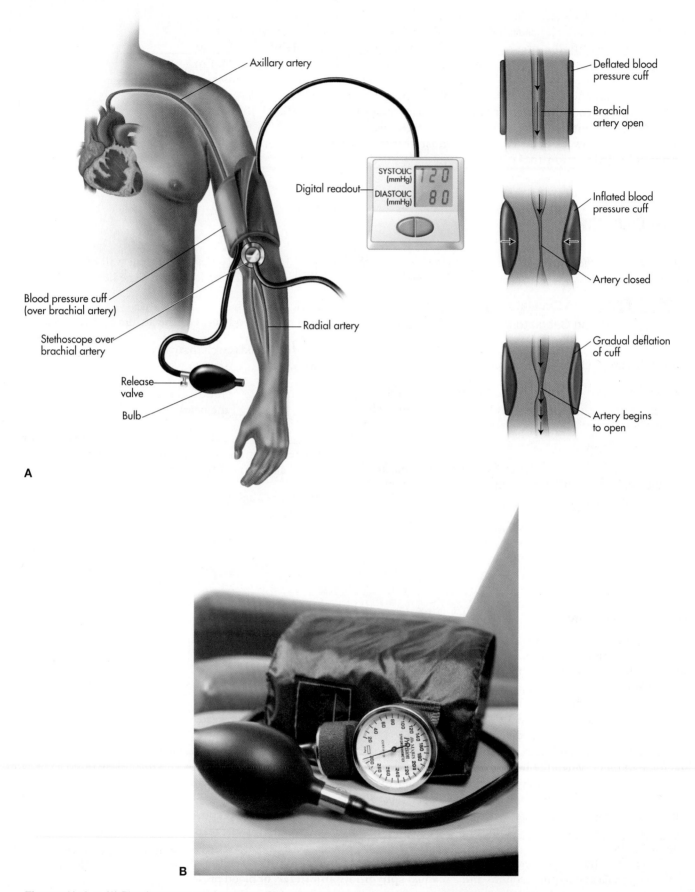

Figure 11-4 ■ (A) Blood pressure measurement; (B) A sphygmomanometer or blood pressure cuff.
Photo credit: Amanda Mills/CDC.

■ TABLE 11-1   BLOOD PRESSURE LEVELS—NORMAL, AT RISK, AND HIGH

Blood Pressure Level	Systolic Measurement (top number)	Diastolic Measurement (bottom number)
Normal	< 120 mm/Hg	<80 mm/Hg
At Risk (prehypertension)	120–139 mm/Hg	80–89 mm/Hg
High (hypertension)	140 mm/Hg or higher	90 mm/Hg or higher

Source: Department of Health and Human Services, Centers for Disease Control and Prevention, www.cdc.gov/dhdsp/data_statistics/fact_sheets/fs_bloodpressure.htm, accessed 12/28/10.

The manual sphygmomanometer contains mercury that provides the unit of measurement for blood pressure, called millimeters of mercury (mm/Hg). ■ Table 11-1 shows normal, at risk, and high blood pressure levels.

Keep in mind that a patient may also have *hypotension*, or low blood pressure, and if it is too low, it could indicate more serious health problems that the physician needs to address.

Physicians diagnose patients with hypertension after taking repeated readings of elevated blood pressure. Sometimes, a patient experiences a temporary elevation of blood pressure, but that does not mean that the patient has hypertension. Be very careful before you assign a hypertension code because the patient's documentation must support hypertension, rather than simply stating *elevated blood pressure*. These are two different diagnoses. Hypertension is divided into two *stages*, on the basis of systolic and diastolic measurements:

*   Stage 1—systolic 140–159, diastolic 90–99
*   Stage 2—systolic 160 or higher, diastolic 100 or higher

Patients can also have **prehypertension**, in which their blood pressure is close to high levels. There are two main types of hypertension, benign and malignant, and several other common types of hypertension that can be classified as benign, malignant, or neither (■ Table 11-2).

■ TABLE 11-2   COMMON TYPES OF HYPERTENSION AND DEFINITIONS

Type of Hypertension	Definition
Prehypertension (also called borderline hypertension or *high normal* blood pressure)	Blood pressure readings are in the at-risk range.
Benign hypertension	Hypertension, also described as mild or moderate, that progresses very slowly; patients often have it for years without any symptoms.
Malignant hypertension	Hypertension with a sudden onset that can cause heart and renal disorders and that often poses an emergent threat to life.
Essential hypertension (also called primary hypertension or hypertension)	Hypertension with no known cause; this is the most common type of hypertension and often has no symptoms (malignant or benign).
Portal hypertension	Hypertension in which blood flow through the liver is obstructed, causing increased pressure in the **portal** vein (neither malignant nor benign).
Renal hypertension	Hypertension with kidney disease (malignant or benign).
Secondary hypertension	Hypertension that another condition caused; it often has no symptoms (malignant or benign).

portal (por′təl)—pertaining to an opening in an organ

proteinuria (pro-te-nu′re-ə)— abnormal condition of excessive protein in the urine

Most people with essential or benign hypertension are asymptomatic until their conditions become severe. Left untreated and uncontrolled, hypertension can cause an MI; stroke; congestive heart failure (CHF); coronary artery disease (CAD); peripheral vascular disease (PVD); ESRD; irreversible damage to the heart, kidneys, blood vessels, brain, and eyes; and even death.

In cases of malignant hypertension, or benign hypertension that becomes severe, symptoms include dangerously high blood pressure, headache, dyspnea, nausea, vomiting, blurred vision, chest pain, and **proteinuria**. Symptoms vary depending on the severity of the patient's condition.

Causes of hypertension include obesity, lack of exercise, smoking, drinking alcohol, eating excess salt, kidney failure, African-American heritage, other hereditary factors, and aging. Physicians diagnose hypertension more quickly when patients have regular blood pressure checks. Treatment for and control of hypertension includes making lifestyle changes including losing weight, getting more exercise, quitting smoking, not drinking alcohol, and eating a healthy diet, including reducing salt intake. Treatment also includes taking medications, including **diuretics**, which help the body to excrete retained fluid through urination, and making regular follow-up visits with a physician to monitor blood pressure and progress.

diuretics (di-u-ret′iks)— agents that promote increased excretion of urine

It is imperative for a patient with hypertension to follow his or her physician's treatment plan to control the disease and maintain normal blood pressure. In uncontrolled and severe cases of hypertension in which blood pressure is dangerously high, treatment varies depending on the patient's situation but many times includes life-saving interventions.

The Hypertension Table

Do you remember from Chapter 3 that you code hypertension using the Hypertension Table in the ICD-9-CM's Index, listed under the main term *hypertension*? In the Hypertension Table (■ FIGURE 11-5), notice that there are various types of hypertension, as shown with nonessential modifiers and subterms. *Read essential modifiers and subterms very carefully* because it is easy to overlook an important word or phrase that leads to correct code assignment.

Remember that the Hypertension Table has columns labeled Malignant, Benign, and Unspecified. In order to code hypertension correctly, you not only have to know the *type* of hypertension that the patient has, but you also have to know whether the hypertension is *malignant, benign,* or *unspecified.* Table 11-2 provides definitions of both malignant and benign hypertension for you to reference. Unspecified hypertension is when the physician does not document the hypertension as either malignant or benign.

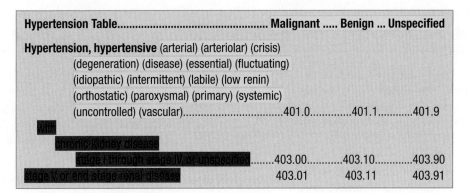

Figure 11-5 ■ Hypertension Table.

Hypertension Table	Malignant	Benign	Unspecified
Hypertension, hypertensive (arterial) (arteriolar) (crisis) (degeneration) (disease) (essential) (fluctuating) (idiopathic) (intermittent) (labile) (low renin) (orthostatic) (paroxysmal) (primary) (systemic) (uncontrolled) (vascular)	401.0	401.1	401.9
with chronic kidney disease stage I through stage IV, or unspecified	403.00	403.10	403.90
stage V or end stage renal disease	403.01	403.11	403.91

Hypertension, Essential Hypertension, or Hypertension Not Otherwise Specified

Recall from Table 11-2 that essential hypertension has no known cause. Assign hypertension (arterial) (essential) (primary) (systemic) (NOS) to category code 401, along with the appropriate fourth digit to indicate malignant (.0), benign (.1), or unspecified (.9) (Figure 11-5). Do not use either 0 *malignant* or 1 *benign* unless the physician specifically states malignant or benign in the medical record. Refer to the following example to code essential hypertension for a patient's encounter:

Example: Mrs. Diaz, a 58-year-old established patient, sees Dr. Hoffman for a biweekly blood pressure check. During the visit, Rhonda, the medical assistant, takes Mrs. Diaz's blood pressure and finds that it is 150/95 mm/Hg. It is the second high reading in a row. Dr. Hoffman performs an examination and diagnoses the patient with hypertension. She is healthy otherwise. Dr. Hoffman prescribes Coreg®, a medication to control hypertension.

To code this case, search the Index for the main term *hypertension*. Because Dr. Hoffman did not document whether Mrs. Diaz's hypertension was malignant or benign, choose the code listed under the *Unspecified* column in the Hypertension Table, which is 401.9 (See Figure 11-5). Then cross-reference code **401.9** to the Tabular (■ Figure 11-6).

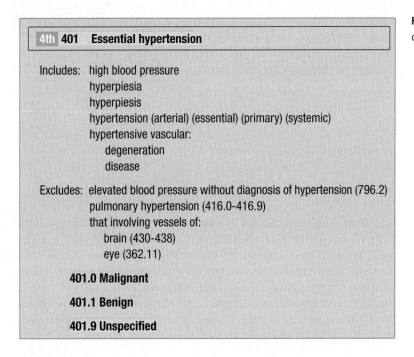

Figure 11-6 ■ Code 401.9 cross-referenced to the Tabular.

4th 401	Essential hypertension

Includes: high blood pressure
hyperpiesia
hyperpiesis
hypertension (arterial) (essential) (primary) (systemic)
hypertensive vascular:
degeneration
disease

Excludes: elevated blood pressure without diagnosis of hypertension (796.2)
pulmonary hypertension (416.0-416.9)
that involving vessels of:
brain (430-438)
eye (362.11)

401.0 Malignant

401.1 Benign

401.9 Unspecified

POINTERS FROM THE PROS: Interview with a Medical Auditor

Kimberly Gallagher works as a medical auditor for a children's hospital. She audits charts for patients who receive evaluation and management (E/M) services. (Most E/M services are face-to-face encounters between a patient and physician.) She compares chart documentation with coded diagnoses and procedures to ensure that the codes are accurate. She also educates physicians, clinicians, coders, and administrators on her findings and on correct coding. Ms. Gallagher holds a Bachelor of Science degree in Health Information Management and is a Registered Health Information Administrator (RHIA), certified by the American Health Information Management Association.

What interests you most about the job that you perform?

- I enjoy being a resource to faculty and staff; I learn something new each time I perform an audit and/or provide education; (and) I'm involved in the clinical environment without actually seeing patients.

What are the most challenging aspects of your job?

- I'd say the most challenging aspect is understanding the complexities of a diagnosis and/or procedure.

I can read about it online and in textbooks, but until a physician describes the risks, complications, and feelings or emotions that a patient is undertaking, it's hard to separate textbook from real life. Medicine is more fascinating than textbooks make it out to be.

What advice would you like to give to coding students to help them prepare to work successfully in the healthcare field?

- Get certified. Physicians do notice this, as do your managers and supervisors. Never stop learning. Challenge yourself, and try to learn as much as you can. Go beyond coding—look at payer policies, reimbursement, and teaching physician rules. So much of the healthcare environment is geared by appropriate coding. The more you know, the more valuable you are as an employee. Remember to be open-minded and understanding of others' thought processes. We all need to teach each other to be successful.

(Used by permission of Kimberly Gallagher.)

Hypertension and Heart Disease

Hypertensive heart disease is a heart condition that hypertension causes. It takes various forms, including CHF, CAD, MI, and ischemic heart disease. Hypertension damages the heart because it causes blood to flow through the arteries with increased force. This makes the heart strain and work harder to pump blood through the arteries, enlarging the heart and causing heart failure and possibly death.

When you code heart disease with hypertension, it is important to carefully read the diagnostic statement to determine whether you need to assign *one* or *two* codes. You should code heart conditions in the following categories under category *402—Hypertensive heart disease* when *there is a relationship* between the heart disease and hypertension, with medical documentation stating "due to hypertension" or "hypertensive heart disease."

- 425.8—Cardiomyopathy in other diseases classified elsewhere
- 429.0—Myocarditis, unspecified
- 429.1—Myocardial degeneration
- 429.2—Cardiovascular disease, unspecified
- 429.3—Cardiomegaly
- 429.8—Other ill-defined heart diseases
- 429.9—Heart disease, unspecified

Causal Relationship between Heart Disease and Hypertension

When a patient has *both* a heart condition and hypertension, assign *one* combination code from category 402—*Hypertensive heart disease* only when there is a **causal relationship**. A causal (also called cause-and-effect) relationship is present when one condition *causes* another. If hypertension caused the heart condition, the physician would document that the heart condition is *due to* hypertension, hypertension *caused* the heart condition, or the patient has *hypertensive* heart disease. The combination code describes both the hypertension and the heart disease that the hypertension caused.

An exception to this rule is when a patient has *heart failure* due to hypertension. In that case, assign *two* codes: a combination code from category 402—*Hypertensive heart disease* for hypertension and heart failure, and an additional code from category 428—*Heart failure.* You can assign more than one code from category 428 if the patient has more than one type of heart failure, such as systolic and congestive heart failure.

When the physician documents heart disease *with* hypertension, or heart disease *and* hypertension, there is no causal relationship unless the physician specifically documents that the hypertension and heart disease are related. You cannot assume that the conditions are related simply because the physician documents both of them in a patient's record. When there is no relationship between hypertension and heart disease, assign *two separate codes* for heart disease and hypertension because the documentation does not show that hypertension caused the heart disease. Sequence codes according to the circumstances of the admission or encounter.

To better understand coding guidelines for hypertension and heart disease, let's review three examples of patients' encounters to determine whether to assign one or two codes.

Example 1: Mr. Reynolds, a 45-year-old established patient, sees Dr. Woods, a cardiologist, for a follow-up appointment to manage his cardiomegaly and benign hypertension.

The diagnostic statement includes the word *and* (*cardiomegaly and benign hypertension*), which does *not* show a causal relationship between hypertension and heart disease. If the documentation included *cardiomegaly due to hypertension*, then there is a causal relationship. Assign *two codes*, cardiomegaly and benign hypertension.

For cardiomegaly, search the Index for the main term *cardiomegaly* and cross-reference code 429.3 to the Tabular to assign the code. For hypertension, search the Index for the main term *hypertension*. Go to the first entry in the Hypertension Table for *hypertension, hypertensive*. Cross-reference the code that you find in the Benign column, 401.1 (Figure 11-5). For Example 1, assign two codes: **429.3** (cardiomegaly) and **401.1** (benign hypertension).

Example 2: Mr. Ellis, a 63-year-old new patient, sees Dr. Woods. Mr. Ellis complains of intermittent **angina** (chest pain) and shortness of breath. Dr. Woods examines the patient, and the patient undergoes a monitored *stress test* (a test that determines how well the patient's heart functions and reveals heart disorders) (■ FIGURE 11-7). Dr. Woods diagnoses the patient with cardiovascular disease due to benign hypertension.

angina (ăn′jĭ-nă)

The diagnostic statement includes the words *due to* (*cardiovascular disease due to benign hypertension*), which establishes a *causal relationship* between benign hypertension and cardiovascular disease. Assign *one code* that includes both hypertension and cardiovascular disease.

Search the Index for the main term *hypertension*, subterm *cardiovascular disease*. Search for the code under the Benign column in the Hypertension Table, which is code 402.10. Then cross-reference code 402.10 to the Tabular (■ FIGURE 11-8). Final code assignment for this example is code **402.10**, which includes both conditions.

Example 3: Mrs. Freeman, a 77-year-old established patient, sees Dr. Woods for a follow-up visit. He diagnoses her with CHF due to benign hypertension.

The diagnostic statement includes the words *due to*, which establishes a causal relationship between hypertension and heart failure. The coding rule tells you that when there is a causal relationship between *heart failure* and hypertension, you should assign two codes—a combination code for hypertension and heart failure, and an additional code for heart failure.

For the first code, search the Index for the main term *hypertension*, subterm *cardiovascular disease*, connecting word *with*, and subterm *heart failure*. Search for the code under the *Benign* column in the Hypertension Table, which is 402.11. Then cross-reference **402.11** to the Tabular (■ FIGURE 11-9).

Figure 11-7 ■ A patient undergoes a stress test.

Photo credit: GWIMages / Shutterstock.com.

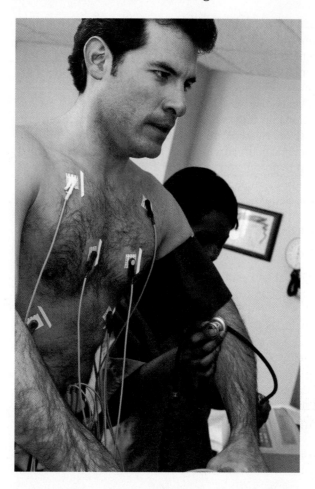

Figure 11-8 ■ Index entry for hypertensive cardiovascular disease, with code 402.10 cross-referenced to the Tabular.

Hypertension Table	Malignant	Benign	Unspecified
Hypertension, hypertensive (arterial) (arteriolar) (crisis) (degeneration) (disease) (essential) (fluctuating) (idiopathic) (intermittent) (labile) (low renin) (orthostatic) (paroxysmal) (primary) (systemic) (uncontrolled) (vascular)	401.0	401.1	401.9
cardiovascular disease (arteriosclerotic) (sclerotic) with	402.00	402.10	402.90
heart failure	402.01	402.11	402.91
renal involvement (conditions classifiable to 403) (see also Hypertension, cardiorenal)	404.00	404.10	404.90

> **4th 402 Hypertensive heart disease**

Includes: hypertensive:
   cardiomegaly
   cardiopathy
   cardiovascular disease
   heart (disease) (failure)
   any condition classifiable to 429.0-429.3, 429.8, 429.9 due to hypertension

Use additional code to specify type of heart failure (428.0-428.43), if known

   5th 402.1 Benign

   402.10 Without heart failure

   402.11 With heart failure

Hypertension Table.. **Malignant ...... Benign ...... Unspecified**

Hypertension, hypertensive (arterial) (arteriolar) (crisis)
        (degeneration) (disease) (essential) (fluctuating)
        (idiopathic) (intermittent) (labile) (low renin)
        (orthostatic) (paroxysmal) (primary) (systemic)
        (uncontrolled) (vascular).................................401.0.............401.1.............401.9

cardiovascular disease (arteriosclerotic) (sclerotic).........402.00............402.10............402.90
   with
      heart failure..402.01............402.11............402.91
      renal involvement (conditions classifiable to 403)
         (see also Hypertension, cardiorenal).............404.00............404.10............404.90

`4th` **402   Hypertensive heart disease**

Includes: hypertensive:
      cardiomegaly
      cardiopathy
      cardiovascular disease
      heart (disease) (failure)
      any condition classifiable to 429.0-429.3, 429.8, 429.9 due to hypertension

Use additional code to specify type of heart failure (428.0-428.43), if known

    `5th` **402.0 Malignant**
        402.00 Without heart failure
        402.01 With heart failure

    `5th` **402.1 Benign**
        402.10 Without heart failure
        402.11 With heart failure

Figure 11-9 ■ Index entry for hypertension with heart failure, with code 402.11 cross-referenced to the Tabular.

Did you notice the *Use additional code* note under category 402 in the Tabular instructing you to assign a code for heart failure? Search the Index for the main term *failure*, subterm *heart*, and subterm *congestive*. Then cross-reference code 428.0 to the Tabular (■ FIGURE 11-10).

Figure 11-10 ■ Index entry for congestive heart failure with code 428.0 cross-referenced to the Tabular.

Failure, failed

    heart (acute) (sudden) 428.9

       congestive (compensated) (decompensated) (see also Failure, heart) 428.0

    `4th` **428   Heart failure**

Code, if applicable, heart failure due to hypertension first (402.0-402.9, with fifth-digit 1 or 404.0-404.9 with fifth-digit 1 or 3)

Excludes: rheumatic (398.91)
      that complicating:
         abortion (634-638 with.7, 639.8)
         ectopic or molar pregnancy (639.8)
         labor or delivery (668.1, 669.4)

      428.0 Congestive heart failure, unspecified
        Congestive heart disease
        Right heart failure (secondary to left heart failure)

      Excludes: fluid overload NOS (276.69)

The ICD-9-CM gave you another coding instruction under category 428 in the Tabular to *Code, if applicable, heart failure due to hypertension first.* For Example 3, assign two codes: **402.11** (congestive heart failure due to benign hypertension), and **428.0** (congestive heart failure).

TAKE A BREAK

That was a lot of information to remember! Let's take a break and then practice assigning codes for hypertension and heart disease.

Exercise 11.2   Hypertension and Heart Disease

Part 1: Theory

Instructions: Refer to Table 11-2 to complete the following definitions by filling in the type of hypertension.

1. Hypertension with a sudden onset that is life threatening and that causes heart and renal disorders is called _____ hypertension.

2. Another condition causes _____ hypertension.

3. When patients are at risk for developing hypertension, their condition is called _____.

4. Hypertension that progresses slowly is called _____ hypertension.

5. Hypertension that is simply known as "hypertension" is also called _____ hypertension.

6. _____ hypertension obstructs blood flow through the liver.

Part 2: Coding

Instructions: Assign diagnosis codes to the following patient cases, using both the Index and Tabular. Refer to the coding guidelines and the examples already discussed for assistance.

1. Dr. Woods, a cardiologist, treats new patient Curtis Trujillo, age 51, for cardiomegaly (heart enlargement) due to benign hypertension.

   Code(s): _____

2. Dr. Woods schedules established patient Eleanor Corn, age 72, for open heart surgery to correct mitral valve stenosis (narrowing) and aortic valve insufficiency. She also has benign hypertension, but it is stable so she is cleared for surgery.

   Code(s): _____

3. Dr. Woods treats new patient Marianne Lail, a 78-year-old, for hypertension, myocardial degeneration, and coronary arteriosclerosis (hardening of the arteries).

   Code(s): _____

4. Established patient Penny Hendon, age 69, sees Dr. Woods for ongoing monitoring and management of left heart failure due to benign hypertension.

   Code(s): _____

5. Jeff Partida, age 46, sees Dr. Hoffman for a follow-up on a series of blood pressure readings that the registered nurse took over the past three months. His readings were 145/90, 150/92, 150/95, and 150/90. Dr. Hoffman tells Mr. Partida that he has benign hypertension. He prescribes an antihypertensive medication and counsels him about changes he should make in his diet, lifestyle, and exercise routine. Dr. Hoffman also recommends that Mr. Partida quit smoking because his tobacco abuse contributes to his hypertension.

   Code(s): _____

6. Mabel Will, a 70-year-old new patient, sees Dr. Woods for intermittent angina. He diagnoses her with atrial **fibrillation** (irregular heartbeat, usually fast) with essential hypertension. He prescribes a beta blocker medication to help regulate her heart rhythm and schedules her for a follow-up visit in three months.

   Code(s): _____

fibrillation (fĭ-brĭ-la′shən)

Hypertensive Chronic Kidney Disease

We have already reviewed hypertension with heart disease; now let's discuss coding guidelines for hypertension with chronic kidney disease when the condition also involves heart disease. Assign a code from category 403—*Hypertensive chronic kidney disease* when a patient has hypertension and

1. *Chronic kidney disease (CKD)* (category 585)

sclerosis (sklə-ro′sis)— hardening

2. *Renal* **sclerosis,** *unspecified* (code 587)

   Unlike hypertension with heart disease, the ICD-9-CM does not assume a causal (cause-and-effect) relationship between hypertension and heart disease. But it does presume a causal relationship between hypertension and chronic kidney disease or renal sclerosis. This means that even if the physician did not document that a patient's CKD is *due to* hypertension, or that hypertension *caused* CKD, as you are coding the case you

DESTINATION: MEDICARE

You learned in Chapter 7 of this book that the CMS website contains the Medicare Learning Network (MLN), which provides training and education on Medicare regulations and issues. In this exercise, your Medicare destination is an MLN's computer-based training module called *Medicare Fraud and Abuse,* which covers information about the coding and billing practices that constitute healthcare provider fraud and abuse. As you learn about diagnosis and procedure coding, it is also important for you to learn and remember fraud and abuse regulations so that you can perform your job duties ethically and legally. Follow these instructions to access the *Medicare Fraud and Abuse* training module:

1. Go to the website: http//:cms.gov.

2. At the top of the screen on the banner bar, choose *Outreach & Education.*

3. Scroll down to *Medicare Learning Network* and choose *MLN Products.*

4. Choose *Web-Based Training (WBT)* on the left side of the screen. Scroll to the right and down the page, and choose *Web-Based Training (WBT) Courses.*

5. You will then see a list of web-based training courses. Click on *Medicare Fraud and Abuse.*

6. Click the link to log in using your ID and password. If you have never accessed the MLN's computer-based training before, you will have to register as a new user. Registration is free and takes a few minutes. You will need your login and password each time you access the computer-based MLN. After registering or logging in, click *Web-based Training Courses* again, and click *Medicare Fraud and Abuse* again.

7. On the next screen, click the radio button for *No credits* or *Continuing Education Units (CEU).* (CMS grants 1 CEU to coders who are certified through the AAPC for scoring 70% or higher on the post-test.) Then click *Take Course.* You will take both a pretest and a post-test so that you can monitor how well you learned the material.

presume a causal relationship anyway. According to the National Kidney Foundation®, hypertension is one of two main causes of CKD; the other is diabetes.

When you presume a causal relationship between hypertension and CKD, it does not mean that you are falling into the trap of assumption coding, in which you make assumptions about what to code on the basis of your personal experiences. It is safe to assume a causal relationship between hypertension and CKD because medical research proves that hypertension causes CKD.

The ICD-9-CM classifies renal sclerosis with hypertension and chronic kidney disease (CKD) with hypertension in category 403—*Hypertensive chronic kidney disease.* Fifth-digit choices for category 403 are as follows:

0—with chronic kidney disease stage I through stage IV, or unspecified

Use additional code to identify the stage of chronic kidney disease (585.1–585.4, 585.9)

1—with chronic kidney disease stage V or end stage renal disease

Use additional code to identify the stage of chronic kidney disease (585.5, 585.6)

When a patient has CKD and hypertension, assign a code from category 403—*Hypertensive chronic kidney disease, and* assign an additional code from category 585—*Chronic kidney disease* to identify the *stage* of CKD (■ FIGURE 11-11).

Figure 11-11 ■ Category 585 with stages of CKD.

4th 585 Chronic kidney disease (CKD)

Includes: Chronic uremia

Code first hypertensive chronic kidney disease, if applicable, (403.00-403.91, 404.00-404.93)

Use additional code to identify:
  kidney transplant status, if applicable (V42.0)
  manifestation as:
    uremic:
      neuropathy (357.4)
      pericarditis (420.0)

585.1 Chronic kidney disease, Stage I

585.2 Chronic kidney disease, Stage II (mild)

585.3 Chronic kidney disease, Stage III (moderate)

585.4 Chronic kidney disease, Stage IV (severe)

585.5 Chronic kidney disease, Stage V

Excludes: chronic kidney disease, stage V requiring chronic dialysis (585.6)

585.6 End stage renal disease
    Chronic kidney disease, stage V requiring chronic dialysis

585.9 Chronic kidney disease, unspecified
    Chronic renal disease
    Chronic renal failure NOS
    Chronic renal insufficiency

Refer to the following example to code hypertension and CKD for a patient's encounter.

Example: Mrs. Crawford, a 55-year-old established patient, sees Dr. Mason, a nephrologist, for a follow-up visit for management of benign hypertension and CKD, Stage I.

According to coding guidelines, assign two codes for Mrs. Crawford's encounter: a code from category 403—*Hypertensive chronic kidney disease* for both hypertension and CKD, and a code from category 585—*Chronic kidney disease* as an additional code to show the *stage of CKD*.

Follow along with your ICD-9-CM manual to code this case. For the first code for hypertensive CKD, search the Index for the main term *hypertension*, connecting word *with*, subterm *chronic kidney disease*, and subterm *stage I through stage IV*. Search for the code under the Benign column, which is 403.10. Then cross-reference **403.10** to the Tabular (■ Figure 11-12).

For the second code, assign the stage of CKD. Search the Index for the main term *disease*, subterm *kidney*, subterm *chronic*, subterm *stage*, subterm *I*. Then cross-reference code **585.1** to the Tabular (■ Figure 11-13).

Hypertensive Chronic Kidney Disease Patients Receiving Dialysis

It is important to note that if a patient with hypertensive CKD receives dialysis, you should also assign a V code to the patient's encounter, regardless of whether the encounter is for dialysis:

- V45.11—*Renal dialysis status.* Assign as an additional code if the patient's encounter is *not* for dialysis, but the patient receives dialysis. (Index entries: *dependence, on, hemodialysis, peritoneal dialysis,* or *renal dialysis machine.*) Assign a code for the patient's condition that indicates that the encounter is the first-listed code.

- V56—*Encounter for dialysis and dialysis catheter care.* Assign a code from category V56 as the first-listed code if the patient's encounter is for dialysis or dialysis catheter care. (Index entries: *admission, for, dialysis.*) Assign an additional code for the patient's condition.

Hypertension Table..	Malignant	Benign	Unspecified

Hypertension, hypertensive (arterial) (arteriolar) (crisis)
    (degeneration) (disease) (essential) (fluctuating)
    (idiopathic) (intermittent) (labile) (low renin)
    (orthostatic) (paroxysmal) (primary) (systemic)
    (uncontrolled) (vascular)...................................401.0...............401.1............401.9

  with
    chronic kidney disease
        stage I through stage IV, or unspecified.....403.00.............403.10..........403.90
        stage V or end stage renal disease............403.01.............403.11..........403.91

4th   **403 Hypertensive chronic kidney disease**

Includes: arteriolar nephritis
    arteriosclerosis of:
        kidney
        renal arterioles
    arteriosclerotic nephritis (chronic) (interstitial)
    hypertensive:
        nephropathy
        renal failure
        uremia (chronic)
    nephrosclerosis
    renal sclerosis with hypertension
    any condition classifiable to 585 and 587 with any condition classifiable to 401

Excludes: acute kidney failure (584.5-584.9)
    renal disease stated as not due to hypertension
    renovascular hypertension (405.0-405.9 with fifth-digit 1)

The following fifth-digit subclassification is for use with category 403:
    0 with chronic kidney disease stage I through stage IV, or unspecified
    Use additional code to identify the stage of chronic kidney disease (585.1-585.4, 585.9)
    1 with chronic kidney disease stage V or end stage renal disease
    Use additional code to identify the stage of chronic kidney disease (585.5, 585.6)

403.0 Malignant
[0-1]

403.1 Benign
[0-1]

403.9 Unspecified
[0-1]

Figure 11-12 ■ Index entry for hypertensive chronic kidney disease, stage I, with code 403.10 cross-referenced to the Tabular.

Hypertensive Heart Disease and Chronic Kidney Disease

When a patient has *both* hypertensive heart disease and chronic kidney disease, assign a combination code from category 404—*Hypertensive heart and chronic kidney disease*. Assume that there is a relationship between hypertension and chronic kidney disease if they are both documented, even if the provider does not state that there is a relationship between them. Assign additional codes as follows:

- Assign an additional code from category 585—*Chronic kidney disease* to identify the *stage* of kidney disease.

- Assign an additional code from category 428, to identify the *type* of heart failure if the patient has heart failure.

Figure 11-13 ■ Index entry for chronic kidney disease Stage I with code 585.1 cross-referenced to the Tabular.

Disease, diseased - see also Syndrome

  kidney (functional) (pelvis) (see also Disease, renal) 593.9
    chronic 585.9
      requiring chronic dialysis 585.6
      stage
        I 585.1
        II (mild) 585.2
        III (moderate) 585.3
        IV (severe) 585.4
        V 585.5

4th **585** **Chronic kidney disease (CKD)**

Includes: Chronic uremia

Code first hypertensive chronic kidney disease, if applicable, (403.00-403.91, 404.00-404.93)

Use additional code to identify:
  kidney transplant status, if applicable (V42.0)
  manifestation as:
    uremic:
      neuropathy (357.4)
      pericarditis (420.0)

      585.1 Chronic kidney disease, Stage I

For this example, assign two codes: 403.10 (hypertensive chronic kidney disease, stage I), and 585.1 (chronic kidney disease, stage I).

Fifth-digit choices for category 404—*Hypertensive heart and chronic kidney disease* are as follows:

0—without heart failure and with chronic kidney disease stage I through stage IV, or unspecified

Use additional code to identify the stage of chronic kidney disease (585.1–585.4, 585.9)

1—with heart failure and with chronic kidney disease stage I through stage IV, or unspecified Use additional code to identify the stage of chronic kidney disease (585.1–585.4, 585.9)

2—without heart failure and with chronic kidney disease stage V or end stage renal disease

Use additional code to identify the stage of chronic kidney disease (585.5, 585.6)

3—with heart failure and chronic kidney disease stage V or end stage renal disease

Use additional code to identify the stage of chronic kidney disease (585.5, 585.6)

Refer to the following example to code hypertensive heart and chronic kidney disease.

Example: Mrs. Ramos, a 52-year-old new patient, sees Dr. Woods, a cardiologist. He examines Mrs. Ramos, conducts testing, and determines that she has CHF due to benign hypertension and CKD, stage II. Dr. Woods discusses several treatment and management options with the patient.

Use your ICD-9-CM to code the following diagnoses in this example:

1. **404.11**—Hypertensive heart and chronic kidney disease, benign, with heart failure and with chronic kidney disease stage I through stage IV (Index entries: *hypertension, cardiorenal, with, chronic kidney disease, stage I through stage IV,* and *heart failure, benign.*)

2. **428.0**—Heart failure

3. **585.2**—Chronic kidney disease, stage II

WORKPLACE IQ

You have been working as a medical assistant for Dr. Fisher, a cardiologist, for one year. Part of your job involves assisting the office manager, Beverly, with coding. Today, Beverly gives you a list of 50 patient names, their demographic information, and their Medicare Health Insurance Claim numbers. She tells you to register all of them in the computer. For each patient's account, Beverly says, you need to enter their diagnoses as *congestive heart failure with benign hypertension* and enter a charge for a high-level office visit on February 15th. She says that when you finish, she will electronically bill Medicare for the patients' services.

You review the list of patient names, none of which you recognize, and you wonder why the charges are on a printed list instead of on encounter forms, as is usually done with patients' visits. You ask Beverly why there are no encounter forms and whether the patients are new or established. She tells you, "Oh, don't worry about that. Just register them, enter the diagnoses and charges, and let me know when you're finished."

What would you do?

TAKE A BREAK

Let's take a break and then practice assigning codes for hypertensive CKD and hypertensive heart and CKD.

Exercise 11.3 Hypertensive Chronic Kidney Disease, and Hypertensive Heart Disease and Chronic Kidney Disease

Instructions: Assign diagnosis codes to the following patient cases, using both the Index and Tabular. Refer to the guidelines and examples that were already discussed for assistance.

1. Dr. Mason, a nephrologist, diagnoses new patient Marsha Smithe, age 76, with hypertensive CKD. The hypertension is benign and the CKD is stage III.

   Code(s): _____

2. Douglas Priest, age 43, sees Dr. Mason, who diagnoses him with hypertensive cardiovascular renal disease.

   Code(s): _____

3. Dr. Hoffman refers Roberta Perea, age 66, to Dr. Mason. She has had benign hypertension for several years, and recent lab tests showed a decreased GFR and the presence of proteinuria (excessive protein in the urine). After reviewing the labs and conducting further testing and examination, Dr. Mason confirms stage I CKD.

   Code(s): _____

4. Florence Stover, a 67-year-old established patient, sees Dr. Mason for management of ESRD with benign hypertension. She also receives renal dialysis three times a week.

   Code(s): _____

5. Dr. Mason diagnoses new patient Jesse Cooksey, age 65, with essential hypertension and renal sclerosis.

   Code(s): _____

6. Stephen Lawlor, an 81-year-old established patient, sees Dr. Woods, a cardiologist, for management of stage II CKD and benign hypertensive heart disease. He has combined chronic systolic and diastolic heart failure.

   Code(s): _____

Coding Additional Types of Hypertension

You have learned how to code hypertension with heart disorders and with CKD. The ICD-9-CM also has specific guidelines for coding several other types of hypertension, along with related disorders, which you should review carefully to ensure that you assign the correct codes. Refer to your ICD-9-CM manual to review the specific categories listed in the guidelines, which are as follows:

1. **Hypertensive Cerebrovascular Disease** If a patient has hypertensive cerebrovascular disease, assign two codes. Sequence first cerebrovascular disease from categories 430–438. Assign an additional code for hypertension from categories 401–405.

2. **Hypertensive Retinopathy** If a patient has hypertensive retinopathy (a retinal disorder), assign two codes. Sequence first a code from subcategory 362.11—*Hypertensive retinopathy*. Assign an additional code for hypertension from categories 401–405.

3. **Hypertension, Secondary** Secondary hypertension is hypertension that another condition caused. The word *secondary* does not mean that you always sequence the hypertension code second. If a patient has secondary hypertension, assign two codes: one for the underlying etiology that caused the hypertension, and the other from category 405—*Secondary hypertension*. Sequence codes according to the circumstances of the admission or encounter.

4. **Hypertension, Transient and Elevated Blood Pressure** *Transient* refers to a situation that comes and goes. When a physician documents *transient hypertension*, do not code hypertension. Instead, assign code 796.2—*Elevated blood pressure reading without diagnosis of hypertension* (main term *elevation*, subterm *blood pressure*, and subterm *reading*). Before you assign code 796.2, carefully read the patient's documentation to check whether the physician diagnosed the patient with hypertension. If he did, assign a code for hypertension.

    For a pregnant patient with transient hypertension, assign a code from subcategory 642.3—*Transient hypertension of pregnancy*. You will learn more about coding pregnancy conditions in Chapter 14 of this book.

    When a physician documents that a patient has elevated blood pressure, assign code 796.2—*Elevated blood pressure reading without diagnosis of hypertension*. Just as in the case of transient hypertension, before you assign code 796.2, carefully read the patient's documentation to check whether the physician diagnosed the patient with hypertension.

5. **Hypertension, Controlled** When a physician documents that a patient has controlled hypertension, it usually means that the physician diagnosed the patient with hypertension at some point, but the condition is now under control through medication and/or other therapy and lifestyle changes. For these patients, assign a hypertension code from categories 401–405.

6. **Hypertension, Uncontrolled** When a physician documents that the patient has uncontrolled hypertension, it means that the patient's hypertension is untreated or is not responding to current treatment. In either case, assign a code from categories 401–405 to designate the stage and type of hypertension.

TAKE A BREAK

Let's take a break and then practice assigning codes for other types of hypertension.

Exercise 11.4 Coding Additional Types of Hypertension

Instructions: Assign diagnosis codes to the following patient cases, using both the Index and Tabular. Refer to the guidelines that were previously discussed for assistance.

1. Dr. Woods, a cardiologist, treats Ellen Estep, age 58, at Williton Medical Center for transient cerebral ischemia and hypertension.

    Code(s): _____

2. Dr. Fisher, an ophthalmologist, diagnoses new patient Russell Bundy, age 73, with hypertensive retinopathy.

    Code(s): _____

3. Dr. Mason, a nephrologist, treats established patient Allan Liddell, age 43, for benign essential hypertension due to polycystic kidney disease, which he has had for most of his life.

    Code(s): _____

4. Joanne Gales, age 59, sees Dr. Hoffman for a follow-up visit on her essential benign hypertension. She has been on medication for several months and tells Dr. Hoffman that she recently started walking a mile a day. She also lost 10 pounds. Dr. Hoffman is pleased to report to Mrs. Gales that the changes to her lifestyle have helped to control her hypertension, and tells her to keep up the good work.

    Code(s): _____

5. Dr. Hoffman sees Ronald Greentree, age 51, for a health examination. His last blood pressure reading was 110/80, and today it is 140/90.

    Code(s): _____

6. At her annual check-up, Dr. Hoffman reviews established patient Susan Sherry's recent elevated blood pressure readings of 140/95 and 140/90.

    Code(s): _____

MYOCARDIAL INFARCTION (MI)

The coronary arteries provide the heart with oxygenated blood that it needs to function properly. The most common cause of an **MI**, also called a heart attack, is when plaque and/or a blood clot (**thrombus**) forms in a coronary artery and occludes (blocks) blood flow, causing necrosis of heart muscle. Plaque, called an **atheroma**, is a combination of cholesterol and the body's proteins and calcium deposited on artery walls. It causes arteries to harden and become weak, a condition called atherosclerosis (■ FIGURES 11-14). Plaque can rupture and cause a thrombus to form.

MIs cause severe damage to muscular heart tissue, which is called myocardium, and can also cause death. Causes of atherosclerosis and resulting MI include hypertension, smoking, type I diabetes mellitus, high cholesterol (**hypercholesterolemia**), being over age 45, being male, stress, lack of exercise, and family history of atherosclerosis.

Symptoms of an MI include chest and arm pain, shortness of breath, weakness, dizziness, dyspnea, syncope, nausea, vomiting, coughing, wheezing, and **diaphoresis** (excessive sweating). Many people ignore these symptoms or think that they are symptoms of something else, not an MI. Physicians diagnose an MI by listening to the heart and to a patient's breathing. They also conduct tests, such as a coronary **angiogram**, an X-ray of the arteries (■ FIGURE 11-15); an **electrocardiogram** (EKG or ECG), a test that measures electrical signals of the heart as it beats (■ FIGURE 11-16), a computed tomography (CT) scan, which produces three-dimensional images of occluded arteries; and blood tests for the presence of cardiac *enzymes* that the body releases after experiencing an MI.

A myocardial infarction is a medical emergency. Treatment includes administering oxygen, giving the patient aspirin (which helps prevent blood clots), providing **nitroglycerin** (which improves arterial blood flow), and giving the patient medications to eliminate chest pain, prevent blood clots, and reduce blood pressure (to lessen the work that the heart is doing). Surgical interventions include **angioplasty**, in which a physician inserts a balloon catheter into a coronary artery, also called balloon angioplasty (■ FIGURE 11-17).

After the catheter has been inserted, the balloon is inflated, pushing plaque against the artery walls, which widens the artery and allows blood to flow through again.

Another surgical intervention is a coronary artery bypass graft (CABG), a procedure in which a physician removes arteries and veins from the body, such as the **saphenous vein** from the leg or the left internal mammary artery. The physician then grafts the vein and artery to a new area to allow blood to flow through and bypass the blocked artery (■ FIGURE 11-18).

thrombus (throm'bəs)
atheroma (ăth'ĕr-ōmă)

hypercholesterolemia
(hi-pər-kə-les'tər-ol-e'me-ə)

diaphoresis (di-a-fō-rē' sĭs)

angiogram (ăn'jē-ō-grăm)
electrocardiogram (e-lek-tro-kahr'de-o-gram')

nitroglycerin (ni-tro-glis'-ər-in)—a pharmaceutical preparation of diluted nitric acid that is used to treat chest pain, heart attack, and high blood pressure

angioplasty (ăn'jĭ-ō-plăs-tē)

saphenous vein (sə-fe'nəs)—the longest vein in the body, extending from the foot to the groin, where it opens into the femoral vein

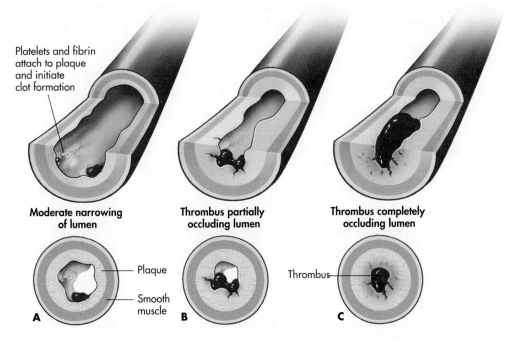

Platelets and fibrin attach to plaque and initiate clot formation

Moderate narrowing of lumen

Thrombus partially occluding lumen

Thrombus completely occluding lumen

Plaque

Smooth muscle

Thrombus

A   B   C

Figure 11-14 ■ Thrombus formation in an atherosclerotic vessel: (A) the initial clot formation, (B) partial occlusion, and (C) complete occlusion.

Figure 11-15 ■ Angiogram of the heart showing obstruction in a major coronary artery.

Photo credit: Zephyr/Photo Researchers, Inc.

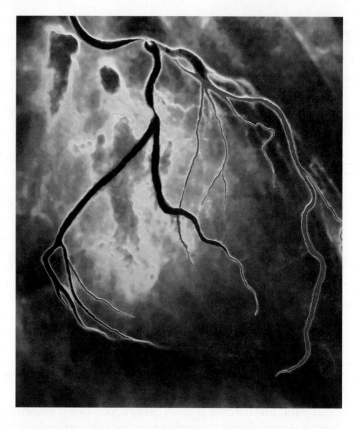

The physician may also insert a stent (small tube) to help keep the artery open permanently (■ FIGURE 11-19).

Patients who survive an MI frequently participate in a *cardiac rehabilitation program,* in which providers help patients develop an exercise program and provide counseling and education.

Coding Acute Myocardial Infarction

ICD-9-CM classifies an AMI in category 410—*Acute myocardial infarction* (main term *infarct, infarction,* and subterm *myocardium, myocardial*). The fourth digit of category 410 designates where the infarction occurred, such as the anterior or inferior heart wall (■ FIGURE 11-20).

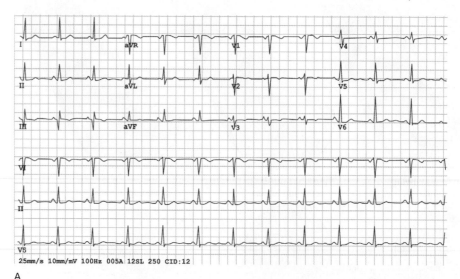

25mm/s 10mm/mV 100Hz 005A 12SL 250 CID:12

A

Figure 11-16 ■ Two electrocardiograms: (A) normal, and (B) showing a myocardial infarction.

Source: yaskii/Shutterstock.com.

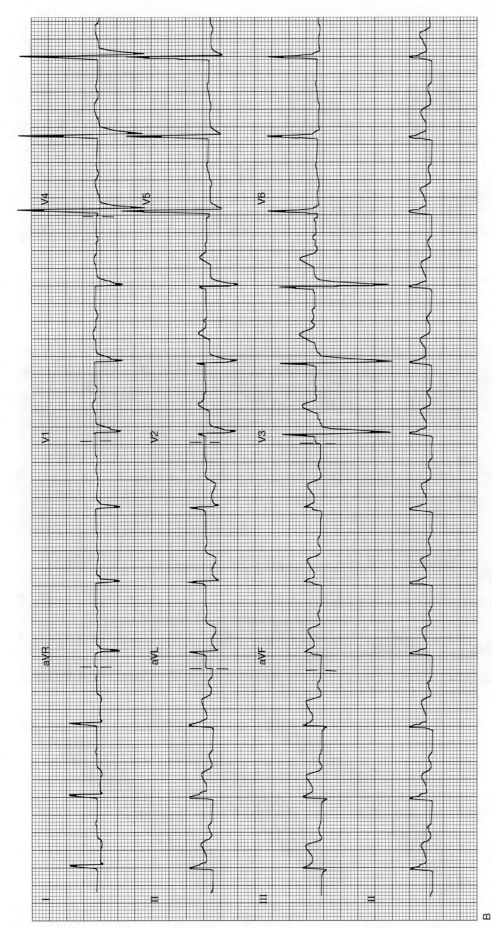

B

Figure 11-16 ■ (continued)

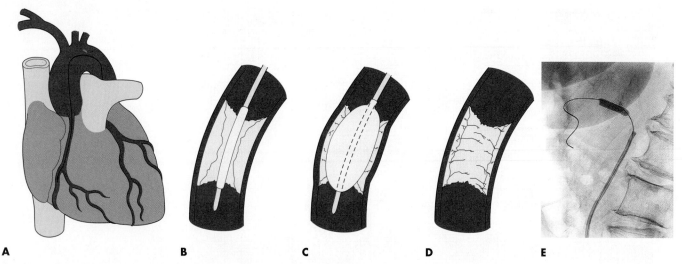

A   B   C   D   E

Figure 11-17 ■ Balloon angioplasty procedure: (A) The balloon catheter is threaded into the affected coronary artery. (B) The balloon is positioned across the area of obstruction. (C) The balloon is then inflated, flattening the plaque against the arterial wall. (D) X-ray angiogram of balloon catheter. (E) Balloon angioplasty.

Photo credit: Du Cane Medical Imaging Ltd. / Photo Researchers, Inc.

Figure 11-18 ■ A physician attaches a healthy artery to a diseased coronary artery during CABG surgery.

Photo credit: beerkoff/Shutterstock. com.

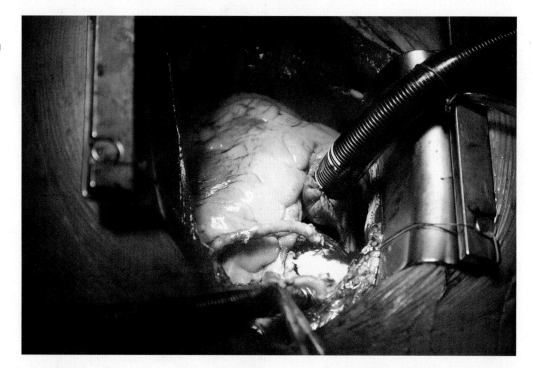

Figure 11-19 ■ Placement of a balloon expandable intracoronary stent: (A) The stainless steel stent is fitted over a balloon-tipped catheter. (B) The stent is positioned along the blockage and expanded. (C) The balloon is deflated and removed, leaving the stent in place.

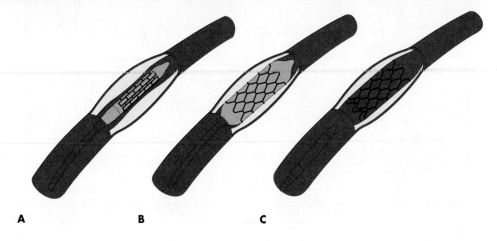

A   B   C

4th 410	**Acute myocardial infarction**

5th 410.0 Of anterolateral wall
[0-2]
> ST elevation myocardial infarction (STEMI) of anterolateral wall

5th 410.1 Of other anterior wall
[0-2]
> Infarction:
> anterior (wall) NOS (with contiguous portion of intraventricular septum)
> anteroapical (with contiguous portion of intraventricular septum)
> anteroseptal (with contiguous portion of intraventricular septum)
> ST elevation myocardial infarction (STEMI) of other anterior wall

5th 410.2 Of inferolateral wall
[0-2]
> ST elevation myocardial infarction (STEMI) of inferolateral wall

5th 410.3 Of inferoposterior wall
[0-2]
> ST elevation myocardial infarction (STEMI) of inferoposterior wall

5th 410.4 Of other inferior wall
[0-2]
> Infarction:
> diaphragmatic wall NOS (with contiguous portion of intraventricular septum)
> inferior (wall) NOS (with contiguous portion of intraventricular septum)
> ST elevation myocardial infarction (STEMI) of other inferior wall

5th 410.5 Of other lateral wall
[0-2]
> Infarction:
> apical-lateral
> basal-lateral
> high lateral
> posterolateral
> ST elevation myocardial infarction (STEMI) of other lateral wall

5th 410.6 True posterior wall infarction
[0-2]
> Infarction:
> posterobasal
> strictly posterior
> ST elevation myocardial infarction (STEMI) of true posterior wall

5th 410.7 Subendocardial infarction
[0-2]
> Non-ST elevation myocardial infarction (NSTEMI)
> Nontransmural infarction

5th 410.8 Of other specified sites
[0-2]
> Infarction of:
> atrium
> papillary muscle
> septum alone
> ST elevation myocardial infarction (STEMI) of other specified sites

5th 410.9 Unspecified site
[0-2]
> Acute myocardial infarction NOS
> Coronary occlusion NOS
> Myocardial infarction NOS

Notice that many subcategory code titles in Figure 11-20 include the terms ST elevation MI (STEMI) and non-ST elevation MI (NSTEMI).

Before you can practice coding AMIs, you need to understand what these terms mean. An EKG is divided into various parts, each of which represents a specific heart function. ST refers to the ST segment, the part of an EKG that shows atrial and ventricular contractions. Think of the EKG as a type of map that shows how the heart functions.

Physicians classify MIs two ways:

- STEMI—The most severe form of MI; the coronary artery is completely occluded, and the heart muscle is dying.

- NSTEMI—A milder form of MI; the coronary artery is partially occluded, and only part of the heart muscle is dying. NSTEMI does not show ST segment elevation on an EKG. Physicians can test for the presence of cardiac enzymes for patients with NSTEMI to determine whether the patient had an MI.

Be sure to refer to your medical dictionary and other medical resources to learn any terms that you do not know when coding AMIs. It is very important for you to understand the information that you code not only to ensure correct code assignment, but to also enable you to query the physician if you need clarification.

Category 410 also includes the following fifth-digit choices, based on the patient's episode of care:

0—episode of care unspecified

Use when the source document does not contain sufficient information for the assignment of fifth-digit 1 or 2.

1—initial episode of care

Use fifth-digit 1 to designate the first episode of care (regardless of facility site) for a newly diagnosed myocardial infarction. The fifth-digit 1 is assigned regardless of the number of times a patient may be transferred during the initial episode of care.

2—subsequent episode of care

Use fifth-digit 2 to designate an episode of care following the initial episode when the patient is admitted for further observation, evaluation or treatment for a myocardial infarction that has received initial treatment, but is still less than 8 weeks old.

Assign a fifth digit of 1 for *initial episode of care* the first time any provider treats the patient for a newly diagnosed MI, regardless of how many times a patient is transferred during the initial episode. Refer to the following example.

> **Example:** Mr. Mills, a 72-year-old, experiences shortness of breath and chest pain. He arrives by ambulance at Strongville Community Hospital. Dr. White, the emergency department physician, diagnoses him with an AMI. Dr. White determines that the patient needs intensive treatment that only a larger hospital can provide. An ambulance transfers Mr. Mills to Williton Medical Center, a large regional hospital.
>
> For each encounter at each hospital, the coder would assign a code from category **410** and add the fifth digit 1 *initial episode of care*. It was the first time the patient was treated at Strongville Community Hospital and the first time he was treated at Williton Medical Center for the same newly diagnosed MI, which means that each facility assigns a fifth digit for an initial episode of care.

Assign a fifth digit of 2 for a *subsequent episode of care* when the patient returns to the same provider for evaluation, treatment, and observation related to the MI that the provider treated during the initial episode. The patient must return within eight weeks of the initial episode of care in order to assign a fifth digit of 2. If a patient returns to the hospital within eight weeks for any procedure or examination related to the initial episode, assign a code from category 410, along with the fifth digit 2.

Refer to the following example to code an MI for a patient's encounter.

Example: Mr. Grant, a 55-year-old, arrives by ambulance at Williton Medical Center with complaints of chest and left arm pain, along with shortness of breath. His wife accompanies him and explains that he experienced symptoms while at home watching television. Dr. Daniels, the emergency physician, assesses Mr. Grant and diagnoses him with an AMI. The patient's EKG shows a STEMI of the **anterolateral** (front and side) wall, and Dr. Daniels admits him for treatment. It is the first time the patient has ever had an AMI.

anterolateral (an-tər-o-lat′ ər-əl)

    Use your ICD-9-CM manual to code this case. Search the Index for the main term *infarct*, subterm *myocardium*, and subterm *anterolateral*, and you will find code 410.0. (Notice that the word *acute* is a nonessential modifier for the subterm *myocardium*.) Refer to the note in the Index that shows fifth-digit choices listed under the subterm *myocardium*. As this is the patient's initial episode, assign the fifth digit of 1 for *initial episode*. Then cross-reference code **410.01** to the Tabular (■ FIGURE 11-21).

TAKE A BREAK

That was a lot of information to remember! Let's take a break and then practice assigning codes for MIs.

Exercise 11.5   MI

Instructions: Assign diagnosis codes to the following patient cases, using both the Index and Tabular.

1. Mrs. Spooner brings her husband Stanley, age 61, to Williton Medical Center's emergency department (ED) due to complaints of chest pain that arose when they were driving. Dr. Daniels orders lab tests and an EKG. He diagnoses Mr. Spooner with an ST elevation MI of the anterolateral wall.

   Code(s): _____

2. An ambulance transports Candace Kirkham, age 78, to Williton Medical Center's ED. She called the ambulance from her home after she experienced sudden chest pain and numbness in her left arm. Dr. Daniels diagnoses a STEMI of the inferolateral (below and side) wall. This is the first time anything like this has happened to Mrs. Kirkham.

   Code(s): _____

3. George Bohn, a 71-year-old, had a posterobasal (back and bottom wall of the heart) STEMI six weeks ago and is again experiencing chest pain. He calls Dr. Woods, his cardiologist, who asks Mr. Bohn to meet him at Williton Medical Center's ED. After conducting an examination and tests, Dr. Woods determines that Mr. Bohn was experiencing angina but has not had another MI.

   Code(s): _____

4. An ambulance rushes Jeffrey Wesley, age 59, to Williton Medical Center's ED for acute chest pain and shortness of breath that Mr. Wesley began to experience when he was shoveling snow. Dr. Daniels administers nitroglycerin and performs an EKG, which does not show ST elevation. Blood tests are also negative, so Dr. Woods rules out an MI. Dr. Woods monitors Mr. Wesley, and there are no further problems. Dr. Woods diagnoses the patient with angina pectoris and releases him with instructions to return to the ED if symptoms return.

   Code(s): _____

5. A helicopter transfers Mario Regan, age 52, from Valley Hospital's ED to Williton Medical Center due to low diastolic arterial pressure and a suspected infarction of the subendocardial, the area between the endocardium (the lining of the heart chambers) and the myocardium (the heart muscle). Valley does not have adequate resources to care for Mr. Regan's conditions. Dr. Woods, the cardiologist on call at Williton, confirms Valley's diagnoses and admits Mr. Regan for treatment. This is the patient's initial episode.

   Code(s): _____

6. Dr. Woods examines new patient Yvette Childress, age 58, due to her complaints of chest pain. An EKG and blood tests rule out an MI. Instead, Dr. Woods diagnoses Mrs. Childress with acute coronary occlusion and benign hypertension.

   Code(s): _____

Infarct, infarction

myocardium, myocardial (acute or with a stated duration of 8 weeks or less) (with hypertension) 410.9

> Note Use the following fifth-digit subclassification with category 410:
>
> | 0 | episode unspecified |
> | 1 | initial episode |
> | 2 | subsequent episode without recurrence |

with symptoms after 8 weeks from date of infarction 414.8
anterior (wall) (with contiguous portion of intraventricular septum) NEC 410.1
anteroapical (with contiguous portion of intraventricular septum) 410.1
anterolateral (wall) 410.0

4th **410** **Acute myocardial infarction**

Includes: cardiac infarction
    coronary (artery):
      embolism
      occlusion
      rupture
      thrombosis
    infarction of heart, myocardium, or ventricle
    rupture of heart, myocardium, or ventricle
    ST elevation (STEMI) and non-ST elevation (NSTEMI) myocardial infarction
    any condition classifiable to 414.1-414.9 specified as acute or with a stated
        duration of 8 weeks or less

The following fifth-digit subclassification is for use with category 410:
    0 episode of care unspecified
      Use when the source document does not contain sufficient information for
        the assignment of fifth-digit 1 or 2.
    1 initial episode of care
      Use fifth-digit 1 to designate the first episode of care (regardless of facility
        site) for a newly diagnosed myocardial infarction. The fifth-digit 1
        is assigned regardless of the number of times a patient may be
        transferred during the initial episode of care.
    2 subsequent episode of care
      Use fifth-digit 2 to designate an episode of care following the initial episode
        when the patient is admitted for further observation, evaluation or
        treatment for a myocardial infarction that has received initial
        treatment, but is still less than 8 weeks old.

    5th **410.0** **Of anterolateral wall**
    [0-2]

        ST elevation myocardial infarction (STEMI) of anterolateral wall

Figure 11-21 ■ Index entry for AMI initial episode with code 410.01 cross-referenced to the Tabular.

A LOOK AHEAD TO ICD-10-CM

Several guidelines for the circulatory system will change in ICD-10-CM. Here are the highlights:

- The Hypertension Table was removed from ICD-10-CM. In the Index, under the main term *hypertension*, malignant and benign have been added as nonessential modifiers.
- Guidelines for essential hypertension and hypertension NOS were removed.
- Guidelines for elevated blood pressure were removed.

- Several revisions exist for coding cerebrovascular accident.
- Guidelines were added for atherosclerotic coronary disease, angina, and subsequent AMI.
- There are specific I-10 guidelines for coding a *subsequent* MI within *four* weeks of an *initial* MI.

Instructions: Assign ICD-10-CM codes to the following cases that you have already coded in ICD-9-CM, using both the ICD-10-CM Index and the Tabular. (Refer to ICD-10-CM Official Guidelines for additional information; directions for accessing the guidelines are located in Appendix A of this text.).

1. Dr. Woods schedules established patient Eleanor Corn, age 72, for open heart surgery to correct mitral valve stenosis and aortic valve insufficiency. She also has benign hypertension, but it is stable so she is cleared for surgery. Code(s):_____

2. Established patient Penny Hendon, age 69, sees Dr. Woods for ongoing monitoring and management of left heart failure due to benign hypertension. Code(s):_____

3. Stephen Lawlor, an 81-year-old established patient, sees Dr. Woods, a cardiologist, for management of stage II CKD and benign hypertensive heart disease. He has combined chronic systolic and diastolic heart failure. Code(s):_____

4. Dr. Mason, a nephrologist, treats established patient Allan Liddell, age 43, for benign essential hypertension due to polycystic kidney disease, which he has had for most of his life. Code(s):_____

5. Mrs. Spooner brings her husband, Stanley, age 61, to Williton Medical Center's emergency department due to complaints of chest pain. Dr. Daniels, orders lab tests and an EKG. He diagnoses Mr. Spooner with a STEMI of the anterolateral wall. Code(s):_____

6. George Bohn, a 71-year-old, had a posterobasal (back and bottom) STEMI six weeks ago and is again experiencing chest pain. He calls Dr. Woods, his cardiologist, who asks Mr. Bohn to meet him at Williton Medical Center's ED. After examination and tests, Dr. Woods determines that Mr. Bohn was experiencing angina but has not had another MI. Code(s):_____

CHAPTER REVIEW

Multiple Choice

Instructions: Circle one best answer to complete each statement.

1. Coronary artery disease is
   a. a general description for any disorder that affects the heart.
   b. a general description for a disorder that affects the heart and related blood vessels.
   c. when plaque forms and clogs an artery, restricting blood flow.
   d. the force of blood pumped through the arteries.

2. Which of the following situations does *not* require two codes?
   a. When a patient has a heart condition that is due to hypertension
   b. When a patient has heart failure that is due to hypertension
   c. When the physician documents heart disease and hypertension
   d. When a patient has hypertension and CKD Stage II

3. You should presume a causal relationship between hypertension and
   a. heart disease.
   b. MI.
   c. ischemia.
   d. CKD.

4. When a patient has *both* hypertensive CKD and hypertensive heart disease, you can assign codes from each of the following categories, *except*
   a. 404—Hypertensive heart and chronic kidney disease.
   b. 585—Chronic kidney disease.
   c. 428—Congestive heart failure.
   d. 405—Secondary hypertension.

5. When a patient has untreated hypertension or the hypertension is not responding to current treatment, the condition is called _____ hypertension.
   a. uncontrolled
   b. controlled
   c. malignant
   d. essential

6. When a physician documents transient hypertension, you should assign a code for
   a. benign hypertension.
   b. elevated blood pressure.
   c. essential hypertension.
   d. hypertensive retinopathy.

7. The most common cause of an MI is
   a. chest and arm pain, shortness of breath, weakness, dizziness, and dyspnea.
   b. administering oxygen, aspirin, and nitroglycerin.
   c. when plaque and/or a blood clot forms in a coronary artery and occludes blood flow.
   d. necrosis of heart muscle.

8. Physicians classify MIs two ways:
   a. STEMI and NSTEMI.
   b. STEMI and NOSTEMI.
   c. NSTEMI and MI.
   d. STEMMI and NSTEMMI.

9. When a patient is admitted for further observation, evaluation, or treatment related to an MI that the physician treated fewer than eight weeks before, it is called a(n) _____ episode of care.
   a. initial
   b. subsequent
   c. old
   d. unspecified

10. Circulatory system disorders include all of the following *except*
    a. rheumatic fever.
    b. diseases of pulmonary circulation.
    c. diseases of veins and lymphatics.
    d. CKD.

Coding Assignments

Instructions: Assign ICD-9-CM code(s) to the following cases, referencing both the Index and Tabular.

1. Tina Burdette, a 48-year-old established patient, sees Dr. Woods, a cardiologist, for management of atherosclerosis and benign hypertension.

   Code(s): _____

2. Dr. Woods diagnoses Stephen Raphael, age 58, with acute on chronic systolic heart failure due to hypertension.

   Code(s): _____

3. Rosie Groom, age 68, sees Dr. Woods for worsening symptoms of increased dyspnea and peripheral edema. Dr. Woods diagnoses Mrs. Groom with chronic cor pulmonale (enlarged right ventricle of the heart). He adjusts her diuretic and prescribes a bronchodilator to help her breathe. He schedules the patient for a return visit in two weeks and states that if she is not better soon, she will have to consider supplemental oxygen.

   Code(s): _____

4. Edward Shears, age 65, arrives at Williton Medical Center via ambulance. He has dyspnea, blurred vision, and a severe headache. His blood pressure is 200/120. Dr. Woods, a cardiologist working in the ED, diagnoses Mr. Shears with malignant hypertension and immediately administers an intravenous vasodilator (medication that widens blood vessels). Mr. Shear's condition stabilizes, and Dr. Woods admits him for monitoring.

   Code(s): _____

5. Dr. Woods treats Anita Norton, a 70-year-old established patient, at Williton for hypertensive acute cerebrovascular insufficiency (lack of blood to the brain). Clinicians are treating her condition and administering further tests.

   Code(s): _____

6. Jesse Garibay, age 61, reports to the Williton Medical Center dialysis center to receive hemodialysis for hypertensive CKD, end-stage. The hypertension is benign.

   Code(s): _____

7. Dr. Mason, a nephrologist, diagnoses Michael Hummel, age 64, with left-side CHF due to hypertensive stage V CKD.

   Code(s): _____

8. Dr. Woods treats Shawn Navarrete, age 35, for uncontrolled hypertension due to Cushing's disease.

   Code(s): _____

9. Dr. Daniels, an ED physician, treats Carl Eyre, age 56, in Williton Medical Center's ED for recurrent chest pain and dyspnea (shortness of breath), following a lateral wall STEMI two weeks ago.

   Code(s): _____

10. Dr. Woods diagnoses Nathan Rollins, a 45-year-old, with benign hypertension and anterolateral STEMI. Dr. Woods admits Mr. Rollins to the coronary care unit at Williton Medical Center for stabilization and treatment.

    Code(s): _____

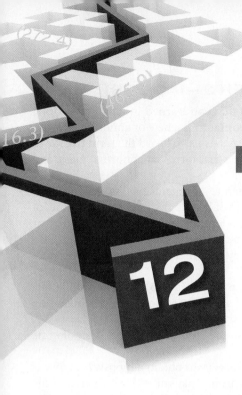

Neoplasms

Learning Objectives

After completing this chapter, you should be able to

- Spell and define the key terminology in this chapter.
- Identify how to use the Neoplasm Table to find various types of neoplasms.
- Define morphology codes and explain how to assign them.
- Discuss when you should assign V codes with neoplasm codes.
- Define malignant neoplasm, identify types of malignant neoplasms, and describe how to code them.
- Explain cancer staging.
- Define a benign neoplasm, and describe how to code a benign neoplasm.
- Discuss neoplasms of uncertain behavior or unspecified.
- Describe which additional coding guidelines you should reference for neoplasm coding.

Key Terms

benign neoplasm
malignant Ca in situ
malignant neoplasm
malignant primary
malignant secondary

neoplasm
tumor
Tumor, Nodes, Metastasis (TNM) classification system
uncertain behavior
unspecified (whether malignant or benign)

INTRODUCTION

Do you remember in Chapter 3 when you reviewed the Neoplasm Table in the Index to find neoplasm codes for specific body sites? Coding neoplasms can often be challenging, especially if the neoplasm has spread to different body sites. If a patient has neoplasms of multiple sites, then you need to determine which neoplasm(s) the physician treated during the encounter so that you code conditions in the correct order. In this chapter, we will review different types of neoplasms, and you will then practice coding them. You already have an advantage because you learned medical terms involving neoplasms and learned how to use the Neoplasm Table in Chapter 3. So let's continue on your journey and enter the world of neoplasms, expanding your skills and further enhancing your coding knowledge!

"Life doesn't require that we be the best, only that we try our best."
—H. JACKSON BROWN, JR.

ICD-9-CM codes in this chapter are from the ICD-9-CM 2012 code set from the Department of Health and Human Services, Centers for Disease Control and Prevention.
ICD-10-CM codes in this chapter are from the ICD-10-CM 2012 Draft code set from the Department of Health and Human Services, Centers for Disease Control and Prevention.

NEOPLASMS (ICD-9-CM CHAPTER 2—140–239)

Let's begin with a brief review of some of the terms that you learned in Chapter 3, along with new terms that you will use in this chapter. A **neoplasm** is a new or abnormal growth, such as a cancerous growth or a benign lesion. You may have also heard the term **tumor** to describe a neoplasm. A tumor is a new growth of tissue that forms an abnormal mass, and it can also involve swelling.

morphology (mor-fol′ə-je)

histology (hĭs-tŏl′ ō-jē)

Morphology is the study of the form and structure of organisms, and **histology** is the study of the structure of microscopic tissue. Think of histology as the *type*, or name, of the neoplasm. The histology might be carcinoma, adenoma, glioblastoma, myoma, or hemangioma—all of these are descriptions of the type of neoplasm the patient has. ICD-9-CM classifies neoplasms by their histology, the body site where the neoplasm is located, and their behavior, such as malignant or benign.

oncology (ŏng-kŏl′ ō-jē)

oncologist (ŏng-kŏl′ ō-jist)

pathologist (pă-thŏl′ ō-jist)

Oncology literally means the study of (-ology) a tumor (onc/o). An **oncologist** is a physician who specializes in the diagnosis, treatment, and prevention of tumors, including malignant neoplasms. *Pathology* literally means the study of (-ology) path/o (disease). A **pathologist** is a physician who studies cells, tissues, and disease behaviors. Pathologists often work in hospital pathology departments.

You may have heard of a physician performing surgery to obtain a biopsy. A biopsy is when a surgeon removes a specimen of tissue or cells from a patient and can then send the specimen to a pathologist for testing (▪ FIGURE 12-1). The pathologist determines the histology (type) and behavior of the specimen (malignant or benign) and reports the findings to the surgeon. When you code neoplasms, you should assign codes based on the *pathology report* because it will list the definitive diagnosis. You will learn how to code pathology services in Chapter 33.

ICD-9-CM categorizes neoplasms as malignant, benign, uncertain behavior, or unspecified behavior. ICD-9-CM also lists neoplasms by body sites. Refer to ▪ TABLE 12-1 to review neoplasm categories from Chapter 2 of the Tabular List.

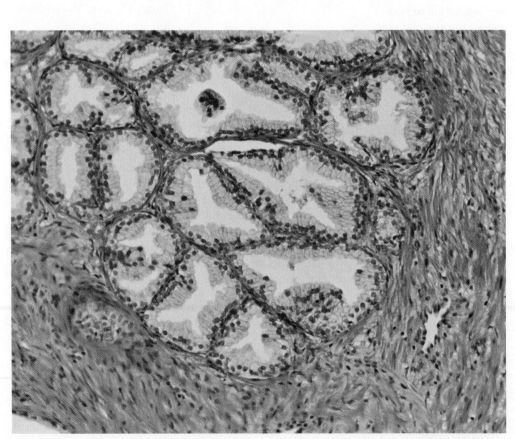

Figure 12-1 ▪ Prostate tissue the physician removed during surgery and sent to pathology.

Photo credit: Custom Medical Stock Photo.

■ TABLE 12-1 ICD-9-CM CHAPTER 2 NEOPLASM CATEGORIES (140–239)

Category	Title
140–149	Malignant Neoplasm of Lip, Oral Cavity, and Pharynx
150–159	Malignant Neoplasm of Digestive Organs and **Peritoneum**
160–165	Malignant Neoplasm of Respiratory and **Intrathoracic** Organs
170–176	Malignant Neoplasm of Bone, Connective Tissue, Skin, and Breast
179–189	Malignant Neoplasm of Genitourinary Organs
190–199	Malignant Neoplasm of Other and Unspecified Sites
200–208	Malignant Neoplasm of Lymphatic and **Hematopoietic** Tissue
209	**Neuroendocrine** Tumors
210–229	Benign Neoplasms
230–234	Carcinoma **in Situ**
235–238	Neoplasms of Uncertain Behavior
239	Neoplasms of Unspecified Nature

peritoneum (per ĭ-to-ne ′əm)—the membrane lining the walls of the abdominal and pelvic cavities

intrathoracic (in-trə-thə-ras′ik)—pertaining to the area within the thorax (chest cavity)

hematopoietic (hem-ə-to-poi-et′ik)—pertaining to the formation and development of blood cells

neuroendocrine (noor-o-en′do-krin)—interactions between the nervous and endocrine systems

in situ (ĭn sī′ too)

metastasis (mě-tăs′ tă-sis)

contiguous (kən-tig′u-əs)

adjunct (ad′junkt)

nevus (ne′vəs)

nevi (nē′ vī)

You will learn many different coding guidelines for neoplasms, which are from the Official Guidelines for Coding and Reporting. It is very helpful to understand neoplasm terminology before reviewing coding guidelines and assigning neoplasm codes. Review ■ TABLE 12-2 for a list of common terms related to neoplasms, along with their definitions.

Neoplasms can occur anywhere on or in the body. When you code neoplasms, search for the histologic type of neoplasm (leukemia, lymphoma, glioblastoma) in the Index, rather than

■ TABLE 12-2 COMMON NEOPLASM TERMS

Term	Definition
Malignant neoplasm, or malignancy	Life-threatening neoplasm or tumor, also called cancer or carcinoma (CA, Ca). Cancer can spread throughout the body.
Malignant primary	Life-threatening neoplasm or tumor that has spread to surrounding tissues within the same organ.
Malignant secondary	Life-threatening neoplasm or tumor that spread from the primary site to a secondary site.
Malignant Ca in situ	Cancer confined to the tissue layer where it originated and *has not spread* to surrounding tissues within the same organ; can become life-threatening; in situ is also called • Intraepithelial • Noninfiltrating • Noninvasive
Benign	Neoplasm that is not life-threatening and does not spread. Benign neoplasms can pose serious health risks if they interfere with normal body functions.
Uncertain behavior	Neoplasm where the pathology report does not indicate whether the neoplasm is benign or malignant, usually due to mixed cell types.
Unspecified (whether malignant or benign)	Neoplasm for which the physician does not document the behavior.
Metastasis, metastases, metastasized, metastatic (abbreviated *mets*)	Cancer that has spread to other organs or structures from its original site.
Contiguous site	Neoplasms in side-by-side sites, such as adjacent organs or structures.
Adjunct therapy	Therapy, in addition to surgery, to treat cancer, such as chemotherapy, radiotherapy, and immunotherapy.
Nevus (plural: nevi)	A lesion containing nevus cells (also called melanocytes), cells that form pigment of the skin, hair, and eyes. Nevi are also called moles.

going directly to the Neoplasm Table to assign codes. At the beginning of the Neoplasms section in Chapter 2 of the Tabular, you will find specific guidelines and definitions to help you code neoplasms. Be sure to review the guidelines before you assign codes from the chapter.

In addition, with some of the categories in Chapter 2, you have to assign a fifth digit to identify specific body sites or note whether the patient's cancer is *in remission* or *in relapse*. In remission is when a patient's symptoms become less severe and the condition improves. In relapse is when a patient's illness improves but then worsens again. Pay close attention to fifth digits to ensure correct code assignment.

TAKE A BREAK

Let's take a break and then review neoplasm terms.

Exercise 12.1 **Neoplasms**

Instructions: Fill in each blank with the best answer, choosing from the list of words and terms provided.

1. The _____ site is the first site where a malignant neoplasm is found and has invaded the tissues within the organ where it started.

2. A _____ neoplasm is not life threatening and does not spread.

3. When the physician does not document the behavior of the neoplasm, it is _____.

4. Cancer that has spread to other organs and structures from the primary site is called _____.

5. The site where metastasis is found is called the _____ site.

6. When the pathology report does not indicate whether the neoplasm's behavior is benign or malignant, it is _____.

7. A _____ is also called a mole.

8. Cancer in which malignant cells are confined to the tissue layer where they originated and have not spread to surrounding tissues within the same organ is called _____.

9. Sites where neoplasms are side-by-side in adjacent organs or structures are called _____ sites.

10. _____ therapy is cancer treatment that is provided in addition to surgery.

adjunct	malignant	oncology	screening
benign	metastasis	pathology	uncertain
contiguous	mixed	primary	unspecified
in situ	nevus	secondary	

NEOPLASM TABLE

Remember from Chapter 3 of this text that you can find the Neoplasm Table under the main term *neoplasm*. The Neoplasm Table uses subterms to show the location of the neoplasm. There are six columns to identify different neoplasm behaviors (■ FIGURE 12-2).

Chapter 2 of the Tabular List contains all malignant neoplasm codes and numerous benign neoplasm codes. Some benign neoplasm codes are located in other chapters of ICD-9-CM. When you are coding neoplasms, first search the Index for the *histologic type* of neoplasm (carcinoma, leukemia, glioblastoma). The histologic type will provide you with a neoplasm code to cross-reference, or it will instruct you to go to the Neoplasm Table to find the code, typically indicating if the neoplasm is malignant or benign, or you will see both the code and an instruction to go to the Neoplasm Table. For example, turn to the Index entry "adenoma" in your ICD-9-CM manual. Notice that "adenoma" has the instruction to *see also Neoplasm, by site, benign*. There are many subterms under "adenoma" for specific body sites, which list neoplasm codes. If the body site you are searching for is not listed as a subterm under "adenoma," then you can go to the Neoplasm Table, search for the body site as a subterm, and go to the *Benign* column to find the code. The Index entry instruction listed "benign" for "adenoma."

The only time that you should search for a code in the Neoplasm Table first, rather than searching for the histology first, is when the physician *does not* document the histologic type of the neoplasm but does document that the patient has a neoplasm and documents the location.

Figure 12-2 ■ Neoplasm Table.

Neoplasm, neoplastic	Malignant Primary	Malignant Secondary	Malignant Ca in situ	Benign	Uncertain Behavior	unspecified
Neoplasm, neoplastic	199.1	199.1	234.9	229.9	238.9	239.9

Notes - 1. The list below gives the code numbers for neoplasms by anatomical site. For each site, there are six possible code numbers according to whether the neoplasm in question is malignant, benign, in situ, of uncertain behavior, or of unspecified nature. The description of the neoplasm will often indicate which of the six columns is appropriate; e.g., malignant melanoma of skin, benign fibroadenoma of breast, carcinoma in situ of cervix uteri.

Where such descriptors are not present, the remainder of the Index should be consulted where guidance is given to the appropriate column for each morphological (histological) variety listed; e.g., Mesonephroma-see Neoplasm, malignant; Embryoma-see also Neoplasm, uncertain behavior; Disease, Bowen's-see Neoplasm, skin, in situ. However, the guidance in the Index can be overridden if one of the descriptors mentioned above is present; e.g., malignant adenoma of colon is coded to 153.9 and not to 211.3 as the adjective "malignant" overrides the Index entry "Adenoma-see also Neoplasm, benign."

2. Sites marked with the sign * (e.g., face NEC*) should be classified to malignant neoplasm of skin of these sites if the variety of neoplasm is a squamous cell carcinoma or an epidermoid carcinoma and to benign neoplasm of skin of these sites if the variety of neoplasm is a papilloma (any type).

	Malignant Primary	Malignant Secondary	Malignant Ca in situ	Benign	Uncertain Behavior	unspecified
abdomen, abdominal	195.2	198.89	234.8	229.8	238.8	239.89
cavity	195.2	198.89	234.8	229.8	238.8	239.89
organ	195.2	198.89	234.8	229.8	238.8	239.89
viscera	195.2	198.89	234.8	229.8	238.8	239.89
wall	173.5	198.2	232.5	216.5	238.2	239.2
connective tissue	171.5	198.89	-	215.5	238.1	239.2
abdominopelvic	195.8	198.89	234.8	229.8	238.8	239.89
accessory sinus- see Neoplasm, sinus						
acoustic nerve	192.0	198.4	-	225.1	237.9	239.7

When you find the histologic type, you will notice that the Index also lists a morphology code, or M code, for the neoplasm. Recall from Chapter 3 that morphology codes describe the morphology of a neoplasm (form and structure). You will learn more about coding morphology codes in the next section.

Use your ICD-9-CM manual to code the following two examples for neoplasm encounters:

Example 1: Mr. Jones, a 42-year-old established patient, has an encounter at Williton Medical Center with Dr. Simmons, an oncologist. The patient's pathology report from a biopsy lists a diagnosis of primary liver cell carcinoma. Dr. Simmons and the patient discuss treatment options.

Carcinoma is the *histologic type* of the neoplasm. You already learned that carcinoma means cancer, and it is a malignant neoplasm. Search the Index for the main term *carcinoma* and subterm *liver cell* (■ Figure 12-3).

> **Carcinoma** (M8010/3) - see also Neoplasm, by site, malignant
>
> liver cell (M8170/3) 155.0

Figure 12-3 ■ Index entry for primary liver cell carcinoma.

The code listed is 155.0. Did you read the note to *see also, Neoplasm, by site, malignant*? This means that you can also go to the Neoplasm Table and search for the subterm *liver* and subterm *primary*, which will take you to the same code, 155.0. Then you can cross-reference code 155.0 to the Tabular for final code assignment (■ FIGURE 12-4).

Figure 12-4 ■ Index entry from the Neoplasm Table for primary liver cell carcinoma with code 155.0 cross-referenced to the Tabular.

	Malignant Primary	Malignant Secondary	Malignant Ca in situ	Benign	Uncertain Behavior	unspecified
Neoplasm, neoplastic	**199.1**	**199.1**	**234.9**	**229.9**	**238.9**	**239.9**
liver	155.2	197.7	230.8	211.5	235.3	239.0
primary	155.0	-	-	-	-	-

> **4th** **155 Malignant neoplasm of liver and intrahepatic bile ducts**

> **155.0 Liver, primary**
>   Carcinoma:
>   liver, specified as primary
>   hepatocellular
>   liver cell
>   Hepatoblastoma

adenocarcinoma
(ad-ə-no-kahr-sĭ-no′mə)

Example 2: Mrs. Rodriguez, a 62-year-old established patient, sees Dr. Simmons at Williton Medical Center to discuss test results from a biopsy. Her pathology report lists her diagnosis as primary **adenocarcinoma** (found in glandular tissue lining the internal organs) of the sigmoid colon (■ FIGURE 12-5). Dr. Simmons and the patient discuss surgical options and palliative (to ease pain) treatment.

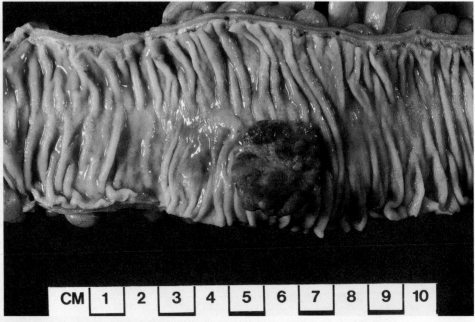

Figure 12-5 ■ Adenocarcinoma in the colon. *Photo credit:* © Medical-on-Line/Alamy.

Adenocarcinoma is the histologic type of neoplasm. You already know that adenocarcinoma is malignant because it has the word *carcinoma* in it. Search the Index for the main term *adenocarcinoma*. If you search for *colon* as the subterm, then you will not find an entry. The Index entry for *adenocarcinoma* does not provide a neoplasm code, only an M code (morphology code), and it instructs you to *see also neoplasm by site, malignant* (■ FIGURE 12-6).

Because there is no code for adenocarcinoma of the colon, you must go to the Neoplasm Table. Search the Index for the main term *neoplasm*, subterm *colon* (■ FIGURE 12-7).

Notice that *sigmoid* is not listed as a subterm under *colon*. However, there is a note to *see also Neoplasm, intestine, large*, and you can then find the code by referencing additional subterms (■ FIGURE 12-8).

Adenocarcinoma (M8140/3) - see also Neoplasm, by site, malignant

Figure 12-6 ■ Index entry for adenocarcinoma.

	Malignant Primary	Malignant Secondary	Malignant Ca in situ	Benign	Uncertain Behavior	unspecified
Neoplasm, neoplastic	**199.1**	**199.1**	**234.9**	**229.9**	**238.9**	**239.9**
colon - see also Neoplasm, intestine,						
large	153.9	197.5	230.3	211.3	235.2	239.0
with rectum	154.0	197.5	230.4	211.4	235.2	239.0

Figure 12-7 ■ Index entry in the Neoplasm Table for neoplasm of the colon.

	Malignant Primary	Malignant Secondary	Malignant Ca in situ	Benign	Uncertain Behavior	unspecified
Neoplasm, neoplastic	**199.1**	**199.1**	**234.9**	**229.9**	**238.9**	**239.9**
intestine, intestinal	159.0	197.8	230.7	211.9	235.2	239.0
large	153.9	197.5	230.3	211.3	235.2	239.0
appendix	153.5	197.5	230.3	211.3	235.2	239.0
caput coli	153.4	197.5	230.3	211.3	235.2	239.0
cecum	153.4	197.5	230.3	211.3	235.2	239.0
colon	153.9	197.5	230.3	211.3	235.2	239.0
and rectum	154.0	197.5	230.4	211.4	235.2	239.0
ascending	153.6	197.5	230.3	211.3	235.2	239.0
caput	153.4	197.5	230.3	211.3	235.2	239.0
contiguous sites	153.8	—	—	—	—	—
descending	153.2	197.5	230.3	211.3	235.2	239.0
distal	153.2	197.5	230.3	211.3	235.2	239.0
left	153.2	197.5	230.3	211.3	235.2	239.0
pelvic	153.3	197.5	230.3	211.3	235.2	239.0
right	153.6	197.5	230.3	211.3	235.2	239.0
sigmoid (flexure)	153.3	197.5	230.3	211.3	235.2	239.0
transverse	153.1	197.5	230.3	211.3	235.2	239.0

Figure 12-8 ■ Index entry in the Neoplasm Table for adenocarcinoma of the sigmoid colon.

The code to cross-reference to the Tabular is 153.3, found under the column for Malignant, Primary. It is important to remember that if the medical documentation does not state if a malignant neoplasm is primary, secondary, or in situ, always code it as primary. Now cross-reference code 153.3 to the Tabular (■ Figure 12-9).

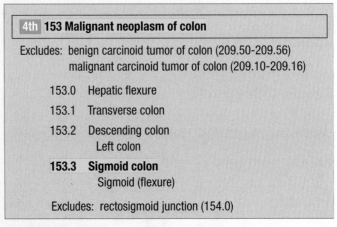

Figure 12-9 ■ Code 153.3 cross-referenced to the Tabular for adenocarcinoma of the sigmoid colon.

You learned in these two examples that when coding a neoplasm, you should search for the histologic type of the neoplasm, unless the physician does not document it. With the histologic type, ICD-9-CM will list a morphology code, a neoplasm code, and/or direct you to the Neoplasm Table. Be extremely careful when assigning neoplasm codes because it is very easy to become confused in the Neoplasm Table when trying to follow subterms for specific body sites. Do not go directly to the Neoplasm Table to code neoplasms. It is better to go to the Index first because the entry in the Index for the histologic type could provide you with the code to cross-reference or give you additional valuable information that will affect your final code assignment.

TAKE A BREAK

Good job! Let's take a break and then practice assigning neoplasm codes.

Exercise 12.2 Neoplasm Table

Instructions: Assign neoplasm codes to the following patient encounters using both the Index and Tabular. Search first for the histologic type of neoplasm in the Index before you refer to the Neoplasm Table.

1. Dr. Simmons, an oncologist, sees Aaron Beatty, age 38, who is experiencing a relapse of hemoblastic leukemia (neoplastic disorder of bone marrow).

   Code(s): _____

2. Jeff Hollingsworth, age 61, meets with Dr. Simmons to review the results of a biopsy, which Dr. Simmons performed because Mr. Hollingsworth had hemorrhaging. Dr. Simmons says that the biopsy is positive for adenocarcinoma in situ in the sigmoid colon. Because Dr. Simmons found the adenocarcinoma early, the prognosis is good.

   Code(s): _____

3. Dr. Simmons diagnoses Vicki Cosgrove, age 78, with primary osteosarcoma (malignant bone tumor) of the hip.

   Code(s): _____

4. Dr. Simmons removes lesions from Mark Gilliard's back, and the pathology report reveals that the lesions are melanoma (form of skin cancer).

   Code(s): _____

TAKE A BREAK *continued*

5. Justin Brinker, age 65, sees Dr. Ferguson, a dermatologist (physician who treats skin disorders), for removal of basal cell adenoma (found in the deepest layers of the epithelium or skin) on his left cheek. Dr. Ferguson asks him to report back in six months for a recheck to ensure that there is no further evidence of the adenoma.

Code(s): _____

6. Carla Hubbell, a 79-year-old, recently had a hysterectomy (removal of the uterus) due to post-menopausal bleeding. A frozen section during surgery (biopsy) shows clear cell adenocarcinoma of the uterus. She meets with Dr, Simmons, who recommends that she begin radiotherapy in a few weeks to treat the adenocarcinoma.

Code(s): _____

MORPHOLOGY CODES

Recall from Chapter 3 that you can also assign a morphology code, or M code, for a neoplasm to show the *type* of cancer that a patient has (like lymphoma, carcinoma, or glioblastoma), along with its behavior (such as malignant, benign, or uncertain). Appendix A of ICD-9-CM, Morphology of Neoplasms, contains morphology codes, which specify types of neoplasms (histologic) and their behaviors.

Providers may use morphology codes to track the number and types of neoplasms that patients have, along with types of treatment. Providers also report morphology codes to cancer registries, organizations that gather and analyze information and statistics about cancer. Information from cancer registries is critical for developing effective cancer prevention and control programs toward specific geographic areas or populations. Cancer registry information is also important for identifying populations who might benefit from enhanced cancer screening efforts and for developing and implementing long-term strategies to ensure that all people have access to adequate diagnostic and treatment services.

Morphology codes begin with the letter M, followed by four numbers that identify the histological type of neoplasm, a slash (/), and then the fifth digit, which indicates the neoplasm's behavior. Review examples of morphology codes in ■ Figure 12-10, along with the descriptions and meanings of their fifth-digit behaviors in ■ Table 12-3.

Whenever you search the Index for the histologic type of a neoplasm, you will find an M code. Cross-reference the M code to Appendix A in the ICD-9-CM manual for final code assignment.

It is important to understand when to assign a neoplasm code and when to assign a morphology code for the neoplasm. You will *always* assign a neoplasm code. You will only assign an M code if the provider for whom you work requires it. Sequence M codes as *additional* codes after the neoplasm code. M codes have no bearing on insurance reimbursement because insurances pay claims based on neoplasm codes. Refer to the following example to assign *both* a morphology code and a neoplasm code for a patient's encounter.

| M912-M916..Blood vessel tumors |
| M9120/0   Hemangioma NOS |
| M9120/3   Hemangiosarcoma |
| M9121/0   Cavernous hemangioma |
| M9122/0   Venous hemangioma |
| M9123/0   Racemose hemangioma |

Figure 12-10 ■ Examples of morphology codes from Appendix A in the ICD-9-CM.

■ TABLE 12-3 **DESCRIPTIONS OF FIFTH-DIGIT BEHAVIORS FOR MORPHOLOGY CODES**

Fifth Digit	Description
/0	Benign
/1	Uncertain whether benign or malignant Borderline malignancy
/2	Carcinoma in situ, also called • Intraepithelial • Noninfiltrating • Noninvasive
/3	Malignant, primary site
/6	Malignant, metastatic (spread to) site Secondary site
/9	Malignant, uncertain whether primary or metastatic site

Example: Lacey Powell, a 9-year-old established patient at Jordan-Fields Cancer Center, suffers from acute leukemia (cancer of white blood cells). She and her mother see Dr. Wallace, an oncologist, to review the progress of her chemotherapy treatments.

The cancer center tracks statistics on patients, so for this case, you will need to assign a neoplasm code and a morphology code. To find the neoplasm code, search the Index for the histologic type, *leukemia* and subterm *acute*, and you will find code 208.0. Review the note listed under the main term *leukemia* instructing you to assign a fifth digit. There is no mention of remission or relapse, so choose fifth digit 0 *without mention of having achieved remission, failed remission.* Then cross-reference code 208.00 to the Tabular (■ FIGURE 12-11).

You will also find the morphology code in the Index under the main term *leukemia* (FIGURE 12-11). Then cross-reference code M9800/3 to Appendix A in ICD-9-CM (■ FIGURE 12-12).

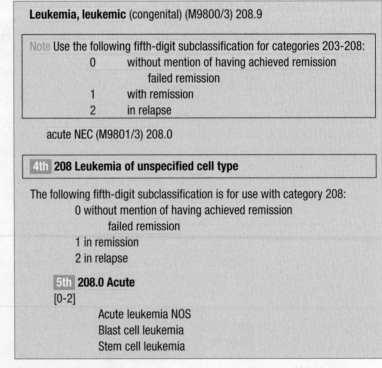

Leukemia, leukemic (congenital) (M9800/3) 208.9

Note Use the following fifth-digit subclassification for categories 203–208:
    0   without mention of having achieved remission
            failed remission
    1   with remission
    2   in relapse

acute NEC (M9801/3) 208.0

4th **208 Leukemia of unspecified cell type**

The following fifth-digit subclassification is for use with category 208:
    0 without mention of having achieved remission
       failed remission
    1 in remission
    2 in relapse

5th **208.0 Acute**
[0-2]
        Acute leukemia NOS
        Blast cell leukemia
        Stem cell leukemia

Figure 12-11 ■ Index entry for acute leukemia with code 208.00 cross-referenced to the Tabular.

Appendix A:

The morphology code numbers consist of five digits; the first four identify the histological type of the neoplasm and the fifth indicates its behavior. The one-digit behavior code is as follows:

/0	Benign
/1	Uncertain whether benign or malignant
	Borderline malignancy
/2	Carcinoma in situ
	Intraepithelial
	Noninfiltrating
	Noninvasive
/3	Malignant, primary site
/6	Malignant, metastatic site
	Secondary site
/9	Malignant, uncertain whether primary or metastatic site

M980 Leukemias NOS

M9800/3	Leukemia NOS
M9801/3	Acute leukemia NOS
M9802/3	Subacute leukemia NOS
M9803/3	Chronic leukemia NOS
M9804/3	Aleukemic leukemia NOS

Figure 12-12 ■ Morphology code M9800/3 cross-referenced to Appendix A in the ICD-9-CM.

Note that you only had one choice for the M code for leukemia, M9800/3. The last digit is a 3 because leukemia is primary, since it is a systemic illness that spreads throughout the body. Code assignments for this example are 208.00 (acute leukemia) and M9800/3 (morphology code for acute leukemia).

TAKE A BREAK

Good work! Let's take a break and then practice assigning morphology codes.

Exercise 12.3   **Morphology Codes**

Instructions: Assign morphology codes only to the following patient encounters, using both the Index and cross-referencing to Appendix A in ICD-9-CM. You will have more practice assigning morphology codes later, along with corresponding neoplasm codes .

1. Dr. Simmons, an oncologist, diagnoses established patient Nora Crotty, age 48, with malignant primary adenocarcinoma of the upper outer quadrant of the right breast.

   Code(s): _____

2. Daniel Rocha, age 50, sees Dr. Simmons for treatment of metastatic malignant adenocarcinoma to the pelvic lymph nodes.

   Code(s): _____

3. Dr. Simmons sees Charles Sprinkle, age 72, for a growth in his bronchus. The pathology report reveals benign adenoma.

   Code(s): _____

4. Dr. Simmons diagnoses new patient Joe Deaton, age 24, with malignant giant cell leukemia.

   Code(s): _____

5. New patient Nellie Darby, age 35, sees Dr. Hoffman for a lump on the back of her neck. Dr. Hoffman diagnoses it as a benign lipoma (tumor made of fat cells) and tells her that she does not need to worry.

   Code(s): _____

6. Dr. Simmons sees new patient, Jacquelyn Benz, age 57, for treatment of intraductal papillary adenocarcinoma (breast cancer of the milk ducts) in situ in the left breast.

   Code(s): _____

POINTERS FROM THE PROS: Interview with a Medical Office Administration Graduate

Stacey Super, CPC-A, holds an Associate in Science degree in Medical Office Administration. During her last quarter in school, she worked as an intern for a cancer center, where she coded, billed, scheduled appointments, and took patients' vital signs. Ms. Super recently passed the certification examination for Certified Professional Coder (CPC) through the American Academy of Professional Coders. She is considered a coding apprentice until she has gained additional coding work experience.

Was there anything that surprised you about your internship?

I worked in the cancer center and expected it to be sad and hard to work there with patients, but it wasn't.

How did your coding education prepare you for your internship?

It helped me be trusted with more responsibility knowing I had the background and showed my intelligence when (I found) a few mistakes made by the physicians.

What advice can you give to coding students when they start working in the healthcare field?

Review what you learned before starting. Always tab your coding book.

What advice can you give to new coders about working with physicians?

Don't be scared of the physician. They make errors, and you need to ask questions to code properly.

(Used by permission of Stacey Super.)

V CODES FOR NEOPLASMS

Remember from Chapter 7 that you can assign V codes from category V10 to show personal history of a malignant neoplasm *only when* the neoplasm is gone, and there is no further treatment for it. For example, a patient had a left breast mastectomy to treat breast cancer, and there is no further evidence of cancer. This patient has a *personal history* of a malignant neoplasm, breast cancer.

Do not assign a V code for personal history of a malignant neoplasm if a physician removes the patient's neoplasm but continues to treat the patient for disease that may still be present. For example, a patient had a left breast mastectomy to treat cancer, and the patient is now receiving chemotherapy to eliminate any additional evidence of disease. This patient will not have a personal history of breast cancer until the cancer is completely eliminated, and the physician is no longer treating it.

Keep in mind that a patient's cancer can be cured in one site (personal history of a malignant neoplasm) but can still spread to another site (secondary neoplasm). If the documentation includes any mention of extension, invasion, or metastasis to another site from the primary site that is now history, then code the metastasis as a secondary malignant neoplasm. The primary malignant neoplasm is personal history. When the physician treats the patient for the secondary malignant neoplasm, it should be the first-listed diagnosis code, and the secondary diagnosis code should be a V10 category code for personal history of a malignant neoplasm, indicating the body site.

For example, a patient had a breast mastectomy to treat breast cancer, which is now gone. A year later, the patient develops brain cancer, which the breast cancer caused. Even though the breast cancer is gone, it still spread to another site. For this case, assign a first-listed code for brain cancer (secondary malignant neoplasm—198.3) and a secondary V code for personal history of a malignant neoplasm of the breast (V10.3).

Do you remember from Chapter 7 that you should also assign a V code as the first-listed code for a patient whose encounter is for chemotherapy (V58.11), radiotherapy (V58.0), or immunotherapy (V58.12) to treat a neoplasm? Then assign the neoplasm code second.

MALIGNANT NEOPLASMS

Malignant neoplasms are cancerous, meaning that they are life-threatening and can spread throughout the body. Cancer is a very common condition, so common in fact that you may know someone with cancer, or you may have had cancer yourself. Several decades ago, when a physician diagnosed a patient with cancer, it was a death sentence. But because there have been numerous advances in cancer treatment, including *cancer screenings* (tests to diagnose cancer in its early stages when it is more treatable), many people survive cancer.

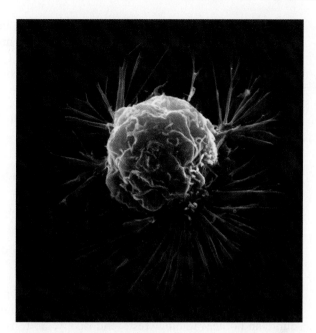

Figure 12-13 ■ A scanning electron microscopic image of invading cancer cells and their characteristic spikes or pseudopodia.

Photo credit: National Cancer Institute.

It may surprise you to know that factors in the environment cause most cancers, rather than heredity. These include cigarette smoking, exposure to chemicals and ultraviolet radiation (UV) from the sun, obesity, consuming a high-fat diet, and exposure to certain viruses, such as the Human Papillomavirus (HPV). This does not mean that everyone who is exposed to these factors will get cancer, but exposure does significantly increase the risk.

You may wonder what cancer actually is and how environmental factors contribute to it. Exposure to certain substances causes **anaplastic** cells to form in the body. Anaplastic, or poorly differentiated, cells (cells that are different from normal cells) are at the root of cancer. They infiltrate the body's healthy cells and take over, stopping healthy cells from performing their normal functions (■ FIGURE 12-13). The anaplastic cells can spread to any site in the body. Left untreated, cancer can cause death.

anaplastic (an-ə-plas′tik)

Cancer does not just happen to humans. It occurs in many other species that are also exposed to environmental toxins (■ FIGURE 12-14).

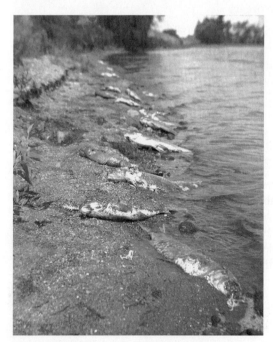

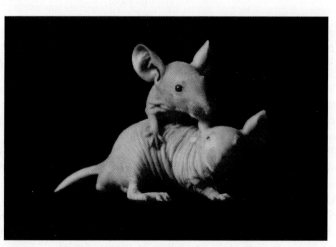

Figure 12-14(A) ■ Dead fish with malignant tumors caused by water pollution.

Photo credit: CDC.

Figure 12-14(B) ■ Cancer in laboratory mice.

Photo credit: National Cancer Institute.

immunology (im u-nol′ə-je)

Cancer **immunology** is the study of how the body's immune system responds to invading cancer cells, including development of vaccines to prevent cancer.

Cancer symptoms vary depending on the type of cancer. Many people have no symptoms until cancer is severe. General symptoms for common types of cancer include

- pain
- hoarseness, persistent cough, and coughing bloody sputum
- indigestion
- difficulty swallowing
- blood in the stool or urine, changes in bowel habits or urination, abnormal menstrual bleeding
- presence of a lump, swollen glands, changes to the shape and color of a mole or wart, sores that do not heal
- headaches, nausea, vomiting, and vomiting blood
- unexplained weight loss

Physicians diagnose cancer in different ways, depending on the type of cancer. Diagnostic methods include examination, X-ray, computed tomography (CT) scan, ultrasound, and other radiology tests, endoscopy, lab tests, and biopsy. Cancer cells can break away from the site of origin, enter the bloodstream or lymphatic system, and spread to other sites in the body. Cancer treatment differs depending on the type of cancer, how far it progressed, and factors related to the individual patient. Treatment includes surgery, medications, chemotherapy (drugs that destroy cancer cells), radiotherapy (radiation that destroys cancer), and immunotherapy (antibodies that fight cancer).

palliative (pal′e-ə-tiv)

Treatment also includes **palliative** pain management, or care to relieve pain and other symptoms of serious disease and hospice care, care that providers typically render to terminally ill patients , including treating the patient's medical, psychological, family, and social needs.

Primary, Secondary, and in Situ Malignant Neoplasms

Recall that malignant neoplasm (cancer) behavior can occur in the following sites:

- *primary*—The first site where the malignant neoplasm was found; and has spread to surrounding tissues within the same organ.
- *secondary*—All sites where the neoplasm has spread to from the primary site, including the second, third, fourth, etc.
- *in situ*—The neoplasm is confined to its original site and has not spread to surrounding tissues within the same organ. This type is also called intraepithelial, noninfiltrating, or noninvasive.

INTERESTING FACT: We Can Prevent 90% of Cancers

Do you know people who have smoked their whole lives and thrived well into old age without any sign of lung cancer? Or do you know of someone who never seemed to go near fruits and veggies but lived a long, full life? When you think of them, you might decide that cancer will come when it comes and there is nothing you can do about it. That is where you would be wrong.

According to Dr. John A. Milner of the National Institutes of Health's National Cancer Institute, about 30%–35% of cancers relate to smoking, and "about 30% to 35% relate to diet. Overall, it's estimated that about 90% of cancers are due to factors in the environment. Something other than our genes are triggers."

Cigarette smoking leads to an estimated 438,000 deaths—or about 1 out of every 5 deaths—each year. People who have poor diets, do not get enough physical activity, or are overweight may be at increased risk of developing several types of cancer. UV radiation, which comes from the sun, sunlamps, and tanning booths, causes skin damage that can lead to skin cancer. People who have certain jobs—such as painters, construction workers, and those in the chemical industry—have an increased risk of cancer from exposure to hazardous chemicals.

(National Institutes of Health, newsinhealth.nih.gov/2008/February/docs/01features_01.htm, accessed 12/30/10.)

It is important to carefully read the diagnostic statement in order to ensure correct code assignment, especially when a patient has cancer affecting multiple body sites, since you have to assign multiple codes.

When the physician does not document the histologic type of malignant neoplasm or the neoplasm's behavior, assign a code for primary *unless* the type of cancer that the patient has cannot ever be in a primary site. Always query the physician if you need clarification.

Let's review the following examples to identify malignant neoplasm sites that are primary, secondary, and in situ.

- **Lung carcinoma (■ Figure 12-15) metastasized to the liver:**

  Primary site: lung, secondary site: liver

- **Liver carcinoma metastatic from the lung:**

  Primary site: lung, secondary site: liver

- **Metastatic carcinoma of the breast to the brain:**

  Primary site: breast, secondary site: brain

- **Adenocarcinoma of the esophagus spread to the lymph nodes:**

  Primary site: esophagus, secondary site: lymph nodes

- **Noninvasive melanoma of the shoulder (■ Figure 12-16):**

  No primary or secondary site; noninvasive means that the cancer is in situ

- **Noninfiltrating squamous cell carcinoma of the lip:**

  No primary or secondary site; noninfiltrating means that the cancer is in situ

squamous cell carcinoma (skwā′mŭs sel kărsĭ-nō′mă) malignant tumor of flat cell epithelial tissue

Sequence codes for primary and secondary neoplasms for the same patient *depending on the circumstances of the encounter* and how the physician documents the patient's information. If the patient has a neoplasm in a primary and secondary site, then this does not mean that you should sequence the code for the primary site first just because it is primary. Sequence first the code for the neoplasm that is treated during the encounter, whether it is in a primary or secondary site. Assign an additional code for the neoplasm of the other site that is documented.

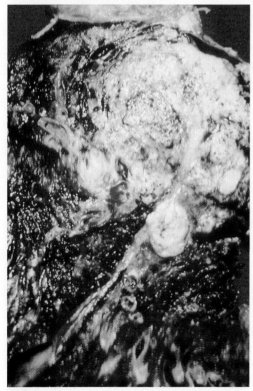

Figure 12-15 ■ Lung carcinoma metastasized to the liver.

Photo credit: National Cancer Institute.

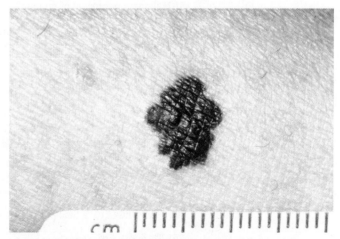

Figure 12-16 ■ Melanoma with an uneven, ragged, border. The ABCDE test is used to detect melanomas: A—Asymmetry, B—Border, C—Color, D—Diameter, E—Elevation/Evolution.

Photo credit: National Cancer Institute.

Refer to the following two examples to code malignant neoplasms of more than one site for the same patient during the same encounter:

Example 1: Mr. Huber, a 53-year-old established patient, sees Dr. Simmons at Williton Medical Center for treatment of stomach cancer in the body of the stomach, which has spread to multiple lymph nodes.

Since the medical documentation lists two diagnoses, determine which code to assign first:

- The encounter was to treat stomach cancer, so assign the code for stomach cancer first. The behavior of the stomach cancer is *malignant primary* because the cancer originated in the stomach and has spread.

- Assign the code for cancer of the lymph nodes second because although the documentation includes cancer of the lymph nodes, the encounter focused on treating the stomach cancer. The behavior of the cancer of the lymph nodes is *malignant secondary* because the stomach cancer spread to the lymph nodes.

To code stomach cancer, search the Index for the main term *carcinoma*. There is no subterm for stomach, so you will need to follow instructions in the Index to *see also Neoplasm, by site, malignant,* and search for the code using the Neoplasm Table. Then cross-reference code 151.4 to the Tabular (■ FIGURE 12-17).

Figure 12-17 ■ Index entry for carcinoma, Index entry for neoplasm of the body of the stomach from the Neoplasm Table, and code 151.4 cross-referenced to the Tabular.

Carcinoma (M8010/3) - see also Neoplasm, by site, malignant

	Malignant Primary	Malignant Secondary	Malignant Ca in situ	Benign	Uncertain Behavior	unspecified
Neoplasm, neoplastic	**199.1**	**199.1**	**234.9**	**229.9**	**238.9**	**239.9**
stomach	151.9	197.8	230.2	211.1	235.2	239.0
antrum (pyloric)	151.2	197.8	230.2	211.1	235.2	239.0
body	151.4	197.8	230.2	211.1	235.2	239.0
cardia	151.0	197.8	230.2	211.1	235.2	239.0
cardiac orifice	151.0	197.8	230.2	211.1	235.2	239.0
contiguous sites	151.8	-	-	-	-	-

4th 151 Malignant neoplasm of stomach

Excludes: benign carcinoid tumor of stomach (209.63)
malignant carcinoid tumor of stomach (209.63)

151.0   Cardiac
Cardiac orifice
Cardio-esophageal junction
Excludes: squamous cell carcinoma (150.2, 150.5)

151.1   Pylorus
Prepylorus
Pyloric canal

151.2   Pyloric antrum
Antrum of stomach NOS

151.3   Fundus of stomach

151.4   Body of stomach

Next, assign the code for cancer of the lymph nodes, secondary site. Search the Index for the main term *carcinoma*. There is no subterm for lymph node, so you will need to follow instructions in the Index to *see also Neoplasm, by site, malignant* and search for the code using the Neoplasm Table. When you search for lymph node as a subterm in the Neoplasm Table, you will find the instruction to *see also Neoplasm, lymph gland*. The only code choice for lymph node is for a primary site, and you need to code it as a secondary site. Next, search for lymph gland of multiple sites, and cross-reference code 196.8 to the Tabular (■ FIGURE 12-18).

Carcinoma (M8010/3) - see also Neoplasm, by site, malignant

	Malignant Primary	Malignant Secondary	Malignant Ca in situ	Benign	Uncertain Behavior	unspecified
Neoplasm, neoplastic	199.1	199.1	234.9	229.9	238.9	239.9
lymph, lymphatic						
node (*see also* Neoplasm, lymph gland)						
primary NEC	202.9					
gland (secondary)	-	196.9	-	229.0	238.8	239.89
multiple sites in categories						
196.0-196.6	-	196.8	-	229.0	238.8	239.89

4th **196 Secondary and unspecified malignant neoplasm of lymph nodes**

Excludes: any malignant neoplasm of lymph nodes, specified as primary (200.0-202.9)
  Hodgkin's disease (201.0-201.9)
  lymphosarcoma (200.1)
  reticulosarcoma (200.0)
  other forms of lymphoma (202.0-202.9)
  secondary neuroendocrine tumor of (distant) lymph nodes (209.71)

 196.8 Lymph nodes of multiple sites

Figure 12-18 ■ Index entry for carcinoma, Index entry for neoplasm of the lymph gland, multiple sites from the Neoplasm Table, and code 196.8 cross-referenced to the Tabular.

Source: Department of Health and Human Services, Centers for Disease Control, National Center for Health Statistics, ICD-9-CM 2010, accessed: ftp://ftp.cdc.gov/pub/Health_Statistics/NCHS/Publications/ICD9-CM/2010/]

Assign two codes for Example 1: 151.4 (neoplasm, stomach, body, malignant primary) and 196.8 (neoplasm, lymph gland, multiple sites, malignant secondary).

Example 2: Mrs. Cooke, a 68-year-old established patient, returns to see Dr. Simmons at Williton Medical Center to review her CT and magnetic resonance imaging (MRI) results of the brain. Dr. Simmons discusses an occipital craniotomy (cutting into the skull) procedure for a brain biopsy. His diagnosis is lung carcinoma, upper lobe, metastasized to the brain.

The lung is the primary malignant neoplasm because that is the site of origin. The brain is the secondary malignant neoplasm because the brain is the site where the lung cancer spread.

Figure 12-19 ■ Neoplasm Table Index entry for neoplasm of the brain, occipital lobe, malignant secondary, with code 198.3 cross-referenced to the Tabular.

	Malignant Primary	Malignant Secondary	Malignant Ca in situ	Benign	Uncertain Behavior	unspecified
Neoplasm, neoplastic	199.1	199.1	234.9	229.9	238.9	239.9
brain NEC	191.9	198.3	-	225.0	237.5	239.6
occipital lobe	191.4	198.3	-	225.0	237.5	239.6

> **4th** **198 Secondary malignant neoplasm of other specified sites**
>
> Excludes: lymph node metastasis (196.0-196.9)
> secondary neuroendocrine tumor of other specified sites (209.79)
>
> **198.0 Kidney**
> **198.1 Other urinary organs**
> **198.2 Skin**
>   Skin of breast
> **198.3 Brain and spinal cord**

Determine the order in which to assign the codes by the reason for the encounter. Dr. Simmons focuses the encounter on treating the brain cancer, so assign the code for brain cancer as the first-listed code. Assign the code for lung cancer second.

For the neoplasm of the brain, search the Index for the main term *carcinoma.* There is no subterm for brain, so you will need to follow instructions in the Index to *see also Neoplasm, by site, malignant,* and search for the code using the Neoplasm Table, subterm *brain,* and subterm *occipital lobe, malignant secondary.* Then cross-reference code 198.3 to the Tabular (■ FIGURE 12-19).

Next, assign the code for the lung neoplasm. Search the Index for the main term *carcinoma.* There is no subterm for lung, so you will need to follow instructions in the Index to *see also Neoplasm, by site, malignant,* and search for the code using the Neoplasm Table, subterm *lung,* and subterm *upper lobe, malignant primary.* Then cross-reference code 162.3 to the Tabular (■ FIGURE 12-20).

Assign two codes for Example 2: 198.3 (secondary malignant neoplasm of the occipital lobe of the brain and 162.3 (primary malignant neoplasm of the upper lobe of the lung).

Cancer Staging

Providers classify cancers according to their stage, which indicates the severity of the cancer and whether it has spread. Providers determine stages from patients' examinations and diagnostic tests. Staging helps to determine the patient's prognosis and treatment options.

Although there are different staging systems for different types of cancer, each system identifies the same basic information, including the primary neoplasm's cell structure, site, and size; the number of neoplasms; and whether the cancer has metastasized to lymph nodes or other sites. One of the most common cancer staging systems is the **Tumor, Nodes, Metastasis (TNM) classification system**. It focuses on the size and/or extent of the tumor **(T)**, how far it has spread to the lymph nodes **(N)**, and whether there is any metastasis to other body sites **(M)**. To use the TNM system, providers add a number to each letter, which represents the primary neoplasm's extent and size, as well as the extent of metastasis.

	Malignant Primary	Malignant Secondary	Malignant Ca in situ	Benign	Uncertain Behavior	unspecified
Neoplasm, neoplastic	**199.1**	**199.1**	**234.9**	**229.9**	**238.9**	**239.9**
lung	162.9	197.0	231.2	212.3	235.7	239.1
azygos lobe	162.3	197.0	231.2	212.3	235.7	239.1
carina	162.2	197.0	231.2	212.3	235.7	239.1
contiguous sites with bronchus or						
trachea	162.8	-	-	-	-	-
hilus	162.2	197.0	231.2	212.3	235.7	239.1
linqula	162.3	197.0	231.2	212.3	235.7	239.1
lobe NEC	162.9	197.0	231.2	212.3	235.7	239.1
lower lobe	162.5	197.0	231.2	212.3	235.7	239.1
main bronchus	162.2	197.0	231.2	212.3	235.7	239.1
middle lobe	162.4	197.0	231.2	212.3	235.7	239.1
upper lobe	162.3	197.0	231.2	212.3	235.7	239.1

4th   162 Malignant neoplasm of trachea, bronchus, and lung

Excludes: benign carcinoid tumor of bronchus (209.61)
          malignant carcinoid tumor of bronchus (209.21)

    162.0   Trachea
          Cartilage of trachea
          Mucosa of trachea

    162.2   Main bronchus
          Carina
          Hilus of lung

    162.3   Upper lobe, bronchus or lung

Figure 12-20 ■ Neoplasm Index entry for neoplasm of the lung, upper lobe, malignant primary, with code 162.3 cross-referenced to the Tabular.

DESTINATION: MEDICARE

      You already completed computer-based training on CMS's MLN. The MLN also has additional resources to help you better interpret Medicare's regulations and guidelines. In the following exercise, you will access an MLN article and answer questions about colorectal cancer screenings. Follow these instructions to access the *MLN Matters* article:

1. Go to the website http://cms.gov/.
2. At the top of screen on the banner bar, choose *Outreach & Education*.
3. Under the *Medicare Learning Network*, click *MLN Matters Articles*.
4. On the left side of the screen, click *2009 MLN Matters Articles*.
5. Under 2009 MLN Matters Articles on the next screen, you will see the message, "The 2009 MLN Matters Articles List has been consolidated with 2009 Transmittals. Please visit the following page: *2009 Transmittals*"
6. Click the link for *2009 Transmittals*.
7. Click Transmittal # in the first column to sort results by transmittal number.
8. Scroll to Transmittal # *R105NCD*, and click on it.

continued

9. Scroll down to Downloads, and click *MM6578*.

10. You will then see the MLN Matters article on *Screening Computed Tomography Colonography (CTC) for Colorectal Cancer.*

Answer the following questions:

1. Will Medicare cover colorectal screening computed tomography **colonography** (CTC)?

2. What types of screening will Medicare cover for colorectal cancer?

3. What criteria does a patient have to meet in order for Medicare to cover colorectal cancer screening?

4. What three organizations recommended that CTC be considered an acceptable option for colorectal cancer screening?

colonography (ko lən-og′rə-fe) imaging of the intestine using computed tomography (CT) or magnetic resonance imaging (MRI)

For example, a patient with breast cancer classified as T3 N2 M0 has a large tumor (T3), which spread to nearby lymph nodes (N2) but has not spread anywhere else (M0). A patient with prostate cancer classified as T3 N0 M0 has a large tumor (T3), which has not spread to any lymph nodes (N0), and has not spread anywhere else (M0).

Cancer has five stages (■ TABLE 12-4). Depending on the type of cancer, the criteria for a specific stage may be different. Many times, a patient's TNM classification correlates to one of the five cancer stages.

■ TABLE 12-4 **STAGES OF CANCER**

Stage	Definition
Stage 0	Carcinoma in situ
Stage I, Stage II, Stage III	Stages I, II, and III determine the extent of cancer. The higher the stage, the greater the extent. These stages can describe large tumor size and/or metastasis to nearby lymph nodes and/or organs that are close to the site of the primary neoplasm.
Stage IV	Carcinoma that has spread to another organ or organs

Source: (National Cancer Institute, www.cancer.gov/cancertopics/factsheet/Detection/staging, accessed 2/26/12.)

TAKE A BREAK

Wow! That was a lot of information to remember! Let's take a break and then practice assigning malignant neoplasm codes and V codes.

Exercise 12.4 **V Codes for Neoplasms and Malignant Neoplasms**

Instructions: For the following patient encounters, answer the questions and assign both neoplasm codes and morphology codes using the Index, Tabular, and Appendix A of ICD-9-CM.

1. Hilda Tabor, age 54, receives chemotherapy at Williton Medical Center for adenocarcinoma of the right breast, lower outer quadrant, which metastasized to the brain.

a. How many codes do you need to assign to this encounter? _____

b. What is the first-listed diagnosis? _____

c. What is the first-listed diagnosis code? _____

d. What is the secondary diagnosis? _____

e. What is the neoplasm code for the secondary diagnosis? _____

f. What is the M code for the secondary diagnosis? _____

TAKE A BREAK *continued*

g. Are there other codes that you need to assign? __
_____

h. If so, what are the condition(s) and the code(s) (including M codes)? _____

2. Della Bumgarner, age 48, sees Dr. Simmons to discuss treatment options for her recently diagnosed gastric adenocarcinoma. The gastric adenocarcinoma metastasized to the abdominal lymph nodes.

a. How many codes do you need to assign to this encounter? _____

b. What is the first-listed diagnosis? _____
_____

c. What is the neoplasm code for the first-listed diagnosis? _____

d. What is the M code for the first-listed diagnosis? _____
_____

e. What is the secondary diagnosis? _____
_____

f. What is the neoplasm code for the secondary diagnosis? _____

g. What is the M code for the secondary diagnosis? _____
_____

h. Are there other codes that you need to assign? __
_____

i. If so, what are the condition(s) and the code(s) (including M codes)? _____

3. Fred Kelso, age 66, reports to Williton Medical Center's outpatient surgery department for a colonoscopy because he has a personal history of colon cancer, which was successfully removed five years ago.

a. How many codes do you need to assign to this encounter? _____

b. What is the first-listed diagnosis? _____
_____

c. What is the first-listed diagnosis code? _____
_____

d. What is the secondary diagnosis? _____
_____

e. What is the secondary diagnosis code? _____
_____

f. Should you also assign a neoplasm code or an M code? _____

g. Why or why not? _____
_____

4. Samuel Helms, age 48, has radiotherapy at Williton Medical Center to treat malignant melanoma of his lungs, which spread from his back.

a. How many codes do you need to assign to this encounter? _____

b. What is the first-listed diagnosis? _____
_____

c. What is the first-listed diagnosis code? _____
_____

d. What is the secondary diagnosis? _____
_____

e. What is the secondary diagnosis code? _____
_____

f. What is the M code for the secondary diagnosis?
_____

g. Are there other codes that you need to assign? __
_____

h. If so, what are the condition(s) and the code(s) (including M codes)? _____

5. Dr. Simmons admits Leon Nelson, age 61, to Williton Medical Center for surgery to remove a malignant brain tumor resulting from metastasis from squamous cell (flat cells of the epithelium) carcinoma of the lung.

a. How many codes do you need to assign to this encounter? _____

b. What is the first-listed diagnosis? _____
_____

c. What is the neoplasm code for the first-listed diagnosis? _____

d. What is the M code for the first-listed diagnosis?
_____

e. What is the secondary diagnosis? _____
_____

f. What is the neoplasm code for the secondary diagnosis? _____

g. What is the M code for the secondary diagnosis?
_____

h. Are there other codes that you need to assign? __
_____

i. If so, what are the condition(s) and the code(s) (including M codes)? _____

6. Jessica Lemus brings her 1-year-old son, Todd, to Dr. Simmons today for results of a liver biopsy performed a week ago. Dr. Simmons states that Todd has stage I hepatoblastoma (malignant liver neoplasm). Two risk factors for the condition are low birth weight and family history. Todd only weighed 950 grams (2 pounds, 2 ounces) at birth, whereas normal birth weight is

continued

TAKE A BREAK *continued*

2,800–4,800 grams (6 pounds, 3 ounces to 10 pounds, 9 ounces). There is a family history of adenomatous polyposis (inherited condition of numerous polyps on the inside walls of the colon). Dr. Simmons explains that with surgery and chemotherapy, Todd's prognosis is good. He states that he would like to start Todd on chemotherapy today, and Mrs. Lemus agrees.

a. How many codes do you need to assign to this encounter? _____

b. What is the first-listed diagnosis? _____

_____

c. What is the neoplasm code for the first-listed diagnosis? _____

d. What is the M code for the first-listed diagnosis? _____

e. What is the secondary diagnosis? _____

_____

f. What is the diagnosis code for the secondary diagnosis? _____

g. Are there other codes that you need to assign? __

_____

h. If so, what are the condition(s) and the code(s) (including M codes)? _____

i. Can you assign a V code for personal history of low birth weight? _____ Why or why not? ____

_____

BENIGN NEOPLASMS

Benign neoplasms are not life threatening, do not spread, and are not cancer. However, they can grow in organs and tissue and interfere with normal body functions, sometimes causing life-threatening complications. Benign neoplasms remain localized to one area and have a fibrous covering that inhibits their ability to spread. Benign neoplasms may also be a precursor (sign) for malignancies that develop later. Examples of benign neoplasms, or tumors, include moles, skin tags (skin flaps) (■ FIGURE 12-21), **lipoma** (neoplasm of fat cells) (■ FIGURE 12-22), and uterine **leiomyoma**, also called a uterine fibroid (neoplasm of smooth muscle—myometrium—of the uterus) (■ FIGURE 12-23).

lipoma (lip-o′mə)

leiomyoma (li o-mi-o′mə)

The causes of benign neoplasm include underlying diseases, exposure to viruses or bacteria, and aging, as with skin tags. Many benign neoplasms have no symptoms. When symptoms are present, they can include pain, swelling, the presence of a lump, inflammation, and itching. Diagnosis includes examination, radiology, and lab tests, including standard cancer screening tests. Many benign neoplasms, such as moles, do not need any treatment. If benign neoplasms do require treatment, physicians can remove them surgically or with topical medications and can also treat them with radiation and chemotherapy.

You cannot find all benign neoplasm codes in Chapter 2 of the Tabular List. ICD-9-CM categorizes some of the codes in other chapters in the Tabular. Refer to the following example to code a benign neoplasm for a patient's encounter.

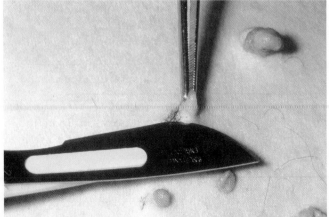

Figure 12-21 ■ Skin tags are a small outgrowth of epidermal and dermal tissue that occur most often on the eyelids, neck, and axillae. Most do not require treatment.

Photo credit: © Medical-on-Line/Alamy.

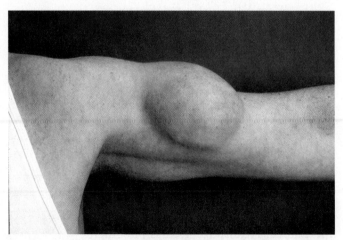

Figure 12-22 ■ Massive lipoma of arm.

Photo credit: © SHOUT/Alamy.

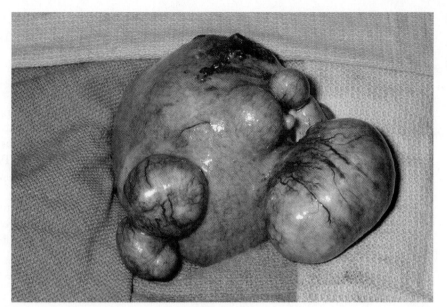

Figure 12-23 ■ Uterus with leiomyomas

Photo credit: MICHAEL ENGLISH, M.D. / Custom Medical Stock Photo.

Example: Ms. Knowles, a 35-year-old established patient, sees Dr. Ferguson, a dermatologist, for removal of moles. Dr. Ferguson excises five benign moles from the patient's neck.

Since there is no histologic type of the neoplasm, go directly to the Neoplasm Table. Search for the subterm *skin* and subterm *neck*, and find the code under the Benign column. Then cross-reference code 216.4 to the Tabular (■ FIGURE 12-24).

Figure 12-24 ■ Index entry for benign neoplasm of the skin of the neck, with code 216.4 cross-referenced to the Tabular.

	Malignant Primary	Malignant Secondary	Malignant Ca in situ	Benign	Uncertain Behavior	unspecified
Neoplasm, neoplastic	199.1	199.1	234.9	229.9	238.9	239.9
skin NEC	173.9	198.2	232.9	216.9	238.2	239.2
neck	173.4	198.2	232.4	216.4	238.2	239.2

4th 216 Benign neoplasm of skin

Includes: blue nevus
dermatofibroma
hydrocystoma
pigmented nevus
syringoadenoma
syringoma
Excludes: skin of genital organs (221.0-222.9)
   216.4   Scalp and skin of neck

Histology for a Benign or Malignant Neoplasm

Be very careful when you are coding neoplasms because many histologic types end with the suffix "-oma," meaning tumor. Just because a word ends in "-oma" does not mean that the condition is cancerous. For example, carcin*oma* is cancerous, but lip*oma* is not. Always consult your medical dictionary or other medical references for medical term definitions before final code assignment. Never guess whether a neoplasm is malignant or benign.

NEOPLASMS OF UNCERTAIN BEHAVIOR OR UNSPECIFIED

Uncertain behavior and unspecified are additional choices for identifying neoplasm behavior which are listed in the last two columns of the Neoplasm Table. **Uncertain behavior** means that the pathologist cannot determine whether the neoplasm is malignant or benign. It may have characteristics of both, or it may be unclear. Typically, the physician will order further testing to determine the neoplasm's behavior or will send the specimen to another pathologist for a second opinion.

Unspecified means that the documentation provides the neoplasm site but not its behavior or histologic type. Assign unspecified as the behavior as a *last resort*. Always query the physician for additional information before you assign an unspecified code.

Behavior Is Known, Site Is Unknown or Unspecified

According to the National Cancer Institute, physicians diagnose thousands of patients with metastatic cancer every year, but they cannot determine the cancer's primary site. When the physician cannot identify the primary site, it is called *carcinoma of unknown primary (CUP)*. Physicians frequently find metastatic cancer in the lymph nodes, liver, lung, or bone but cannot identify the primary source. Documentation typically states "metastatic lung cancer" or "bone metastasis," identifying the secondary site (lung or bone) but not the primary site.

It is important to note that the Neoplasm Table lists a subterm for *unknown site or unspecified* with a code in each of the six columns identifying neoplasm behavior. Assign codes from *unknown site or unspecified* when the physician documents the neoplasm's behavior (malignant primary, malignant secondary) but the neoplasm site is unknown or not specified in the documentation.

Note that the codes listed under the subterm *unknown site or unspecified* are the same codes listed under the main term *neoplasm* in the Neoplasm Table (■ FIGURE 12-25).

Refer to the following example to code a patient encounter for a neoplasm of an unknown site.

> **Example 1:** Mr. Gilliam, a 58-year-old established patient, returns for a follow-up visit to Dr. Simmons at Williton Medical Center. Mr. Gilliam has metastatic bone cancer in the spine.
>
> Assign two codes for this encounter, the first for the bone cancer, malignant secondary, which is the reason for the encounter. Assign a second code for the unknown primary site, malignant.
>
> For bone cancer, search the Index for the main term *carcinoma*. There is no subterm for bone, so you will need to follow instructions in the Index to *see also Neoplasm, by site, malignant,* and search for the code using the Neoplasm Table, subterm *bone* and subterm *spine, malignant secondary*. Then cross-reference code 198.5 to the Tabular (■ FIGURE 12-26).

Figure 12-25 ■ Neoplasm Table showing codes for unknown site or unspecified in each of the six columns.

	Malignant Primary	Malignant Secondary	Malignant Ca in situ	Benign	Uncertain Behavior	unspecified
Neoplasm, neoplastic	**199.1**	**199.1**	**234.9**	**229.9**	**238.9**	**239.9**
unknown site or unspecified	199.1	199.1	234.9	229.9	238.9	239.9

	Malignant Primary	Malignant Secondary	Malignant Ca in situ	Benign	Uncertain Behavior	unspecified
Neoplasm, neoplastic	**199.1**	**199.1**	**234.9**	**229.9**	**238.9**	**239.9**
bone (periosteum)	170.9	198.5	-	213.9	238.0	239.2
spine, spinal (column)	170.2	198.5	-	213.2	238.0	239.2
coccyx	170.6	198.5	-	213.6	238.0	239.2
sacrum	170.6	198.5	-	213.6	238.0	239.2

`4th` **198 Secondary malignant neoplasm of other specified sites**

Excludes: lymph node metastasis (196.0-196.9)
           secondary neuroendocrine tumor of other specified sites (209.79)

198.5 Bone and bone marrow

Figure 12-26 ■ Index entry for neoplasm of the spine, malignant secondary from the Neoplasm Table, with code 198.5 cross-referenced to the Tabular.

Next, assign the code for an unspecified neoplasm, primary site. If you search the Index under *carcinoma*, you will find that there is no subterm for unspecified site. Instead, go to the Neoplasm Table and find the subterm for *unknown site or unspecified*, then find the code under the *Malignant Primary* column. Cross-reference code 199.1 to the Tabular. You can also find the same entry under the main term *neoplasm* without checking any additional subterms (■ FIGURE 12-27).

	Malignant Primary	Malignant Secondary	Malignant Ca in situ	Benign	Uncertain Behavior	unspecified
Neoplasm, neoplastic	**199.1**	**199.1**	**234.9**	**229.9**	**238.9**	**239.9**
unknown site or unspecified	199.1	199.1	234.9	229.9	238.9	239.9

`4th`   **199 Malignant neoplasm without specification of site**

Excludes: malignant carcinoid tumor of unknown primary site (209.20)
              malignant (poorly differentiated) neuroendocrine carcinoma, any site (209.30)
              malignant (poorly differentiated) neuroendocrine tumor, any site (209.30)
              neuroendocrine carcinoma (high grade), any site (209.30)

    199.0   Disseminated
            Carcinomatosis unspecified site (primary) (secondary)
            Generalized:
              cancer unspecified site (primary) (secondary)
              malignancy unspecified site (primary) (secondary)
            Multiple cancer unspecified site (primary) (secondary)

    199.1   Other
            Cancer unspecified site (primary) (secondary)
            Carcinoma unspecified site (primary) (secondary)
            Malignancy unspecified site (primary) (secondary)

Figure 12-27 ■ Index entry unknown site of a neoplasm, malignant primary, from the Neoplasm Table, with code 199.1 cross-referenced to the Tabular.

WORKPLACE IQ

You have worked for one month as a coding specialist for Dr. Simmons, an oncologist. The senior coder, Jamie, trains you and reviews your work for accuracy. Today, Jamie asks you to code an encounter for a follow-up visit for Mrs. Bales, a patient who had breast cancer, underwent a total right breast mastectomy, and then had chemotherapy. Dr. Simmons found no further evidence of cancer. Jamie tells you that coding the encounter presents a challenge because you need to assign two V codes. She asks you to give her the two codes that you would assign so that she can check them for accuracy.

What two V codes would you assign?

TAKE A BREAK

Way to go! Let's take a break and then practice assigning codes for neoplasms that are benign, of uncertain behavior, or unspecified.

Exercise 12.5 Benign Neoplasms and Neoplasms of Uncertain Behavior or Unspecified

Instructions: Assign neoplasm codes to the following patient encounters, using the Index and the Tabular. Do not assign morphology codes.

1. Albert Dominguez, a 33-year-old new patient, sees Dr. Grisham, an orthopedist, for a lump behind his knee. After evaluation, Dr. Grisham diagnoses Mr. Dominguez with osteochondroma (benign tumor of bone and cartilage). Dr. Grisham states that Mr. Dominguez will not need to have surgery unless the lump causes pain.

   Code(s): _____

2. Terry Theobald, age 58, sees Dr. Simmons, an oncologist, for a follow-up visit to learn his test results. Dr. Simmons diagnoses Mr. Theobald with malignant metastasis in the lung, but the tests do not reveal the primary site.

   Code(s): _____

3. Bobby Patino, age 63, sees Dr. Hoffman for a follow-up on a benign islet cell (pancreas cell) neoplasm of the pancreas.

   Code(s): _____

4. Dr. Nathan, an interventional radiologist, performs **interventional radiology** surgery on Rosalie Sheppard, age 42, at Williton Medical Center for embolization of uterine leiomyoma (benign neoplasm of smooth muscle).

   Code(s): _____

5. Dr. Hoffman treats Daniel Trinh, a 71-year-old, for prostatic (pertaining to the prostate) adenoma.

   Code(s): _____

6. Earl Jaquez, a 64-year-old new patient, sees Dr. Ariss, a podiatrist, for a thickening between the third and fourth toes on his left foot. Dr. Ariss diagnoses Mr. Jaquez with Morton's neuroma (benign neoplasm between toes) and discusses possible treatment options.

   Code(s): _____

ADDITIONAL GUIDELINES FOR CODING NEOPLASMS

interventional radiology—a specialty branch of medicine in which physicians insert catheters into arteries to diagnose and treat specific disorders

You have already learned some of the neoplasm coding guidelines from the ICD-9-CM Official Guidelines for Coding and Reporting. ICD-9-CM also contains additional guidelines for coding neoplasms that you should review and reference as you continue to code neoplasms in the next exercise. Here are the additional guidelines:

1. When an admission or encounter is for management of anemia associated with a malignant neoplasm, and the treatment is only for anemia, assign a code for anemia (such as code 285.22—*Anemia in neoplastic disease*) as the principal diagnosis. Assign second code(s) for the malignant neoplasm.

2. If a physician treats the patient for a malignant neoplasm, and the patient also has anemia, then assign a code for the neoplasm as the first-listed diagnosis and assign a code for anemia second.

3. If the physician documents both *anemia in neoplastic disease* and *anemia due to antineoplastic chemotherapy*, code for both conditions.

4. Sequence first the code for anemia when the admission or encounter is for management of anemia associated with chemotherapy, immunotherapy, or radiotherapy, and the only treatment is for anemia. Assign a code for the neoplasm as an additional code.

5. Sequence first a code for dehydration when the admission or encounter is for management of dehydration due to a malignant neoplasm, therapy for the neoplasm, or a combination of both, and only the dehydration is being treated (through intravenous rehydration). Assign a code for the neoplasm as an additional code.

6. When the admission or encounter is to treat a complication resulting from a surgical procedure, sequence first the complication if treatment is intended to resolve the complication.

7. Assign a neoplasm code as the first-listed diagnosis when an episode of care involves the surgical removal of a neoplasm, primary or secondary site, followed by adjunct chemotherapy or radiation treatment during the same episode of care. Assign codes from categories 140–198 or 200–203.

8. When a patient is admitted for radiotherapy, immunotherapy, or chemotherapy and develops complications, such as uncontrolled nausea and vomiting or dehydration, the principal or first-listed diagnosis is V58.0—*Encounter for radiotherapy*, or V58.11—*Encounter for antineoplastic chemotherapy*, or V58.12—*Encounter for antineoplastic immunotherapy* followed by any codes for the complications. Assign a secondary code for the complication treated, and assign a third code for the neoplasm.

9. Sequence first the primary malignancy or metastatic site when the reason for an admission or encounter is to determine the extent of the malignancy or for procedures such as **paracentesis** or **thoracentesis**, even though the provider administers chemotherapy or radiotherapy.

10. Code a malignant neoplasm of a transplanted organ as a transplant complication. Assign first the appropriate code from subcategory 996.8—*Complications of transplanted organ*, followed by code 199.2—*Malignant neoplasm associated with transplanted organ*. Assign an additional code for the specific malignancy.

paracentesis (păr ă-sĕn-tē′sĭs)—surgical puncture of a body cavity to remove fluid

thoracentesis (thō ră-sĕn-tē′sĭs)—surgical puncture of the chest wall to remove fluid

hyponatremia (hī pō-nā-trē′mē-ə)

TAKE A BREAK

Good job! Let's take a break and then practice assigning more neoplasm codes using the additional guidelines.

Exercise 12.6 Additional Guidelines for Coding Neoplasms

Instructions: Assign codes to the following patient encounters, using the Index and the Tabular. Do not assign morphology codes.

1. Dr. Mills treats Teresa Pritchard, age 65, at Williton Medical Center's ED for anemia, which is due to Hodgkin's lymphoma. (lymphatic system cancer—part of the immune system.)

Code(s): _____

2. Thomas Dressler, age 76, sees Dr. Simmons, an oncologist, for a follow-up appointment to discuss treatment options for colon cancer. Mr. Dressler can adequately manage his pain, and Dr. Simmons says that he should continue his medication for the neoplasm-associated anemia.

Code(s): _____

continued

TAKE A BREAK *continued*

3. Madeline Barner, age 81, collapses at home. An ambulance transports her to Williton Medical Center. In the ED, Dr. Mills diagnoses her with dehydration and **hyponatremia** (low level of sodium in the blood) due to chemotherapy. She was undergoing treatment for ovarian cancer of the right side, which has metastasized to several other sites. Dr. Mills starts the patient on IV fluids and admits her. (Hint: This case also requires an E code.)

Code(s): _____

4. Antonio Aguiar, age 60, reports to the outpatient radiology department at Williton Medical Center for a series of CT scans to determine the extent of metastasis from pancreatic cancer.

Code(s): _____

5. Dr. Simmons discharges Jill Roderick, age 43, from Williton Medical Center after a lumpectomy due to cancer in the upper outer quadrant of the right breast. She also had an initial round of chemotherapy. She will report back as an outpatient for chemotherapy in three weeks.

Code(s): _____

6. Dr. Simmons sees established patient Eddie Heiser, age 5, for management of anemia, which is due to acute lymphocytic leukemia (cancer of the white blood cells). Dr. Simmons also administers chemotherapy.

Code(s): _____

↳ A LOOK AHEAD TO ICD-10-CM

ICD-10-CM includes several new guidelines for neoplasms (C00–D49). It also has revised guidelines pertaining to anemia and a malignant neoplasm and to a malignant neoplasm of a transplanted organ.

Instructions: Refer to the ICD-10-CM Official Guidelines for additional information. (Instructions for accessing the guidelines are in Appendix A of this text.) Then assign codes from ICD-10-CM referencing both the Index and the Tabular.

1. Jeff Hollingsworth, age 61, meets with Dr. Simmons to review the results of a biopsy, which Dr. Simmons performed because Mr. Hollingsworth had hemorrhaging. Dr. Simmons says that the biopsy is positive for adenocarcinoma in situ in the sigmoid colon. Because Dr. Simmons found the adenocarcinoma early, the prognosis is good. Code(s):_____

2. Justin Brinker, age 65, sees Dr. Ferguson, a dermatologist, for removal of basal cell adenoma on his left cheek. Dr. Ferguson asks him to report back in six months for a recheck to ensure that there is no further evidence of the adenoma. Code(s):_____

3. Hilda Tabor, age 54, receives chemotherapy at Williton Medical Center for adenocarcinoma of the right breast, lower outer quadrant, which metastasized to the brain. Code(s):_____

4. Dr. Simmons admits Leon Nelson, age 61, to Williton Medical Center for surgery to remove a malignant brain tumor resulting from metastasis from squamous cell carcinoma of the lung. Code(s):_____

5. Dr. Mills treats Teresa Pritchard, age 65, at Williton Medical Center's ED for anemia, which is due to Hodgkin's lymphoma. Code(s):_____

6. Madeline Barner, age 81, collapses at home. An ambulance transports her to Williton Medical Center. In the ED, Dr. Mills diagnoses her with dehydration and hyponatremia due to chemotherapy. She was undergoing treatment for ovarian cancer of the right side, which has metastasized to several other sites. Dr. Mills starts the patient on IV fluids and admits her. Code(s):_____

CHAPTER REVIEW

Multiple Choice

Instructions: Circle one best answer to complete each statement.

1. Which of the following is not a column on the Neoplasm Table?
   a. Primary
   b. Secondary
   c. Unknown
   d. Benign

2. Histology refers to the _____ of a neoplasm.
   a. history
   b. type
   c. behavior
   d. metastasis

3. When you are coding a neoplasm, you should first search the Index for the _____ of the neoplasm.
   a. site
   b. history
   c. histology
   d. behavior

4. Morphology codes are used by
   a. cancer registries to analyze statistics about cancer.
   b. insurance companies to determine payment for malignant neoplasms.
   c. physicians to get higher reimbursement for cancer treatment.
   d. all of the above

5. When a patient is being treated for cancer after a malignant tumor was removed, and the medical documentation does not state the neoplasm behavior, you should assign a code for
   a. personal history of malignant neoplasm.
   b. primary malignant neoplasm.
   c. secondary malignant neoplasm.
   d. cancer in situ.

6. When a patient is receiving treatment directed at a metastatic site, the principal diagnosis should be
   a. primary malignant neoplasm.
   b. secondary malignant neoplasm.
   c. cancer in situ.
   d. uncertain behavior.

7. Providers describe primary neoplasm cell structure, site, size, number of neoplasms, and metastasis as
   a. screening.
   b. behavior.
   c. adjunct therapy.
   d. staging.

8. Which of the following is *not* true of benign neoplasms?
   a. They remain localized to one area.
   b. They may be a precursor for malignancies that occur later.
   c. They are life threatening.
   d. They can be caused by an underlying disease, exposure to viruses or bacteria, or aging.

9. A histologic type of neoplasm ending in "-oma" means
   a. cancer.
   b. malignant.
   c. a tumor.
   d. benign.

10. When the physician does not document the site of cancer, you should assign a code for
    a. unknown site.
    b. unspecified behavior.
    c. uncertain behavior.
    d. in situ.

Coding Assignments

Instructions: Assign neoplasm codes and codes for any additional diagnoses using both the ICD-9-CM Index and Tabular. Do not assign morphology codes unless directed.

1. Caroline Newberry, age 15, undergoes limb-salvage surgery to remove the remaining osteosarcoma in her thigh. She completed chemotherapy three weeks earlier, which was successful in shrinking the tumor. Assign both a neoplasm code and a morphology code.

   Code(s): _____

2. Ronald Oxley, age 56, sees Dr. Simmons, an oncologist, for management of multiple myeloma (cancer of plasma cells—a type of white blood cell). After conducting an examination and reviewing test results, Dr. Simmons delivers the good news that the disease is in remission.

   Code(s): _____

3. Randy Krug, age 27, sees Dr. Ferguson, a dermatologist, for removal of a malignant melanoma on his forehead.

   Code(s): _____

4. Misty Gunther, a 32-year-old, sees Dr. Simmons regarding the biopsy report of a lesion on her breast that he removed a week ago. He confirms that it is a malignant neoplasm in situ. He states that he believes that he removed all of the lesion.

   Code(s): _____

5. Steve Doane, age 44, receives chemotherapy at Williton Medical Center for pancreatic cancer, which has metastasized. Because the disease is so advanced, the prognosis is not good, but Dr Simmons tells Mr. Doane that he feels that chemotherapy could be beneficial.

Code(s): _____

6. Dr. Evora, a pediatric (pertaining to children) oncologist, meets with the parents of Lisa Woodham, age 3, to discuss treatment options for the child's recently diagnosed malignant juvenile cystic astrocytoma (brain neoplasm), which was found in the cerebrum. Assign both a neoplasm code and a morphology code.

Code(s): _____

7. Dr. Mills, ED physician, admits Jack Ferrante, age 63, to Williton Medical Center for treatment of complications from chemotherapy, including anemia and severe dehydration with **hypernatremia** (high level of sodium in the blood). He received the first infusion of chemotherapy three days ago for widely metastasized adenocarcinoma of the bladder.

Code(s): _____

hypernatremia (hī-per-nā-trē′-mē-ə)

8. Katrina Huynh, age 36, sees Dr. Simmons to review the results of blood work and a thoracic CT scan after she complained of dyspnea and hemoptysis (coughing blood). She had a mastectomy a year ago due to breast cancer, and there has been no recurrence in the breast. However, Dr. Simmons tells her that tests show metastasis to the lung, and he discusses options for treatment.

Code(s): _____

9. Grace Batton, age 55, receives chemotherapy at Williton Medical Center for malignant **ependymoma** of the spinal cord (central nervous system tissue tumor).

Code(s): _____

10. Harriet Fenwick, age 46, undergoes surgery for removal of a mixed **meningioma** (tumor of the meninges, the membrane surrounding the brain and spinal cord). She previously complained of double vision and headaches and had a CT scan, which detected the benign tumor. Dr. Lombard, a neurologist, tells the patient that she may need radiation therapy to remove all of the tumor.

Code(s): _____

ependymoma (ep-en-də-mō′-mə)

meningioma (mə-nin-jē-′ō-mə)

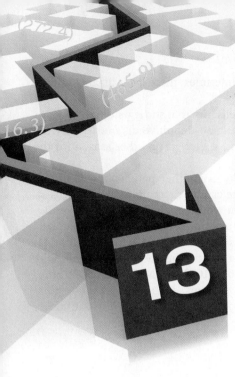

Signs, Symptoms, Ill-Defined Conditions, and Surgical or Medical Complications

13

Learning Objectives

After completing this chapter, you should be able to

- Spell and define the key terminology in this chapter.
- Define signs and symptoms, and describe how to code signs, symptoms, and ill-defined conditions.
- Describe types of surgical and medical complications and how to code them.
- Explain additional coding guidelines for coding complications of care.

Key Terms

ill-defined and unknown causes of morbidity and mortality

nonspecific abnormal findings

medical or surgical complications

INTRODUCTION

In Chapter 4, you learned how to code encounters for patients with signs and symptoms. You will have the opportunity for more coding practice in this chapter and will also learn to code medical and surgical complications. You may also notice that there are not as many new medical terms in this chapter because you have learned many of them in previous chapters. Some of the coding exercises in this chapter will ask you to define medical terms that you already learned. Also, continue to practice pronouncing medical terms so that you will be better prepared to work in healthcare when communicating with physicians and other clinicians. Remember, the more you practice, the more valuable your coding skills will be when you work for a healthcare provider!

"Practice does not make perfect, perfect practice makes perfect."

—VINCE LOMBARDI

SYMPTOMS, SIGNS, AND ILL-DEFINED CONDITIONS (ICD-9-CM CHAPTER 16—780–799)

Remember that you can assign codes for symptoms and signs when the provider has not established (confirmed) a related definitive diagnosis. A *sign* is objective evidence of disease that the physician discovers, commonly through an examination and testing. A *symptom* is subjective evidence of disease that the patient reports to the physician. In the physician's medical documentation of the patient's encounter, he will document signs,

ICD-9-CM codes in this chapter are from the ICD-9-CM 2012 code set from the Department of Health and Human Services, Centers for Disease Control and Prevention.

ICD-10-CM codes in this chapter are from the ICD-10-CM 2012 Draft code set from the Department of Health and Human Services, Centers for Disease Control and Prevention.

symptoms, and a definitive diagnosis, if one exists. Sometimes, there is no diagnosis, only a sign or a symptom.

For example, if Dr. Hoffman sees a patient who tells him that she is nauseated (symptom) and Dr. Hoffman cannot determine why, there is no definitive diagnosis, only the *symptom* of nausea. You would then code nausea because there is no other reason for the patient's encounter.

During a physical examination and discussion with another patient, Dr. Hoffman observes that the patient has memory loss (sign), but he cannot determine why. There is no definitive diagnosis, only the *sign* of memory loss. You would code memory loss because there is no other reason for the patient's encounter. Many times, when patients show signs and symptoms without definitive diagnoses, physicians treat the sign or symptom and then order additional tests or refer the patient to a specialist to find the underlying condition.

Signs and symptoms are classified to Chapter 16 in ICD-9-CM, as well as in other chapters of ICD-9-CM pertaining to specific organ systems, such as a gastrointestinal hemorrhage, a sign that you learned to code in Chapter 10 of this book. You can locate signs and symptoms in the Index by searching for the name of the condition.

Coding Signs and Symptoms

Do not assign codes for signs and symptoms that are an integral to (associated routinely with) a disease process, unless you are otherwise instructed by the classification in ICD-9-CM. This means that you should not assign codes for signs and symptoms which are part of a definitive diagnosis. It is assumed that if a patient has a specific diagnosis, then the patient also has the signs and symptoms that are typically associated with it, so you do not need to report them. If you are not sure whether signs and symptoms documented in the patient's chart are part of the specific diagnosis, then you should consult your medical references and query the physician for clarification.

For example, heartburn, arm pain, and shortness of breath are all symptoms of an MI. A patient with a definitive diagnosis of MI would not need additional codes assigned for heartburn, arm pain, and shortness of breath because it is known that these are common *symptoms* of the definitive diagnosis. It would be redundant to code these signs and symptoms of the MI. However, if a patient had the symptom of heartburn but the physician found no evidence of an MI or any other condition causing heartburn, then you *would* code heartburn because it is not associated with any other condition.

If a patient has other signs or symptoms that are *unrelated* to the definitive diagnosis, then you should code those signs and symptoms separately. For example, a patient complains to his physician that he has heartburn and a sore, swollen ankle. After an examination, the physician cannot find a cause for the heartburn but diagnoses the patient with an ankle sprain. He prescribes medication for heartburn, puts strapping on the ankle, and gives at-home care instructions for the ankle. In this case, heartburn is a symptom that you should code. The physician treated the patient for it, and it is unrelated to the definitive diagnosis of ankle sprain. You would also assign a code for the ankle sprain because the physician also treated it. You would not assign separate codes for the sore, swollen ankle because these are *symptoms* of the ankle sprain. It is understood that a patient with an ankle sprain has soreness and swelling. Again, when you are not sure if signs and symptoms are related to a disease, you should consult your medical references and query the physician.

Chapter 16 Guidelines for Signs and Symptoms

Chapter 16 in ICD-9-CM contains the following categories of symptoms, signs, and ill-defined conditions:

- 780–789—Symptoms
- 790–796—Nonspecific Abnormal Findings (signs)
- 797–799—Ill-defined and Unknown Causes of Morbidity and Mortality (signs and symptoms)

■ TABLE 13-1   **COMMON SIGNS AND SYMPTOMS FROM CHAPTER 16 OF ICD-9-CM**

Subcategory/Code	Sign/Symptom
780.2	Syncope
781.94	Facial droop
782.0	Numbness/tingling
783.5	Polydipsia
784.0	Headache
785.0	Tachycardia
786.05	Shortness of breath
787.0	Nausea and vomiting
788.31	Urge **incontinence**
789.0	Abdominal pain

incontinence (ĭn-kən′ tĭn-əns)—the inability to control urination or defecation

Pay close attention to the Excludes notes throughout Chapter 16 directing you elsewhere in ICD-9-CM. It is also important to refer to the note at the beginning of Chapter 16 because it provides valuable information on how to code for signs and symptoms, outlined as follows:

1. In general, categories 780–796 include the more ill-defined conditions and symptoms that point with equal suspicion to two or more diseases, or to two or more systems of the body, and without the necessary study of the case to make a final diagnosis.

2. Practically all the categories in this group could be designated as "not otherwise specified," "unknown etiology," or "transient."

3. Consult the Alphabetic Index to determine which symptoms and signs to code from Chapter 16 and which to code in more specific sections of ICD-9-CM.

4. Use residual subcategories ending in 9 for other relevant symptoms which are not classified in any other chapters.

5. The conditions and signs or symptoms included in categories 780–796 consist of

   - cases when the physician cannot render a more specific diagnosis, even after investigating all of the facts of the case.
   - signs or symptoms that existed at the time of the initial encounter but that proved to be transient and whose causes could not be determined.
   - cases when the physician made a provisional (temporary) diagnosis in a patient who left after the encounter and failed to return for further investigation or care.
   - cases that were referred elsewhere for investigation or treatment before the physician made a diagnosis.
   - cases in which a more precise diagnosis was not available for any other reason.
   - certain symptoms which represent important problems in medical care, which can be coded in addition to a definitive diagnosis.

Let's review each category of codes for signs and symptoms and then practice coding exercises.

Refer to ■ TABLE 13-1 for a list of subcategories and codes of common signs and symptoms from Chapter 16.

Refer to the following examples of patient encounters to determine whether to code symptoms.

Example 1: A symptom that is an integral part of another condition.
A patient with seizures has an encounter for an EEG, and the physician diagnoses the patient with epilepsy.

A seizure is a *symptom* of epilepsy, so you would not need to code the seizure. Only assign a code for epilepsy.

INTERESTING FACT: Ovarian Cancer Causes Common Signs and Symptoms

Each year, approximately 20,000 women in the United States get ovarian cancer. In the U.S., ovarian cancer is the eighth most common cancer and the fifth leading cause of cancer deaths. About 90% of women who get ovarian cancer are older than 40 years of age, with the greatest number of cases occurring in women aged 60 years or older. There is no way to predict who will have ovarian cancer, but there are often signs and symptoms, including:

✔ Pain in the pelvic or abdominal area

✔ Back pain

✔ Constant fatigue

✔ Bloating in the area below the stomach, which swells or feels full

✔ Changes in urinary habits, such as the frequent and immediate urge to pass urine

✔ Upset stomach or heartburn

✔ Abnormal vaginal bleeding or discharge (also common with cervical, uterine, and vaginal cancer)

✔ Constipation or diarrhea

(Department of Health and Human Services, Centers for Disease Control and Prevention, www.cdc.gov/cancer/ovarian/basic_info/symptoms.htm, www.cdc.gov/cancer/ovarian/, accessed 1/3/11.)

Example 2: A symptom without a definitive diagnosis. A patient experiences dizziness, and after examination, the physician cannot make a definitive diagnosis.

Assign a code for the symptom of dizziness, since it is the only reason for the encounter, and there is no definitive diagnosis.

Example 3: Symptoms related to a definitive diagnosis, and another symptom that is unrelated. A patient experiences an acute cough, sore throat, fatigue, and diarrhea. After examination, the physician determines that the patient has an upper respiratory infection but cannot explain the diarrhea. He treats the patient for both conditions.

Acute cough, sore throat, and fatigue are all *symptoms* of an upper respiratory infection, so you would not code them. Instead, assign a code for the upper respiratory infection. Assign an additional code for diarrhea, a symptom that is unrelated to the definitive diagnosis.

TAKE A BREAK

Good job! Let's take a break and then practice coding encounters with signs and symptoms.

Exercise 13.1   Symptoms, Signs, and Ill-Defined Conditions

Instructions: Review each patient's encounter, and determine the signs and/or symptoms. Then assign the appropriate codes to signs, symptoms, and/or the definitive diagnosis, referencing both the Index and the Tabular.

1. A new patient, Ruby Overby, age 16, sees Dr. Hoffman due to repeated seizures. Dr. Hoffman cannot determine the cause and refers Ruby to a neurologist.

   Code(s): _____

2. In 2009, Dr. Hoffman saw established patient Chad Ahmed, age 23, who complained of nausea, vomiting, and diarrhea. After testing, Dr. Hoffman diagnoses him with novel H1N1.

   Code(s): _____

3. Mildred Meekins, a 27-year-old established patient, sees Dr. Hoffman about daily headaches that she has had for quite some time. Dr. Hoffman says they might be migraines and refers her to a neurologist for further testing and evaluation.

   Code(s): _____

4. Jason Coon, age 62, sees his cardiologist, Dr. Woods, for congestive heart failure and says he has recently experienced shortness of breath. Dr. Woods notes that Mr. Coon has edema in his legs and decides to increase the dosage of the patient's diuretic.

   Code(s): _____

TAKE A BREAK *continued*

5. Dr. Hoffman sees established patient Nathan Cato, age 45, who complains of polydipsia, polyuria, and difficulty sleeping. His most recent blood test shows hyperglycemia (excessive sugar in the blood). Dr. Hoffman diagnoses Mr. Cato with diabetes. He also gives the patient an educational brochure with tips to promote better sleeping.

Code(s): _____

6. Mr. Leavitt takes his wife Arlene, age 62, to Williton Medical Center's ED after she complained of an irregular heartbeat, chest pain, and lightheadedness. Dr. Daniels, the ED physician, says that the cause is atrial fibrillation, for which she already takes medication. Dr. Daniels stabilizes her and recommends that she follow up with her cardiologist, Dr. Bergin, for a possible medication adjustment to regulate her heartbeat.

Code(s): _____

Nonspecific Abnormal Findings (790–796)

Nonspecific abnormal findings are test results that are unusual or irregular, including lab and radiology tests, **function studies**, blood pressure, and reflex tests. Examples of codes for nonspecific abnormal findings are listed next:

function studies (funk'shən)—a group of laboratory tests designed to give information about how an organ or body system functions

- 790.21—Elevated fasting glucose
- 790.91—Abnormal arterial blood gases
- 791.0—Proteinuria
- 793.80—Abnormal mammogram, unspecified
- 795.01—Papanicolaou smear of cervix with atypical squamous cells of undetermined significance [ASC-US]

Turn to categories 790–796 in the Tabular List of your ICD-9-CM manual to review more codes for nonspecific abnormal findings. Typically when patients' tests reveal nonspecific abnormal findings, the physician will order additional tests and/or examinations to determine a definitive diagnosis. When there is a definitive diagnosis, you should code it, rather than code nonspecific abnormal findings. If you are in doubt, then query the physician. There may also be nonspecific abnormal findings that do not require further testing, depending on the patient's situation. ICD-9-CM also classifies elevated or abnormal findings to other chapters in the Tabular List, besides Chapter 16.

You can locate codes for nonspecific abnormal findings in the Index under *Findings, (abnormal), without diagnosis,* or search under *Abnormal* or *Elevation.* ■ FIGURE 13-1 shows

Findings, (abnormal), without diagnosis (examination) (laboratory test) 796.4
  17-ketosteroids, elevated 791.9
  acetonuria 791.6
  acid phosphatase 790.5
  albumin-globulin ratio 790.99
  albuminuria 791.0
  alcohol in blood 790.3

Elevation
  17-ketosteroids 791.9
  acid phosphatase 790.5
  alkaline phosphatase 790.5
  amylase 790.5
  antibody titers 795.79
  basal metabolic rate (BMR) 794.7
  blood pressure (see also Hypertension) 401.9
      reading (incidental) (isolated) (nonspecific), no diagnosis of hypertension 796.2
  blood sugar 790.29
  body temperature (of unknown origin) (see also Pyrexia) 780.60

Figure 13-1 ■ Index entries for code 791.9.

code 791.9 for elevation of 17-ketosteroids, which you can find under the main terms *Findings* or *Elevation*. You can also search under the name of the condition that is abnormal (example: proteinuria) or the name of the test performed that showed abnormal results (example: mammographic).

TAKE A BREAK

Good work! Let's take a break and then practice coding encounters with nonspecific abnormal findings.

Exercise 13.2   Nonspecific Abnormal Findings

Instructions: Review each patient's encounter, and identify nonspecific abnormal findings. Then assign the appropriate codes to nonspecific abnormal findings or the definitive diagnosis, referencing both the Index and the Tabular.

1. Established patient Arthur Pauley, age 26, is concerned that he was exposed to HIV and requests a blood test from Dr. Hoffman. When he later meets with Dr. Hoffman to review the result, Dr. Hoffman says that it is inconclusive and that Mr. Pauley will need to undergo further testing.

   Code(s): _____

2. Dr. Hoffman tells Catheryne Ricketts, a 48-year-old established patient, that her mammogram is abnormal because it shows microcalcifications (small calcium deposits).

   Code(s): _____

3. Dr. Hoffman sees Sheila Emory, age 56, to review results of previous blood work (tests). He notes that her cholesterol is 239 mg/dL (milligrams per deciliter of blood), which is elevated. Dr. Hoffman discusses the results of her LDL and HDL levels (which refer to two types of cholesterol in the blood). After discussing

Mrs. Emory's lifestyle, Dr. Hoffman suggests that she make some changes, including losing weight, exercising more, and changing her dietary habits. They create a plan for improvement, and Mrs. Emory is to return for a follow-up visit and testing in three months.

   Code(s): _____

4. Sarah Lovelace, a 61-year-old new patient, sees Dr. Hoffman for an annual examination. The medical assistant measures Mrs. Lovelace's blood pressure at 140/100. Because the reading is high, Dr. Hoffman also measures the patient's blood pressure. The second reading is 145/100, and Dr. Hoffman documents it in the patient's record.

   Code(s): _____

5. Christine Hulse, age 50, sees Dr. Hoffman to review her recent lab work. Everything is normal except that Mrs. Hulse has low levels of Vitamin D. Dr. Hoffman says that there is no cause for alarm, but he asks her to take 50,000 IU (international units) of Vitamin D each week and to return for a recheck in eight weeks.

   Code(s): _____

6. Betti Thiel, age 24, sees Dr. Hoffman for follow up of an abnormal cervical Pap test result. He says that there is cytologic (pertaining to cells) evidence of a malignancy and suggests a retest to compare the findings.

   Code(s): _____

Ill-defined and Unknown Causes of Morbidity and Mortality (797–799)

Morbidity refers to illness, and mortality means death. **Ill-defined and unknown causes of morbidity and mortality** represent general descriptions of conditions that caused a patient's illness or death but do not provide specific information. Refer to the list that follows for examples of ill-defined and unknown causes. Then turn to categories 797–799 in your ICD-9-CM manual to review all of the conditions. Assign these codes as a *last resort*, only when there is no definitive diagnosis.

senility (sə-nil′ĭ-te)
- 797—**Senility** (mental and physical deterioration from aging) without mention of psychosis

- 798.0—Sudden infant death syndrome

asphyxia (as-fik′-sē-ə)
- 799.01—**Asphyxia** (lack of oxygen, too much carbon dioxide)

hypoxemia (hi pok-se′me-ə)
- 799.02—**Hypoxemia** (decreased oxygen in blood)

- 799.22—Irritability

- 799.24—Emotional **lability** (mood change)
- 799.3—**Debility** (weakness), unspecified
- 799.4—**Cachexia** (wasting away)
- 799.81—Decreased **libido** (sexual drive)

lability (lə-bil′ə-te)

debility (də-bil′ĭ-te)

cachexia (kə-kek′-se-ə)

libido (lĭ-be′do)

You can find these conditions in the Index by searching for the name of the condition (*irritability*) or description of the condition (*decreased libido*).

We have now reviewed all of the categories in Chapter 16 of the Tabular List: symptoms, nonspecific abnormal findings, and ill-defined and unknown causes of morbidity and mortality. Complete the next exercise, and we will then move on to coding surgical and medical complications.

TAKE A BREAK

Let's take a break and then practice coding encounters with ill-defined and unknown causes of morbidity and mortality.

Exercise 13.3 Ill-Defined and Unknown Causes of Morbidity and Mortality

Instructions: Review each patient's encounter, and assign codes for ill-defined and unknown causes of morbidity and mortality, referencing both the Index and Tabular.

1. Dr. Vader, a medical examiner, determines that one-month-old Latoya Hyder died of sudden infant death syndrome.

   Code(s): _____

2. Nellie Salgado, age 71, arrives at Williton's ED with various symptoms. Dr. Daniels examines Mrs. Salgado and orders tests. He determines that she is suffering from hypoxemia and hypotension, but he is unable to determine the cause.

   Code(s): _____

3. Dr. Hoffman sees Janet Ulmer, a 91-year-old established patient, and finds that she is in good health, aside from senility and generalized osteoarthritis due to aging.

   Code(s): _____

4. A neighbor finds Timothy Craig, age 54, dead in his apartment. He died alone of unknown causes, according to Dr. Vader, the medical examiner.

   Code(s): _____

5. An ambulance transports emaciated (severely thin) Daniel Lemoine, age 38, to Williton's ED after he collapsed at home. When his sister arrives in the ED, she tells Dr. Mills, the ED physician, that Mr. Lemoine's health has declined over the past year, since his wife died. He has lost interest in all activities, barely makes it to work each day, and has practically stopped eating. Mr. Lemoine dies in the ED, and Dr. Mills cannot find a cause. He documents cachexia in the patient's record.

   Code(s): _____

6. Martin Morris, age 29, sees Dr. Hunter, a psychiatrist, for extreme nervousness and irritability, which has continued for several weeks. Dr. Hunter schedules Martin for various tests to try to determine the underlying cause.

   Code(s): _____

COMPLICATIONS OF SURGICAL AND MEDICAL CARE, NOT ELSEWHERE CLASSIFIED (ICD-9-CM CHAPTER 17—996–999)

We already reviewed guidelines and coding for specific conditions in Chapter 17 of the Tabular List, such as various types of injuries and poisonings. We will now review surgical and medical complications that are also included in Chapter 17. It is important to understand that the **medical or surgical complications** classified to categories 996–999 are *unexpected* problems from surgery or medical care that are not classified anywhere else in ICD-9-CM. Keep in mind that ICD-9-CM classifies some complications in other chapters in addition to Chapter 17. Problems can be the result of medical negligence or incompetence and include infection, illness, disease, pain, or other symptoms. Keep in mind that all surgeries and medical procedures involve common complications and risks, which physicians should explain to patients before they receive care or undergo procedures. However, there are also complications that physicians and other clinicians do not anticipate, and these complications can cause serious problems for patients, even death.

You should assign codes for complications based on the provider's documentation of the relationship between the condition and the care or procedure. The guideline extends to any complications of care, regardless of the chapter in which the code is located. It is important to note that not all conditions that occur during or following medical care or surgery are classified as complications. There must be a cause-and-effect relationship between the care provided and the condition, and an indication in the documentation that it is a complication. Query the provider for clarification if the provider does not clearly document the complication.

When you are coding medical or surgical complications, you will need to identify whether a condition is *unexpected*, which the medical care or surgery caused (cause-and-effect), because it is then considered to be a complication, or whether it is a condition *common to* the care or surgery because it is then not considered to be a complication. Always query the physician to clarify any unclear medical documentation so that you can assign correct codes. Refer to the following examples to better understand the difference between conditions that patients may commonly experience after a procedure and unexpected complications.

> **Example 1:** A patient has surgery for a hernia repair. Common conditions following surgery include pain, infection, and fever. An unexpected complication is nerve damage.

mitral valve (mī′ trăl vălv)—the valve between the left atrium and left ventricle of the heart

> **Example 2:** A patient has **mitral valve** replacement surgery. Common conditions following surgery include nausea and vomiting. An unexpected complication is death.

appendectomy (ăp-ĕn-dĕk′ tō-mē)—surgical removal of the appendix

> **Example 3:** A patient has an **appendectomy**. Common conditions following surgery include infection of the surgical wound site and fever. An unexpected complication is excessive postoperative bleeding.

Keep in mind that medical/surgical complications do not have to occur *immediately after* a procedure. For example, if providers mistakenly left a surgical instrument inside a patient, then the patient may not have an immediate unexpected complication. It may take several days before the patient's body reacts to the foreign object.

To assign complication codes, search the Index for the main term describing the condition or search under the main term *complications* (■ FIGURE 13-2).

Figure 13-2 ■ Index entry for Complications.

Complications
  abortion NEC - see categories 634-639
  accidental puncture or laceration during a procedure 998.2
  amniocentesis, fetal 679.1
  amputation stump (late) (surgical) 997.60
    traumatic - see Amputation, traumatic
  anastomosis (and bypass) - see also Complications, due to (presence of) any device, implant, or graft classified to 996.0-996.5 NEC
    hemorrhage NEC 998.11
    intestinal (internal) NEC 997.4
      involving urinary tract 997.5
    mechanical - see Complications, mechanical, graft
    urinary tract (involving intestinal tract) 997.5
  anesthesia, anesthetic NEC (see also Anesthesia, complication) 995.22

You may also need to assign an additional code to more fully describe the patient's condition if the complication code is too general. Follow the *Use additional code* notes carefully, and also follow any Excludes notes in case you need to assign a code from elsewhere in ICD-9-CM.

In addition, you may need to assign an E code to further describe the patient's complication to show why it happened. You can locate E codes in the Index to External Causes of Injury and Poisoning by searching for the main term *reaction* and subterm *abnormal to or following medical or surgical procedure*. You can also search for the main term *reaction* or *misadventure*.

Search for *complications* in your ICD-9-CM manual to review the conditions listed to become more familiar with them. ICD-9-CM classifies surgical and medical complications to four different categories (996–999), outlined as follows, along with examples under each category:

996—Complications Peculiar to Certain Specified Procedures

Examples include mechanical complications of a

- cardiac pacemaker
- dialysis catheter
- urethral indwelling catheter.

997—Complications Affecting Specified Body Systems, Not Elsewhere Classified

Examples include

- cardiac arrest, during or resulting from a procedure
- ventilator-associated pneumonia
- intestinal obstruction due to a procedure
- infection of amputated stump.

998—Other Complications of Procedures, Not Elsewhere Classified

Examples include

- postoperative shock during or resulting from a surgical procedure
- accidental puncture or laceration during a procedure
- wound **dehiscence**
- acute reaction to foreign substance accidentally left in the patient during a procedure.

dehiscence (dē-hĭs′ ĕns)—separation or bursting open of a surgical wound

999—Complications of Medical Care, Not Elsewhere Classified

Examples include

- an embolism following **infusion**, **perfusion**, or **transfusion**
- an infection following infusion, injection, transfusion, or vaccination
- an incompatible blood transfusion
- other and unspecified misadventure of medical care.

infusion (in-fu′zhən)—introducing a substance, other than blood, into a vein

perfusion (pur-fŭ′ zhŭn)—passing of a fluid through spaces

transfusion (trăns-fū′ zhŭn)—transferring blood directly into the bloodstream

POINTERS FROM THE PROS: Interview with a Billing/Coding Specialist

Tonya McCall has worked for over a year for an orthopedic practice and surgery center where she codes fractures, consultations, and surgery center admissions. She also performs insurance billing, which requires her to understand Medicare's billing, coding, and reimbursement guidelines. Ms. McCall holds a certificate in coding and billing from a one-year postsecondary-school certificate program.

What are the most challenging aspects of your job?

Sometimes writing appeal letters for bills that have been denied because of certain procedure codes. You have to be very informative and explain why you billed certain procedure codes together and why it should be paid. Also, coding can be a challenge, as sometimes there are procedures I have not seen before, and I need to research and figure out what the best code would be for that particular procedure performed.

What advice would you like to give to coding students about working with different personalities?

I think it is the same in any place you are working, really, whether it is coding or billing or anything (else). You may have a personality you clash with, but my feeling is you are there to work, not to make a best friend. Be nice and respectful, but it is your job (to) do the best that you can.

What advice would you like to give to coding students to help them prepare to work successfully in the healthcare field?

Go into it with an open mind and ready to learn more because working gives you the experience that will make you a better coder.

(Used by permission of Tonya McCall.)

ADDITIONAL GUIDELINES FOR CODING COMPLICATIONS OF CARE

ICD-9-CM has additional guidelines for coding complications of care, which are as follows:

1. As with all procedural or postprocedural complications, base your code assignment on the provider's documentation of the cause-and-effect relationship between the condition and the procedure.

2. Assign codes under subcategory 996.8—*Complications of transplanted organ* for both complications and rejection of transplanted organs:

   • Only assign a transplant complication code if the complication affects the function of the transplanted organ.

   • Assign two codes to fully describe a transplant complication, a code from subcategory 996.8—*Complications of transplanted organ*, and a secondary code that identifies the complication.

   • Do not code complications as pre-existing conditions or conditions that develop after a transplant unless they affect the function of the transplanted organs.

3. Patients who have undergone a kidney transplant may still have some form of CKD because the kidney transplant may not fully restore kidney function. But just because the patient has CKD, this does not mean that the CKD is a *transplant complication*.

WORKPLACE IQ

You work as a medical coder for Dr. Sims, a family care physician. Today, you need to code an encounter for Mrs. Fitzwilliams, a 53-year-old established patient, who presents with complaints of headache, nausea, tinnitus, tingling of the left arm, and dizziness. After examination and discussion with the patient, Dr. Sims diagnoses the patient with labyrinthitis. He does not find any cause for the arm tingling and does not treat the patient for arm tingling.

What code(s) would you assign?

- Do not assign code 996.81—*Complications of transplanted organ, kidney* for post-kidney transplant patients who have CKD, unless the physician documents that CKD is a transplant complication, stating that the patient has transplant failure or rejection because of CKD.

- If the patient has a kidney transplant and CKD but the physician *does not document* that CKD is a transplant complication, then first assign a code from category 585—*Chronic kidney disease (CKD)* to identify the patient's stage of CKD. Then assign code V42.0 *Organ or tissue replaced by transplant, kidney* as an additional code. Assign additional codes for any other conditions that the patient has.

- Assign code 996.81—*Complications of transplanted organ, kidney* when the physician documents complications of a kidney transplant, such as transplant failure or rejection, or other transplant complication. Assign an additional code that more specifically describes the complication, such as CKD. Assign additional codes for any other conditions that the patient has.

- Query the provider if the documentation is unclear as to whether the patient has a complication of the transplant.

4. Assign code 997.31—*Ventilator associated pneumonia* only when the provider documents ventilator-associated pneumonia (VAP), pneumonia as the result of the patient's reliance on a mechanical ventilator for breathing (■ FIGURE 13-3):

- Assign an additional code to identify the organism (e.g., *Pseudomonas aeruginosa*, code 041.7).

- Do not assign an additional code from categories 480–484 to identify the type of pneumonia.

- Do not assign code 997.31—*Ventilator associated pneumonia* for a patient with pneumonia who is on a mechanical ventilator unless the provider states that the pneumonia is VAP. If the provider does not document VAP, assign a code from categories 480–484 to identify the type of pneumonia.

- Query the provider if the documentation is unclear as to whether the patient's pneumonia is a complication from the mechanical ventilator.

- A patient may be admitted with one type of pneumonia (e.g., code 481—*Pneumococcal pneumonia*) and subsequently develop VAP. In this instance, assign the principal diagnosis code from categories 480–484 for the pneumonia that was diagnosed at the time of admission. Assign code 997.31—*Ventilator associated pneumonia* as an additional code when the provider also documents the presence of VAP. Also assign codes for the organism that caused pneumonia.

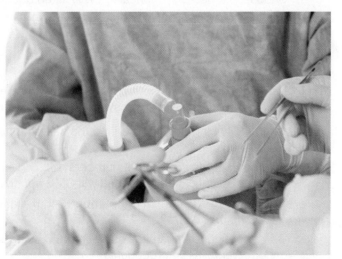

Figure 13-3 ■ Patient on ventilation.

Photo credit: Dmitriy Shironosov/Shutterstock.com.

TAKE A BREAK

Way to go! Let's take a break and then practice coding surgical and medical complications.

Exercise 13.4   Complications of Surgical and Medical Care, Not Elsewhere Classified, and Additional Guidelines for Coding Complications of Care

Instructions: Assign codes for medical and surgical complications, referencing both the Index and the Tabular. Include any applicable E codes. Refer to the guidelines outlined for assistance.

1. Physicians at Williton Medical Center treat Bryan Dotson, age 52, for hemorrhaging following an accidental puncture of his colon during a colonoscopy. (Hint: This case requires an E code.)

   Code(s): _____

2. Cheryl Shope, age 48, sees Dr. Ladwig, a plastic surgeon, due to leakage from her prosthetic breast.

   Code(s): _____

3. Mike Woodruff, a 65-year-old, sees Dr. Dew, an orthopedic surgeon, for monitoring a *Staphylococcus* infection at the site where Dr. Drew recently amputated the patient's great toe, a complication of peripheral autonomic diabetic neuropathy (diabetes complication causing nerve damage and possible amputation). The patient suffers from uncontrolled type II diabetes mellitus.

   Code(s): _____

4. Physicians at Williton Medical Center treat Lola Linares, age 47, for postoperative shock after she lost a large amount of blood during a hysterectomy. (Hint: This case requires an E code.)

   Code(s): _____

5. Dr. Mason, a nephrologist, admits George Danner, age 35, to Williton Medical Center for stage V CKD, which is a result of his body's rejection of a transplanted kidney.

   Code(s): _____

6. Dr. Daniels, an ED physician, admits Misty Driver, an 83-year-old, to Williton Medical Center for pneumococcal pneumonia and puts her on a mechanical ventilator. Her condition worsens, and Dr. Daniels documents that she also has VAP due to *Pseudomonas*.

   Code(s): _____

DESTINATION: MEDICARE

For the Medicare exercise, you will review surgical procedures in Medicare program transmittals from Medicare's National Coverage Determinations Manual. Program transmittals communicate new or changed policies and/or procedures that are incorporated into a specific program manual. Follow these instructions to access the specific manual:

1. Go to the website http://www.cms.gov.

2. From the top banner bar, choose *Regulations & Guidance*.

3. Choose *Manuals* from the options listed under *Guidance*.

4. Choose *Internet-Only Manuals (IOMs)* listed under *Manuals*.

5. Scroll down to *Publication #,* and choose *100-03 Medicare National Coverage Determinations (NCD) Manual*.

6. Scroll down to *Downloads*, and choose *Chapter—Coverage Determinations, Part 2*.

7. Use the search box at the top of the screen to type in the transmittal numbers that you need to review to answer the following questions.

Answer the following questions, using the search function (Ctrl + F) to find information that you need:

1. According to transmittal numbers 140.6, 140.7, and 140.8, under what three specific circumstances will CMS *not* cover services?

2. According to transmittal number 140.6, what is CMS's definition of a *wrong procedure*?

3. According to transmittal number 140.6, what is the definition of a *surgical or other invasive procedure*?

A LOOK AHEAD TO ICD-10-CM

ICD-10-CM classifies Symptoms, Signs, and Abnormal Clinical and Laboratory Findings, Not Elsewhere Classified (R00–R99) to Chapter 18. It classifies Complications of Surgical and Medical Care, Not Elsewhere Classified (T80–T88) to Chapter 19 (Injury, Poisoning, and Certain Other Consequences of External Causes).

ICD-10-CM added these guidelines for Complications of care, including:

- Pain due to medical devices
- Complication codes that include the external cause

Instructions: Refer to ICD-10-CM Official Guidelines for additional information. (Instructions for accessing the guidelines are in Appendix A of this text.) Then assign codes from ICD-10-CM, referencing both the Index and the Tabular.

1. A new patient, Ruby Overby, age 16, sees Dr. Hoffman due to repeated seizures. Dr. Hoffman cannot determine the cause and refers Ruby to a neurologist. Code(s):_____

2. A neighbor finds Timothy Craig, age 54, dead in his apartment. He died alone of unknown causes, according to Dr. Vader, the medical examiner. Code(s):_____

3. Betti Thiel, age 24, sees Dr. Hoffman for follow up of an abnormal cervical Pap test result. He says that there is cytologic evidence of a malignancy and suggests a retest to compare the findings. Code(s):_____

4. Dr. Vader, a medical examiner, determines that one-month-old Latoya Hyder died of sudden infant death syndrome. Code(s):_____

5. Cheryl Shope, age 48, sees Dr. Ladwig, a plastic surgeon, due to leakage from her prosthetic breast. Code(s):_____

6. Dr. Daniels, an ED physician, admits Misty Driver, an 83-year-old, to Williton Medical Center for pneumococcal pneumonia and puts her on a mechanical ventilator. Her condition worsens, and Dr. Daniels documents that she also has VAP due to *Pseudomonas.* Code(s):_____

CHAPTER REVIEW

Multiple Choice

Instructions: Circle one best answer to complete each statement.

1. You should assign codes for signs and symptoms when
   a. the provider documents them.
   b. they are an integral part of a disease process.
   c. the provider has not established a definitive diagnosis.
   d. the provider discovers them through a physical examination.

2. If you are not sure whether signs and symptoms documented in the patient's chart are part of the specific diagnosis, then you should
   a. query the physician.
   b. not code them.
   c. assign only the diagnosis.
   d. assign the signs, symptoms, and diagnosis.

3. The conditions and signs or symptoms included in categories 780–796 consist of all of the following *except*
   a. signs or symptoms existing at the time of the initial encounter that proved to be transient and whose causes could not be determined.
   b. cases referred elsewhere for investigation or treatment before the physician made a diagnosis.
   c. certain symptoms which represent important problems in medical care which can be coded in addition to a definitive diagnosis.
   d. signs and symptoms that should be coded as part of a definitive diagnosis.

4. Which of the following symptoms is *not* related to an upper respiratory infection?
   a. Acute cough
   b. Diarrhea
   c. Fatigue
   d. Sore throat

5. Test results that are unusual or irregular are classified as
   a. function studies.
   b. nonspecific abnormal findings.
   c. definitive diagnoses.
   d. signs and symptoms.

6. An example of an ill-defined and unknown cause of morbidity and mortality is
   a. elevated fasting glucose.
   b. polydipsia.
   c. VAP.
   d. sudden infant death syndrome.

7. All of the following are examples of mechanical complications *except*
   a. VAP.
   b. breast implant.
   c. cardiac pacemaker.
   d. dialysis catheter.

8. An unexpected complication of surgery for a hernia repair would be
   a. pain.
   b. infection.
   c. nerve damage.
   d. fever.

9. You should assign a code for VAP when
   a. a patient with pneumonia is also on a mechanical ventilator.
   b. the infectious organism is *Pseudomonas aeruginosa*.
   c. the patient's pneumonia is caused by poor ventilation.
   d. the provider documents pneumonia as a result of the patient's reliance on a mechanical ventilator.

10. You should code *complications of transplanted organ, kidney* when
    a. the physician documents a transplant complication, such as transplant failure or rejection.
    b. CKD is present.
    c. the patient has a pre-existing condition.
    d. all of the above.

Coding Assignments

Instructions: Assign ICD-9-CM code(s) to the following cases, referencing both the Index and Tabular. Many of the coding cases contain E codes.

1. Dr. Nichols treats Roy Shipley, age 56, at Williton Medical Center's pain management clinic for pain related to adenocarcinoma of the stomach.

   Code(s): _____

2. Daniel Lemoine, a 35-year-old patient, sees Dr. Hoffman due to epigastric (over the stomach) pain, but Dr. Hoffman cannot determine the cause. He refers Mr. Lemoine to a gastroenterologist.

   Code(s): _____

3. Dr. Lightner, a pulmonologist, sees Lula Sparks, age 21, to review an X-ray of her right lung, which reveals a shadow. He is not sure what the shadow represents and states that he will monitor her over the coming months to determine its exact cause or if it dimishes.

   Code(s): _____

4. Tony Hancock, a 61-year-old, sees Dr. Hoffman to discuss the abnormal results from his liver function test.

   Code(s): _____

5. Rosemary McCombs brings her daughter Marie, age four, to Dr. Flynn, a pediatrician, due to nausea and vomiting that has lasted more than 24 hours.

   Code(s): _____

6. Dr. Flynn sees Anita Ruano, 18 months old, for a fever of 105° that started the day after she received a DTaP immunization (a vaccine that protects against *diphtheria*—a contagious, often fatal respiratory disease; *tetanus*—a rare, fatal disease caused by bacteria, often entering the body through a puncture wound; and *pertussis*—whooping cough). Dr. Flynn determines that the vaccination caused the fever (also called postvaccination fever).

   Code(s): _____

7. Dr. Moir, a urologist, sees Chris Larkins, age 70, for hematuria, pressure in the abdomen, and burning during urination. Dr. Moir determines that Mr. Larkins has acute cystitis (an infection or inflammation of the urinary bladder). Symptoms began after the patient underwent a catheterization procedure. The cause of the patient's cystitis is bacteria introduced by a Foley catheter (a flexible, hollow tube inserted into a body cavity to introduce or withdraw fluid, also called an indwelling catheter).

   Code(s): _____

8. Dr. Dunford, a general surgeon at Williton, calls for the code team (a group of clinicians trained in life-saving measures, including advanced cardiac life support) when William Hambrick, age 78, goes into cardiac arrest during an open cholecystectomy (gall bladder removal). After much time and effort, they are able to resuscitate him.

   Code(s): _____

9. Dr. Galindo, a thoracic surgeon, sees Jill Byrne, age 69, due to chest pain and oozing from her sutures following a mitral valve repair (repair of heart valve). After conducting an examination, Dr. Galindo states that Ms. Byrne's internal sternotomy (incision into the sternum, or breastbone) closure has burst due to poor healing. He immediately admits her to Williton Medical Center.

   Code(s): _____

10. Brandon Gonzalez, age 37, sees Dr. Hoffman for pain in his leg following an infusion procedure. Dr. Hoffman determines that the pain is due to thrombophlebitis (inflammation of a vein with a thrombus—blood clot) in the femoral vein (largest vein in the groin).

    Code(s): _____

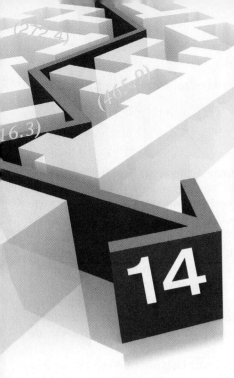

Complications of Pregnancy, Childbirth, and the Puerperium, Perinatal Conditions, Congenital Anomalies

14

Learning Objectives

After completing this chapter, you should be able to

- Spell and define the key terminology in this chapter.
- Describe the phases of pregnancy and labor.
- Discuss how to code complications of pregnancy, childbirth, and the puerperium.
- Explain how to code normal and complicated deliveries on the mother's record.
- Describe how to code for the birth status of an infant on the infant's record.
- Discuss how to code perinatal conditions on the infant's record.
- Explain how to code congenital anomalies on the infant's record.
- Explain when to assign V codes for obstetrics cases and related conditions.
- Review ICD-9-CM Official Guidelines for complications of pregnancy, childbirth, and the puerperium, perinatal conditions, and congenital anomalies.

Key Terms

amniotic sac
delivery
fetus
gestation
labor

placenta
pregnancy
prenatal
trimesters
zygote

INTRODUCTION

Recall from Chapter 10 that you learned about obstetrics and gynecology when you reviewed the female reproductive system and related diagnoses. In this chapter, you will take those skills a step further; in fact, you will use all of your previous coding skills! Coding complications of pregnancy and childbirth can be very challenging because there are many different guidelines and rules to follow, including correct fifth-digit assignment, as well as assigning multiple codes to one episode of care or encounter. It is important to take time to carefully review ICD-9-CM Official Guidelines that pertain to assigning codes for these complications. You will learn to assign codes to both the mother's record and the infant's record. If this sounds like a lot to learn, then you are right—it is! Look at how far you have progressed already and how much you know!

ICD-9-CM codes in this chapter are from the ICD-9-CM 2012 code set from the Department of Health and Human Services, Centers for Disease Control and Prevention.
ICD-10-CM codes in this chapter are from the ICD-10-CM 2012 Draft code set from the Department of Health and Human Services, Centers for Disease Control and Prevention.

"They can conquer who believe they can. He has not learned the first lesson in life who does not every day surmount a fear."—RALPH WALDO EMERSON

PREGNANCY

embryo (em′bre-o)

Pregnancy occurs when a male sperm fertilizes a female ovum (egg), and it is implanted in the uterine lining. Refer to Figure 10-22 in Chapter 10 to review the female reproductive system. The fertilized egg is called a **zygote**. A zygote becomes an **embryo** (an early stage of development) within two weeks and remains an embryo for up to eight weeks (■ FIGURE 14-1).

The embryo is referred to as a **fetus** from week eight until birth. The **placenta** (a membrane that lines the uterine wall and contains the fetus) produces the hormone human chorionic gonadotropin (hCG), which causes pregnancy symptoms. The placenta provides blood to the fetus, carrying oxygen and nutrients to it through the umbilical cord. The fetus grows within an **amniotic sac** containing amniotic fluid. The temperature inside the sac is higher than the mother's body temperature, and the sac protects the fetus throughout development.

Pregnancy, also called the period of **gestation**, typically lasts about 40 weeks, or 9 ½ months. Pregnancies are measured in three-month increments called **trimesters**, which represent continued stages of development.

amenorrhea (ă-mĕn ō-rē′ a)

Symptoms of pregnancy include delayed menstruation or **amenorrhea** (absence of menstruation), spotty bleeding, fatigue, tender or swollen breasts, nausea (morning sickness), backaches, headaches, frequent urination, and craving specific foods. Physicians diagnose pregnancy through an examination; obtaining the patient's history, including information about her menstrual cycle; and reviewing urine and blood tests to determine the presence and quantity of the hCG hormone and ultrasound to view the fetus.

Pregnant patients schedule regular **prenatal** (before birth) visits with their obstetrician/gynecologists (OB/GYNs). During these visits, the provider examines the patient, monitors vital signs of mother and fetus; discusses the mother's diet, exercise, and medications; checks the fetal position inside the uterus; and determines if there are any complications for either the mother or fetus. During prenatal visits, physicians also perform

Figure 14-1 ■ A 30-day-old human embryo. During the fifth week, the eyes and ear structures start to form, the brain develops into five areas, some cranial nerves become visible, and the arm and leg buds become visible.

Photo credit: Christopher Meade/ Shutterstock.com.

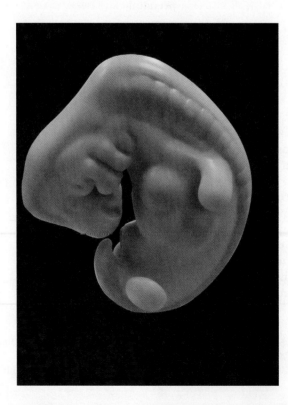

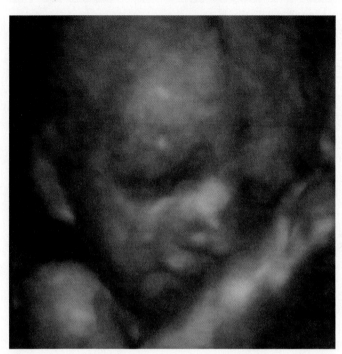

Figure 14-2 ■ Colored 3-D ultrasound scan of a fetus.
Photo credit: Science Photo Library/Custom Medical Stock Photo.

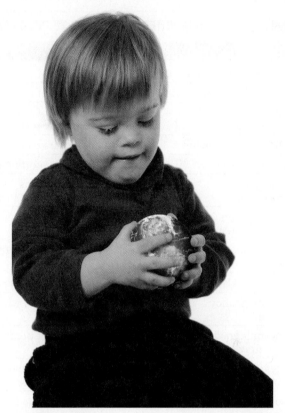

Figure 14-3 ■ Child with Down syndrome. The main physical features are slanted eyes, a flat nose on a round head, and abnormalities of the palms of the hands and the soles of the feet. Children with Down syndrome usually have a below-average I.Q. of 30 to 80.
Photo credit: R. Gino Santa Maria/Shutterstock.com.

ultrasounds to assess the rate of growth of the fetus and discover any abnormalities (■ FIGURE 14-2). They can also perform **amniocentesis**, a test where the physician removes amniotic fluid from the uterus and tests it to determine if the fetus has abnormalities, such as Down's syndrome (■ FIGURE 14-3) and **spina bifida**.

amniocentesis (ăm-nĭ-ō -sĕn-tĕ′ sĭs)

spina bifida (spi′nə bif'-ə-də)—a congenital opening in the spinal column from which the spinal membranes and/or spinal cord protrude

    Labor begins when the cervix dilates (opens), and the uterus contracts, which leads to **delivery**, when the fetus is born. Labor has three stages:

- Stage 1—The cervix dilates until it is fully dilated at 10 centimeters.
- Stage 2—The fetus moves through the birth canal and vagina, and birth occurs.
- Stage 3—The placenta separates from the uterine wall and is expulsed through the vagina, along with the remains of the umbilical cord (also called afterbirth).

    A **neonatologist** is a physician specializing in newborn care, and a **pediatrician** is a physician specializing in the care of infants, children, and adolescents.

neonatologist (ne-o-na-tol′ə-jist)

pediatrician (pe-de-ə-trĭ′shən)

COMPLICATIONS OF PREGNANCY, CHILDBIRTH, AND THE PUERPERIUM (ICD-9-CM CHAPTER 11—630–679)

ICD-9-CM classifies conditions that are related to pregnancy, childbirth, and the **puerperium** (the first six weeks after delivery) to Chapter 11. Before you begin coding these conditions, it is important to become familiar with common terms and their definitions (■ TABLE 14-1). You will find many of the terms in medical documentation, as well as in Chapter 11. Refer to Table 14-1 as you read coding instructions in this chapter and as you work through the coding exercises.

puerperium (pu-ər-pēr′e-əm)

■ **TABLE 14-1** **COMMON TERMS RELATED TO PREGNANCY, CHILDBIRTH, AND THE PUERPERIUM**

Term	Definition
abortion—illegally induced	The premature end of a pregnancy using illegal methods
abortion—legally induced	The premature end of a pregnancy using legal methods
abortion—missed	The premature end of a pregnancy where the fetus dies and the fetus and placenta remain in the uterus; can cause serious complications for the patient
abortion—spontaneous	Abortion that occurs naturally (miscarriage)
abortion—threatened	Uterine bleeding or spotting that is serious but does not terminate the pregnancy
cephalopelvic disproportion	When the mother's pelvis cannot expand enough for the baby to fit through the pelvis, or the baby's head is misaligned in such a way that it cannot fit through the pelvis
cesarean section (c-section) (sə-zar′e-ən)	Surgical delivery of the fetus through an incision into the abdominal cavity and the uterus
congenital anomaly (kən-jen′ĭ-təl ə-nom′ə-le)	An abnormality (anomaly) that is present at birth (congenital)
eclampsia (ĕ-klămp′ sē-ă)	Convulsions and coma during or immediately after pregnancy
ectopic pregnancy (ĕk-tŏp′ĭk)	A pregnancy that occurs when the fertilized egg is implanted outside the uterus
elderly multigravida (mul-te-grav′ĭ-də)	Second or subsequent pregnancy in a woman who will be 35 years or older at the time of delivery
elderly primigravida (pri-mĭ-grav′ĭ-də)	First pregnancy in a woman who will be 35 years or older at the time of delivery
episiotomy (ə-piz-e-ot′o-me)	Surgical incision into the perineum and vagina to prevent traumatic tearing during delivery
false labor	Pains resembling normal labor pains that occur at irregular intervals and are not accompanied by dilation of the cervix
fetal lie	The position of the fetus within the uterus, specifically, the angle of the fetus's spine in relation to the mother's spine. If both spines are at the same angle, it is called a cephalic lie. If the angle of the fetus's spine is different from the angle of the mother's spine, it is called an unstable lie.
fetal manipulation	When the physician moves the fetus to facilitate delivery
full term	Gestational duration of 37–40 completed weeks
grand multiparity (mul-te-par′ĭ-te)	A woman who has had five or more pregnancies, all of which resulted in viable fetuses
gravida (also called gravid, gravidarum, examples: multigravida, gravida 1, gravida 2) (grăv′ ĭ-dă)	Used to record a patient's obstetrical history to indicate the number of pregnancies, including the current one
habitual aborter (hə-bich'-ə wəl)	Spontaneous abortion in three or more consecutive pregnancies
hyperemesis gravidarum (hī-pĕr-ĕm′ ĕ-sĭs grav-ə-dar'-əm)	Excessive vomiting during pregnancy
in utero (u′tər-o)	Inside the uterus
intrapartum	During delivery
intrauterine (ĭn-tră-ū′ tĕr-ĭn)	Within the uterus
labor—threatened	Labor after 22 weeks but before 37 completed weeks of gestation, without delivery
lactation	The period of time that the mother produces and secretes milk
large-for-dates (also called large for gestational age—LGA)	Any infant who is above the 90th percentile for gestational age in head circumference, body weight, or length

■ **TABLE 14-1**   *continued*

Term	Definition
light-for-dates (also called small for gestational age—SGA)	Any infant who is below the 10th percentile for gestational age in head circumference, body weight, or length
low birthweight (LBW)	An infant weighing less than 2,500 grams (5 pounds, 8 ounces) at birth
malposition	An abnormal position of the top of the fetus' head relative to the mother's pelvis
malpresentation	Any position of the fetus during labor other than vertex (back of head down and forward)
molar pregnancy	Pregnancy in which the placenta transforms into an abnormal mass of cysts, rather than a pregnancy
neonate	Newborn infant of 28 days or fewer
obstructed labor	Labor that is hindered by a structure or other physical element
para (also called parity, examples: multipara, para 1, para 2, para 1-0-0-1) (par′ə)	Designation of the number of pregnancies that have resulted in the birth of viable infants
perinatal (per-i-na′tal)	The time period of approximately five months before birth to one month following birth
perineal laceration (per-ĭ-ne′əl)	A tear in the area between the vulva and anus
peripartum	Time period from the last month of pregnancy to five months after delivery
placenta previa (prē′vē-ă)	An obstetric condition in which the placenta is improperly implanted in the lower portion of the uterus
postpartum	Time period beginning just after delivery and continuing for six weeks
post-term	A pregnancy of more than 40 completed weeks of gestation
pre-eclampsia (prē ē-klămp′ sē-ă)	A serious complication of pregnancy characterized by increasing hypertension, proteinuria, and edema
presentation	The position of the fetus in the birth canal
presentation—breech	During labor, presentation of the buttocks or feet of the fetus, instead of the head
presentation—brow	Presentation of the forehead of the fetus during labor
presentation—cephalic (sə-fal′ik)	Presentation of any part of the fetal head during labor, including occiput (back of the head), forehead, or face
presentation—occipital (ok′sĭ-pət əl)	Presentation of the back of the fetal head during labor
presentation—shoulder	Presentation of the shoulder of the fetus during labor
presentation—transverse or oblique (o-blek′)	Presentation when the position of the fetus is at approximately a 45-degree angle to the long axis of the mother
preterm (premature)	A pregnancy of fewer than 37 completed weeks of gestation
primigravida (gravida 1) (pri-mi-grăv′ ĭ-dă)	A woman who is pregnant for the first time
primipara (para 1) (pri-mip′ə-rə)	A woman who has had one pregnancy that resulted in a viable infant
prolonged	Labor lasting more than 18 hours
retained placenta	A placenta that is not delivered after the birth of the infant
term	A specific period of time, usually 37–40 weeks when used to refer to pregnancy
toxoplasmosis (tŏks-ō-plăs-mō′sĭs)	An infection by a protozoan organism, with few or no symptoms in the mother; can be transmitted to the fetus through the placenta, potentially causing serious damage to the central nervous system
true labor	Expulsion of the fetus from the uterus, through the vagina, into the outside world

Fifth-Digit Assignments for Episode of Care

In order to code many complications of pregnancy, childbirth, and the puerperium, you have to add a fifth digit for the episode of care. Remember from Chapter 1 that an episode of care is when a patient receives care, such as an individual office visit or a hospital admission from the date of the admission to the date of discharge. For several categories of complications, you need to assign fifth digits to show the patient's current episode of care for which you are assigning codes. The following categories require fifth digits to show the current episode of care:

- 640–649—Complications Mainly Related to Pregnancy
- 651–659—Normal Delivery, and Other Indications for Care in Pregnancy, Labor, and Delivery
- 660–669—Complications Occurring Mainly in the Course of Labor and Delivery
- 670–676—Complications of the Puerperium
- 678–679—Other Maternal and Fetal Complications

To choose the correct fifth digit, first determine whether the delivery occurred during the current episode of care. If it did, then choose from fifth digits 1 or 2. If it did not, then choose from fifth digits 0, 3, or 4. Fifth digit choices for the episode of care are as follows:

0—unspecified as to episode of care or not applicable

- The medical documentation does not state the episode of care, or the episode of care does not apply to the patient's condition.

1—delivered, with or without mention of antepartum condition

antepartum (an-te-pahr′təm)

- *The delivery occurred* during the current episode of care. The medical documentation may also describe an **antepartum** condition (before delivery), but it does not have to in order to assign 1. Delivery means that the physician delivered the baby during the episode of care that you are coding. You cannot assign a fifth digit of 1 for *subsequent* episodes of care because the delivery only happens once.

2—delivered, with mention of postpartum complication

The delivery occurred during the current episode of care, and the physician also documented a postpartum condition (after delivery). Delivery means that the physician delivered the baby during the episode of care that you are coding. You cannot assign a fifth digit of 2 for *subsequent* episodes of care because the delivery only happens once.

3—antepartum condition or complication

The delivery did not occur during the current episode of care. The patient has an antepartum condition or complication.

4—postpartum condition or complication

The delivery did not occur during the current episode of care. The patient has a postpartum condition or complication.

You cannot choose from all of the available fifth digits for every subcategory code. ICD-9-CM lists fifth-digit choices in brackets underneath each subcategory (■ FIGURE 14-4).

Note that codes in Figure 14-4 from category 640 were for hemorrhage *in early pregnancy* with fifth-digit choices for the episode of care of 0, 1, or 3. You could never assign a fifth digit of 2 or 4 to these conditions because 2 is for a delivery encounter with a postpartum complication, and 4 is for a postpartum condition. Be very careful before assign-

---

4th **640 Hemorrhage in early pregnancy**

Requires fifth digit; valid digits are in [brackets] under each code. See beginning of section 640-
    649 for definitions.
Includes: hemorrhage before completion of 22 weeks' gestation

5th **640.0**   **Threatened abortion**
[0,1,3]

5th **640.8**   **Other specified hemorrhage in early pregnancy**
[0,1,3]

5th **640.9**   **Unspecified hemorrhage in early pregnancy**
[0,1,3]

Figure 14-4 ■ Fifth-digit choices for subcategories 640.0–640.9.

---

ing fifth digits to ensure that you first review the choices available for each subcategory
and completely understand the meaning of medical terms .

TAKE A BREAK

*Wow! There were a lot of terms! Let's take a break and then
review common terms related to pregnancy, childbirth, and the
puerperium.*

Exercise 14.1   Complications of Pregnancy, Childbirth, and the Puerperium

Instructions: Fill in each blank with the best answer, choosing from the list of words and terms provided.

1. _____ designates the number of pregnancies that have resulted in the birth of a viable infant.

2. _____ is a serious complication of pregnancy that is characterized by increasing hypertension, proteinuria, and edema.

3. Uterine bleeding or spotting that is serious but does not terminate the pregnancy is called _____.

4. A _____ is a malformation that is present at birth.

5. _____ refers to any position of the fetus during labor other than vertex.

6. Labor lasting more than 18 hours is considered to be _____.

abortion—spontaneous	gravida
abortion—threatened	malpresentation
eclampsia	obstructed labor
congenital anomaly	para
disproportion	post term
episiotomy	pre-eclampsia
malposition	prolonged

Sequence Chapter 11 Codes First

For complications of pregnancy, childbirth, or the puerperium, Chapter 11 codes in the Tabular List take precedence over codes in other ICD-9-CM chapters. This means that when coding complications of pregnancy, childbirth, or the puerperium, you will always assign codes from Chapter 11 first to the mother's record, followed by codes from other chapters, as needed. Never assign Chapter 11 codes for the newborn's record. Turn to Chapter 11 of the Tabular List in your ICD-9-CM manual to become familiar with the conditions listed.

For example, sometimes Chapter 11 describes conditions in a general way, not a specific one. You still need to assign the general code from Chapter 11, and then you will need to assign additional codes from elsewhere in ICD-9-CM that represent the *specific* condition. Note that when the physician documents a complication, it must be related to pregnancy, childbirth, or the puerperium in order for you to sequence first a code from Chapter 11.

Refer to the following example of a pregnancy complication to better understand when to assign two codes.

Example: Mrs. O'Neil, a 28-year-old established patient, sees Dr. Wooten, an OB/GYN, for a prenatal visit to discuss the results of her complete blood count (CBC) lab test. Dr. Wooten diagnoses the patient with iron deficiency anemia, which the pregnancy caused. He tells the patient that she does not have enough iron in her diet, and he suggests an iron supplement.

Iron deficiency anemia is a common pregnancy complication. Without taking iron supplements, it is unlikely that the mother will receive enough iron from her diet alone. When you code this encounter, you need to ensure that the code for anemia indicates that it is related to the pregnancy, which means first assigning a code from Chapter 11.

To find iron deficiency anemia, search the Index for the main term *anemia*, subterm *iron deficiency*, and subterm *of or complicating pregnancy*, then cross-reference code 648.2 to the Tabular (■ FIGURE 14-5). Note that you can also find pregnancy complications by searching under *Pregnancy, complicated (by)*.

Notice that code 648.2 requires a fifth digit, with the range of 0–4 listed in brackets under the code. You can find fifth-digit choices at the beginning of the section for categories 640–649. You already reviewed these choices earlier in this chapter (■ FIGURE 14-6).

Remember that when choosing a fifth digit for a complication, first determine whether the encounter involved a delivery (fifth digits 1 and 2). In this case it did not, so you can eliminate fifth digits 1 and 2. Next, determine if the encounter was

---

Anemia 285.9

    iron (Fe) deficiency 280.9
        due to blood loss (chronic) 280.0
            acute 285.1
        of or complicating pregnancy 648.2
        specified NEC 280.8

| 4th | **648 Other current conditions in the mother classifiable elsewhere, but complicating pregnancy, childbirth, or the puerperium** |

Use additional code(s) to identify the condition

Requires fifth digit; valid digits are in [brackets] under each code. See beginning of section 640-649 for definitions.

Includes: the listed conditions when complicating the pregnant state, aggravated by the pregnancy, or when a main reason for obstetric care

Excludes: those conditions in the mother known or suspected to have affected the fetus (655.0-655.9)

    5th **648.2 Anemia**
    [0-4]
        Conditions classifiable to 280-285

Figure 14-5 ■ Index entry for iron deficiency anemia of pregnancy with code 648.2 cross-referenced to the Tabular.

The following fifth-digit subclassification is for use with categories 640-649 to denote the current episode of care:

0 unspecified as to episode of care or not applicable

1 delivered, with or without mention of antepartum condition

Antepartum condition with delivery

Delivery NOS (with mention of antepartum complication during current episode of care)

Intrapartum

obstetric condition (with mention of antepartum complication during current episode of care)

Pregnancy, delivered (with mention of antepartum complication during current episode of care)

2 delivered, with mention of postpartum complication

Delivery with mention of puerperal complication during current episode of care

3 antepartum condition or complication

Antepartum obstetric condition, not delivered during the current episode of care

4 postpartum condition or complication

Postpartum or puerperal obstetric condition or complication following delivery that occurred:

during previous episode of care

outside hospital, with subsequent admission for observation or care

Figure 14-6 ■ Fifth-digit choices for code 648.2.

for an antepartum or postpartum condition. Since the condition happened during pregnancy, it is an antepartum condition, and the fifth digit is 3. The final code assignment from Chapter 11 is 648.23.

But you cannot stop coding there. Remember that for a complication of pregnancy, childbirth, or the puerperium, codes from Chapter 11 take precedence over all other codes in ICD-9-CM, meaning that you sequence Chapter 11 codes first. For Mrs. O'Neil's pregnancy complication, sequence first code 648.23 from Chapter 11. However, 648.23 does not fully describe the patient's condition. It only describes *anemia*, not *iron deficiency anemia*. You will need to assign an *additional code* that describes iron deficiency anemia.

Notice in Figure 14-5 that there is an instruction under category 648 to *Use additional code(s) to identify the condition,* and there is another instruction under code 648.2 which shows that the anemia is *Conditions classifiable to 280–285.* This range of categories is where you can find iron deficiency anemia. Go back to Figure 14-5 to the Index entry for anemia. Notice the subterm for iron deficiency, which lists code 280.9. Let's cross-reference code 280.9 to the Tabular. Category 280 represents iron-deficiency anemias, so check all codes listed under category 280 to ensure that you choose the correct code (■ FIGURE 14-7).

Code 280.1 represents the fact that the patient does not have enough iron in her diet, which correlates to the medical documentation.

For this encounter, assign two codes, 648.23 (anemia, complicating pregnancy, antepartum condition) and 280.1 (iron deficiency anemia secondary to inadequate dietary intake). Keep in mind that if Chapter 11 contained a code for *iron deficiency* anemia, then you would only need to assign *one* code to the patient's encounter. It is because of the fact that code 648.23 in Chapter 11 is *not specific enough* that you need to assign an *additional code* with greater specificity to show that the anemia is iron deficiency.

Figure 14-7 ■ Codes listed under category 280 for iron deficiency anemias.

4th 280 Iron deficiency anemias

Includes: anemia:
    asiderotic
    hypochromic-microcytic
    sideropenic

Excludes: familial microcytic anemia (282.49)

280.0 Secondary to blood loss (chronic)
    Normocytic anemia due to blood loss

Excludes: acute posthemorrhagic anemia (285.1)

280.1 Secondary to inadequate dietary iron intake

280.8 Other specified iron deficiency anemias
    Paterson-Kelly syndrome
    Plummer-Vinson syndrome
    Sideropenic dysphagia

280.9 Iron deficiency anemia, unspecified
    Anemia:
        achlorhydric
        chlorotic
        idiopathic hypochromic
        iron [Fe] deficiency NOS

TAKE A BREAK

Good job! Let's take a break and then practice coding pregnancy complications. Take your time while you review and code these exercises to ensure that you code correctly.

Exercise 14.2 **Sequence Chapter 11 Codes First**

Instructions: Assign codes for pregnancy complications to the following patient encounters, using the Index and the Tabular. These encounters *do not involve deliveries.* Be sure to determine if the patient's condition is antepartum, postpartum, or unspecified before choosing the fifth digit.

1. Della Ryan, age 35, gravida 3, para 2, sees Dr. Wooten, her OB/GYN, near the end of her second trimester with vaginal bleeding. After examination, Dr. Wooten states that she has placenta previa and hemorrhage. He tells her to stay home in bed and states that he will closely monitor her care, adding that she may need to deliver by cesarean section.

   Code(s): _____

2. Tanya Oberg, age 21, gravida 1, para 0, sees Dr. Wooten for a prenatal visit. She is 12 weeks pregnant and has long-standing essential hypertension. Dr. Wooten says that he needs to monitor her blood pressure closely while she is pregnant. He adjusts the dosage of her hypertension medication.

   Code(s): _____

3. During a postpartum visit with Cora Stanley, age 32, Dr. Wooten finds an abscess of her right breast. He prescribes an antibiotic and says he will monitor the abscess to see if surgery will be necessary.

   Code(s): _____

4. Dr. Wooten diagnoses Sylvia Whitcomb, a 23-year-old, with postpartum deep venous phlebothrombosis in the tibial vein of her left leg.

   Code(s): _____

5. Marilyn Delacruz, age 30, gravida 2, para 1, sees Dr. Wooten for a prenatal visit in her 12th week. He is following her pernicious anemia, and blood work shows that it is under control.

   Code(s): _____

6. Deanna Westmoreland, age 24, gravida 1, para 0, is in her 28th week of pregnancy and sees Dr. Wooten for Rhesus isoimmunization (Rh incompatibility) because she has Rh-negative blood and her fetus has Rh-positive blood. Dr. Wooten explains that this means that the patient's immune system will produce antibodies to attack the fetal blood cells as foreign bodies. If this

TAKE A BREAK *continued*

happens, then the infant will be born with Rhesus disease, which causes serious health problems. Treatment is for Mrs. Westmoreland to receive immune globulin that will stop her body from producing antibodies against the Rh-positive blood of her fetus. The patient agrees to receive Rho(D) immune globulin treatment on Monday.

Code(s): _____

DELIVERY

A delivery encounter occurs when the mother *actually delivers* the baby *during* the episode of care that you are coding. Remember that you only code a delivery once because it only happens once.

When you are coding a delivery encounter and there is a liveborn infant, assign codes for the delivery on the mother's (maternal) record and for the birth on the infant's (newborn) record. You also need to determine whether either patient had a complication and then assign code(s) for complication(s).

Coding Delivery on the Mother's Record

When coding a mother's chart for a delivery encounter, first determine whether the delivery was normal or complicated. A normal delivery means that the mother is admitted for a full-term normal delivery. She delivers a single, healthy infant without any complications antepartum, during the delivery, or postpartum, during the delivery episode. A normal delivery meets the following criteria:

- Requires minimal or no assistance
- Occurs with or without an episiotomy
- Occurs without fetal manipulation or instrumentation
- Is spontaneous
- Features a **cephalic** presentation (head first)   cephalic (sə-fal′-ik)
- Is vaginal
- Produces a full-term, *single* liveborn

If any of these criteria are not met, it is a complicated delivery. For example, deliveries by c-section, deliveries that produce multiple births, and birth presentations other than cephalic are all complicated deliveries.

Follow these guidelines to code a delivery for the mother's record:

- Sequence first a code from Chapter 11 which represents *either a normal delivery* (650) or *a delivery complication* (630–676). You can never code both a normal delivery and a complication during the same encounter because the patient can only have one or the other.

- For a normal delivery, sequence any additional codes to identify conditions affecting the patient that are not related to the pregnancy or to a delivery complication. For a delivery complication, sequence any additional codes to identify further complications.

- In cases of cesarean delivery (complicated), the principal diagnosis should be the condition that is established after study to be responsible for the patient's admission. If the patient is admitted with a condition that causes the c-section delivery, then that condition is the principal diagnosis. If the patient is admitted with a condition that is *unrelated* to the problem that causes the c-section delivery, then the principal diagnosis is the reason for the admission. The principal diagnosis is not the reason for the c-section.

- You can still assign code 650 (normal delivery) as the principal diagnosis if the patient had a complication at some point during her pregnancy, but the complication is not present at the time of the admission for delivery.

Figure 14-8 ■ Category V27—*Outcome of delivery.*

> **4th** | **V27 Outcome of delivery**
>
> Note: This category is intended for the coding of the outcome of delivery on the mother's record.
> V27.0 Single liveborn
> V27.1 Single stillborn
> V27.2 Twins, both liveborn
> V27.3 Twins, one liveborn and one stillborn
> V27.4 Twins, both stillborn
> V27.5 Other multiple birth, all liveborn
> V27.6 Other multiple birth, some liveborn
> V27.7 Other multiple birth, all stillborn
> V27.9 Unspecified outcome of delivery
> routine prenatal care (V22.0-V23.9)

- For every delivery encounter, sequence an additional code from category V27 that represents the *outcome of delivery* (infants born) (■ FIGURE 14-8). Assign codes from category V27 once on the mother's record, never on the infant's record.

- Code V27.0 (single liveborn) is the *only* outcome of delivery code that you can assign with code 650 for a normal delivery. Remember, multiple births mean that there is a complication, and the delivery is not considered to be a normal one.

Coding Mother's Record—Normal Delivery, No Complications   Refer to the following example to code the mother's record for an episode of care for a *normal delivery without complications.*

Example: Ms. Hyde, a 24-year-old, gives birth vaginally to a full-term single live-born at Williton Medical Center. Dr. Wooten delivers the infant without complications for the mother or infant.

Assign two codes to the mother's record, one representing a normal delivery, and the other representing the outcome of delivery (single liveborn). For the first code, search the Index for the main term *delivery* and subterm *completely normal case*, which refers you to category 650 in the Tabular (■ FIGURE 14-9). (For a delivery complica-

> **Delivery**
>
> completely normal case - see category 650
>
> ---
>
> **650   Normal delivery**
>
> Delivery requiring minimal or no assistance, with or without episiotomy, without fetal manipulation [e.g., rotation version] or instrumentation [forceps] of a spontaneous, cephalic, vaginal, full-term, single, live-born infant. This code is for use as a single diagnosis code and is not to be used with any other code in the range 630-676.
> Use additional code to indicate outcome of delivery (V27.0)
> Excludes: breech delivery (assisted) (spontaneous) NOS (652.2)
> delivery by vacuum extractor, forceps, cesarean section, or breech extraction, without specified complication (669.5-669.7)

Figure 14-9 ■ Index entry for a normal delivery with category 650 cross-referenced to the Tabular.

```
Outcome of delivery
     multiple birth NEC V27.9
          all liveborn V27.5
          all stillborn V27.7
          some liveborn V27.6
          unspecified V27.9
     single V27.9
          liveborn V27.0
          stillborn V27.1
     twins V27.9
          both liveborn V27.2
          both stillborn V27.4
          one liveborn, one stillborn V27.3


     ┌──────────────────────────────────────────────┐
     │ 4th  V27  Outcome of delivery                  │
     └──────────────────────────────────────────────┘

     Note:   This category is intended for the coding of the outcome of delivery on the
             mother's record.

             V27.0 Single liveborn
```

Figure 14-10 ■ Index entry for outcome of delivery with category V27 cross-referenced to the Tabular.

tion, search the Index for *delivery, complicated by* or *delivery,* and a subterm for the type of delivery.)

Next, assign an additional code for the outcome of delivery. ICD-9-CM lists a *use additional code* note under category 650 instructing you to assign a code from subcategory V27.0. You can also search in the Index for the main term *outcome of delivery,* subterm *single,* and subterm *liveborn* (■ FIGURE 14-10).

Category V27 provides you with a note that reminds you that you should only assign codes from V27 to the mother's record. For this episode of care, assign two codes, 650 (normal delivery) and V27.0 (single liveborn).

Coding Mother's Record—Delivery with Complications   A complication of pregnancy, childbirth, or the puerperium is a condition that affects the pregnancy or a condition that the pregnancy affects or causes. Refer to the following example to code the mother's record for an episode of care for a *complicated delivery.*

Example: Mrs. McMahon, a 30-year-old, spontaneously gives birth to liveborn twins at Williton Medical Center. Dr. Wooten delivers the infants.

You can immediately tell that this delivery is a complicated one because the patient gave birth to twins. A normal delivery is for a single liveborn, not twins. Instead of assigning code 650 (normal delivery) as the first code, assign a code representing the complication (twins). Then assign an additional code to show the outcome of delivery (twins, both liveborn).

For the first code, search the Index for the main term *delivery* and subterm *twins.* Then cross-reference code 651.0 to the Tabular (■ FIGURE 14-11).

Assign a fifth digit of 1 to indicate *delivered, with or without mention of antepartum condition,* since the episode of care involved a delivery, and there was no mention of an antepartum condition. Code 651.01 is the final code assignment for the complication.

Next, assign an additional code for the outcome of delivery. Search the Index for the main term *outcome of delivery,* subterm *twins,* and subterm *both liveborn,* and cross-reference code V27.2 to the Tabular (■ FIGURE 14-12).

For this episode of care, assign two codes, 651.01 (delivery of twins) and V27.2 (twins, both liveborn).

Delivery

twins NEC 651.0
    with fetal loss and retention of one fetus 651.3
    delayed delivery (one or more mates) 662.3
    following (elective) fetal reduction 651.7
    locked mates 660.5

The following fifth-digit subclassification is for use with categories 651-659 to denote the current episode of care:
    0 unspecified as to episode of care or not applicable
    1 delivered, with or without mention of antepartum condition
    2 delivered, with mention of postpartum complication
    3 antepartum condition or complication

4th 651 Multiple gestation

    5th 651.0 Twin pregnancy
    [0,1,3]
    Excludes: fetal conjoined twins (678.1)

Figure 14-11 ■ Index entry for delivery of twins with code 651.0 cross-referenced to the Tabular.

Outcome of delivery
    multiple birth NEC V27.9
        all liveborn V27.5
        all stillborn V27.7
        some liveborn V27.6
        unspecified V27.9
    single V27.9
        liveborn V27.0
        stillborn V27.1
    twins V27.9
        both liveborn V27.2
        both stillborn V27.4
        one liveborn, one stillborn V27.3

4th V27 Outcome of delivery

Note: This category is intended for the coding of the outcome of delivery on the mother's record.

    V27.0 Single liveborn

    V27.1 Single stillborn

    V27.2 Twins, both liveborn
For this episode of care, assign two codes: 651.01 (delivery of twins), and V27.2 (twins, both liveborn).

Figure 14-12 ■ Index entry for outcome of delivery, twins, with code V27.2 cross-referenced to the Tabular.

TAKE A BREAK

Good work! Let's take a break and then practice coding normal and complicated deliveries on the mother's record.

Exercise 14.3 Delivery

Instructions: Assign codes for normal and complicated deliveries to the mothers' records, referencing both the Index and the Tabular. Identify any antepartum or postpartum conditions which will affect your fifth digit assignment. Refer to the guidelines we previously discussed, as well as the examples for normal and complicated deliveries.

1. Under the supervision of Dr. Wooten, her OB/GYN, Candy Fields, age 25, gives birth to baby boy William, who makes a cephalic presentation and quick delivery. Aside from requesting an epidural injection (pain medication injected into the spine) and having an episiotomy, she has no problems. William's Apgar scores★ are 7 and 9.

   ★The Apgar score, invented by Dr. Virginia Apgar, is a method for evaluating newborns on five criteria: Activity, Pulse, Grimace, Appearance, and Respiration. Newborns are evaluated twice, once at one minute after birth, and again at five minutes after birth. Scores range from 0 to 10.

   Code(s): _____

2. Dr. Wooten performs a cesarean section on Danielle Fix, age 31, gravida 2, para 2. She had a c-section with her first child, and the second child presents with cephalopelvic disproportion. Cassandra, a healthy baby girl, is born.

   Code(s): _____

3. Dr. Wooten attends the labor and delivery of Mary Rose, age 23. Labor is obstructed due to a brow presentation of the baby (instead of the baby holding his head tucked down on his chest, his head is slightly extended). Dr. Wooten successfully converts the presentation to cephalic. Mrs. Rose then vaginally delivers Brandon, a healthy boy. Brandon's Apgars are 7 and 9. Dr. Wooten transfers the mother and baby to the postpartum department in good condition.

   Code(s): _____

4. Maryann Avila, age 32, gravida 1, para 3, gives birth to Marcus, Martin, and Marcella. Dr. Wooten delivers the infants, who are all alive and healthy.

   Code(s): _____

5. Carolyn Smith, age 29, successfully gives birth to baby Carl vaginally, with Dr. Wooten's supervision. She then begins hemorrhaging due to a retained placenta.

   Code(s): _____

6. Dr. Wooten admits Laurie Ferrell, a 33-year-old, for severe pre-eclampsia and premature labor in her 32nd week of pregnancy. He delivers a healthy baby, Lawrence, via c-section.

   Code(s): _____

BIRTH STATUS OF THE INFANT

Recall that coding deliveries involves assigning codes to both the mother's record and the infant's record. The infant has to be liveborn in order for you to code the record. Whereas you always assign a V code to the mother's record as an *additional* code, always assign a V code to the infant's record as the *first* code. When a delivery results in a liveborn infant, sequence first a code from category V30–V39 to show the circumstances or status of birth (single liveborn; twin, mate liveborn, etc.) (■ FIGURE 14-13).

Figure 14-13 ■ Categories
V30–V39—*Liveborn infants.*

LIVEBORN INFANTS ACCORDING TO TYPE OF BIRTH (V30-V39)

Note: These categories are intended for the coding of liveborn infants who are consuming health care [e.g., crib or bassinet occupancy].

The following fourth-digit subdivisions are for use with categories V30-V39:
  0 Born in hospital
  1 Born before admission to hospital
  2 Born outside hospital and not hospitalized

The following two fifths-digits are for use with the fourth-digit .0, Born in hospital:
   0 delivered without mention of cesarean delivery
   1 delivered by cesarean delivery

V30	Single liveborn
V31	Twin, mate liveborn
V32	Twin, mate stillborn
V33	Twin, unspecified
V34	Other multiple, mates all liveborn
V35	Other multiple, mates all stillborn
V36	Other multiple, mates live- and stillborn
V37	Other multiple, unspecified
V39	Unspecified

Categories V30–V39 also require a *fourth digit* to identify *where* the infant was born:

0 Born in hospital

1 Born before admission to hospital

2 Born outside hospital and not hospitalized

In addition, for hospital deliveries (fourth digit 0), you also need to assign a *fifth digit* to identify if the delivery was cesarean:

0 delivered without mention of cesarean delivery

1 delivered by cesarean delivery

For every infant's chart, assign the first code from category V30–V39. Assign additional codes from

- ICD-9-CM Chapter 15—Certain Conditions Originating in the Perinatal Period (760–779) for perinatal conditions
- ICD-9-CM Chapter 14 —Congenital Anomalies (740–759) for problems diagnosed at birth

Coding Infant's Record—Normal Birth, No Complications

To better understand how to code a birth *without complications* on the infant's record, let's revisit Ms. Hyde's episode of care for delivery in the following example.

Example: Ms. Hyde, a 24-year-old, gives birth vaginally to a single liveborn at Williton Medical Center. Dr. Wooten delivers the infant without complications. The infant has no perinatal conditions or congenital anomalies.

You already coded the mother's record. For the infant's record, search the Index for the main term *newborn*, subterm *single*, and subterm *born in hospital (without mention of cesarean delivery or section)*. Then cross-reference code V30.00 to the Tabular (■ FIGURE 14-14).

Newborn (infant) (liveborn)
  single
    born in hospital (without mention of cesarean delivery or section) V30.00
      with cesarean delivery or section V30.01
    born outside hospital
      hospitalized V30.1
      not hospitalized V30.2

Figure 14-14 ■ Index entry for single liveborn born in the hospital with code V30.00 cross-referenced to the Tabular.

LIVEBORN INFANTS ACCORDING TO TYPE OF BIRTH (V30-V39)

Note: These categories are intended for the coding of liveborn infants who are consuming health care [e.g., crib or bassinet occupancy].

The following fourth-digit subdivisions are for use with categories V30-V39:
    0 Born in hospital
    1 Born before admission to hospital
    2 Born outside hospital and not hospitalized

The following two fifths-digits are for use with the fourth-digit .0, Born in hospital:
    0 delivered without mention of cesarean delivery
    1 delivered by cesarean delivery

V30	Single liveborn
V31	Twin, mate liveborn
V32	Twin, mate stillborn
V33	Twin, unspecified
V34	Other multiple, mates all liveborn
V35	Other multiple, mates all stillborn
V36	Other multiple, mates live- and stillborn
V37	Other multiple, unspecified
V39	Unspecified

Notice that you assign the *fourth digit 0* to show that the infant was born in the hospital, and the *fifth digit 0* to show that the delivery was not by cesarean section. The final code assignment is V30.00 with no additional codes assigned because the infant was normal and had no diagnosed conditions (complications).

Now that you coded a normal birth for the infant's record, you will next learn how to code births with perinatal conditions and congenital anomalies.

TAKE A BREAK

Let's take a break and then practice assigning codes to the infant's record for normal births without complications.

Exercise 14.4 Birth Status of the Infant

Instructions: Assign codes for normal births to the infants' records only (not the mothers' records), referencing both the Index and the Tabular. Refer to the previous example for assistance.

1. Dr. Wooten decides to perform cesarean delivery for Jennie Solano, age 20, due to the unstable lie of baby girl, Jeannie. Jeannie's Apgars are 7 and 8. The infant has no perinatal conditions or congenital anomalies.

  Code(s): _____

2. Brandi Gilmer, a 26-year-old, delivers baby boy Bruce and his brother Bob vaginally after occipital presenta-

continued

TAKE A BREAK *continued*

tions. Bruce's Apgars are 8 and 10, and Bob's are 8 and 9. The infants have no perinatal conditions or congenital anomalies.

Code(s): _____

3. Dr. Wooten supervises the delivery of baby boy Jesse to Jessica Essex, age 28, after obstructed labor due to transverse presentation (shoulder or back down). Baby Jesse experiences no problems as a result of the difficult labor.

Code(s): _____

4. Dr. Wooten performs a cesarean section on Carrie Newton, age 31, due to a previous c-section and high risk for cephalopelvic disproportion. Twins are born, Cassandra and Maxwell.

Code(s): _____

5. Dr. Wooten delivers a healthy boy, Adam. His mother, Carolyn Williams, age 23, gives birth vaginally, and Dr. Wooten uses forceps for assistance due to shoulder presentation. Adam's Apgars are 7 and 9. Dr. Wooten transfers the mother and baby to the postpartum department in good condition.

Code(s): _____

6. Wanda Terrazas, a 25-year-old, is traveling in a taxi when she goes into labor. On the way to Williton Medical Center, the taxi driver, Ronald, stops because Ms. Terrazas is about to deliver. With assistance from a 911 dispatcher, Ronald delivers a baby boy who makes a cephalic presentation, and it is a quick delivery. Ronald then drives mother and baby to Williton, where they are both admitted. Mrs. Terrazas decides to name the baby Ronald.

Code(s): _____

CERTAIN CONDITIONS ORIGINATING IN THE PERINATAL PERIOD (ICD-9-CM CHAPTER 15—760–779)

Chapter 15 contains codes for perinatal conditions, which can begin within five months before or within a month after birth. Many times, the mother's condition or activities that she performs cause perinatal conditions in the fetus. Examples include hypertension and malnutrition, drinking alcohol, smoking, or taking prescribed or illegal drugs, which can create medical problems for the fetus or infant. Perinatal conditions include premature birth, injuries that occur at birth (cerebral or intracranial trauma), apnea, infections, hemorrhage, and tachycardia. Perinatal conditions are *not* congenital anomalies, which are birth defects, discussed later in this chapter. ICD-9-CM divides Chapter 15 into the following two sections of categories:

- 760–763—Maternal Causes of Perinatal Morbidity and Mortality—Assign codes from these categories when the mother has a condition that affects the fetus or infant, and the physician documents the fetus or newborn condition.

- 764–779—Other Conditions Originating in the Perinatal Period—Assign codes from these categories when the physician documents a condition in the fetus or infant, which the mother did not cause.

There is an *Includes* note at the beginning of Chapter 15 in ICD-9-CM which states that conditions included in the chapter originate in the perinatal period, even though death or morbidity occurs later. There is also a *Use additional code* note instructing you to assign an additional code to further specify any condition in the chapter that is described too generally.

When perinatal conditions are present *at delivery*, assign codes for the conditions *secondary* to the V code (V30–V39) showing birth status (single liveborn; twin, mate liveborn, etc.).

Coding Infant's Record—Birth Status with Perinatal Conditions

Refer to the following example to code an infant's record for an episode of care involving delivery and perinatal conditions.

Example: Mrs. Hewitt, a 22-year-old, vaginally delivers an infant, John, at Williton Medical Center. The infant is premature at 30 weeks and weighs 1,500 grams (3 pounds, 5 ounces). (Normal birth weight for a full-term infant is 2,800–4,800 grams (6 pounds, 3 ounces to 10 pounds, 9 ounces). Dr. Wooten diagnoses the infant with mild jaundice.

Jaundice is a condition where the infant's blood contains too much bilirubin, a yellow pigment found in red blood cells. The liver produces bilirubin and it excretes in **bile**. Too much bilirubin in the bloodstream causes jaundice, a yellowing of the skin and sclera (whites of the eyes), which can lead to additional medical problems. Jaundice commonly occurs in premature infants because their livers are not fully developed enough to properly excrete bilirubin.

jaundice (jawn′ dĭs)

bile—a yellow or greenish fluid the liver secretes, which drains into the small intestine

Coding the episode of care for infant John's record involves assigning four different codes, including *three codes* for perinatal conditions:

- Sequence first a code from V30–V39 to show birth status (single liveborn)
- Sequence second a code for prematurity, including low birthweight
- Sequence third a code for weeks of gestation
- Sequence last a code for jaundice

Birth Status

You already know how to code the birth status. For the first code, search the Index for the main term *newborn*, subterm *single*, subterm *born in hospital (without mention of cesarean delivery or section)*. Then cross-reference code V30.00 to the Tabular for final code assignment.

Prematurity/Low Birth Weight

Sequence second a code for prematurity by searching the Index for the main term *premature*, subterm *birth*, then cross-reference code 765.1 to the Tabular (■ FIGURE 14-15).

Notice that you need to assign a fifth digit to show the birth weight. For this infant, the birth weight was 1,500 grams, so assign fifth digit 6. The final code assignment for prematurity is 765.16.

Did you see the *Use additional code* note under subcategory 765.1? It reminds you to assign an additional code for the weeks of gestation from codes 765.20–765.29. Let's look at assigning this code next.

Weeks of Gestation

Sequence third a code showing 30 weeks of gestation for the premature infant. You can go directly to 765.20–765.29, or search the Index for the main term *newborn*, subterm *gestation*, subterm *29–30 completed weeks*. Then cross-reference code 765.25 to the Tabular for final code assignment (■ FIGURE 14-16).

Jaundice

Sequence last a code for jaundice by searching in the Index for the main term *jaundice*, subterm *fetus or newborn*, subterm *due to*, and subterm *preterm delivery*, then cross-reference code 774.2 to the Tabular (■ FIGURE 14-17).

Final code assignments for this infant's record are as follows:

1. V30.00 (birth status—single liveborn, born in hospital, without cesarean)
2. 765.16 (prematurity/low birth weight—preterm infant, 1,500 grams)
3. 765.25 (weeks of gestation—30 weeks)
4. 774.2 (jaundice—newborn, associated with preterm delivery)

Premature - see also condition
  beats (nodal) 427.60
    atrial 427.61
    auricular 427.61
    postoperative 997.1
    specified type NEC 427.69
    supraventricular 427.61
    ventricular 427.69
birth NEC 765.1

OTHER CONDITIONS ORIGINATING IN THE PERINATAL PERIOD (764-779)

The following fifth-digit subclassification is for use with category 764 and codes 765.0 and 765.1 to denote birthweight:
    0 unspecified [weight]
    1 less than 500 grams
    2 500-749 grams
    3 750-999 grams
    4 1,000-1,249 grams
    5 1,250-1,499 grams
    6 1,500-1,749 grams
    7 1,750-1,999 grams
    8 2,000-2,499 grams
    9 2,500 grams and over

`4th`   **765 Disorders relating to short gestation and low birthweight**

Requires fifth digit. See beginning of section 764-779 for codes and definitions.
Includes: the listed conditions, without further specification, as causes of mortality, morbidity, or additional care, in fetus or newborn

`5th`   **765.0**   **Extreme immaturity**
[0-9]
Note: Usually implies a birthweight of less than 1,000 grams.

Use additional code for weeks of gestation (765.20-765.29)

`5th`   **765.1**   **Other preterm infants**
[0-9]
Note: Usually implies birthweight of 1,000-2,499 grams.
    Prematurity NOS
    Prematurity or small size, not classifiable to 765.0 or as "light-for-dates" in 764
Use additional code for weeks of gestation (765.20-765.29)

Figure 14-15 ■ Index entry for premature birth with code 765.1 cross-referenced to the Tabular.

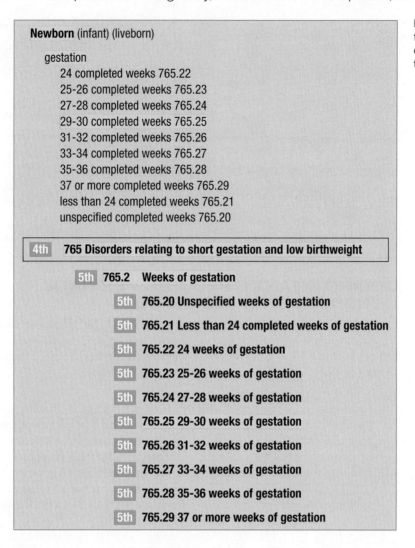

Figure 14-16 ■ Index entry for 30 weeks gestation with code 765.25 cross-referenced to the Tabular.

Newborn (infant) (liveborn)

gestation
    24 completed weeks 765.22
    25-26 completed weeks 765.23
    27-28 completed weeks 765.24
    29-30 completed weeks 765.25
    31-32 completed weeks 765.26
    33-34 completed weeks 765.27
    35-36 completed weeks 765.28
    37 or more completed weeks 765.29
    less than 24 completed weeks 765.21
    unspecified completed weeks 765.20

4th   **765 Disorders relating to short gestation and low birthweight**

    5th **765.2** **Weeks of gestation**

      5th **765.20 Unspecified weeks of gestation**

      5th **765.21 Less than 24 completed weeks of gestation**

      5th **765.22 24 weeks of gestation**

      5th **765.23 25-26 weeks of gestation**

      5th **765.24 27-28 weeks of gestation**

      5th **765.25 29-30 weeks of gestation**

      5th **765.26 31-32 weeks of gestation**

      5th **765.27 33-34 weeks of gestation**

      5th **765.28 35-36 weeks of gestation**

      5th **765.29 37 or more weeks of gestation**

Figure 14-17 ■ Index entry for newborn jaundice with code 774.2 cross-referenced to the Tabular.

Jaundice (yellow) 782.4
    acholuric (familial) (splenomegalic) (see also Spherocytosis) 282.0
        acquired 283.9
    breast milk 774.39
    catarrhal (acute) 070.1
        with hepatic coma 070.0
        chronic 571.9
        epidemic - see Jaundice, epidemic
    cholestatic (benign) 782.4
    chronic idiopathic 277.4
    epidemic (catarrhal) 070.1
        with hepatic coma 070.0
        leptospiral 100.0
        spirochetal 100.0
    febrile (acute) 070.1
        with hepatic coma 070.0
        leptospiral 100.0
        spirochetal 100.0
    fetus or newborn 774.6
        due to or associated with

            preterm delivery 774.2

Figure 14-17 ■ *continued*

> **4th** **774 Other perinatal jaundice**
>
> **774.2 Neonatal jaundice associated with preterm delivery**
> Hyperbilirubinemia of prematurity
> Jaundice due to delayed conjugation associated with preterm delivery
>
> Final code assignments for this infant's record are as follows:
>
> 1. V30.00 (birth status - single liveborn, born in hospital, without cesarean)
>
> 2. 765.16 (prematurity/low birth weight - preterm infant, 1,500 grams)
>
> 3. 765.25 (weeks of gestation - 30 weeks)
>
> 4. 774.2 (jaundice - newborn, associated with preterm delivery)

CODING INFANT'S RECORD—PERINATAL CONDITION ONLY (NO BIRTH)

An infant can be born with a perinatal condition and continue to receive treatment for the condition during subsequent encounters, for weeks, months, or years. Therefore, you can still assign codes from Chapter 15 for a perinatal condition even if the patient's encounter did not involve birth. Refer to the following example.

fetal alcohol syndrome—birth defects, often including facial disfigurement, mental retardation, and central nervous system problems, that are seen in infants whose mothers consumed large volumes of alcohol while pregnant

Example: Miss Workman takes her 10-month-old baby, Rachel, to see Dr. Wooten for the first time. The mother is concerned that her baby has developmental problems. After an interview with the mother, Dr. Wooten finds that she drank alcohol while pregnant. Dr. Wooten examines the child and diagnoses her with **fetal alcohol syndrome**. He discusses recommendations for more testing to further diagnose additional disorders.

To code Rachel's condition, search the Index for the main term *syndrome* and subterm *fetal alcohol*, and cross-reference code 760.71 to the Tabular.

TAKE A BREAK

That was a lot to remember! Let's take a break and then practice assigning codes to the infant's record for perinatal conditions.

Exercise 14.5 Certain Conditions Originating in the Perinatal Period

Instructions: Assign codes to infants' records only (not the mothers' records) for episodes or care for births with perinatal conditions, and for encounters for perinatal conditions only. Reference both the Index and the Tabular. Refer to previous examples for assistance.

1. Gina Holbrook, age 21, goes into labor at 34 weeks gestation. Dr. Wooten has been treating her for pre-eclampsia and decides to deliver via cesarean section because the baby is not receiving enough oxygen. Dr. Wooten documents a premature birth. Baby Gerald weighs 1,990 grams (4 pounds, 6 ounces) and has Apgars of 6 and 7. A nurse takes him to the NICU (Neonatal Intensive Care Unit) for evaluation of breathing and provides continuous positive airway pressure (CPAP) to help him breathe.

   Code(s): _____

2. Andrea Hussey is born four weeks early to Alice, age 25, via vaginal delivery with Dr. Wooten in attendance. She weighs 2,176 grams (4 pounds, 13 ounces) and has jaundice as a result of her preterm delivery. Dr. Wooten orders phototherapy (light therapy treatment for jaundice) for Andrea and expects a full recovery for both with discharge in a day.

   Code(s): _____

3. Dr. Wooten performs a cesarean section on Regina Wilkie, age 29, who is a heroin addict. Baby Richard is diagnosed with drug withdrawal syndrome and needs to be weaned off heroin. (Hint: This case involves a poisoning.)

   Code(s): _____

4. During labor, Pam Fonseca's full-term fetus develops bradycardia (slow heart rate). Dr. Wooten uses forceps to assist in the delivery of baby Paul. The birth is successful without further incident, but baby Paul is taken

TAKE A BREAK *continued*

to the NICU for monitoring and treatment of his heart rate, which continues to be low.

Code(s): _____

5. Monique Cotton, age 20, brings three-week-old baby, Michael, to see Dr. Flynn, a pediatrician, due to foul-smelling urine. Dr. Flynn diagnosis Michael with a urinary tract infection due to *E. coli*.

Code(s): _____

6. Dr. Flynn sees baby Douglas Fogg in the office for neonatal diabetes. Douglas was born two weeks ago via vaginal delivery in the hospital.

Code(s): _____

CONGENITAL ANOMALIES (ICD-9-CM CHAPTER 14—740–759)

Chapter 14 of ICD-9-CM contains codes for congenital anomalies, mental or physical problems that the infant has at birth. You may also hear people refer to congenital anomalies as birth defects. Congenital anomalies can occur for a variety of reasons, including a condition that the mother developed during pregnancy, and it negatively affects the infant, such as an infection, hereditary factors, drinking alcohol, smoking, or other problems that were the result of a complicated pregnancy. Common congenital anomalies include **cleft palate**, Down's syndrome, **polydactyly** (■ FIGURE 14-18), and hydrocephalus. Congenital anomalies are not perinatal conditions, which can occur before, during, or after birth, such as a hemorrhage or an infection. Many times, congenital anomalies result in a physical change, such as extra or missing fingers or toes, or an organ that is not completely formed, like the heart.

cleft palate (kleft pal'ət)—a congenital anomaly; an elongated opening through the roof of the mouth into the nasal cavity

polydactyly (pol-e-dak'tə -le)—a congenital anomaly of having more than the normal number of fingers or toes

POINTERS FROM THE PROS: Interview with a Patient Financial Services Director and Consultant

Patricia Zubritzky is a Certified Professional Coder (CPC) who worked as a Director of Patient Financial Services for hospitals for several years, overseeing insurance and patient billing and collections. Ms. Zubritzky spent nearly a decade as a healthcare consultant, helping hospitals and physician groups charge and code procedures and services correctly.

What interested you in coding when your work background was more on the patient accounting side of healthcare?

Because of Patient Financial Service's dependence on coding, I felt it was imperative that I had a better understanding of how codes were selected and applied. Becoming a Certified Coder has not only expanded my understanding of the codes themselves, but also allows me to have a better grasp of what is needed to accurately code claims.

What did you find rewarding about working as a healthcare consultant?

The best part for me had to be the relief (and anticipation) often seen on the faces of the client's staff when they realized you were there to help them. Too often they recognized the problems, and sought correction, but because they were employees of the facility or practice, no one listened to them. I think it helped, too, that I had been on their side of the fence once and could relate to their frustration!

What advice can you give to coders who would someday like to enter the consulting field?

You are in an excellent position to make such a transition. Your expertise would be invaluable to a consulting firm. One suggestion would be to try and familiarize yourself with all aspects of the revenue cycle processes. It will broaden your understanding of the financial continuum and give you a better understanding of the importance and impact of what you do now.

(Used by permission of Patricia Zubritzky.)

Figure 14-18 ■ Polydactyly, a congenital anomaly. Notice that the feet have extra toes.

Photo credit: Dr. James Hanson/ CDC.

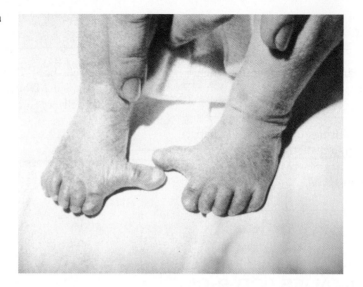

It is also important to understand the difference between a condition that is congenital and one that is acquired. Congenital means present at birth, while acquired means a condition that the patient developed after birth. For example, an infant who was born without a right thumb has a congenital condition or anomaly, but an infant who lost a thumb in a car accident has an acquired condition.

Physicians may diagnose a congenital anomaly at birth or after the infant is born because signs and symptoms occur later, even though the condition was present at birth. Patients with congenital anomalies may receive continued treatment for their conditions for weeks, months, or years. Therefore, you may code an encounter for a birth with a diagnosed congenital anomaly, or you may only code a congenital anomaly when the encounter does not involve the birth.

ICD-9-CM's Chapter 14 contains one section of categories, 740–759, with conditions arranged by type and body site.

Coding Infant's Record—Birth with a Congenital Anomaly

Refer to the following example to code an infant's record when a birth occurred, and the infant has a congenital anomaly.

Example: Mrs. Levine, a 42-year-old, vaginally delivers a single liveborn male at Williton Medical Center. Dr. Wooten diagnoses infant Paul Levine with Down's syndrome, which he discovered previously through amniocentesis prenatal testing at 19 weeks gestation.

For this case, you will assign two codes to the infant's record: birth status (V30–V39) and the congenital anomaly of Down's syndrome. You already know how to assign a code for birth status. For the first code, search the Index for the main term *newborn*, subterm *single*, subterm *born in hospital (without mention of cesarean delivery or section)*, and cross-reference code V30.00 to the Tabular for final code assignment.

Next, assign second a code for Down's syndrome by searching the Index for the main term *syndrome*, subterm *Down's*, and then cross-reference code 758.0 to the Tabular for final code assignment.

Final code assignment for infant Paul Levine's record is

1. V30.00 (birth status, single liveborn, born in hospital, no cesarean)

2. 758.0 (congenital anomaly—Down's syndrome)

INTERESTING FACT: Mice Can Injure or Kill Unborn Babies

Lymphocytic choriomeningitis virus (LCMV) causes infection in animals and humans. Wild mice can carry LCMV and infect other rodents, such as hamsters, mice, and guinea pigs. People can be infected through contact with urine, blood, saliva, droppings, or nesting materials of infected animals. A person can become infected by

✔ inhaling (breathing in) dust or droplets while sweeping up droppings from an infected rodent.

✔ touching infected rodent urine or droppings and then touching the eyes or the inside of the nose or mouth.

✔ being bitten by an infected rodent.

If a woman has an LCMV infection while she is pregnant, the unborn baby can also become infected. LCMV infection can cause severe birth defects or loss of the preg-

nancy. Although the risk of LCMV infection is low, there is no treatment available. Women who are pregnant or planning to become pregnant should avoid contact with wild or pet rodents, hamsters, pet mice, and guinea pigs. To reduce the risk of LCMV infection during pregnancy,

✔ Exterminate mice in your home.

✔ Avoid vacuuming or sweeping rodent urine, droppings, or nesting materials. Wash hands thoroughly after any contact.

✔ Ask a friend or family member who does not live with you to care for pet rodents.

(Department of Health and Human Services, Centers for Disease Control and Prevention, www.cdc.gov/ncbddd/pregnancy_gateway/ infections-LCMV.html, accessed 1/4/11)

Coding Infant's Record—Congenital Anomaly Only (No Birth)

Patients with congenital anomalies may continue to receive treatment for their conditions indefinitely, including throughout their lives. Refer to the following example to code an encounter for a nine-month-old with a congenital anomaly.

Example: Mrs. Beach brings her nine-month-old daughter, Kelly, to Dr. McCray, a hand surgeon, for an evaluation. Dr. McCray diagnoses Kelly with radial polydactyly (extra thumb) and discusses surgical treatment options.

Search the Index for the main term *polydactylism, polydactyly*, and subterm *fingers*, and cross-reference code 755.01 to the Tabular for final code assignment (■ FIGURE 14-19).

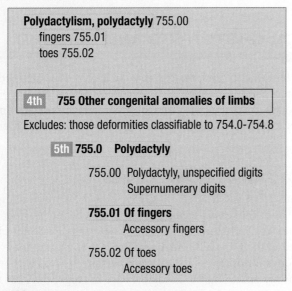

Figure 14-19 ■ Index entry for polydactyly of the fingers with code 755.01 cross-referenced to the Tabular.

TAKE A BREAK

Good job! Let's take a break and then practice coding congenital anomalies.

| Exercise 14.6 | **Congenital Anomalies** |

Instructions: Assign codes to infants' records only (not the mothers' records) for episodes or care for births with congenital anomalies and for encounters for congenital anomalies only. Reference both the Index and the Tabular.

1. Theresa Acosta, age 30, sees Dr. Woods, a cardiologist, for Marfan syndrome (genetic disorder of excessive height and long extremities), which she has had since birth. He discusses the need for mitral valve replacement in the near future.

   Code(s): _____

2. Caleb Reynolds was born yesterday to Charlotte Mattison at Washington Bryant Memorial Hospital via cesarean section. Today, clinicians transfer him to Williton Medical Center for treatment for congenital hydrocephalus. Assign codes for the encounter at Washington Bryant.

   Code(s): _____

3. Dr. Wooten performs a cesarean section on Jodi Martins, a 40-year-old, who gives birth to baby Julie. Through antepartum genetic testing Jodi and her husband, James, knew that there was a high possibility that Julie could have Down's syndrome. Julie's physical appearance at birth and subsequent neonatal testing at Williton confirm trisomy 21 Down's syndrome.

   Code(s): _____

4. Margie Spriggs delivers baby Manuel vaginally with no maternal complications. Manuel has an incomplete cleft lip on his left side (lack of lip tissue). Dr. Wooten supervises the birth.

   Code(s): _____

5. Dr. Tanner, a neonatologist, meets with Victoria Bradberry, age 24, in the hospital to discuss test results for baby Victor, who was born via cesarean section. Victor has significant hypotonia (muscle weakness), so Dr. Wooten called Dr. Tanner for evaluation and tests. A blood test, FISH (fluorescent in situ hybridization), is positive for Prader-Willi Syndrome, which results from the deletion of paternal chromosome 15. The condition causes developmental delays. Dr. Tanner discusses the progression of the disease and management options with Mrs. Bradberry.

   Code(s): _____

6. Dr. Mason, a nephrologist, admits Suzanne Walters, 22 days old, to Williton Medical Center for a single congenital renal cyst.

   Code(s): _____

V CODES FOR OBSTETRICS AND RELATED CONDITIONS

Do you remember learning in Chapter 7 that there are V codes for specific encounters for obstetrics and related conditions? You also reviewed various coding examples and practiced assigning V codes to these types of encounters, which you can find in ■ TABLE 14-2. Review the V codes to be sure that you understand when to assign them.

ICD-9-CM OFFICIAL GUIDELINES

There are numerous ICD-9-CM Official Guidelines for coding complications of pregnancy, childbirth, and the puerperium, as well as coding perinatal conditions and congenital anomalies. You have already learned many of the guidelines in this chapter, but there are more listed in the Official Guidelines. Refer to the guidelines for assistance when you are assigning codes for other conditions that pertain to areas with which you are unfamiliar. (Instructions for accessing the guidelines are in Appendix A of this text). This will give you practice reviewing the guidelines and interpreting them. If you cannot find specific guidelines for a condition, then always follow the coding conventions in the ICD-9-CM manual.

■ TABLE 14-2   V CODES FOR OBSTETRICS AND RELATED CONDITIONS

Category, Subcategory, Subclassification	Title	Main Term/Subterm
V20.2	Routine infant or child health check	Examination, child care
V22	Normal pregnancy	Pregnancy, supervision
V22.2	Pregnant state, incidental	Pregnancy, incidental
	Assign V22.2 as an additional code when the encounter is for a condition that is unrelated to the pregnancy.	
V23	Supervision of high-risk pregnancy	Pregnancy, supervision
	Assign a code from V23 if the patient has poor obstetric history or is age 35 or older.	
V24	Postpartum care and examination	Postpartum
V25	Encounter for contraceptive management	Admission, for
	Exception: V25.0x	
	(See Official Guidelines, Section I.C.18.d.11, Counseling)	
V26	Procreative management	Management
	Exception: V26.5x, Sterilization status, V26.3 and V26.4	
	(See Official Guidelines, Section I.C.18.d.11., Counseling)	
V27	Outcome of delivery	Outcome of delivery (mother's record)
V28	Encounter for antenatal screening of mother	Screening
V29	Observation and evaluation of newborns and infants for suspected condition not found	Observation, condition, newborn
V30-V39	Birth status (infant's record)	Newborn
V91	Multiple gestation placenta status	Gestation

TAKE A BREAK

That was a lot of information to absorb! Let's take a break and then practice assigning V codes to encounters and assigning codes to the same types of encounters listed in the Official Guidelines.

Exercise 14.7   V Codes for Obstetrics and Related Conditions, ICD-9-CM Official Guidelines

Instructions: Assign V codes for obstetrics and related conditions. Also assign codes for the same types of encounters listed in the Official Guidelines for complications of pregnancy, childbirth, and the puerperium, referencing both the Index and the Tabular. For some of these cases, you will need to refer to the Official Guidelines for assistance.

1. Joanne Bozeman, a 31-year-old, arrives at Williton Medical Center's emergency department (ED) in an ambulance. She has a broken leg. She is 38½ weeks pregnant with twins and was trying to walk down steep basement steps when she fell. She also complains of labor symptoms lasting for the past two weeks. Dr. Burns, an ED physician, states that her tibia shaft is fractured. He applies a cast and decides to keep her under observation in the ED to monitor her for threatened labor. He discharges her home the next day.

   Code(s): _____

2. Dr. Wooten, an OB/GYN, admits Joanne Bozeman, the same patient who fell and broke her leg a few days ago, to Williton Medical Center because she is in true labor at 39 weeks. Dr. Wooten delivers twins Jolene and Joseph, with no complications. Assign code(s) to the mother's record.

   Code(s): _____

3. Gloria Warrick, age 35, sees Dr. Wooten for her first prenatal visit at 10 weeks. She is gravida 1, para 0.

   Code(s): _____

continued

TAKE A BREAK *continued*

4. Valerie Lagasse, age 24, is 14 weeks pregnant when she hurts her shoulder while lifting bags of mulch to spread in her flower beds. She is able to drive herself to Williton Medical Center's ED, where Dr. Mills examines her. He states that her right shoulder is sprained, applies ice, and places her arm in a sling. He tells her to follow up with Dr. Hoffman, her primary care physician, in a week to evaluate her to determine if she still needs the sling.

Code(s): _____

5. Shelly Sommerville, age 27, sees Dr. Wooten for a routine prenatal check-up in her 25th week. She has no complaints, but Dr. Wooten performs a glucose test and diagnoses her with gestational diabetes.

Code(s): _____

6. Dr. Mills admits Molly Andrews, age 18, to the labor and delivery unit through the ED at Williton Medical Center. She attempted self-induced abortion at 28 weeks, but was unsuccessful and went into labor (early delivery). Dr. Wooten meets her in the delivery room where he delivers a liveborn infant. Assign code(s) to the mother's record.

Code(s): _____

WORKPLACE IQ

You work as a coder for Williton Medical Center, and today you need to code both the mother's record and infants' records for a delivery encounter with multiple births. Dr. Wooten delivered Mrs. Lancaster's quintuplets by c-section. The patient suffered pelvic fractures three years ago in a car accident, and Dr. Wooten determines that it would be beneficial to deliver the infants by c-section. The infants were at 37 weeks gestation (premature). Baby Jean weighed 1,247 grams; baby Doug weighed 1,190 grams ; baby Anna weighed 1,162 grams; baby Kate weighed 1,134 grams; and baby Ralph weighed 992 grams. Dr. Wooten diagnosed each infant with jaundice and anemia. Mr. Lancaster attended the surgery and had to be taken to the ED for treatment for fainting and dizziness. He was released later the same day.

1. What code(s) would you assign to Mrs. Lancaster's record?

_____

2. What code(s) would you assign to each infant's record?

Jean Lancaster _____

Doug Lancaster _____

Anna Lancaster _____

Kate Lancaster _____

Ralph Lancaster _____

3. What code(s) would you assign to Mr. Lancaster's record?

_____

DESTINATION: MEDICARE

For this Medicare exercise, you will review surgical procedures in Medicare program transmittals from Medicare's National Coverage Determinations Manual. Program transmittals communicate new or changed policies and/or procedures that are incorporated into a specific program manual. Follow these instructions to access the specific manual:

1. Go to the website http://www.cms.gov.

2. In the search field on the top right of the screen, type Coding Policy Manual and Change Report 2011, and then hit Enter.

3. From the list of choices, click the option for 2004400 October 2004.

4. You will then see the document entitled *Medicare National Coverage Determinations (NCD) Coding Policy Manual and Change Report January 2011.*

5. Use the search field at the top of the screen, or hit the Ctrl key and the F key, to locate the diagnoses referenced in the questions.

Answer the following questions:

1. Does the Medicare program cover ICD-9-CM diagnoses of *Legally induced abortion, complicated by delayed or excessive hemorrhage*?
2. What are the code ranges listed for *Legally induced abortion, complicated by delayed or excessive hemorrhage*?
3. Does the Medicare program cover ICD-9-CM diagnoses of *Infection of amniotic cavity*?
4. What are the code ranges listed for *Infection of amniotic cavity*?
5. Does the Medicare program cover ICD-9-CM diagnoses of *Malposition or chronic inversion of uterus*?
6. What are the code ranges listed for *Malposition or chronic inversion of uterus*?

A LOOK AHEAD TO ICD-10-CM

ICD-10-CM classifies Pregnancy, Childbirth, and the Puerperium (O00–O9A) to Chapter 15, Certain Conditions Originating in the Perinatal Period (P00–P96) to Chapter 16, and Congenital Malformations, Deformations, and Chromosomal Abnormalities (Q00–Q99) to Chapter 17. There were many additions, revisions, and deletions within these chapters from ICD-9-CM to ICD-10-CM, including adding a character to the ICD-10-CM code to identify the trimester.

Instructions: Refer to ICD-10-CM Official Guidelines for additional information. (Instructions for accessing the guidelines are in Appendix A of this text.) Then assign codes from ICD-10-CM referencing both the Index and the Tabular.

1. Della Ryan, age 35, gravida 3, para 2, sees Dr. Wooten, OB/GYN, near the end of her second trimester with vaginal bleeding. After examination, Dr. Wooten states that she has placenta previa and hemorrhage. He tells her to stay home in bed and states that he will closely monitor her care, adding that she may need to deliver by cesarean section. Code(s): _____

2. Marilyn Delacruz, age 30, gravida 2, para 2, sees Dr. Wooten for a prenatal visit in her 12th week. He is following her pernicious anemia, and blood work shows that it is under control. Code(s): _____

3. Under the supervision of Dr. Wooten, Candy Fields, age 25, gives birth to baby boy William, who makes a cephalic presentation and quick delivery. Aside from requesting an epidural injection (pain medication injected into the spine) and having an episiotomy, she has no problems. William's Apgar scores are 7 and 9.

   Mother's chart code(s): _____

   Baby's chart code: _____

4. Dr. Wooten admits Laurie Ferrell, a 33-year-old, for severe pre-eclampsia and premature labor in her 32nd week of pregnancy. He delivers a healthy baby, Lawrence, via c-section.

   Mother's chart code(s): _____

5. Dr. Wooten performs a cesarean section on Jodi Martins, 40, who gives birth to baby Julie. Through antepartum genetic testing, Jodi and her husband James knew that there was a high possibility that Julie could have Down's syndrome. Julie's physical appearance at birth and subsequent neonatal testing at Williton confirm trisomy 21 Down's syndrome. The type of Down's syndrome is nonmosaic. (Hint: Nonmosaic Down's syndrome occurs when the patient has an extra copy of chromosome 21 in every cell of his body. The disease accounts for 98% of all cases of Down's syndrome.) Assign ICD-10-CM codes for the baby's birth status and diagnosis.

   Baby's chart code(s): _____

6. Gloria Warrick, 35, sees Dr. Wooten for her first prenatal visit at 10 weeks. She is gravida 1, para 0. (Hint: When you are coding, be careful to distinguish between the capital letter O and the number zero, 0.) Code(s): _____

CHAPTER REVIEW

Multiple Choice

Instructions: Circle one best answer to complete each statement.

1. _____ occurs when the placenta separates from the uterine wall and is expulsed through the vagina, along with the remains of the umbilical cord.
   a. Labor
   b. Delivery
   c. Afterbirth
   d. Complication

2. In ICD-9-CM's Chapter 11, fifth digits describe the mother's
   a. episode of care.
   b. trimester.
   c. weeks of gestation.
   d. previous pregnancies.

3. How should you sequence codes for complications of pregnancy, childbirth, or the puerperium?
   a. Always assign code(s) from other chapters first, followed by code(s) from Chapter 11.
   b. Always assign code(s) from Chapter 11 first, followed by code(s) from other chapters.
   c. Always assign code(s) in the same order that the conditions are mentioned in the medical record.
   d. Always assign code(s) from Chapter 11 instead of codes from any other chapter(s).

4. All of the following can be present in a delivery coded as normal (650) *except*
   a. episiotomy.
   b. vaginal delivery.
   c. fetal rotation.
   d. cephalic presentation.

5. Where should you assign a code from category V27—*Outcome of delivery?*
   a. On the mother's record, for all births
   b. On the mother's record, for live births only
   c. On the baby's record
   d. On both the mother's and baby's record

6. For every infant's chart, assign the first code from
   a. Chapter 14—Congenital Anomalies (740–759) for problems diagnosed at birth.
   b. Chapter 15—Certain Conditions Originating in the Perinatal Period (760–779) for perinatal conditions.
   c. category V27—*Outcome of delivery.*
   d. category V30–V39 for newborn birth status.

7. Perinatal conditions can be present within _____ birth.
   a. five months before or within a month after
   b. five months before or after
   c. 28 days before or after
   d. nine months before

8. Which of the following conditions should you code as a perinatal condition for the infant?
   a. Cleft palate
   b. Polydactyly
   c. Hydrocephalus
   d. Jaundice

9. A congenital anomaly is
   a. always diagnosed before birth.
   b. coded for only the first year of the child's life.
   c. coded for as long as the child receives treatment.
   d. all of the above

10. According to the ICD-9-CM guidelines, how should you code puerperal sepsis?
    a. Assign code 670.2x—*Puerperal sepsis* with a secondary code to identify the causal organism.
    b. Assign a code to identify the causal organism with a secondary code of 670.2x *Puerperal sepsis.*
    c. Assign a code from category 038—*Septicemia.*
    d. Assign code 995.91—*Sepsis.*

Coding Assignments

Instructions: Assign ICD-9-CM code(s) to the following cases, referencing both the Index and Tabular.

1. Christy Mauney, age 22, gravida 2, para 1, sees Dr. Wooten, OB/GYN, who diagnoses her with an ectopic pregnancy in her right fallopian tube.

   Code(s): _____

2. Dr. Wooten sees Velma Potter, gravida 1, para 0, for prenatal supervision. She is in her 10th week and is expected to deliver a month before her 16th birthday.

   Code(s): _____

3. Taniesha Monti brings in Daniel, a two-week-old, to see Dr. Flynn, a pediatrician. She is concerned because Daniel is constantly spitting up. Dr. Flynn diagnoses the baby with a congenital esophageal ring (a ring of fibrous tissue surrounding the esophagus, causing reflux).

   Code(s): _____

4. Dr. Wooten meets Heather Goodwin, age 23, in the labor suite where she is having difficulty. Due to her severe obesity, she has obstructed labor due to cephalopelvic disproportion. Dr. Wooten decides to perform a cesarean delivery, which results in the birth of baby Tyrell. (Hint: This case requires several codes.)

Mother's chart code(s): _____

5. Dr. Wooten sees Sonia Mayes, age 31, in the office for size/date discrepancy (difference between the uterus size and last menstrual period, indicating that the fetus is developing faster or slower than anticipated). Mrs. Mayes also reports that she has not felt her baby move in the past 24 hours.

Code(s): _____

6. Paula Delorenzo, age 19, sees Dr. Wooten for a prenatal visit. She is 20 weeks pregnant and is HIV positive.

Code(s): _____

7. Toni Rahn, age 22, is full term at 40 weeks and sees Dr. Wooten in his office. He determines that the baby has an unstable lie (baby continues to change position), and he is concerned that it could cause serious complications. Mrs. Rahn agrees to a c-section. Dr. Wooten tells her to meet him at Williton Medical Center at 3 pm when he will perform surgery. Assign the diagnosis code for the office visit.

Code(s): _____

8. Dr. Wooten admits Valerie Elmore, age 18, to Williton Medical Center for delivery at 38 weeks gestation. Dr. Wooten delivers a stillborn fetus due to a placental infarction (inadequate blood supply to the placenta).

Code(s): _____

9. Dr. Wooten delivers Carlos Geiger to Carlotta, age 22, via c-section. Dr. Wooten diagnoses baby Carlos with Meckel's diverticulum (bulge in the small intestine) and pyloric stenosis (narrow opening between the stomach and intestines).

Baby's chart code(s): _____

10. Miranda Strange, age 33, delivers baby Peter under the direction of Dr. Wooten at Williton Medical Center. Dr. Wooten diagnoses Peter with meconium obstruction (inability to pass the first stools) and a congenital hiatal hernia (the stomach protrudes through the diaphragm).

Baby's chart code(s): _____

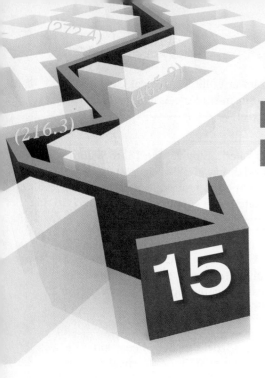

Inpatient Coding, Medicare Reimbursement

15

Learning Objectives

After completing this chapter, you should be able to

- Spell and define the key terminology in this chapter.
- Describe the differences between first-listed and principal diagnoses.
- Explain how coding relates to Medicare reimbursement to physicians, outpatient hospitals, and inpatient hospitals.
- Define the meaning of Present on Admission (POA).
- Identify the role of Medicare Administrative Contractors (MACs).
- Define Medicare's three-day payment window (72-hour rule).
- Discuss ICD-9-CM Official Guidelines for the selection of the principal diagnosis.
- List the general rules for reporting other (additional) diagnoses.

Key Terms

admitting diagnosis
diagnostic workup
Inpatient Prospective Payment System (IPPS)
length of stay (LOS)

Medicare Physician Fee Schedule (MPFS)
Medicare Severity DRGs (MS-DRGs)
Outpatient Prospective Payment System (OPPS)
Present on Admission (POA) Indicator
resource-based relative value scale (RBRVS)

INTRODUCTION

This chapter presents Sections II and III of the ICD-9-CM Official Guidelines. You already reviewed Section I for Conventions, General Coding Guidelines, and Chapter-Specific Coding Guidelines, as well as Section IV for Reporting Diagnoses for Outpatient Services. Section II covers Selecting the Principal Diagnosis for Inpatients, and Section III covers Reporting Additional Diagnoses in Inpatient Settings. You will learn how to determine the principal diagnosis and how to code various types of conditions in inpatient settings. Remember that in your career in healthcare, you may work for any type of provider, including an acute care hospital. Learning how to code for inpatients will help you to become even more of a skilled coder.

During this last stop of your journey for diagnosis coding, you now have the opportunity to apply all of the information that you learned to coding a new type of record. When you complete exercises in this chapter, you will notice that they require you to analyze specific elements and apply previously learned coding skills.

But before you can begin learning about coding inpatient records, you need to understand how Medicare pays inpatient claims, because the diagnosis codes that you assign, and the order in which you assign them, directly affect Medicare reimbursement. Remember that coding involves not only knowing code set guidelines, but also knowing Medicare's

CPT-4 codes in this chapter are from the CPT-4 2012 code set. CPT is a registered trademark of the American Medical Association.

ICD-9-CM codes in this chapter are from the ICD-9-CM 2012 code set from the Department of Health and Human Services, Centers for Disease Control and Prevention.

ICD-10-CM codes in this chapter are from the ICD-10-CM 2012 Draft code set from the Department of Health and Human Services, Centers for Disease Control and Prevention.

coding and billing regulations, as well as regulations from other insurances, so that you can code correctly and ensure correct reimbursement. Enjoy this stop of the journey, and add the information that you learn to your ever-growing repertoire of coding skills!

"Develop a passion for learning. If you do, you will never cease to grow."
—Anthony J. D'Angelo

FIRST-LISTED AND PRINCIPAL DIAGNOSES

When you are sequencing codes, it is important to understand the order in which you should assign them. Remember that the first-listed diagnosis is the primary diagnosis and reason for the encounter in an outpatient setting, and the principal diagnosis is the reason for the inpatient admission in an inpatient setting.

In an inpatient setting, a patient has an **admitting diagnosis,** the diagnosis that the physician documents to show why he is admitting the patient. However, the admitting diagnosis could be different from the *principal* diagnosis, which you determine at the time of the patient's *discharge* from the hospital. At the time of admission, the patient may have one diagnosis to justify the admission, but may need further lab or radiology testing or additional examinations.

Later, after the *attending physician* (the physician who oversees the patient's care) reviews the patient's test results and discusses findings with other examining physicians, he may determine that the reason for the admission is another condition, which then requires further inpatient treatment. In fact, an admitting diagnosis may be for a sign or symptom because the definitive diagnosis has not yet been established.

MEDICARE REIMBURSEMENT TO PROVIDERS

Before learning how to assign codes in an inpatient setting, it is important for you to understand how Medicare's regulations apply to code assignment for all settings. Let's review more about Medicare reimbursement next. You already coded many different diagnoses for patient encounters with physicians in various locations—physician offices, clinics, and hospitals. You learned the importance of establishing medical necessity on claims that providers send to insurances, including ensuring that the diagnosis code justifies the procedure code.

Medicare and other payers reimburse physician services and procedures based on medical necessity and the Current Procedural Terminology (CPT) or Healthcare Common Procedural Coding System (HCPCS) codes. It is crucial that you code encounters correctly to ensure that insurances pay not only based on medical necessity, but also based on correct assignment of diagnosis and procedure codes.

Providers submit inpatient and outpatient *hospital* claims on the UB-04 (CMS-1450) claim form, which you reviewed in Chapter 1 of this text. Refer to Figure 1-2 to review the UB-04 blocks for ICD-9-CM codes:

- Block 67 contains the principal diagnosis code.
- Blocks 67A–Q contain additional diagnosis codes.
- Block 69 contains the admitting diagnosis code.
- Block 74 contains the principal inpatient procedure code.
- Blocks 74a–e contain additional procedure codes.

It really helps to understand where the codes appear on the claim form so that you know how the work that you perform directly relates to billing and reimbursement.

Medicare Reimbursement to Physicians

Medicare pays physicians through the **Medicare Physician Fee Schedule (MPFS),** which Medicare created in 1983 and updates yearly. A fee schedule is a complete listing

CPT-4 Code	Modifier	Short Description	Carrier Locality	Non-Facility Price	Facility Price	Conversion Factor
99201	—	Office/outpatient visit new	0000000	$41.11	$25.82	33.9764
99201	—	Office/outpatient visit new	0051200	$16.31	$16.31	33.9764
99201	—	Office/outpatient visit new	0052013	$16.31	$16.31	33.9764

of fees that Medicare uses to pay physicians or other providers or suppliers for services and procedures. The fee corresponds to a Current Procedural Terminology (CPT) or Healthcare Common Procedural Coding System (HCPCS) code (■ FIGURE 15-1). Medicare has a fee schedule search tool on its website where you can search for a fee based on the CPT or HCPCS code of the service or procedure. The CMS developed fee schedules for physicians, ambulance services, clinical laboratory services, and durable medical equipment, including prosthetics, orthotics, and supplies.

The provider submits a claim on the CMS-1500 form to the *Medicare carrier/ Medicare Administrative Contractor (MAC),* an insurance company that Medicare pays to process physician claims. A *carrier* is the old name for the company that processed physician claims for Medicare, and MACs replaced carriers. You will still see the term *carrier* referenced in Medicare regulations and still hear it mentioned within the healthcare industry.

You reviewed the CMS-1500 form for physician services in Chapter 1 and can refer to it again in Figure 1-1. Physicians submit the form with ICD-9-CM diagnosis codes and CPT-4 or HCPCS procedure codes to the carrier/MAC, and the MAC pays physicians according to the Medicare Physician Fee Schedule. Payment amounts are different for each procedure code. Fee schedule amounts also differ according to the geographic location of the provider because costs to provide services vary from region to region. This payment variation is called a *geographic practice cost index (GPCI).* Medicare calculates a fee schedule payment that is based on the GPCI and a **resource-based relative value scale (RBRVS)** for a procedure or service. The RBRVS is a calculation of the cost that the physician incurs for

- Physician work involved in providing a service
- Expense to provide the service (other clinicians involved, utilities, equipment)
- Malpractice expense should the physician make an error

Medicare uses a conversion factor, a number that is used for calculating actual payments to providers (see Figure 15-1). It is very important to not only assign diagnosis and procedure codes to show medical necessity, but it is also important to understand that Medicare's fee schedule reimbursement is directly based on any CPT or HCPCS codes that you assign.

So providers send physician claims to the MAC on a CMS-1500 form, and the MAC pays providers from a fee schedule. Let's now review how Medicare reimburses outpatient hospitals.

Medicare Reimbursement to Outpatient Hospitals

Medicare pays outpatient hospitals through the **Outpatient Prospective Payment System (OPPS),** which it updates yearly. OPPS is also called the Hospital Outpatient Prospective Payment System (HOPPS). In the OPPS system, Medicare pays a set amount for a service or procedure according to a specific classification, called the *Ambulatory Payment Classification (APC).* Every procedure code is classified into an APC group, with an APC group number, along with similar procedures in that same group.

CPT-4 Code	Short Descriptor	Status Indicator	APC	Relative Weight	Payment Rate
22999	Abdomen surgery procedure	T	0049	22.9744	$1,582.38
23000	Removal of calcium deposits	T	0021	18.0784	$1,245.17
23020	Release shoulder joint	T	0051	47.3213	$3,259.30
23030	Drain shoulder lesion	T	0008	20.1996	$1,391.27
23031	Drain shoulder bursa	T	0008	20.1996	$1,391.27
23035	Drain shoulder bone lesion	T	0049	22.9744	$1,582.38
23040	Exploratory shoulder surgery	T	0050	32.2439	$2,220.83

Figure 15-2 ■ Excerpt from the OPPS status indicators, APC numbers, and payment rates per CPT-4 code for 2011.

Source: Centers for Medicare and Medicaid Service, Current Procedural Terminology copyright American Medical Association.

Medicare reviews the procedure code on the claim, determines the APC group the code belongs to, then pays the amount assigned to that APC group. There is also a *status indicator (SI)* assigned to each APC which represents the type of service (■ FIGURE 15-2). Medicare does not pay based on the *individual* procedure code, as is paid with physician services. Instead, Medicare pays a set amount for a procedure within a similar grouping of procedures. Medicare does not use the same criteria used for the physician fee schedule to determine payments to outpatient hospitals. Medicare will not pay hospitals for unnecessary services, such as routine tests whose results have nothing to do with the patient's definitive diagnosis.

The provider submits outpatient hospital claims to *Fiscal Intermediaries (FIs)/MACs,* insurance companies that Medicare pays to process outpatient hospital claims. A *fiscal intermediary* is the old name for an insurance company that processes outpatient hospital claims. MACs replaced fiscal intermediaries, but you will still hear the term *fiscal intermediary* used within the healthcare industry. Providers list both ICD-9-CM codes, along with CPT and HCPCS codes, on outpatient claims. MACs use Medicare's *Integrated Outpatient Code Editor (I/OCE)* computer software to process claims for all outpatient institutional providers. The OCE performs three major functions:

1. Edit the data to identify errors and return a series of edit flags so that the provider can correct them.

2. Assign an Ambulatory Payment Classification (APC) number for each service covered under OPPS and returns information to a computerized *Pricer program,* which determines the Medicare payment amount.

3. Assign an Ambulatory Surgical Center (ASC) payment group for services on claims from certain non-OPPS hospitals.

CMS also developed the *National Correct Coding Initiative (NCCI),* a method to identify procedure codes that should not be reported together. *NCCI edits* are rules incorporated into a computer software program that automatically flag procedures that are incompatible. CMS added NCCI edits to the OCE, so when a provider submits a claim to Medicare, the OCE will identify codes which are incorrectly reported together. The purpose of NCCI edits is to prevent improper Medicare payments when providers report incorrect code combinations. NCCI edits do not apply to ICD-9-CM diagnosis codes, only to CPT-4 and HCPCS codes.

For example, you should not report codes together if one of the codes is normally an integral part of the other code. If a provider performs two procedures that cannot be reported together, but it was necessary to perform each separately, then the provider can still report both codes to Medicare. The difference is that the provider will have to add a modifier to the procedure code of the second service, giving additional information to justify why the provider performed it separately. You will learn more about modifiers in Chapter 18 of this text.

As with physician services and procedures, it is not only very important to assign diagnosis codes and procedure codes that meet medical necessity to outpatient hospital records, but to also assign correct procedure codes to ensure correct Medicare reimbursement according to the APC group number. You also need to ensure that you do not report incorrect procedure codes together so that CMS's OCE does not deny payment based on NCCI edits. You can check the Medicare website for files which show procedure code pairs that you should not report together.

So providers send outpatient hospital claims to the MAC on a UB-04 form, and the MAC pays providers from the OPPS using APC numbers for each procedure or service. Let's now review how Medicare reimburses inpatient hospitals.

Medicare Reimbursement to Inpatient Hospitals

Medicare pays acute care inpatient hospital stays under the **Inpatient Prospective Payment System (IPPS)**. Unlike physician and outpatient hospital payments, the IPPS pays once the patient is discharged. Medicare calculates payments based on the diagnosis or diagnoses that a coder assigns to the patient's episode of care, the order in which the codes are assigned, the patient's age, the patient's gender, the principal procedure, and additional procedures. The principal procedure should relate to the principal diagnosis and is not a diagnostic test. It is a procedure (such as surgery) for treating the principal diagnosis and can occur within various hospital departments, depending on the patient's case.

Providers submit inpatient hospital claims on the UB-04 claim form to FIs/MACs, listing the principal diagnosis code, additional diagnosis codes, and ICD-9-CM Volume 3 codes for the principal procedure and additional procedures. In Chapter 16 of this text, you will learn more about how to code inpatient procedures using ICD-9-CM Volume 3. You will also learn more about the new system for coding procedures, the International Classification of Diseases, Tenth Revision, Procedure Coding System (ICD-10-PCS).

Medicare Severity Diagnosis Related Group Under IPPS, Medicare pays a set amount for specific diagnoses, or groups of diagnoses, for a specific case, regardless of how long the patient is hospitalized. Refer to ■ FIGURE 15-3 to review the average length of hospital stays for specific diagnoses. Medicare reviews the principal and secondary diagnoses on the patient's claim, along with any other diagnoses for complications and comorbidities, principal and additional procedures, and patient demographics, then assigns the patient's hospital stay to a specific category, called the **Medicare Severity Diagnosis-Related Group (MS-DRG)**.

The MS-DRG classification system assigns beneficiaries to one of over 700 categories of diagnosis related groups (DRGs). Generally, hospitals receive Medicare IPPS payment on a per discharge or per case basis for Medicare beneficiaries with inpatient stays. Related therapeutic outpatient department services that are provided within three days prior to admission are included in the payment for the inpatient stay and may not be separately

Figure 15-3 ■ Average length of hospital stays according to diagnoses.

Source: Department of Health and Human Services, Centers for Disease Control, http://www.cdc.gov/mmwr/preview/mmwrhtml/mm5427a6.htm.

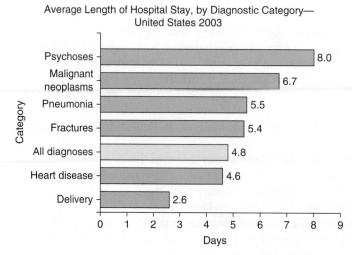

billed. Discharges are assigned to a DRG, which groups similar clinical conditions (diagnoses) and the procedures furnished by the hospital during the stay. The beneficiary's principal diagnosis and up to eight secondary diagnoses that indicate comorbidities and complications will determine the DRG assignment. DRG assignment can be affected by up to six procedures that are furnished during the stay.

CMS reviews the DRG definitions annually to ensure that each group continues to include cases with clinically similar conditions that require comparable amounts of inpatient resources. When the review shows that subsets of clinically similar cases within a DRG consume significantly different amounts of resources, they may be assigned to a different DRG with comparable resource use or a new DRG may be created.

MS-DRGs classify the severity of a patient's case. There are three levels of severity in the MS-DRGs, based on the following types of *secondary* diagnosis codes:

*   Major Complication/Comorbidity (MCC)—highest level of severity
*   Complication/Comorbidity (CC)—next level of severity
*   Non-complication/comorbidity (non-CC)—lowest level of severity; does not affect severity of illness and resources used

The IPPS per-discharge payment is based on two national base payment rates or "standardized amounts," for operating expenses and capital expenses. These payment rates are adjusted to account for

*   The costs associated with the beneficiary's clinical condition and related treatment relative to the costs of the average Medicare case (i.e., the DRG relative weight, as described in the "How Payment Rates Are Set" section that follows); and
*   Market conditions in the facility's location relative to national conditions.

Major Diagnostic Categories (MDCs)

MS-DRGs are divided into broad categories of conditions called *major diagnostic categories (MDCs)*. Each MDC has a number from 0 to 25 that groups diagnoses of a specific organ system or medical specialty. For example, MDC 6 represents the digestive system, and MDC 11 represents the kidney and urinary tract. In general, cases are assigned to an MDC based on the beneficiary's principal diagnosis *before assignment* to a MS-DRG. However, there are several MS-DRGs to which cases are directly assigned based on ICD-9-CM procedure codes. The principal diagnosis determines MDC assignment. Within most MDCs, cases are divided into surgical and medical MS-DRGs.

Each IPPS claim is assigned to one MS-DRG that determines the payment for the inpatient stay. The MS-DRG payment amount may be more or less than the actual cost of the stay (■ FIGURE 15-4).

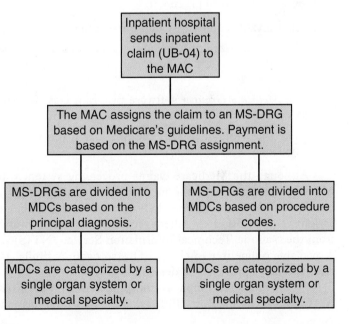

Figure 15-4 ■ Diagram of IPPS reimbursement.

Are you wondering how correct coding relates to Medicare's IPPS payments? Review the following example so that you will better understand the coding/payment relationship.

Example: A patient is hospitalized for a mitral valve replacement and has a principal diagnosis of mitral valve prolapse, a secondary diagnosis of congestive heart failure (CHF), and a third diagnosis of diabetes mellitus type II, along with a procedure of mitral valve replacement.

Medicare would pay the provider one set amount for the patient's case, according to the MS-DRG. Medicare determines DRG payments based on the average amount of time and resources that a hospital uses to treat patients with the same diagnoses, in the same order reported.

But if the coder incorrectly listed diabetes type II as the principal diagnosis, CHF secondary, and mitral valve prolapse third, then the MS-DRG assignment and payment would be different, even if Medicare pays the claim. A principal diagnosis of diabetes mellitus type II does not justify performing a mitral valve replacement. Therefore, it is crucial for you to ensure that when you code diagnoses for an inpatient claim, you not only assign the correct codes, but that you report them in the correct order.

Additional Medicare Payments for Inpatient Hospitals Paying hospitals a set amount for each patient's episode of care encourages hospitals to work efficiently because Medicare will not pay them more money if they increase the patient's **length of stay (LOS)** (time spent hospitalized). Medicare also pays additional money if the inpatient hospital

- Treats a high percentage of low-income patients, then it receives an add-on payment, called a *disproportionate share hospital (DSH) adjustment.*
- Is an approved teaching hospital, then it receives a percentage add-on payment for each case paid through IPPS, called an *indirect medical education (IME) adjustment.*
- Treats patients who have unusually costly cases, known as *outlier cases,* and Medicare pays *outlier payments.* This additional payment is designed to protect the hospital from suffering large financial losses due to unusually expensive cases.

Inpatient Claims Processing After the FI/MAC receives the provider's claim, it follows these steps to process it:

1. The FI/MAC enters the claim into a computerized claim processing system.
2. The computerized processing system edits the beneficiary's diagnoses, procedure(s), discharge status, and demographic information, using a tool called the *Medicare Code Editor (MCE).*
3. The *Medicare Grouper* software program classifies the claim into the appropriate MS-DRG, using data elements that the hospital reported on the claim.
4. Once the Grouper assigns the MS-DRG, the Pricer software calculates the DRG payment.

Although the Medicare claims processing system will automatically calculate the MS-DRG and payment amount for each claim, hospitals may be interested in knowing how much Medicare will pay before they file the claim. Inpatient coders may have to assign the MS-DRG to inpatient records. Grouper software is available on magnetic tape from the National Technical Information Service (NTIS) website. A Pricer software tool is available online free of charge. This software is similar to the program that FI/MACs have and helps providers to determine payment.

So providers send inpatient hospital claims to the MAC on a UB-04 form, and the MAC pays providers from IPPS using the MS-DRG classification.

TAKE A BREAK

Let's take a break and then review common terms related to coding and Medicare reimbursement to providers.

Exercise 15.1   **Medicare Reimbursement to Providers**

Instructions: Fill in each blank with the best answer, choosing from the list of terms provided.

1. The provider or physician submits a claim on the CMS-1500 form to the _____.

2. Medicare pays outpatient hospitals through the _____.

3. Medicare pays acute care inpatient hospital stays under the _____.

4. Medicare calculates a fee schedule payment based on the _____ and a _____ for a procedure or service.

5. CMS developed the _____, a method that identifies procedure codes that should not be reported together.

6. Medicare reviews the principal and secondary diagnoses on the patient's claim, along with any other diagnoses for complications and comorbidities, principal and additional procedures, and patient information, then assigns the patient's hospital stay into a specific category called a(n) _____.

APC	LOS	NCCI
GPCI	MAC	OPPS
I/OCE	MDC	RBRVS
IPPS	MS-DRG	

PRESENT ON ADMISSION

To group diagnoses into the proper MS-DRG, Medicare also needs to capture a **Present on Admission (POA) Indicator**, information about the patient's principal and secondary diagnoses at the time of admission to an acute care hospital, as opposed to new diagnoses that occur during the inpatient episode of care. Medicare will not pay inpatient hospitals additional payments for cases when selected conditions are acquired during hospitalization (not present on admission). Medicare will not pay for treating diagnoses that the provider could have avoided, such as injuries to the patient during the inpatient stay, hospital-acquired infections, or any other conditions that the provider caused.

Assign the POA Indicator according to the principal and secondary diagnoses documented in the patient's record. The POA Indicator appears on the UB-04 claim form with each diagnosis code reported. The admitting diagnosis code does not need a POA Indicator. Review ■ TABLE 15-1 for a list of POA Indicators and definitions. Refer to Appendix I of the ICD-9-CM Official Guidelines for further direction on assigning the POA indicator. (Instructions for accessing the guidelines are located in Appendix A of this text.)

■ TABLE 15-1   **CMS POA INDICATORS AND DEFINITIONS**

Code	Reason for Code
Y	Diagnosis was present at time of inpatient admission.
	CMS will pay claims with "Y" for the POA Indicator.
N	Diagnosis was not present at time of inpatient admission.
	CMS will **not** pay claims with "N" for the POA Indicator.
U	Documentation insufficient to determine if the condition was present at the time of inpatient admission.
	CMS will **not** pay claims with "U" for the POA Indicator.
W	Clinically undetermined. Provider is unable to clinically determine whether the condition was present at the time of inpatient admission.
	CMS will pay claims with "W" for the POA Indicator.
1	Unreported/Not used.

MEDICARE ADMINISTRATIVE CONTRACTORS

You already learned that MACs replaced fiscal intermediaries for processing hospital claims and replaced carriers for processing physician claims. You also need to know that MACs contract with Medicare to process claims for physicians and hospitals throughout the U.S., based on geographic region. For example, a MAC that processes claims for providers in Montana may not also process claims in Pennsylvania. Some MACs process claims for multiple states or large areas within one state.

MACs process claims according to Medicare's national regulations on coding, billing, and reimbursement. However, as regional companies, they have authority to set local policies, which differ from Medicare's national regulations. National regulations are called National Coverage Determinations (NCDs), and local policies are called Local Coverage Determinations (LCDs), as you learned in Medicare website exercises in previous chapters. It is your responsibility to ensure that you not only follow Medicare's national regulations, but that you also follow local regulations for your provider.

MEDICARE'S THREE-DAY PAYMENT WINDOW (72-HOUR RULE)

Medicare's three-day payment window guideline, also called the *72-hour rule*, states that if a patient has outpatient services and is admitted within 72 hours for *related reasons*, then the provider should combine the services into one inpatient claim. You have to be aware of this rule in case you are faced with coding both an outpatient claim and related inpatient claim for one patient's services within 72 hours. Combine the outpatient and inpatient claim when the ICD-9-CM code for the outpatient services and principal diagnosis for the inpatient stay are the same code, according to Medicare regulations. When the outpatient claim and inpatient claim that occur within 72 hours of each other *do not* have the same diagnosis code, then the provider should submit two separate claims to Medicare. However, MACs that process Medicare claims for a specific region may follow different guidelines, so it is best to check both national and local regulations.

DESTINATION: MEDICARE

In this exercise, you will review additional information about the Correct Coding Initiative (CCI) and correct coding edits in the Medicare Claims Processing Manual Chapter 23. Follow the instructions listed next to access Chapter 23:

1. Go to the website http://www.cms.gov.
2. Click on the *Regulations and Guidance* tab in the banner at the top of the page.
3. On the left column under *Guidance*, choose *Manuals*.
4. On the left side of the screen, under *Manuals*, choose *Internet-Only Manuals (IOMs)*.
5. Scroll down to Publication # *100-04 Medicare Claims Processing Manual*, and click *100-04*.
6. Scroll down to the list of Downloads, and choose *Chapter 23—Fee Schedule Administration and Coding Requirements*.

Answer the following questions, using the search function (Ctrl + F) to find information that you need:

1. How often does Medicare update correct coding edits?
2. Why did CMS develop the CCI?
3. Does Medicare notify a Medicare beneficiary if a provider incorrectly codes and bills procedures that are not allowed to be reported together? If yes, then how? If no, then why not?

TAKE A BREAK

Good job! Let's take a break and then review common terms related to POA Indicators, MACs, and the 72-hour rule.

Exercise 15.2 POA Indicators, MACs, and Medicare's 72-Hour Rule

Instructions: On the line preceding each statement, write T for True or F for False.

1. _____ Medicare will not pay for treating diagnoses that the provider could have avoided, such as injuries to the patient during the inpatient stay, hospital-acquired infections, or any other conditions that the provider caused.

2. _____ The admitting diagnosis code does not need a POA Indicator.

3. _____ MACs are prohibited from setting local policies, which are different from Medicare's national regulations.

4. _____ MACs are Medicare offices located in each state.

5. _____ Medicare's 72-hour rule states that if a patient has outpatient services and is admitted within 72 hours, then the provider should combine all the services, regardless of reason, into one inpatient claim.

6. _____ When the outpatient claim and inpatient claim that occur within 72 hours of one another do not have the same diagnosis code, the provider should submit two separate claims to Medicare.

ICD-9-CM OFFICIAL GUIDELINES—SELECTION OF PRINCIPAL DIAGNOSIS

When you are coding the principal diagnosis, determine the reason for the patient's admission and hospital stay, just as you determined the reason for the patient's encounter in an outpatient setting. Sometimes, it is not easy to determine the reason for admission, so ICD-9-CM created Official Guidelines for assigning the principal diagnosis, along with guidelines for assigning additional diagnoses, which are outlined next. Follow the guidelines very carefully before coding a patient's episode of care. You will have the chance to practice coding diagnoses using the rules from the guidelines.

Circumstances of Inpatient Admission

The circumstances of inpatient admission always govern the selection of principal diagnosis. This means that the principal diagnosis is the reason that the patient receives treatment during the length of stay. Sometimes there can be more than one diagnosis that you can choose for the principal diagnosis.

The principal diagnosis is defined in the Uniform Hospital Discharge Data Set (UHDDS) as "that condition established after study to be chiefly responsible for occasioning the admission of the patient to the hospital for care." The UHDDS is the format that hospitals use to classify types of hospital discharges, including the patient's age, race, gender, address, diagnoses, procedures, and length of stay.

Hospitals use the UHDDS definitions to report inpatient data elements in a standardized manner. (You can find the data elements and their definitions in the July 31, 1985, Federal Register, Vol. 50, No. 147, pp. 31038–40.) Since 1985, UHDDS definitions expanded to include all nonoutpatient settings (acute care, short-term care, long-term care, and psychiatric hospitals; home health agencies; rehabilitation facilities; nursing homes, etc.).

When determining the principal diagnosis, the coding conventions in ICD-9-CM, Volumes I and II, take precedence over these official coding guidelines.

Codes for Symptoms, Signs, and Ill-Defined Conditions

Do not assign codes for symptoms, signs, and ill-defined conditions from Chapter 16 of ICD-9-CM (Symptoms, Signs, and Ill-defined Conditions) as the principal diagnosis when the provider establishes a related definitive diagnosis. You learned about coding for signs and symptoms in the outpatient setting when you studied Official Guidelines for Outpatients in Chapter 5 of this text.

Refer to the following example of an inpatient stay to assign the principal diagnosis when signs and symptoms are present. Remember that Medicare determines the MS-DRG assignment and payment based on the *order* of diagnoses coded, procedures performed, and additional patient information at the time of discharge.

Example: Olivia Dale, a 22-year-old, presents to Williton Medical Center's ED with complaints of right lower quadrant abdominal pain, vomiting, and diarrhea. Dr. Mills, the emergency physician, examines and assesses the patient. Lab work shows an elevated white blood count (WBC), and urinalysis rules out a urinary tract infection. A color Doppler ultrasound reveals an inflamed appendix. Dr. Mills admits the patient with acute appendicitis, and she undergoes a laparascopic appendectomy (appendix removal using a laparoscope). The length of stay is two days.

Principal diagnosis: acute appendicitis (540.9)

Abdominal pain, vomiting, and diarrhea are all symptoms of appendicitis, and you should not code them.

pneumococcal (noo-mo-kok′ əl)—type of bacterium that causes pneumonia

TAKE A BREAK

That was a lot of information to cover! Let's take a break and then practice assigning principal diagnoses with symptoms, signs, and ill-defined conditions.

Exercise 15.3 **ICD-9-CM Official Guidelines— Selection of Principal Diagnosis**

Instructions: Review each patient's episode of care, and assign codes for the principal diagnosis, along with any other diagnoses. Reference both the Index and Tabular when assigning codes.

1. Dr. Mills admits Lula Newton, age 37, to Williton Medical Center with dyspnea, a fever of 102.5°, and vomiting. He orders a chest X-ray and sputum culture, which are positive for (indicate) **pneumococcal** pneumonia.

Dr. Mills orders intravenous (IV) antibiotics and fluids for the patient. After two days, he discharges her home with orders to continue oral antibiotics.

Code(s): _____

2. Eugene Shepard, age 64, arrives at Williton's ED with complaints of chest pain, left arm numbness, and dizziness. Dr. Mills orders a series of tests, which reveal a STEMI of the inferolateral wall of the heart. Dr. Mills admits the patient for further treatment. This is the first time that the patient has experienced these problems.

Code(s): _____

Two or More Interrelated Conditions

nitrates (ni′trāts)

Lasix (la′siks)

packed blood cells—blood from which the plasma has been removed

When there are two or more interrelated conditions (such as diseases in the same ICD-9-CM chapter, or manifestations characteristically associated with a certain disease) potentially meeting the definition of principal diagnosis, sequence either condition first, *unless* the circumstances of the admission, the therapy provided, the Tabular List, or the Alphabetic Index indicate otherwise. To better understand this guideline, review cases for patients' episodes of care listed in Exercise 15.4, and then answer the questions pertaining to each case.

TAKE A BREAK

Good work! Let's take a break and then review cases with two or more interrelated conditions.

Exercise 15.4   Two or More Interrelated Conditions

Instructions: Review each case and then answer the questions that follow. Reference both the Index and Tabular when assigning codes.

Case 1

An ambulance transports David Finch, a 17-year-old, to Williton Medical Center's ED. He was driving on State Route 50 and was involved in a motor vehicle accident where another car hit him in the driver's side. Dr. Mills examines the patient and orders CT scans and an MRI. The patient has a closed fracture of the neck (base) of the femur and multiple closed pelvic fractures involving the ischium and pubis, which disrupt the pelvic circle. Dr. Burt, an orthopedic surgeon, performs an open reduction internal fixation (ORIF) (■ FIGURE 15-5) for femur fracture repair and open reductions with external fixations to repair the pelvic fractures. The patient remains at Williton for three weeks.

a. What are the two diagnoses for the patient?
_____ and _____

b. Are the diagnoses interrelated? (Hint: The same surgeon treated each diagnosis, and each diagnosis was responsible for the hospital admission.) _____

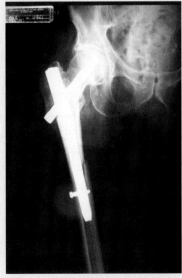

Figure 15-5 ■ Colored x-ray (front view) of the pelvis of a patient, showing open reduction internal fixation (ORIF). The thigh bone (femur) suffered a fracture and was surgically immobilized by inserting long metal pins (dynamic hip screws).

Photo credit: R.C.Hall—Medical Media / Custom Stock Medical Photo.

c. What is the ICD-9-CM code for each of the two diagnoses? _____ and _____

d. According to the guideline, which of the two diagnoses is the principal diagnosis? _____

e. On what information did you base your decision? ___ _____

f. What E code(s) would you assign to this patient's case? _____

Case 2

Dr. Woods, a cardiologist, admits Candace Nguyen, age 69, to Williton with unstable angina and acute CHF. He treats the angina with **nitrates** (salt) and orders **Lasix®** (a diuretic, a drug that helps remove excess fluid from the body) to manage the heart failure. After four days, he discharges her home in stable condition.

a. What are the two diagnoses for the patient?
_____ and _____

b. Are the diagnoses interrelated? (Hint: The same physician treated each diagnosis, and each diagnosis was responsible for the hospital admission.) _____

c. What is the ICD-9-CM code for each of the two diagnoses? _____ and _____

d. According to the guideline, which of the two diagnoses is the principal diagnosis? _____

e. On what information did you base your decision? _____

Case 3

Dr. Hoffman admits Josalyn Early, a 25-year-old, to Williton Medical Center. She complains of heavy menstrual bleeding for two days and reports severe abdominal pain. Dr. Robbins, the attending physician, orders blood work that shows anemia due to acute blood loss. He orders pain medication and **packed blood cells** for the anemia. The patient stabilizes, and Dr. Robbins discharges her to home.

a. What are the two diagnoses for the patient?
_____ and _____

b. Are the diagnoses interrelated? (Hint: The same physician treated each diagnosis, and each diagnosis was responsible for the hospital admission.) _____

c. What is the ICD-9-CM code for each of the two diagnoses? _____ and _____

d. According to the guideline, which of the two diagnoses is the principal diagnosis? _____

e. On what information did you base your decision? _____

hemostasis (hē-mə-stā′-səs)—to stop bleeding

pyelonephritis (pi-ə-lo-nə-fri′tis)—a bacterial infection of the kidney and renal pelvis

echocardiogram (ek-o-kahr′de-ō-gram)—an image of the heart using ultrasound

electrophysiological (i-lek-trō-fiz- ē-äl-ə′-jē-kal)—electrical activity within the heart or other organ

anti-arrhythmic medications (an-ti-ə-rith′mik)

spondylosis (spon-də-lo′sis)

Two or More Diagnoses that Equally Meet the Definition for Principal Diagnosis

In the unusual instance when two or more diagnoses equally meet the criteria for principal diagnosis as determined by the circumstances of admission, diagnostic workup, and/or therapy provided, sequence any of the diagnoses first. A **diagnostic workup** is a series of laboratory and/or radiology tests that the physician orders for the patient to help determine the patient's diagnosis(es). Be sure to refer to the Alphabetic Index, Tabular List, or other coding guidelines, because they may provide you with directions for sequencing the codes.

In the previous exercise, you answered questions and coded diagnoses for cases with interrelated conditions that potentially met the definition of a principal diagnosis. For this guideline, the diagnoses may not be related, but the patient receives testing and treatment for them, and the patient is admitted because of them. When this situation occurs, you can sequence any of the diagnoses first. Review cases for patients' episodes of care listed in Exercise 15.5, and then answer the questions pertaining to each case.

TAKE A BREAK

Let's take a break and then review cases with two or more diagnoses that meet the definition of principal diagnosis.

Exercise 15.5 Two or More Diagnoses That Equally Meet the Definition for Principal Diagnosis

Instructions: Review each case and then answer the questions that follow. Reference both the Index and Tabular when assigning codes.

Case 1

Mr. Whitfield, a 38-year-old, arrives at Williton Medical Center's ED by ambulance after he suffered a fall from a building while working at a construction site. Dr. Mills examines the patient, who has been unconscious for 45 minutes. His Glasgow Coma Scale (GCS) score is 9 (a score that assesses traumatic brain injuries). CT scans and MRI reveal that the patient has a depressed skull fracture, with subarachnoid, subdural, and extradural hemorrhage, and a right ruptured globe. The patient undergoes surgery for elevation of the depressed skull fracture and treatment of hemorrhage to achieve **hemostasis**, as well as repair of the ruptured globe. The patient's length of stay is 10 days.

a. What are the diagnoses for the patient? _____

_____

b. Are the diagnoses interrelated? _____ If yes, which diagnoses? _____

c. What ICD-9-CM codes would you assign for each diagnosis? _____

d. Which of the diagnoses is the principal diagnosis? ___

_____

e. On what information did you base your decision? ___

_____

f. What E code(s) would you assign to this patient's case? _____

Case 2

Dr. Robbins admits Vincent Abramson, age 56, to Williton Medical Center for acute **pyelonephritis** and atrial fibrillation. He evaluates the infection and treats it with IV antibiotics. Dr. Robbins requests a consultation (opinion) from Dr. Woods, a cardiologist, for the atrial fibrillation. Dr. Woods orders an **echocardiogram** and **electrophysiological** studies, then treats the fibrillation with **anti-arrhythmic medications** (medications that stabilize the heartbeat). After two days, Dr. Robbins is satisfied with Mr. Abramson's progress and discharges him home with oral antibiotics and anti-arrhythmics. The patient will follow up with Dr. Woods in four weeks.

a. What are the diagnoses for the patient? _____

_____

b. Are the diagnoses interrelated? _____ If yes, which diagnoses? _____

c. What ICD-9-CM codes would you assign for each diagnosis? _____

d. Which of the diagnoses is the principal diagnosis? ___

_____

e. On what information did you base your decision? ___

_____

Case 3

Dr. Robbins assesses the case of David Wieland, age 35, an inpatient at Williton Medical Center. He calls in Dr. Reilly, an orthopedic spinal surgeon, for a consultation on

TAKE A BREAK *continued*

Mr. Wieland's back pain from lumbosacral **spondylosis** (spinal osteoarthritis). He also requests a consultation from Dr. Drimond, a gastroenterologist, for Mr. Wieland's acute gastroenteritis. Mr. Wieland improves after receiving medication for both conditions. Dr. Robbins discharges him home after three days.

a. What are the diagnoses for the patient? _____
_____

b. Are the diagnoses interrelated? _____ If yes, which diagnoses? _____

c. What ICD-9-CM codes would you assign for each diagnosis? _____

d. Which of the diagnoses is the principal diagnosis? ____
_____

e. On what information did you base your decision? ____
_____

Two or More Comparative or Contrasting Conditions

In those rare instances when two or more contrasting or comparative diagnoses are documented as "either/or" (or similar terminology), code the diagnoses as though they have been confirmed. Comparative means that the physician compares conditions to each other, or the conditions may contrast, or be different from, each other. The physician is not sure which diagnosis is more accurate. Sequence the diagnoses according to the circumstances of the admission. Sequence either diagnosis first if it is not possible to confirm which diagnosis should be principal.

This guideline means that when a patient has two conditions, and the physician documents the diagnoses as *either* one condition *or* the other, you can sequence either condition first. This situation is not common, and typically, there is one principal diagnosis that the provider treats, which is the reason for the patient's admission, and there may also be other diagnoses that are secondary to the principal. It may be more likely that you will find a situation with comparative or contrasting diagnoses at the time of admission, prior to any lab or radiology test results or further examinations, which then more accurately determine a principal diagnosis and additional diagnoses.

Read the next coding guideline, which is very closely related to the one that you just reviewed, and then review cases for patients' episodes of care listed in Exercise 15.6, answering the questions for each case.

Symptom(s) Followed by Contrasting/Comparative Diagnoses

When a symptom(s) is followed by contrasting/comparative diagnoses, sequence the symptom first. Code all contrasting/comparative diagnoses as additional diagnoses.

infarction (in-fahrk′shən)—death of tissue because blood flow was obstructed, often by a clot

creatine phosphokinase (kre′ə-tin fos′fo-ki-nāse)—a blood test that is used to determine if a person has had a heart attack or other muscle damage

cholecystitis (ko′lə-sis-ti′tis)—inflammation of the gall bladder

pancreatitis (pan′kre-ə-ti′tis)—inflammation of the pancreas

hemoptysis (he-mop′tĭ-sis)—coughing up blood

pulmonary thromboembolism (pool′mo-nar-e thrombo-em′bo-liz-əm)—a blood clot in the lung

Churg-Strauss syndrome (chərg-straus)—growths of inflamed tissue in the lung

TAKE A BREAK

Let's take a break and then review cases with symptoms and comparative or contrasting diagnoses.

Exercise 15.6 Two or More Comparative or Contrasting Conditions, Symptom(s) Followed by Contrasting/Comparative Diagnoses

Instructions: Review each case and then answer the questions that follow. Reference both the Index and Tabular when assigning codes.

Case 1

Mr. Clements, a 56-year-old, arrives at Williton Medical Center's ED by ambulance with chest pain. The patient has a history of gastroesophageal reflux disease (GERD) and anxiety attacks. His family history is positive for myocardial **infarction** (MI). Dr. Mills admits the patient and orders lab tests to determine troponin and **creatine phosphokinase** levels and a complete blood count (CBC). He also orders an echocardiogram (ECG). The results of all

continued

TAKE A BREAK *continued*

the tests are normal. The patient receives antacids and anti-anxiety medication to treat the GERD and his anxiety. Dr. Mills documents the patient's diagnoses as chest pain from GERD *or* anxiety. The patient's length of stay is two days.

a. What are the diagnoses for the patient? _____
_____

b. Which of the diagnoses is a symptom? _____
_____

c. Should you assign an ICD-9-CM code for the symptom? _____

d. Why or why not? _____
_____

e. In what order should you sequence the diagnoses? ___
_____

f. On what information did you base your decision? ___
_____

g. What ICD-9-CM diagnosis codes would you assign to the patient's record? _____
_____

Case 2

Dr. Robbins admits Ralph Telles, age 27, to Williton Medical Center for abdominal pain. Several days of testing prove inconclusive. Dr. Robbins discharges Mr. Telles on the fourth day with a diagnosis of acute abdominal pain due to acute **cholecystitis** or acute **pancreatitis**.

a. What are the diagnoses for the patient? _____
_____

b. Which of the diagnoses is a symptom? _____
_____

c. Should you assign an ICD-9-CM code for the symptom? _____

d. Why or why not? _____
_____

e. In what order should you sequence the diagnoses? ___
_____

f. On what information did you base your decision? ___
_____

g. What ICD-9-CM diagnosis codes would you assign to the patient's record? _____
_____

Case 3

Dr. Mills admits Ron Meador, age 43, to Williton because he reports coughing up large amounts of blood for over a week. Dr. Mills calls Dr. Rutner, a pulmonologist, for a consultation. Dr. Rutner performs a complete workup including blood work, sputum culture, X-rays, and a CT scan. He controls the bleeding through medication and discharges Mr. Meador. The cause is uncertain, and further testing is scheduled. The final diagnosis is **hemoptysis**, **pulmonary thromboembolism**, or **Churg-Strauss** syndrome.

a. What are the diagnoses for the patient? _____
_____

b. Which of the diagnoses is a symptom? _____
_____

c. Should you assign an ICD-9-CM code for the symptom? _____

d. Why or why not? _____
_____

e. In what order should you sequence the diagnoses? ___
_____

f. On what information did you base your decision? ___
_____

g. What ICD-9-CM diagnosis codes would you assign to the patient's record? _____
_____

WORKPLACE IQ

You are working as a coder at Williton Medical Center in the Health Information Management Department. You are cross-trained to code both outpatient encounters and inpatient stays. Today, your manager, Sandy, asks you to sit with Tina, a new coder, and explain the differences between Medicare's OPPS and IPPS.

Sandy admits that Medicare's guidelines can be confusing, but she asks you to help Tina by using basic language, in your own words, that makes the information easy to understand.

What would you do?

Original Treatment Plan Not Carried Out

Sequence as the principal diagnosis the condition which, after study, occasioned the admission to the hospital, even though treatment may not have been carried out due to unforeseen circumstances. For example, if a patient is scheduled for surgery to treat a specific condition but experiences a complication which would make the surgery dangerous for the patient (a contraindication), then you would still code the *reason for surgery* as the principal diagnosis. Assign a code for the complication that cancelled the surgery as an *additional diagnosis*.

   You will also assign a third code to show that the physician did not perform the surgery due to a complication. To locate this code, search the Index for the main term, *surgery, not done because of.* Review cases for patients' episodes of care listed in Exercise 15.7, answering the questions for each case.

endoscopic biopsy (en-do-skop′ik bi′op-se)

ureteritis (u-re-tər-i′tis)

TAKE A BREAK

Let's take a break and then review cases when the patient's original treatment plan is not carried out.

Exercise 15.7 Original Treatment Plan Not Carried Out

Instructions: Review each case and then answer the questions that follow. Reference both the Index and Tabular when assigning codes.

Case 1

Mr. Emerson, a 68-year-old, is scheduled for CABG surgery due to chronic coronary artery disease with hypertension. Prior to surgery, the patient's blood pressure is 200/110. The surgeon decides to cancel surgery until the patient's blood pressure is stable.

   a. Why does the patient need to have CABG surgery? __

   _____

   b. What was the complication that caused the physician to cancel surgery?_____

   c. How many codes should you assign to this patient's record? _____

   d. In what order should you assign the codes? _____

   _____

   e. What ICD-9-CM codes should you assign?_____

   _____

Case 2

Dr. Stuart, an orthopedic surgeon (a physician who treats bone disorders), admits Lena Conn, age 72, to Williton Medical Center for a total left knee replacement due to osteoarthritis. While clinicians prepare her for surgery, she complains of chest pain, so Dr. Stuart cancels the procedure. Lena remains in the hospital for testing and evaluation of her chest pain by Dr. Woods, a cardiologist.

   a. Why does the patient need to have a knee replacement? _____

   b. What was the complication that caused Dr. Stuart to cancel the knee replacement?_____

   c. How many codes should you assign to this patient's record? _____

   d. In what order should you assign the codes? _____

   _____

   e. What ICD-9-CM codes should you assign?_____

   _____

Case 3

Dr. Moir, a urologist (a physician who treats disorders of the urinary system), schedules Jason Colquitt, age 43, for an **endoscopic biopsy** (biopsy performed with an endoscope) of the left ureter due to severe **ureteritis** (inflammation of a ureter). During the procedure, Dr. Moir passes the endoscope through the urethra and into the urinary bladder, but cannot proceed up the ureter due to a blockage. He withdraws the endoscope, and the patient is taken to the recovery room. (Hint: A blockage is also called an obstruction.)

   a. Why does the patient need to have endoscopic biopsy?

   _____

   b. What was the complication that caused the physician to cancel the endoscopic biopsy? _____

   c. How many codes should you assign to this patient's record? _____

   d. In what order should you assign the codes? _____

   _____

   e. What ICD-9-CM codes should you assign? _____

   _____

POINTERS FROM THE PROS: Interview with a Medical Biller

Jarron Sherman works for a large coding, billing, and collections company, performing insurance billing, charge entry, diagnosis coding, and patient customer service. He verifies diagnosis codes for claims that he sends to insurances, which includes reviewing medical documentation for clarification.

What are the most challenging aspects of your job?

Taking specific calls from patients over the phone. It can be very challenging because no calls are exactly alike. I never know what could be coming my way when taking calls to help people out, whether it is about their bill or (outstanding) balance.

What type of training/education did you receive for your job (e.g., coursework, on-the-job training, industry publications, membership in professional organizations)?

I received a one-year certificate in Medical Billing/Coding. I was also trained step-by-step on my actual job. I also had a 160-hour (employer-sponsored) internship. I highly recommend internships; there is no better way of learning than on-the-job, hands-on training.

What advice can you give to new coders to help them succeed in the healthcare field?

The best thing I can offer through my experience is practice, practice, and practice. I was intimidated by this at first, no doubt about it. However, the only way to overcome these things is do not be scared; be willing to dig in and get your feet wet. In life, I see no way around this. Knowing how to communicate with other people in this field is a must. You also want to be thick-skinned, and you can't be surprised how people react to you, whether it is positive or negative.

(Used by permission of Jarron W. Sherman.)

Complications of Surgery and Other Medical Care

hysterectomy (his-tər-ek′tə-me)

salpingo-oophorectomy (sal-ping-go-o-of-ə-rek′tə-me)

When a patient is admitted for treatment of a complication *resulting from* surgery or other medical care, sequence the complication code as the *principal diagnosis*. If the complication is classified to categories 996–999 and the code lacks the necessary specificity in describing the complication, then assign an *additional* code for the specific complication.

When you are coding a complication, search the Index for the main term *complication*. Review cases for patients' episodes of care listed in Exercise 15.8, answering the questions for each case.

TAKE A BREAK

Let's take a break and then review cases for complications of surgery and other medical care.

Exercise 15.8 Complications of Surgery and Other Medical Care

Instructions: Review each case and then answer the questions that follow. Reference both the Index and Tabular when assigning codes.

Case 1

Christine Rutledge, a 56-year-old, is admitted to Williton Medical Center for internal wound dehiscence (■ FIGURE 15-6) after a total abdominal **hysterectomy** (removal of the uterus) and bilateral **salpingo-oophorectomy** (removal of the fallopian tubes and ovaries) for uterine cancer. She is undergoing outpatient chemotherapy to treat uterine cancer.

a. What is the patient's complication? _____

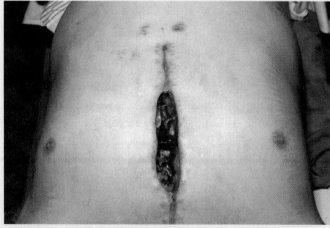

Figure 15-6 ■ Dehiscence (opening) of a surgical wound of the sternum

Photo credit: MICHAEL ENGLISH, M.D. / Custom Medical Stock Photo.

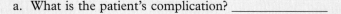

TAKE A BREAK *continued*

b. What is the ICD-9-CM code(s) for the complication? _____

c. What additional diagnosis should you code? _____

d. What is the ICD-9-CM code for the additional diagnosis? _____

e. In what order should you assign the codes? _____

f. On what information did you base your decision? ___

Case 2

Arthur Vanhoose was discharged from Williton Medical Center last week after having a **resection** of the **sigmoid colon** for rupture and **diverticulitis**. Dr. Stark, a general surgeon, readmits him today due to a postoperative **staphylococcal** infection of the surgical site. Dr. Stark

orders antibiotics for the infection and Dr. Drimond, a gastroenterologist, monitors the diverticulitis. Dr. Stark discharges Mr. Vanhoose to home after three days with instructions for postoperative follow-up.

a. What is the patient's complication? _____

b. What is the ICD-9-CM code(s) for the complication? _____

c. What additional diagnosis should you code? _____

d. What is the ICD-9-CM code for the additional diagnosis? _____

e. In what order should you assign the codes? _____

f. On what information did you base your decision? ___
_____

Uncertain Diagnosis

If the diagnosis *at the time of discharge* is documented as "probable," "suspected," "likely," "questionable," "possible," "still to be ruled out," or other similar terms indicating uncertainty, then code the condition as if it existed or was established. The basis for this guideline is that the diagnostic workup, arrangements for further workup or observation, and initial therapeutic approach are the same for a suspected diagnosis as for the established diagnosis.

In the inpatient setting, when the physician orders tests or further examinations for a patient with an uncertain diagnosis, the amount of work performed for the tests and exams (workup) is the same as when the patient has a definitive diagnosis. Therefore, it is important for you to code probable or suspected conditions as though they were definitive diagnoses only when the physician documents them as probable or suspected at the time of discharge.

Keep in mind that the physician can add documentation to a patient's record several times during the patient's stay. The physician may document a condition as probable when he admits the patient and at the time of discharge, he may document a definitive diagnosis. Be careful to only assign codes for probable or suspected conditions if the physician documents them at discharge in a discharge note or a discharge summary report.

It is important to note that this inpatient guideline is completely different from the *outpatient guideline* that you learned about in Chapter 5, which states that when documentation of a patient's encounter describes a diagnosis as "probable," "suspected," "questionable," "rule out," or "working diagnosis," you *cannot* code the diagnosis as though it were confirmed. Instead, code the main reason for the encounter, including symptoms, signs, abnormal test results, or other reasons. So in the inpatient setting, you can code an uncertain diagnosis as though it is confirmed, but in the outpatient setting, you cannot.

resection (re-sek′shən)— excision or removal

sigmoid colon (sig′moid)— the S-shaped portion of the large intestine that lies above the rectum

diverticulitis (di-vər-tik-u-li′tis)—inflammation of the folds or pouches of the lining of an organ

staphylococcal (staf-ə-lo-kok′əl)—pertaining to a bacterial organism that can cause a variety of infections

TAKE A BREAK

Let's take a break and then review cases for uncertain diagnoses.

Exercise 15.9 Uncertain Diagnosis

Instructions: Review each case and then answer the questions that follow. Reference both the Index and Tabular when assigning codes.

Case 1

Dr. Mills admits Susan Bright, a 74-year-old, to Williton Medical Center through the ED due to an acute headache, scalp tenderness, fatigue, and fever. Workup includes

continued

TAKE A BREAK *continued*

erythrocyte sedimentation rate (ESR), complete blood count (CBC), **liver function test (LFT), color duplex sonography,** and temporal artery biopsy. The physician's discharge summary includes suspected **giant cell arteritis.**

a. What is the patient's principal diagnosis? _____

b. What is the ICD-9-CM code(s) for the principal diagnosis? _____

c. Should you code the patient's symptoms? _____

d. Why or why not? _____

Case 2

Dr. Grisham, an orthopedist, admits Gwen Engstrom, age 42, to Williton Medical Center with complaints of severe low back pain and weakness in the left leg. Dr. Grisham orders X-rays, which show no fractures, and an MRI, which shows some inflammation at L4–L5 (lumbar vertebrae). Dr. Grisham prescribes a **morphine** PCA (patient-controlled analgesia) until her pain is under control, then switches her to oral Vicodin®. He also orders a **cortisone** injection. Dr. Grisham documents his diagnosis of a probable herniated **intervertebral disc.**

a. What is the patient's principal diagnosis? _____

b. What is the ICD-9-CM code(s) for the principal diagnosis? _____

c. Should you code the patient's symptoms? _____

d. Why or why not? _____

Case 3

Paul Blair, age 31, has a seizure at home, and Dr. Lombard, a neurologist (a physician who treats nerve disorders), admits him to Williton Medical Center to rule out epilepsy. Dr. Lombard conducts a series of tests and determines that epilepsy is questionable. There are no further incidents, and Dr. Lombard discharges Mr. Blair home with instructions to follow up if there are any more occurrences.

a. Should you code for a condition that is questionable? _____

b. Why or why not? _____

c. What is the patient's principal diagnosis? _____

d. What is the ICD-9-CM code(s) for the principal diagnosis? _____

e. Should you code the patient's symptoms? _____

f. Why or why not? _____

---

liver function test—a standard group of tests used to diagnose and monitor liver diseases

color duplex sonography (doo'-pleks sə-nog'rə-fe)—a type of ultrasound that uses both real-time and Doppler methods

giant cell arteritis (ahr-tə-ri'tis)—a chronic vascular disease that may affect the carotid or temporal arteries and that often includes widespread inflammation, fever, fatigue, and weight loss

morphine (mor'fēn)—an opiate drug used for pain relief

cortisone (kor'tĭ-sōn)—an anti-inflammatory agent

intervertebral disc (in-tər-vur'tə-brəl)—soft cartilage between each pair of vertebra or spinal bones

Hospital Admissions from an Observation Unit or Outpatient Surgery

Review the following guidelines for determining the principal diagnosis when a patient is admitted to a hospital from observation or following an outpatient surgery.

1. *Admission following medical observation*—When a patient is admitted to an observation unit for a medical condition, which either worsens or does not improve, and is then admitted as an inpatient to the same hospital for this same medical condition, the principal diagnosis is the medical condition that led to the hospital admission. Sequence additional codes for other conditions that the physician documents as related to the episode of care.

2. *Admission following postoperative observation*—When a patient is admitted to an observation unit to monitor a condition (or complication) that develops following outpatient surgery, and is then admitted as an inpatient to the same hospital, you should apply the UHDDS definition of principal diagnosis as "that condition established after study to be chiefly responsible for occasioning the admission of the patient to the hospital for care." Sequence additional codes for other conditions that the physician documents as related to the episode of care.

3. *Admission from outpatient surgery*—When a patient receives surgery in the hospital's outpatient surgery department and is then admitted for continuing inpatient

care at the same hospital, refer to the following guidelines to select the principal diagnosis for the inpatient admission:

a. If the reason for the inpatient admission is a *complication*, then assign the *complication as the principal diagnosis.*

b. If no *complication* or other condition is documented as the reason for the inpatient admission, then assign the *reason for the outpatient surgery as the principal diagnosis.*

c. If the reason for the inpatient admission is another condition that is *unrelated* to the surgery, then assign the *unrelated condition as the principal diagnosis.*

Sequence additional codes for other conditions that the physician documents as related to the episode of care.

Review cases for patients' episodes of care listed in Exercise 15.10, answering the questions for each case.

TAKE A BREAK

Let's take a break and then review cases for hospital admissions from observation or outpatient surgery.

Exercise 15.10 **Hospital Admissions from an Observation Unit or Outpatient Surgery**

Instructions: Review each case and then answer the questions that follow. Reference both the Index and Tabular when assigning codes.

Case 1

Trudy Fields, a 75-year-old, has outpatient surgery for senile cataract (■ FIGURE 15-7) removal on her right eye and obtains an intraocular lens (IOL) implant. She develops hypertension postoperatively and is admitted for observation.

When the hypertension exacerbates, the attending physician admits her to the hospital as an inpatient.

a. Why does the attending physician admit Mrs. Fields as an inpatient (principal diagnosis)? _____

_____

b. What is the ICD-9-CM code for the principal diagnosis? _____

c. Are there any other conditions that you should code? _____

d. If so, what are the condition(s), and what ICD-9-CM code should you assign? _____

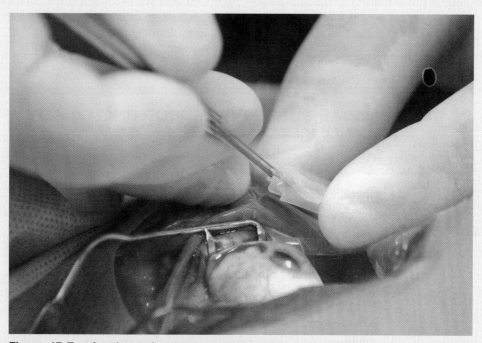

Figure 15-7 ■ A patient undergoes cataract surgery.
Photo credit: Bork / Shutterstock.com.

continued

TAKE A BREAK *continued*

Case 2

Bruce Roland, age 52, reports to outpatient surgery at Williton Medical Center for a colonoscopy and polypectomy to treat colon polyps. Dr. Fitzpatrick completes the procedure without complications, but when Mr. Roland stands up afterward, he feels weak and lightheaded. The nurse takes his blood pressure, which is 90/50, and calls Dr. Fitzpatrick. The doctor admits him to the hospital with **orthostatic hypotension** (a drop in blood pressure when standing). Dr. Fitzpatrick monitors Mr. Roland and releases him the following day.

a. Why does the attending physician admit Mr. Roland as an inpatient (principal diagnosis)? _____

_____

b. What is the ICD-9-CM code for the principal diagnosis? _____

c. Are there any other conditions that you should code?

_____

d. If so, what are the condition(s), and what ICD-9-CM code should you assign? _____

Case 3

Dr. Stark, a general surgeon, performs a laparoscopic cholecystectomy for Gwendolyn Keil at Williton Medical Center's outpatient surgery center. After the procedure, she experiences atrial fibrillation, and Dr. Stark admits her.

a. Why does the attending physician admit Ms. Keil as an inpatient (principal diagnosis)? _____

b. What is the ICD-9-CM code for the principal diagnosis? _____

c. Are there any other conditions that you should code?

_____

d. If so, what are the condition(s), and what ICD-9-CM code should you assign? _____

INTERESTING FACT: Cataracts Cause Blindness throughout the World

A cataract is a clouding of the eye's lens from protein deposits and is the leading cause of blindness worldwide and the leading cause of vision loss in the United States. Cataracts can occur at any age, are due to a variety of causes, and can also be present at birth. Although treatment for the removal of a cataract is widely available, access barriers, such as lack of insurance coverage and ability to pay, or lack of awareness, prevent many people from receiving the proper treatment. An estimated 20.5 million (17.2%) Americans 40 years and older have a cataract in one or both eyes, and 6.1 million (5.1%) have had their lens removed operatively. The total number of people who have cataracts is estimated to increase to 30.1 million by 2020.

orthostatic hypotension
(or-tho-stat'ik)

GENERAL RULES FOR REPORTING OTHER (ADDITIONAL) DIAGNOSES

For reporting purposes, the definition of *other diagnoses* is interpreted as *additional conditions that affect patient care* in terms of requiring

- clinical evaluation; or
- therapeutic treatment; or
- diagnostic procedures; or
- extended length of hospital stay, or
- increased nursing care and/or monitoring

The UHDDS defines other diagnoses as:

- all conditions that coexist at the time of admission
- conditions that develop subsequent to the admission
- or conditions that affect the treatment received and/or the length of stay

Do not report other diagnoses that relate to an earlier episode of care, which have no bearing on the *current* hospital stay.

Apply guidelines for coding previous conditions and abnormal findings when determining *other diagnoses* and neither the Alphabetic Index nor the Tabular List in the ICD-9-CM provides direction. We will review those guidelines next.

Codes for Previous Conditions

If the provider includes a diagnosis in the final diagnostic statement, such as in the discharge summary or the face sheet (record of documentation), then you should code it. Some providers include in the diagnostic statement *resolved* conditions or diagnoses, and status-post procedures from *previous* admissions, *that have no bearing on the current stay.* Do not code these conditions unless the hospital's policy requires it. However, you can assign history codes (V10–V19) as secondary codes if the historical condition or family history has an impact on current care or influences treatment.

Review cases for patients' episodes of care listed in Exercise 15.11, answering the questions for each case.

hemiplegia (hem-i-plē′-jē-ə)

TAKE A BREAK

Let's take a break and then determine whether to code previous conditions.

Exercise 15.11 General Rules for Reporting Other (Additional) Diagnoses

Instructions: Review each case and then answer the questions that follow. Reference both the Index and Tabular when assigning codes.

Case 1

Mr. Sharpe, a 68-year-old, has a two-day inpatient stay due to chest pain. The physician documents in his discharge summary that after further study and workup, the patient had no evidence of an MI, and the discharge diagnosis is acute anxiety with panic attack. He also documents that the patient has a history of MI, mitral valve replacement, and cholecystectomy.

a. What are the principal diagnosis and ICD-9-CM code for the patient? Principal diagnosis:_____ ICD-9-CM code:_____

b. Should you assign an additional code for myocardial infarction? _____

c. Why or why not? _____
_____

d. What additional diagnosis code(s) should you assign for personal history? _____

Case 2

Dr. Robbins admits Wayne Bonds to Williton Medical Center from the nursing home for cellulitis in his left leg (infection or inflammation of connective tissue). Dr. Robbins administers IV antibiotics and elevates the patient's leg. A culture shows that the cellulitis is due to *Staphylococcus*. Upon discharge, Dr. Robbins notes that Mr. Bonds previously experienced urinary retention due to benign prostatic hyperplasia, now resolved, and also had pneumonia three months ago.

a. What are the principal diagnosis and ICD-9-CM code(s) for the patient? Principal diagnosis:_____ ICD-9-CM code: _____

b. Should you assign any additional codes? Why or why not? _____

c. Should you assign codes for personal history of any condition? _____

Case 3

Dr. Lombard, a neurologist, admits Katrina Najera, age 62, to Williton due to left **hemiplegia** (paralysis on one side of the body) and blurriness of vision. She has a history of migraines and GERD. Dr. Lombard orders a CT scan and a neurological workup. Test results are negative for any new problems. Dr. Lombard prescribes medication for migraines. The patient's symptoms improve, and Dr. Lombard discharges her with follow-up instructions. Dr. Lombard documents a final diagnosis of hemiplegic migraine.

a. What are the principal diagnosis and ICD-9-CM code(s) for the patient? Principal diagnosis:_____ ICD-9-CM code:_____

b. Should you assign any additional codes? Why or why not? _____

c. Should you assign codes for personal history of any condition?_____

Abnormal Findings

Do not code abnormal findings (laboratory, X-ray, pathologic, and other diagnostic results) unless the provider indicates their clinical significance. If the findings are outside the normal range, and the attending provider orders other tests to evaluate the condition or prescribes treatment, then it is appropriate to ask the provider if you should code the abnormal findings. Note that this coding guideline is different from outpatient coding guidelines, which instruct you to code abnormal test results in the absence of a definitive diagnosis.

It is important to become familiar with abnormal findings, especially if the physician documents an abnormal lab test result without using the words *elevated, abnormal,* or *decreased.* Remember that coding is not as simple as reviewing medical documentation and picking out diagnoses and procedures to code. You must understand the information that you read, not only to code correctly, but to also be able to query the physician when you are unsure of the information that you review. Refer to Appendix C of this text to review Normal Lab Values and Vital Signs and then answer the questions outlined in Exercise 15.12. You may also need to refer to your medical references and Internet searches to answer additional questions.

albumin (ăl-bū′ mĭn)

TAKE A BREAK

Let's take a break and then answer questions about abnormal findings.

Exercise 15.12 Abnormal Findings

Instructions: Answer the following questions about codes for abnormal findings.

1. The physician documents that a patient's **albumin** (protein) level is 4.0 g/dL. Is this an abnormal finding? _____

2. What information can a physician determine from a patient's albumin level? _____

3. A patient's GFR is 12 mL/min/1.73 m². Is this an abnormal finding? _____

4. What information can a physician determine from a patient's GFR? _____

5. The physician documents that a patient's total cholesterol level is 300 mg/dL. Is this an abnormal finding? _____

6. What types of diseases could elevated total cholesterol cause a patient to develop? _____

7. A patient's oral temperature is 105°F. Is this an abnormal temperature? _____

8. An adult patient's respiratory rate is 15 breaths/minute. Is this an abnormal rate? _____

9. An adult patient's pulse rate is 120 beats per minute (BPM). Is this an abnormal rate? _____

10. After reviewing a patient's inpatient record, you find documentation of a potassium deficiency, elevated prothrombin time (PT), and normal partial thromboplastin time (PTT), along with IV administration of a Vitamin K supplement. Should you query the physician about coding the abnormal lab results? _____

11. On what information did you base your decision? ___ _____ _____

A LOOK AHEAD TO ICD-10-CM

The ICD-9-CM and ICD-10-CM guidelines for Selection of Principal Diagnosis and Reporting Additional Diagnoses remain the same. However, in ICD-10-CM, code complications of surgical and medical care to T80–T88 if they are not classified elsewhere in ICD-9-CM. Appendix I—Present on Admission Reporting Guidelines in the ICD-9-CM guidelines do not exist in the ICD-10-CM guidelines.

Instructions: Assign codes from ICD-10-CM, referencing both the Index and the Tabular.

1. Eugene Shepard, age 64, arrives at Williton's ED with complaints of chest pain, left arm numbness, and dizziness. Dr. Mills orders a series of tests, which reveal STEMI of the inferolateral wall. Dr. Mills admits the patient for further treatment. This is the first time that the patient has experienced these problems. Code(s): _____

2. Dr. Hoffman admits Josalyn Early, a 25-year-old, to Williton Medical Center. She complains of heavy menstrual bleeding for two days and reports severe abdominal pain. Dr. Robbins, the attending physician, orders blood work that shows anemia due to acute blood loss. He orders pain medication and packed blood cells for the anemia. The patient stabilizes, and Dr. Robbins discharges her to home. Code(s): _____

3. Dr. Robbins assesses the case of David Wieland, age 35, an inpatient at Williton Medical Center. He calls in Dr. Reilly, an orthopedic spinal surgeon, for a consultation on Mr. Wieland's back pain from lumbosacral spondylosis. He also requests a consultation from Dr. Drimond, a gastroenterologist, for Mr. Wieland's acute gastroenteritis. Mr. Wieland improves after receiving medication for both conditions. Dr. Robbins discharges him home after three days. Code(s): _____

4. Dr. Robbins admits Ralph Telles, age 27, to Williton Medical Center for abdominal pain. Several days of testing prove inconclusive. Dr. Robbins discharges Mr. Telles on the fourth day with a diagnosis of acute abdominal pain due to acute cholecystitis or acute pancreatitis. Code(s): _____

5. Dr. Stuart, an orthopedic surgeon, admits Lena Conn, age 72, to Williton Medical Center for a total left knee replacement due to osteoarthritis. While clinicians prepare her for surgery, she complains of chest pain, so Dr. Stuart cancels the procedure. Lena remains in the hospital for testing and evaluation of her chest pain by Dr. Woods, a cardiologist. Code(s): _____

6. Bruce Roland, age 52, reports to outpatient surgery at Williton Medical Center for a colonoscopy and polypectomy to treat colon polyps. Dr. Fitzpatrick completes the procedure without complications, but when Mr. Roland stands up afterward, he feels weak and lightheaded. The nurse takes his blood pressure, which is 90/50, and calls Dr. Fitzpatrick. The doctor admits him to the hospital with orthostatic hypotension (a drop in blood pressure when standing). Dr. Fitzpatrick monitors Mr. Roland and releases him the following day. Code(s): _____

CHAPTER REVIEW

Multiple Choice

Instructions: Circle one best answer to complete each statement.

1. The diagnosis that the physician documents to show why he is admitting the patient is called the _____ diagnosis.
   a. principal
   b. rule out
   c. admitting
   d. first-listed

2. Providers submit _____ claims on the UB-04.
   a. physician
   b. pharmacy
   c. inpatient and outpatient hospital claims
   d. urgent care clinic

3. The RBRVS is a calculation of the cost that the physician incurs for all of the following *except*
   a. physician work involved in providing a service.
   b. geographic practice cost index.
   c. expense to provide the service.
   d. malpractice expense.

4. Outpatient hospitals are paid based on
   a. a set amount for a procedure.
   b. "just in case" testing.
   c. the average length of hospital stays for specific diagnoses.
   d. the cost of similar procedures in the same APC group.

5. Medicare pays additional money to inpatient hospitals for all the following *except*
   a. treating a high percentage of low-income patients.
   b. treating hospital-acquired infections.
   c. being an approved teaching hospital.
   d. treating patients who have unusually costly cases.

6. Assign codes for symptoms, signs, and ill-defined conditions from Chapter 16 of ICD-9-CM as the principal diagnosis (inpatient) when
   a. the provider establishes a related definitive diagnosis.
   b. when a symptom(s) is followed by contrasting/comparative diagnoses.
   c. there are two or more interrelated conditions that potentially meet the definition of principal diagnosis.
   d. the diagnosis at the time of discharge is documented using terms indicating uncertainty.

7. When the original treatment plan is not carried out, the principal diagnosis should be
   a. a code to show that the physician did not perform the surgery due to a complication.
   b. the original treatment planned.
   c. comparative or contrasting diagnoses at the time of admission.
   d. the condition, which after study, occasioned the admission to the hospital.

8. When the admission is for treatment of a complication resulting from surgery or other medical care, the principal diagnosis should be the
   a. complication.
   b. original condition treated.
   c. presenting symptoms.
   d. E code describing the cause.

9. Assign a code for an uncertain diagnosis for an inpatient when
   a. you do not understand the documentation.
   b. two or more diagnoses equally meet the criteria for principal diagnosis.
   c. the diagnosis documented at the time of discharge is qualified as "probable," "suspected," or "likely."
   d. the original treatment is not carried out due to unforeseen circumstances.

10. When should you assign codes for abnormal findings?
    a. Only when the provider indicates their clinical significance
    b. Whenever findings are outside the normal range
    c. Only when the physician orders additional tests to evaluate the condition
    d. Only on outpatient records

Coding Assignments

Instructions: Assign ICD-9-CM code(s) to the following cases, referencing both the Index and Tabular.

1. Cathy Foltz, age 34, is admitted to Williton Medical Center with abdominal pain. After a workup, Dr. Valencia, a gastroenterologist, narrows the possible conditions down to gastroenteritis or **diverticulosis**. He is able to help Ms. Foltz manage the pain through medication. The discharge diagnosis is listed as abdominal pain due to gastroenteritis or diverticulosis.

   Code(s): _____

2. Dana Leahy brings her son Tyler, a 6-year-old, to Williton Medical Center's ED due to a high fever. Dr. Daniels, an emergency physician, believes that the patient may have **bacteremia** (bacteria in the blood) and admits him. This diagnosis is later confirmed. Dr. Daniels immediately administers IV antibiotics.

   Code(s): _____

3. Tim Boykins, a 78-year-old, has severe CHF. Dr. Bergin, a cardiologist, admits him to Williton Medical Center because of nocturnal dyspnea and orthopnea. The patient also has type II diabetes mellitus and takes Diabinese®. During his stay, his blood glucose increases sharply, so Dr. Bergin calls in Dr. Mayhew, an endocrinologist, who administers insulin. This brings Mr. Boykins's sugar back under control. He also takes **Accupril**® for hypertension due to his diabetes. His discharge diagnosis is CHF; type II diabetes, uncontrolled; and diabetic nephrosis with hypertension.

   Code(s): _____

4. Dorothy Volk, age 41, is status post mastectomy due to breast cancer and receives chemotherapy. Dr. Simmons, an oncologist, admits her to Williton Medical Center for anemia due to chemotherapy. He administers packed blood cells. She also receives her weekly chemotherapy while she is admitted. Dr. Simmons discharges her in good condition.

   Code(s): _____

5. Dr. Petty, a urologist, admits Wilbur Walton, age 76, to Williton Medical Center for evaluation of overflow incontinence. Mr. Walton complains that he leaks urine continuously, but he never feels an urge to urinate and never feels like his bladder is completely empty. After several days of testing, Dr. Petty rules out benign prostatic hyperplasia, urinary stones, and **neurogenic** bladder.

   Code(s): _____

6. Dr. Robbins admits Craig Rodney, age 50, to Williton Medical Center for testing because of numerous gastrointestinal symptoms. After several rounds of diagnostic testing, Dr. Robbins believes that Mr. Rodney could have acute pancreatitis or acute **cholangitis**.

   Code(s): _____

7. Dr. Robbins admits Jonathan Headley, age 62, to Williton Medical Center with acute low back pain and an acute exacerbation of asthma. Dr. Robbins evaluates both conditions and orders Vicodin® for back pain and steroids for asthma. Both conditions stabilize after three days, and Dr. Robbins discharges him home.

   Code(s): _____

8. Dr. Valencia, a gastroenterologist, sees Janet Laddel, age 64, for a routine screening colonoscopy. When he begins the procedure, he cannot advance the endoscope past the sigmoid colon due to a blockage. He notes that the bowel was not adequately evacuated (cleared), so he cannot perform the procedure.

   Code(s): _____

9. Anita Fishman, age 66, sees Dr. Hoffman for nausea and vomiting. She states that she has been unable to eat and can barely stand up on her own. Dr. Hoffman says that she is dehydrated and immediately admits her to Williton Medical Center for rehydration IV fluids and nourishment. After three days, she improves, and she is discharged home.

   Code(s): _____

10. Raymond Vestal, age 52, presents to Williton Medical Center's ED with a severe headache. A workup reveals a ruptured berry aneurysm (a sac in a cerebral artery that resembles a berry) and Dr. Daniels admits him for surgery.

    Code(s): _____

diverticulosis (di′vər-tik′u-lo′sis)—abnormal bulges, pouches, and pockets in an organ lining, especially the colon

bacteremia (bak′tər-e′me-ə)

Accupril® (ak′u-pril′)—a drug used to treat hypertension

neurogenic (noor′o-jen′ik)—any condition that originates in the nervous system

cholangitis (ko′lan-ji′tis)—inflammation of one or more bile ducts

Vicodin® (vi′ko-din′)—a pain medication derived from codeine that contains acetaminophen

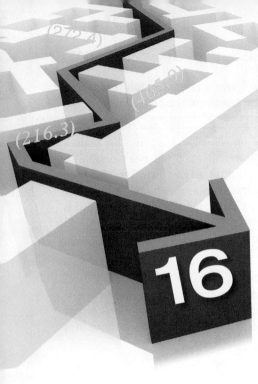

Inpatient Hospital Procedures: ICD-9-CM and ICD-10-PCS

16

Learning Objectives

After completing this chapter, you should be able to

- Spell and define the key terminology in this chapter.
- Define an inpatient hospital procedure.
- Discuss the background and structure of ICD-9-CM procedure codes.
- Explain how to use the ICD-9-CM Volume 3 Tabular List and Alphabetic Index.
- Describe coding conventions in ICD-9-CM Volume 3.
- Assign procedure codes using the ICD-9-CM Alphabetic Index and Tabular List.
- Discuss the background, organization, and structure of the ICD-10-PCS code set.
- Review how to use the ICD-10-PCS Index and Tables to assign procedure codes.

Key Terms

category
chapter
characters
Index to Procedures
inpatient hospital procedure
principal procedure

subcategory
subclassification
synchronous procedure
Tables
Tabular List
values

INTRODUCTION

Just as you learned the rules of the road for coding diagnoses, you will also learn the rules of the road for coding inpatient procedures. Remember that hospitals use ICD-9-CM Volume 3 inpatient procedure codes to bill insurances for inpatient procedures on the UB-04. Physicians and outpatient hospitals use CPT-4 and HCPCS procedure codes to bill insurances on the CMS-1500 (physicians) or on the UB-04 (outpatient hospitals). You will learn more about CPT-4 and HCPCS codes later in this text. In this chapter, we will focus only on coding hospital inpatient procedures. Also remember that there are two different code sets for inpatient procedures, and you will learn how to use both ICD-9-CM Volume 3 procedure codes, which are effective currently, and ICD-10-PCS codes, which will take effect later. We will follow a series of steps to learn the code sets so that you will feel comfortable with them. Let's begin learning about inpatient procedure coding!

"The secret of getting ahead is getting started. The secret of getting started is breaking your complex overwhelming tasks into small manageable tasks, and then starting on the first one."—MARK TWAIN

INPATIENT HOSPITAL PROCEDURE CODES

An **inpatient hospital procedure** is a therapeutic service, such as a surgical operation, or a diagnostic service that is performed for a patient admitted to an inpatient hospital, including an acute care facility. Do you remember reviewing ICD-9-CM Volume 3 inpatient procedure codes in Chapter 2? You learned that inpatient procedure codes are two digits followed by a decimal point, and then up to two more digits. Here are some examples:

- 62.0—Incision of testis
- 85.12—Open biopsy of the breast
- 31.61—Suture of laceration of larynx

ICD-9-CM Volume 3 procedure codes are all numeric; they do not contain any alphabetic characters. The code numbers range from 00.01 to 99.99.

When a patient has more than one procedure, assign codes for each procedure, depending on the circumstances of the patient's admission and episode of care. Read and follow the instructional notes and conventions in your ICD-9-CM manual. The **principal procedure** is the procedure that correlates to the patient's principal diagnosis; it may also be a procedure that the physician performs for a complication. A principal procedure is typically performed to treat a condition, rather than to diagnose it. Assign secondary codes for additional procedures, including those for treatment or diagnosis.

BACKGROUND OF ICD-9-CM PROCEDURE CODES

WHO, American Hospital Association (AHA), and CMS created ICD-9-CM Volume 3 inpatient procedure codes together. Inpatient hospitals and insurance companies in the U.S. have used these codes since 1979. Volume 3 code structures follow WHO's ICD-9 codes structures. CMS and NCHS maintain the code set, updating codes twice a year, on April 1 and October 1. The major revision occurs on October 1, the same time that revisions for ICD-9-CM diagnosis codes go into effect.

Publishers print two versions of the ICD-9-CM manual: Physician offices use the version that contains Volumes 1 and 2, and inpatient hospitals use the version that contains all three volumes. You can also obtain the manual electronically, on CD-ROM, or in a web-based version. Different versions may contain different symbols, colors, or special notes and instructions to help you to assign codes correctly.

Volume 3 has two parts: the **Index** to Procedures (an alphabetic index) and the **Tabular List**, which are structured similarly to Volumes 1 and 2 of ICD-9-CM. The codes represent medical procedures, including diagnostic procedures (to diagnose a condition), such as biopsy, and therapeutic procedures (to treat a condition), such as a repair or organ transplant. There are no ICD-9-CM Official Guidelines for Volume 3 procedure codes, but there are coding conventions that you should follow before final code assignment. We will review the conventions later in this chapter.

ICD-9-CM VOLUME 3 TABULAR LIST

The Tabular List for ICD-9-CM Volume 3 procedure codes contains 17 chapters, starting with 0, which are divided by body system (■ TABLE 16-1). The Tabular List is located after the Index to Procedures (alphabetic index).

Procedure codes in the Tabular List have a minimum of three digits and a maximum of four. They are categorized as follows:

- **Chapter**—a group of two-digit categories that represent related procedures for the same body system(s), procedures that are not elsewhere classified, or miscellaneous procedures.
- **Category**—a two-digit code that represents the *type of procedure*, such as 18—*Operation on external ear* or 87—*Diagnostic radiology*. A category code can never stand alone and will need additional digits before final code assignment.

■ TABLE 16-1   VOLUME 3 PROCEDURE CODES TABULAR LIST CHAPTERS

Chapter	Title	Code Range
0	Procedures and interventions, not elsewhere classified	00
1	Operations on the nervous system	01–05
2	Operations on the endocrine system	06–07
3	Operations on the eye	08–16
3A	Other miscellaneous diagnostic and therapeutic procedures	17
4	Operations on the ear	18–20
5	Operations on the nose, mouth, and pharynx	21–29
6	Operations on the respiratory system	30–34
7	Operations on the cardiovascular system	35–39
8	Operations on the hemic and lymphatic system	40–41
9	Operations on the digestive system	42–54
10	Operations on the urinary system	55–59
11	Operations on the male genital organs	60–64
12	Operations on the female genital organs	65–71
13	Obstetrical procedures	72–75
14	Operations on the musculoskeletal system	76–84
15	Operations on the integumentary system	85–86
16	Miscellaneous diagnostic and therapeutic procedures	87–99

- **Subcategory**—a three-digit code providing further specification for a category, including variations of a procedure or specifying an anatomic site, such as 18.0—*Incision of external ear* or 87.2—*X-ray of spine*. You may assign a three-digit subcategory code as the final code when a four-digit code is not available.

- **Subclassification**—a four-digit code that is the highest level of specificity; *it further* describes the procedure and anatomic site, such as 18.01—*Piercing of ear lobe* or 87.21—*Contrast myelogram*.

Turn to the Volume 3 Tabular List in your ICD-9-CM coding manual to become more familiar with code divisions. When you want to find the correct code, you begin at the category level (two digits), then move to the subcategory level (three digits), and then move to the subclassification level (four digits) if one exists, to assign the most specific code available. You are already familiar with this process from diagnosis coding. It is called coding to the *highest level of specificity*, meaning that you need to assign the *highest level* of a code that exists.

■ FIGURE 16-1 shows the divisions in the Tabular List for a chapter, category, subcategory, and subclassification, along with the code title, for code 53.00.

Code 53.00 describes the procedure for a unilateral repair of an inguinal hernia. To assign code 53.00, you would have to read the patient's documentation to first determine the type of procedure that the physician performed, such as an inguinal **herniorrhaphy**. You would start coding from the category of *Repair of hernia* and then code further to the subcategory and finally the subclassification, which includes the phrase *inguinal herniorrhaphy* under the code title.

herniorrhaphy (hur-ne-or′ ə-fe)—surgical repair and suture of a hernia

Coding Inpatient Procedures to the Highest Level of Specificity in the Tabular List

Follow these steps to help you code inpatient procedures to the highest level of specificity:

1. When you review a category, you will see subcategory options indented below the category, and you will need to review the subcategories.

9. OPERATIONS ON THE DIGESTIVE SYSTEM (42-54) ← **Chapter number and code range - 2 digits**

53 **Repair of hernia** ← **Category - 2 digits**

Includes: hernioplasty

herniorrhaphy

Code also any application or administration of an adhesion barrier substance (99.77)

Excludes: manual reduction of hernia (96.27)

53.0 **Other unilateral repair of inguinal hernia** ← **Subcategory - 3 digits**

Excludes: laparoscopic unilateral repair of inguinal hernia (17.11-17.13)

53.00 **Unilateral repair of inguinal hernia,** ← **Subclassification - 4 digits**
not otherwise specified

Inguinal herniorrhaphy NOS

Figure 16-1 Tabular list entry in Volume 3 for code 53.00.

2. Determine if the subcategories are further divided into subclassifications indented underneath, which you will also need to review. In other words, do not stop coding at the subcategory level if there is a subclassification. Coding to the highest level of specificity is *mandatory*, not optional.

3. If your coding manual contains symbols that direct you to assign additional digits, then review and apply them in the Tabular List, whether you are referencing the code set in a manual, electronic, or web-based version. Review the symbols to identify whether a three-digit subcategory or a fourth-digit subclassification code is available.

ICD-9-CM VOLUME 3 INDEX TO PROCEDURES

You can find the **Index to Procedures** (alphabetic index) at the beginning of Volume 3 before the Tabular List. The Index lists names and descriptions for all therapeutic and diagnostic procedures, arranged in alphabetical order by main terms, subterms that modify main terms, and subterms that modify other subterms (■ FIGURE 16-2).

Depending on the ICD-9-CM manual that you use, main terms may be listed in bold. Subterms are always indented underneath main terms. Main terms generally describe the *type* of procedure, and subterms describe a *variation* of the procedure or the *anatomic site* of the procedure.

To locate a code in the Index, review the patient's medical documentation to find the procedure that the physician performed. Then search for the procedure in the Index as a main term, and review related subterms. To find an eponym (a procedure named after a person), search for the eponym. Another option is to search under the main term *operation* or the type of procedure and then search for a subterm that is the eponym. Body sites are not typically listed as main terms. Pay attention to any coding conventions, which we will review next. Then cross-reference the procedure code to the Tabular List for additional clarification and final code assignment. *Never code directly from the Index.*

Ablation ← **Main term**
  biliary tract (lesion) by ERCP 51.64 ← **Subterm modifying main term**
  endometrial (hysteroscopic) 68.23 ← **Subterm modifying main term**
  inner ear (cryosurgery) (ultrasound) 20.79 ← **Subterm modifying main term**
    by injection 20.72 ← **Subterm modifying another subterm**

Figure 16-2 ■ Index to Procedures in Volume 3.

CODING CONVENTIONS

Many of the coding conventions in the Index and Tabular List of Volume 3 have the same meaning as they do in Volumes 1 and 2 when you code diagnoses, conventions that you learned in Chapter 4. The difference is that the meanings of the conventions apply to procedures, not to diagnoses. Refer to ▪ TABLE 16-2 for a list of coding conventions and their meanings. You can also review the Official Guidelines for more information (instructions for accessing the guidelines are in Appendix A of this text).

Next we will discuss several additional conventions that you will only find in the Tabular List or the Index. They include the following:

- **Code also**—Tabular List
- **Omit code**—Index
- **Synchronous procedure**—Index

Code Also—Tabular List

The instructional note "Code also" is used in two ways in the Volume 3 Tabular List:

1. Code also
2. Code also any (includes *Code also any synchronous*—performed at the same time—procedure)

1. "Code also" instructs you to assign a code for additional procedures that the physicians perform in addition to the primary procedure (▪ FIGURE 16-3).

    Notice that a lung transplant is the primary procedure, and a cardiopulmonary bypass is a separate procedure that the physician performs along with the lung transplant. The convention "Code also" applies to procedures that are performed with another procedure, called a component procedure. If the physician does not document that she performed a component procedure, you should not assign a code for it.

2. "Code also any" instructs you to assign a code for an adjunct (additional) procedure or a synchronous procedure (done at the same time), if it is performed, or for a medical supply or equipment if it is used (▪ FIGURE 16-4). Do not assign a code listed under "Code also any" unless the physician documents that he performed the procedure or dispensed the supply or equipment. It is important to note that "Code also any" could list more than one procedure, supply, or equipment, and any one or more of them can be present in the medical documentation. If more than one procedure is present, then you should assign a code for each one, in addition to the code for the primary procedure.

    This "Code also any" note means that if the physician performs an endarterectomy, then the note to "Code also any" instructs you to assign additional codes for any of the additional procedures listed underneath, if the physician performed them.

Omit Code—Index

The note "omit code" after an Index entry identifies procedures or services that are included in *another* larger procedure or service. This note describes procedures that you

---

33.5 Lung transplant
Note: To report donor source - *see* codes 00.91-00.93

Excludes: combined heart-lung transplantation (33.6)

Code also cardiopulmonary bypass [extracorporeal circulation] [heart-lung machine] (39.61)

Figure 16-3 ▪ Volume 3 Tabular List entry for "Code also."

■ **TABLE 16-2 CODING CONVENTIONS IN VOLUME 3**

CONVENTIONS FOR ICD-9-CM Volume 3

1. Format—Index and Tabular List

Volume 3 uses an indented format for ease of reference. The Index to Procedures contains main terms and subterms in alphabetical order with subterms indented under main terms. Cross-reference codes in the Index to the Tabular List, which also uses an indented format.

2. Abbreviations

Index and Tabular List abbreviations

NEC—Not elsewhere classifiable	Medical documentation specifies the procedure, but there is no specific code in ICD-9-CM.
NOS—Not Otherwise specified	Medical documentation is insufficient to allow for a more accurate code assignment.

3. Punctuation—Index and Tabular List

Brackets [ ]	Used in Tabular List to enclose synonyms, alternative wording, or explanatory phrases. Used in the Index to identify additional codes that you should sequence second, called **synchronous procedures** (performed at the same time).
Parentheses ( )	Used in the Tabular List and the Index to enclose words or terms that may or may not be present in the diagnostic statement (called nonessential modifiers).
Colon :	Used in the Tabular List and Index after an incomplete term to list more information after the colon.

4. Includes Notes, Excludes Notes, Inclusion Terms, Note—Tabular List or Index

Includes	Appears after a category, subcategory, or subclassification in the Tabular List and lists terms included in the code.
Excludes	Appears after a category, subcategory, or subclassification in the Tabular List and lists terms excluded from the code.
Inclusion Terms	Lists terms included under codes in the Tabular List.
Note	Used in Tabular List and Index to provide additional information about conditions and how to code them, including additional codes to report and subclassification code choices.

5. Other and Unspecified Codes—Tabular List and Index

a. "Other" or "Other specified" codes

Medical documentation specifies the procedure, but there is no specific code in ICD-9-CM.

b. "Unspecified" codes

Medical documentation is insufficient to allow for a more accurate code assignment.

6. "And"—Tabular List

When the word "and" appears in a code title, it can mean either "and," but it can also mean "or."

7. "With"—Index

- In the Index, refer to the word "with" immediately following a main term, which connects the main term to a subterm.
- "With" is not listed in alphabetical order with subterms.
- You may also see the terms *from, for, and, as, in, by,* or *of* connecting a main term to a subterm.
- When there is more than one connecting term in the Index, you will see them arranged alphabetically, such as *by* and *with*.

8. "See," "See Also," and "See Category"—Index or Tabular List

- The word "see" in the Tabular List or after a main term or subterm in the Index means to look elsewhere.
- The phrase "see also" after a main term or subterm in the Index means to also reference another main term or subterm.
- The phrase "see category" appears in the Tabular List or after a main term in the Index. It means to look for information under a specific category in the Tabular List.

Figure 16-4 ■ Volume 3
Tabular List entry for "Code
also any."

38.1 Endarterectomy

[0-6,8]

        Endarterectomy with:
          embolectomy
          patch graft
          temporary bypass during procedure
          thrombectomy
Code also any:
        number of vascular stents inserted (00.45-00.48)
        number of vessels treated (00.40-00.43)
        procedure on vessel bifurcation (00.44)

should *not* code separately, such as a surgical incision that is part of the beginning of a surgical procedure, or closure of an incision (wound), which is part of the end of a surgical procedure. The incision is the approach to the procedure, the way that the physician gains access to the surgical site. You should not code it separately because it is a normal part of the procedure, just as the wound closure is part of the procedure. Refer to the following example to review more about the "omit code" note.

Example: Dr. Dunford, a general surgeon, performs a laparotomy with appendectomy on Susan Simmons, age 8, due to a ruptured appendix. (Laparotomy is the incision into the abdomen that is required to perform the procedure.)

Refer to your Volume 3 ICD-9-CM manual, and search for *laparotomy* in the Index. You will then see a note listed under laparotomy, "as operative Approach—omit code" (■ FIGURE 16-5).

This means that if the physician uses a laparotomy as the surgical approach, then you should omit, or leave out, a separate code for the approach because the approach is included in the procedure. In this example, you should only code for the appendectomy. However, there are situations when you should assign a separate code for a laparotomy, including cases when it is the primary procedure, such as in exploratory surgery.

Laparotomy NEC 54.19
    as operative Approach -- *omit code*
    exploratory (pelvic) 54.11
    reopening of recent operative site (for control of hemorrhage) (for exploration) (for incision
        of hematoma) 54.12

Figure 16-5 ■ Example of an Index entry for "omit code."

Synchronous Procedure—Index

A synchronous procedure is a component of another procedure, and you should assign an additional code for a synchronous procedure when it is performed. In the Index, a synchronous procedure code will follow a code for a primary procedure. You will see the synchronous procedure code enclosed in square brackets. This means that you should assign the code in brackets as an additional code (■ FIGURE 16-6).

In Figure 16-6, notice that there are two codes listed for bladder **anastomosis** (a procedure to join two structures that are not normally connected) with an isolated segment of the intestine, codes 57.87 and 45.50. A physician could perform this procedure for a patient with bladder cancer to remove part of the urinary bladder and reconstruct it

anastomosis (ə-nas-tə-moʹsis)

57.87 Reconstruction of urinary bladder
   Anastomosis of bladder with isolated segment of ileum
   Augmentation of bladder
   Replacement of bladder with ileum or sigmoid [closed ileal bladder]

Code also resection of intestine (45.50-45.52)

45.5 Isolation of intestinal segment
   Code also any synchronous:
      anastomosis other than end-to-end (45.90-45.94)
      enterostomy (46.10-46.39)

45.50 Isolation of intestinal segment, not otherwise specified
   Isolation of intestinal pedicle flap
   Reversal of intestinal segment

Figure 16-7 ■ Codes 57.87 and 45.50 in the Tabular List.

Anastomosis
   bladder NEC 57.88
      with
         isolated segment of intestine 57.87 [45.50]
            colon (sigmoid) 57.87 [45.52]
            ileum 57.87 [45.51]

Figure 16-6 ■ Example of Index entry for a synchronous procedure.

with part of the intestine. Code 57.87 represents *Reconstruction of urinary bladder,* which you should assign first, and code 45.50 represents *Isolation of intestinal segment, not otherwise specified,* which you should assign as an additional code because it is listed in brackets. You will also find "Code also" and "Code also any" notes in the Tabular List next to codes that require you to assign an additional code. (■ FIGURE 16-7).

TAKE A BREAK

Let's take a break and then review the Tabular List, Index, and coding conventions.

Exercise 16.1   ICD-9-CM Volume 3 Tabular List and Index to Procedures, Coding Conventions

Instructions: On the line preceding each statement, write T for True or F for False.

1. _____ Volume 3 procedure code categories may be two, three, or four digits in length.

2. _____ Most of the conventions in Volume 3 are similar to coding conventions in Volumes 1 and 2.

3. _____ "Code also any" instructs you to assign a code for a special adjunct procedure, supply, or equipment.

4. _____ Body sites are listed as main terms in the Index.

5. _____ You can find the abbreviation NEC in both the Index and Tabular.

6. _____ You can find parentheses ( ) only in the Index.

7. _____ The "code also" instruction means that it is optional to code a secondary procedure.

8. _____ The "omit code" note means that you should not assign more than two procedure codes for each patient's episode of care.

9. _____ Brackets [ ] are only used in the Tabular List.

10. _____ "Code also any synchronous" instructs you to assign one code for all components of a procedure.

CODING A PROCEDURE

Just like coding a diagnosis, to code a procedure, you will also locate the main term in the Index and cross-reference it to the Tabular List, which we will review next. Locate a procedure code in Volume 3 Index by first identifying the main term, based on the procedure documented in the medical record, a process that is similar to locating main terms for

Figure 16-8 ■ Index entry for O'Donoghue operation.

> **OCT** (optical coherence tomography) (intravascular imaging)
>   coronary vessel(s) 38.24
>   non-coronary vessel(s) 38.25
> **O'Donoghue** operation (triad knee repair) 81.43
> **Odontectomy** NEC -- *see also* Removal, tooth, surgical 23.19

diagnosis codes in the Volume 2 Index. Turn to the Volume 3 Index to review the types of main terms listed which will be one of the following:

- Name or type of procedure (lipectomy, manipulation, fitting, repair, removal)
- Eponym (Browne operation, McBride operation)
- Acronym, or abbreviation (ALIF—anterior lumbar interbody fusion, ERG—electroretinogram)

Note that body sites are not typically listed as main terms, so you should not begin your search with a body site. You should also pay attention to any coding conventions in the Index that will direct you. All main terms are arranged alphabetically, without regard to punctuation. For example, the main term *O'Donoghue* is alphabetized as though the apostrophe is not present (■ FIGURE 16-8).

The Index arranges procedures with Roman numerals (I, II, III) before alphabetized procedures.

Now, let's find a main term in the Index in the following example, along with a procedure code that we can cross-reference to the Tabular.

> **Example:** Dr. Stark, a general surgeon, performs an open repair of a left direct inguinal hernia (a hernia that protrudes through the muscle wall into the opening between an artery and muscle). The patient is Scott Bohn, age 45, and Dr. Stark uses a synthetic mesh prosthesis to help support the abdominal wall.
>
> What is the main term to search based on this documentation? If you answered *repair,* then you are correct! To locate the procedure code, search the Index for the main term *repair,* subterm *hernia,* subterm *inguinal,* subterm *direct,* subterm *with prosthesis or graft* (■ FIGURE 16-9). Not all main terms and subterms are listed in Figure 16-9, but you can find them in your ICD-9-CM manual.
>
> You need to carefully follow the various levels of indented subterms because it is easy to become confused trying to follow all of the indentations. You can use a ruler to create a straight edge down the page to ensure that you follow the appropriate column when referencing main terms and subterms.

> **Repair**
>   abdominal wall 54.72
>   adrenal gland 07.44
>   alveolus, alveolar (process) (ridge) (with graft) (with implant) 24.5
>   anal sphincter 49.79
>
>   hernia NEC 53.9
>   anterior abdominal wall NEC (laparoscopic without graft or prosthesis) 53.59
>   with prosthesis or graft
>   laparoscopic 53.63
>   other and open 53.69
>   colostomy 46.42
>
>   inguinal (unilateral) 53.00
>
>   direct (unilateral)
>   with prosthesis or graft 53.03

Figure 16-9 ■ Index entry for direct inguinal hernia repair.

Notice that you start with the main term *repair* to find the hernia code. If you instead start with *hernia* as the main term, you will not find an entry. You will see entries for **Hernioplasty**, *Herniorrhaphy*, and *Herniotomy*, but next to each entry you will see the instruction "*see* Repair, hernia."

Now, let's cross-reference code 53.03 to the Tabular List (■ FIGURE 16-10).

You should also follow coding conventions in the Tabular for correct code assignment. Notice also that there are instructional notes for category 53 and subcategory 53.0 that you should review before final code assignment. In addition, there may be main terms in the Index that do not appear in code titles when you cross-reference a code to the Tabular. You have also seen this situation when coding diagnosis codes. This is done to save space in the Tabular. If the main term in the Index does not match the code title in the Tabular, then double-check your answer first, and then always trust the Index to provide you with the correct code.

hernioplasty (hur′ne-o-plas-tē)—surgical repair of a hernia, often using synthetic mesh

---

53   Repair of hernia

Includes: hernioplasty
              herniorrhaphy

Code also any application or administration of an **adhesion barrier substance** (99.77)
Excludes: manual reduction of hernia (96.27)

53.0   Other unilateral repair of inguinal hernia

Excludes: laparoscopic unilateral repair of inguinal hernia (17.11-17.13)

> **53.00 Unilateral repair of inguinal hernia, not otherwise specified**
>   Inguinal herniorrhaphy NOS
>
> **53.01 Other and open repair of direct inguinal hernia**
>   Direct and indirect inguinal hernia
>
> **53.02 Other and open repair of indirect inguinal hernia**
>
> **53.03 Other and open repair of direct inguinal hernia with graft or prosthesis**

Figure 16-10 ■ Code 53.03 cross-referenced to the Tabular List.

ileostomy (il-e-os′tə-me)

duodenum (doo-o-de′nəm)

craniotomy (kra-ne-ot′ə-me)

TAKE A BREAK

Great job! Let's take a break and then practice coding procedures in Volume 3.

| Exercise 16.2 | **Coding a Procedure**

Instructions: Review each description of a service or procedure. Underline the main term for the procedure(s) and assign the code, using both the Index and the Tabular.

1. Dr. Lombard, a general surgeon, performs an **ileostomy** (a procedure that creates a new opening in the abdominal wall to eliminate waste) with synchronous resection of the **duodenum** (the first segment of the small intestine), without complications.

The patient is Clarence Neace, age 61, who needs the procedure due to adenocarcinoma of the small intestine.

Code(s): _____

2. Rachel Briggs, age 12, suffers from a ruptured appendix. Dr. Stark, a general surgeon, performs an appendectomy via a laparotomy.

Code(s): _____

3. Dr. Newton, a neurologist, performs a **craniotomy** (incision into the cranium) with an open biopsy of

continued

TAKE A BREAK *continued*

the brain for Pearl Land, age 73, who has a brain tumor.

Code(s): _____

4. Eugene Ingham, age 55, has a detached retina. Dr. Fitzpatrick, an ophthalmologist, performs **scleral buckling** to reattach the retina.

Code(s): _____

5. Dr. Drimond, a gastroenterologist, performs a colonoscopy with polypectomy of the large intestine for Steven Freed, age 57, due to colon polyps.

Code(s): _____

6. Dr. Fairfield, an OB/GYN, repairs a **cystocele** and **rectocele** for Margarita Cepeda, age 32. He also applies a prosthesis made from **allogenic** material.

Code(s): _____

scleral buckling (sklēr′ əl)—wrapping a band, also called a buckle, around all or part of the sclera to push it toward the middle of the eye and ease the tension on the detached retina in the back of the eye

cystocele (sis′to-sēl)—a hernia or protrusion of the urinary bladder through the vaginal wall

rectocele (rek′to-sēl)—a hernia or protrusion of the rectum into the vagina

allogenic (al-o-jen′ik)—tissue from another human

Well done! You learned how to assign inpatient procedure codes using Volume 3 in ICD-9-CM. The journey through the rest of this chapter will teach you how to assign inpatient procedure codes using the new code set, ICD-10-PCS. You will soon be ready to code inpatient procedures using both code sets. Let's keep going!

DESTINATION: MEDICARE

This Medicare exercise will familiarize you with procedure and diagnosis information that appears on the UB-04 (CMS-1450) claim form. Refer to Figure 1-2 to review the form as you complete the exercise. Numbered fields on the form are called form locators (FL). Each numbered FL (FL1, FL66) contains specific information that is necessary for Medicare and other payers to process the hospital's claim. Follow the instructions listed next to access Chapter 25 of the Medicare Claims Processing Manual:

1. Go to the website http://www.cms.gov.

2. At the top of the screen on the banner bar, choose *Regulations and Guidance*.

3. Under Guidance, choose *Manuals*.

4. On the left side of the screen, under *Manuals*, choose *Internet-Only Manuals (IOMs)*.

5. Scroll down to Publication # *100-04 Medicare Claims Processing Manual*, and click *100-04*.

6. Scroll down to the list of Downloads, and choose *Chapter 25—Completing and Processing the Form CMS-1450 Data Set*.

Answer the following questions, using the search function (Ctrl + F) to find information that you need.

1. Identify the FLs that contain the following information:

Principal procedure code and date: _____ Additional diagnosis codes: _____

Principal diagnosis code: _____ Additional diagnosis codes: _____

2. What does the diagnosis and procedure code qualifier in FL66 represent? _____

3. What information should you report in FL69? _____

4. In what FL(s) should you report the code "Y" to indicate that the patient authorized the provider to release medical information to the insurance?

CHARACTERISTICS OF ICD-10-PCS CODES

Several years ago, CMS hired an outside organization, 3M Health Information Systems, to create the ICD-10-PCS code set from a list of guidelines that CMS provided. Since the completion of the code set, CMS oversees code updates to incorporate new technologies and procedures, and the U.S. is the only country that will use ICD-10-PCS codes. The ICD-10-PCS code set has four major characteristics:

1. *Completeness*—Each procedure has its own unique code. In ICD-9-CM, the *same code* is sometimes used to describe procedures on *different body parts*, with *different approaches*, or using *different methods*, which leads to confusion and lack of detail.

2. *Expandability*—There is enough room in the ICD-10-PCS code set to add new procedures as they become available. The ICD-9-CM procedure code set does not allow much room for expansion.

3. *Multi-axial Structure*—Multi-axial means that each position or character within a code has a designated meaning that is the same for all related codes, such as a character that represents a specific anatomic site. You will learn about the designated meanings of each position or character later in this chapter. In ICD-9-CM Volume 3, there is no particular meaning attached to each character within a code.

4. *Standardized Terminology*—The ICD-10-PCS code set includes definitions of medical terminology, and each term has only one meaning. In addition, ICD-10-PCS minimizes the use of eponyms and Latin-based medical terms. The names of operations in ICD-10-PCS use basic contemporary words, such as *repair,* rather than Latin-based medical terms. But ICD-9-CM Volume 3 does not define medical terms, and sometimes one term has more than one meaning.

Review ■ TABLE 16-3, which compares the two code sets.

Organization of the ICD-10-PCS Manual

Depending on the ICD-10-PCS manual that you use, you will find an **Index** and **Tables** which are outlined next:

- **Index**—Lists all procedures in alphabetical order and tells you which Table to use to build the code by listing at least the first three characters of the code.

- **Tables**—Contain reference tables or grids that you use to build each ICD-10-PCS code by selecting the body system, type of procedure, operative approach, body part, and other characteristics. Tables appear in alphanumeric order and are based on the first three characters of the code.

You may also see an introduction or preface, ICD-10-PCS draft coding guidelines, coding conventions, term definitions, reference material, code examples, and a glossary in

---

■ TABLE 16-3   **COMPARISON OF ICD-9-CM WITH ICD-10-PCS INPATIENT PROCEDURE CODES**

ICD-9-CM Volume 3	ICD-10-PCS
Follows ICD-9 structure (designed for diagnosis coding).	Follows a new structure for greater specificity of codes.
Codes are fixed and finite, appearing in list form.	Codes are constructed from flexible code components (values) using tables, and the code set can accommodate additional codes for modern technology and procedures.
Codes are numeric.	Codes are alphanumeric.
Codes are three or four digits long.	Codes are seven characters long.
Uses combination codes to describe two or more procedures with one code.	Limits the use of combination codes to describe two or more procedures with one code.

INTERESTING FACT: Old Name for CMS

CMS created the HCPCS codes. CMS was previously called the Health Care Financing Administration (HCFA) and changed to CMS in 2001. You will still hear CMS referred to as HCFA (pronounced "hick-fa") while working in the healthcare field. It is also interesting to note that the CMS-1500 claim form used to be called the HCFA-1500 claim form, reflecting the old name for CMS. Some providers still call the CMS-1500 form the HCFA-1500 or simply "the HCFA."

your manual. You can obtain all of these elements, in addition to the Index and Tables, on the CMS website at http://www.cms.gov by accessing the ICD-10-PCS Reference Manual. You can find instructions for accessing the guidelines in Appendix A of this text.

TAKE A BREAK

Good job! Let's take a break and then review characteristics of ICD-10-PCS codes.

Exercise 16.3 Characteristics of ICD-10-PCS Codes

Instructions: Fill in each blank with the best answer, choosing from the list of words and terms provided.

1. The _____ code set has room to add new procedures as they become available.

2. _____ means that each position or character within a code should have a designated meaning

3. The _____ code set includes medical terminology definitions.

4. _____ codes are numeric.

5. ICD-10-PCS codes consist of _____ characters.

6. Coders build a code using _____ to select the body system, type of procedure, operative approach, body part, and other characteristics.

three	ICD-9-CM
seven	ICD-10-PCS
transitional	alphanumeric characters
multi-axial	Tables

ICD-10-PCS CODE STRUCTURE

Let's review how individual codes are structured and created in the Tables before you assign a complete code. Because there are numerous code options in ICD-10-PCS, our discussion will focus on the Medical and Surgical section of procedures.

ICD-10-PCS codes have a logical, consistent structure. This means that the process of assigning codes in ICD-10-PCS is also logical and consistent:

- Select individual letters and numbers, called **values**, in a standard order, one at a time.
- Values occupy the seven spaces or positions of the code, called **characters**.
- Each character represents a specific aspect of the procedure, and each of the 34 values has a specific meaning within each character.

Characters

ICD-10-PCS codes consist of seven characters, or positions, each of which has a purpose. The options and values for any character vary based on the first character of the code, called a *section*. The section is a broad procedure category. Characters in the Medical and Surgical Section are defined as follows:

- *Character 1* defines the Section, or broad procedure category.
- *Character 2* defines the Body System in which the procedure is performed.

- *Character 3* defines the Root Operation or the objective of the procedure.
- *Character 4* defines the Body Part, or specific anatomical site where the physician performed the procedure.
- *Character 5* defines the Approach, the technique used to reach the procedure site.
- *Character 6* defines the Device, if any, left in place at the end of the procedure.
- *Character 7* defines a Qualifier for the code which represents additional information about the procedure. Not all procedures have qualifiers.

■ TABLE 16-4 illustrates the purpose of each character for codes within the Medical and Surgical Section.

■ **TABLE 16-4   CODE CHARACTERS FOR THE MEDICAL AND SURGICAL SECTION**

Character →	1	2	3	4	5	6	7
Description →	Section	Body system	Root operation	Body part	Surgical approach	Implanted device	Qualifier

Now you will take a journey through each character of the code. The definitions we will discuss next for each character are specific to the Medical and Surgical Section. However, the techniques for assigning a code are the same no matter what section you choose for a code. Think of each character as a pit stop, where you pick up additional information that will lead you to the final code assignment. Fasten your seat belt!

Character 1: Section   The first character in the code describes the Section, or the category of procedure the physician performs. It can be a number or a letter. The largest section is the Medical and Surgical section. Other Sections describe other medical specialties, such as Obstetrics or Chiropractic, or the type of service, such as Nuclear Medicine. ■ TABLE 16-5 lists the 16 section choices for character 1.

■ **TABLE 16-5   CHARACTER 1: 16 SECTIONS**

Value	Section
0	Medical and Surgical
1	Obstetrics
2	Placement
3	Administration
4	Measurement and Monitoring
5	Extracorporeal Assistance and Performance
6	Extracorporeal Therapies
7	Osteopathic
8	Other Procedures
9	Chiropractic
B	Imaging
C	Nuclear Medicine
D	Radiation Oncology
F	Physical Rehabilitation and Diagnostic Audiology
G	Mental Health
H	Substance Abuse Treatment

Character 2: Body System   Remember that there are 16 different sections, and character 2 has different values in each of those sections. Character 2 in the Medical and Surgical Section defines the body system or anatomical site involved, such as central nervous system or heart and great vessels (■ TABLE 16-6).

■ **TABLE 16-6   CHARACTER 2: BODY SYSTEM, MEDICAL AND SURGICAL**

Value	Body System
0	Central Nervous System
1	Peripheral Nervous System
2	Heart and Great Vessels
3	Upper Arteries
4	Lower Arteries
5	Upper Veins
6	Lower Veins
7	Lymphatic and Hemic System
8	Eye
9	Ear, Nose, Sinus
B	Respiratory System
C	Mouth and Throat
D	Gastrointestinal System
F	Hepatobiliary System and Pancreas
G	Endocrine System
H	Skin and Breast
J	**Subcutaneous** Tissue and **Fascia**
K	Muscles
L	Tendons
M	Bursae and Ligaments
N	Head and Facial Bones
P	Upper Bones
Q	Lower Bones
R	Upper Joints
S	Lower Joints
T	Urinary System
U	Female Reproductive System
V	Male Reproductive System
W	Anatomical Regions, General
X	Anatomical Regions, Upper Extremities
Y	Anatomical Regions, Lower Extremities

subcutaneous (sub-ku-ta′ ne-əs)—below the skin

fascia (fash′e-ə)—fibrous tissue surrounding muscles or organs

Other sections also use character 2 to describe a body system, but some sections use character 2 to describe only an anatomical region or the type of service, such as rehabilitation.

Character 3: Root Operation   Character 3 in the Medical and Surgical Section, and also in most other sections, defines the root operation, which is the objective of the procedure, such as excision, destruction, or extraction. Root operations do not contain diagnoses in their descriptions. Character 3 has different values, depending on the section to which you assign a code. It is very important to remember that root operations are also main terms in the Index, so you will want to become familiar with their names and definitions (see Table 16-8).

In the Medical and Surgical Section, root operations are divided into nine groups that share similar characteristics, and each group contains specific types of root operations (■ TABLE 16-7).

■ **TABLE 16-7   CHARACTER 3: MEDICAL AND SURGICAL ROOT OPERATION GROUPS WITH SPECIFIC ROOT OPERATIONS**

Medical and Surgical Root Operation Group	Root Operations
1. Removes some/all of a body part	Excision Resection Detachment Destruction Extraction
2. Removes solids/fluids/gases from a body part	Drainage Extirpation Fragmentation
3. Involves cutting or separation only	Division Release
4. Puts in/puts back, or moves some/all of a body part	Transplantation Reattachment Reposition
5. Alters the diameter/route of a tubular body part	Restriction Occlusion Dilation Bypass
6. Always involves a device	Insertion Replacement Supplement Change Removal Revision
7. Involves examination only	Inspection Map
8. Includes other repairs	Repair Control
9. Includes other objectives	Fusion Alteration Creation

Notice that Table 16-7 is divided into nine general categories of procedures (Medical and Surgical Root Operation Group), and the specific procedures are listed within each category (Root Operations). The group makes it easier for you to find the *general type of operation* and then identify the *specific* root operation within the group. The Medical and Surgical section contains 31 different root operations, which you can review in ■ TABLE 16-8.

Select a root operation based on its definition. You can find complete definitions of root operations in the ICD-10-PCS manual and on the CMS website. Be sure to follow the ICD-10-PCS root operation definitions because many terms sound similar or are spelled almost the same. For example, sometimes you will find that the words *excision* and *resection* are used interchangeably, but ICD-10-PCS defines them in specific ways. Excision is cutting off *a portion* of a body part, while resection is cutting off *all* of a body part. Regardless of the word that the physician uses to describe a procedure, you need to assign the root operation based on the definition in the ICD-10-PCS manual.

■ TABLE 16-8 **CHARACTER 3: ROOT OPERATIONS AND DEFINITIONS, MEDICAL AND SURGICAL (ALPHABETICAL ORDER)**

Value	Root Operation	Definition
0	Alteration	Modifying the anatomic structure of a body part without affecting the function of the body part
1	Bypass	Altering the route of passage of the contents of a tubular body part
2	Change	Taking out or off a device from a body part and putting back an identical or similar device in or on the same body part without cutting or puncturing the skin or a mucous membrane
3	Control	Stopping, or attempting to stop, postprocedural bleeding
4	Creation	Making a new genital structure that does not take over the function of a body part
5	Destruction	Physically eradicating all or a portion of a body part by the direct use of energy, force or a destructive agent
6	Detachment	Cutting off all or part of the upper or lower extremities
7	Dilation	Expanding an orifice or the lumen of a tubular body part
8	Division	Cutting into a body part without draining fluids and/or gases from the body part in order to separate or transect a body part
9	Drainage	Taking or letting out fluids and/or gases from a body part
B	Excision	Cutting out or off, without replacement, a portion of a body part
C	Extirpation	Taking or cutting out solid matter from a body part
D	Extraction	Pulling or stripping out or off all or a portion of a body part by the use of force
F	Fragmentation	Breaking solid matter in a body part into pieces
G	Fusion	Joining together portions of an articular body part, rendering the articular body part immobile
H	Insertion	Putting in a nonbiological appliance that monitors, assists, performs, or prevents a physiological function but does not physically take the place of a body part
J	Inspection	Visually and/or manually exploring a body part
K	Map	Locating the route of passage of electrical impulses and/or locating functional areas in a body part
L	Occlusion	Completely closing an orifice or the lumen of a tubular body part
M	Reattachment	Putting back in or on all or a portion of a separated body part to its normal location or other suitable location
N	Release	Freeing a body part from an abnormal physical constraint by cutting or by using force
P	Removal	Taking a device out of or off a body part
Q	Repair	Restoring, to the extent possible, a body part to its normal anatomic structure and function
R	Replacement	Putting in or on biological or synthetic material that physically takes the place and/or function of all or a portion of a body part
S	Reposition	Moving to its normal location or other suitable location all or a portion of a body part
T	Resection	Cutting out or off, without replacement, all of a body part
V	Restriction	Partially closing an orifice or lumen of a tubular body part
W	Revision	Correcting, to the extent possible, a portion of a malfunctioning device or the position of a displaced device
U	Supplement	Putting in or on biological or synthetic material that physically reinforces and/or augments the function of a body part
X	Transfer	Moving, without taking out, all or a portion of a body part to another location to take over the function of all or a portion of a body part
Y	Transplantation	Putting in or on all or a portion of a living body part taken from another individual or animal to physically take the place and/or function of all or a portion of a similar body part

■ TABLE 16-9   **CHARACTER 4: BODY PART VALUES FOR THE LOWER EXTREMITIES, MEDICAL AND SURGICAL SECTION**

Value	Body Part	Value	Body Part
0	Buttock, Right	J	Lower Leg, Left
1	Buttock, Left	K	Ankle Region, Right
5	Inguinal Region, Right	L	Ankle Region, Left
6	Inguinal Region, Left	M	Foot, Right
7	Femoral Region, Right	N	Foot, Left
8	Femoral Region, Left	P	1st Toe, Right
9	Lower Extremity, Right	Q	1st Toe, Left
A	Inguinal Region, Bilateral	R	2nd Toe, Right
B	Lower Extremity, Left	S	2nd Toe, Left
C	Upper Leg, Right	T	3rd Toe, Right
D	Upper Leg, Left	U	3rd Toe, Left
E	Femoral Region, Bilateral	V	4th Toe, Right
F	Knee Region, Right	W	4th Toe, Left
G	Knee Region, Left	X	5th Toe, Right
H	Lower Leg, Right	Y	5th Toe, Left

Character 4: Body Part   Character 4 in the Medical and Surgical Section defines the body part or specific anatomic site where the physician performed the procedure. When you combine character 4 (Body Part) with character 2 (Body System), they provide a precise description of the procedure. Most sections in ICD-10-PCS use character 4 for Body Part. The definition of each Body Part value in the Medical and Surgical Section is unique to each Body System. As an example, ■ TABLE 16-9 shows the Body Part values that are used for the lower extremities.

Character 5: Approach   Character 5 in the Medical and Surgical Section defines the approach, or the technique used to reach the procedure site (■ TABLE 16-10). Sections other than Medical and Surgical use character 5 for different reasons; for example, the Imaging Section uses it for contrast.

Character 6: Device   Character 6 in the Medical and Surgical Section defines any device that is left in place at the end of the procedure. Device values fall into four basic categories: grafts and prostheses, implants, simple or mechanical appliances, and

■ TABLE 16-10   **CHARACTER 5: APPROACH, MEDICAL AND SURGICAL**

Value	Approach
0	Open
3	Percutaneous
4	Percutaneous Endoscopic
7	Via Natural or Artificial Opening
8	Via Natural or Artificial Opening Endoscopic
F	Via Natural or Artificial Opening Endoscopic with Percutaneous
	Endoscopic Assistance
X	External

electronic appliances. Sections other than Medical and Surgical use character 6 for different reasons; for example, the Osteopathic Section uses it for method, and the Radiation Oncology Section uses it for isotope.

Character 7: Qualifier   Character 7 in the Medical and Surgical Section defines a qualifier for the code. A qualifier specifies an additional characteristic of a procedure, such as allogenic or diagnostic. When no qualifier applies, assign the value Z for character 7.

TAKE A BREAK

Wow! That was a lot of information to cover! Let's take a break and review the structure of ICD-10-PCS codes.

Exercise 16.4   **ICD-10-PCS Code Structure**

Instructions: Fill in each blank with the best answer.

1. The _____ character in the code determines the broad procedure category, or section, where the code is found.

2. The _____ character defines the Root Operation or objective of the procedure.

3. The _____ character defines the Approach or technique used to reach the procedure site.

4. The definition of the Root Operation _____ is cutting out or off, without replacement, a portion of a Body Part.

5. The definition of the Root Operation _____ is restoring, to the extent possible, a Body Part to its normal anatomic structure and function.

6. The definition of the Root Operation _____ is cutting out or off, without replacement, all of a Body Part.

POINTERS FROM THE PROS: Interview with a Medical Record Auditor

Mary Motznik is an acute care Medical Record Auditor for a national consulting company. She has worked in healthcare for 17 years and is a Registered Health Information Technician (RHIT) and Certified Coding Specialist (CCS) through AHIMA.

Please describe your job duties, including whether or not you perform coding. If you do not perform coding directly, then describe how coding impacts your work:

I perform DRG validation (before billing insurance), and retroactive DRG compliance/DRG validation (after insurance is billed). This requires complete review of all reported diagnosis/procedure codes and physician/clinician documentation within the medical record, including being mindful of all outside regulatory agencies, especially CMS–Medicare.

What interests you the most about the job that you perform?

Being able to apply clinical knowledge (anatomy/physiology) against documentation in the record to determine the most appropriate DRG assignment.

What are the most challenging aspects of your job?

Keeping up to date with coding changes, guidelines, and new medical technology (diagnostic and treatment modalities) in order to provide the highest level of quality review for the client. In the end, all of these things can financially impact reimbursement for the client.

What advice can you give to new coders to help them to communicate effectively with physicians, since physicians can sometimes be intimidating?

Make sure you present any questions in relation to clarification in their "language." Be knowledgeable of anatomy/physiology. Be able to interpret labs, X-rays, or results in relation to treatment and medical planning. Realize that we all share the same goal, patient care/good documentation to ensure financial viability of the organization you both work for. Last, physicians are people too! Be confident in your abilities, don't let them intimidate you, and you may be pleasantly surprised at their reaction.

(Used by permission of Mary Motznik.)

ICD-10-PCS INDEX

Now that you are familiar with the structure of an ICD-10-PCS code, you will learn how to locate a code in the Index, which is the first step for assigning a code. You will also cross-reference the code to a Table a little later. Let's start with the Index. The Index is organized alphabetically based on two types of main terms:

* the value of the third character, such as root operation, and
* common procedure names, excluding eponyms.

Under the main terms are alphabetized subterms that describe the anatomical site or other variation of the root operation. After the subterm, you will find the first three to five characters of the code, which is a *partial code*. The first three characters of the partial code direct you to the appropriate Table that you should use, which we will review later in this chapter.

The terminology used for root operations may be different from what ICD-9-CM uses or what physicians use. For example, in ICD-9-CM, the word *repair* describes a broad range of surgical procedures, such as repairing a hernia with a **mesh prosthesis** or without one. In ICD-10-PCS, there is one specific definition for the Root Operation *repair*: *Restoring, to the extent possible, a body part to its normal anatomic structure and function*. Other procedures that traditionally are called *repair* may be classified under a different Root Operation in ICD-10-PCS. For example, the Root Operation for a *hernia repair with mesh* is classified as a *Supplement*, because a supplemental device (the mesh) is permanently left in the patient.

The Index provides cross-references, such as the *see* instruction, to guide you to another place if you look up a word other than a Root Operation. Let's go back to a previous example we reviewed for the patient, Scott Bohn, to help you better understand how to use the ICD-10-PCS Index to code his procedure. Follow along with your ICD-10-PCS manual while you review the example.

> mesh prosthesis (präs-thē′-səs)—a sterile, woven material used for support during surgical procedures

> **Example:** Dr. Stark, a general surgeon, performs an open repair of a left direct inguinal hernia with a synthetic mesh prosthesis to help support the abdominal wall for Scott Bohn, age 45.
>
> To code this case, let's work through the following steps, referencing Tables 16-7 and 16-8 to help you:
>
> 1. For help in identifying the Root Operation to search for in the Index, refer to Table 16-7 and review the nine general types of Medical and Surgical Root Operations and their definitions. Although you might immediately want to select *repair* because the patient had a hernia repair, remember that each operation has a specific meaning.
>
> 2. *Repair* is defined in Table 16-8 as *Restoring, to the extent possible, a body part to its normal anatomic structure and function*. Remember that Dr. Stark also applied a mesh prosthesis, which is a *device* in ICD-10-PCS. In Table 16-7, under the column for *Medical and Surgical Root Operation Group*, search for operations in the category *Always includes a device*.
>
> 3. In Table 16-7, review the root operations listed under *Always includes a Device* (insertion, replacement, supplement, change, removal, revision). Then look up their definitions using Table 16-8.
>   * Can you identify the root operation in Mr. Bohn's example? ICD-10-PCS classifies applying the mesh prosthesis as a *supplement*, which is defined in Table 16-8 as *putting in or on biological or synthetic material that physically reinforces and/or augments the function of a body part*. Therefore, the root operation and main term is *supplement*.
>
> 4. Search for the main term *supplement* in the ICD-10-PCS Index (■ FIGURE 16-11).

Supplement *continued*
Gingiva *continued*
  Upper **OCU5**
Glenoid Cavity
  Left **OPU8**
  Right **OPU7**
Hand
  Left **OXUK**
  Right **OXUJ**
Head **OWU0**
Heart **02UA**
Humeral Head
  Left **OPUD**
  Right **OPUC**
Humeral Shaft
  Left **OPUG**
  Right **OPUF**
Hymen **OUUK**
Ileocecal Valve **ODUC**
Ileum **ODUB**
Inguinal Region
  Bilateral **OYUA**
  Left **OYU6**
  Right **OYU5**
Intestine
  Large **ODUE**
  Left **ODUG**
  Right **ODUF**
  Small **ODU8**
Iris
  Left **08UD**
  Right **08UC**

Figure 16-11 ■ ICD-10-PCS Index entry for supplement.

Under *supplement*, locate the subterm for the anatomical site *inguinal region*. Under *inguinal region*, you will see additional subterms for *bilateral*, *left*, and *right*. Choose *left*, since the patient had a repair of the left direct inguinal hernia. Next to *left* is the partial code 0YU6. This is the partial code that directs you to the appropriate Table, but wait a minute before you turn to the Tables in the ICD-10-PCS manual.

What would have happened if you had not done your research before determining that *supplement* was the main term? What if, instead, you had looked up hernia, as you did in ICD-9-CM? You would not have found an entry, but you might have noticed the main term *herniorrhaphy*, the Latin-based name of a hernia repair (■ FIGURE 16-12).

When you look under the main term herniorrhaphy, you find the phrase *with synthetic substitute*, which is what the patient received. Notice the instruction underneath *with synthetic substitute* directing you to see the main term *supplement* and then the anatomical region of the procedure to begin your search. You already searched for *supplement* as the main term to find the partial code 0YU6. Once again, the coding manual tells you what to do! You just have to "listen" to its instructions.

> **Herniorrhaphy**
>   *see* Repair, Anatomical Regions, General **0WQ**
>   *see* Repair, Anatomical Regions, Lower Extremities **0YQ**
> with synthetic substitute
>   *see* Supplement, Anatomical Regions, General **0WU**
>   *see* Supplement, Anatomical Regions, Lower Extremities **0YU**

Figure 16-12 ■ ICD-10-PCS Index entry for herniorrhaphy.

We will stop here for an exercise before reviewing Tables and cross-referencing the partial code 0YU6 to a Table for Mr. Bohn's case.

TAKE A BREAK

That was a lot of information to review! Let's take a break and then practice using the ICD-10-PCS Index.

Exercise 16.5 ICD-10-PCS Code Index

Instructions: Complete the following three steps for each patient's case, which you coded previously using Volume 3 in ICD-9-CM.

Step 1. Use Tables 16-7 and 16-8 to locate the root operation and its definition for the following cases. Remember to select the root operation based on the definition of the operation, rather than on terms that may appear in the case.

Step 2. Identify the organ or anatomical site for the procedure.

Step 3. Use the ICD-10-PCS Index to locate the partial code (the three to five characters listed after the main term or subterm).

1. Dr. Lombard, a general surgeon, performs an ileostomy with synchronous resection of the duodenum without complications for Clarence Neace, age 61, due to adenocarcinoma of the small intestine. (*Hint:* Dr. Lombard created a new opening through the abdominal wall to empty the ileum, and he also removed the duodenum.)
   a. An ileostomy involves altering the route of passage of the contents of a tubular body part. Circle the root operation that is the main term: bypass change detachment
   b. What organ did Dr. Lombard treat? _____
   c. Locate the root operation in the Index and then identify the appropriate subterm for the body part. What is the partial code listed in the Index? _____
   d. A synchronous resection of the duodenum involves cutting out or off, without replacement, all of a body part. Circle the root operation that is the main term: detachment removal resection

TAKE A BREAK *continued*

e. What organ did the physician remove? _____
f. Locate the root operation in the Index and then identify the appropriate subterm for the body part. What is the partial code listed in the Index? _____

2. Rachel Briggs, age 12, suffers from a ruptured appendix. Dr. Stark, a general surgeon, performs an appendectomy via a laparotomy.
   a. An appendectomy involves cutting out or off, without replacement, all of a body part. Circle the root operation that is the main term:
      excision   removal   resection
   b. What organ does Dr. Stark remove? _____
   c. Locate the root operation in the Index and then identify the appropriate subterm for the organ. What is the partial code listed in the Index? _____

3. Dr. Newton, a neurologist, performs a craniotomy with an open biopsy of the brain for Pearl Land, age 73, who has a brain tumor.
   a. A biopsy involves cutting out or off, without replacement, a portion of a body part. Circle the root operation that is the main term:
      excision   release   resection
   b. What organ does Dr. Newton biopsy? _____
   c. Locate the root operation in the Index and then identify the appropriate subterm for the organ. What is the partial code listed in the Index? _____

4. Eugene Ingham, age 55, has a detached retina. Dr. Fitzpatrick, an ophthalmologist, performs scleral buckling to reattach the retina. (*Hint:* Scleral buckling is wrapping a band—a buckle—around all or part of the sclera to push it toward the middle of the eye and ease the tension on the detached retina in the back of the eye.)

a. Scleral buckling involves putting in or on biological or synthetic material that physically reinforces and/or augments the function of a body part. Circle the root operation that is the main term:
   alteration   change   supplement
b. What part of the eye is detached? _____
c. Locate the root operation in the Index and then identify the appropriate subterm for the body part. What is the partial code listed in the Index? _____

5. Dr. Drimond, a gastroenterologist, performs a colonoscopy with polypectomy of the large intestine for Steven Freed, age 57, due to colon polyps.
   a. A polypectomy involves cutting out or off, without replacement, a portion of a body part. Circle the Root Operation that is the main term:
      excision   extraction   inspection
   b. What organ is affected? _____
   c. Locate the root operation in the Index and then identify the appropriate subterm for the organ. What is the partial code listed in the Index? _____

6. Dr. Fairfield, an OB/GYN, repairs a cystocele and rectocele for Margarita Cepeda, age 32. He also applies a prosthesis made from allogenic material.
   a. A repair with an allogenic prosthesis involves putting in or on biological or synthetic material that physically reinforces and/or augments the function of a body part. Circle the Root Operation that is the main term: insertion repair supplement
   b. What part of the body is affected? _____
   c. Locate the root operation in the Index and then identify the appropriate subterm for the organ. What is the partial code listed in the Index? _____

ICD-10-PCS TABLES

After you locate the appropriate procedure in the Index, cross-reference the appropriate Table for the procedure using the partial code listed in the Index. Recall that in ICD-9-CM, you learned that you *never* assign a code directly from the Index. This is also true in ICD-10-PCS. In fact, it is *impossible* to assign a code from the ICD-10-PCS Index alone because the Index provides only *partial* codes. The complete code requires *seven characters*, and the Index rarely lists more than three or four characters. There are no shortcuts in this coding journey!

Review the following three steps to find a PCS code in the Tables:

1. Search for the Table that matches the first three characters of the code. The Tables are organized in alphanumeric order by Section, the first character of a code. Tables beginning with the numbers 0 through 9 appear first, followed by Tables beginning with the letters B–D, then letters F–H. Within each Section, Tables are then sequentially arranged according to the value of the second character, Body System. You will

Figure 16-13 ■ Three-character code 0YU in a Table.

0YU			
Section 0 Medical and Surgical			
Body System Y Anatomical Regions, Lower Extremities			
Operation U Supplement: Putting in or on biological or synthetic material that physically reinforces and/or augments the function of a portion of a Body Part			

Body Part	**Approach**	**Device**	**Qualifier**
0 Buttock, Right **1** Buttock, Left **5** Inguinal Region, Right **6** Inguinal Region, Left **7** Femoral Region, Right **8** Femoral Region, Left **9** Lower Extremity, Right **A** Inguinal Region, Bilateral **B** Lower Extremity, Left **C** Upper Leg, Right **D** Upper Leg, Left **E** Femoral Region, Bilateral **F** Knee Region, Right **G** Knee Region, Left **H** Lower Leg, Right **J** Lower Leg, Left **K** Ankle Region, Right	**0** Open **4** Percutaneous Endoscopic	**7** Autologous Tissue Substitute **J** Synthetic Substitute **K** Nonautologous Tissue Substitute	**Z** No Qualifier

notice that the first three characters of the code and the definition of each character are listed at the top of the Table, as shown in ■ FIGURE 16-13 for the three-character code 0YU for Mr. Bohn's procedure.

2. Select one value for characters 4–7, using each column in the Table that describes the procedure. The Table consists of a grid that lists the available options for these characters: the first column of the grid is for Body Part (Character 4); the second column is for Approach (Character 5); the third column is for Device (Character 6); and the fourth column is for Qualifier (Character 7). You cannot use any value that is not listed on the specific Table that you cross-referenced from the Index. You must select one, and only one, value from each column.

3. Review each character of the code to verify that it accurately describes the procedure. Always double-check your work for accuracy when you are writing or entering a code into practice management software. Because ICD-10-PCS codes are alphanumeric, it is easy to transpose characters or to interpret zero (0) for the letter O, which would result in an incorrect code.

We have now covered the three steps for assigning a code from the Tables: search for the Table that matches the first three characters of the code, select one value from each of the four columns in the Table, and check your work for accuracy. We used the Medical and Surgical Section, but there are many other Tables for many other Sections. In addition, they may not have the same headings as the Medical and Surgical Tables, so follow the column headings closely to ensure that you assign the correct values from each column.

Let's continue to build the procedure code for Mr. Bohn's case, following the three steps that we discussed. Remember that Dr. Stark performed an open repair of a left direct inguinal hernia with a synthetic mesh prosthesis to help support the abdominal wall. We found a partial code of 0YU6, using the Index entries for the main term *supplement,* subterm *inguinal region*, and subterm *left*. The entry in the Index directs you to Table 0YU (Figure 16-13).

Step 1: Locate Table 0YU alphanumerically in the Tables section in your ICD-10-PCS manual. Verify that the Table that you select has the heading 0YU with these definitions for Section, Body System, and Operation:

   0 Medical and Surgical

   Y Anatomical Regions, Lower Extremities

   U Supplement

Step 2: Select the appropriate value for characters 4-7 from each of the columns in the grid (■ FIGURE 16-14), as follows:

OYU

Section	0	Medical and Surgical
Body System	Y	Anatomical Regions, Lower Extremities
Operation	U	Supplement: Putting in or on biological or synthetic material that physically reinforces and/or augments the function of a portion of a Body Part

Body Part	Approach	Device	Qualifier
0 Buttock, Right **1** Buttock, Left **5** Inguinal Region, Right **6** Inguinal Region, Left **7** Femoral Region, Right **8** Femoral Region, Left **9** Lower Extremity, Right	**0** Open **4** Percutaneous Endoscopic	**7** Autologous Tissue Substitute **J** Synthetic Substitute **K** Nonautologous Tissue Substitute	**Z** No Qualifier

Figure 16-14 ■ Code 0YU60JZ in the ICD-10-PCS Table, OYU.

- • **Character 4—Body Part: Select the value** *6 Inguinal Region, Left.*
- • **Character 5—Approach: Select the value** *0 Open.*
- • **Character 6—Device: Select the value** *J Synthetic Substitute* for the mesh.
- • **Character 7—Qualifier: Select the value** *Z No Qualifier.* This is your only option, since there are no additional characteristics of the procedure to describe.

Now, combine the first three character values from the top of the Table (0YU) with the four character values you just identified in the grid (60JZ), and you will arrive at the final code of *0YU60JZ* (Figure 16-14).

Review the overall meaning of the code to be sure that it is accurate. The characters of the code are

   0 Medical and Surgical

   Y Anatomical Regions, Lower Extremities

   U Supplement

   6 Inguinal Region, Left

   0 Open

   J Synthetic Substitute

   Z No Qualifier

Code 0YU60JZ accurately describes the procedure, an open repair of a left direct inguinal hernia with mesh prosthesis. Congratulations, you have just constructed your first ICD-10-PCS code!

WORKPLACE IQ

You are working as a coder at Williton Medical Center in the Health Information Management (HIM) Department. Your manager developed a series of worksheets to help train all the coders on the ICD-10-PCS code set. One of the worksheets, which your manager gives to you, covers the process of assigning a code using the Tables. She asks you to verify that the worksheet is valid by completing the exercise and then updating her on the result. The worksheet is listed next for you to complete.

ICD-10-PCS Training Worksheet—Williton Medical Center HIM Department

Dr. Carroll, a neurologist, performs a craniotomy with an open biopsy of the brain for Robert Miles, age 52. The patient suffers from a brain tumor.

1. What are the first three digits of the partial code from the Index? _____
   (Locate the Table that matches these characters.)

2. Character 4—Body Part: What Body Part is affected, and what is its value? _____

3. Character 5—Approach: What is the Approach of the procedure, and what is its value? _____

4. Character 6—Device: What Device did the physician use (if any), and what is its value? _____

5. Character 7—Qualifier: What is the Qualifier, and what is its value? (*Hint:* A biopsy is done in order to diagnose a condition.) _____

6. What is the final code assignment? _____

CHAPTER REVIEW

Multiple Choice

Instructions: Circle one best answer to complete each statement.

1. An inpatient procedure is a therapeutic service, such as a surgical operation, or diagnostic service, that is performed for a patient who
   a. has been treated by a physician.
   b. has received any hospital service.
   c. has been admitted to an inpatient hospital, including an acute care facility.
   d. all of the above

2. The principal procedure code is the surgical operation or service that is most closely related to the
   a. principal diagnosis.
   b. secondary diagnosis.
   c. reason for the office visit.
   d. complication of surgery.

3. Which of the following is *not* an ICD-9-CM inpatient procedure code?
   a. 00.01—Therapeutic ultrasound of vessels of head and neck
   b. 00.10—Intracranial pressure monitoring
   c. 65.13—Laparoscopic biopsy of ovary
   d. 650—Normal delivery

4. Main terms in the ICD-9-CM Volume 3 Index can be
   a. the name of the procedure.
   b. a disease.
   c. an anatomical site.
   d. the body system.

5. Which convention in the ICD-9-CM Volume 3 Index identifies procedures or services that are included in *another* larger procedure or service?
   a. Essential modifiers
   b. Nonessential modifiers
   c. See category
   d. Omit code

6. This ICD-10-PCS characteristic means that the structure of the code set allows new procedures to be easily incorporated as they become available.
   a. Completeness
   b. Expandability
   c. Multi-axial
   d. Standardized

7. The section of the ICD-10-PCS manual that contains the grids that are used to build each ICD-10-PCS code is called the
   a. Index.
   b. Tables.

c. Root Operations.

d. Appendices.

8. Medical and Surgical is the largest ICD-10-PCS

a. Section.

b. Root Operation.

c. Approach.

d. Qualifier.

9. The ICD-10-PCS root operation represents the _____ of the procedure.

a. anatomic site

b. objective

c. approach

d. complication

10. The Tables in ICD-10-PCS enable you to select characters _____ of the code.

a. 1 through 7

b. 1, 2, and 3

c. 4 through 7

d. 5 through 7

Coding Assignments

Part One—ICD-9-CM Volumes 1, 2, and 3

Instructions: Assign both ICD-9-CM diagnosis and ICD-9-CM procedure codes to the following cases.

1. Dr. Wooten, an obstetrician, supervises the manually assisted vaginal delivery of baby Heidi to Heather Downes, age 21. Code for Ms. Downes' delivery encounter.

   a. ICD-9-CM diagnosis code(s): _____

   b. ICD-9-CM procedure code(s): _____

2. Veronica Pisano, age 72, has primary degenerative osteoarthritis localized to the knee and has extreme difficulty walking. Dr. Stuart, an orthopedic surgeon, performs a total **arthroplasty** of the left knee and inserts a **synthetic** total knee prosthesis.

   arthroplasty (ahr′thro-plas-te)—surgical repair or replacement of a joint to relieve pressure on the lower extremities

   synthetic (sin-thet′ik)—artificial

   a. ICD-9-CM diagnosis code(s): _____

   b. ICD-9-CM procedure code(s): _____

3. Leonard Rhodes, age 67, has a gangrenous left foot as a result of uncontrolled type II diabetes. The foot cannot be saved, so Dr. Carver, an orthopedic surgeon, amputates the left foot at the ankle. (*Hint:* An amputation through the ankle is called a **disarticulation**.)

   a. ICD-9-CM diagnosis code(s): _____

   b. ICD-9-CM procedure code(s): _____

Part Two—ICD-10-CM and ICD-10-PCS

Instructions: Assign ICD-10-CM and ICD-10-PCS codes to the same cases.

4. Dr. Wooten, an obstetrician, supervises the manually assisted vaginal delivery of baby Heidi to Heather Downes, age 21. Code for Ms. Downes' delivery encounter.

   a. ICD-10-CM diagnosis code(s): _____

   b. ICD-10-PCS procedure code(s): _____

5. Veronica Pisano, age 72, has primary degenerative osteoarthritis localized to the knee and has extreme difficulty walking. Dr. Stuart, an orthopedic surgeon, performs a total arthroplasty of the left knee and inserts a synthetic total knee prosthesis. (*Hint:* This is a knee replacement.)

   a. ICD-10-CM diagnosis code(s): _____

   b. ICD-10-PCS procedure code(s): _____

6. Leonard Rhodes, age 67, has a gangrenous left foot as a result of uncontrolled type II diabetes. The foot cannot be saved, so Dr. Carver, an orthopedic surgeon, amputates the left foot at the ankle. (*Hint:* The root operation is detachment.)

   a. ICD-10-CM diagnosis code(s): _____

   b. ICD-10-PCS procedure code(s): _____

disarticulation (dis-är-tik-yə-lā′-shən)—amputation at a joint

CPT-4 and HCPCS Coding and Coding with Modifiers

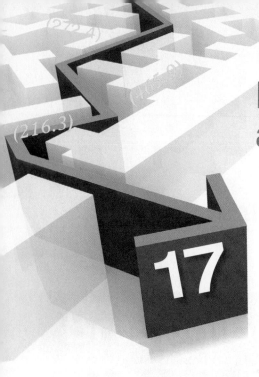

Introduction to CPT-4 and HCPCS Coding

17

Learning Objectives

After completing this chapter, you should be able to

- Spell and define the key terminology in this chapter.
- Describe HCPCS Level I and Level II codes.
- Describe the information that Category I codes represent.
- Discuss instructions for using the CPT® index and cross-referencing to sections.
- Explain the CPT code descriptor formats.
- Describe how and where to apply CPT coding guidelines.
- Discuss CPT code symbols and the information that each symbol represents.
- Describe when to use codes for unlisted procedures and services.
- Explain when to use modifiers.
- Describe the information that Category II codes represent.
- Discuss the information that Category III codes represent.

Key Terms

category
Category I codes
Category II codes
Category III codes
code descriptions
coding guidelines and instructions
indented description

index
section
stand-alone description
subcategory
subheading
subsection
unlisted codes

INTRODUCTION

Your coding journey for coding diagnoses and inpatient procedures has now come to an end. You are embarking on a new course, one that will take you around a significant bend in the road where you will learn how to code services, procedures, medical equipment, drugs, and supplies using *two* different code sets. Coding for procedures and services is very different from coding diagnoses, and the coding exercises may feel awkward at first, but if you keep practicing, then you will gain more knowledge and a higher level of confidence. You are already familiar with the procedure code sets because you learned about them in Chapter 2.

Just as you learned the rules of the road for coding diagnoses, you will also learn the rules of the road for coding services and procedures. The rules are different because you are traveling to a completely new destination, using different roads, somewhat like traveling to a new city and taking roads that you never drove on before! Keep in mind that when you work for a physician, you will typically work for a physician or physicians who concentrate on one specialty (primary care, orthopedics, gastroenterology) or physicians in

CPT-4 codes in this chapter are from the CPT-4 2012 code set. CPT is a registered trademark of the American Medical Association.

ICD-9-CM codes in this chapter are from the ICD-9-CM 2012 code set from the Department of Health and Human Services, Centers for Disease Control and Prevention.

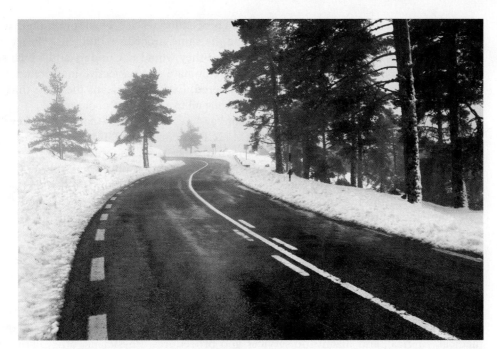

Figure 17-1 ■ The second half of your coding journey.

Photo credit: Carlos Caetano/Shutterstock.com.

related specialties (obstetrics and gynecology). Unless you code for a hospital or consulting company, your job probably will not involve coding for several different specialties. However, we will review how to assign codes from various specialties to prepare you to work for *any type* of provider.

One important point to remember is that when you code procedures and services, you must completely understand their meanings. There can be many variations of the same procedure, and if you do not know what the procedure is or how the physician performed it, then you will only be guessing at the correct code. If you do not understand a procedure, it is best to consult your medical references, such as your medical dictionary, reference books, and Internet searches. Remember that in coding, you will have to communicate with physicians and other clinicians about documentation, and you first need to understand what you are coding so that you know what questions to ask for clarification.

Work slowly and carefully through the examples and exercises in this chapter so that you are ready to apply your newly acquired skills to remaining chapters. Let's begin the second half of your journey and turn that bend in the road (■ FIGURE 17-1) so that you can learn how to correctly code procedures and services!

"Wherever we are, it is but a stage on the way to somewhere else, and whatever we do, however well we do it, it is only a preparation to do something else that shall be different."—ROBERT LOUIS STEVENSON

HEALTHCARE COMMON PROCEDURAL CODING SYSTEM CODE SETS

The Healthcare Common Procedural Coding System (HCPCS) has two divisions, or levels, of codes, which represent two different code sets:

- Level I—Current Procedural Terminology, Fourth Edition (CPT-4) codes
- Level II—National Healthcare Common Procedure Coding System (HCPCS) codes (pronounced "hick-picks")

All providers and insurances in the U.S. use Level I CPT-4 codes for physicians' services and procedures and for other types of services and procedures. Providers, Medicare, and Medicaid use Level II HCPCS codes for supplies, equipment, and drugs, and so do many other payers.

Codes represent a written description of a procedure, service, or supply. If there were no codes, then each provider might describe the same procedure differently in written form. Insurances may become confused because they would not understand which service or procedure the patient received. Codes eliminate any subjective interpretation of the service or procedure that the provider rendered. Each code means the same thing to each provider and to each insurance because they all use the same code sets.

In the healthcare field, providers do not say "Level I HCPCS codes" or "Level II HCPCS codes." Instead, they refer to Level I HCPCS codes as CPT-4 codes and Level II HCPCS codes as simply HCPCS codes, which is what we will do throughout the rest of this text. Remember from Chapter 1 when you learned that physicians submit claims using the CMS-1500 form? Refer to Figure 1-1 again to see that both CPT-4 and HCPCS codes appear on the form in block 24D, lines 1–6. For outpatient hospitals and some other outpatient providers that bill insurances with the UB-04 form, both CPT-4 and HCPCS codes appear on the form in FL44, lines 1–22 (Figure 1-2).

Level I—Current Procedural Terminology, Fourth Edition (CPT-4) Codes

The American Medical Association (AMA) created CPT-4 codes in 1966 to classify physicians' procedures and services (performed in inpatient or outpatient settings) and other medical, surgical, and diagnostic services and procedures. Physicians, other clinicians, and outpatient providers use CPT-4 codes. The AMA maintains CPT-4 codes by implementing revisions, additions, and deletions; updating codes in January for implementation six months later and in July for implementation six months later.

Structure of CPT-4 Codes   Level I CPT-4 codes can be either five digits or four digits followed by the letter F or T, as shown here:

- 71010—Chest X-ray, one view
- 3470F—Rheumatoid arthritis (RA) disease activity, low (RA)[5]
- 0142T—Pancreatic **islet** cell transplantation through portal vein, open

islet (i′let)—one of the islets of Langerhans cells scattered throughout the pancreas

Level II—National Healthcare Common Procedural Coding System (HCPCS) Codes

CMS, which oversees Medicare and Medicaid programs, wanted a classification system for various services, supplies, equipment, and drugs, which are *not included* in CPT-4. In the 1980s, the AMA worked with CMS to develop a new set of codes, Level II HCPCS codes. Examples of services, supplies, and items with Level II HCPCS codes include ambulance services, medical and surgical supplies, drugs, nutrition therapy, durable medical equipment, orthotic and prosthetic procedures, hearing and vision services, some physician services, and many other types of services that are excluded from CPT-4.

Initially, providers only assigned HCPCS codes for Medicare patients; however, many other insurances found HCPCS codes to be very useful and began to require providers to use HCPCS codes. It is best to check individual insurance coding requirements to ensure that you report HCPCS codes on claims when applicable. CMS is in charge of maintaining Level II HCPCS codes through yearly revisions, additions, and deletions.

Structure of Level II HCPCS Codes   HCPCS codes are made up of a letter followed by four numbers and are grouped by similar items. For example, HCPCS codes beginning with the letter J represent drugs and are called J codes, and codes beginning with the letter A represent ambulance services and are called A codes. HCPCS codes represent supplies, equipment, drugs, and some services. Examples of codes and what they represent are as follows:

- J2270—Injection, morphine sulfate, up to 10 mg
- V2756—Eye glass case

- A4206—Syringe with needle, sterile, 1 cc or less, each
- E0130—Walker, rigid (pickup), adjustable or fixed height

Providers from various specialties and facilities, including physicians, hospitals, outpatient clinics, and urgent care centers, can assign HCPCS codes for patients' encounters. Other providers who assign HCPCS codes include pharmacies, ambulance services, and durable medical equipment suppliers. You will learn more about Level II HCPCS codes and how to assign them in Chapter 35 of this text, so we will focus on learning CPT-4 coding in this chapter.

Latest Versions of HCPCS Level I and Level II Codes

When you are coding from CPT-4 or HCPCS, always make sure that you use the coding manual for the current year. You can also obtain both coding manuals in a hard-copy format, electronic format, or on CD-ROM. If you work for a provider who uses older versions of the coding manuals, then ask if they can order the newest ones. Many people do not think that much information changes in the code sets from year to year, but there are often significant additions, deletions, and revisions that could affect reimbursement. Assigning old codes that insurances no longer recognize could mean denied claims. Remember that providers receive money to operate typically from two main sources: insurances and patients. It is much easier to code and bill services correctly the first time and avoid having to appeal denied claims or rebill claims later, which would delay payment.

TAKE A BREAK

Let's take a break and then review HCPCS Level I and Level II code sets.

Exercise 17.1   Healthcare Common Procedural Coding System (HCPCS) Code Sets

Instructions: Fill in each blank with the best answer, choosing from the list of words and terms provided.

1. Both CPT-4 and HCPCS codes represent a _____ description of a procedure or service.

2. _____ created CPT-4 codes in 1966 to classify physicians' services and procedures and outpatient medical, surgical, and diagnostic services and procedures.

3. _____ codes represent supplies, equipment, drugs, and some services.

4. _____ codes can be either five digits, or four digits followed by the letter F or T.

5. V2756—*Eye glass case* is an example of a(n) _____ code.

6. There are often significant additions, deletions, and revisions to codes, which could affect _____.

AMA	Level II HCPCS
CMS	reimbursement
electronic	subjective
information	written
Level I CPT-4	

CURRENT PROCEDURAL TERMINOLOGY, FOURTH EDITION CODES

The CPT-4 coding manual divides services and procedures into three categories, which contain codes for any type of service or procedure that you can imagine, including surgical, medical, and diagnostic. There are even generic codes to use when you have to code a procedure that is not specifically named in the code set, which are called **unlisted codes**. You will learn more about them later. Here is a list of the three categories with services and procedures that they represent:

Category I (00100–99607)

Category I codes, the largest category in CPT-4, are five digits long and are separated into six sections, starting at the beginning of the coding manual. In order for a service or procedure to be listed under Category I, many providers have to perform it, it has to be proven to be effective, and the Food and Drug Administration (FDA) has to approve it (when appropriate). Refer to your CPT-4 coding manual or electronic version to find each of the following six sections, or chapters, in Category I, beginning with the first section located at the beginning of the coding manual:

1. *Evaluation and Management (E/M) (99201–99499)*—face-to-face services between a physician and patient that typically involve the following three components:

    - Obtaining the patient's personal, family, and social histories
    - Examining the patient
    - Determining the patient's diagnosis and developing a treatment plan, if appropriate

    There are exceptions where physicians perform E/M services that do not include the three components, or physicians do not meet with the patient *face-to-face* during an encounter.

2. *Anesthesia (00100–01999)*—services that represent various types of anesthesia administered to a patient during a procedure, monitoring a patient during and after anesthesia administration, and other related services.

3. *Surgery (10021–69990)*—surgical procedures arranged by body system.

4. *Radiology (70010–79999)*—radiology procedures, such as X-rays, CT scans, and ultrasounds.

5. *Pathology and Laboratory (80047–89398)* laboratory tests including biopsies and tests on various body fluids.

6. *Medicine (90281–99607)*—This section contains a variety of other services and procedures that are not classified to any of the other five sections.

You will learn more about coding in each of the six sections in additional chapters in this text. For the most part, the CPT-4 coding manual arranges codes in numeric order except for the E/M section. Notice that the E/M codes start with the number 9 but are the first section of the coding manual. This is because providers use these codes so often that they have been placed at the beginning of the manual for easy access. Throughout the manual, there are other codes which are not arranged in numeric order because the AMA resequenced codes.

Category II (0001F–7025F)

Category II codes (four numbers and the letter F) are supplemental tracking and performance measurement codes, which providers can assign in addition to Category I codes. Providers may want to track specific criteria about patients, such as whether they use tobacco, which is represented by code 1000F. You can find Category II codes listed directly after the last Category I code in the Medicine section.

Category III (0019T–0259T)

Category III codes (four numbers and the letter T) follow Category II codes in the coding manual. They are temporary codes that represent new technology, services, and procedures. Codes remain in Category III for up to five years and can become Category I codes if they meet Category I criteria, including approval from the FDA, evidence that many providers perform the service or procedure, and it is proven to be effective. Category III codes also may be dropped from the Category III if providers do not use them. The AMA updates Category III codes twice a year. When providers assign Category III codes and bill insurances, they have to send medical documentation (special reports) with insurance claims to justify the Category III procedure and further explain why the provider performed it.

Providers Who Assign CPT Codes

The CPT code set is for physician services and services that other qualified health care professionals render, like physician assistants, physical therapists, and psychologists. The

CPT code set is also the designated code set for organizational or facility providers, such as hospitals, ASCs, outpatient clinics, urgent care centers, and offices of other healthcare practitioners. The CPT coding manual uses the term *nonfacility* to describe services that a facility *cannot* code and bill.

Many times, physicians or other qualified health care professionals provide services within facilities, like hospitals. When this happens, both the physician or other qualified health care professional and the facility can each bill the patient's insurance for the same service. The facility wants to be paid for the service because the physician performed it there and used the facility's equipment and resources, and the physician also wants to be paid for performing the service.

Some CPT codes include specific places of service in their descriptors that will help you to assign the correct code. For example, evaluation and management codes are specific to various settings, like a physician's office or inpatient hospital. Other services and procedures may include coding instructions that are specific to the place of service. It is important to pay close attention to the medical documentation to ensure that you assign a code with the appropriate place of service.

Providers can assign CPT codes from any specialty in the coding manual. For example, just because the code for an X-ray is listed in the radiology section does not mean that a primary care physician cannot assign it if he interpreted an X-ray. The same is true for the other sections in the coding manual.

TAKE A BREAK

That was a lot of information to absorb! Let's take a break and then review terms related to HCPCS codes.

Exercise 17.2 **Current Procedural Terminology, Fourth Edition (CPT-4) Codes**

Instructions: Fill in each blank with the best answer, choosing from the list of words and terms provided.

1. In order for a service or procedure to be listed under _____, many providers have to perform it, it has to be proven to be effective, and the Food and Drug Administration has to approve it (when applicable).

2. _____ codes start with the number 9 but are the first section of the coding manual.

3. _____ are temporary codes that represent new technology, services, and procedures.

4. _____ are supplemental tracking and performance measurement codes.

5. Some CPT codes include a specific _____ in their descriptors.

6. For the most part, the CPT-4 coding manual arranges codes in _____ order.

alphabetical	E/M	medicine
Category I	facility	nonfacility
Category II	HCPCS	place of service
Category III	CPT	numerical

STRUCTURE OF THE CPT-4 CODING MANUAL

You will next learn the structure of the CPT-4 manual, professional edition, including where to find specific information, along with guidelines and terms. The CPT Professional Edition coding manual is categorized in the following order:

- Front Matter
- Table of Contents
- Introduction
- Illustrated Anatomical and Procedural Review
- Evaluation and Management (E/M)
- Anesthesia
- Surgery
- Radiology

- Pathology and Laboratory
- Medicine
- Category II codes
- Category III codes
- Appendices
- Index

Front Matter and Table of Contents

The Front Matter includes various AMA divisions who created and review the CPT coding manual, including the CPT Editorial Panel. The Front Matter also includes place-of-service codes for professional claims (CMS-1500). Providers list a place of service code on the CMS-1500 form to show the type of provider that rendered a service. (Refer to Figure 1-1, block 24B.) The Table of Contents will help guide you through the CPT manual, so refer to it often to navigate through the manual.

Introduction to CPT

The Introduction includes basic information about CPT codes, section numbers, and their sequences, along with many types of guidelines and terms that help you travel through the coding manual. The AMA updates CPT nomenclature, or medical language, to reflect current medical procedures and services. It encourages providers to suggest changes to descriptors, codes, and index entries. Providers and other organizations can submit suggestions directly to the AMA.

Illustrated Anatomical and Procedural Review

The Illustrated Anatomical and Procedural Review is a quick reference guide to medical terminology and anatomy. It provides locations of various illustrations for anatomy and procedures. It is also important to keep your medical references handy, such as a medical dictionary, and to utilize them as you code from the CPT manual.

You will learn more about the remaining categories in CPT as you work through the rest of this chapter.

INSTRUCTIONS FOR USING THE INDEX

CPT includes instructions for using the index on the first page that appears before the index. The **index**, found in the last part of the CPT manual, contains procedures and services. Main terms in the index in the CPT manual are arranged alphabetically by procedures and services, body sites, synonyms, eponyms, abbreviations, and some diagnoses. Each page of the index is divided into three columns. You will see entries listed on each page in bold at the top left and at the top right. Information printed on the top left is the first entry on that page. Information on the top right is the last entry on that page. This helps you to quickly locate main terms (■ FIGURE 17-2).

Main terms appear in bold font with corresponding *subterms*, or modifying terms, listed underneath. Subterms may also have additional subterms, which are indented (■ FIGURE 17-3).

Each main term can stand alone, or it can have up to three modifying subterms. In the manual, the first subterm is *not* indented, but additional subterms are indented under the subterms that they modify. There are four types of main terms to search for to locate codes to cross-reference to CPT sections in the first part of the manual:

1. *Procedure or service*

   Examples: endoscopy, repair, anesthesia

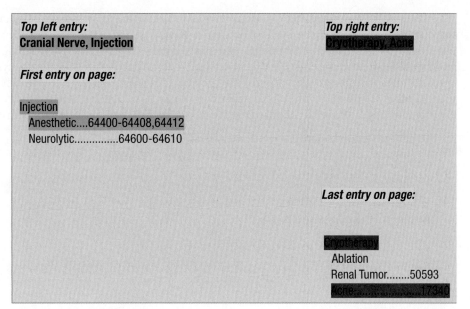

Figure 17-2 ■ Index entries.
The middle column is not shown.

2. *Organ or other anatomic site*

   Examples: tibia, fibula, acetabulum

3. *Condition*

   Examples: abscess, tetralogy of Fallot, tumor

4. *Synonyms, eponyms, or abbreviations*

   Examples: EEG, CPK, CT scan, Seddon-Brookes procedure, phalanx (finger)

Note: Not every procedure that has an abbreviation is listed under its abbreviation in the index. Instead, it is listed under its full descriptions.

Keep in mind that there are many different ways to locate the same code in the index, based on the main term for which you search. If you do not find the information that you are searching for under the *procedure name* as the main term, then you can go to the *anatomic site*, or search under another option, like an *abbreviation or synonym*. Sometimes the same word can serve as a main term or as a subterm, depending on where you begin your search in the index. As you continue to practice finding main terms in the index, you will also find faster ways of locating the information that you need.

For example, a patient's medical documentation stated that the patient had an EGD, and you searched for the abbreviation EGD in the index, but found nothing. You would then need to search under esophagogastroduodenoscopies (EGDs), and you would find the direction to *See Endoscopy, Gastrointestinal, Upper.* You would then have to start your search under *endoscopy* as the main term, and search subterms *gastrointestinal* and *upper*. But the next time you need to assign a code for an EGD, you will know that there is no index entry for EGD, and you will go directly to *endoscopy* to locate the codes to cross-reference.

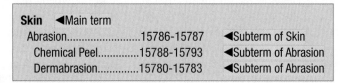

Figure 17-3 ■ Index entry for the main term *Skin* with subterms, or modifying terms.

Chevron (shev′-rən)—
surgical procedure to correct a
bunion (bulging of the joint at
the base of the great toe) in
which a v-shaped hole is made
in the outside bone of the arch
across the foot

orbital contents—the eyeball

test tube fertilization—
removing a woman's egg from
her body, to mate it with a
sperm in the laboratory, then
placing it into the uterus

vagotomy (va-got′ə-me)—
surgical cutting into the vagus
nerve(s), the tenth pair of
cranial nerves originating in
the brain

The first step in identifying a main term is to find it in the medical documentation, searching for the procedure performed or the service rendered. Once you identify the procedure or service in the documentation, locate it in the CPT index by searching for one word or term that represents the procedure, service, anatomic site, condition, synonym, eponym, or abbreviation. You should also review any subterms that are modifying the main term to help you to find the correct code to cross-reference. Review the following examples of main terms (highlighted) to search in the index to find the procedure code:

Repair of skin avulsion

Mole excision

Intravenous infusion

Biopsy of left breast tissue

Revision of aqueous shunt

Skin graft

In some cases, you would also be able to locate the procedure by first searching for the body site and then locating the procedure as a subterm.

TAKE A BREAK

Good job! Let's take a break and then complete practice exercises for finding main terms.

Exercise 17.3 Instructions for Using the Index

Instructions: Review each description of a service or procedure, and underline the main term.

1. **Chevron** procedure

2. Removal of the **orbital contents** of the eye

3. Closed treatment of elbow dislocation

4. **DTaP immunization**

5. **Test tube fertilization**

6. Abdominal **vagotomy**

7. Sinus endoscopy

8. Repair of electrodes for a pacemaker

9. Surgical arthroscopy of the knee

10. Hypothermia, externally generated

11. Cardiopulmonary resuscitation

12. Evaluation and management office visit

DTap immunization—
vaccine to prevent diphtheria,
tetanus, and pertussis
(whooping cough)

CODE OPTIONS IN THE INDEX

When you find a main term and any modifying terms in the index, you will see one of the following types of code choices:

* one code
* more than one code separated by a comma
* code ranges of continuous numbers separated by a hyphen, and more than one code range can be listed
* code(s) separated by commas, along with a code range separated by a hyphen

Refer to ■ FIGURE 17-4 to review different code options for main terms and subterms and options for searching for codes in the index. Main terms appear in bold.

Notice in Figure 17-4 the cross-reference to "See Aortography." When you find the *cross-reference "see,"* it means that you are in the wrong place to find the procedure you are searching for, and you must instead look elsewhere for it.

When the index provides more than one code choice, or a code range, it is *not an option* to choose just one of the codes listed. Instead, you must cross-reference *all* of the codes listed to ensure correct code assignment. Just as you learned with ICD-9-CM to never code directly from the Index, never code directly from the CPT index, either. *Always*

Figure 17-4 ■ Examples of code choices when referencing main terms in the index.

Esophagus	◀**Main term**
Reconstruction............43300, 43310, 43313	◀**Subterm**

OR

Reconstruction	◀**Main term**
Esophagus................43300, 43310, 43313	◀**Subterm**

Debridement	◀**Main term**
Burns............01951-01953, 16020-16030	◀**Subterm**

OR

Burns	◀**Main term**
Debridement.........................01951-01953,	◀**Subterm**
15002-15005, 16020-16030	

Abdomen	◀**Main term**
Abdominal Aorta	
Angiography.....................................75635	◀**Subterm**

OR

Angiography	◀**Main term**
See Aortography	
Abdomen.......74175, 74185, 75635, 75726	◀**Subterm**

cross-reference codes in the index to one or more of the six sections of the CPT coding manual, also called the main text. Even if there is only one code choice, it does not mean that the code is the correct one. You must still cross-reference it, read additional notes, and follow any coding instructions before final code assignment because it may lead you to a completely different code.

SPACE-SAVING CONVENTIONS

As a *space-saving convention*, certain terms in the index have a specific meaning, even though the meaning is not printed to save space. In the index, you may see the following types of information:

Knee ◀ Main term

Incision ◀ Subterm

In this example, the word *incision* actually means *incision of*. The word *of* is not printed in the index to save space, but it is inferred, or understood. Refer to the next example:

Pancreas ◀ Main term

Anesthesia ◀ Subterm

In this example, the word *anesthesia* actually means *anesthesia for procedures on the pancreas*. The words *for procedures on the pancreas* are not printed to save space, but they are inferred.

TAKE A BREAK

Let's take a break and then review more about code options and space-saving conventions.

Exercise 17.4   Code Options in the Index, Space-Saving Conventions

Instructions: Fill in each blank with the best answer.

1. When you are in the wrong place to find the procedure you are searching for, and you must instead look elsewhere, the CPT index includes a note that instructs you to _____.

2. A _____ convention is when certain words have specific meaning, even though the meaning is not printed to save space.

3. When the index provides more than one code choice, or a code range, you must cross-reference _____ of the codes listed to ensure correct code assignment.

4. Even if there is _____ code choice(s) listed in the index, it does not mean that the code(s) is correct.

5. When you search for the main term *knee*, subterm *incision*, the word incision really means _____.

6. The index entry *See* Aortography is an example of a _____.

CODE DESCRIPTIONS

When you cross-reference codes in the CPT coding manual to various sections, it is crucial that you know how to read the code descriptors. In order to find codes and their descriptors, you first have to navigate through sections in the manual. Pay attention to codes printed at the top of pages, which show the code range of codes printed on the page, and to codes printed along the sides of pages, which show code ranges that you can find using various side tabs. You can also place your own tabs and labels in your code book to navigate faster and find the codes you are cross-referencing.

Once you find the code that you are searching for, you will need to review its code descriptor to interpret its meaning. There are two different types of **code descriptions**, also called descriptors, for codes:

- Stand-alone code description
- Indented code description

A **stand-alone description** is a full description of a code, and it is not indented. Code 71010 has a stand-alone description. Notice that it is not indented:

71010	Radiologic examination, chest; single view, frontal	◀ Stand-alone description
71015	stereo, frontal	◀ Indented description

An **indented description** is a *partial* description that has no meaning if you read it by itself. If you read the indented description for code 71015 as *stereo, frontal*, it does not mean anything. You have to *combine the partial description with a stand-alone description* in order to obtain the full description of the code. Follow these four steps for obtaining the full description when a code's description is indented:

1. For any indented description, go to the *first* stand-alone description listed before the indented description.

2. Read the first part of the stand-alone description up to the semicolon, then stop. Drop the information listed after the semicolon.

3. Add the indented description.

4. The first part of the *full description up to the semicolon* plus the *indented description* will give you the full description of the indented code.

For example, let's review code 71015 and follow the four steps to obtain the full description:

71010   Radiologic examination, chest; single view, frontal

71015   stereo, frontal

1. Go to the first stand-alone description that you can find listed before the indented description, which is the stand-alone description for 71010:

71010   Radiologic examination, chest; single view, frontal

2. Read the first part of the stand-alone description *up to the semicolon,* then stop. Drop the information listed after the semicolon:

71010   Radiologic examination, chest| single view, frontal

3. Add the indented description:

71015   stereo, frontal

4. The first part of the *full description up to the semicolon* plus the *indented description* will give you the full description of code 71015:

71015   Radiologic examination, chest; stereo, frontal

Note that the semicolon becomes part of the full description for code 71015. Also, when you borrow the first part of a stand-alone description, you *do not also assign the code of the stand-alone description.* Therefore, when the full description in this example is *Radiologic examination, chest; stereo, frontal,* it is only for code 71015. *Do not assign both codes 71010 and 71015* because it would mean there were *two* procedures performed, not one. The AMA implemented the indented descriptions in order to save space. Refer to the next example to obtain the full description of code 70558:

70557 Magnetic resonance (e.g., proton) imaging, brain (including brain stem and skull base), during open intracranial procedure (e.g., to assess for residual tumor or residual vascular malformation); without contrast material

70558   with contrast material(s)

1. Go to the first stand-alone description listed before the indented description, which is the stand-alone description for 70557:

70557 Magnetic resonance (e.g., proton) imaging, brain (including brain stem and skull base), during open intracranial procedure (e.g., to assess for residual tumor or residual vascular malformation); without contrast material

2. Read the first part of the stand-alone description *up to the semicolon,* then stop. Drop the information listed after the semicolon:

70557 Magnetic resonance (e.g., proton) imaging, brain (including brain stem and skull base), during open intracranial procedure (e.g., to assess for residual tumor or residual vascular malformation)| without contrast material

3. Add the indented description:

70558   with contrast material(s)

4. The first part of the *full description up to the semicolon* plus the *indented description* will give you the full description of the code:

70558 Magnetic resonance (e.g., proton) imaging, brain (including brain stem and skull base), during open intracranial procedure (e.g., to assess for residual tumor or residual vascular malformation)| with contrast material(s)

Note that the full description includes any information listed in parentheses because it is still part of the meaning.

TAKE A BREAK

Good work! Let's take a break and then review code descriptions.

Code Descriptions

Instructions: Write the full description of each code listed. Be sure to include the semicolon and any information listed in parentheses as part of the full description.

1. 57283

_____

_____

_____

2. 43887

_____

_____

_____

3. 87045

_____

_____

4. 41155

_____

_____

_____

5. 83662

_____

_____

_____

6. 78011

_____

_____

CPT CLASSIFICATIONS

Recall from earlier in the chapter that there are six sections, or chapters, in the first part of the CPT manual. **Sections** are the first classifications in CPT, and CPT further divides sections into additional classifications:

- Subsection
- Subheading
- Category
- Subcategory

It is important to understand classifications for specific procedures and services to help you to locate them in CPT. In the manual, all classifications appear in bold font but are in different colors. The font becomes smaller as the classifications further subdivide. Refer to the beginning of the Surgery section next, starting with code 10021 (■ FIGURE 17-5), to better understand the following explanations of classifications:

Figure 17-5 ■ Classifications in the Surgery section.

Surgery ◀**Section**

General (10021-10022) ◀**Subsection**

Integumentary System ◀**Subsection**

Skin, Subcutaneous and Accessory Structures ◀**Subheading**

Incision and Drainage (10040-10180) ◀**Category**

Debridement (11000-11047) ◀**Category**

Paring or Cutting (11055-11057) ◀**Category**

■ **TABLE 17-1   EXAMPLES OF CLASSIFICATIONS OF CPT CODES**

CPT Code	Section	Subsection	Subheading	Category	Subcategory	Additional Classification
61580	Surgery	Nervous System	Skull, Meninges, and Brain	Surgery of Skull Base	Approach Procedures	Anterior Cranial Fossa
64400	Surgery	Nervous System	Extracranial Nerves, Peripheral Nerves, and Autonomic Nervous System	Introduction/Injection of Anesthetic Agent (Nerve Block), Diagnostic or Therapeutic	Somatic Nerves	None
65400	Surgery	Eye and Ocular Adnexa	Anterior Segment	Cornea	Excision	None

- Surgery is the name of the section, and the word *Surgery* is in large bold black font.

- **Subsections** break down sections by type and/or anatomic sites. The first subsection of Surgery is *General*, which appears in bold green font. General surgery has no further divisions. At the top of each page for a specific section, you will see the section name followed by the subsection on that page (Surgery/General). The second subsection of Surgery is *Integumentary System* (skin), appearing in bold green font.

- **Subheadings** further divide subsections. Subheadings group procedures by location within a body system. The subsection Integumentary System is further divided into the subheading *Skin, Subcutaneous, and Accessory Structures,* appearing in smaller bold red font.

- **Categories** further divide subheadings. Categories show specific methods for completing procedures. The subheading Skin, Subcutaneous, and Accessory Structures is further divided into categories: The first category is *Incision and Drainage,* the second is *Debridement,* and the third is *Paring or Cutting.* All categories appear in smaller bold blue font.

- Some categories are further divided into **subcategories**, which provide more specific information about the procedure or service. Subcategories appear in even smaller bold black font. Subcategories can also subdivide into additional classifications appearing in italics.

Refer to ■ TABLE 17-1 for more examples of classifications for specific CPT codes, and turn to your manual to review them.

TAKE A BREAK

Let's take a break and then review CPT classifications.

Exercise 17.6   **CPT Classifications**

Instructions: Locate each CPT code listed for specific procedures, then write the section, subsection, subheading, category, and subcategory to which the procedure is classified.

1. 52204—Cystourethroscopy, with biopsy(s)

   Section: _____

   Subsection: _____

   Subheading: _____

   Category: _____

   Subcategory: _____

2. 35452—Transluminal balloon angioplasty, open; aortic

   Section: _____

   Subsection: _____

   Subheading: _____

   Category: _____

   Subcategory: _____

3. 44180—Laparoscopy, surgical, enterolysis (freeing of intestinal adhesion) (separate procedure)

   Section: _____

   Subsection: _____

   Subheading: _____

   Category: _____

   Subcategory: _____

CPT CODING GUIDELINES AND INSTRUCTIONS

The AMA includes many different **coding guidelines and instructions** for sections, subsections, subheadings, categories, subcategories, and many individual codes. Guidelines and instructions provide specific information about when and how to assign codes, how providers perform procedures, which codes can and cannot be reported together, and other details related to coding.

Think of the guidelines and instructions as the Dos and Don'ts road signs as you navigate the CPT coding manual. You could not operate a vehicle effectively without road signs to guide you, and CPT coding works the same way. Just as you should not ignore road signs while driving, you should not ignore CPT's additional guidelines that help you along your way to choosing the correct code. Review the guidelines and instructions for each section, subsection, subheading, category, and subcategory *before* assigning codes within that classification. Many new coders skip the guidelines and instructions, thinking they may take too long to read or that they are unnecessary. Do not make the mistake of ignoring guidelines and instructions because they will help you to better understand when to assign certain codes and how providers perform services and procedures. Reading the guidelines could certainly affect your final code assignment and whether the insurance company pays for a service!

Each of the six sections, or chapters, within CPT has its own unique *section guidelines*, which provide information about assigning codes within that section. *Section guidelines* appear before the first code in the section and are printed on green pages in the Professional Edition of the CPT-4 manual. Review ■ FIGURE 17-6, which shows part of the guidelines from the Pathology and Laboratory section.

Notice how the Pathology and Laboratory guidelines provide you with additional information, depending on what services/procedures you need to code. Refer to ■ FIGURE 17-7 to

Figure 17-6 ■ Part of the section guidelines for Pathology and Laboratory.

Pathology and Laboratory

Pathology and Laboratory Guidelines

Items used by all physicians in reporting their services are presented in the Introduction. Some of the commonalities are repeated here for the convenience of those physicians referring to this section on **Pathology and Laboratory**. Other definitions and items unique to Pathology and Laboratory are also listed.

Services in Pathology and Laboratory

Services in Pathology and Laboratory are provided by a physician or by technologists under responsible supervision of a physician.

Figure 17-7 ■ Subsection guidelines for Organ or Disease-Oriented Panels in Pathology and Laboratory.

Organ or Disease-Oriented Panels (80047-80076)

These panels were developed for coding purposes only and should not be interpreted as clinical parameters. The tests listed with each panel identify the defined components of that panel.

These panel components are not intended to limit the performance of other tests. If one performs tests in addition to those specifically indicated for a particular panel, those tests should be reported separately in addition to the panel code.

Do not report two or more panel codes that include any of the same constituent tests performed from the same patient collection. If a group of tests overlaps two or more panels, report the panel that incorporates the greater number of tests to fulfill the code definition and report the remaining tests using individual test codes (eg, do not report 80047 in conjunction with 80053).

92081	Visual field examination, unilateral or bilateral, with interpretation and report; limited examination (eg, tangent screen, Autoplot, arc perimeter, or single stimulus level automated test, such as Octopus 3 or 7 equivalent)
92082	intermediate examination (eg, at least 2 isopters on Goldmann perimeter, or semiquantitative, automated suprathreshold screening program, Humphrey suprathreshold automatic diagnostic test, Octopus program 33)
92083	extended examination (eg, Goldmann visual fields with at least 3 isopters plotted and static determination within the central 30°, or quantitative, automated threshold perimetry, Octopus program G-1, 32 or 42, Humphrey visual field analyzer full threshold programs 30-2, 24-2, or 30/60-2)
	(Gross visual field testing (eg, confrontation testing) is a part of general ophthalmological services and is not reported separately.)

Figure 17-8 ■ Coding instructions shown for code 92083.

review guidelines for the first subsection in the Pathology and Laboratory section, Organ or Disease-Oriented Panels.

Note that the subsection guidelines provide you with specific information to review *before* assigning codes 80047–80076. You can also find specific guidelines for subheadings, categories, subcategories, and individual codes, which are listed in parentheses, as shown for code 92083 in ■ FIGURE 17-8.

TAKE A BREAK

Good job! Let's take a break and then review CPT guidelines and instructions.

Exercise 17.7   CPT Coding Guidelines and Instructions

Instructions: Review coding guidelines listed to answer the following questions. Turn to the Table of Contents before each section in your CPT manual to find locations of specific subsections, subheadings, categories, and subcategories.

1. Turn to the section guidelines for Anesthesia.

   What code should you assign for supplies that are over and above those usually included with a service? _____

   _____

2. Refer to the section guidelines for Surgery.

   What type of service may require a special report?

   _____

3. Turn to the guidelines listed in the Surgery section, subsection Musculoskeletal System, subheading Endoscopy/Arthroscopy.

   A surgical endoscopy/arthroscopy always includes what type of service? _____

4. Review the guidelines listed in the Surgery section, subsection Digestive System, subheading Vestibule of Mouth.

   What is the definition of the vestibule of the mouth?

   _____

   _____

5. Refer to the guidelines following code 53665.

   If a provider performs dilation of a urethra under local anesthesia, then what codes should you review?

   _____

6. Review the guidelines following code 96416.

   What codes should you review for refilling and maintenance of an implantable infusion pump for drug delivery? _____

INTERESTING FACTS: **Cardiovascular Procedures are More Common for Men; Digestive System Procedures are More Common for Women**

In 2002, 42.5 million procedures were performed on hospital inpatients nationally. The rate was 1,481 procedures per 10,000 people. For males, the rate was 1,197 procedures per 10,000 people, and for females, it was 1,753 procedures per 10,000 people.

✔ About one-quarter of all procedures performed on females were obstetrical. Repair of current obstetric laceration (1.2 million), followed by cesarean section (1.1 million), were the most frequent obstetrical procedures performed.

✔ Almost one-quarter of all procedures performed on males were cardiovascular. The rate of cardiovascular procedures performed on males was 282 per 10,000 people.

✔ Males had more cardiovascular procedures than females (4.0 million versus 2.8 million), and females had more operations on the digestive system than males (3.2 million versus 2.4 million).

✔ Frequent procedures for males were arteriography and angiocardiography, removal of coronary artery obstruction and insertion of stent(s), cardiac catheterization, respiratory therapy, endoscopy of small intestine, coronary artery bypass graft, and diagnostic ultrasound.

✔ Frequent procedures for females were repair of current obstetric laceration, cesarean section, arteriography, angiocardiography, artificial rupture of membranes, episiotomy, hysterectomy, and endoscopy of small intestine.

(Department of Health and Human Services, Centers for Disease Control and Prevention, www.cdc.gov/nchs/data/ad/ad342.pdf, accessed 2/4/11.)

CODE SYMBOLS

CPT uses *code symbols* to provide you with additional information about codes, including code and descriptor changes from the previous year to the current year. You can find code symbols listed at the bottom of each page of the CPT manual to remind you of what the symbols mean. The CPT Professional Edition also includes a quick reference of code symbols on the inside cover. You will see code symbols throughout the manual, and they are printed beside or after codes to which they refer. Review ■ TABLE 17-2 for a list of symbols, along with their descriptions and meanings, and the appendices, where you can find all codes with the symbol listed.

■ TABLE 17-2 **CPT CODE SYMBOLS, DESCRIPTIONS, AND MEANINGS**

Symbol	Description	Meaning	Figure
⊘	Modifier -51 Exempt	Modifier -51 is added to a CPT code to show that a code was an additional procedure the provider performed. Never add modifier -51 to codes that are Modifier -51 exempt (Appendix E).	17-9
⊙	Moderate Sedation	Code includes moderate sedation, so do not code sedation separately (Appendix G).	17-10
+	Add-on Code	Add-on codes describe additional work associated with a primary procedure (Appendix D). Add-on codes include phrases in the descriptor such as "each additional" or "(List separately in addition to primary procedure)." Add-on codes are always performed in addition to the primary service or procedure and must never be reported alone.	17-11
⚹	FDA approval pending	Codes for vaccines that are pending approval for use from the FDA (Appendix K). Even though the FDA has not approved a vaccine, a provider is still permitted to give the vaccine to patients. However, the provider should review with the patient the fact that the vaccine is not yet FDA approved and obtain the patient's written permission to receive the vaccine.	17-12
▲	Revised Code	The code's descriptor changed from last year (Appendix B).	17-13

continued

■ TABLE 17-2   *continued*

Symbol	Description	Meaning	Figure
●	New Code	A new procedure/service that did not exist last year (Appendix B).	17-14
○	Reinstated/ Recycled Code	A code the AMA has reinstated this year because the code was previously deleted.	17-15
#	Resequenced Code	A code that is not listed in numerical order (Appendix N). Resequencing allows the AMA to include coding concepts in appropriate locations within the families of codes, regardless of the availability of numbers for sequential numerical placement. There are also notes throughout CPT alerting you that codes are out of sequence and directing you to the correct place to find them.	17-16
▷◁	New or Revised Text (facing triangles)	Text for the descriptor is new or revised since last year, or there are new or revised instructions for assigning a code.	17-16
⊘●	References to AMA coding materials	The symbol ● means that you can find more information about the code in a specific issue of the *CPT Assistant* monthly newsletter and/or *CPT Changes: An Insider's View*, an annual book with all of the coding changes for the current year. The symbol ● means that you can find more information about the code in the quarterly newsletter *Clinical Examples in Radiology*. Providers can purchase these publications from the AMA.	17-17

⊘**17004**   Destruction (eg, laser surgery, electrosurgery, cryosurgery, chemosurgery, surgical curettement), premalignant lesions (eg, actinic keratoses), 15 or more lesions

Figure 17-9 ■ Code that is exempt from modifier -51.

⊙▲**35471**   Transluminal balloon angioplasty, percutaneous; renal or visceral artery

⊙**35472**   aortic

Figure 17-10 ■ Codes that include moderate sedation.

11100   Biopsy of skin, subcutaneous tissue and/or mucous membrane (including simple closure), unless otherwise listed; single lesion

+**11101**   each separate/additional lesion (List separately in addition to code for primary procedure)
(Use 11101 in conjunction with 11100)

Figure 17-11 ■ Add-on code that can never be reported alone.

↗●**90664**   Influenza virus vaccine, pandemic formulation, live, for intranasal use

Figure 17-12 ■ Code for a vaccine with pending FDA approval.

▲**50250**   Ablation, open, 1 or more renal mass lesion(s), cryosurgical, including intraoperative ultrasound guidance and monitoring, if performed

Figure 17-13 ■ Revised code.

●**53860**   Transurethral radiofrequency micro-remodeling of the female bladder neck and proximal urethra for stress urinary incontinence

Figure 17-14 ■ New code.

○**0058T**   Cryopreservation; reproductive tissue, ovarian

Figure 17-15 ■ Reinstated/recycled code.

▲**11042**   Debridement, subcutaneous tissue (includes epidermis and dermis, if performed); first 20 sq cm or less

▶(For debridement of skin [ie, epidermis and/or dermis only], see 97597, 97598)◀

#+●**11045**   each additional 20 sq cm, or part thereof (List separately in addition to code for primary procedure)

▶(Use 11045 in conjunction with 11042)◀

Figure 17-16 ■ New or revised text (11042, 11045) and resequenced code (11045).

77080   Dual-energy X-ray absorptiometry (DXA), bone density study, 1 or more sites; axial skeleton (eg, hips, pelvis, spine)
➲ *CPT Changes: An Insider's View* 2007;
➲ *Clinical Examples in Radiology* Fall 2007:11

Figure 17-17 ■ References to AMA coding materials.

Deleted Codes and Text

Any time that you see a line drawn through codes or text, it means that the codes and text have been deleted. The text appears so that you will know the exact information that was deleted (Figure 17-18).

Resequencing Notes

When a code appears out of sequence, you will see a note that provides you with this information (Figure 17-19).

~~93556 pulmonary angiography, aortography, and/or selective coronary angiography including venous bypass grafts and arterial conduits (whether native or used in bypass)~~

Figure 17-18 ■ Deleted code and deleted text.

⁄●**90664**   Influenza virus vaccine, pandemic formulation, live, for intranasal use

90665 ▶ Code is out of numerical sequence. See 90476-90749

⁄●**90666**   Influenza virus vaccine, pandemic formulation, split virus, preservative free, for intramuscular use

⁄●**90667**   Influenza virus vaccine, pandemic formulation, split virus, adjuvanted, for intramuscular use

⁄●**90668**   Influenza virus vaccine, pandemic formulation, split virus, for intramuscular use

#**90665**   Lyme disease vaccine, adult dosage, for intramuscular use

Figure 17-19 ■ Resequencing note.

TAKE A BREAK

Good work! Let's take a break and then review code symbols.

Exercise 17.8   Code Symbols

Instructions: Match the code symbol to its meaning by writing the letter of the meaning on the line preceding each symbol.

1. _____ ○
2. _____ ✗
3. _____ ⊙
4. _____ ▶◀
5. _____ #
6. _____ ▲
7. _____ +
8. _____ ●
9. _____ ⊝⊙
10. _____ ⊘

a. Add-on code describing additional work associated with a primary procedure
b. A new procedure/service
c. Exempt from adding modifier −51 to show an additional procedure
d. References to AMA coding materials
e. A code not listed in numerical order
f. Codes for vaccines that are pending FDA approval
g. Code includes moderate sedation
h. The code's descriptor changed from last year
i. A reinstated/recycled code
j. New or revised text

WORKPLACE IQ

You are working as a new coder for a neurologist, Dr. Fisher. One of your colleagues, Becky, is training you, and today, as you read a patient's chart, you find a procedure for chemodenervation of eccrine glands. You have no idea what this procedure is, let alone eccrine glands, and you are too embarrassed to ask Becky because you do not want her to think that you do not know.

What would you do?

CPT APPENDICES A–N

CPT Appendices are listed in the back of the coding manual, immediately following Category III codes. You already learned about information in many of the appendices from Table 17-2. ▪ TABLE 17-3 provides a comprehensive list of each appendix and the information that it contains. Turn to each appendix as you review Table 17-3.

TAKE A BREAK

Let's take a break and then review more about CPT appendices.

Exercise 17.9   CPT Appendices A–N

Instructions: Read each statement, and write a T for True or an F for False on the line preceding each statement.

1. _____ Appendix A is a list of codes that are exempt from modifier -51.

2. _____ Appendix I is a list of modifiers for genetic testing codes.

3. _____ Types of nerves included in nerve conduction studies tests are included in Appendix L.

4. _____ Groups of artery branches are listed in Appendix J.

5. _____ The AMA is no longer deleting and resequencing codes.

6. _____ Motor nerves carry impulses from the brain and spinal cord to muscles.

■ TABLE 17-3 **CPT APPENDICES AND DESCRIPTIONS**

Appendix	Title	Description
A	**Modifiers**	A modifier is added to a CPT code to give additional information about a service or procedure. Modifiers are covered in more detail later in this chapter.
B	**Summary of Additions, Deletions, and Revisions**	A list of all additions, deletions, and revisions for the new year of CPT. The summary changes every year.
C	**Clinical Examples**	A list of medical record chart examples for evaluation and management (E/M) services that help you to better understand when to assign specific E/M codes.
D	**Summary of CPT Add-on Codes**	A list of codes that cannot be used alone and must be reported with another service.
E	**Summary of CPT Codes Exempt from Modifier -51**	A list of codes that are exempt from adding modifier -51 (multiple procedures).
F	**Summary of CPT Codes Exempt from Modifier -63**	A list of codes that are exempt from adding modifier -63 (a procedure performed on infants weighing less than 4 kgs).
G	**Summary of CPT Codes That Include Moderate (Conscious) Sedation**	A list of codes that include moderate (conscious) sedation, so you should not report sedation separately.
H	**Alphabetical Clinical Topics Listing (AKA - Alphabetical Listing)**	Appendix H was removed from CPT. It was a list of Category II codes (for performance and tracking purposes) and their meanings. Because the list is ever-changing, the AMA made it available on its website.
I	**Genetic Testing Code Modifiers**	A list of modifiers to add to codes relating to laboratory genetic testing (tests to determine the presence of a disease or disorder or predict whether a person may someday contract the disease or disorder). Modifiers are made up of a number that classifies the type of disease and a letter that that classifies the type of gene.
J	**Electrodiagnostic Medicine Listing or Sensory, Motor, and Mixed Nerves**	Electrodiagnostic medicine involves nerve conduction studies, tests which measure how nerves respond to stimulation to assess the level of nerve functioning and presence of disorders or diseases. Appendix J provides types of nerves (sensory, motor, and mixed) included with codes for nerve conduction studies.
		Sensory nerves are connected to the central nervous system (CNS), the brain and spinal cord. Motor nerves carry impulses from the brain and spinal cord to muscles. Mixed nerves are made up of both sensory and motor fibers.
K	**Product Pending FDA Approval**	A list of vaccines waiting for approval from the FDA. The AMA updates the list on its website.
L	**Vascular Families**	A vascular family is a group of connected arteries that branch out from the aorta, like branches of a tree. In order to code certain procedures that involve movement through the arteries, such as a heart catherization, you have to understand where arteries are located and how they connect. Appendix L provides a breakdown of artery branches and their connections.
M	**Deleted CPT Codes**	A list of deleted and resequenced codes from 2007–2009, along with the current code to use for a deleted code. This list will not change because the AMA no longer deletes and resequences codes.
N	**Summary of Resequenced CPT Codes**	A list of codes that are not listed numerically with other codes.

UNLISTED PROCEDURES AND SERVICES

Many codes in CPT Category I have very general descriptions, which are intended to cover a variety of services and procedures. They are called *unlisted codes* meaning that you use them whenever you code a procedure or service for which there is no specific CPT code in either Category I or Category III (■ FIGURE 17-20).

The AMA designated many unlisted codes in the six sections of CPT that you can assign for reporting unlisted procedures, including procedures that providers do not often perform, procedures that are experimental, or new procedures that do not yet have a spe-

68899	Unlisted procedure, lacrimal system
79999	Radiopharmaceutical therapy, unlisted procedure
89698	Unlisted reproductive medicine laboratory procedure

Figure 17-20 ▪ Examples of unlisted codes in CPT.

cific Category I or Category III code. There are reporting guidelines associated with many unlisted procedures, which you can find in the guidelines before each section and after the unlisted code. You should review and understand the guidelines before reporting the unlisted code.

A comprehensive list of all the unlisted codes in a section appear in the guidelines before each section. You can find unlisted codes at the end of specific subsections, sub-headings, categories, and subcategories. Unlisted codes end with the numbers 98 or 99. Descriptions of services that you report with unlisted codes should be included in block 19 of the CMS-1500 form. You should only assign unlisted codes as a *last resort*, after checking for a more specific Category I or Category III code, because you have to send a special report along with the claim and it will take an insurance longer to pay the claim. We will discuss special reports next.

SPECIAL REPORTS

For services that providers rarely perform, services that are unusual, or services that are reported with unlisted codes, insurances typically require *special reports*, including medical documentation or letters from clinicians to justify the medical necessity of a procedure and provide greater detail about the procedure performed. Providers send special reports with claims for Category I unlisted codes and Category III codes. Special reports include the definition or description of the nature, extent, and need for the procedure, as well as the time, effort, and equipment used to provide the service. Be aware that when you have to send additional information with claims, insurances typically take longer to process them because they spend more time reviewing the additional information before process-ing the claim.

TAKE A BREAK

Good work! Let's take a break and then review more about unlisted procedures and special reports.

Exercise 17.10 **Unlisted Procedures and Services**
Special Reports

Instructions: Answer each question, using the CPT coding manual as directed.

1. Refer to code 97799 in your CPT coding manual. What type of procedure would a patient need to have in order for you to assign this unlisted code? _____

2. Review code 60699 in your CPT coding manual. What type of procedure would a patient need to have in order for you to assign this unlisted code? _____

3. Why should you only assign an unlisted code as a last resort? _____

4. Why did the AMA create unlisted codes? _____

5. What is a special report? _____

6. What categories of CPT codes should you first check before assigning an unlisted code from Category I? _____

MODIFIERS

A modifier is composed of two letters, two numbers, or a letter and a number. You should add, or append, a modifier to the end of a CPT or HCPCS code to provide additional information about the procedure or service. Insurances require you to append modifiers in specific circumstances in order to process claims. Insurances require different modifiers, so it is best to check with each individual insurance to determine its modifier requirements. You do not need to append modifiers to every CPT code that you assign; it just depends on the situation. Here are some examples of modifiers:

- LT—a procedure performed on the left side
- RT—a procedure performed on the right side
- 50—a procedure performed on both sides, or a bilateral procedure

If the patient has a procedure performed on the left side of the body, you should append modifier LT to the end of the CPT code to further specify information about the procedure, such as *73620-LT* (Radiologic exam, foot; two views—left foot).

One modifier may apply to many different codes in various CPT sections. Modifiers exist to save space in the CPT manual because the code set would be too large if there were separate codes to identify every possible scenario for each code and corresponding modifier.

Often you will see modifiers printed with a hyphen in front of them, such as -51 or -26. The hyphen helps you to differentiate the modifier from the CPT code. When you work in the healthcare field, many modifiers are already programmed into a provider's practice management software, so you do not need to enter the hyphen with the modifier.

Modifiers appear in block 24D of the CMS-1500 form, following the CPT/HCPCS code. (Refer to Figure 1-1 in Chapter 1 of this text.) There is room in block 24D for up to four modifiers. You can append as many modifiers to a CPT code as are necessary to completely describe a service or procedure.

There are two types of modifiers: Level I HCPCS—CPT-4 modifiers (two numbers) and Level II HCPCS—HCPCS modifiers (two letters or a letter and a number). Appendix A of CPT contains CPT-4 modifiers listed in ascending order and a partial list of HCPCS modifiers, presented in alphanumeric order. Appendix A also provides modifiers related to anesthesia services and modifiers approved for ASC hospital outpatient use. Turn to Appendix A to review full definitions of modifiers and descriptions of circumstances of when you should assign them. The CPT Professional Edition includes a quick reference to the modifiers on the inside cover. You can find the full list of HCPCS modifiers with the HCPCS code set.

You may be wondering how you will know when to append a modifier to a CPT code. The best way to know is to first become familiar with modifiers and their definitions, and then you will learn more through practice and experience. You will have the chance to learn more about modifiers and practice appending them in Chapter 18 of this text.

TAKE A BREAK

Let's take a break and then review more about modifiers.

Exercise 17.11   **Modifiers**

Instructions: Refer to Appendix A of the CPT manual to answer the following questions about CPT-4 and HCPCS modifiers.

1. What modifier would you append to a CPT code for a procedure performed on the great toe (big toe) of the left foot? _____

2. What modifier would you append to a CPT code for a lab procedure performed by a party other than the treating or reporting physician? _____

3. Which modifier should you append to an evaluation and management CPT code that resulted in an initial decision to perform surgery? _____

4. What modifier should you append to an anesthesia CPT code to show that the patient has a severe systemic disease? _____

5. What modifier would you append to a CPT code for a procedure performed on the fifth digit of the right hand? _____

6. What modifier should you append to a CPT code for a surgery to show that a surgical assistant was present? _____

SERVICES AND PROCEDURES THAT INCLUDE TIME

CPT contains many codes that use time as the basis for the code selection. Be very careful when the code descriptor involves time to ensure that you assign the correct code. CPT defines time as the amount of time the physician spends face-to-face with the patient. There are specific services that also include time that the physician spends performing duties related to the patient's encounter but are not face-to-face, such as time spent coordinating other care for the patient or time spent meeting with family members or caregivers about the patient. Be sure to follow the guidelines included for time-based services to better understand what activities are included in the total time for a service. Refer to the following CPT guidelines that apply when time is part of the code descriptor:

1. When you see a phrase such as "interpretation and report" in the code descriptor, it means that the provider interpreted and reported on a specific service, test, or procedure. Just because the descriptor shows "interpretation and report" does not mean that time spent interpreting and reporting is *included in the total time* for all the services, tests, or procedures.

2. Code descriptors outline time in increments, such as 15 minutes, 30 minutes, or 60 minutes, among others. When you compare the medical documentation time to the code descriptor time, you have to make sure that you are not coding time inaccurately. A unit of time is attained when the midpoint of the time unit has passed, unless the guidelines for the code state otherwise.

   - For example, if the medical documentation shows that the total time is 45 minutes, but the code descriptor time is an hour, you can still assign the code for the hour. This is because the total time documented is past the midpoint (30 minutes), so you can round the time up to an hour.

3. When the total service time is between two times with two different codes, assign the code with the time that is closest to the total service time.

4. When a provider performs two services for the same patient, including one that is time-based and one that is not, the total time calculated is just for the time-based service. Do not add the time spent on the service that is not time-based.

You will learn more about coding for time-based services as you work through additional chapters in this text, and you can find more information about the guidelines in your CPT manual.

ASSIGNING A CATEGORY I CODE

Now that you learned how to locate a code in the index and learned the formats of various sections in CPT and the structure of the CPT manual, let's review how to assign a CPT code following the examples listed next. Turn to your CPT manual to code along with the examples.

Example 1: Dr. Hoffman writes an order for Joseph Barlow, age 45, to have a chest X-ray at Williton Medical Center. The hospital's radiology department performs a two-view chest X-ray, frontal and lateral, and sends it back to Dr. Hoffman to interpret, which you will now code.

To code the chest X-ray for this case, search the index for the main term *X-ray*, subterm *chest* (■ FIGURE 17-21).

Notice in Figure 17-21 that there are several subterms listed under *X-ray, Chest*, but Example 1 did not provide any additional information that matches any of the subterms. Remember, you cannot assign a code for a service or procedure that the physician did not document. So you have to cross-reference the code range 71010–71035, which is listed next to the subterm *Chest*, to find the two-view chest X-ray.

Cross-reference this code range to the Radiology section in your CPT manual, which includes codes beginning with the number 7. There are many code options in the range of 71010–71035, so let's start with the first code, 71010. Code 71010

X-ray

Chest	71010-71035
Complete (Four Views)	
with Fluoroscopy	71034
Insert Pacemaker	71090
Partial (Two Views)	
with Fluroscopy	71023
Stereo	71015
with Computer-Aided	
Detection	0174T-0175T
with Fluroscopy	71090

Figure 17-21 ■ Index entry for chest X-ray.

71020	Radiologic examination, chest, 2 views, frontal and lateral;
71021	with apical lordotic procedure
71022	with oblique projections
71023	with fluoroscopy

Figure 17-22 ■ Codes 71020–71023 cross-referenced to the Radiology section.

represents a *chest x-ray, single view, frontal,* which was not the service performed. The second code represents *chest x-ray, stereo, frontal,* which was not the service, either. The next code, 71020, represents a *two-view chest x-ray, frontal and lateral,* which is the procedure that you are searching for. But take a look at the other code options for a two-view chest X-ray before final code assignment, codes 71021–71023 (■ FIGURE 17-22).

When you review all four codes, you find that Example 1 did not refer to any information listed in descriptors for codes 71021–71023, so *you have to assign code 71020 because it matches the medical documentation* of a two-view chest X-ray, frontal and lateral. This code also requires modifier -26 (professional component), which we will discuss in Chapter 18.

trimalleolar (trī-mə-lē′-ə-lər)

Example 2: Dr. Velaquez, an orthopedic surgeon, performs closed treatment (no skin is broken) of a **trimalleolar** ankle fracture (fractured in three areas) without manipulation (without placing bones back into position) and applies an ankle brace. The patient is Maggie Rocha, age 32, who fractured her ankle after falling during a hiking trip.

To code this case, let's start by searching the index for the main term *fracture,* subterm *ankle.* You will notice several code options listed under *fracture, ankle* (■ FIGURE 17-23).

Fracture

Ankle	
Bimalleolar	27808-27814
Closed	27816-27818
Lateral	27786-27814, 27792
Medial	27760-27766, 27808-27814
Posterior	27767-27769, 27808-27814
Trimalleolar	27816-27823
with Manipulation	27818
without Manipulation	27816

Figure 17-23 ■ Index entry for ankle fracture.

| 27816 | Closed treatment of trimalleolar ankle fracture; without manipulation |

Figure 17-24 ■ Code 27816 cross-referenced to the Surgery section.

When you review the options for an ankle fracture, notice that there are sub-terms for *trimalleolar* (27816–27823), *closed* (27816–27818), and *without manipulation* (27816), which were all part of the documentation. We will need to review code options for all three subterms in order to find the code that we need. Fortunately, each subterm starts with the same code, 27816, which is a good place to start. Cross-reference code 27816 to the Surgery section of your CPT manual (■ Figure 17-24).

Did you notice that code 27816 contains all of the information documented for the patient's procedure? Dr. Velaquez performed *closed* treatment of a *trimalleolar ankle fracture without manipulation*. All of this information is covered in the descriptor for code 27816. There is no more information left to code, and the descriptor does not contain any information that is not documented.

But just as a precaution, let's review the code descriptors for the other codes we were going to cross-reference for the subterms that we found, 27818–27823. Notice that code 27818 includes *with manipulation*, which was not done, and codes 27822 and 27823 include *open treatment*, which also was not done. So our final code assignment is code 27816 which completely matches the chart documentation.

arthroscopy (ahr-thros′k-pe)—visual examination of the inside of a joint using a viewing instrument

synovial (sĭ-no′ve-əl)—connective tissue membrane that lines joints and other structures and secretes fluid

osseous (os′e-əs)—bony

acupuncture (ak′u-punk char)—a form of traditional Chinese medicine that involves inserting fine needles into specific body sites for pain relief, anesthesia, and other therapeutic purposes

saphenous (saf′-ə-nəs)—the vein in the center and back part of the thigh near the skin

saphenopopliteal (sa-fe-no pop-lit′e-əl)—point where the saphenous vein (at the back of the thigh) joins the popliteal vein (at the back of the knee)

TAKE A BREAK

Good job! Let's take a break and then practice assigning Category I CPT codes, including time-based services and procedures.

Exercise 17.12   **Services and Procedures that Include Time: Assigning a Category I Code**

Instructions: For each service or procedure, underline the main term to search in the index to find the code(s) to cross-reference. *Hint: Recall that you can locate main terms by searching for the procedure, service, organ, anatomic site, condition, synonym, eponym, or abbreviation. There can be more than one main term for a procedure.* Then assign the codes, using the index and cross-referencing to the sections of CPT.

1. Diagnostic knee **arthroscopy**, without **synovial** biopsy:

   Code: _____

2. Vaginal hysterectomy with removal of tubes and ovaries, for uterus greater than 250 g.

   Code: _____

3. X-ray, bone, **osseous** survey, complete.

   Code: _____

4. **Acupuncture**, 3 needles, without electrical stimulation, 25 minutes, with reinsertion of needles.

   Code: _____

5. Physician standby services, 50 minutes.

   Code: _____

6. Ligation and division of short **saphenous** vein, at **saphenopopliteal** junction performed as a separate procedure.

   Code: _____

CATEGORY II CODES

Remember that CPT also contains Category II codes, which are made up of four numbers and the letter F. Providers use Category II codes for tracking services and reporting statistical information, rather than for billing insurances. You can find main terms for Category II codes in the index and then cross-reference codes to Category II, which follows Category I codes in the CPT manual. Using Category II codes, providers can generate computerized reports showing the frequency and types of services that patients receive, such as assessing a patient's tobacco use (code 1000F). Providers can report Category II codes in block 24D of the CMS-1500 form. (Refer to Figure 1-1 in Chapter 1 of this text.)

Physician Quality Reporting System

Providers can earn *additional* money from CMS which offers a bonus payment program to physicians for reporting specific services using Category II codes. The bonus payment program is called the *Physician Quality Reporting System (PQRS)*, and the goal is for providers to monitor the type and quality of care that they provide to patients with specific diagnoses (such as diabetes) and to report the results to CMS, using Category II codes when they are available. Examples of measurements reported with Category II codes are 3075F to show measurement of a patient's systolic blood pressure of 130–139 mm Hg and 3080F to show measurement of a patient's diastolic blood pressure greater than or equal to 90 mm Hg.

By reviewing a provider's Category II codes and performance measurements, CMS determines the type and frequency of services that providers render and assesses how well they perform. It is important for you to understand the reporting process under PQRS because you may need to assign Category II codes for reporting services to CMS for patients with specific conditions.

CMS created PQRS because the *2006 Tax Relief and Health Care Act (TRHCA) (P.L. 109-432)* required CMS to establish a physician quality reporting system, including an incentive payment for eligible professionals who satisfactorily report data on quality measures for covered professional services that are furnished to Medicare beneficiaries. PQRS was formerly called the Physician Quality Reporting Initiative (PQRI).

To participate in PQRS, eligible professionals report information on individual Physician Quality Reporting measures using one of three methods, reporting to:

1. CMS on their Medicare Part B (CMS-1500 form) claims
2. A qualified Physician Quality Reporting registry
3. CMS through a qualified electronic health record (EHR) program

CMS developed a PQRS list of 194 measures for physicians to track and report specific services for patients (Category II codes) with certain conditions (ICD-9-CM codes). Each year, CMS identifies specific conditions for performance measurement and acceptable Category II codes to report for those conditions, like diabetes mellitus, coronary artery disease, major depressive disorder, and primary open angle glaucoma. Every measure in the list includes a reporting frequency requirement.

In 2012, eligible professionals who met criteria for satisfactory submission of Physician Quality Reporting quality measures data through one of the three reporting methods qualified to earn a Physician Quality Reporting incentive payment. The payment is equal to 1.0% of the provider's total estimated Medicare Part B Physician Fee Schedule (PFS) allowed charges for covered professional services that are furnished during that same reporting period. A group practice (one with multiple providers) may also potentially qualify to earn a Physician Quality Reporting incentive payment equal to 1.0% of the group practice's total estimated Medicare Part B PFS allowed charges.

Although it may seem like a lot of extra work to assign Category II tracking codes, it means that an individual provider or group practice could potentially receive several hundreds or thousands of dollars more from CMS for reporting specific measures for patients' conditions! In addition, providers have extra incentive to comply with PQRS because in 2015, CMS will impose a negative payment adjustment (financial penalty) of 1.5% to providers who do not comply with PQRS, which will increase to 2% in 2016. Therefore, it is in a provider's best interest to comply with PQRS performance measures.

CMS tracks each provider's performance measures reporting through their national provider identifier (NPI) number, which you learned in Chapter 2 is a unique 10-digit number assigned to each provider for electronic transmissions. PQRS will become even more important when CMS integrates the PQRS measures with the electronic health record (EHR) meaningful use incentive payment program, part of the American Recovery and Reinvestment Act, which you also learned about in Chapter 2. The *Affordable Care Act* required CMS to create an implementation plan by January 1, 2012, to integrate PQRS

DESTINATION: MEDICARE

In this exercise, your Medicare destination is an MLN computer-based training module called *PQRI and E-Prescribing.*, which covers more information about PQRI, now called PQRS. In addition, you will also learn more about E-Prescribing, also called eRx, a separate financial incentive program that CMS oversees as part of the Medicare Improvements for Patients and Providers Act of 2008 (MIPPA). The program is separate from PQRS and pays providers additional money if they electronically transmit patients' prescriptions to pharmacies (which can be done through many EHRs) and also report additional information to CMS about the patients' conditions, prescriptions, and insurance authorization requirements. You may be involved with reporting eRx information to Medicare, so it will be very helpful for you to learn more about the program.

1. Go to the website http://www.cms.gov.
2. At the top of screen on the banner bar, choose *Outreach & Education.*
3. Scroll down to *Medicare Learning Network (MLN)* and choose *MLN Products.*
4. Choose *Web-Based Training (WBT).*
5. Under *Related Links,* click on *Web-Based Training (WBT) Courses.* You will then see a list of web-based training courses. Click on *PQRI and E-Prescribing (October 2011).*
6. Click the link to Login using your previously created Login ID and Password. If you never accessed the MLN's computer-based training, then you will have to register as a new user. Registration is free and takes a few minutes. Once registered, you will only need your login and password each time you access the computer-based MLN. After registering or logging in, click *Web-Based Training (WBT) Courses*, and click *PQRI and E-Prescribing* again.
7. On the next screen, click the radio button for *No credits* or *Continuing Education Units* (CEU). (CMS grants 1 CEU to coders who are certified through the American Academy of Professional Coders (AAPC); for scoring 70% or higher on the post-test.) Then click *Take Course.* You will take both a pretest and post-test so that you can monitor how well you learned the material.

with the EHR. Medicare providers will need to ensure that they meet all of the goals of each program and can integrate performance measures reporting with the EHR. There are also HCPCS G codes that providers use for PQRS, along with several different modifiers. You can find more information about the PQRS process on the CMS website at www.cms.gov/pqri, and you will also learn more in the above *Destination: Medicare* exercise.

TAKE A BREAK

Let's take a break to review more about Category II codes.

Exercise 17.13   Category II Codes

Part 1 Theory

Instructions: Read each question, and write your answer in the space provided.

1. What is the goal of the PQRS program?

_____

2. What three methods can providers choose to report Physician Quality Reporting measures?

_____

_____

_____

_____

continued

TAKE A BREAK *continued*

3. How do Category II codes relate to the PQRS program?

_____

4. When will CMS impose financial penalties to providers for noncompliance with the PQRS program?

_____

5. What information do Category II codes represent?

_____

6. Besides Category II codes, what other types of codes can providers assign for the PQRS program?

_____

Part 2—Coding

Instructions: For each service or procedure, underline the main term (one word) to search in the index to find the Category II code(s). Then assign Category II codes, cross-referencing to the Category II section of CPT.

1. Antibiotic administration, prescribed.

Code: _____

2. Performance measure reporting of stage II colon cancer.

Code: _____

3. Hemodialysis **Kt/V** level greater than or equal to 1.7.

Code: _____

4. Performance measure reporting of blood pressure reading, 150/100. (Hint: the first blood pressure number is systolic, the second is diastolic.)

Code: _____

5. Performance measure reporting of **wound compression therapy** prescribed.

Code: _____

6. Performance measure reporting of hepatitis C **quantitative RNA testing** documented as performed at 12 weeks from initiation of **antiviral** treatment.

Code: _____

Kt/V—measurement to assess the efficiency of hemodialysis; K is the volume of fluid completely cleared of urea in milliliters per minute, t is the amount of time in the dialysis session, and V is the urea distribution volume

wound compression therapy—treatment of poor circulation to wounds by applying pressure, such as with elastic compression stockings or an elastic bandaging strap

CATEGORY III CODES

Recall that Category III codes (four numbers and the letter T) follow Category II codes in the CPT manual. They are temporary codes that represent new technology, services, and procedures. Providers send special reports with insurance claims containing Category III codes to establish medical necessity for services. You can find main terms for Category III codes in the index of the CPT manual. Like Category II codes, providers can also generate computerized reports for Category III codes for statistics and tracking. But unlike Category II codes, providers can submit Category III codes to insurances for reimbursement. If a Category III code is available, then the provider must assign it, rather than assigning an unlisted Category I code. Category III codes also appear in block 24D of the CMS-1500 form. (Refer to Figure 1-1 in this text.)

TAKE A BREAK

Let's take a break to practice assigning Category III codes.

Exercise 17.14 Category III Codes

Instructions: For each service or procedure, underline the main term (one word) to search in the index to find the Category III code(s). Then assign Category III codes, cross-referencing to the Category III section of CPT. Be sure to use your medical references to look up terms that you do not understand.

1. **Endovascular** repair of abdominal aortic aneurysm involving superior mesenteric vessel, using fenestrated modular bifurcated prosthesis, radiological supervision and interpretation.

Code: _____

2. Islet cell transplantation through portal vein, open.

Code: _____

TAKE A BREAK *continued*

3. **Transforaminal** epidural injection of steroid into L3, L4, and L5 using ultrasound guidance.

   Code: _____

4. **Transcatheter** placement of **extracranial** vertebral carotid artery stents for two vessels, including radiologic supervision and interpretation, **percutaneous.**

   Code: _____

5. Laparoscopic replacement of **gastric stimulation electrodes** in the lesser curvature of the stomach.

   Code: _____

6. **Computer aided detection (CAD)** of **digitized** chest radiograph with further physician review for interpretation and report, performed remote from primary interpretation.

   Code: _____

POINTERS FROM THE PROS: Interview with a Coding Manager

Suzan Berman is a Senior Manager for Coding Education and Documentation Compliance for a large teaching hospital and medical center. She has 20 years of experience in the coding field and is a certified coder for physicians, the emergency department (ED), and evaluation and management, through the American Academy of Professional Coders. Ms. Berman manages a group of physician educators and auditors. They review medical documentation to ensure that it is thorough and appropriate for services rendered and educate physicians on the relationship between coding and documentation.

What type of training or education did you receive for your job (e.g., coursework, on-the-job training, industry publications, membership in professional organizations)?

Most of my training was on the job. I learned as I went along. I used documentation, textbooks, magazines, newsletters, the Internet, and professional organization networks to gain the knowledge I now have. However, the real-world situations are what will keep you on top of your game.

Please give an example of a time when you educated a physician on coding processes or any other procedures, and the outcome:

One of the first physicians I worked with was known to be difficult with all levels of nonclinicians. I was to shadow this physician, Dr. G., the entire morning and then provide education immediately after. At first, the face-to-face

time was difficult. He didn't want a "regulations" person hanging around. And being new, I didn't want confrontation this early on. As the day went on, we started talking about baseball in between patients, a little about documentation, and more about day-to-day routines. The air turned, and we really had a wonderful morning. When I presented to a group of his colleagues a few weeks after, he was my strongest supporter. He encouraged all of the physicians to let me shadow them. He felt it was a very useful tool in his desires to do the right thing. It made me feel great knowing I had that impact, and it certainly gave me the much-needed confidence to press forward with the other physicians. Now 10 years later, he is retired, but calls on me often just to see how I am.

What advice would you like to give to coding students about working with different personalities?

Communicate on a level you and the providers (clinicians) are comfortable. Shadow the providers so that you understand their environment. Understand how your world fits into their world. Understand that coding is only a minor piece of their day and their patient care; although vital for financial survival, their knowledge of disease states, anatomy, and patient care are extremely important. You are there as a resource; do not expect the providers to know as much as you do about the codes, the process, the guidelines, and the requirements.

(Used by permission of Suzan Berman.)

---

quantitative RNA testing—laboratory test for hepatitis C that detects and measures the number of viral ribonucleic acid (ri′bo-noo-kle-ik) (RNA) particles in the blood

percutaneous (pur′ku-ta′ne-əs)—through the skin

antiviral (an′ti-vi-rəl)—acting against a virus

transcatheter (tranz-kath′-ə-tər)—through a catheter

gastric stimulation electrodes—small discs that transmit electric current to stomach tissue

endovascular (en-do-vas′ku-lər)—within a blood vessel

extracranial (eks-trə-kra′ne-əl)—outside the skull

computer aided detection (CAD)—computer scanning of an X-ray to detect abnormalities

transforaminal (tranz-fo-ra′mən-əl)—into the opening (foramen) in the side of the spine where a nerve root exits

digitized—computer imagery

CHAPTER REVIEW

Multiple Choice

Instructions: Circle one best answer to complete each statement.

1. Category II codes are used for
   a. services approved by the Food and Drug Administration.
   b. new technology, services, and procedures.
   c. performance measurement reporting.
   d. supplies and nonphysician services.

2. Temporary codes that represent new technology, services, and procedures are _____ codes.
   a. Category I
   b. Category II
   c. Category III
   d. Category IV

3. Face-to-face services between a physician and patient are reported with codes from the _____ section of the CPT manual.
   a. Medicine
   b. Surgery
   c. Radiology
   d. Evaluation and Management

4. Two numbers, a letter and a number, or two letters are called _____, and you _____ them to a CPT or HCPCS code.
   a. qualifiers, append
   b. modifiers, remove
   c. modifiers, append
   d. qualifiers, remove

5. The following index entry represents what formatting convention?
   Esophagus
   Reconstruction............43300, 43310, 43313
   a. Stand-alone code
   b. Codes separated by a comma
   c. Add-on code
   d. Cross-referencing

6. When the index provides more than one code choice, or a code range,
   a. you have the option to choose any one of the codes listed.
   b. you should use all of the codes listed to fully describe the procedure.
   c. it means that you are in the wrong place to find the procedure that you are searching for and you must instead look elsewhere.
   d. you should always cross-reference each code choice in the index to the main text (sections).

7. The first part of the stand-alone description of one code, plus the indented description of another code, will give you the full description of a(n) _____ code.
   a. unlisted
   b. indented
   c. stand-alone
   d. temporary

8. For services that providers rarely perform, or services that are unusual, insurances may require
   a. special reports.
   b. proof of reimbursement.
   c. Level II modifiers.
   d. performance measurement reports.

9. Appendix A of the CPT manual contains
   a. genetic testing modifiers.
   b. modifier -63 exempt codes.
   c. modifier -51 exempt codes.
   d. modifiers.

10. _____ group procedures by location within a body system.
    a. Subsections
    b. Subheadings
    c. Subcategories
    d. Subclassifications

Coding Assignments

Instructions: Assign CPT-4 procedure code(s) to the following cases, referencing both the index and CPT sections. Optional: Also assign ICD-9-CM diagnosis codes using both the Index and Tabular for additional practice.

1. Dustin Carney, age 28, arrives at Williton Medical Center's ED with complaints of headaches, vomiting, and memory loss over the past month. Dr. Burns, an ED physician, performs an evaluation and management service, including an examination with further work-up. He calls in Dr. Foreman, a neurosurgeon (a physician who specializes in treating disorders involving nerves), who determines that the patient has a glioblastoma (aggressive malignant brain tumor) in the temporal lobe, which is inoperable. Assign a procedure code for the ED exam, which involved a comprehensive history and exam and medical decision-making of high complexity.

   Diagnosis code(s): _____

   Procedure code(s): _____

2. Dr. Vinson, an oncologist, excises a malignant tumor from the **mandible** (jaw bone) for patient John Forbes, age 58.

   Diagnosis code(s): _____

   Procedure code(s): _____

3. Dr. Whitley, a cardiologist (a physician who prevents, diagnoses, and treats heart disorders) performs a diagnostic evaluation with interpretation and report of 64 lead EKG (an EKG with 64 sensors rather than the usual 12), with graphic presentation and analysis. The patient is Helmet Vang, a 64-year-old who suffers from ventricular tachycardia (rapid heart rate from heart ventricles).

   Diagnosis code(s): _____

   Procedure code(s): _____

4. Christine Guthrie, age 52, arrives at Williton Medical Center's ED. Dr. Mills, the ED physician, diagnoses her with severe dehydration and administers intravenous IV hydration for three hours.

   Diagnosis code(s): _____

   Procedure code(s): _____

5. Dr. Langley, an anesthesiologist (a physician specializing in anesthesia), administers anesthesia during Edna Haney's total hip arthroplasty (hip replacement with an artificial hip). The patient, age 72, suffers from osteoarthritis and diabetes. Assign a procedure code only for the anesthesia.

   Diagnosis code(s): _____

   Procedure code(s): _____

6. Williton Medical Center's lab performs a quantitative analysis of **calculi** removed from the **bile duct**. The patient is SuLyn Yang, age 48.

   Diagnosis code(s): _____

   Procedure code(s): _____

7. Dr. Sargent, a urologist (a physician who prevents, diagnoses, and treats urological disorders), performs a **cystourethroscopy,** with **balloon dilation** for treatment of **ureteral stricture** for Larry Nieves, age 62.

   Diagnosis code(s): _____

   Procedure code(s): _____

8. Maria Sosa, age 41, arrives at Williton Medical Center's ED with right elbow pain and swelling. Dr. Mills orders an X-ray of the elbow, with two views: anteroposterior (AP) (front to back) and lateral. The X-ray does not reveal a fracture, so Dr. Mills will order a CT scan for more definitive information. Assign codes for this case before the patient has the CT scan.

   Diagnosis code(s): _____

   Procedure code(s): _____

9. Williton Medical Center tracks performance measurements for various situations. Assign a code for performance measurement reporting of documentation of hydration status as dehydrated.

   Procedure code(s): _____

10. Beverly Franks, age 60, suffers from uncontrolled primary open-angle glaucoma (an eye disorder marked by elevated intraocular pressure). Dr. Rasmussen, an ophthalmologist, inserts an **aqueous drainage device** into the anterior (front) segment of the eye, without **extraocular reservoir**, external approach.

    Diagnosis code(s): _____

    Procedure code(s): _____

---

mandible (man′dĭ-bəl)

calculi (kal′-ku-lī)—hard deposits of mineral salts

bile duct—a vessel that moves bile, a greenish-yellowish fluid, in and out of the liver

cystourethroscopy (sis-to-u-re-thros′kə-pe)—visual examination of the urethra and urinary bladder with a viewing instrument

balloon dilation (di-la′shən)—stretching a body cavity or vessel by inserting a sac and filling it with air or gas

ureteral stricture (u-re′tər-əl strik′chər)—abnormal narrowing of the ureters, the tubes that carry urine from the kidney to the urinary bladder

aqueous drainage device (a′kwe-əs)—a technique to relieve pressure in the eye by attaching a shunt or tube to the eye to drain fluid

extraocular reservoir (eks-trə-ok′u-lər)—a collection tube placed outside the eye to drain fluid

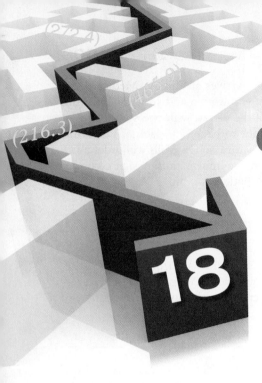

Coding with Modifiers

18

Learning Objectives

After completing this chapter, you should be able to

- Spell and define the key terminology in this chapter.
- Identify the two main types of modifiers.
- Explain and apply guidelines for coding with CPT modifiers.
- Define the Charge Description Master (CDM) and modifiers.
- Discuss billing, coding, and payment regulations for modifiers.
- Describe the global surgical package and modifiers.
- Identify the circumstances when you should use each CPT modifier.

Key Terms

Charge Description Master (CDM)
CPT modifiers
global period
global service

global surgical package
HCPCS modifiers
modifier
professional component
technical component

INTRODUCTION

In this chapter, you will learn about modifiers that both physicians and hospitals use and practice appending modifiers to patients' cases. Recall that a **modifier** is composed of two letters, two numbers, or a letter and a number, which you append to a CPT or HCPCS code to provide additional information about the procedure or service. You will practice appending modifiers to procedure codes for patients' cases. Once you learn when you should append specific modifiers to procedure codes, you will be better able to assign modifiers throughout the remaining chapters in this text. Think of the modifiers as a new beginning which will further advance your coding skills. Let's continue along your coding journey, following the path to modifiers!

"He who chooses the beginning of a road chooses the place it leads to. It is the means that determine the end." —HENRY EMERSON FOSDICK

MODIFIERS

You already learned a little about modifiers in Chapter 17. Insurances require you to append modifiers to codes in specific circumstances in order to process claims. Modifiers provide more information about services and procedures. Not all insurances require the same modifiers, so it is best to check with each individual insurance to determine its modifier requirements. You do not need to append modifiers to every CPT code that you assign; it just depends on the situation.

Here are some examples of modifiers:

- LT—a procedure performed on the left side
- RT—a procedure performed on the right side
- 50—a procedure performed on both sides, or bilateral procedure

If the patient has a procedure performed on the left side of the body, then you should append modifier LT to the end of the CPT code to further specify information about the procedure, such as *73620-LT* (Radiologic exam, foot; two views—left foot).

One modifier may apply to many different codes in various CPT sections. Modifiers exist to save space in the CPT manual because the code set would be too large if there were separate codes to identify every possible scenario for each code and corresponding modifier.

Often you will see modifiers printed with a hyphen in front of them, such as -51 or -26. The hyphen helps you to differentiate the modifier from the CPT code. When you work in the healthcare field, many modifiers are already programmed into a provider's practice management software, so you do not need to enter the hyphen with the modifier.

Modifiers appear in block 24D of the CMS-1500 form, following the CPT/HCPCS code. (See Figure 1-1 in Chapter 1 of this text.) You can append as many modifiers to a CPT code as are necessary to completely describe a service or procedure, but there is only room for four modifiers on the CMS-1500 form in block 24D. When there are five or more modifiers for a CPT or HCPCS code, append modifier -99 to the code, which means that there are multiple modifiers. Then list the code and all of the applicable modifiers in block 19 of the CMS-1500.

There are two types of modifiers:

1. Level I HCPCS—**CPT modifiers** (two numbers appended to a CPT or HCPCS code)
2. Level II HCPCS—**HCPCS modifiers** (two letters or a letter and a number appended to a CPT or HCPCS code)

As you learned in Chapter 17, Appendix A in the CPT manual contains CPT-4 modifiers listed in ascending order and a partial list of HCPCS modifiers, presented in alphanumeric order. Modifiers are also printed on the inside cover of the CPT Professional Edition. You can find the full list of HCPCS with the HCPCS code set.

The best way to know when to append a modifier is to become familiar with modifiers and their definitions and then to learn more through practice and experience. For example, you may wonder when you should append modifier -LT, -RT, or -50 to a procedure, such as a skin laceration repair. Left, right, and bilateral apply to paired organs or structures, or organs or structures that are different on the left side from the right side, such as the right leg or left leg, or the right eye or left eye. Left and right do not apply to structures like skin, muscle, or fascia, which have no left or right. For example, can you tell the difference between the skin on your left arm and the skin on your right arm? You cannot differentiate left skin from right skin, so you do not need to append an -LT, -RT, or -50 to procedures the physician performs on the skin. You will learn more about when to append specific modifiers as you work through this chapter.

An important point to remember is that you should not append modifiers to unlisted procedure codes. A modifier's purpose is to provide more information about a procedure's descriptor. Unlisted codes do not have specific descriptors, so modifiers do not apply.

TYPES OF MODIFIERS

The CPT manual contains 32 CPT modifiers (■ TABLE 18-1) and 48 HCPCS modifiers (■ TABLE 18-2). There are many more HCPCS modifiers, but CPT only contains the most common ones. You can find a list of all HCPCS modifiers in Appendix D of this text. Various types of outpatient providers append modifiers to CPT and HCPCS codes. Thirteen modifiers are approved for ASC hospital outpatient use, some of which are also listed under CPT modifiers (■ TABLE 18-3).

In this chapter, we will review CPT modifiers. You will learn more about HCPCS modifiers in Chapter 35 of this text.

■ TABLE 18-1   **CPT MODIFIERS**

Modifier	Description
22	Increased procedural services
23	Unusual anesthesia
24	Unrelated evaluation and management service by the same physician during a postoperative period
25	Significant, separately identifiable evaluation and management service by the same physician on the same day of the procedure or other service
26	Professional component
32	Mandated services
33	Preventive service
47	Anesthesia by surgeon
50	Bilateral procedure
51	Multiple procedures
52	Reduced services
53	Discontinued procedure
54	Surgical care only
55	Postoperative management only
56	Preoperative management only
57	Decision for surgery
58	Staged or related procedure or service by the same physician during the postoperative period
59	Distinct procedural service
62	Two surgeons
63	Procedure performed on infants less than 4 kgs
66	Surgical team
76	Repeat procedure or service by same physician or other qualified health care professional
77	Repeat procedure or service by another physician or other qualified health care professional
78	Unplanned return to the operating/procedure room by the same physician or other qualified health care professional following initial procedure for a related procedure during the postoperative period
79	Unrelated procedure or service by the same physician during the postoperative period
80	Assistant surgeon
81	Minimum assistant surgeon
82	Assistant surgeon (when qualified resident surgeon not available)
90	Reference (outside) laboratory
91	Repeat clinical diagnostic laboratory test
92	Alternative laboratory platform testing
99	Multiple modifiers

■ **TABLE 18-2   HCPCS MODIFIERS INCLUDED IN THE CPT MANUAL**

Modifier	Description
A1	Principal Physician of Record
BL	Special acquisition of blood and blood products
CA	Procedure payable only in the inpatient setting when performed emergently on an outpatient who expires prior to admission
CR	Catastrophe/disaster related
E1	Upper left eyelid
E2	Lower left eyelid
E3	Upper right eyelid
E4	Lower right eyelid
FA	Left hand, thumb
F1	Left hand, second digit
F2	Left hand, third digit
F3	Left hand, fourth digit
F4	Left hand, fifth digit
F5	Right hand, thumb
F6	Right hand, second digit
F7	Right hand, third digit
F8	Right hand, fourth digit
F9	Right hand, fifth digit
FB	Item provided without cost to provider, supplier, or practitioner, or full credit received for replaced device (examples, but not limited to covered under warranty, replaced due to defect, free samples)
FC	Partial credit received for replaced device
GA	Waiver of liability statement on file
GG	Performance and payment of a screening mammogram and diagnostic mammogram on the same patient, same day
GH	Diagnostic mammogram converted from screening mammogram on same day
LC	Left circumflex, coronary artery
LD	Left anterior descending coronary artery
LT	Left side (used to identify procedures performed on the left side of the body)
P1	Physical status modifier for anesthesia—a normal healthy patient
P2	Physical status modifier for anesthesia—a patient with mild systemic disease
P3	Physical status modifier for anesthesia—a patient with severe systemic disease
P4	Physical status modifier for anesthesia—a patient with severe systemic disease that is a constant threat to life
P5	Physical status modifier for anesthesia—a moribund (near death) patient who is not expected to survive without the operation
P6	Physical status modifier for anesthesia—a declared brain-dead patient whose organs are being removed for donor purposes
Q0	Investigational clinical service provided in a clinical research study that is in an approved clinical research study
Q1	Routine clinical service provided in a clinical research study that is in an approved clinical research study
QM	Ambulance service provided under arrangement by a provider of services
QN	Ambulance service furnished directly by a provider of services
RC	Right coronary artery

continued

■ TABLE 18-2 *continued*

Modifier	Description
RT	Right side (used to identify procedures performed on the right side of the body)
TA	Left foot, great toe
T1	Left foot, second digit
T2	Left foot, third digit
T3	Left foot, fourth digit
T4	Left foot, fifth digit
T5	Right foot, great toe
T6	Right foot, second digit
T7	Right foot, third digit
T8	Right foot, fourth digit
T9	Right foot, fifth digit

■ TABLE 18-3 **CPT MODIFIERS APPROVED FOR AMBULATORY SURGERY CENTER HOSPITAL OUTPATIENT USE INCLUDED IN THE CPT MANUAL**

Modifier	Description
25	Significant, separately identifiable evaluation and management service by the same physician on the same day of the procedure or other service
27	Multiple outpatient hospital evaluation and management (E/M) encounters on the same date
50	Bilateral procedure
52	Reduced services
58	Staged or related procedure or service by the same physician during the postoperative period
59	Distinct procedural service
73	Discontinued outpatient hospital/ambulatory surgery center (ASC) procedure prior to the administration of anesthesia
74	Discontinued outpatient hospital/ambulatory surgery center (ASC) procedure after administration of anesthesia
76	Repeat procedure or service by same physician or other qualified health care professional
77	Repeat procedure or service by another physician or other qualified health care professional
78	Unplanned return to the operating or procedure room by the same physician or other qualified health care professional following initial procedure for a related procedure during the postoperative period
79	Unrelated procedure or service by the same physician during the postoperative period
91	Repeat clinical diagnostic laboratory test

THE CHARGE DESCRIPTION MASTER AND MODIFIERS

Remember that different insurances, or payers, have different billing, coding, and payment regulations regarding modifiers. You have to check individual payer regulations to ensure that you append the correct modifiers to specific CPT and/or HCPCS codes because it can affect insurance reimbursement. Many providers can enter coding and billing information, including modifiers, directly into computer software.

The **Charge Description Master (CDM)**, also called a chargemaster, is a database of information in a physician's or hospital's software program. The CDM contains a list of every service and procedure that the provider offers, called line items, including the associated CPT or HCPCS code, a description of the service/procedure, and the current charge for the service/procedure. The CDM also typically has an individual number associated with every service/procedure, which the provider can enter into the computer software to charge a patient's account for the procedure. Hospitals' CDMs also contain revenue codes for every line item showing what department generated the charge to the patient (■ FIGURE 18-1). Revenue codes appear on the UB04 claim form in block 42. (See Figure 1-2 in Chapter 1.)

You may wonder what the CDM has to do with coding modifiers. The CDM also has the capability of containing specific modifiers for specific services and procedures. For example, a CDM can contain a line item for an X-ray, with the associated procedure code, and can also contain line items for that same X-ray with the -LT modifier, for an X-ray performed on the patient's left side, or a line item with the -RT modifier, for an X-ray performed on the patient's right side. The modifiers are already part of the line item, so the person entering charges would only need to enter the date of service and the line item number of the appropriate service. Having the line item information already built into the CDM eliminates the need to individually enter the modifier and saves time. However, it does require that the person entering charges is very careful about choosing the correct line item.

As codes and modifiers change each year, and as the provider updates charges, the provider also makes changes to the line items of the CDM to reflect current codes, modifiers, and charges. The CDM can also be integrated with coding software so that coders can assign codes to patients' records using software that links directly to the CDM for charging. Coders can also have the ability to verify the accuracy of codes that are already entered in the software during the charge entry process, before the provider bills the patient's insurance.

A CDM can also list more than one procedure code for a specific service/procedure, depending on an individual payer's requirements. For example, for the same service, one payer may require a HCPCS code, but another payer may require a CPT code. Many CDMs have the capability of containing *both* the HCPCS and the CPT codes for the same service. If the coder assigns the CPT code to the patient's service, but the patient has insurance that requires the HCPCS code, then the software can automatically bill the HCPCS code to the insurance. The same is true for modifiers; the CDM can be programmed to generate charges with specific modifiers to specific insurances, depending on the situation.

Line Item Number	Description	Hospital Revenue Code	CPT Code	HCPCS Code	Modifier	Charge
457219	Emergency Department E/M Level 1	450	99281	-	-	$200.00
457220	Emergency Department E/M Level 2	450	99282	-	-	$225.00
457221	Emergency Department E/M Level 3	450	99283	-	-	$250.00
457222	Emergency Department E/M Level 4	450	99284	-	-	$275.00
457223	Emergency Department E/M Level 5	450	99285	-	-	$300.00

Figure 18-1 ■ Example of line items from a hospital's Charge Description Master.

TAKE A BREAK

Let's take a break and then review more about modifiers.

The Charge Description Master (CDM) and Modifiers

Instructions: Fill in each blank with the best answer.

1. Modifiers such as left, right, and bilateral apply to paired _____ or _____ .

2. The _____ contains a list of every service and procedure that the provider offers, called line items, including the associated CPT or HCPCS code, a description of the service/procedure, and the current charge for the service /procedure.

3. _____ codes do not have specific descriptors, so modifiers do not apply.

4. _____ provides more information about a code's description.

5. _____ modifiers have two numbers.

6. _____ modifiers have two letters or a letter and a number.

BILLING, CODING, AND PAYMENT REGULATIONS FOR MODIFIERS

As you know, Medicare is one of the largest payers in the U.S., so it is very important to become familiar with the CMS regulations for coding, including how coding applies to billing and reimbursement. Many other insurances also follow CMS guidelines.

CMS has various regulations for coding with modifiers, and you will learn more about many of them in this chapter. You already learned about some CMS regulations in this text, including the National Correct Coding Initiative (NCCI) in Chapter 15. CMS has many different coding, billing, and payment regulations, including NCCI edits; or part of a National Coverage Determination (NCD); Medicare's national regulations; Local Coverage Determinations (LCDs) from Medicare Administrative Contractors (MACs); or other regulations. You will learn about many different CMS regulations in this chapter and throughout this text, but CMS regulations change frequently, so it is always best to research the most current regulations on the CMS website at www.cms.gov.

THE GLOBAL SURGICAL PACKAGE

An important part of understanding when to append specific modifiers is knowing which modifiers relate to a **global surgical package**. A global surgical package, which insurances created, represents a group, or package, of services that all relate to a *single surgery*. The insurance specifies a time frame, called the **global period**, during which the provider must render all of the services related to the surgery. The insurance will issue *one payment* to the provider to cover the multiple services that the provider renders during the global period, instead of issuing individual payments for each service.

CPT and Medicare

The CPT manual contains the CPT definition of a surgical package, which you can find in the Surgery section guidelines if you need to review additional information. The surgical package includes specific types of anesthesia, one related evaluation and management (E/M) encounter on the date immediately prior to or on the date of the procedure (including history and physical) after the decision is made for surgery, postoperative care, writing orders, an evaluation of the patient in the postanesthesia recovery area, and typical postoperative follow-up care.

The following services are included in Medicare's global surgical package (Medicare Claims Processing Manual, Chapter 12, publication #100-04): preoperative visits *after the decision is made to operate*, starting on the day *before* surgery for major procedures and the day *of surgery* for minor procedures (includes examination and workup to determine if the patient is healthy enough for surgery), intra-operative services (performing the surgical procedure), complications following surgery that do not require additional trips to the operating room, postoperative visits related to recovery from the surgery (including wound checks and overall health of the patient), postsurgical pain management, supplies, miscellaneous services (dressing changes; staples; lines; wires; tubes; drains; casts; splints; insertion, irrigation and removal of urinary catheters, routine peripheral intravenous lines, and nasogastric and rectal tubes; and changes and removal of tracheostomy tubes).

Physicians who perform the patient's surgery and render all of the usual pre- and postoperative services code and bill Medicare and other payers for the global package with one CPT code *for the surgical procedure only*. Insurances do not allow providers to bill individual services with individual charges for visits or other services that are included in the global package. Instead, providers should report code 99024 with *no charge* to show that the service was related to the surgery and was within the postoperative period (main term: *post-op visit*):

99024—Postoperative follow-up visit, normally included in the surgical package, to indicate that an evaluation and management service was performed during a postoperative period for a reason(s) related to the original procedure

Medicare classifies surgeries as major, with a 90-day postoperative period, or minor, with a 10-day postoperative period or a zero-day postoperative period. Other payers may or may not have the same postoperative periods for the same surgeries. It is best to check with individual payers for additional information on surgical package postoperative periods.

Specific modifiers relate to the global surgical package and give the insurance further information about procedures rendered during the global period. You will learn more about when to append modifiers related to the global surgical package later in this chapter.

Services Excluded from the Medicare Global Surgical Package

Medicare carriers *do not include* many different services in the global surgical package payment, and Medicare *may pay* for these services separately:

- The surgeon's initial consultation or evaluation of the patient's condition to determine the need for surgery. Please note that this policy only applies to *major surgical procedures*. The initial evaluation is *always included* in the allowance *for a minor* surgical procedure.
- Services of *other physicians*, except where the surgeon and the other physician(s) agree on the transfer of care.
- Visits that are *unrelated to the diagnosis for which the surgical procedure is performed*, unless the visits occur due to complications *of the surgery*.
- *Treatment for the underlying condition, or an added* course of treatment, which is *not part* of normal recovery from surgery.
- Diagnostic tests and procedures, including diagnostic radiological procedures.
- Clearly distinct surgical procedures during the postoperative period, which are not re-operations or treatment for complications. (A new postoperative period begins with the subsequent procedure.)
- Treatment for postoperative complications, which *requires a return trip to the operating room* (OR). An OR for this purpose is defined as a place of service that is specifically equipped and staffed for the sole purpose of performing procedures. Examples include a cardiac catheterization suite, a laser suite, and an endoscopy suite. An OR is *not* a patient's room, a minor treatment room, a recovery room, or an intensive care unit (unless the patient's condition was so critical that there would be insufficient time for transportation to an OR).
- If a less extensive procedure fails, and a more extensive procedure is required, then Medicare pays the second procedure separately.

- For certain services that are performed in a physician's office, separate payment can no longer be made for a surgical tray (code A4550). However, splints and casting supplies are separately payable.

- Immunosuppressive therapy for organ transplants.

- Critical care services (codes 99291 and 99292) that are *unrelated to the surgery* when a seriously injured or burned patient is critically ill and requires the physician's constant attendance.

TAKE A BREAK

Wow! That was a lot of information to remember! Let's take a break and then review more about insurance regulations and the global surgical package.

Exercise 18.2 Billing, Coding, and Payment Regulations for Modifiers; the Global Surgical Package

Instructions: On the line preceding each statement, write T for True or F for False.

1. _____ MACs create LCDs, and Medicare creates NCDs.

2. _____ The insurance will issue separate payment to the provider to cover multiple services that the provider renders during the global period.

3. _____ The CPT surgical package includes one visit on the date immediately prior to the procedure or on the date of the procedure.

4. _____ Medicare's global package includes all additional medical or surgical services that are required of the surgeon during the postoperative period after the surgery because of complications which do not require additional trips to the operating room.

5. _____ Providers should report CPT code 99024 when they need to charge for postoperative visits that are related to the initial surgery.

6. _____ Medicare will not pay for treatment for a return trip to the operating room for postoperative complications.

CPT MODIFIERS

You will next learn about specific CPT modifiers including their definitions, examples, Medicare regulations related to them, and practice exercises. Refer to Table 18-1 as a quick reference, and refer to Appendix A in your CPT manual to review each modifier's definition.

Modifier -22—Increased Procedural Services

Append modifier -22 to a surgical procedure code when the physician's work involved to perform the procedure is substantially greater than is typically required. The physician must document in the patient's medical record the reason(s) why the work that he performed exceeded the work that is normally required. These reasons may include

- increased intensity

- additional time

- technical difficulty of the procedure

- severity of the patient's condition, which causes greater surgical difficulty, danger to the patient, and additional physical and mental effort for the physician.

A procedure is not considered unusual if the physician decides to perform more complex surgery when simpler surgery would have been successful. Every procedure has an average range of difficulty. It may be *slightly* more or less difficult and still meet the criteria of the description of the procedure. Do not append modifier -22 to a surgical procedure code if you can instead assign an additional procedure code to capture the increased services. Here are some examples of patient circumstances that could warrant using modifier -22, including a patient who

- is morbidly obese, and the condition complicates surgery or causes the need for additional work and time to perform surgery.

- has comorbidities or anomalies, which create surgical complications and cause additional work or time to manage.

- suffers trauma that is serious enough to cause surgical complications.

- has other conditions, such as neoplasms, malformations, or scarring, that cause surgical complications or additional effort and/or time to manage.

- undergoes a procedure that is significantly more complex than the CPT code's descriptor, and there is no other CPT code to describe it.

- experiences excessive blood loss during the procedure.

- has conditions or comorbidities, which cause the surgeon to utilize a complex and/or difficult surgical approach.

- undergoes revisions or removals following prior surgery that are complex or difficult to perform.

Note: Modifier -22 applies to procedure codes in the surgery section. Do not append modifier -22 to procedure codes that are classified in the E/M, Anesthesia (use modifier -23—unusual anesthesia), Radiology, Pathology, or Medicine sections. Modifier -22 applies to both major procedures with a 90-day postoperative period and minor procedures with a 10-day postoperative period (or a zero day postoperative period).

Providers who submit claims to insurances for procedures with modifier -22 should also increase the procedure charge because the work that the provider performed was greater than usual. Providers also typically send medical documentation with the claim, including

1. A copy of the operative report where the physician documented why the procedure was unusual, including the amount of time and extra effort required to perform the procedure and any complications and risks.

2. A letter from the physician providing additional information about the patient's case to justify why the insurance should increase reimbursement, or a statement from the physician including this information documented within the operative report. Documentation should include the normal time, effort, and level of complexity required for the procedure compared to the extra time, effort, and complexity required for this patient's case.

3. Any other medical documentation that helps to support the unusual procedure, including lab test results.

   If the insurance agrees that the provider justifiably performed additional work and that appending modifier -22 was correct, then they will issue additional payment. The additional insurance reimbursement is approximately 25% more than the usual payment for the procedure, but insurances could pay more or less, depending on individual payer policies. Insurances could also manually review the claim and ask the provider additional questions or request more information before processing it.

   Be careful when you append modifier -22 because you should not append it if the procedure is only *slightly* more difficult, or if the surgeon took only *a few extra minutes* on the patient's case. Append modifier -22 when it is clear in the medical documentation that the surgeon performed work and/or took time that was above and beyond what is normally required for the procedure. When in doubt, always query the physician for clarification.

Modifier -23—Unusual Anesthesia

Occasionally, because of unusual circumstances, a procedure which usually requires *local, regional, or no anesthesia* must be done under *general anesthesia*. When this occurs, append modifier -23 to the procedure code of the basic service for the anesthesia. Refer to the anesthesia definitions listed next, which will help you to better understand this situation:

Local and regional anesthesia—An anesthetic drug that prevents patients from experiencing pain in a specific body site; regional anesthesia affects a larger body site than local anesthesia. Under local and regional anesthesia, the patient remains awake and can communicate with the physician and also remember circumstances of the procedure. Examples of procedures requiring local or regional anesthesia include skin or tissue biopsies; cesarean section childbirth; procedures that are performed on the arms, legs, hands, feet, urinary tract, or sexual organs; and some types of cosmetic surgery.

General anesthesia—An anesthetic drug which prevents patients from experiencing pain from major surgical procedures. The patient's entire body, including the brain, is anesthetized. The patient is unconscious, cannot communicate with the physician, and remembers nothing about the surgery. Examples of procedures requiring general anesthesia include major orthopedic procedures, like a knee replacement; various general surgeries; cardiac surgery; neurosurgery; and pediatric surgery.

You may wonder why a patient would need general anesthesia for a procedure that normally requires local, regional, or no anesthesia. Refer to the following examples:

- A patient needs to undergo various dental procedures and fears being awake during the procedures.
- A mentally ill patient is physically abusive to clinicians in the operating room.
- A child is uncooperative during a procedure.
- A trauma patient will not stop yelling and swinging his arms and legs when physicians try to repair his skin lacerations.

Providers who bill procedures with unusual anesthesia must also include supporting documentation with the insurance claim, including reasons why the patient required general anesthesia. You will learn more about the specialty of anesthesia in Chapter 20 of this text.

Modifier -24—Unrelated Evaluation and Management (E/M) Service by the Same Physician During a Postoperative Period

Append modifier -24 to an evaluation and management service when the physician performs an E/M service during the patient's global surgery period (postoperative), but the service is unrelated to the patient's surgery. Recall that providers report code 99024 for postoperative visits that are related to the original surgery's global period. Code 99024 has no associated charge, and the insurance does not pay for it separately because the insurance makes *one payment* for all services related to a surgery, including preoperative, intra-operative, and postoperative care. However, when the patient visits the surgeon within the global period for a reason that is *unrelated to the surgery*, you have to append modifier -24 to the evaluation and management code so that the insurance knows that the service is *unrelated to the original surgery* and will then process the claim for payment. The patient's diagnosis for the unrelated service must also justify the visit.

If the patient has a postoperative visit to the surgeon and the surgeon also assesses the patient for *another reason*, then assign both the no-charge code of 99024 and the E/M visit for the other reason, appending modifier -24.

General Ophthalmological Services, codes 92002–92014, are also considered evaluation and management services, even though they are located in the Medicine section, and you can also append modifier -24 to these codes.

Modifier -25—Significant, Separately Identifiable Evaluation and Management Service by the Same Physician on the Same Day of the Procedure or Other Service

A patient can receive more than one type of service from the same provider on the same day, including an E/M service, along with another service or procedure. When the physician performs a procedure for the same patient on the same day as a separate E/M service, you can code and bill for *both* the procedure and the E/M service. Append modifier -25 to the E/M service to show the insurance that the E/M was separate from the other procedure.

The provider's medical documentation must justify performing the separate E/M service. The patient's symptom or condition may cause the provider to perform a separate E/M service.

A provider may also perform two E/M services for the same patient on the same day. If this situation occurs, then append modifier -25 to the *second* E/M service to show that it was a separate and distinct service from the first E/M.

Review these additional Medicare guidelines when appending modifier -25:

- Medicare carriers pay for an E/M service that is provided on the day of a procedure with a global fee period if the physician indicates that the service is for a significant, separately identifiable E/M service that is above and beyond the usual pre- and post-operative work of the procedure.

- Different diagnoses are not required for reporting the E/M service on the same date as the procedure or other service.

- The provider must appropriately and completely document both the medically necessary E/M service and the procedure to support the claim for the services, even though the provider does not need to submit supporting documentation with the claim unless the Medicare carrier requests it.

Append modifier -25 to the E/M service when the physician decides to perform a minor surgery on the same day. For major surgeries, see modifier -57.

Modifier -26—Professional Component

A *professional component* is the part of a service that represents the work that the physician performs, including supervision and interpretation of a service, such as interpreting a test result. In order to better understand the professional component, you must first understand that specific services can be one of three types:

1. **Professional component**—The professional component represents the physician's work involved in a service and can include the supervision and interpretation of the service (also called S and I), such as interpreting a radiology test. Services with both

POINTERS FROM THE PROS: Interview with a Billing and Coding Specialist

Tammy Trombetta has worked for a physician group practice for the past seven years. She bills insurance claims electronically for four doctors and a nurse practitioner. This includes patients seen in the office, in nursing homes, at the hospital, and at home. The clinicians assign procedure codes to the services that they render, and Ms. Trombetta assigns ICD-9-CM codes.

Please give an example of a time when you educated a physician on processes of coding or any other procedures, and the outcome.

The most basic example, which occurs often with internal medicine physicians, is suture/staple removal. Our physicians were simply using the suture removal code which (insurances) paid $10, at best. If the patient's vitals are taken, along with a brief medical review, a low-level 99212 can be used, and insurances typically pay $54.

What advice would you like to give to coding students about working with different personalities?

I have always approached my work with the goal of learning something new every day. I frequently train extern students in billing/coding as part of their education requirements. Some are interested, some not . . . some have good work ethics, some don't . . . some have an interest in learning; some are taking up space . . . but even the laziest students have taught me a new approach or short-cut. So even when our personalities might not work well together, I remain patient and open-minded to learning from them.

What advice would you like to give to coding students to help them prepare to work successfully in the healthcare field?

An eye for detail is helpful. Keeping updated yearly with new codes or deleted (codes), proper use of modifiers, and use of specified codes (vs. diagnostic codes ending in .9 that are unspecified) can mean a higher reimbursement for your physicians. This, in turn, can result in bonus or salary compensation for the employee.

(Used by permission of Tammy Trombetta.)

a professional and technical component can be specific radiology services and some services in other sections of CPT, including Medicine. Append modifier -26 to the procedure code to show the professional component.

2. **Technical component**—The technical component of a service is separate from the professional component and represents the use of the room to perform the service, as well as equipment, supplies, and staff, like a technician, for services performed at hospitals or other facilities where the physician who performed the professional component of the same service is not an employee of the facility or hospital. Append modifier -TC (technical component) to the procedure code to show the technical component.

3. **Global service**—When a service is global, it means that *both* the professional and technical components were performed in one provider location, which codes and bills for the service. Do not append a modifier to the procedure code of a global service. (A global service is unrelated to a global surgery period.)

Review the following example to better understand professional and technical components.

> **Example:** Dr. Stuart, an orthopedic surgeon, sees a new patient in his office, Mr. Nielson, a 58-year-old, for possible rib fractures. Dr. Stuart conducts an examination and writes an order for a bilateral X-ray of the ribs, posteroanterior chest, four views.
>
> The patient brings the X-ray order to Brandyburg Radiology, an outpatient radiology clinic. The X-ray technician takes the X-ray and sends it to Dr. Stuart to review and interpret. Dr. Stuart then determines that the patient has multiple rib fractures involving two ribs. The X-ray is a service with both a professional component (reading and interpreting), and a technical component (equipment, supplies, technician, and room).
>
> - Dr. Stuart's coder assigns code 71111 for the X-ray of bilateral ribs and appends modifier -26 to show the insurance that Dr. Stuart performed the *professional component* of the service, 71111-26.
> - The coder at Brandyburg Radiology also assigns code 71111 for the X-ray of bilateral ribs and appends modifier -TC to show the insurance that the clinic performed the *technical component* of the service, 71111-TC.
> - The insurance then sends payment to Dr. Stuart for reading and interpreting the X-ray (professional component) and also sends a separate payment to Brandyburg Radiology for the use of their room, equipment, supplies, and technician to perform the X-ray (technical component).
> - The insurance pays each provider a separate amount for the X-ray because each provider rendered a separate part of the service that has both a professional and technical component.

Some CPT codes already contain the professional component for supervision and interpretation as part of their descriptors. When this occurs, you *do not* need to append modifier -26 to the CPT code because the service is already a professional service. Refer to the following examples:

cisternography (sis-tər-ˈnäg-rə-fē)—radiography of the brain's basal cisterns (spaces)

70015—**Cisternography**, positive contrast, radiological supervision and interpretation

70170—**Dacryocystography, nasolacrimal** duct, radiological supervision and interpretation

dacryocystography (daˈ-crēo-sis-täg-rə-fē)—radiography of the lacrimal sacs

70170—**Dacryocystography, nasolacrimal** duct, radiological supervision and interpretation

nasolacrimal (nāzo-lakˈ-rə-məl)—pertaining to the lacrimal (tear) duct and the nose

Coding and Billing a Global Service   If one provider codes and bills for *both* the professional component and technical component of a service, then it means that the same provider performed both the professional and technical components, typically at one location. When you are coding a global service, do not append any modifier to the

CPT code. Without a modifier, the insurance knows that the procedure is a global procedure that includes *both* a professional and technical component. The insurance issues one payment for *both components* of the service because the provider rendered a global service.

In the example of Mr. Nielsen's rib X-ray, if neither provider appended a modifier to the procedure code for the X-ray, then the insurance would pay the first claim it received as a global service and would most likely deny the second claim as a duplicate service.

Hospitals and the Technical Component   An important point to remember is that when a hospital renders the technical component of a service, do not assign modifier -TC to the procedure code because it is *understood* that the hospital provides the technical component of specific services, including the use of rooms, equipment, and supplies. Physicians will code and bill for the professional component of services that they render in hospitals, and hospitals will code and bill for the technical component.

The hospital component, also called a technical component, represents the following hospital resources used during a procedure:

- hospital staff, including nurses, surgical technicians, nurses' aides, and ancillary (assisting) hospital staff
- space, equipment, and supplies, such as operating rooms; surgical instruments; X-ray, MRI, and CT equipment; surgical supplies; and linens
- overhead, including utilities and operating expenses.

Just because a physician performs a procedure at a hospital does not mean that the hospital codes the procedure and bills the patient's insurance for *both* the physician and hospital components of the service. Some physicians do not work *for* a hospital but work *within* a hospital. Many physicians own their own practice or are employees of or own a group practice. The hospital does not employ them. This means that the physician's practice staff codes the professional component of a service and bills the patient's insurance for the professional service (on a CMS-1500 claim form). The hospital's staff codes the technical component and bills the patient's insurance for resources that the hospital used during the same procedure (on a UB-04 claim form).

Physicians want to be paid for the work they perform for the procedure, and hospitals want to be paid for the use of their resources during the procedure. Insurances process two different claims for the same service: a CMS-1500 for the physician component, and the UB-04 for the hospital component.

Now that you understand that some services have both a professional component and technical component (typically radiology services and other specific laboratory, medicine, and surgical services within the CPT code set), it is important to also understand that many other services *do not* have both a professional and technical component. When physicians perform most services in an outpatient or inpatient hospital, physicians still bill insurances separately from the hospitals. Physicians' staff code and bill insurances for procedures and services that physicians perform at the hospitals, and hospitals' staff code and bill insurances for using their facility, including assigning Volume 3 inpatient procedure codes.

cholecystectomy
(kō-lə-sis-tek′-tə-mē)
cholelithiasis (kō-li-lith-′ī- ə-səs)

TAKE A BREAK

Great job! You have done well. Let's take a break and then practice coding with modifiers and assigning diagnosis codes.

Exercise 18.3   Modifiers -22, -23, -24, -25, -26

Instructions: Review each patient's case, answer questions about the case, and assign codes for the procedure(s), appending a modifier when appropriate. Optional: For additional practice, assign diagnosis(es) codes.

Case 1

At Williton Medical Center, Dr. Valencia, a gastroenterologist, performs a **cholecystectomy** (gall bladder removal) on Mr. Bird, a 56-year-old, 330-lb. patient. Mr. Bird suffers from **cholelithiasis** (gall stones) (■ FIGURE 18-2). He previously underwent abdominal surgery, developing adhesions in his upper abdomen. The adhesions made it

continued

TAKE A BREAK *continued*

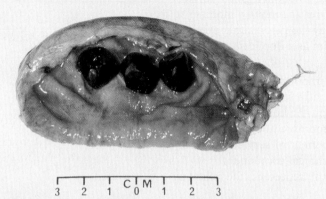

Figure 18-2 ■ Excised gall bladder with three gall stones (black). Gall stones are hard masses composed of cholesterol, bile, and calcium salts that form when the chemical composition of bile changes.

Photo credit: © SPL / Photo Researchers, Inc.

extremely difficult for Dr. Valencia to remove the patient's gallbladder because it adhered to the liver. The amount of time that Dr. Valencia spent in surgery was *nearly double* the amount of time needed under normal circumstances.

1. What procedure code and modifier should you assign to Mr. Bird's cholecystectomy? _____

2. What diagnosis code should you assign for cholelithiasis? _____

Case 2

At Williton Medical Center, Dr. Lindsay, an ophthalmologist, performs an endothelial corneal transplant from a cadaver donor for Mr. Downs, a 48-year-old patient. Mr. Downs suffers from severe corneal edema from an old corneal injury, and he insists before surgery that he wants to be asleep because surgeries make him very nervous. The patient's procedure normally requires local anesthesia. Dr. Kirkland, the anesthesiologist (a physician specializing in anesthesia care), oversees the patient's case, administers general anesthesia, and monitors Mr. Downs' progress throughout the surgery.

1. What procedure code should you assign for the corneal transplant? _____

2. What procedure code and modifier should you assign for the anesthesia? _____

3. What is the diagnosis code(s) for the patient's condition? _____

Case 3

Dr. Valencia sees Mr. Bird for a postoperative visit to check wound healing and overall health, conducted during the global period for his cholecystectomy. Mr. Bird

states that he is constipated, and Dr. Valencia explains that it is a common side effect of his surgery. He advises Mr. Bird to drink more water and reiterates the diet that he should follow.

Mr. Bird then discusses a new problem that is unrelated to his surgery. He states that lately, he has been feeling nauseated after drinking milk or eating cheese. After further examination and assessment, Dr. Valencia diagnoses the patient with lactose intolerance and prescribes Lactaid® to help him digest lactose. Dr. Valencia documents that the E/M office visit regarding the lactose intolerance included a problem-focused history, problem-focused examination, and straightforward medical decision making.

1. What no-charge procedure code should you assign to Mr. Bird's postoperative visit to check his wound and overall health? _____

2. What procedure code and modifier should you assign to Mr. Bird's E/M office visit (established patient) where Dr. Valencia addressed the lactose intolerance? _____

3. What diagnosis code should you assign for lactose intolerance? _____

Case 4

Dr. Daniels sees Mrs. Slater, a 72-year-old, in the emergency department at Williton Medical Center. Dr. Daniels performs an intermediate 20-cm laceration repair to the skin of the scalp. The patient suffered the scalp wound when she fell down the front steps of her home. When Dr. Daniels questions the patient, she seems to be confused, so he admits her to observation (an E/M service) and orders additional tests. The observation service includes a detailed history, detailed examination, and straightforward medical decision making.

1. What procedure code should you assign for the laceration repair? _____

2. What initial observation code and modifier should you assign to show that this E/M service was separate from the laceration repair? _____

3. What diagnosis code would you assign for the scalp wound? _____

4. What diagnosis code would you assign for the confusion? _____

5. What E code(s) should you assign to the patient's case? _____

TAKE A BREAK *continued*

Case 5:

Dr. Stuart sees Mrs. Mooney, an 82-year-old new patient, for possible hip fractures from a fall in her bedroom. The patient's daughter accompanies her to the appointment. Dr. Stuart conducts an examination and orders a bilateral hip X-ray, with two views of each hip, and an anteroposterior view of the pelvis.

The patient brings the X-ray order to Brandyburg Radiology, where the X-ray technician takes the X-ray and sends it to Dr. Stuart to review and interpret. Dr. Stuart then determines that the patient suffers from bilateral pelvic fractures with disruption of the pelvic circle.

1. What procedure code and modifier should you assign for Dr. Stuart's professional services? _____

2. What procedure code and modifier should you assign for Brandyburg Radiology's technical services? _____

3. What is the diagnosis code for the patient's condition? _____

4. If a hospital took the patient's X-ray and sent it to Dr. Stuart to review and interpret, what procedure code would you assign for the hospital's service? _____

5. Would you also assign a modifier? _____ Why or why not? _____

Modifier -32—Mandated Services

Mandated services are services or consultations that a third party requires for the patient, including an insurance company, federal or state government, or other regulatory agency. For example, a worker's compensation or disability insurance may dispute a patient's claim that he is ill or dispute his cause of an injury, and may request a second opinion to determine the patient's condition.

Append modifier -32 to codes for procedures or services that a third party mandates for the patient, and bill the third party that mandated the service. Because a third party mandates the service, providers expect to be paid the full amount of charges billed. *Do not* append modifier -32 to services or procedures that a physician, other clinician, patient, or patient's family requests, because these are not mandated services.

Consultations as Mandated Services Typically, mandated services include consultations. *Consultations* occur when a physician, other clinician, or third party (such as an insurance company) requests that a physician examine and assess a patient to provide an opinion about the patient's condition. It could be a second opinion if the patient already saw another provider for the same condition. Not all consultations involve second opinions.

A consultation is an E/M service that a physician provides to examine and assess a patient and possibly assume continued care for the patient, depending on the situation. A physician consultant may also provide or order additional diagnostic and/or therapeutic services during the consultation or during a subsequent visit.

The party requesting the consultation, like an insurance company, should document the written or verbal request for the consultation, and the consulting physician should also document it. After the consultation, the consulting physician must document the results in the patient's record, including further tests and treatment, and send a written report with his findings to the party who requested the consultation.

If a third party, such as an insurance company, mandates the consultation, then append modifier -32 to the evaluation and management consultation code. Do not assign a consultation procedure code and append modifier -32 for a service that the patient or patient's family requests. Instead, assign a code for an E/M office visit, home service, or domiciliary/rest home care, as appropriate, and do not append modifier -32.

Modifier -33—Preventive Service

A preventive service is designed to identify an illness as early as possible so that the patient can receive treatment, such as identifying, or screening, patients for hypertension, breast cancer, or cervical cancer. The U.S. Preventive Services Task Force (USPSTF) is a panel of healthcare experts, including providers, that reviews many types of care to determine whether it is preventive. The task force created a list of preventive services and assigned each an A or B rating, depending on how much a preventive service will benefit the patient, including whether it is a substantial benefit or moderately substantial benefit. When providers code these services, they can append modifier -33 to show the insurance that the service was preventive and should be paid. Under the Patient Protection and Affordable Care Act of 2010, in-network insurances must cover specific preventive services in full, without passing any of the cost on to the patient. Modifier -33 appended to the procedure code identifies these services. You can review the services that are rated with an A or B at www.healthcare.gov. Note that you do not need to append modifier -33 to services that are inherently *screening* services, such as a screening mammogram, where the CPT code descriptor already includes the word "screening." Medicare and other payers do not recognize modifier -33 and will not reimburse services that include modifier -33. It is best to check with individual payers for specific coverage.

Modifier -47—Anesthesia by Surgeon

Recall that an anesthesiologist or Certified Registered Nurse Anesthetist (CRNA) can administer anesthesia to a patient, while a surgeon performs the procedure. Sometimes a surgeon performs the procedure *and* administers the anesthesia without an anesthesiologist or CRNA. An example is an obstetrician who administers regional anesthesia (such as an **epidural** to relieve pain) to a patient in labor.

epidural (ep-ĭ-doo′rəl)— outside the dura mater, the tough outer layer of the membranes over the brain and spinal cord

Modifier -47 applies only to cases when the surgeon performs the surgery and administers regional or general anesthesia. Modifier -47 does not include local anesthesia. When the surgeon performs surgery and administers regional or general anesthesia, assign codes for the procedure to report on the insurance claim. Assign a code for the procedure, assign the code for the procedure again, and append modifier -47 to the second code to show that the surgeon also administered the anesthesia. The insurance will process the claim for the procedure itself and for the anesthesia the surgeon administered during the procedure. *Note:* Do not append modifier -47 to anesthesia procedure codes.

Some insurances will not pay separately for anesthesia when the surgeon administers it. Insurances that reimburse surgeons for anesthesia services base their payments on the amount of time that the surgeon spent administering and monitoring the patient on anesthesia.

Modifier -50—Bilateral Procedure

When a procedure is bilateral, or performed on both sides, it means that the physician performed the procedure on paired organs (lungs, kidneys) or paired body structures (ears, eyes, extremities). Append modifier -50 to the diagnostic, radiology, or surgical procedure code when the physician performed the procedure bilaterally during the same operative session.

Modifier -50 eliminates the need to code the same procedure twice, once with the -LT modifier for the left side and again with the -RT modifier for the right side. Appending modifier -50 means assigning one procedure code. Assign modifiers -LT or -RT for one procedure that is performed on *either* the left or right side of the body.

vasotomy (vā-zät′-ə-mē)— incision of the vas deferens, the duct that carries sperm

cannulization (kanu-l-za′shn)—inserting a tube into a space

fontanelle (fon-tə-nel′)—a soft area between two bones, covered by membrane

Some CPT codes already contain the word *bilateral* in their descriptors, so do not append modifier -50 to these codes because the procedures are *already bilateral*. Other code descriptors contain the words *unilateral or bilateral*, so the procedures can either be performed on one side *or* both sides. Do not append modifier -50 to these procedures because they are *already bilateral* or unilateral. Examples of procedures that do not need modifier -50 include:

27158—Osteotomy, pelvis, bilateral (e.g., congenital malformation)

55200—Vasotomy, cannulization with or without incision of vas, unilateral or bilateral (separate procedure)

61000—Subdural tap through **fontanelle**, or suture, infant, unilateral or bilateral; initial

Insurance Reimbursement for Bilateral Procedures   Insurances, including Medicare, typically reimburse providers *more* for bilateral procedures because the physician performed more work than described for the CPT code. For specific bilateral procedures, Medicare pays either 150% of the Medicare Physician Fee Schedule (MPFS) amount (one side is reimbursed at 100% and the other side is reimbursed at 50%) *or* the provider's charge, whichever is less. For other bilateral procedures, Medicare pays either 100% of the MPFS amount for each side of the body or the provider's charge, whichever is less.

Medicare recognizes three different types of bilateral procedures:

1. Conditional bilateral—a procedure with a descriptor that does *not* contain the word *bilateral* or the phrase *unilateral or bilateral*. The procedure is considered bilateral if modifier -50 is appended to it.

2. Inherent bilateral—a procedure with a descriptor that contains the word *bilateral* or the phrase *unilateral or bilateral*. Modifier -50 is unnecessary.

3. Independent bilateral—a procedure with a descriptor that does *not* contain the word *bilateral* or the phrase *unilateral or bilateral*. The procedure is considered bilateral if modifier -50 is appended to it.

Billing Bilateral Procedures to Insurances   Recall that as *a* coder, you typically *also* do not bill insurances unless you work for a small provider. Larger providers have coders who perform diagnosis and procedure coding and billers who bill claims to insurances. However, both coders and billers must communicate regularly to discuss claims that are denied because of incorrect or invalid codes or changes to insurance regulations that affect how providers code and bill claims. When you append modifier -50 to a procedure code, it means that one bilateral procedure will be billed to the insurance company on the CMS-1500 claim form unless the insurance has special requirements.

Some insurances require special coding and billing for a bilateral procedure on the CMS-1500 claim form, and the Charge Description Master (CDM) in the practice management software can be programmed to perform this task to bill the insurance correctly. For example, XYZ Insurance requires that providers submit bilateral procedures with two codes, one code without modifier -50 and the same code with modifier -50. As the coder, you can code the procedure only once and append modifier -50. The CDM can be programmed to recognize that the patient has XYZ Insurance and will then split the procedure that you coded into two procedures on the claim form, appending modifier -50 to the second procedure. Refer to the following example:

Example: A female patient has a bilateral breast **mastectomy** (■ FIGURE 18-3). Assign code 19305, and append modifier -50 to show that the procedure was bilateral. Enter the code and modifier into the practice management software.

mastectomy (ma-stek'-tə-mē)—partial or total breast removal

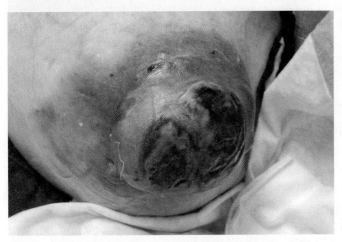 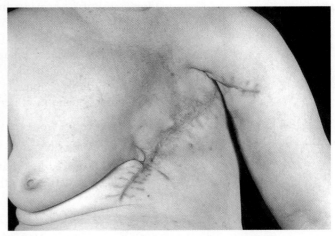

Figure 18-3 ■ (A) Infected, fungating stage IV left breast malignancy. (B) The patient after a left breast mastectomy to remove a fungating malignancy.

Photo credits: (A) © Medical-on-Line / Alamy; (B) Slaven/Custom Medical Stock Photo.

The patient has XYZ Insurance. The software recognizes that when a procedure code with modifier -50 is entered on a patient's account with XYZ Insurance, it should bill the insurance this way:

19305

19305-50

You only had to assign one code with modifier -50, and the software's CDM performed the rest of the work, adding another line item with the same procedure code. This process is called a *charge line item explode,* when you enter one procedure into the software, and the CDM "explodes" the procedure into multiple procedures, based on the insurance's billing requirements.

Both you and the insurance billing staff will need to determine which insurances require special billing for bilateral procedures and then program the CDM to explode the line item, or work with an information technology (IT) professional who can program the CDM.

Programming the CDM to explode line items saves you from having to remember various insurance's billing specifications for bilateral procedures every time you code, and it saves you from performing double work.

Some insurances do not recognize modifier -50 and may require that instead of billing one procedure code with modifier -50, you instead must bill the procedure code twice, once with modifier -LT and once with modifier -RT. Depending on the type of software that the provider has, the CDM may also be able to be programmed to explode one procedure with modifier -50 into two procedure codes with modifiers -LT and -RT and only bill those two line items to the specific insurance that requires it. This way, you, as the coder, enter the procedure code with modifier -50, and the software correctly bills it to the insurance as two line items, one with the code and modifier -LT, and the other with the code and modifier -RT.

Modifier -51—Multiple Procedures

Append modifier -51 when the same provider performs multiple procedures for the same patient during the same encounter or session. Append modifier -51 to all procedure codes except to the first one reported. The purpose of modifier -51 is to notify the insurance that the patient had multiple procedures done, because the insurance will reduce payment on all procedures after the first one. Insurances typically reimburse the first procedure at a higher rate than subsequent procedures because subsequent procedures require less time, effort, and cost to provide during the same session.

You can use modifier -51 along with other modifiers, except for modifier -50 (bilateral procedure). Modifier -51 does not apply to E/M services, physical medicine and rehabilitation services, or supplies (such as vaccines). Do not confuse modifier -51 with modifier -59, which should be used for a distinct procedural service, which you will learn about later in this chapter.

Do not append modifier -51 to

- add-on codes (codes with a + symbol in front of them),
- modifier -51 exempt codes (codes with a $\oslash$ symbol in front of them), or
- bilateral procedures that require modifier -50, because insurances already know to reduce payment, since the physician performed two procedures.

Types of Multiple Procedures A physician can perform different types of multiple procedures on the *same patient* during the *same encounter* or *session*, as shown in the following examples:

1. The physician performs the *same procedure* on *different anatomic sites:*

   12034—Intermediate repair of wounds of the *scalp*, 8.0 cm

   12041—Intermediate repair of wounds of the *neck*, 2.0 cm

2. The physician performs *different related procedures* on *the same anatomic site:*

   11606—Excision, malignant lesion, trunk, excised diameter over 4 cm

   12032—Intermediate repair (layer closure) of wounds of trunk, 5.0 cm

3. The physician performs the *same procedure* on the *same anatomic site, multiple times*:

   28080—Arthrotomy, with exploration, drainage, or removal of loose or foreign body; interphalangeal joint, *each*

   28080—Arthrotomy, with exploration, drainage, or removal of loose or foreign body; interphalangeal joint, *each*

For example, the physician performs the procedure on *three* interphalangeal joints. Report code 28080 three times, appending modifier -51 to the second and third procedure, or report it once and add *x 3* to show three interphalangeal joints:

28080, 28080-51, 28080-51 *or*

28080 *x* 3

Insurances may request that you report modifier -51 with the second and third procedures or report the procedure code *x 3* units. Other insurances may instead request the HCPCS modifier for the anatomic site (refer to Table 18-2), so you will need to check with individual payers to determine how to report and bill multiple procedures. Again, many software CDMs can be programmed to bill line items a specific way to specific insurances.

Ranking Multiple Procedures for Coding and Billing   When you code multiple procedures for the same patient, from the same provider, during the same encounter, you not only have to understand when to append modifier -51, but you also have to place the procedure codes in the correct order to bill the insurance on the CMS-1500 form. Insurances, including Medicare, process different payments for claims with multiple procedures. Medicare pays the first procedure reported at 100% of the Medicare Fee Schedule (MFS) amount or the provider's charge, whichever is less. For each subsequent procedure, Medicare then pays 50% of the MFS amount or the provider's charge, whichever is less.

Medicare will only pay for five procedures for the same patient on the same day with the same provider. If the provider's claim includes six or more procedures, then Medicare will suspend payment on the sixth and subsequent procedures. Medicare will then conduct a manual review of the procedures (reviewed by a person) and possibly request that the provider submit medical documentation to justify the services. Then Medicare will determine whether to pay for the sixth and subsequent procedures.

Keep in mind that *not all* procedures are subject to a payment reduction. It just depends on the procedure. Many insurances follow the same multiple procedure payment guidelines as Medicare, and other insurances follow different guidelines, reducing the third procedure's payment to less than the second procedure. Some insurances also do not require you to append modifier -51 to multiple procedures. They can process the claim with multiple procedures without modifier -51. It is best to check with individual payers to determine their coding guidelines for multiple procedures.

So how do you know what order to report multiple procedures that you code? You always have to report the procedure with the highest charge first, because the insurance will pay more for the first procedure reported. Then list remaining procedures in descending charge order to ensure that the lower reimbursement will apply to the lower charges. It is important for healthcare providers to regularly update their charges in their software's CDM to ensure correct reimbursement. If a provider's charge is *less than* the MFS amount, or any other payer's fee schedule amount, then the provider only receives payment for the procedure which is equal to their charge, instead of receiving higher reimbursement, because the MFS amount would have been more.

TAKE A BREAK

You are doing great! Let's take a break and then practice coding with more modifiers and assigning diagnosis codes.

Exercise 18.4   Modifiers -32, -33, -47, -50, -51

Instructions: Review each patient's case, answer questions about the case, and assign codes for the procedure(s), appending a modifier when appropriate. Optional: For additional practice, assign diagnosis(es) codes.

Case 1

Dr. Reilly, an orthopedic spinal surgeon, sees Mr. Donovan, a 36-year-old, in his office for a mandated consultation. Mr. Donovan's worker's compensation insurance company requested the consultation for a second opinion related to Mr. Donovan's symptoms of lower back pain and numbness in his legs. Dr. Reilly conducts a full examination and various assessments. The consultation includes a comprehensive history, comprehensive examination, and high-complexity medical decision making. Dr. Reilly diagnoses the patient with lumbar **radiculopathy** and sends a written report of his findings to the worker's compensation insurance.

1. What procedure code and modifier should you assign for the patient's consultation? _____

2. What is the diagnosis code for the patient's condition? _____

Case 2

Sandra Shelton, age 40, has a bilateral screening mammogram for breast cancer, which her insurance covers as a preventive service. The mammogram does not show any evidence of abnormalities.

1. What procedure code and modifier should you assign for the patient's service? _____

2. What is the diagnosis code for the patient's condition? _____

Case 3

Dr. Wooten, an obstetrician/gynecologist, administers an epidural to Mrs. Mayer, a 28-year-old patient, during labor at Williton Medical Center. Mrs. Mayer then vaginally delivers baby John, a full-term infant. Neither Mrs. Mayer nor baby John experience complications. Dr. Wooten oversees the vaginal delivery and provides postpartum care.

1. What procedure code should you assign for the vaginal delivery and postpartum care? _____

2. What procedure code and modifier should you assign for the anesthesia that Dr. Wooten administered during the patient's procedure? _____

3. What diagnosis code(s) should you assign to Mrs. Mayer's chart for her normal delivery? _____

4. What diagnosis code(s) should you assign to baby John's chart? _____

Case 4

Dr. Fitzpatrick, an ophthalmologist, performs a bilateral upper eyelid blepharoplasty on Mrs. Guy, a 61-year-old, to improve her vision. Mrs. Guy suffers from ptosis of her upper eyelids. Her insurance requires that the provider bill her procedure as one line item on the 1500 form with the correct modifier for both eyelids appended to the procedure code.

1. What procedure code and modifier should you assign for the bilateral blepharoplasty? _____

2. What diagnosis code should you assign to Mrs. Guy's chart? _____

Case 5

Dr. Hoffman, a family practitioner, sees Jonathan Fry, an 8-year-old established patient, for multiple facial skin lacerations and an external ear laceration that he suffered after falling at the neighborhood playground. Dr. Hoffman performs a simple repair of a 6.2-cm facial wound ($25), a simple repair of a 3.2-cm wound of the right ear ($15), and an intermediate repair of a 5.3-cm wound of the face ($40).

1. Assign procedure codes to the three procedures that Jonathan had. Include modifier-51 where applicable. Rank the procedures in the correct order to bill the insurance.

_____

2. What diagnosis code(s) should you assign to Jonathan's chart? Include any applicable E code(s). _____

_____

radiculopathy (rə -dic- u-läp′- ə-thē)—disorder of the nerves

Modifier -52—Reduced Services

Sometimes a physician does not perform the full procedure outlined in the CPT code descriptor, and there is not another CPT code to describe the *reduced*, or lesser, procedure. When this situation occurs, append modifier -52 to the procedure code to show *reduced services*. Refer to the following examples of reduced services:

DESTINATION: MEDICARE

This Medicare exercise will help you to better understand Medicare's National Correct Coding Initiative (NCCI). Follow the instructions listed next to access an educational document called How to Use the National Correct Coding Initiative (NCCI) Tools:

1. Go to the website http://www.cms.gov.
2. At the top of the screen on the banner bar, choose *Medicare.*
3. Scroll down to *Coding,* and choose *National Correct Coding Initiative Edits.*
4. Scroll down to downloads, and choose *How to Use the National Correct Coding Initiative (NCCI) Tools.*

Review the document to answer the following questions:

1. What is the difference between NCCI code pair edits and MUEs?
2. Explain the difference between codes in Column 1 and codes in Column 2 of the code pair edit tables.
3. In the code pair edit tables, which modifier indicator in the modifier indicator table column is allowed with a specific code pair?

- **58200**—Total abdominal **hysterectomy**, including partial **vaginectomy**, with para-aortic and pelvic lymph node sampling, with or without removal of tube(s), with or without removal of ovary(s).

    The physician performed the components of the procedure to treat a patient's cancer, *except for* a partial vaginectomy, because the patient did not have cancer of the vagina. Append modifier -52 to the procedure code because there is not another CPT code to describe the reduced services: 58200-52.

- **92551**—Screening test, pure tone, air only

    The CPT guidelines for this **audiologic** service state that the code descriptor applies to *both* ears. The physician only performed the test on *one ear* because the patient is deaf in the other ear. Append modifier -52 to the procedure code because there is not another CPT code to describe the reduced service: 92551-52.

- **99173**—Screening test of visual acuity, quantitative, bilateral

    The descriptor for code 99173 states *bilateral.* The physician only performed the test on one eye because the patient is blind in the other eye. Append modifier -52 to the procedure code because there is not another CPT code to describe the reduced service: 99173-52.

hysterectomy (histr-ek't-me)—surgical removal of the uterus

vaginectomy (vaj-ĭ-nek'tə-me)—surgical removal of the vagina

audiologic (aw-de-ol'ə-jik)—pertaining to hearing

Modifier -52 may also apply to a partially completed procedure that the physician terminated and replaced with another procedure. For example, a physician begins a procedure, completes part of it, but then stops it because he determines that he will not succeed, based on his additional findings during the procedure. Instead, he decides to complete a *different procedure*, which is successful. Append modifier -52 to the partially completed procedure, and code the second procedure without a modifier.

For any reduced procedure, the physician should document in the patient's record the reason(s) why the procedure was reduced, and the provider should submit supporting medical documentation with the claim to the insurance.

Do not append modifier -52 to E/M codes or to codes that are time-based, outlining a specific amount of time included for the procedure. If the physician reduces time-based services, then code them with an unlisted procedure code, and submit medical documentation with the claim to show the payer the reason(s) for reduced services.

Many insurances reduce payments for procedures with modifier -52, so providers should bill reduced services to insurances for their total charges. Providers should not reduce charges because insurances will then reduce payment on the reduced charge. Not all insurances will pay less for reduced services. It depends on each individual case and how far the physician progressed with the procedure.

Note: For hospital outpatient procedures that were partially reduced or cancelled prior to or after anesthesia administration, see modifiers -73 or -74.

Modifier -53—Discontinued Procedure

Append modifier -53 to surgical or diagnostic procedure codes when the physician begins a procedure but terminates it because continuing would threaten the well-being of the patient. Reasons for discontinuing a procedure may include

- severe hypertension or hypotension
- hemorrhage
- cardiac arrest
- reaction to anesthesia
- airway obstruction

The beginning of the procedure is defined as administering anesthesia and/or preparing the patient for the procedure in the *operating suite*, the area where the procedure will be performed, which may be located in a hospital, clinic, or physician's office. Do not append modifier -53 to procedures that are electively cancelled *prior to* the patient's anesthesia induction and/or surgical preparation in the operating suite. For any discontinued procedure, the physician should document in the patient's record the reason(s) why the procedure was discontinued, and the provider should submit the documentation to the payer to review and process the provider's claim. Do not append modifier -53 to E/M or time-based services.

Note: For hospital outpatient procedures that were partially reduced or cancelled prior to or after anesthesia administration, see modifiers -73 or -74.

Modifiers -54, -55, and -56—Components of a Surgical Package

Recall that there are three components of a global surgical package: preoperative (before surgery), intra-operative (during surgery), and postoperative (after surgery) care. There are a specific number of total days for the global period when all three components occur. Many times, the same physician provides *all three* types of services to the patient. However, there may be occasions when different physicians provide different components of the surgical package, or one physician transfers the patient's care to another physician. Refer to the following example.

- Mr. Reine sees Dr. Newton, a gastroenterologist, for preoperative services for gallbladder removal. Dr. Newton performs the surgery. Mr. Reine is in the process of moving to another city, and a new physician, Dr. Miller, assumes his postoperative care after he is discharged from the hospital. Dr. Newton transfers the patient's care to Dr. Miller.

A transfer of care occurs when one physician transfers the responsibility of care for the patient to another physician. It may occur for various reasons, including complications that the patient has that another physician could more effectively monitor. The patient, patient's family member, or physician can decide that the patient needs a transfer of care. The physician must notify the patient of the transfer and document in the patient's record the reasons for the transfer. Physicians can use a *transfer of care agreement* to document transfer of care from one physician to another and state whether the transfer is permanent or temporary, depending on the patient's situation. Both physicians sign the transfer of care agreement and keep a copy of it in the patient's record.

Append the following modifiers to surgical procedure codes when different physicians perform different components of a procedure:

- **-54—Surgical Care Only:** Append modifier -54 to the procedure for the physician who performs a surgical procedure.
- **-55—Postoperative Management Only:** Append modifier -55 for the physician who performs the postoperative management of the patient after surgery.
- **-56—Preoperative Management Only:** Append modifier -56 for the physician who performed the preoperative care and evaluation before surgery.

Recall that insurances issue one payment to providers to cover all services related to the surgical package. Physicians who provide only *part* of the surgical package submit claims with the procedure code for the surgery and modifier -54, -55, or -56 appended. When insurances receive claims with procedures containing modifiers -54, -55, and -56, they know that they must split the global surgical package payment between different providers, rather than paying the full amount to one provider. Each payer has its own guidelines for paying components of the surgical package to different physicians. Payment is typically a specific percentage of the full payment and is based on the number of days after surgery that the transfer of care takes place. In general, reimbursement is higher for the physician who provides intra-operative services than it is for physicians who provide preoperative and postoperative care. Some insurances do not allow these modifiers because they will not separate payments in a surgical package.

Do not append modifiers -54, -55, and -56 when different physicians who are working in the same group practice provide different components of the surgical package to a patient. In this case, the group practice will bill the insurance claim with the procedure code and no modifier. The provider will also list the name of the physician who provided intra-operative services in block 31 of the CMS-1500 form (Figure 1-1). The insurance will issue *one payment* for the surgical package to the group practice.

Modifier -57—Decision for Surgery

Append modifier -57 to an E/M service when the physician decides to perform surgery. You can also append modifier -57 to ophthalmological service codes 92002–92014. Modifier -57 tells the insurance that they should process payment for the E/M service, rather than including it as preoperative services in the surgical package payment. Payers develop their own guidelines for appending modifier -57 to E/M services, so you will need to check with individual payers for specific directions. Refer to the following important points for appending modifier -57 to E/M services for Medicare patients (Medicare Claims Processing Manual, Chapter 12, Physicians/Nonphysician Practitioners):

- Evaluation and management services on the *day before* major surgery (90-day global period) or on the *day of* major surgery that result in the initial decision to perform the surgery are *not included in the global surgery payment* for the major surgery.
- Providers can code and bill the E/M services separately.
- Providers should append modifier -57 (decision for surgery) to identify an E/M visit which results in the initial decision to perform major surgery.
- If E/M services occur on the day of a minor surgery (10-day global period or no global period), append modifier -25, not modifier -57, to the E/M service.

Modifier -58—Staged or Related Procedure or Service by the Same Physician during the Postoperative Period

Append modifier -58 to a procedure or service that occurs during the postoperative period when the procedure was planned or staged. Planned or staged procedures occur after an initial procedure to allow the patient time to heal or time for an infection to subside. Planned procedures also apply to situations where patients cannot withstand multiple procedures performed at the same operative session. Modifier -58 includes procedures that are

- planned or anticipated (staged),
- more extensive than the original procedure,
- for therapy following a surgical procedure.

Note: For treatment of a problem that requires a return to the operating or procedure room (unanticipated clinical condition), see modifier -78.

Here are some examples of staged or planned procedures:

- multiple surgical procedures for **scar revision**, or skin grafting, with procedures performed at various stages of healing
- weight loss surgery, where the physician performs the first procedure, such as **laparoscopic sleeve gastrectomy**, to help the patient lose enough weight to prepare for the second procedure, such as **gastric bypass**
- two-stage **tympanotomy** procedures to treat **cholesteatoma**
- various procedures to remove excess skin after weight loss, with a specific number of days between procedures
- procedures to treat pressure ulcers, including an initial procedure to debride necrotic tissue, and a subsequent reconstruction procedure later after the ulcer heals
- diagnostic biopsy where the physician discovers a malignancy, followed by a second procedure to remove the malignancy

When you append modifier -58 to a procedure, it tells the insurance that the provider performed a new, subsequent procedure. The new procedure typically has its own global period, separate from the first surgery that the physician performed.

It is important to understand that some CPT codes already include the first procedure and subsequent procedures in their descriptors. Do not append modifier -58 to these codes. Here are some examples:

65855—**Trabeculoplasty** by laser surgery, 1 or more sessions (defined treatment series)

66762—**Iridoplasty** by photocoagulation (1 or more sessions) (eg, for improvement of vision, for widening of anterior chamber angle)

67101—Repair of retinal detachment, 1 or more sessions; **cryotherapy** or **diathermy**, with or without drainage of subretinal fluid

---

scar revision—surgery to improve or reduce the appearance of scars

laparoscopic sleeve gastrectomy (lap-ə-ro-skop′ik gas-trek′t-me)—removal of the lower part of the stomach, which leaves the remaining part shaped like a sleeve, done through a laparoscope

gastric bypass (gas′trik)—surgical division of the stomach near the top that joins it to the small intestine

tympanotomy (tim-pə-not′ə-me)—creating a hole in the membrane of the eardrum

cholesteatoma (ko-lə-ste-ə-to′mə)—a tumor in a small space such as the middle ear

trabeculoplasty (trə-bek′u-lo-plas-tē)—an eye operation that treats open-angle glaucoma

iridoplasty (ir′-ī-do plas-te)—an eye operation that treats angle-closure glaucoma

cryotherapy (kri-o-ther′ə-pe)—applying cold for therapeutic purposes

diathermy (di′ə-thur-me)—using low electrical currents to heat tissues

otorhinolaryngologist (ōt′-ō-rī-nō-lar-ən-gäl-ə-jəst)

TAKE A BREAK

Keep up the good work! Let's take a break and then practice coding with modifiers and assigning diagnosis codes.

Exercise 18.5 Modifiers -52, -53, -54, -55, -56, -57, and -58

Instructions: Review each patient's case, answer questions about the case, and assign codes for the procedure(s) and diagnosis(es), appending a modifier when appropriate. Optional: For additional practice, assign diagnosis(es) codes.

Case 1

Dr. Rosa, an **otorhinolaryngologist** (a physician who diagnoses, treats, and prevents ear, nose, and throat disorders)

sees Mr. Hooper, a 47-year-old established patient. Mr. Hooper suffers from tinnitus in his right ear and sees Dr. Rosa for audiologic function testing. Dr. Rosa administers pure tone audiometry, air and bone conduction testing to the patient's right ear, and diagnoses the patient with subjective tinnitus.

1. What procedure code and modifier should you assign to the patient's service? _____

2. What diagnosis code(s) should you assign to Mr. Hooper's case? _____

TAKE A BREAK *continued*

Case 2

Mr. Duffy, a 58-year-old established patient with coronary artery disease, arrives at Williton Medical Center for a right heart catheterization to measure cardiac output, an outpatient procedure. He is anesthetized and prepped for surgery in the operating room. As Dr. Woods, the cardiologist, begins the procedure, the patient's blood pressure drops significantly. Dr. Woods discontinues the procedure because of the threat to the patient's health from severe hypotension. Dr. Woods and emergency physicians render treatment to the patient and admit him to observation.

1. What procedure code and modifier should you assign to the patient's service? _____

2. What diagnosis code(s) should you assign to Mr. Duffy's case? _____

Case 3

Dr. Manfred, an oncologist, provides preoperative services to Mr. Brown, a 71-year-old, for a partial colectomy to treat colon carcinoma, which metastasized to the liver. Dr. Manfred has to go out of town for several weeks, so he transfers Mr. Brown's care, including the surgery (intra-operative) and postoperative care to Dr. Steele, documenting the transfer of care in the patient's record.

1. What procedure code and modifier should you assign to Mr. Brown's chart for Dr. Manfred's preoperative services? _____

2. What procedure code and modifier(s) should you assign to Mr. Brown's chart for Dr. Steele's intra-operative and postoperative care? _____

3. What diagnosis code(s) should you assign for the patient's condition? _____

Case 4

Dr. Woods, a cardiologist, sees established patient, Mr. Franco, a 54-year-old, who suffers from **sinus bradycardia**. During the patient's E/M visit, Dr. Woods discusses recent test results with the patient and recommends that he undergo a pacemaker insertion to regulate his heart (■ FIGURE 18-4). The E/M office visit includes an expanded problem-focused history and examination and medical decision making of low complexity.

The medical assistant schedules Mr. Franco for surgery the following day, verifying his insurance coverage and benefits. Mr. Franco's insurance considers pacemaker insertion to be a major procedure.

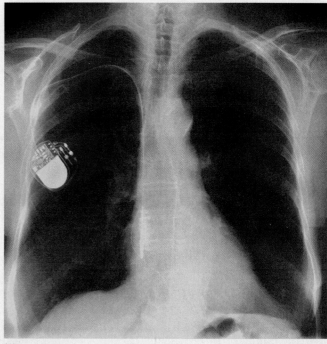

(A)

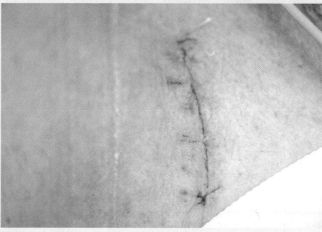

(B)

Figure 18-4 ■ (A) Colored frontal X-ray of a chest with a heart pacemaker (yellow, upper left). The heart is the orange mass at lower right, in between the lungs (red). A pacemaker is a device that supplies electrical impulses to a malfunctioning heart so that it beats normally. (B) Scar from pacemaker insertion.

Photo credits: (A) © Science Photo Library/Alamy; (B) Keith/Custom Medical Stock Photo.

1. What procedure code and modifier should you assign to Mr. Franco's record for Dr. Woods' E/M services?

_____

2. What diagnosis code(s) should you assign for the patient's condition? _____

continued

TAKE A BREAK *continued*

Case 5

Dr. Pickett, a cardiothoracic surgeon, performs planned chest wall reconstruction involving an **omental flap** on Mrs. McKay, a 48-year-old. Dr. Pickett performed previous surgery on Mrs. McKay to remove **necrotizing fasciitis** (flesh-eating disease) that was also in the abdominal wall, which Group A *Streptococcus* caused (■ FIGURE 18-5).

1. What procedure code and modifier should you assign to Mrs. McKay's chart for her reconstructive surgery?

   _____

2. What diagnosis code(s) should you assign for the patient's condition? _____

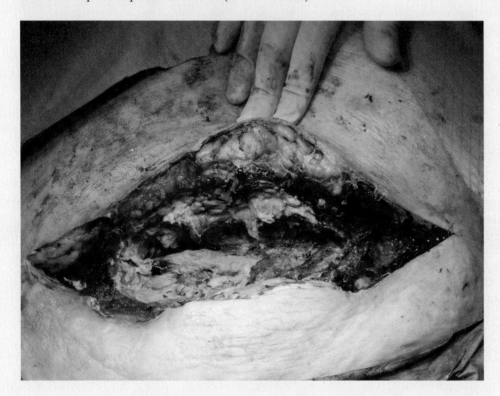

Figure 18-5 ■ A patient with necrotizing fasciitis, a bacterial infection of connective tissue, affecting the abdominal wall.

Photo credit: Slaven/Custom Medical Stock Photo.

sinus bradycardia (si′nəs brad-e-kahr′de-ə)—a heart rate of less than 60 beats per minute

omental flap (o-men′təl)—a piece of tissue from the omentum, a tissue connecting several abdominal organs

necrotizing fasciitis (nek-rə-tī′-ziη fash-ē-īt′-əs)

Modifier -59—Distinct Procedural Service

Append modifier -59 to identify procedures or services that are distinct or independent from other *non-E/M* services performed on the same day. Modifier -59 applies to procedures or services that are *not normally reported together* but that are appropriate under certain circumstances. Documentation must support a different session or encounter, different procedure or surgery, different site or organ system, separate incision or excision, separate lesion, or separate injury (or area of injury in extensive injuries) that is *not ordinarily encountered or performed on the same day by the same provider.*

Do not use modifier -59 when another modifier is more appropriate. Do not append modifier -59 to an E/M service. Instead, to report a separate and distinct E/M service with a *non-E/M service performed on the same date*, use modifier -25.

Modifier -59 helps the insurance know that the provider performed a separate procedure from procedures that would normally be bundled together under one code. Some procedures already contain the words "separate procedure" in their descriptors, alerting you to the fact that the procedures are separate from other procedures performed and that modifier -59 is appropriate:

38100—Splenectomy; total (separate procedure)

38101—partial (separate procedure)

Also remember that CMS has NCCI code pair edits to show which procedures providers should not report together. Modifier -59 alerts CMS that the provider performed two separate procedures, which should not be subject to code pair edits. For example, code 11719 and 11720 have a mutually exclusive edit and providers should *not* report them together:

11719—Trimming of nondystrophic nails, any number

11720—Debridement of nail(s) by any method(s); 1 to 5

CMS does not allow providers to report both codes together for the same patient, same anatomic site, and at the same session. However, if the provider performs both services, then you can append modifier -59 to one of the services to bypass the CMS edit which prohibits both procedures from being reported together. The mutually exclusive edit will then no longer apply because of the presence of modifier -59.

Do not append modifier -59 to procedures when the physician performs them with other procedures included in the same code descriptor. The descriptor is for a primary procedure and can also include additional procedures, which are incidental to, or part of, the primary procedure. Refer to the following example:

19302—Mastectomy, partial (eg, lumpectomy, tylectomy, quadrantectomy, segmentectomy); with axillary lymphadenectomy

Code 19302 describes two procedures: mastectomy and **axillary lymphadenectomy**. You do not need to assign separate codes for each procedure when the physician performs both of them because *both procedures are included*, or bundled, into code 19302. Remember that coding and billing bundled procedures separately is called unbundling. Insurances typically pay more for individual procedures that are coded and billed separately than they would pay if the procedures were bundled together under one code. Unbundling can be considered fraud or abuse, depending on the reason the codes were unbundled.

axillary lymphadenectomy (ak′sĭ-lar-e lim-fad-ə-nek′tə-me)—surgical removal of lymph nodes under the arm

Modifier -62—Two Surgeons

For some surgeries, two surgeons of different or the same specialties work together as primary surgeons performing distinct part(s) of a procedure. Each surgeon bills the insurance the same procedure code for the surgery with modifier -62 appended. Modifier -62 tells the insurance to pay each surgeon for the work performed during the surgery. CMS reimburses each surgeon a specific percentage of the Medicare global surgery fee schedule amount for the procedure. It is important to understand that when two surgeons are primary surgeons for a procedure, each surgeon's coder must code the *same procedure code* and append modifier -62 to the code.

An example of two surgeons working as primary surgeons include a complex condition, such as a trauma patient's lengthy time in surgery, causing the surgeons to take turns working in shifts. Each primary surgeon can also perform a specific component of the same procedure; for example, a general surgeon may prepare a surgical site, another surgeon may perform the surgery, and the general surgeon may close the surgical site. Each surgeon documents the procedure in the patient's record, and payers require documentation to support medical necessity.

The following Medicare billing procedures apply to claims for a surgical procedure or procedures that required two surgeons or a team of surgeons:

- Documentation of medical necessity for two surgeons is required for certain procedures that Medicare specifies.

- Modifier -62 does not apply to team surgery. If a *team* of surgeons (three or more surgeons of different specialties) is required to perform a specific procedure, then each surgeon bills for the procedure with modifier -66 (surgical team).

- If surgeons of different specialties each perform a different procedure (with specific CPT codes), then neither cosurgery nor multiple surgery rules apply (even if the procedures are performed through the same incision). If one of the surgeons performs multiple procedures, then the multiple procedure rules apply to that surgeon's services.

Modifier -63—Procedure Performed on Infants Less Than 4 kgs

Procedures that physicians perform on neonates and infants weighing up to 4 kg (8.8 pounds) may involve significantly increased complexity and physician work. Append modifier -63 to procedures in the 20000–69990 code series for neonates and infants up to 4 kg unless CPT coding instructions prohibit appending modifier -63. Do not append modifier -63 to CPT codes for Evaluation and Management Services, Anesthesia, Radiology, Pathology/Laboratory, or Medicine.

Modifier -66—Surgical Team

Under some circumstances, highly complex and difficult procedures require a surgical team, including three or more physicians, often of different specialties; other highly skilled clinicians (physician assistants, registered nurses, or technicians); and the use of complex surgical equipment. When this situation occurs, each physician on the surgical team documents the procedure in the patient's record. Coders for each physician code the procedure, appending modifier -66. Modifier -66 notifies the insurance that the physician was part of a surgical team, and insurances pay each physician on the surgical team a specific amount for the procedure, rather than paying one physician the full amount.

Examples of procedures requiring team surgery include multistage transplant surgery and some types of cardiac surgery, where each physician performs a unique function requiring special skills that are integral to the total procedure. Each physician is engaged in a level of activity that is different from *assisting* the surgeon in charge of the case. Physicians of different specialties may also be necessary during surgery because the patient has multiple conditions requiring diverse, specialized medical services. For example, a patient's cardiac condition may require a cardiologist to join the surgical team to monitor the patient's condition during abdominal surgery.

Modifiers -76 and -77—Repeat Procedures

Append modifier -76 to a procedure or service that was repeated by the same physician. Modifier -76 is used for a repeat procedure or service that occurs after the original procedure performed by the *same physician* or other qualified health care professional. A physician could repeat a procedure because the patient did not respond well after the first procedure, or because the first procedure was unsuccessful. Modifier -76 alerts the insurance that the repeat procedure is *not the same procedure* performed the first time. For example, the insurance processes the claim for the first procedure code and pays the provider. If you do not append modifier -76 to the repeat procedure code, then the insurance will think that you are rebilling the *same service* that they already paid. **Note**: Do not append modifier -76 to E/M services.

Modifier -77 is used for a repeat procedure or service that occurs after the original procedure performed by *another physician* or other qualified health care professional. Append modifier -77 to a procedure or service that was repeated. Modifier -77 also notifies the insurance that the repeat procedure is not the same as the procedure performed the first time, so they will not deny payment for the repeat procedure as a duplicate service.

When billing insurance for any repeat procedures, providers should attach medical documentation to establish medical necessity.

Modifier -78—Unplanned Return to the Operating/Procedure Room

Modifier -78 represents an unplanned return to the operating/procedure room for a related procedure during the postoperative period of an initial procedure. The same physician or other qualified health care professional performs the unplanned procedure. The unplanned procedure can be the result of a complication that the initial surgery caused and is not considered to be a repeat procedure (see modifiers -76 and -77).

Append modifier -78 to the unplanned procedure code when it is related to the first procedure and requires the use of an operating or procedure room. Operating or procedure rooms, where physicians typically perform procedures, are also called *surgical suites*. They contain the equipment necessary to perform the procedure and to care for the patient.

Medicare defines an OR as a place of service that is specifically equipped and staffed for the sole purpose of performing procedures. It can be a cardiac catheterization suite, a laser suite, or an endoscopy suite. An OR is not a patient's room, a minor treatment room, a recovery room, or an intensive care unit (unless the patient's condition is so critical that there is insufficient time for transportation to an OR).

Modifier -78 tells the payer that the unplanned procedure occurred within the first procedure's global period. Insurances typically reimburse unplanned related procedures the same amount as they pay for intra-operative services of the surgical package. A new global period *does not begin with the unplanned related procedure* because it is typically from a complication that is *related to the original procedure*. However, if the unplanned return to the OR for a complication occurred *after* the global period for the first procedure, then a new global period would begin for the unplanned procedure.

Modifier -79—Unrelated Procedure or Service by the Same Physician during the Postoperative Period

Sometimes when patients have surgery, they need to return to the operating room during the postoperative period for another procedure by the same physician, which is *unrelated* to the initial surgery. When this situation occurs, append modifier -79 to the unrelated procedure code. Modifier -79 tells the insurance that the second procedure is *not related* to the initial surgery and that a new global period should begin for the second procedure.

Scheuermann's disease (shoΙ′-ər-mänz)—a spinal disorder in children consisting of exaggerated roundness or hump in the upper back; also called kyphosis

anterior arthrodesis (an-tēr′e-ər ahr-thro-de′sis)—surgical immobilization or fusing together of vertebrae from the front

spinal instrumentation (spi′nəl)—surgically attaching devices, such as hooks, rods, and wire to stabilize the spine after surgery

bone grafting—placing new bone or replacement material into spaces between or around broken bone

TAKE A BREAK

Let's take a break and then practice coding with modifiers and assigning diagnosis codes.

Exercise 18.6   Modifiers -59, -62, -63, -66, -76, -77, -78, and -79

Instructions: Review each patient's case, answer questions about the case, and assign codes for the procedure(s), appending a modifier when appropriate. Optional: Assign diagnosis(es) codes.

Case 1

Mr. Jackson, a 68-year-old Medicare patient, visits Williton Rehabilitation Clinic for physical therapy with Regina Jones, a physical therapist. Mr. Jackson suffers from low back pain. He receives a total of 30 minutes of physical therapy, including 15 minutes of manual therapy techniques (97140) and 15 minutes of therapeutic activities (97530). CMS has a mutually exclusive edit, which prohibits providers from reporting both codes together for the same patient during the same session *unless* the patient receives each service during a *different* 15-minute interval. The medical documentation shows that Mr. Jackson's total therapy time was 30 minutes, and he received manual therapy for the first 15 minutes and therapeutic activities for the last 15 minutes.

1. What procedure codes and modifier should you assign to Mr. Jackson's chart for his physical therapy? _____

2. What diagnosis code(s) should you assign for the patient's condition? _____

Case 2

Dr. Reilly, an orthopedic spinal surgeon, and Dr. Stark, a general surgeon (a physician who is experienced in performing various procedures), work as cosurgeons on a procedure for Tyler Lynn. The patient is a 16-year-old with **Scheuermann's disease**. Dr. Reilly performs definitive surgery of an **anterior arthrodesis** for the patient's spinal deformity (three vertebral segments). Dr. Stark opens and closes for the procedure. Dr. Reilly also performs additional procedures of **spinal instrumentation** and **bone grafting**, but Dr. Stark is not considered a cosurgeon for these procedures.

1. What procedure code and modifier should you assign to Tyler Lynn's chart for Dr. Reilly's part of the definitive procedure?_____

2. What procedure code and modifier should you assign to the patient's chart for Dr. Stark's part of the definitive procedure?_____

continued

TAKE A BREAK *continued*

3. According to CPT coding guidelines, what code range should you refer to for reporting additional instrumentation procedures? _____

4. What code range should you refer to for reporting additional procedures for bone grafting, per CPT guidelines? _____

5. Is it appropriate to append modifier -62 to instrumentation procedures or bone grafting? _____ How do you know? _____

6. What is the patient's diagnosis code? _____

Case 3

Baby Jamie Bonner, a neonate weighing 3.2 kg, suffers from **tetralogy of Fallot**. Dr. Lott, a cardiothoracic surgeon, performs tetralogy of Fallot repair with **transannular** patch.

1. What procedure code and modifier should you assign to the neonate's chart?_____

2. What is the patient's diagnosis code? _____

Case 4

At Williton Medical Center, Dr. Holder, a vascular surgeon, performs an endovascular repair of abdominal aortic aneurysm on Mr. Mayo, a 70-year-old patient. Mr. Mayo had a recent myocardial infarction and suffers from angina and acute renal failure. Dr. Benjamin, a cardiologist, and Dr. Stein, a nephrologist, work with Dr. Holder as part of the surgical team.

1. What procedure code and modifier should you assign to the patient's chart for Dr. Holder's part of the procedure? _____

2. What procedure code and modifier should you assign to the patient's chart for Dr. Benjamin's part of the procedure? _____

3. What procedure code and modifier should you assign to the patient's chart for Dr. Stein's part of the procedure? _____

4. What are the patient's diagnosis code(s)? _____

Case 5

Dr. Lindsay, an ophthalmologist at Williton Medical Center, performs a repeat procedure for an intraocular lens (IOL) placement in the right eye for Mrs. Osborn, a 62-year-old patient. Mrs. Osborn suffers from **presbyopia**. Two days earlier, Dr. Lindsay performed the IOL placement, but the IOL shifted, and he had to repeat the procedure.

1. What procedure code and modifier(s) should you assign to Mrs. Osborn's chart for the repeat procedure that Dr. Lindsay performed? _____

2. If another ophthalmologist performed the repeat procedure, then what code and modifier(s) would you assign? _____

3. What is the patient's diagnosis code(s)? _____

4. If the same physician repeated only part of the original procedure, then what additional modifier should you assign to the procedure code? _____

Case 6

Mrs. Stout, a 42-year-old established patient, experiences wound dehiscence (opening of incision site) following abdominal surgery that Dr. Valencia performed a week earlier. Dr. Valencia finds that the patient has a necrotizing postoperative infection. In the operating room, he debrides the wound of the abdominal wall, including the skin, subcutaneous tissue, muscle, and fascia. The procedure falls within Mrs. Stout's insurance's global period for the initial abdominal surgery.

1. What procedure code and modifier(s) should you assign to Mrs. Stout's chart for the unplanned procedure? _____

2. What is the patient's diagnosis code(s)? _____

Case 7

Mrs. McNeil, a 62-year-old, undergoes a sling operation (the physician fastens a sling around the urethra to return it to its regular position) to treat stress urinary incontinence. Dr. Petty, a urologist, performed the surgery. During the global period for the procedure, Mrs. McNeil returns to the operating room because of **nephrolithiasis** (kidney stones, also called calculi). Dr. Petty performs a **nephrolithotomy** (incision into the kidney to remove calculi).

1. What procedure code and modifier should you assign to Mr. McNeil's chart for the nephrolithotomy? _____

2. What is the patient's diagnosis code? _____

3. Does a new global period begin with the nephrolithotomy, or is it part of the global period for the sling operation? _____

Modifiers -80, -81, and -82—Assistant at Surgery Services

An assistant surgeon is a physician who actively assists an operating, or principal, surgeon to perform a procedure. The principal surgeon is in charge of the patient's case. Assistants are often necessary because of the complex nature of the procedure(s) or the patient's condition. The assistant surgeon performs medical functions *under the direct supervision* of the operating physician. The assistant is generally in the same specialty as the principal surgeon.

The principal surgeon submits the procedure code for the surgery to the patient's insurance. Append one of the assistant surgeon modifiers to the procedure code for the assistant surgeon's services. Modifiers for an assistant surgeon include

- **-80—Assistant Surgeon:** The assistant surgeon assists during an *entire* procedure.

- **-81—Minimum Assistant Surgeon:** The assistant surgeon assists during *part* of a procedure.

- **-82—Assistant Surgeon (when qualified resident surgeon is not available):** The assistant surgeon assists the principal surgeon because a medical resident was not available to assist.

Other nonphysician clinicians can also assist with surgeries; however, the assistant surgeon modifiers are for procedures involving a *physician*. Medicare and other payers that consider assistant surgeon claims for payment require providers to obtain *preauthorization* (approval before the service is rendered). Preauthorization involves contacting the payer to provide documentation supporting medical necessity and the appropriateness of an assistant surgeon. Any staff member working for the provider may be responsible for obtaining preauthorizations for patients' procedures and services.

The reimbursement amount to an assistant surgeon depends on the individual payer, and insurances typically pay the assistant surgeon a percentage of the total reimbursement amount for the surgery, with a lower percentage paid to a *minimum* assistant surgeon.

Refer to the following guidelines to better understand Medicare's policies involving assistant surgeon services:

- Medicare will not pay assistant surgeons for surgical procedures in which a physician assists with surgery in *fewer than five percent* of the cases for that procedure nationally.

- Physicians cannot bill Medicare beneficiaries for balances remaining after Medicare pays for assistant at surgery services.

- Medicare will not pay for an assistant surgeon when payment for either two surgeons (modifier -62) or team surgeons (modifier -66) is appropriate.

Modifier -82 represents an assistant surgeon's services when a qualified *resident* surgeon is not available. Residents have finished medical school and completed their internships working in hospitals. They are physicians who are receiving additional training in their medical specialties. They work in teaching hospitals, hospitals that work with medical schools to provide training programs for physicians, which attending physicians supervise. Each teaching hospital has different requirements and guidelines for the total number of residents allowed, their qualifications, job duties, and the types of surgeries they can perform.

Medicare *does not pay* for assistant surgeons in a teaching hospital when a qualified resident is available to perform the service. However, there are occasions when Medicare will consider payment because a qualified resident *is not* available, including the following situations:

- No resident was available because they were involved in other activities.

- The surgery was too complex for a resident's skill level.

- There were not enough residents in the residency program.

- The patient experienced exceptional medical circumstances (emergency, life-threatening situations, such as multiple traumatic injuries) which required immediate treatment.

tetralogy of Fallot (tĕ-tral'ə-je fal-ōz')—a combination of four congenital heart defects

transannular (trans an'u-lər)—across the ring of the pulmonary valve

presbyopia (pres-be-o'pe-ə) —difficulty of focusing near vision

nephrolithiasis (nef-ro-lī-thi'ə-sis)

nephrolithotomy (nef-ro-lī-thot'ə-me)

· The primary surgeon has an across-the-board policy of never involving residents in the preoperative, operative, or postoperative care of patients.

Medicare carriers will process assistant at surgery claims for services furnished in teaching hospitals as long as the provider submits the procedure with modifier -82 and includes a certification statement that no qualified resident was available to assist and the reason(s) why.

Modifier -90—Reference (Outside) Laboratory

Append modifier -90 to laboratory and pathology procedures when a reference, or outside laboratory, performs the lab test, rather than the treating or reporting physician. Physicians who do not perform lab tests can still collect specimens for lab tests and then send the specimens to a reference lab. The reference lab performs the test and bills the physician for the service.

The physician bills the patient's insurance for the lab procedure, along with shipping and handling charges to send the specimen. The physician appends modifier -90 to the lab procedure code to show the insurance that the physician collected the specimen and sent it to an outside lab for testing. The insurance pays the physician the amount that the physician paid to the reference lab.

Medicare will not pay physicians for lab services that they refer to an outside lab. However, Medicare does allow labs to append modifier -90 to lab services that they refer to *other labs* (Medicare Claims Processing Manual, Chapter 16, Laboratory Services). It is best to check individual payer guidelines to determine how they interpret modifier -90.

Modifier -91—Repeat Clinical Diagnostic Laboratory Test

In the course of treatment of the patient, it may be necessary to repeat the same laboratory test on the same day for the same patient to obtain subsequent (multiple) test results. When this situation occurs, append modifier -91 to the subsequent laboratory test to show the insurance that the subsequent test was necessary and should not be denied as a duplicate service.

Do not append modifier -91 to tests that are rerun to confirm initial results due to testing problems with specimens or equipment, or for any other reason when a normal, one-time, reportable result is all that is required. Do not append modifier -91 when other code(s) describe a series of test results (such as glucose tolerance tests or evocative/suppression testing).

Modifier -92—Alternative Laboratory Platform Testing

Append modifier -92 to a laboratory procedure code to identify a lab test in the form of a kit or transportable instrument that wholly or in part consists of a single use, disposable analytical chamber. The test does not require permanent dedicated space to perform it. A clinician can hand-carry the test or transport it to another place for testing. An antibody HIV-1 test is an example of alternative laboratory platform testing.

WORKPLACE IQ

You are working as a coder at Williton Medical Center in the Health Information Management Department. You are cross-trained to code both outpatient encounters and inpatient stays. Your manager asks you to prepare an overview of modifiers -80, -81, and -82 to educate a group of physicians. The information that you prepare should be brief and easy to follow.

What would you do?

INTERESTING FACT: Over Half of the U.S. Adult Population Has Never Had an HIV Test

In the U.S., an estimated 1.2 million people are living with HIV, and as many as 1 in 5 do not know that they are infected. About 55% of adults aged 18–64 years have never been tested for HIV. Even among people who are at higher risk for HIV infection, 28% have never been tested. The Centers for Disease Control recommends routine HIV testing in healthcare settings. People need to get tested so that they can get treated and not infect others. Being tested will save their lives and the lives of other people.

(Department of Health and Human Services, Centers for Disease Control and Prevention, www.cdc.gov/VitalSigns/HIVtesting/index.html, accessed 2/7/2010, and www.cdc.gov/nchhstp/newsroom/docs/Vital-Signs-Fact-Sheet.pdf, accessed 3/23/2012.)

Modifier -99—Multiple Modifiers

Under certain circumstances, you may append two or more modifiers to fully describe a procedure or service. When this situation occurs, append modifier -99 first (multiple modifiers), followed by all other applicable modifiers. Some insurances require providers to bill procedures with multiple modifiers by listing modifier -99 in the MODIFIER field of block 24D of the CMS-1500, and listing all other modifiers in block 19, along with the appropriate CPT/HCPCS code. (See Figure 1-1 in Chapter 1 of this text.) Other payers require different reporting for multiple modifiers or do not require providers to append modifier -99 when there are two or more other modifiers.

Neither the AMA nor CMS offers guidelines for the order in which to append multiple CPT or HCPCS modifiers to the same code. The best approach is to first list modifiers that directly affect insurance reimbursement, such as -26 (professional component), -50 (bilateral procedure), and -53 (discontinued procedure), followed by the modifiers that provide *additional information* but do not necessarily affect reimbursement, such as -LT (left) or -RT (right). It is best to check with individual payers to determine their rules for the order in which to append multiple modifiers to the same code because rules can be different, depending on the payer.

Ambulatory Surgery Center (ASC) Hospital Outpatient Modifiers

You already learned about most of the ASC hospital outpatient modifiers because they are CPT modifiers that we already reviewed. Here are the three additional ASC modifiers that we did not discuss yet:

- -27—Multiple outpatient hospital E/M encounters on the same date
- -73—Discontinued outpatient hospital/ASC procedure *prior to* anesthesia administration
- -74—Discontinued outpatient hospital/ASC procedure *after* anesthesia administration

Modifier -27—Multiple Outpatient Hospital E/M Encounters on the Same Date   Append modifier -27 to a subsequent, separate, and distinct E/M encounter when a patient has more than one E/M encounter in the hospital on the same day (with different physicians). The E/M services can be within various hospital departments, such as the ED or a hospital-based clinic. When the same physician provides multiple E/M services to the same patient on the same day, do not append modifier -27. Instead, use modifier -25. Medicare will process claims with E/M codes with modifier -27, and it is best to check individual payer guidelines on reimbursement involving modifier -27.

Modifier -73 and -74—Discounted Outpatient Hospital/ASC Procedures Modifier -73 represents a discontinued outpatient procedure that is terminated *before* anesthesia administration. Append modifier -73 to the surgical procedure code to indicate that a surgical or diagnostic procedure requiring anesthesia was terminated due to extenuating circumstances that threatened the well-being of the patient, after the patient had been prepared for the procedure and taken to the procedure room. Do not append modifier -73 when the patient elects to cancel a procedure.

Anesthesia includes:

- Local
- Regional block(s)
- General anesthesia

Modifier -74 represents a discontinued outpatient procedure that is terminated *after* anesthesia administration (local, regional block(s), general). Append modifier -74 to the procedure code to indicate that a surgical or diagnostic procedure requiring anesthesia was terminated after the induction of anesthesia, or after the physician started the procedure, such as the incision made, intubation started, or endoscope inserted. Do not append modifier -74 when the patient elects to cancel a procedure.

Medicare pays 50% of the Outpatient Prospective Payment System (OPPS) payment amount for a discontinued procedure. Append modifier -53 to a procedure code for physician reporting of a discontinued procedure (not the outpatient hospital or ASC).

assay (as-ā′)—test to determine the presence and quantity of a substance

TAKE A BREAK

Let's take a break and then practice coding with modifiers and assigning diagnosis codes.

Exercise 18.7 Modifiers -80, -81, -82, -90, -91, -92, -99, -27, -73, and -74

Instructions: Review each patient's case, answer the questions about the case, and assign codes for the procedure(s) and diagnosis(es), appending a modifier when appropriate. Optional: Assign diagnosis(es) codes.

Case 1

Dr. Carver, an orthopedic surgeon, performs a total knee replacement for Mr. Santana, a 70-year-old patient who suffers from osteoarthritis of the knee (■ FIGURE 18-6). Dr. Gould, also an orthopedic surgeon, provides assistance at surgery services throughout the entire procedure.

1. What procedure code should you assign to Mr. Santana's chart for Dr. Carver's services? _____

2. What procedure code and modifier should you assign to Mr. Santana's chart for Dr. Gould's services? _____

3. If Dr. Gould only assisted during *part* of the procedure, then what modifier would you append to the procedure code? _____

4. What is the patient's diagnosis code? _____

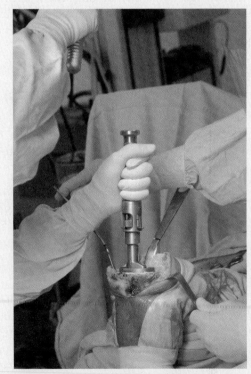

Figure 18-6 ■ Close-up of surgeons performing a total knee replacement. The worn knee joint is shown at center. The patient suffers from severe osteoarthritis of the knee.

Photo credit: Reflekta/Shutterstock.com.

TAKE A BREAK *continued*

Case 2

Dr. Hoffman's office staff sends a lab specimen (blood) to Minnington Labs to perform a drug **assay** to test doxepin levels for Mrs. Howe, a 38-year-old established patient, who suffers from depression. Minnington Labs charges Dr. Hoffman's office $150 for the lab procedure, and the office incurs an additional $25 for shipping and handling.

1. What procedure code and modifier should you assign to Mrs. Howe's chart for the lab test? _____

2. What is the total charge that Dr. Hoffman's staff should bill to the insurance? _____

3. What is the patient's diagnosis code? _____

Case 3

Minnington Labs performs a lab test for a blood cell count of hematocrit (percentage of blood containing red blood cells) twice in the same day for the same patient. The first test shows elevated hematocrit levels, and the patient's physician determines that the patient is dehydrated. The patient then receives hydration therapy, and the second lab test reveals normal hematocrit levels.

1. What procedure code and modifier should you assign to the patient's chart for the first lab test and subsequent lab test? _____

2. What is the patient's diagnosis code? _____

Case 4

With the patient's blood sample collected in the office by venipuncture, Dr. Hoffman administers an antibody HIV-1 test to Mrs. Gamble, a 30-year-old established patient. The test is negative for HIV infection.

1. What procedure code and modifier should you assign to Mrs. Gamble's chart for the antibody HIV-1 test? _____

2. What diagnosis code should you assign for the screening test? _____

3. Should you assign a code for an HIV infection? _____

   Why or why not? _____

4. If more medical documentation were provided showing that Dr. Hoffman reviewed the patient's history, examined the patient, and rendered medical decision making, what other service(s) could you code? _____

Case 5

Mrs. Dixon, a 43-year-old new patient, sees Dr. Woods, a cardiologist, due to repeated angina. The encounter is at the outpatient cardiology clinic within Williton Medical Center. Dr. Woods examines and assesses the patient and orders additional tests. The E/M service includes a comprehensive history, comprehensive exam, and medical decision-making of moderate complexity.

After the patient leaves the cardiology clinic, she experiences severe angina and goes to Williton's ED, where Dr. Mills examines her. His E/M service within the ED has an expanded problem-focused history and exam, with moderate medical decision-making.

1. What procedure code should you assign for Dr. Wood's E/M service? _____

2. What procedure code and modifier should you assign for Dr. Mills' E/M service? _____

3. What is the patient's diagnosis code for both services? _____

Case 6

Mr. Peck, a 23-year-old, is prepped and taken to the operating room for an appendectomy to treat acute appendicitis (■ FIGURE 18-7). Before he receives anesthesia, he develops severe hypertension, and Dr. Stark cancels the procedure.

1. What procedure code and modifier should you assign for the appendectomy? _____

2. What diagnosis code(s) should you assign? _____

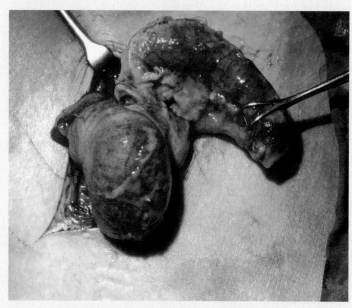

Figure 18-7 ■ An inflamed appendix removed from a patient with acute appendicitis.

Photo credit: © SHOUT / Alamy.

CHAPTER REVIEW

Multiple Choice

Instructions: Circle one best answer to complete each statement.

1. Which of the following is *not* part of the CPT global surgical package?
   a. Local infiltration, metacarpal/metatarsal/digital block, or topical anesthesia
   b. General anesthesia
   c. Immediate postoperative care, including dictating operative notes, talking with the family, and consulting with other physicians
   d. Evaluating the patient in the postanesthesia recovery area

2. Which of the following is *not* part of the Medicare global surgical package?
   a. Preoperative visits
   b. Intra-operative services
   c. Postsurgical pain management
   d. Complications that require additional trips to the operating room

3. Examples of circumstances that could warrant using modifier -22 include all the following patients *except* a patient who
   a. is hearing impaired and requires an interpreter during the E/M visit when the decision for surgery is made.
   b. is morbidly obese, and the condition complicates surgery or causes additional work and time to perform surgery.
   c. has other conditions, such as neoplasms, malformations, or scarring, that cause surgical complications or additional effort and/or time to manage.
   d. experiences excessive blood loss during the procedure.

4. When a radiologist provides only the supervision and interpretation of an X-ray, you should use a modifier for the
   a. professional component.
   b. technical component.
   c. increased procedure.
   d. global service.

5. Append modifier -47 *Anesthesia by Surgeon* to services that _____ perform.
   a. anesthesiologists
   b. CRNAs
   c. surgeons
   d. all of the above

6. Append modifier -50 *Bilateral Procedure* when
   a. a physician performs a procedure on both sides, and the code descriptor does *not* contain the word *bilateral* or the phrase *unilateral or bilateral*.
   b. a physician performs a procedure on both sides, and the code descriptor contains the word *bilateral* or the phrase *unilateral or bilateral*.
   c. a physician performs a procedure on only one of two paired organs or structures, and the code descriptor does *not* contain the word *bilateral* or the phrase *unilateral or bilateral*.
   d. a physician provides the supervision and interpretation for a bilateral procedure.

7. When using modifier -51 *Multiple Procedures* you should
   a. report the procedures in the order in which the physician performed them.
   b. report the procedures in numerical order.
   c. report procedures from lowest charge to highest charge.
   d. report procedures from highest charge to lowest charge.

8. How should providers bill procedures when physicians from different group practices provide services in the global surgical package?
   a. The surgeon who performs the procedure bills the entire service, then reimburses the other surgeons.
   b. The surgeon who performs the postoperative care bills the entire service, then reimburses the other surgeons.
   c. Each surgeon submits the same procedure code and appends a modifier indicating the component of the surgical package that he provided.
   d. The surgical package does not apply when physicians from different group practices provide services in the global surgical package.

9. Do not report modifier -57 *Decision for Surgery* when the physician provides E/M services
   a. on the day before a major surgery.
   b. which result in the initial decision to perform major surgery.
   c. that occur on the day of major surgery.
   d. that occur on the day of minor surgery.

10. Append modifier _____ to represent an unplanned return to the operating/procedure room by the same physician for a related procedure, after the initial procedure, during the postoperative period.
    a. -59   b. -77
    c. -78   d. -79

Coding Assignments

Instructions: Assign CPT-4 procedure code(s) to the following cases, referencing both the index and CPT sections. Optional: For additional practice, assign ICD-9-CM diagnosis codes using both the Index and Tabular.

1. Dr. Rippon, a radiologist, has a contract with Williton Medical Center to provide professional services for the hospital's radiology department. Today, he interprets an X-ray for Gary Hutchison, age 25, with two views of the left foot. The X-ray shows a stress fracture of the first **metatarsal** (bone segment of the great toe closest to the foot).

   Diagnosis code(s) for Dr. Rippon's services:

   _____

   Procedure code(s) for Dr. Rippon's services:

   _____

2. The radiology technician at Williton Medical Center takes X-rays of both knees for Joyce McGruder, age 53, in the standing **anteroposterior** (from front to back) position. Dr. Stuart, an orthopedist, ordered the X-rays due to Ms. McGruder's osteoarthritis. Dr. Stuart asks the radiology department to send the X-rays to him for interpretation.

   Diagnosis code(s) for Williton Medical Center's services: _____

   Procedure code(s) for Williton Medical Center's services: _____

3. Arlene Ball, age 21, is on vacation when she breaks her leg during a fall from a high rock while rock climbing. Her boyfriend brings her to Williton Medical Center's ED where Dr. Carver, the orthopedic surgeon on call, determines that she has fractured the **medial malleolus** (rounded bony prominence) on the **distal** (far, bottom) end of the right tibia. He determines that the patient needs surgery. Dr. Carver provides the surgical service only. He performs open treatment of the fracture of weight-bearing **articular surface** (the curved portion on the bottom of the medial malleolus) of the distal tibia, with internal fixation. (*Hint:* The fracture is closed, but requires an open treatment.) An orthopedist in the patient's home town will provide postoperative follow-up care.

   Diagnosis code(s) for Dr. Carver's services:

   _____

   Procedure code(s) for Dr. Carver's services:

   _____

4. Arlene Ball returns home after Dr. Carver treated her medial malleolus of her right tibia. She sees Dr. Cosgrove, an orthopedic surgeon in her home town, for postoperative follow-up. The insurance allows 90 global days for her surgery. Dr. Cosgrove reviews the operative report from Dr. Carver, the original surgeon, and assigns the same diagnosis and procedure codes. However, he uses a different modifier.

   Diagnosis code(s) for Dr. Cosgrove's services:

   _____

   Procedure code(s) for Dr. Cosgrove's services:

   _____

5. The next day, Arlene Ball slips while getting out of her boyfriend's pick-up truck and braces herself with her arms. She thinks that she sprained her right wrist and calls Dr. Cosgrove. Dr. Cosgrove does not believe that the injury is serious enough to go to the local hospital's ED, so he suggests that Ms. Ball visit the office for an evaluation. Dr. Cosgrove examines her wrist and concludes that it has a slight sprain. He wraps it and tells her to keep ice on it for a day. The visit includes an expanded problem-focused examination and straightforward medical decision making.

   Diagnosis code(s) for Dr. Cosgrove's services:

   _____

   Procedure code(s) for Dr. Cosgrove's services:

   _____

6. Juanita Slate, age 43, has uterine fibroids, which obstruct her urethra and cause a slow and intermittent (start and stop) urine flow. Her gynecologist recommends a hysterectomy. Before her insurance will pay for the surgery, they require a consultation for a second opinion (E/M service). Ms. Slate then sees Dr. Wooten, an OB/GYN, for the first time. He conducts a detailed history and examination and renders medical decision making of low complexity. He agrees that a hysterectomy is appropriate and sends his report to the insurance company.

   Diagnosis code(s) for Dr. Wooten's services:

   _____

   Procedure code(s) for Dr. Wooten's services:

   _____

7. Stephen Strader, age 50, presents to Williton Medical Center's outpatient procedure center for a colonoscopy. Dr. Valencia, a gastroenterologist, administers **Versed** (a central nervous system depressant) for moderate sedation. Mr. Strader immediately goes into acute respiratory distress, so Dr. Valencia discontinues the anesthesia and administers an **antidote** (an agent that reverses the effect). The patient's symptoms subside, but Dr. Valencia cancels the procedure for today in the best interest

of the patient. Dr. Valencia tells Ms. Strader that he will reschedule the procedure using a different anesthetic. (*Hint:* CPT indexes a colonoscopy as an exploratory endoscopy.)

Diagnosis code(s) for Dr. Valencia's services:

_____

Procedure code(s) for Dr. Valencia's services:

_____

8. Dr. Ferguson, a dermatologist, removes two lesions from the skin on Tamara Kilpatrick's back. The first lesion is on the upper right quadrant and is 2.2 cm in diameter. The second lesion is on the upper left quadrant and is 1.5 cm in diameter. The pathology report indicates that both lesions are melanomas.

Diagnosis code(s) for Dr. Ferguson's services:

_____

Procedure code(s) for Dr. Ferguson's services:

_____

metatarsal (met-ə-tahr′səl)

anteroposterior
(an-ər-o-pos-tēr′e-ər)

medial malleolus
(me′de-əl mə-le′o-ləs)

distal (dis′təl)

articular surface
(ahr-tik′u-lər)

Versed (ver-sed′)

antidote (an′tī-dōt)

9. Dr. Drimond, a gastroenterologist, repairs an incarcerated umbilical (navel region) hernia on newborn Benjamin Britt. Benjamin was born prematurely and weighs 3,500 grams (7.7 pounds).

Diagnosis code(s) for Dr. Drimond's services:

_____

Procedure code(s) for Dr. Drimond's services:

_____

10. Dr. Hoffman sees Diana Delossantos, age 57, for her annual preventive medicine examination (E/M service). She is an established patient. Dr. Hoffman draws blood by venipuncture for a CBC but cannot process the specimen because his equipment is broken. He sends it to Minnington Labs for processing of an automated CBC. Dr. Hoffman will pay Minnington Labs and bill Ms. Delossantos' insurance for the cost.

Diagnosis code(s) for Dr. Hoffman's services:

_____

Procedure code(s) for Dr. Hoffman's services:

_____

(465.9)

(216.3)

(272.4)

(296.2)

Evaluation and Management (E/M) Coding and Anesthesia Coding

(787.91)

(789.07)

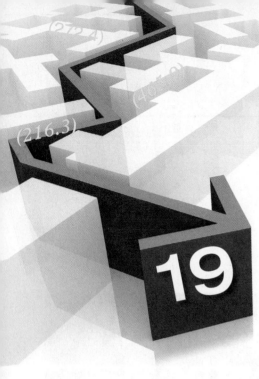

Evaluation and Management (E/M)

19

Learning Objectives

After completing this chapter, you should be able to

- Spell and define the key terminology in this chapter.
- Define evaluation and management (E/M) services.
- Identify the three factors of E/M services.
- Discuss the importance of evaluation and management (E/M) documentation.
- Describe information contained in the E/M guidelines in the CPT manual.
- Identify the seven components of E/M services and discuss the information contained in each.
- Demonstrate how to assign codes to patient encounters within each E/M category.

Key Terms

chief complaint (CC)
coordination of care
counseling
examination
history

medical decision-making (MDM)
nature of the presenting problem
patient status
place of service
time
type of service

INTRODUCTION

During this next stop on your coding journey, you will learn how physicians and other providers assign E/M codes. E/M coding is difficult because you have to review many different criteria from the patient's documentation and analyze it thoroughly before you can assign the correct code. The analysis takes various forms and follows many steps. It is not as straightforward as simply finding the main term in the index and cross-referencing it to the E/M section. Understanding E/M coding is a long process, so take your time as you work through this chapter, and do not get discouraged! As with everything you learned so far, it is hard at first but becomes easier with practice. And think of the satisfaction you will have when you finish the chapter knowing that you have mastered yet another coding skill!

"For they conquer who believe they can."—JOHN DRYDEN

EVALUATION AND MANAGEMENT CODING

Evaluation and Management (E/M) services are the most common services that providers perform, and you can find codes for them in the front of the CPT manual. An E/M service is also called a *professional service*. Recall from Chapter 17 that an E/M service is a face-to-face service between a physician and patient that typically includes a history, examination, and medical decision-making. However, there are some exceptions when E/M services do not involve face-to-face time with a patient.

Providers Who Assign E/M Codes

In this chapter, you will learn how physicians assign E/M codes, and other *nonphysician practitioners (NPPs)* can also assign some of the E/M codes, depending on their scope of practice for the state in which they provide services. NPPs cannot perform all of the same services that physicians perform. NPPs include:

- physician assistants (PAs)
- nurse practitioners (NPs)
- clinical nurse specialists (CNSs)
- certified nurse midwives (CNMs)

In this chapter, the word *physician* can refer to physicians and/or NPPs.

Different Locations for E/M Services

Physicians provide E/M services in many different locations, including an outpatient office or clinic, inpatient hospital, ED, or the patient's home. One physician may render E/M services in multiple settings, such as in an office and in a nursing home. Physicians record E/M services on a paper or electronic encounter form for each patient, and they also document the service in the patient's record. Recall from Chapter 1 that an encounter form (Figure 1-15) is a preprinted form that includes basic patient demographic information, along with a list of commonly performed services and procedure codes and a list of common diagnoses and diagnosis codes. Providers also call an encounter form a superbill, charge slip, or charge ticket.

When a physician provides E/M services *outside the office*, the facility where the physician sees the patient does not typically bill for the patient's services. The physician's office staff code and bill for the service. However, in some cases, when the facility employs the physician, such as certain hospitals, the facility performs the coding and billing. When physicians who own their own practice or are part of a group practice see patients outside the office, they turn in an encounter form to their office staff. The encounter form shows the E/M service provided and the patient's diagnosis. The physician assigns the code, and you, as the coder, audit the patient's medical documentation and compare it to the E/M level on the encounter form. Remember that medical documentation must support codes assigned before you can bill the insurance.

Auditing and Coding E/M Services

When auditing an E/M service, if you find discrepancies between the code that the physician assigned and the patient's medical documentation, you should always review them with the physician. For example, the medical documentation may support a higher level code than the one that the physician assigned, or the documentation may only support a lower level code than the one the physician assigned. When you review E/M services in the CPT manual, notice that many of the codes in a given group are in sequential order (Office or Other Outpatient Services—99201, 99202, 99203, 99204, 99205). For many E/M services, the higher the code number in a given group of codes, the higher the level of service. For example, code 99205 is a higher level than code 99201, just as 99205 is a higher number than 99201. Not all E/M codes in a given group are listed in sequential order, so a higher code number does not necessarily represent a more complex service. Carefully read code descriptors and CPT guidelines to interpret the codes correctly.

You should never change information that the physician documented in the record or alter an encounter form. The physician must make these changes, if appropriate. Once the E/M code is correct and matches the medical documentation, the coder or other employee, such as a billing specialist, enters the E/M visit into the patient's account in the computer system so that the office can bill the patient's insurance.

In larger physician offices or group practices, it may not be feasible for a coder to audit every E/M code that a physician assigns. Coders may instead perform *periodic chart audits* for a group of records to determine coding discrepancies and then provide physician education when needed. Depending on the provider, some physicians do not assign E/M codes. Instead, coders abstract patient medical information to assign E/M codes.

If you understand the processes that the physician must follow to assign E/M codes, then you will be able to identify documentation or code assignment problems and make recommendations for improvements. It is important to have excellent communication skills for successful interactions with physicians and other clinicians. You must also be very sure that you do not make mistakes when comparing documentation to codes assigned, because you have to provide physicians with correct information and recommendations to improve coding and documentation processes.

THREE FACTORS OF E/M SERVICES

Now that we reviewed some background information about E/M coding, let's review the steps that physicians follow to assign E/M codes. The beginning steps are basic because CPT classifies E/M services by three broad factors. Before the physician assigns an E/M code, he must first review the three factors to determine the place of service, type of service, and the patient's status:

1. **Place of service**—location of the facility where the physician provides an E/M service, such as an office, hospital, or nursing home

2. **Type of service**—specific service the physician provides, such as an office visit, consultation, hospital admission, hospital discharge, initial (first) service, or subsequent (following the first) service

3. **Patient status**—type of patient the physician treats, such as new patient, established patient, inpatient, or outpatient

Recall the following terms from earlier chapters, which will help you to better understand patient status:

- *New patient*—a patient who has not received any professional services within the past three years from the physician or another physician of the same specialty or subspecialty who belongs to the same group practice

- *Established patient*—a patient who has received professional services within the past three years from the physician or another physician of the same specialty or subspecialty who belongs to the same group practice

- *Inpatient*—a patient who is typically hospitalized for more than 24 hours, but it can be less

- *Outpatient*—a patient who returns home or to another facility the same day after receiving a service or procedure at a hospital or another provider; an outpatient is also a patient admitted for observation or an ED patient.

CPT divides the E/M section into categories representing the place or type of service, such as office visits, hospital visits, and consultations. Most categories further divide into two or more subcategories of E/M services, including the patient's status.

For example, the Office or Other Outpatient Services category is divided into two subcategories, New Patient and Established Patient. Hospital Inpatient Services is a category that is divided into subcategories, Initial Hospital Care and Subsequent Hospital Care. Note that the categories and subcategories of the E/M section differ from classifications that you learned in Chapter 17, including subsection, subheading, and category. Turn to the E/M section in your CPT manual to review classifications outlined in ■ TABLE 19-1 and find the services listed under each category or subcategory. Then identify the three factors of E/M services as you read them in the code descriptors—place of service, type of service, and patient status. In Table 19-1, categories appear in bold, and subcategories are italicized. You can find the same information in the table of contents before the E/M guidelines in your CPT manual.

You can find E/M services in the index by searching under *Evaluation and Management*, and then the subterm for the category, such as *Critical Care* (■ FIGURE 19-1). Notice

■ **TABLE 19-1   CATEGORIES AND SUBCATEGORIES OF E/M SERVICES**

Categories and Subcategories of E/M Services	Code Range
Office or Other Outpatient Services	**99201–99215**
New Patient	99201–99205
Established Patient	99211–99215
Hospital Observation Services	**99217–99226**
Observation Care Discharge Services	99217
Initial Observation Care—New or Established Patient	99218–99220
Subsequent Observation Care	99224–99226
Hospital Inpatient Services	**99221–99239**
Initial Hospital Care—New or Established Patient	99221–99223
Subsequent Hospital Care	99231–99239
Observation or Inpatient Care Services (Including Admission and Discharge Services)	99234–99236
Hospital Discharge Services	99238–99239
Consultations	**99241–99255**
Office or Other Outpatient Consultations—New or Established Patient	99241–99245
Inpatient Consultations—New or Established Patient	99251–99255
Emergency Department Services—New or Established Patient	**99281–99288**
Other Emergency Services	99288
Critical Care Services	**99291–99292**
Nursing Facility Services	**99304–99318**
Initial Nursing Facility Care—New or Established Patient	99304–99306
Subsequent Nursing Facility Care	99307–99310
Nursing Facility Discharge Services	99315–99316
Other Nursing Facility Services	99318
Domiciliary, Rest Home (e.g., Boarding Home), or Custodial Care Services	**99324–99337**
New Patient	99324–99328
Established Patient	99334–99337
Domiciliary, Rest Home (e.g., Assisted Living Facility), or Home Care Plan Oversight Services	**99339–99340**
Home Services	**99341–99350**
New Patient	99341–99345
Established Patient	99347–99350
Prolonged Services	**99354–99365**
With Direct (Face-to-Face) Patient Contact	99354–99357
Without Direct (Face-to-Face) Patient Contact	99358–99359
Physician Standby Services	99360–99365
Case Management Services	**99363–99368**
Anticoagulant Management	99363–99365
Medical Team Conferences—With or Without Direct (Face-to-Face) Contact With Patient and/or Family	99366–99368

continued

■ TABLE 19-1 *continued*

Categories and Subcategories of E/M Services	Code Range
Care Plan Oversight Services	**99374–99380**
Preventive Medicine Services	**99381–99429**
New Patient	99381–99387
Established Patient	99391–99397
Counseling Risk Factor Reduction and Behavior Change Intervention	99401–99429
New or Established Patient	99401–99412
Other Preventive Medicine Services	99420–99429
Non-Face-to-Face Physician Services	**99441–99444**
Telephone Services	99441–99443
On-Line Medical Evaluation	99444
Special Evaluation and Management Services	**99450–99456**
Basic Life and/or Disability Evaluation Services	99450
Work-Related or Medical Disability Evaluation Services	99455–99456
Newborn Care Services	**99460–99465**
Delivery/Birthing Room Attendance and Resuscitation Services	99464–99465
Inpatient Neonatal Intensive Care Services and Pediatric and Neonatal Critical Care Services	**99466–99480**
Pediatric Critical Care Patient Transport	99466–99467
Inpatient Neonatal and Pediatric Critical Care	99468–99476
Initial and Continuing Intensive Care Services	99477–99480
Other Evaluation and Management Services (unlisted E/M service)	**99499**

Figure 19-1 ■ Index entry for Evaluation and Management services.

Another entry for Evaluation →	**Evaluation**
	Aneurysm Pressure 93982
	Cine 74230
	Treatment 92526
	Video 74230
E/M entry →	Evaluation and Management
	Assistive Technology
	Assessment 97755
	Athletic Training
	Evaluation 97005
	Re-evaluation 97006
	Basic Life and/or Disability Evaluation
	Services 99450
	Care Plan Oversight Services 99339-99340, 99374-99380
	Home Health Agency Care 99374
	Home or Rest Home Care 99339-99340
	Hospice 99377-99378
	Nursing Facility 99379-99380
	Case Management Services 99366-99368
	Consultation 99241-99255
	Critical Care 99291-99292
	Interfacility Pediatric
	Transport 99466-99467

in Figure 19-1 that there are other main terms for *Evaluation,* so be sure to find *Evaluation and Management* to begin your search. You can also search for categories as main terms, like *Office and/or Other Outpatient Services* or *Hospital Services.*

E/M Levels

You learned about the three factors, categories, and subcategories of E/M services. Once the physician determines each of the three factors, he can then review medical documentation to choose an E/M level. This process can be detailed and difficult because the physician has to review documentation and compare it to E/M guidelines for choosing the correct level of service. We will review these steps and guidelines throughout this chapter. Let's first review some general information about E/M code levels.

Codes in ranges for specific categories or subcategories are higher if the E/M level of service is more complex, where the physician performs more work during the service. Turn to the E/M section of codes in your CPT manual. Notice the codes listed for place of service category Office or Other Outpatient Services, subcategory New Patient. Codes range from 99201 to 99205. Code 99201 represents the lowest level in the range, and code 99205 represents the highest. The amount of physician work involved in a service determines the code level. Physician work includes

- Discussing the patient's current condition and/or symptoms
- Obtaining and reviewing the patient's past medical, family, and social history
- Examining the patient, which could involve several organ systems and body areas
- Reviewing and interpreting test results and/or additional medical documentation
- Assessing and diagnosing the patient
- Recommending treatment options
- Determining follow-up visits or additional services needed

The nature and amount of physician work varies according to the place of service, type of service, and patient status. Levels of E/M services are not interchangeable across categories or subcategories. For example, code 99201, the first level of Office or Other Outpatient Services for New Patient, is not interchangeable with code 99211, the first level of Office or Other Outpatient Services for Established Patient.

TAKE A BREAK

Let's take a break and then review more about E/M services.

Exercise 19.1   Evaluation and Management Coding; Three Factors of E/M Services

Instructions: On the line preceding each statement, write T for True or F for False.

1. _____ Only physicians can assign E/M codes.

2. _____ Physicians provide E/M services in many different locations, including an outpatient office or clinic, inpatient hospital, and ED.

3. _____ When a physician provides E/M services outside the office, the facility where the physician sees the patient typically bills for the patient's services.

4. _____ CPT classifies E/M services by three broad factors: place of service, type of service, and length of service.

5. _____ The nature and amount of physician work varies according to the place of service, type of service, and patient status.

6. _____ Levels of E/M services are not interchangeable across categories or subcategories.

EVALUATION AND MANAGEMENT DOCUMENTATION

Medical record documentation is required to record pertinent facts, findings, and observations about an individual's health history, including past and present illnesses, examinations, tests, treatments, and outcomes. Assigning E/M levels to patients' encounters is a complex process that requires physicians to document medical information accurately, clearly, and completely. You previously learned that clear and concise medical record documentation is critical to providing patients with quality care. An appropriately documented medical record reduces claims processing problems, errors, and denials. It also serves as a legal document to verify care provided to the patient. Medical documentation should accurately identify the following:

- place of service
- medical necessity and appropriateness of the diagnostic and/or therapeutic services provided
- all services provided, and body areas examined and tested

Medical record documentation also

- chronologically reports the care a physician rendered to a patient
- assists physicians and other health care professionals to evaluate and plan the patient's immediate treatment and monitor the patient's health care over time
- helps physicians and other healthcare professionals to communicate and ensure continuity of care for the patient
- allows for accurate and timely claims review and payment
- ensures appropriate utilization review and evaluation of the quality of care
- enables collection of data that may be useful for research and education

1995 and 1997 Documentation Guidelines for E/M Services

CMS and AMA created guidelines for physicians to follow when documenting and determining the level of patients' E/M services. They developed the first set of guidelines in 1995 and revised them in 1997. The 1995 guidelines are more general, and the 1997 guidelines provide greater specificity for E/M services for medical specialties. Both the 1995 and 1997 guidelines share many of the same criteria for choosing E/M codes.

Physicians can follow *either* the 1995 or 1997 guidelines to assign an E/M code, rather than a combination of both sets of guidelines. Payers review claims with E/M services using guidelines that the physician follows for *either* 1995 or 1997. In this chapter, you will learn more about *both* sets of guidelines, but you will use 1995 guidelines to determine the level of an E/M code. You can find directions for accessing both sets of guidelines in Appendix A of this text. It is important to note that individual payers may have variations of the guidelines that they require for E/M documentation, so it is always best to verify guidelines with each payer.

Principles of Documentation

Providers should ensure that medical record documentation for all E/M services is appropriate. The following are principles of documentation from the 1995 E/M guidelines:

1. The medical record should be complete and legible.
2. The documentation of each patient encounter should include
   - The reason for the encounter and relevant history, physical examination findings, and prior diagnostic test results
   - An assessment, clinical impression, or diagnosis
   - A medical plan of care
   - The date and legible identity of the provider
3. If the physician does not document the reason for ordering diagnostic tests and other services, then the person reading the record should be able to find the rationale somewhere within the documentation.
4. The treating and/or consulting physician should be able to easily access past and present diagnoses.

5. The physician should identify appropriate health risk factors.

6. The physician should document the patient's progress, response to treatment, and changes in treatment, and document a revised diagnosis when appropriate.

7. The medical documentation should support the diagnosis and procedure codes that the provider reports on the health insurance claim form.

In addition, in order to maintain an accurate medical record, the physician should document services during the patient's encounter or as soon as possible after the encounter to avoid forgetting to document any information.

E/M GUIDELINES IN CPT

The E/M section in CPT contains guidelines for assigning E/M levels, which you should read to become familiar with common terms and factors for choosing various levels. You can find additional guidelines within categories and subcategories in the E/M section to help you correctly choose codes. Some common terms include the following:

- *Chief complaint*—A **chief complaint** is a brief statement in the patient's words, documented in the record, that describes the patient's symptom(s), problem(s), condition(s), or reason(s) for the encounter.

- *Concurrent care*—Concurrent care is when different physicians provide similar care to the same patient on the same day, as with some hospitalized patients who receive treatment from more than one physician.

- *Transfer of care*—The physician treating the patient and managing care transfers care to another physician; transfer of care is not a *consultation* (a physician's opinion about a patient's condition, which we will cover later in this chapter).

- *Counseling*—The physician discusses and educates a patient and/or family regarding test results, the patient's prognosis (future), benefits and risks of treatment options, treatment instructions, follow-up services needed, and how to reduce the risk of developing a condition or problem.

- *Family history*—The physician reviews health status information about a patient's family, including diseases, causes of death, and any hereditary factors that could pose a health risk to the patient.

- *History of present illness*—The physician documents the chronological progression of a patient's illness, from the time it began to the present.

You can also refer to the E/M tables in the Professional Edition of the CPT manual, which will help you to assign E/M codes.

TAKE A BREAK

Good job! Let's take a break and then review more about E/M documentation and guidelines.

Exercise 19.2 Evaluation and Management Documentation, E/M Guidelines in CPT

Instructions: Fill in each blank with the best answer.

1. Medical documentation should accurately identify _____ and _____ of the diagnostic and/or therapeutic services provided.

2. The 1995 guidelines are more _____, and the 1997 guidelines provide greater _____ for E/M services for medical specialties.

3. The documentation of each patient encounter should include the _____ for the encounter and relevant history, physical examination findings, and prior diagnostic test results.

4. _____ is a brief statement in the patient's words, documented in the record, that describes the patient's symptom(s), problem(s), condition(s), or reason(s) for the encounter.

5. _____ occurs when the physician treating the patient passes care on to another physician.

6. CMS and the AMA developed the _____ and the _____ guidelines for assigning E/M codes.

SEVEN COMPONENTS OF E/M SERVICES

E/M services are complex to code because they contain many different components, or parts, which each represent different information that the physician obtains during the E/M service. ■ TABLE 19-2 shows the seven components of an E/M service, including three key components: history, examination, and medical decision-making, and four contributing components: counseling, coordination of care, nature of presenting problem, and time. Each of the three key components is divided into four types, depending on the complexity of the service and the physician work performed.

You can find types of the three key components in the code descriptors for many of the E/M services. You will also see the number of key components that must be present in the service to assign the code. An average time is identified for many services, and time is a contributing component (■ FIGURE 19-2).

Three Key Components

Three key components—history, examination, and medical decision-making—are the main classifications of information that physicians use to determine an E/M level and code. Each key component is divided into four different types (Table 19-2) based on the complexity of a service. Before a physician can choose an E/M code, he must first review the patient's medical documentation to determine the *type* of each of the three key components. Remember from earlier in the chapter that the physician also needs to consider the place of service, type of service, and/or patient status before choosing an E/M code.

■ TABLE 19-2   **SEVEN COMPONENTS OF E/M SERVICES**

Three Key Components	
History—Four Types: • *Problem-focused* • *Expanded problem-focused* • *Detailed* • *Comprehensive*	Subjective information that the patient provides, including four elements: 1. Chief complaint 2. History of present illness 3. Review of systems 4. Past, family, and/or social history
Examination—Four Types: • *Problem-focused* • *Expanded problem-focused* • *Detailed* • *Comprehensive*	Objective information that the physician finds during the examination of specific body areas and/or organ systems.
Medical Decision-Making—Four Types: • *Straightforward* • *Low* • *Moderate* • *High*	The physician renders a diagnosis and makes recommendations for treatment. Medical decision-making includes reviewing and analyzing the • number of possible diagnoses and/or number of management options • amount and/or complexity of medical records, diagnostic tests, and/or other information • risk of significant complications, morbidity, and/or mortality, and comorbidities

Four Contributing Components	
Counseling	The physician provides counseling to a patient and/or family members regarding the patient's diagnosis, treatment, and follow-up.
Coordination of Care	The physician coordinates the patient's care with other healthcare providers or agencies.
Nature of Presenting Problem	A symptom, complaint, condition, illness, disease, sign, finding, or injury that represents the reason for the patient's encounter.
Time	Face-to-face time the physician spends with the patient for office or other outpatient services, and unit/floor time for hospital and other inpatient services.

99203	Number of key components needed to assign code →	Office or other outpatient visit for the evaluation and management of a new patient, which requires these 3 key components:	
		• A detailed history; • A detailed examination; and • Medical decision making of low complexity.	←Key components
		Counseling and/or coordination of care with other providers or agencies are provided consistent with the nature of the problem(s) and the patient's and/or family's needs.	←Contributing components
		Usually, the presenting problem(s) are of moderate severity. Physicians typically spend 30 minutes face-to-face with the patient and/or family.	←Contributing components

Figure 19-2 ■ Description for code 99203 from the CPT manual.

Turn to the E/M section in your CPT manual to review the types of key components. Refer to the category Office or Other Outpatient Services (place of service), subcategory New Patient (patient status). Notice the types of the three key components for code 99201: problem-focused history, problem-focused examination, and straightforward medical decision-making. These are the lowest types of the three key components. Now review the types for code 99205: comprehensive history, comprehensive examination, and medical decision-making of high complexity. These are the highest types of the three key components. Note that the higher the E/M code, the higher the types of the three key components.

Four Contributing Components

The three key components make up each E/M service *except* when counseling and/or coordination of care represent more than 50% of the total visit time, or the 50% rule. This exception is when you should consider contributing components, counseling, coordination of care, nature of presenting problem, and time, rather than key components, to choose an E/M code. You will review more about contributing components later in this chapter. You will next learn processes for determining each type of the three key components.

TAKE A BREAK

Let's take a break and then review the seven components of E/M services.

Exercise 19.3   Seven Components of E/M Services

Instructions: Fill in each blank with the best answer.

1. Each of the three key components is divided into four types, depending on the _____ of the service and the physician work performed.

2. The key component of _____ describes subjective information that the patient provides.

3. The key component of _____ describes objective information that the physician finds during the assessment of specific body areas and/or organ systems.

4. In the key component of _____, the physician renders a diagnosis and makes recommendations for treatment.

5. The four contributing components are _____ _____.

6. The three key components make up each E/M service except for E/M services when counseling and/or coordination of care represent more than _____ of the total visit time.

HISTORY

History is the first of the three key components of an E/M service. The patient's **history** consists of *subjective* information that the patient provides to the physician and other clinicians, which can be verbal and may come from the patient's health history form. Remember from Chapter 1 that the health history form is where the patient lists information about his current and past medical, family, and social history, including allergies and current medications (Figure 1-8). Even if another clinician, such as the medical assistant, records part of the patient's history in the medical record, the physician must still review the information for accuracy and may also validate the information with the patient. The physician documents in the record that he reviewed the information and confirmed it, and he also provides any additional documentation.

The purpose of the history is for the physician to obtain information about the patient's current condition and overall health so that he will know where to focus his attention for the examination and assessment (medical decision-making). There are four types of history that you will see when you review many E/M services:

- Problem-focused
- Expanded problem-focused
- Detailed
- Comprehensive

The complexity of the history that the physician reviews, and the amount of information that he documents in the record, determines the type of history assigned. The lowest history type, problem-focused, is the least complex and requires the least amount of documentation. The highest history type, comprehensive history, is the most complex and requires the most documentation. In order to choose the type of history, you must review the *history elements* that the physician documents in the patient's record. A physician may document information about some or all of the elements of history, depending on the individual patient's case.

The history consists of *four elements*: **chief complaint (CC)**, history of present illness (HPI), review of systems (ROS), and past family and/or social history (PFSH). Three of the elements, HPI, ROS, and PFSH, are divided into specific types, or levels, according to the amount and complexity of information that the physician reviews and documents. The four elements and types are as follows:

1. CC
2. HPI (8 elements)—*Two types:*
   - Brief
   - Extended
3. ROS (14 body systems)—*Three types:*
   - Problem-pertinent
   - Extended
   - Complete
4. PFSH—*Two types:*
   - Pertinent
   - Complete

Next, you will review more about each of the four elements.

Chief Complaint

The CC is the first element of a patient's history. A CC is a concise statement that describes the patient's symptom, problem, condition, diagnosis, or reason for the patient encounter. The patient usually states the CC in his own words. Examples of chief complaints are an

■ TABLE 19-3   **HPI ELEMENTS**

HPI Element	Question to Ask the Patient	Examples
1. Location	*Where is the problem/condition located?*	left leg, stomach, elbow, head
2. Quality	*Can you describe how the condition feels?*	aching, burning, radiating pain, raw, itching
3. Severity	*What is the level of sensation or pain on a scale of 1 to 10, with 1 being the least severe and 10 being the most severe?*	10 on a pain scale of 1 to 10
4. Duration	*How long have you had the condition; when did it begin?*	started three days ago; condition has lasted two weeks
5. Timing	*When does the condition occur?*	constant, or comes and goes
6. Context	*Does the condition appear when you are engaging in a certain activity or at a certain time of the day?*	pain occurs when lifting large objects at work; pain is worse upon awakening
7. Modifying factors	*What factors improve or worsen the condition?*	pain decreases when heat is applied; pain increases when standing up
8. Associated signs and symptoms	*Are there any other problems that occur along with the condition?*	numbness in toes also occurs with leg pain

upset stomach, aching joints, sore throat, or constant fatigue. The physician or another clinician documents the CC in the patient's record.

History of Present Illness

The HPI, the second element of a patient's history, is a chronological description of the development of the patient's present illness from the first sign and/or symptom, or from the previous encounter to the present encounter. Physicians can document *eight HPI elements* for patients' conditions. Physicians obtain information about the history of present illness from the patient's health history form, from documentation in the record that another clinician recorded (like the medical assistant), and by asking the patient questions about his condition. Physicians must also document on the health history form that they reviewed it. Each patient's case is different, so physicians do not document all of the HPI elements for every patient. ■ TABLE 19-3 lists the eight HPI elements, along with questions that the physician can ask the patient about each element.

There are *two types* of the HPI, brief or extended, depending on the total number of HPI elements that the physician documents:

- *Brief HPI*—includes documentation of one to three HPI elements

> **Example:** Patient complains of a dull earache pain (CC) lasting for 24 hours. This example is a brief HPI that contains *three* HPI elements: location (ear), quality (dull pain), and duration (24 hours).

- *Extended HPI*—describes four or more HPI elements or associated comorbidities (other conditions that contribute to the condition)

> **Example:** Patient complains of a dull earache pain (CC) lasting for 24 hours. Patient states that the pain began after he went swimming two days ago. Symptoms are somewhat relieved by warm compress and ibuprofen. This example of an extended HPI contains *five* HPI elements: location (ear), quality (dull pain), duration (24 hours), context (happened while swimming), and modifying factors (pain relief with warm compress and ibuprofen).

TAKE A BREAK

Wow! That was a lot of information to absorb! Let's take a break and then review more about history, including the first two elements—CC and HPI.

Exercise 19.4 History—Chief Complaint and History of Present Illness

Instructions: On the line preceding each statement, write T for True or F for False.

1. _____ If another clinician records part of the patient's history in the medical record, then the physician does not need to review the information.

2. _____ The HPI is a chronological description of the development of the patient's past health experiences.

3. _____ There are three types of the HPI depending on the total number of HPI elements that the physician documents: Brief, Problem-Focused, and Extended.

4. _____ The HPI element of location asks the question, *Where is the problem/condition located?*

5. _____ The HPI element of severity asks the question, *How long have you had the condition; when did it begin?*

6. _____ The HPI element of modifying factors asks the question, *Are there any other problems that occur along with the condition?*

Review of Systems

An ROS, the third element of a history, occurs when the physician reviews information about the patient's body systems by asking the patient a series of questions to identify past or current signs and/or symptoms. *The ROS is not the physician's examination of the patient.* Like the HPI, physicians obtain information related to the review of systems from the patient's health history form and by asking the patient questions about his condition. Physicians must also document their review of the health history form.

There are 14 body systems listed under the ROS, and the total number that the physician reviews depends on the patient's condition(s). Physicians can document positive responses within a body system when the patient admits to having a specific problem, using the phrase "positive for." They can document negative responses within a body system when the patient states that he does not have a specific problem, using phrases such as "patient denies" or "negative for." The 14 body systems in the ROS, along with examples of signs and symptoms that the physician documents, are as follows:

1. *Constitutional Symptoms*—symptoms that affect the entire body, including fever, vomiting, chills, and weight loss

2. *Eyes (ophthalmology)*—vision changes (double vision, blurred vision), corrective lenses, pain, flashing lights, floaters, cataract, glaucoma, infection, redness, inflammation, frequency of eye exams

3. *Ears, Nose, Mouth, Throat (otorhinolaryngology)*
   - *Ears*—deafness, hearing loss, tinnitus, dizziness, pain, discharge
   - *Nose and sinuses*—pain, discharge, **epistaxis,** inflammation, infection, obstructive breathing
   - *Mouth and throat*—tooth pain, swelling, sore throat, dental caries, gum problems, hoarseness, redness, dysphagia, frequency of dental exams

4. *Cardiovascular*—chest pain, palpitations, tachycardia, bradycardia, hypertension, dizziness, difficulty exercising, edema of extremities

5. *Respiratory*—chest pain, shortness of breath, coughing (sputum, blood), dyspnea, wheezing, asthma, emphysema

epistaxis (ep-i-stak′sis)— bleeding from the nose

6. *Gastrointestinal*—appetite, dietary habits, change in bowel habits, nausea, vomiting, diarrhea, indigestion, **flatus**, hemorrhoids, constipation, melena

7. *Genitourinary*

   • *Genital tract (female)*—menstrual periods (frequency, flow, pain), discomfort, discharge, contraception, pain, pregnancies, abortions, lesions, **venereal** disease, menopause, frequency of Pap smears

   • *Genital tract (male)*—pain, discomfort, discharge, lesions, venereal disease, hernia

   • *Urinary*—**hematuria**, dysuria, nocturia, incontinence, changes to urine frequency or color, infection

8. *Musculoskeletal*—joint or muscle pain, discomfort, edema, deformity, functional limitations, **crepitus**, redness, arthritis, cramps

9. *Integumentary (skin and/or breast)*—pain, laceration, lesion, bruise, discoloration, edema, moles, ulcers, dryness, scaling, breast lump, nipple discharge

10. *Neurological*—loss of memory, disorientation, syncope, seizures, stroke, **hemiplegia, hemiparesis**

11. *Psychiatric*—disorientation, depression, mood swings, anxiety, loss of memory, phobias (irrational fears), sleep habits, personality changes

12. *Endocrine*—polyuria, polydipsia, polyphagia, sensitivity to hot or cold, **goiter, exophthalmos**

13. *Hematologic/Lymphatic*—swollen or painful lymph nodes, fatigue, anemia, bruises

14. *Allergic/Immunologic*—sensitivity to substances, foods, environmental factors, frequency of illness, sneezing, itching, watery eyes, skin redness or lesions

There are *three types of an ROS*, depending on the total number of body systems that the physician reviews and documents:

• *Problem-pertinent*—1 system

• *Extended*—2 to 9 systems

• *Complete*—10 or more systems

Problem-pertinent ROS—The physician asks the patient about the system directly related to the problem identified in the HPI and then documents related symptoms and signs.

> **Example:** The patient's CC is an earache. The ROS is positive for left ear pain. The patient denies tinnitus or a feeling of fullness in the ear. In this example, the physician reviews one system, the ear.

Extended ROS—The physician asks the patient about the system that is directly related to the problem(s) identified in the HPI and also asks about additional systems, for a review of a total of *two to nine* systems. The physician documents symptoms and signs related to each system.

> **Example:** The patient's CC (reason for the encounter) is a follow-up visit after a cardiac catheterization. The patient states, "I feel great." The patient denies chest pain, syncope, palpitations, and shortness of breath. In this example, the physician reviews two systems, cardiovascular, and respiratory.

Complete ROS—The physician asks the patient about the system(s) directly related to the problem(s) identified in the HPI and also asks about a *minimum of 10 additional* systems. The physician then documents symptoms and signs related to each system.

---

flatus (flāt'əs)—gas in the stomach or intestines

venereal (və-nēr'e-əl)—transmitted through sexual contact

hematuria (hem-ə-tu're-ə)—blood in the urine

crepitus (krep'ĭ-təs)—discharge of gas from the anus

hemiplegia (hem-e-ple'jə)—paralysis affecting only one side of the body

hemiparesis (hem-e-pə-re'sis)—weakness or partial paralysis affecting only one side of the body

goiter (goi'tər)—enlargement of the thyroid gland with edema in the front of the neck

exophthalmos (ek-sof-thal'mos)—abnormal bulging of the eyeball

In a complete ROS, the physician must document the patient's positive or negative responses for problems or conditions within each body system. The physician is permitted to document in the patient's record, "all other systems are negative" without individually documenting that each additional system is negative.

Example: The patient's CC is having a "fainting spell." The ROS includes the following:

- *Urinary:* Denies incontinence, frequency, urgency, nocturia, pain, or discomfort.
- *Constitutional:* Weight is stable, positive for fatigue.
- *Eyes:* Positive for loss of peripheral vision.
- *Ear, Nose, Mouth, Throat:* No complaints.
- *Cardiovascular:* Positive for palpitations; denies chest pain; denies calf pain, pressure, or edema.
- *Respiratory:* Positive for shortness of breath on exertion.
- *Gastrointestinal:* Appetite good, denies heartburn and indigestion. Positive for episodes of nausea. Bowel movement daily; denies constipation or loose stools.
- *Skin:* Positive for clammy, moist skin.
- *Neurological:* Positive for fainting; denies numbness, tingling, and tremors.
- *Psychiatric:* Denies memory loss or depression. Mood is pleasant.

In this example, the physician reviews 10 body systems and documents related signs and symptoms.

Past, Family, and/or Social History

PFSH is the fourth and final element of a history. It consists of a review of three areas of the patient's history:

1. *Past medical history*—includes the patient's experiences with illnesses, surgeries, injuries and treatments, current medications, and allergies.
2. *Family medical history*—includes the health history of family members (parents, siblings, children), such as diseases or conditions they have or had, including the patient's current problem(s) and if family members are living or deceased; also includes a review of medical hereditary conditions that may place the patient at risk for developing specific conditions.
3. *Social history*—includes an age-appropriate review of the patient's past and current activities, such as occupation, education, marital status, smoking, drinking alcohol, and drug use.

The two types of PFSH, pertinent and complete, depend on the amount of information that the physician documents:

- *Pertinent PFSH* This type of PFSH reviews the PFSH areas that are directly related to the problem(s) identified in the HPI. The physician must document *at least one* item from any of the three history areas.

Example: The patient's HPI is coronary artery disease. The PFSH includes a coronary artery bypass graft in 1992. Recent cardiac catheterization demonstrates 50% occlusion of a vein graft to the **obtuse marginal artery**. In this example of a pertinent PFSH, the physician reviews one history area, past medical history, including surgical history related to the HPI.

obtuse marginal artery (äb-tüs' mahr'jin-el ahr'tə-re)—an artery along the left edge of the heart

- *Complete PFSH*—This type of PFSH reviews *two or all three* of the PFSH areas, depending on the category of the E/M service. Some E/M services require the physician to review two history areas, while other E/M services require the physician to review three history areas to qualify for a complete PFSH.

Example: The patient's HPI is congestive heart failure.

Past medical history reveals the following information:

- The patient was diagnosed with diabetes five years ago.
- The patient was diagnosed with congestive heart failure three months ago.
- The patient was in a motor vehicle accident 10 years ago, suffering a lacerated cornea and multiple pelvic fractures. Treatment included five eye surgeries.

Family history reveals the following information:

- Maternal grandparents—Both were positive for congestive heart failure; grandfather deceased at age 69 due to congestive heart failure; grandmother is age 72, living.
- Paternal grandparents—Grandmother is positive for diabetes, hypertension, age 68, living; grandfather was positive for a heart attack at age 55, living.
- Parents—Mother is positive for obesity, diabetes, age 51, living; father was positive for a heart attack at age 51, deceased at age 57 of heart attack.
- Siblings—Sister is positive for diabetes, obesity, hypertension, age 39, living; brother was positive for a heart attack at age 45, living.

Social history reveals the following information:

- Patient has worked as a laborer for the past 25 years, which requires heavy lifting. Patient smokes a pack of cigarettes a week, and drinks beer at least once a week.

In this example of a complete PFSH, the physician reviews all three PFSH areas—the patient's past medical, family, and social histories.

The physician must document at least one specific item from *two of the three PFSH areas* for a complete PFSH for the following categories of E/M services:

- Office or Other Outpatient Services, Established Patient
- Emergency Department Services
- Nursing Facility Services, Subsequent Nursing Facility Care
- Domiciliary, Rest Home, or Custodial Care Services, Established Patient
- Home Services, Established Patient

The physician must document at least one specific item from *each of the three PFSH areas* for a complete PFSH for the following categories of E/M services:

- Office or Other Outpatient Services, New Patient
- Hospital Observation Services
- Hospital Inpatient Services, Initial Hospital Care
- Nursing Facility Services, comprehensive assessments
- Domiciliary, Rest Home, or Custodial Care Services, New Patient
- Home Services, New Patient

TAKE A BREAK

Good job! Now hang in there because you are making great progress! Let's take a break and then review the third and fourth history elements, ROS and PFSH.

Exercise 19.5 Review of Systems, Past, Family, and/or Social History

Instructions: Fill in each blank with the best answer.

1. The ROS is not the physician's _____ of the patient.

2. Physicians can document *negative responses* within a body system when the patient states that he does not have a specific problem, using phrases such as _____ or _____.

3. _____ symptoms affect the entire body, including fever, vomiting, chills, and weight loss.

4. In a(n) _____ ROS, the physician asks the patient about the system that is directly related to the problem(s) identified in the HPI and also asks about additional systems, for a review of a total of two to nine systems.

5. _____ history includes an age-appropriate review of the patient's past and current activities, such as occupation, education, marital status, smoking, alcohol use, and drug use.

6. The physician must document at least one specific item from _____ PFSH areas for a complete PFSH for Office or Other Outpatient Services, Established Patient.

Summary of History

You learned about each of the four history elements and that three of the elements have additional types, depending on the amount of medical documentation for the patient. To review, the history elements are as follows:

1. CC
2. HPI (8 elements)—*Two types:*
   - Brief
   - Extended
3. ROS (14 body systems)—*Three types:*
   - Problem-pertinent
   - Extended
   - Complete
4. PFSH—*Two types:*
   - Pertinent
   - Complete

After you review medical documentation to determine the *number* of history elements the physician documents, you can then determine each type of history. Once you know each type of history, you can determine the history level, or type, for the E/M service. The levels are as follows, from the lowest type to the highest:

- Problem-focused
- Expanded problem-focused
- Detailed
- Comprehensive

■ TABLE 19-4 lists elements required for each history type. The number of elements that the physician reviews depends on each patient's case. Note that as the history type

■ TABLE 19-4 **TYPE OF HISTORY AND REQUIRED ELEMENTS**

Type of History	CC	HPI	ROS	PFSH
Problem-focused	Required	Brief (1–3 elements)	N/A	N/A
Expanded problem-focused	Required	Brief (1–3 elements)	Problem-pertinent (current problem = 1 system)	N/A
Detailed	Required	Extended (4+ elements)	Extended (current problem and additional systems—total of 2–9 systems)	Pertinent (1 area)
Comprehensive	Required	Extended (4+ elements)	Complete (current problem and additional systems—total of 10 or more systems)	Complete (2–3 areas)

becomes more complex, the elements that are required to meet the type of history also become more complex. *Choose the history type according to the lowest type of history that the physician documents in the medical record.* For example, if the HPI is problem-focused, the ROS is expanded problem-focused, and the PFSH is not applicable, assign problem-focused as the history type, the lowest type documented.

Additional Points on History Documentation

Review the following guidelines for additional information on documenting the patient's history:

1. The physician may list the CC, ROS, and PFSH as separate elements of history or he can include them in the description of the history of the present illness.

2. If the physician obtained an ROS and/or PFSH during an earlier encounter, then he does not need to record them again if he reviews and updates the previous information. This situation may occur when a physician updates his own record or in an institutional setting or group practice where many physicians use a common record. The review and update may be documented by

   • Describing any new ROS and/or PFSH information or noting there has been no change in the information; and

   • Noting the date and location of the earlier ROS and/or PFSH.

3. If the physician is unable to obtain a history from the patient or other source (such as family), then the physician should describe the patient's condition or other circumstance and note why there is no history documented.

WORKPLACE IQ

You are working as a coder at Williton Medical Center in the Health Information Management (HIM) department. Today, your manager asks you to prepare documentation on E/M Critical Care Services to help educate two new coders. She asks you to address the following issues by researching the E/M CPT guidelines for Critical Care Services and then explain your findings to the coders:

1. Definition of critical care
2. Definition of a critical illness or injury
3. Two codes used for critical care
4. How to determine which services are part of critical care

What would you do?

TAKE A BREAK

Let's take a break and then practice what you learned so far about a patient's history.

Exercise 19.6 **Summary of History, Additional Points on History Documentation**

Instructions: Review each patient's case to determine the type of HPI, ROS, and PFSH that applies. Then identify the history type. Use the information outlined in this section and in Tables 19-3 and 19-4 to help you.

1. Mrs. Walker, a 35-year-old new patient, sees Dr. Hoffman with a chief complaint of a sore throat that started three days ago. She describes the pain as "raw" and says it is worse when she wakes in the morning and at bedtime. The patient is positive for fever and denies any other symptoms related to her throat pain. Dr. Hoffman reviews the patient's health history form, which includes past medical history, family history, and social history.

   a. Total number and type(s) of HPI elements reviewed: _____

   b. Type of HPI (brief, extended): _____

   c. Total number and type(s) of body systems reviewed: _____

   d. Type of ROS (problem-pertinent, extended, complete): _____

   e. PFSH reviewed: _____

   f. Type of PFSH (pertinent, complete): _____

   g. History type (problem-focused, expanded problem-focused, detailed, comprehensive): _____

2. Established patient Arthur Tapp, age 31, sees Dr. Hoffman with a complaint of low back pain which he has had for the past week. The patient states that he is not aware of anything that he did that initially caused the pain, and this is the first time it occurred. He states that he "was hoping it would get better, but it hasn't." Mr. Tapp describes the pain as "dull and achy," but it sometimes turns into a "sharp stab." The patient also states that he has experienced left leg pain along with the back pain. He states that he tried to use a heating pad, but it does not seem to help and that Tylenol helps a little to relieve the pain. The patient denies joint or muscle pain in his right leg, neck, and arms and denies paralysis in his extremities. He is a manager with a desk job and gets little exercise.

   a. Total number and type(s) of HPI elements reviewed: _____

   b. Type of HPI (brief, extended): _____

   c. Total number and type(s) of body systems reviewed: _____

   d. Type of ROS (problem-pertinent, extended, complete): _____

   e. PFSH reviewed: _____

   f. Type of PFSH (pertinent, complete): _____

   g. History type (problem-focused, expanded problem-focused, detailed, comprehensive): _____

3. Madeline Perkins, age 57, is an established patient with Dr. Hoffman and sees him for a cough and chest congestion that she has had for three days. She states that she "feels worse each morning and decided to come in." She denies fever, nausea, vomiting, and diarrhea. She states that she has a productive cough that is "yellow-greenish" in color and feels "some tightness" in her chest. She does not smoke. She does experience seasonal allergies and is allergic to penicillin.

   a. Total number and type(s) of HPI elements reviewed: _____

   b. Type of HPI (brief, extended): _____

   c. Total number and type(s) of body systems reviewed: _____

   d. Type of ROS (problem-pertinent, extended, complete): _____

   e. PFSH reviewed: _____

   f. Type of PFSH (pertinent, complete): _____

   g. History type (problem-focused, expanded problem-focused, detailed, comprehensive): _____

4. Sandy Scales brings her daughter Robin, age 10, to see Dr. Rosa, an otorhinolaryngologist, after Dr. Hoffman referred her due to chronic tonsillitis. Mrs. Scales

TAKE A BREAK *continued*

states that Robin has had a "sore and swollen throat for several days" and this is the fifth time it has occurred in the past year. The mother also reports that Robin has had a fever, nasal congestion, and runny nose. The patient denies nausea or vomiting. Mrs. Scales says past prescriptions of antibiotics have not seemed to help.

a. Total number and type(s) of HPI elements reviewed: _____

b. Type of HPI (brief, extended): _____ _____

c. Total number and type(s) of body systems reviewed: _____

d. Type of ROS (problem-pertinent, extended, complete): _____

e. PFSH reviewed: _____ _____

f. Type of PFSH (pertinent, complete): _____ _____

g. History type (problem-focused, expanded problem-focused, detailed, comprehensive): _____ _____

EXAMINATION

The **examination** is the second of the three key components of an E/M service. It involves *objective* information that the physician finds during the patient's encounter. Recall that CMS has two versions of the E/M documentation guidelines, 1995 and 1997. You already learned the 1995 guidelines for determining the type of history, and next you will learn about the 1995 guidelines for determining the examination level. The most substantial differences between the 1995 and 1997 versions occur in the examination documentation section; because the 1995 guidelines are not always clear, so providers sometimes have difficulty interpreting them. The 1997 guidelines provide more definitive information for providers to follow. Providers can use either version of the documentation guidelines for documenting E/M services but cannot use a combination of both.

Physicians document examinations based on body areas and/or organ systems that they evaluate through a hands-on exam. The ***body areas*** are as follows:

1. Head, including the face
2. Neck
3. Chest, including breasts and **axillae**

axillae (ak-sil′ə)—the armpits

4. Abdomen
5. Genitalia, groin, and buttocks
6. Back, including spine
7. Each extremity

The ***organ systems*** are as follows:

1. Constitutional (vital signs, general appearance)
2. Eyes (ophthalmologic)
3. Ears, nose, mouth, and throat (otolaryngologic)
4. Cardiovascular
5. Respiratory
6. Gastrointestinal
7. Genitourinary
8. Musculoskeletal
9. Skin (integumentary)
10. Neurologic
11. Psychiatric
12. Hematologic/lymphatic/immunologic

The types of examinations are based on the number of body areas and organ systems that the physician reviews, depending on the complexity level of the patient's case. The more body areas and organ systems reviewed, the higher the type of exam. The four exam types have the same titles as history types, which are as follows:

- **Problem-Focused**—*limited* examination of the affected body area or organ system related to the chief complaint.
- **Expanded Problem-Focused**—*limited* examination of the affected body area or organ system and other symptomatic or related organ system(s). The total exam includes 2–7 organ system(s), including the affected body area(s) or organ system.
- **Detailed**—*extended* examination of the affected body area(s) or organ system and other symptomatic or related organ system(s). The total exam includes 2–7 organ system(s), including the affected body area(s) or organ system.
- **Comprehensive**—general multisystem examination or complete examination of a single organ system. The physician's documentation should include an exam of eight or more of the 12 organ systems.

An examination may involve several organ systems or a single organ system. The type and extent of the examination that the physician performs is based on his clinical judgment, the patient's history, and the nature of the presenting problem(s). Recall that the physician uses the patient's subjective information to determine where and how to focus the examination.

Notice that the exam types include a *limited* exam and *extended* exam. The 1995 guidelines do not define the difference between a limited and extended exam, which can leave providers confused. Think of a limited exam as limited to the patient's chief complaint; the physician only examines organ systems that are related to the chief complaint. An extended exam goes beyond organ systems related to the chief complaint; the physician examines other organ systems that could relate to the chief complaint. Be careful when you are counting organ systems to ensure that you do not count a body area and then count it again as an organ system. For example, if a physician examines a patient's abdomen, then you should not also count the gastrointestinal system.

Review these additional points related to the 1995 guidelines to better understand the information that physicians document for patients' exams:

- The physician should document specific abnormal and relevant negative findings of the examination of the affected or symptomatic body area(s) or organ system(s). Documentation is insufficient if the physician simply states "abnormal" without providing additional information.
- The physician should describe abnormal or unexpected findings of the examination of the unaffected or asymptomatic body area(s) or organ system(s).
- A brief statement or notation indicating "negative" or "normal" is sufficient to document normal findings that are related to unaffected area(s) or asymptomatic organ system(s).
- The medical record for a general multisystem examination should include findings related to eight or more of the 12 organ systems.

Although many payers follow 1995 or 1997 guidelines, some payers may follow E/M documentation guidelines that are different from the 1995 and 1997 guidelines. It is best to check with each payer for additional information. Refer to ■ TABLE 19-5 for a summary of exam types, and then review the example to determine the type of exam.

Example: Mrs. Tillman, a 75-year-old established patient, sees Dr. Hoffman with a chief complaint of a persistent cough and wheezing, which started two days ago. In addition, she complains of an upset stomach, which started about the same time. Dr. Hoffman's exam involves the patient's respiratory system, gastrointestinal system, and constitutional (vital signs).

■ TABLE 19-5   **TYPE OF EXAM AND REQUIRED ELEMENTS**

Type of Exam	Affected Body Area(s) or Organ System(s)	Examination	Total Number of Body Area(s) and Organ System(s) Reviewed
Problem-focused	Required	*limited* examination of the affected body area or organ system related to the chief complaint	1
Expanded problem-focused	Required	*limited* examination of the affected body area or organ system and other symptomatic or related organ system(s)	2–7 organ systems, including affected body area(s) or system(s)
Detailed	Required	*extended* examination of the affected body area(s) or organ system, and other symptomatic or related organ system(s)	2–7 organ systems, including affected body area(s) or system(s)
Comprehensive	Required	general multisystem examination or complete examination of a single organ system	8 or more of the 12 organ systems

In this example, the physician reviewed and documented three systems: respiratory, gastrointestinal, and constitutional. His exam focused on her chief complaints: cough, wheezing, and upset stomach, resulting in a limited exam. Refer to Table 19-5 to review that a limited exam with three body systems qualifies as an expanded problem-focused exam.

TAKE A BREAK

Let's keep going! You have come a long way in learning about the key components! Let's take a break and then assign examination types.

<table><tr><td>Exercise 19.7</td><td>Examination</td></tr></table>

Instructions: Review each patient's case where you previously assigned the history level. Determine the body area(s) or organ system(s) related to the CC, along with additional organ system(s) reviewed. Then assign the type of exam. Use the information outlined in this section and in Table 19-5 to help you.

1. Mrs. Walker, a 35-year-old new patient, sees Dr. Hoffman with a chief complaint of a sore throat that started three days ago. She describes the pain as "raw" and says it is worse when she wakes in the morning and at bedtime. The patient is positive for fever and denies any other symptoms related to her throat pain.

   Dr. Hoffman reviews the patient's health history form, which includes past medical history, family history, and social history. Dr. Hoffman also reviews the patient's vital signs; notes that she has a fever; examines her mouth, and throat, and takes a rapid strep throat culture. He observes white spots on her tonsils and notes that lymph nodes in her neck are swollen. She is negative for any respiratory problems.

a. Body area(s) or organ system(s) related to the chief complaint: _____

b. Total number and type(s) of additional organ system(s) reviewed: _____

c. Type of exam (problem-focused, expanded problem-focused, detailed, comprehensive): _____
   _____

2. Established patient Arthur Tapp, age 31, sees Dr. Hoffman with a complaint of low back pain which he has had for the past week. The patient states that he is not aware of anything that he did that initially caused the pain, and this is the first time it occurred. He states that he "was hoping it would get better, but it hasn't." Mr. Tapp describes the pain as "dull and achy," but it sometimes turns into a "sharp stab." The patient also states that he has experienced left leg pain along with the back pain. He states that he tried to use a heating pad, but it does not seem to help and that Tylenol helps a little to relieve the pain. The patient denies joint or muscle pain in his right leg, neck, and arms and denies paralysis in his extremities. He is a manager with a desk job and gets little exercise.

   During the examination, Dr. Hoffman documents the following information: The lumbar spine is

continued

TAKE A BREAK *continued*

sensitive to palpation (feeling with hands). Reflexes are good. Patient limps when walking. Extremities are negative for edema and redness. Skin is warm and dry. Patient exhibits limited range of motion in the left leg and has limited strength in left leg but no problems in the right leg or either arm. Vision and hearing negative (for problems).

a. Body area(s) or organ system(s) related to the chief complaint: _____

b. Total number and type(s) of additional organ system(s) reviewed: _____

c. Type of exam (problem-focused, expanded problem-focused, detailed, comprehensive): _____

3. Madeline Perkins, age 57, is an established patient with Dr. Hoffman and sees him for a cough and congestion that she has had for three days. She states that she "feels worse each day and decided to come in." She denies fever, nausea, vomiting, or diarrhea. She states that she has a productive cough that is "yellow-greenish" in color and feels "some tightness" in her chest. She does not smoke. She does experience seasonal allergies and is allergic to penicillin.

Upon examination, Dr. Hoffman documents the following information: BP 130/80, temperature 98.5°, pulse 80, respirations 16. Neck is supple and nontender. PERRLA.* Ears, nose, and throat are clear. Breathing is equal, no rales or wheezes. Heart is negative. Abdomen is soft, not tender, bowel sounds in all four quadrants. Skin is warm and dry. Pulses are equal in the extremities.

a. Body area(s) or organ system(s) related to the chief complaint: _____

b. Total number and type(s) of additional organ system(s) reviewed: _____

c. Type of exam (problem-focused, expanded problem-focused, detailed, comprehensive): _____

_____

4. Sandy Scales brings her daughter Robin, age 10, to see Dr. Rosa, an **otorhinolaryngologist**, after Dr. Hoffman referred her due to chronic tonsillitis. Mrs. Scales states that Robin has had a "sore and swollen throat for several days" and this is the fifth time it has happened in the past year. The mother also reports that Robin has had a fever, nasal congestion, and runny nose. The patient denies nausea or vomiting. Mrs. Scales says past prescriptions of antibiotics have not seemed to help.

Dr. Rosa reviews information that the medical assistant documented, including a temperature of 101.9°. Upon examination, Dr. Rosa notes the following information: Swollen cervical lymph nodes and a raw red throat. Negative for any other lymphadenopathy. Ears and nose are clear. Lungs are clear to auscultation. Reflexes are normal.

a. Body area(s) or organ system(s) related to the chief complaint: _____

b. Total number and type(s) of additional organ system(s) reviewed: _____

c. Type of exam (problem-focused, expanded problem-focused, detailed, comprehensive): _____

_____

_____

*PERRLA—Pupils are equal, round, reactive to light and accommodation (able to focus near and far).

POINTERS FROM THE PROS: Interview with a Primary Care Physician

Anthony Colangelo, M.D., specializes in family practice and emergency medicine and has worked as a physician for 25 years.

What do you find the most challenging about obtaining correct insurance reimbursement?

It seems insurance companies deliberately delay payment by repeatedly requesting additional information from the patient and/or physician regarding coordination of benefits (which insurance to bill first) and pre-existing conditions.

What advice can you give to coding students to help them to prepare to work successfully with physicians?

Pay attention to detail, be willing to research a condition or procedure, and keep up with insurance company guidelines to educate staff.

What qualities do you look for when hiring any member of your team?

Flexibility, team player, detail-oriented, and willingness to learn.

(Used by permission of Ellwood Family Medicine.)

MEDICAL DECISION-MAKING

Medical decision-making (MDM) is the third and final key component of an E/M service. Medical decision making is the last part of an E/M service where the physician establishes the patient's diagnosis, decides on a treatment plan, and decides whether any follow-up tests or exams are necessary. The level of complexity of medical decision-making depends on the severity of the patient's condition(s) and the amount of information that the physician reviews to establish the diagnosis and management options.

Physicians determine the level of medical decision-making based on the following three elements:

1. The number of possible diagnoses and/or the number of management options that the physician considers (minimal, limited, multiple, or extensive)

2. The amount and/or complexity of medical records, diagnostic tests, and/or other information that the physician obtains, reviews, and analyzes (minimal/low, limited, moderate, or extensive)

3. The risk of significant complications, morbidity, and/or mortality, comorbidities associated with the patient's presenting problem(s), diagnostic procedure(s), and/or possible management options (minimal, low, moderate, or high)

There are four types, or levels, of medical decision-making: straightforward, low complexity, moderate complexity, and high complexity. As the information in the three elements becomes more complex, so does the level of medical decision-making. ■ TABLE 19-6 shows the elements for each type of medical decision-making. To qualify for a given type, *two of the three elements* must either meet or exceed the requirements.

For example, if the number of diagnoses or management options is moderate complexity, the amount or complexity of data is low complexity, and the risk is low complexity, the type of medical decision-making is low complexity. Two of the three elements (amount or complexity of data and risk) met the requirements for low complexity.

You will next learn about each of the three elements that determine the level of medical decision-making.

Number of Diagnoses and/or Management Options

The first element of MDM is the number of diagnoses and/or management options. Recall that there are four types of diagnoses/management options (Table 19-6):

- Minimal—1 or none
- Limited—2
- Multiple—3
- Extensive—4 or more

otorhinolaryngologist (ōt-ō-rī-nō-lar-ən-gäl′-ə-jəst)—physician who specializes in the diagnosis and treatment of ear, nose, and throat disorders

■ TABLE 19-6   **TYPE OF MEDICAL DECISION-MAKING AND REQUIRED ELEMENTS**

Type of Medical Decision-Making	Number of Diagnoses or Management Options	Amount and/or Complexity of Data To Be Reviewed	Risk of Significant Complications, Morbidity, and/or Mortality
Straightforward	Minimal (1 or none)	Minimal	Minimal
Low Complexity	Limited (2)	Limited	Low
Moderate Complexity	Multiple (3)	Moderate	Moderate
High Complexity	Extensive (4 or more)	Extensive	High

The number of possible diagnoses and/or the number of treatment/management options are based on the following information:

* number and types of problems addressed during the encounter
* complexity of establishing a diagnosis
* management decisions that the physician makes regarding the patient's condition

Refer to the following guidelines to better understand factors that make up the number of diagnoses/management options:

* Decision-making for a diagnosed problem is easier than decision-making for an identified but undiagnosed problem.
* The number and type of diagnostic tests may indicate the number of possible diagnoses.
* Problems that are improving or resolving are less complex than problems that are worsening or failing to change as expected.
* The need to seek advice from other providers is another indicator of the complexity of diagnostic or management problems.

For each encounter, the physician should document an assessment, clinical impression, or diagnosis. These can also be implied by reviewing the physician's documented decisions regarding management plans and/or further evaluation. In addition, the physician should also refer to the following points when documenting the number of diagnoses and management options:

1. For a presenting problem *with* an established diagnosis, the record should reflect whether the problem is
   * improved, well-controlled, resolving, resolved, or
   * inadequately controlled, worsening, or failing to change as expected.
2. For a presenting problem *without* an established diagnosis, the physician can document the assessment or clinical impression in the form of a differential diagnosis (two or more possible conditions) or as "possible," "probable," or "rule out" (R/O) diagnoses.
3. The physician should also document the initiation of or changes in treatment. Treatment includes a wide range of management options, including patient instructions, nursing instructions, therapies, and medications.
4. If the physician refers the patient to another provider, including for a consultation, or seeks advice from another provider, then he should document to whom and/or where he referred the patient, or from whom he requested the advice.

Amount and/or Complexity of Data

The second element of MDM is the amount and/or complexity of data to review. There are four types of the amount and/or complexity of data:

* Minimal/Low
* Limited
* Moderate
* Extensive

Neither the 1995 nor the 1997 guidelines defines the amount of information that must be present to qualify for each of the four types of the amount and/or complexity of data. The amount of information the physician reviews and its complexity depend on many factors because each patient's case is different. Refer to the following guidelines to better understand the types of information the physician reviews and documents related to the amount and/or complexity of data:

1. The amount and complexity of data the physician analyzes depend on the number and types of diagnostic tests that he orders and reviews.

2. The amount and complexity of data increase when the physician obtains and reviews prior medical records from other providers and/or obtains history information from sources other than the patient.

3. When the physician discusses contradictory or unexpected test results with the physician who performed or interpreted the test, it is also a factor for determining the complexity level of data reviewed.

4. Occasionally, the physician who ordered a test may personally review the image or specimen from the physician who prepared the test report or interpretation and/or already interpreted the data.

5. If the physician orders, plans, or schedules a diagnostic service (a test or procedure, such as lab work or radiology) at the time of the E/M encounter, then he should document the type of service that the patient should receive.

6. The physician should document his review of lab, radiology and/or other diagnostic tests. An entry in a progress note such as "WBC elevated" or "chest X-ray unremarkable" is acceptable. The physician may also document the review of results by initialing and dating the report containing the test results.

7. The physician should document a decision to obtain old records or to obtain additional history from the family, caretaker, or other source to supplement information that the patient provides. The physician should also document the review of old records and/or the receipt of additional history from another source. If there is no relevant information in addition to the information that the physician already obtained, then he should document this fact. A notation of "old records reviewed" or "additional history obtained from family" without elaboration is insufficient documentation.

8. The physician should document the results of his discussion of laboratory, radiology or other diagnostic tests with the physician who performed or interpreted the study.

Risk of Significant Complications, Morbidity, and/or Mortality

The third and final element of MDM is the risk of significant complications, morbidity, and/or mortality. It is based on the risks associated with the presenting problem(s), the diagnostic procedure(s), possible management options, and the patient's outcome if the physician does not treat the patient's condition. Refer to the following guidelines to better understand the types of information the physician reviews and documents to determine the risk:

1. The physician should document comorbidities, underlying diseases, or other factors that increase the patient's risk of complications, morbidity, and/or mortality.

2. The physician should document the type of surgical or invasive diagnostic procedure (such as laparoscopy) that he orders, plans, schedules, or performs at the time of the E/M encounter.

3. The physician should document, or the documentation should imply, a referral for or decision to perform a surgical or invasive diagnostic procedure on an urgent basis.

Review ■ TABLE 19-7 to determine the level of the risk: minimal, low, moderate, or high. The table includes common clinical examples that you can use as a guide. The assessment of risk of the presenting problem(s) is based on the risk that is related to the disease process anticipated between the present encounter and the next one. The assessment of risk of selecting diagnostic procedures and management options is also based on the risk during, and immediately following, any procedures or treatment. *The highest level of risk in any one category*—presenting problem(s), diagnostic procedure(s), or management options—determines the overall risk.

tinea corporis (tin′e-ə cor′pə ris)—a fungal infection of the skin in areas other than hands and feet, also called ringworm

KOH prep—a laboratory test for fungal infection

cystitis (sis-ti′tis)—inflammation of the urinary bladder

allergic rhinitis (ə-lur′jik ri-ni′tis)—runny nose due to allergies

pyelonephritis (pi-ə-lo-nə-fri′tis)—inflammation of the kidney and renal pelvis (the juncture of the kidney and ureters)

pneumonitis (noo-mo-ni′tis)—inflammation of the lungs

colitis (ko-li′tis)—inflammation of the colon

lumbar puncture (lum′bər pungk′chər)—removing fluid from the space between the vertebrae in the lower region of the spine

culdocentesis (kul-do-sen-te′sis)—puncturing the wall of the vagina with a needle to remove fluid from the space between the rectum and uterus

discography (dis-kog′rə-fe)—X-ray of a disc in the spinal column after injecting a colored dye

■ **TABLE 19-7** **LEVEL OF RISK FOR MEDICAL DECISION-MAKING**

Level of Risk	Presenting Problem(s)	Diagnostic Procedure(s) Ordered	Management Options Selected
Minimal	One self-limited or minor problem (cold, insect bite, **tinea corporis**)	Laboratory tests requiring venipuncture Chest X-rays EKG or EEG Urinalysis Ultrasound (echocardiography) **KOH prep**	Rest Mouth gargles Elastic bandages Superficial dressings
Low	Two or more self-limited or minor problems One stable, chronic illness (well-controlled hypertension, noninsulin-dependent diabetes, cataract, benign prostatic hyperplasia) Acute uncomplicated illness or injury (**cystitis**, **allergic rhinitis**, simple sprain)	Physiologic tests not under stress (pulmonary function tests) Noncardiovascular imaging studies with contrast (barium enema) Superficial needle biopsies Clinical laboratory tests requiring arterial puncture Skin biopsies	Over-the-counter drugs Minor surgery with no identified risk factors Physical therapy Occupational therapy IV fluids without additives
Moderate	One or more chronic illnesses with mild exacerbation, progression, or side effects of treatment Two or more stable chronic illnesses Undiagnosed new problem with uncertain prognosis (lump in breast) Acute illness with systemic symptoms (**pyelonephritis, pneumonitis, colitis**) Acute complicated injury (head injury with brief loss of consciousness)	Physiologic tests under stress (cardiac stress test, fetal contraction stress test) Diagnostic endoscopies with no identified risk factors Deep needle or incisional biopsy Cardiovascular imaging studies with contrast and no identified risk factors (arteriogram, cardiac catheterization) Obtain fluid from body cavity (**lumbar puncture**, thoracentesis, **culdocentesis**)	Minor surgery with identified risk factors Elective major surgery (open, percutaneous, or endoscopic) with no identified risk factors Prescription drug management Therapeutic nuclear medicine IV fluids with additives Closed treatment of fracture or dislocation without manipulation
High	One or more chronic illnesses with severe exacerbation, progression, or side effects of treatment Acute or chronic illnesses or injuries that pose a threat to life or bodily function (multiple trauma, acute myocardial infarction, pulmonary embolus, severe respiratory distress, progressive severe rheumatoid arthritis, psychiatric illness with potential threat to self or others, peritonitis, acute renal failure) An abrupt change in neurologic status (seizure, transient ischemic attack, weakness, sensory loss)	Cardiovascular imaging studies with contrast with identified risk factors Cardiac electrophysiological tests Diagnostic endoscopies with identified risk factors **discography**	Elective major surgery (open, percutaneous, or endoscopic) with identified risk factors Emergency major surgery (open, percutaneous, or endoscopic) Parenteral controlled substances Drug therapy requiring intensive monitoring for toxicity Decision not to resuscitate or to de-escalate care because of poor prognosis

Refer to Table 19-7 as you review the following example to determine the level of risk.

Example: Miss Richmond, a 15-year-old established patient, sees Dr. Hoffman for an office visit. Miss Richmond's chief complaint is acne on her face, shoulders, and back. She is experiencing redness and soreness of the affected areas. Dr. Hoffman instructs the patient to use 10% benzoyl peroxide (nonprescription) in the morning and at bedtime. Dr. Hoffman establishes that the HPI and exam are both problem-focused.

In this example, under the category of Presenting Problem(s) in Table 19-7, the patient has one self-limited minor problem, acne, which is *minimal* risk. Under the category Diagnostic Procedures Ordered, Dr. Hoffman did not order any diagnostic procedures, so there is no risk under this category. Under the category Management Options Selected, Dr. Hoffman advised the patient to use an over-the-counter medication, which falls under *low* risk. Referring to Table 19-7, the *highest* level of risk in any category determines the overall risk. The highest level for this patient out of the three categories is *low*.

You can assign the level of MDM once you know the three elements:

- Type of diagnoses/management options
- Type of amount and/or complexity of data
- Level of risk

Refer to Table 19-6 again to see how you determine the level of medical decision-making after you have reviewed the three elements.

streptococcal pharyngitis
(strep'-to-kok'əl far-ən-jīt'-əs)

sciatica (sī-at'-i-kə)—pain
and numbness from the sciatic
nerve, originating in the spine

TAKE A BREAK

You are doing very well! That was a lot of information to grasp! Let's take a break and then assign types of medical decision-making.

Exercise 19.8 Medical Decision-Making

Instructions: Review each patient's case where you previously assigned the history and exam levels. Determine the number of diagnoses or management options, amount and/or complexity of data to review, and risk. Then assign the type of medical decision-making. Use the information outlined in this section and in Tables 19-6 and 19-7 to help you.

1. Mrs. Walker, a 35-year-old new patient, sees Dr. Hoffman with a chief complaint of a sore throat that started three days ago. She describes the pain as "raw" and says it is worse when she wakes in the morning and at bedtime. The patient is positive for fever and denies any other symptoms related to her throat pain. Dr. Hoffman reviews the patient's health history form, which includes past medical history, family history, and social history. Dr. Hoffman also reviews the patient's vital signs; notes that she has a fever; examines her mouth, and throat, and takes a rapid strep throat culture. He observes white spots on her tonsils and notes that lymph nodes in her neck are swollen. She is negative for any respiratory problems.

Dr. Hoffman diagnoses the patient with **streptococcal pharyngitis** (sore throat caused by *Streptococcus* bacteria) (■ FIGURE 19-3). He prescribes antibiotics. The patient is to follow up within a week if her condition does not improve or worsens.

Refer to Table 19-6:

a. Number of diagnoses and/or management options (minimal, limited, multiple, extensive): _____

_____

b. Amount and/or complexity of data to review (minimal, limited, moderate, extensive): _____

_____

Refer to Table 19-7:

c. Risk: Presenting Problem(s) (minimal, low, moderate, high): _____

_____

Diagnostic Procedures Ordered (minimal, low, moderate, high): _____

continued

TAKE A BREAK *continued*

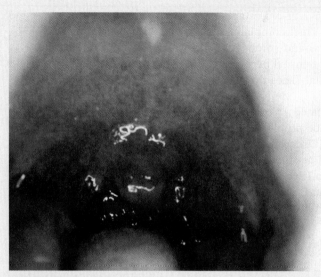

Figure 19-3 ■ Strept throat.
Photo credit: CDC.

Management Options Selected (minimal, low, moderate, high): _____

d. Level of risk (minimal, low, moderate, high): ____
_____

Refer to Table 19-6:

e. Type of medical decision-making (Table 19-6—straightforward, low complexity, moderate complexity, high complexity): _____

f. Optional coding practice: What is the patient's diagnosis code? _____

2. Established patient Arthur Tapp, age 31, sees Dr. Hoffman with a complaint of low back pain which he has had for the past week. The patient states that he is not aware of anything that he did that initially caused the pain, and this is the first time it occurred. He states that he "was hoping it would get better, but it hasn't." Mr. Tapp describes the pain as "dull and achy," but it sometimes turns into a "sharp stab." The patient also states that he has experienced left leg pain along with the back pain. He states that he tried to use a heating pad, but it does not seem to help and that Tylenol helps a little to relieve the pain. The patient denies joint or muscle pain in his right leg, neck, and arms and denies paralysis in his extremities. He is a manager with a desk job and gets little exercise.

During the examination, Dr. Hoffman documents the following information: The lumbar spine is sensitive to palpation (feeling with hands). Reflexes are good. Patient limps when walking. Extremities are negative for edema and redness. Skin is warm and dry. Patient exhibits limited range of motion in the left leg and has limited strength in left leg but no

problems in the right leg or either arm. Vision and hearing are negative.

Dr. Hoffman documents that the patient's diagnosis could be a sprain, herniated disc, or **sciatica**. He prescribes pain medication and requests a consultation from Dr. Lombard, a neurologist.

Refer to Table 19-6:

a. Number of diagnoses and/or management options (minimal, limited, multiple, extensive): ____
_____

b. Amount and/or complexity of data to review (minimal, limited, moderate, extensive): _____

_____

Refer to Table 19-7:

c. Risk: Presenting Problem(s) (minimal, low, moderate, high): _____
_____

Diagnostic Procedures Ordered (minimal, low, moderate, high): _____

Management Options Selected (minimal, low, moderate, high): _____

d. Level of risk (minimal, low, moderate, high): ____
_____

Refer to Table 19-6:

e. Type of medical decision-making (Table 19-6—straightforward, low complexity, moderate complexity, high complexity): _____

f. Optional coding practice: What is the patient's diagnosis code? _____

TAKE A BREAK *continued*

3. Madeline Perkins, age 57, is an established patient with Dr. Hoffman and sees him for a cough and congestion that she has had for three days. She states that she "feels worse each day and decided to come in." She denies fever, nausea, vomiting, or diarrhea. She states that she has a productive cough that is "yellow-greenish" in color and feels "some tightness" in her chest. She does not smoke. She does experience seasonal allergies and is allergic to penicillin.

Upon examination, Dr. Hoffman documents the following information: BP 130/80, temperature 98.5°, pulse 80, respirations 16. Neck is supple and nontender. PERRLA. Ears, nose, and throat are clear. Breathing is equal, no rales or wheezes. Heart is negative. Abdomen is soft, not tender, bowel sounds in all four quadrants. Skin is warm and dry. Pulses are equal in the extremities.

Dr. Hoffman takes a chest X-ray in the office and it is negative for pneumonia. He rules out the possibility that her symptoms are due to allergies. His final diagnosis is acute bronchitis, and he prescribes an antibiotic. He instructs the patient to call him if she is not doing better within a week, or sooner *prn* (pro re nata—as needed).

Refer to Table 19-6:

a. Number of diagnoses and/or management options (minimal, limited, multiple, extensive): _____

_____

b. Amount and/or complexity of data to review (minimal, limited, moderate, extensive): _____

_____

Refer to Table 19-7:

c. Risk: Presenting Problem(s) (minimal, low, moderate, high): _____

_____

Diagnostic Procedures Ordered (minimal, low, moderate, high): _____

Management Options Selected (minimal, low, moderate, high): _____

d. Level of risk (minimal, low, moderate, high): _____

_____

Refer to Table 19-6:

e. Type of medical decision-making (Table 19-6—straightforward, low complexity, moderate complexity, high complexity): _____

f. Optional coding practice: What is the patient's diagnosis code? _____

4. Sandy Scales brings her daughter Robin, age 10, to see Dr. Rosa, an otorhinolaryngologist, after Dr. Hoffman referred her due to chronic tonsillitis. Mrs. Scales states that Robin has had a "sore and swollen throat for several days" and that this is the fifth time it has occurred in the past year. The mother also reports that Robin has had a fever, nasal congestion, and runny nose. The patient denies nausea or vomiting. Mrs. Scales says past prescriptions of antibiotics have not seemed to help.

Dr. Rosa reviews information that the medical assistant documented, including a temperature of 101.9°. Upon examination, Dr. Rosa notes the following information: Swollen cervical lymph nodes and a raw red throat. Negative for any other lymphadenopathy. Ears and nose are clear. Lungs are clear to auscultation. Reflexes are normal.

Dr. Rosa reviews the past incidence and frequency of tonsillitis, medications and their effectiveness, her parents' concerns, and the risks and benefits of surgery vs. continued medical treatment. Because of Robin's history with tonsillitis and unresponsiveness to treatment, Dr. Rosa recommends a tonsillectomy. She discusses the procedure in detail with Mrs. Scales and also talks with Robin. Mrs. Scales states that she will talk to her husband tonight and call Dr. Rosa back tomorrow with a decision.

Refer to Table 19-6:

a. Number of diagnoses and/or management options (minimal, limited, multiple, extensive): _____

_____

b. Amount and/or complexity of data to review (minimal, limited, moderate, extensive): _____

_____

Refer to Table 19-7:

c. Risk: Presenting Problem(s) (minimal, low, moderate, high): _____

_____

Diagnostic Procedures Ordered (minimal, low, moderate, high): _____

Management Options Selected (minimal, low, moderate, high): _____

d. Level of risk (minimal, low, moderate, high): _____

_____

Refer to Table 19-6:

e. Type of medical decision-making (Table 19-6—straightforward, low complexity, moderate complexity, high complexity): _____

f. Optional coding practice: What is the patient's diagnosis code? _____

INTERESTING FACT: Three Seasons Carry Strep Throat

Strep throat, the most common throat infection, usually occurs in the late fall, winter, and early spring. People spread strep throat by direct contact with saliva or fluids from the nose of an infected person. Most people do not get group A *Streptococcus* infections from casual contact with others. A crowded environment like a dormitory, school, or nursing home can make it easier for the bacteria to spread. There have also been reports of contaminated food, especially milk and milk products, causing infection. You can get sick within three days of exposure. After you have been infected, you can pass the infection to others for two to three weeks, even if you do not have symptoms. After taking antibiotics for 24 hours, you will no longer spread the bacteria.

(National Institute of Allergy and Infectious Diseases: www.niaid.nih.gov/topics/strepThroat/Pages/treatment.aspx, accessed 3/5/11)

SUMMARY OF THREE KEY COMPONENTS

You have now learned about assigning each of the three key components to an E/M service: history, exam, and medical decision-making! Coding E/M services is probably the most difficult of all CPT codes because there is so much information that you must review before you can even begin to assign E/M codes. Keep in mind that it took a long time to learn the three key components because you had to learn about each step in the process and practice with exercises. You will become more efficient with more time and practice. Once you know each level of the three key components, you can choose the correct E/M code.

The E/M CPT guidelines at the beginning of the E/M section list the number of key components that must be met in order for you to assign a specific E/M code. Turn to the guidelines and look under the heading *Select the Appropriate Level of E/M Services Based on*

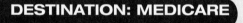

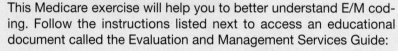

DESTINATION: MEDICARE

This Medicare exercise will help you to better understand E/M coding. Follow the instructions listed next to access an educational document called the Evaluation and Management Services Guide:

1. Go to the website http://www.cms.gov.
2. At the top of the screen on the banner bar, choose *Outreach & Education*.
3. Under the Medicare Learning Network (MLN), choose *MLN Educational Web Guides*.
4. On the left side of the screen, choose *Documentation Guidelines for Evaluation and Management (E/M) Services*.
5. Scroll down to Downloads, and choose *Evaluation and Management Services Guide*.

Review the document to answer the following questions:

1. How does medical record documentation assist physicians and other healthcare professionals?
2. How should you use the volume of documentation to determine the E/M level?
3. What is an NPP?
4. What two criteria must an NPP meet in order to bill E/M services to Medicare?
5. Whose responsibility is it to make sure that E/M codes correlate to medical documentation?

the Following. The guidelines state that for the following categories/subcategories (place of service/patient status), *all three* of the key components must meet or exceed the stated requirements to qualify for a specific level of E/M service:

- Office, new patient
- Hospital observation services
- Initial hospital care
- Office consultations
- Initial inpatient consultations
- Emergency department services
- Initial nursing facility care
- Domiciliary care, new patient
- Home, new patient

For the following categories/subcategories (place of service/patient status), only *two of the three* key components must meet or exceed the stated requirements:

- Office, established patient
- Subsequent hospital care
- Subsequent nursing facility care
- Domiciliary care, established patient
- Home, established patient

Code descriptors also state the number of key components that must be met in order to assign the code. It is a good idea to note beside each category/subcategory in your CPT manual whether two or three components are required so that you can quickly identify the number of components.

Refer to the following example for assistance with assigning E/M levels using the three key components.

Example: Dr. Hoffman sees a *new patient in the office* for an E/M service with the following levels of the key components:

- expanded problem-focused history
- expanded problem-focused exam
- straightforward MDM

Because this is a new patient office visit, *all three key components must meet or exceed* the code requirements. You can find E/M codes in the CPT index by searching under *evaluation and management* and the appropriate subterm, such as *office and other outpatient.* Turn to the E/M codes for office visit, new patient (99201–99205). In this example, the code is **99202** because all three key components meet the requirements of 99202.

Review the next example for a patient encounter that is a bit more challenging to code.

Example: Dr. Hoffman sees a new patient in the office for an E/M service with the following levels of the key components:

- problem-focused history
- expanded problem-focused exam
- straightforward MDM

In this example, the patient's history is *problem-focused,* and only *two* of the three components meet the requirements for 99202, so you cannot assign 99202. Instead, you have to go back to code **99201** because the history for 99201 is problem-focused.

Notice that the medical decision-making for 99201 is also *straightforward*, the same as for 99202. Even though the exam for 99202 is expanded problem-focused, you cannot assign 99202 because *all three components* must meet the requirements for 99202. Assigning 99202 would be upcoding, giving the history a higher level than what actually exists. Remember that the medical documentation must always support the code assignment. If the documentation does not support a higher level history, then you cannot assign the code with the higher history.

Appendix C in the CPT manual contains Clinical Examples of documentation from various medical records and the E/M codes that the documentation supports. Turn to Appendix C to review the examples and compare the documentation to correlating codes.

Recall from Chapter 1 that coders can also work as chart auditors for providers or other organizations, such as consulting firms, where they review medical documentation and compare it to codes assigned. Auditors use E/M audit forms that are based on the 1995 or 1997 guidelines and record the types of information the physician documented in the record. Many Medicare Administrative Contractors (MACs) also have their own E/M audit forms that they use when auditing providers' E/M levels for coding accuracy. Providers can develop their own audit forms or use the MACs' audit forms to help them choose the correct E/M code. You can find many of the audit forms on the MACs' websites. In addition, the CPT Professional Edition includes Evaluation and Management Tables, quick references to assist you in choosing the correct E/M code.

You will next learn when to use *contributing components*, rather than the three key components, to assign an E/M code.

TAKE A BREAK

Way to go! Give yourself a pat on the back! Let's take a break and then combine all of the key components that you learned to assign E/M codes.

Exercise 19.9 Summary of Three Key Components

Instructions: Turn to the E/M codes in your CPT manual, or start in the index under Evaluation and Management and search for the place of service or type of service as a subterm to locate specific codes. For each patient's case, review the level of history, exam, and medical decision-making; place of service; type of service; and patient status. Next, determine whether all three or two out of three of the key components must be met to assign a specific E/M code. Then assign the E/M procedure code.

1. Dr. Hoffman sees an established patient for an office visit with these levels: detailed history, detailed exam, MDM high.

   Does this service need to meet 3/3 or 2/3 of the key components? _____

   What is the E/M code? _____

2. Dr. Hoffman admits a patient to the hospital. The E/M service has these levels: comprehensive history, comprehensive exam, MDM high.

   Does this service need to meet 3/3 or 2/3 of the key components? _____

   What is the E/M code? _____

3. Dr. Mills, the ED physician, sees a patient for an E/M service with these levels: expanded problem-focused history, detailed exam, MDM moderate.

   Does this service need to meet 3/3 or 2/3 of the key components? _____

   What is the E/M code? _____

4. Dr. Hoffman sees a patient in a skilled nursing facility (SNF) during the third day of her stay. The E/M service has these levels: problem-focused history, expanded problem-focused exam, MDM low.

   Does this service need to meet 3/3 or 2/3 of the key components? _____

   What is the E/M code? _____

5. Dr. Hoffman makes a house call to a new patient. The E/M service has these levels: expanded problem-focused history, detailed exam, MDM moderate.

   Does this service need to meet 3/3 or 2/3 of the key components? _____

   What is the E/M code? _____

6. Dr. Barrett sees a new patient in Williton's outpatient clinic for an E/M service with these levels: expanded problem-focused history, detailed exam, MDM low.

   Does this service need to meet 3/3 or 2/3 of the key components? _____

   What is the E/M code? _____

FOUR CONTRIBUTING COMPONENTS

There are times when you do not need to review the three key components to determine the E/M level. Remember the 50% rule? If the physician documents that counseling and/or coordination of care took more than 50% of the total visit time, then you can use time as the sole determining factor for the E/M level. Take a look at the E/M services again in your CPT manual. Notice that many of them include a paragraph that specifies the typical total visit time. You will use these times to assign E/M codes when counseling and/or coordination of care comprise more than 50% of the service. The nature of the presenting problem, counseling, coordination of care, and time make up the four contributing components of an E/M service. Let's review them next.

Nature of Presenting Problem

The first contributing component for choosing an E/M level is the **nature of the presenting** problem. The AMA defines a presenting problem as a "disease, condition, illness, injury, symptom, sign, finding, complaint, or other reason for encounter, with or without a diagnosis being established at the time of the encounter." E/M codes recognize five types of presenting problems that the AMA defines as follows:

- *Minimal:*   A problem that may not require the presence of the physician. Another clinician working under the physician's supervision, such as a physician assistant or certified registered nurse practitioner, may treat the patient. **Examples**: patient who has a blood pressure reading, or a patient who requires a medication refill.

- *Self-limited or minor:*   A problem that runs a definite and prescribed course, is transient in nature, and is not likely to permanently alter health status or has a good prognosis with management/compliance. **Examples**: low-risk patient with gastroenteritis, or a patient who experiences leg cramps after exercise.

- *Low severity:*   A problem where the risk of morbidity without treatment is low, there is little to no risk of mortality without treatment, and full recovery without functional impairment is expected. **Examples**: patient with a leg sprain, or a patient who experiences anxiety attacks.

- *Moderate severity:*   A problem where the risk of morbidity without treatment is moderate, there is moderate risk of mortality without treatment, and there is an uncertain prognosis or an increased probability of prolonged functional impairment. **Examples**: patient with a respiratory infection, or a patient with rheumatoid arthritis (FIGURE 19-4).

- *High severity:*   A problem where the risk of morbidity without treatment is high to extreme, and there is a moderate to high risk of mortality without treatment or a high probability of severe, prolonged functional impairment. **Examples**: AIDS patient, or a patient who requires an organ transplant.

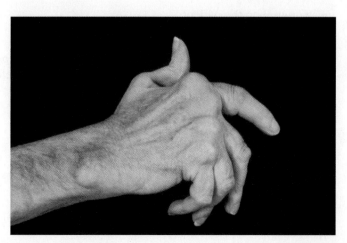

Figure 19-4 ■ Rheumatoid arthritis caused severe deformities in this patient's right hand.

Photo credit: SIU BIOMED COMM / Custom Medical Stock.

Counseling

Counseling, the second contributing component, occurs when the physician talks with the patient and family members about the patient's condition. Examples of counseling include

- Management of a condition or disease
- Treatment for a condition or disease
- Prognosis (future outcome) for a condition or disease
- Medication management
- Preparation for surgery and/or testing, including risk assessment
- Treatment recommendations
- Test results
- Disease prevention and risk factor reduction
- Caring for a family member.

Coordination of Care

Coordination of care is the third contributing component. It occurs when the physician discusses the patient's case with other providers or agencies and arranges for additional services, which can include

- Home health nursing, skilled nursing, or assisted living
- Physical, occupational, or speech therapy
- Durable medical equipment
- Social services (such as an area agency on aging)
- Other physician specialty services.

Time

Time is the fourth and last contributing component. The AMA includes total visit times with E/M codes to help physicians determine the *average time* for a specific visit. The actual visit time for each patient may be more or less, depending on the patient's case.

The AMA defines *intraservice time* (time spent delivering an E/M service) in two ways: face-to-face time spent between a physician and patient for office and other outpatient visits, and unit/floor time for hospital and other inpatient visits, which are both included in the E/M service time.

Face-to-Face Time   Office and other outpatient face-to-face time includes

- Obtaining the patient's history
- Performing the exam
- Counseling the patient
- Coordinating the patient's care

Physicians also spend *non-face-to-face time,* also called *pre-* and *post-encounter time,* for office or other outpatient services, which is time spent before and/or after the patient's service performing the following tasks:

- Reviewing medical records
- Analyzing test results
- Planning additional services
- Communicating and following up with other providers and the patient in writing or by phone.

Non-face-to-face time is *excluded* from the total time specific to an E/M code.

Unit/Floor Time   Unit/floor time includes the time that the physician is present on the patient's hospital unit and time that the physician renders bedside services. Unit/floor time includes

- Establishing and/or reviewing the patient's chart
- Examining the patient
- Writing notes in the chart
- Communicating with other professionals and the patient's family members.

Physicians also spend *pre- and post-visit time* off of the patient's floor before and after the patient's service reviewing radiology, laboratory, and pathology test results; reading and documenting in the patient's record, and planning or ordering additional services. Pre- and postvisit time is *excluded* from the total visit time.

Coding Based on Time   In order to use time associated with an E/M code as the sole factor, the physician must spend more than 50% of the total visit time counseling the patient and/or coordinating the patient's care. The physician must document the total encounter time or the start and end times of the visit and indicate how much time he spent on counseling and/or coordination of care, including the activities that he performed. Code descriptors list the average time spent on the service, and you should only use this information when assigning a code that is based on time, rather than the three key components. Refer to the following examples for guidance on coding an E/M service based on time.

> **Example 1:** Dr. Hoffman sees John Miller, age 57, for a follow-up appointment to discuss his PSA levels. Mr. Miller suffers from advanced prostate cancer and is terminally ill. Dr. Hoffman documents that he spent the entire 40 minutes of the visit counseling the patient and his wife on managing his disease and working with a hospice agency for palliative care.
>
> In this example, Mr. Miller is an established patient whom Dr. Hoffman sees in his office. Refer to the established patient codes for Office or Other Outpatient Services. Time is the sole factor for choosing the E/M code because Dr. Hoffman spent more than 50% (40 minutes) of the total visit time (40 minutes) counseling the patient. Assign code **99215**, which is for 40 minutes.

> **Example 2:** Dr. Hoffman sees established patient Fred Jackson, age 62, to discuss his newly diagnosed diabetes. Mr. Jackson's wife accompanies him to the appointment. Dr. Hoffman documents that he spent 20 minutes discussing diabetes management, dietary needs, and medication schedule with Mr. and Mrs. Jackson. He also documents a total visit time of 30 minutes.
>
> Refer to the established patient codes for Office or Other Outpatient Services. Time is the sole factor for assigning the E/M level because Dr. Hoffman spent more than 50% (20 minutes) of the total visit time (30 minutes) counseling the patient and his wife. Review the E/M codes to determine if there is a code with a total visit time of 30 minutes. Code 99214 is for 25 minutes, and code 99215 is for 40 minutes, but there is no code for 30 minutes. You will need to review the code that is *closest to the time* that you are searching, 30 minutes, which is 99214 for 25 minutes. If you choose 99215 for 40 minutes, then you are upcoding, since Dr. Hoffman did not see the patient for 40 minutes. Your final code assignment is **99214**.

It is important to note that there are several E/M services that are solely based on time, such as critical care services. To code these services, you have to choose a code that is based on the total service time, rather than on the three key components. You should carefully review code descriptors and CPT guidelines for specific information on using time for specific codes.

TAKE A BREAK

You are doing great! You finished learning how to code E/M services! Let's take a break and then assign E/M codes using the four contributing components.

| Exercise 19.10 | **Four Contributing Components** |

Instructions: Turn to the E/M codes in your CPT manual. Use the information presented in this chapter to determine the E/M procedure code to assign.

1. Dr. Hoffman sees established patient Mrs. Gregory, age 52, for an office visit. The patient suffers from hypertension and needs maintenance medication for the disease. Dr. Hoffman documents that he spent 12 minutes counseling the patient on medication management and dietary changes. He also documents that the total visit time is 20 minutes.

   E/M code: _____

2. John Miller, age 57, returns to Dr. Hoffman for another visit for management of advanced prostate cancer. Dr. Hoffman spends time calling Mr. Miller's oncologist for a progress report and treatment discussion. He recommends to the patient that he obtain a stair lift so that he can move easily up and down the stairs of his home. Dr. Hoffman states that his office manager will review the insurance benefits for the stair lift. Documentation includes 20 minutes of counseling and coordination of care. The visit lasted 35 minutes, which is documented.

   E/M code: _____

3. Mrs. Rodriquez, age 22, is a new patient who sees Dr. Hoffman for a physical. During the exam, she states that she has felt depressed for the past six months, and she provides details of her marriage and family life that contribute to the problem. Dr. Hoffman counsels the patient on managing stress and recommends that she see a psychologist for therapy. He documents the total visit time of 45 minutes with 30 minutes counseling the patient. The visit includes a comprehensive history.

   E/M code: _____

E/M CATEGORIES

Remember that physicians provide E/M services in a variety of settings. We already reviewed and coded E/M services for some of these settings. It is important to become familiar with each setting and the code choices available for E/M services to ensure correct code assignment. Categories of E/M services can represent the place of service (office), type of service (case management), or both (ED services—place is emergency department and type is emergency). There are 19 categories of E/M services, which we will review together as we work through this section:

1. Office or Other Outpatient Services
2. Hospital Observation Services
3. Hospital Inpatient Services
4. Consultations
5. Emergency Department Services
6. Critical Care Services
7. Nursing Facility Services
8. Domiciliary, Rest Home (e.g., Boarding Home), or Custodial Care Services
9. Domiciliary, Rest Home (e.g., Assisted Living Facility), or Home Care Plan Oversight Services
10. Home Services
11. Prolonged Services
12. Case Management Services
13. Care Plan Oversight Services
14. Preventive Medicine Services
15. Non-Face-to-Face Physician Services
16. Special Evaluation and Management Services
17. Newborn Care Services

18. Inpatient Neonatal Intensive Care Services and Pediatric and Neonatal Critical Care Services

19. Other Evaluation and Management Services

Most categories also have subcategories that divide the services into greater detail. Refer to Table 19-1 to review the categories and subcategories, along with their code ranges. Turn to your CPT manual, and refer to each category of codes as you read about them in this section. Note that some of the categories have separate subcategories with code ranges for a new patient and for an established patient. With other categories, there is only one code range, regardless of whether the patient is new or established.

Also note that the E/M categories have CPT guidelines that you should always review when assigning codes from each category. It may be tempting to skip the guidelines because some of them are very long, but you should instead read them carefully and thoroughly. They contain important information that can affect your final code assignment. We will cover some of the information in the guidelines but will not review every point in each set of guidelines for every category.

Let's review the categories next, which are outlined for you in the form of tables so that you can easily reference them. The three key components are not separately defined in each table for each type of face-to-face E/M service. You can refer to the E/M code descriptors to determine if they include the three key components of history, exam, and medical decision-making. Note that the levels of the key components are different based on each E/M category.

Also note that Medicare regulations are not included in the tables for E/M services because there are numerous billing and coding requirements, as well as reimbursement regulations, which can change regularly. It is best to check the Medicare website and review the most current guidelines and regulations and check with MACs for local regulations for your geographic region.

1—Office or Other Outpatient Services (99201–99215)

Patient Status	Outpatient, New or Established (code ranges are separate for new and established patients)
Location	Office, outpatient clinic, ambulatory facility
Description of Services	Examination and assessment of patients Most frequently used E/M codes in a physician's office. E/M services for new patients have a higher charge than E/M services for established patients because there is more physician work involved.
Time Based	Yes, only when counseling and/or coordination of care take more than 50% of total visit time.
Subcategories	• *New Patient*—A patient who has not received any professional services (face-to-face) within the past three years from the physician or another physician of the same specialty who belongs to the same group practice. • *Established Patient*—A patient who has received professional services (face-to-face) within the past three years from the physician or another physician of the same specialty who belongs to the same group practice.
Key Components	3/3—New Patient 2/3—Established Patient
Additional Points to Remember—Dos and Don'ts	✓ Do report code 99211 (established patient service—lowest level) for services that nurses provide (blood pressure check, vitamin injection). The presence of a physician is not required, although the physician must be on site to supervise and review the work performed. (Physicians can also report code 99211.) ✓ Do not report an E/M office/outpatient visit code if, in the course of the encounter, the patient is admitted to the hospital the same day. Instead, report a code for Initial Inpatient Hospital Care. The E/M office/outpatient visit is bundled into the initial hospital care. ✓ Do not assign an E/M office/outpatient visit code if the visit is a postoperative follow up that is included in the global surgical package. Instead, assign code 99024 (Post-op follow-up visit). ✓ Do not assign an E/M office/outpatient visit code for preventive care services, ED services, or hospital observation services, even though they are outpatient services. Instead, assign codes from each of the individual categories for these services.

2—Hospital Observation Services (99217–99226)

Patient Status	Outpatient, New or Established (code ranges combine new and established patients)
Location	Hospital observation unit, hospital floor or unit, ED
Description of Services	Assessments and reassessments of patients admitted to observation who typically begin in a hospital's ED, but; a physician within the community can also refer a patient to observation. There is not enough information about the patient's condition to either admit the patient to the hospital as an inpatient or to discharge the patient to home or another facility.
	The supervising physician admits the patient for observation to assess the patient's progression or regression, administer tests, develop a treatment plan, and determine the next steps for admission or discharge. Observation stays are typically 48 hours or less.
Time Based	Yes, only when counseling and/or coordination of care take more than 50% of total visit time. *Exception:* Observation discharge services are the day of discharge.
Subcategories	*Initial Observation Care*—First day in observation. Report once.
	Subsequent Observation Care—Second and subsequent days in observation. Report for each day in observation, other than day of admit and discharge.
	Observation Care Discharge Services—Last day in observation. Report once for the physician responsible for the patient's observation care. Assign for patients discharged from observation on a day other than the admit date. (For admit/discharge on the same date, see codes 99234–99236.) Services include final patient exam, discussion of stay, discharge instructions (continuing care), and preparing discharge records.
	(These subcategories are in a different order in the CPT manual.)
Key Components	3/3—Initial Observation Care
	2/3—Subsequent Observation Care
Additional Points to Remember—Dos and Don'ts	✓ Do report a code for Initial Inpatient Hospital Care when the patient is in observation and
	• admitted the same day
	• admitted on a subsequent day
	✓ Do not report a separate code for observation. The observation services are bundled into the initial hospital care services.
	✓ Do not assign separate E/M codes for E/M services related to the observation, such as ED services. Instead, report only the observation code, which bundles all other services.
	✓ Do not assign an observation code for post-operative recovery if the service is part of the global surgical package. Instead, report code 99024 (Post-op follow-up visit).
	✓ Do not report observation discharge (99217) when a patient is discharged from observation in order to be admitted as an inpatient. Observation services are bundled into the inpatient services.

3—Hospital Inpatient Services (99221–99239)

Patient Status	Inpatient, New or Established (code ranges combine new and established)
Location	Hospital floor or unit, partial hospitalization (psychiatry)
Description of Services	Hospital care provided to an inpatient for acute care services. The stay typically lasts 24 hours or more but can be less than 24 hours. The admitting physician admits the patient to the hospital. An *attending physician* (also called an *attending*) oversees and is legally responsible for the patient's care while the patient is in the hospital. Many different physicians and other providers can render care during the stay (called concurrent care). An attending is trained in a specialty area, including family practice, and can supervise medical students and residents.
Time Based	Yes, only when counseling and/or coordination of care take more than 50% of total visit time (not hospital discharge). *Exception:* Codes for admit and discharge on same day are not time based—99234–99236.
Subcategories	*Initial Hospital Care*—First day in hospital. Report once. For use only by admitting physician, who can be the patient's physician working outside the hospital, a physician who works within the hospital, or an ED physician, depending on the hospital's procedures. *Subsequent Hospital Care*—Second and subsequent days in hospital. Report for each day as an inpatient, other than the day of admit and discharge. For use by physicians overseeing the patients care. Includes review of medical records, test results, changes to physical condition, and responses to treatment. Three codes are available, and each descriptor lists the patient's condition (e.g., stable/recovering, not responding to therapy, unstable). *Hospital Discharge Services*—Last day in hospital. Report once. For use only by the attending physician for 30 minutes or less or more than 30 minutes. If the physician does not document time, then report the code for 30 minutes or less. The time does not have to be continuous. Services include final patient exam, discussion of stay, discharge instructions (continuing care), and preparing discharge records. Concurrent care providers should report other codes (subsequent hospital care, consultation). *Admit and Discharge on Same Day*—Report for patients admitted to and discharged from the hospital on the same day. Also report for patients admitted to and discharged from observation on the same day. E/M services related to the admission and discharge, and their complexity levels, are bundled into this service. Do not code them separately. (These subcategories are in a different order in the CPT manual.)
Key Components	3/3—Initial Hospital Care 2/3—Subsequent Hospital Care

Additional Points to Remember—Dos and Don'ts	✓ Do report a code for Initial Inpatient Hospital Care when the patient is in observation and
	  • admitted the same day
	  • admitted on a subsequent day
	✓ Do not report a separate code for observation. The observation services are bundled into the initial hospital care services.
	✓ Do not assign separate E/M codes for E/M services related to the admission, such as ED services. Instead, report only the initial hospital care code, which bundles all other services.
	✓ Do not report a code from Hospital Inpatient Services when physicians make postoperative follow up visits while the patient is hospitalized if the procedure has a global surgical package. Instead, report code 99024 (Post-op follow-up).

4—Consultations (99241–99255)

Patient Status	Outpatient or Inpatient, New or Established (code ranges combine new and established patients)
Location	*Outpatient:* office, outpatient clinic, ambulatory facility, hospital observation, home, domiciliary (residence, home), rest home, ED *Inpatient:* hospital floor or unit, partial hospitalization (psychiatry), nursing facility
Description of Services	Examination and assessment to provide an opinion about a patient's condition, which could be a second opinion if the patient already saw another provider for the same condition. A physician, other clinician, or third party (insurance company) can request consultations. If a patient or family member requests the consultation, assign codes from Office or Other Outpatient Services or from another appropriate E/M category. Do not use consultation codes. The consulting physician, or consultant, may assume continued care for the patient, depending on the situation. A consultant may also provide or order additional diagnostic and/or therapeutic services during the consultation or during a subsequent visit. Both the requesting party and consultant document the written or verbal request for the consultation. After the consultation, the consultant documents the results in the patient's record, including further tests and treatment, and sends a written report with findings to the requesting party.
Time Based	Yes, only when counseling and/or coordination of care take more than 50% of total visit time.
Subcategories	*Office or Other Outpatient Consultations*—Report once per consultation. It is acceptable to report codes more than once for requested consultations for the same patient for the same or different condition. Report follow-up visits using codes for Office or Other Outpatient Services. *Inpatient Consultations*—Report once per inpatient stay. Report separately from an inpatient admission. Report follow-up visits using codes for subsequent hospital or nursing facility services.
Key Components	3/3—Office or Other Outpatient, Inpatient
Additional Points to Remember—Dos and Don'ts	✓ Do append modifier -32 to a consultation code if a third party mandates the consultation. ✓ Do not assign consultation codes when a requesting physician *transfers* the patient's care to another physician. The second physician then assumes care of the patient. The exception is if the physician cannot agree to assume the patient's care until she performs a consultation. Then you should report a consultation code. ✓ Do not confuse a request for consultation with a *referral*. A referral typically occurs when one physician refers a patient to another physician for evaluation and treatment, not for a consultation. Some providers use the term "referral for consultation," which is the same as a request for consultation.

5—Emergency Department Services (99281–99288)

Patient Status	Outpatient, New or Established (code ranges combine new and established patients)
Location	Hospital-based facility, open 24 hours, which provides immediate care
Description of Services	Examination, assessment, and treatment for unscheduled patients with presenting problems of various severity levels, including self-limited or minor, low to moderate, moderate, and high severity, which can be life-threatening problems.
	Patients with acute conditions can be admitted to the hospital from the ED.
	Depending on the hospital, there are different procedures to designate specific physicians who can admit patients from the ED. Examples include the ED physician, internist working in the ED, a specialist called upon to assess or treat the patient in the ED, another physician within the hospital, an outside physician who referred the patient or needs to approve an admission, and a *hospitalist*, an inpatient-based attending physician.
	Any physician who renders E/M services in the ED, not just the ED physician, can report Emergency Department Services codes.
Time Based	No. These services include many different types of care, and physicians may see patients multiple times during an encounter. It is often difficult to determine total face-to-face time.
Key Components	3/3
Subcategories	*Other Emergency Services*—Report when a physician in the ED or critical care unit communicates with ambulance or rescue clinicians to direct emergency care procedures (see CPT guidelines) or advanced life support for a patient transported to the ED.
Additional Points to Remember—Dos and Don'ts	✓ Do report Critical Care codes for critical care services rendered in the ED.
	✓ Do not use these codes to report services that physicians provide at an urgent care clinic, which is not an ED.
	✓ Do not assign separate Emergency Department Services codes for services related to an inpatient or observation admission. Instead, report only the initial hospital care code or the initial observation care code, which bundles all other services.

6—Critical Care Services (99291–99292)

Patient Status	Inpatient, New or Established (codes do not specify new or established patient)
Location	Hospital units for intensive care, coronary care, respiratory care, or emergency care
Description of Services	Critical care assessment and treatment to a critically ill or critically injured patient (over 71 months old) with a life-threatening condition, such as a severe malfunction of vital organ systems.
	Critical care codes include specific bundled procedures (see critical care services in CPT guidelines). Report separate codes for procedures performed in critical care that are not on the list of bundled procedures.
Time Based	Yes. Report one or both critical care codes, per day (see Critical Care Example outlined after this table):
	• 99291—first 30 to 74 minutes
	• +99292—each additional 30 minutes (add-on code)
	Report another E/M code when critical care time is less than 30 minutes. Do not report a critical care code.
	Documented time includes time at the patient's bedside or floor or unit time (reviewing test results and records, discussing the patient with another clinician or family). Time does not have to be continuous, but during critical care services, the physician must devote *all time* to one specific patient.
	Critical care time *excludes*:
	• Activities performed outside the unit or off the floor (meetings, phone calls)
	• Time spent in critical care performing separately reportable procedures (excluded from critical care list of bundled services in CPT guidelines)
Key Components	Not applicable
Subcategories	Not applicable
Additional Points to Remember—Dos and Don'ts	✓ Do report separate E/M codes for patients who are not critically ill but who are placed in a critical care unit.
	✓ Do refer to specific payer guidelines for required modifiers, including modifier -25 (separate E/M service).
	✓ Do report pediatric critical care codes (99471–99476) for critical care to patients 29 days to 71 months old.
	✓ Do report neonatal critical care codes (99468–99469) for critical care to neonates (28 days old or younger).
	✓ Do report critical care codes (99291–99292) for pediatric and neonatal (up to 71 months old) when critical care is provided in an outpatient setting (ED).

Critical Care Example: On Monday, Wayne Castro, age 52, is in a motor vehicle accident, and an ambulance transports him to Williton Medical Center. After ED assessments, physicians transfer the patient to the critical care unit (CCU). Dr. Miles, an intensivist (specialist in critical care), provides critical care services, which he documents last two hours. Services include pulse oximetry, blood gases, gastric intubation, and chest X-rays, among other services excluded from bundled critical care services.

To code critical care services for this case, turn to your CPT manual and perform the following steps:

Search the index for the main term *evaluation and management*, subterm *critical care*, which lists codes 99291–99292. You can also turn directly to the Critical Care Services category in the E/M section. The easiest way to code critical care is to use the Total Duration of Critical Care table in the CPT manual that appears before the codes. Turn to the table to review the choices. Notice that the table lists critical care time in minutes, not hours.

Convert the patient's critical care time of two hours to minutes, which is 120. The total minutes of 120 falls between the range of 105–134 minutes listed in the table. This range lists code **99291** (first 30–74 minutes) and **99292** (each additional 30 minutes) × 2, which is the final code assignment.

7—Nursing Facility Services (99304–99318)

Patient Status	Inter-Facility, New or Established (codes do not specify new or established patients)
Location	Nursing facility, also called a skilled nursing facility, nursing home, or long-term care facility; intermediate care facility; psychiatric residential treatment center (living environment staffed 24 hours)
Description of Services	Evaluation and assessment of nursing facility residents, visiting the resident on site, including reviewing medical care plans and participating in development of treatment plans with multi-disciplinary teams (multiple medical disciplines or specialties). (Review the CPT guidelines for more information on resident assessments.) Nursing facilities (NFs) follow federal, state, and local regulations, including licensure. Two types of NFs include • Skilled nursing facility (SNF), also called a long term care facility—(LTCF) - A separate facility or a unit of a hospital that provides 24-hour skilled medical care for patients whose conditions are not acute enough for inpatient hospitalization, but not mild enough for the patients to be discharged. Care includes nursing, rehabilitation, treatment, physician attendance and supervision, and recreation. Care can be temporary or long term. • Intermediate care facility (ICF) - A separate facility or a unit of a hospital or skilled nursing facility that provides both inpatient care and skilled nursing supervision.
Time Based	Yes, only when counseling and/or coordination of care take more than 50% of total visit time. *Exception:* Nursing Facility Discharge Services are solely time based.
Key Components	3/3—Initial Nursing Facility Care 2/3—Subsequent Nursing Facility Care 3/3—Other Nursing Facility Services
Subcategories	*Initial Nursing Facility Care:* First day in an NF. Report once for an NF admission or readmission. The admitting physician should include other E/M services related to the admission (office visit) with the Initial Nursing Facility Care code. *Exception:* When an inpatient or observation patient is discharged from the hospital, report *both* the discharge code and the NF admission code. *Subsequent Nursing Facility Care:* Report per day for a physician assessment after the admission. Includes review of records, diagnostic tests, and changes in the patient's condition or responses to treatment. *Nursing Facility Discharge Services:* Last day in an NF. Report once. Two codes are available: for 30 minutes or less or more than 30 minutes. If the physician does not document time, then report the code for 30 minutes or less. The time does not have to be continuous. Services include final patient exam, discussion of stay, discharge instructions (continuing care), and preparing discharge records. *Other Nursing Facility Services:* Report for an annual assessment. NFs who want to participate in Medicare must ensure that residents receive an annual assessment.
Additional Points to Remember—Dos and Don'ts	✓ Do not report NF codes when nursing facility residents see physicians in the office. Instead, report the appropriate E/M code, such as Office or Outpatient Services or Preventive Care Services.

TAKE A BREAK

Wow! What a lot of information to remember! Let's take a break and then practice coding from various categories.

Exercise 19.11 E/M Categories 1–7

Instructions: Assign procedure code(s) to the following cases, referencing both the index and CPT sections. Refer to the CPT manual and tables provided for specific information on each category.

1. Dr. Mayhew, an endocrinologist, sees new patient Victor Magness, age 48, at his office for management of uncontrolled diabetes due to chronic pancreatitis. The physician performs and documents a comprehensive history and examination and medical decision-making of high complexity. He spends 25 minutes of the 60-minute visit counseling Mr. Magness on diet management and other lifestyle changes that are needed to prevent serious diabetic manifestations.

   Code(s): _____

2. Dr. Hoffman sees Scott Creighton, age 51, at his hospital bedside. Dr. Hoffman admitted Mr. Creighton yesterday. The patient has a history of alcohol abuse and currently has liver **cirrhosis** (scarring, typically from alcohol abuse). Dr. Hoffman conducts and documents a detailed history, detailed examination, and medical decision-making of high complexity.

   Code(s): _____

3. Dr. Hoffman admits Daniel Siegel, age 25, to Williton Medical Center at 7 a.m. on Monday due to hematuria and severe pain in the lower pelvic region. He performs and documents a detailed history, comprehensive examination, and medical decision-making of low complexity. He diagnoses Mr. Seigel with ureteral calculi (stones in the ureters). Dr. Hoffman orders pain medicine and administers fluids. Mr. Seigel passes the stones

   spontaneously, and the pain subsides. Dr. Hoffman discharges Mr. Siegel on Monday evening at 9 p.m.

   Code(s): _____

4. Dr. Hoffman refers Tracy Bumgarner, age 48, to Dr. Simmons, an oncologist, for an office consultation regarding her recently diagnosed gastric adenocarcinoma. Dr. Simmons conducts and documents a comprehensive history and exam. He reviews imaging studies and lab reports and discusses a variety of treatment options with Mrs. Bumgarner. He tells her that the gastric adenocarcinoma has metastasized to the abdominal lymph nodes. Medical decision-making is of high complexity due to the severity of the illness and the need for multiple types of treatment. Dr. Simmons documents the consultation and findings and sends the report to Dr. Hoffman.

   Code(s): _____

5. Alice Poisson, age 81, collapses at home, and an ambulance brings her to Williton Medical Center's ED. Dr. Burns, the ED physician, conducts and documents a detailed history and examination and orders a number of lab tests. Medical decision-making is of moderate complexity, as he reviews multiple lab reports and risk factors. He diagnoses dehydration and **hyponatremia** (sodium deficiency) and begins IV hydration. Mrs. Poisson's condition stabilizes and Dr. Burns discharges her home.

   Code(s): _____

6. Dr. Lambert, an intensivist, provides two hours and 20 minutes of critical care at Williton for Jeff Lavin, age 36, who experiences **hypovolemic** shock due to severe diarrhea and dehydration.

   Code(s): _____

cirrhosis (sə-rō′-səs)

hyponatremia (hi-po-nə-tre′me-ə)

hypovolemic (hi-po-vo-le′mik)—an abnormally low volume of blood circulating throughout the body

8—Domiciliary, Rest Home (e.g., Boarding Home), or Custodial Care Services (99324–99337)

Patient Status	Inter-Facility or Home, New or Established (code ranges are separate for new and established patients)
Location	Facility that provides domiciliary (home), rest home, boarding home (also called assisted living), and custodial care (nonmedical) services
Description of Services	Evaluation and assessment of residents at a supervised facility that provides room, board, and various types of nonmedical personal assistance, such as activities of daily living (ADLs), medications, meals, housekeeping, shopping, transportation, and recreation. Residents are not completely independent due to their conditions, including the elderly and mentally and physically disabled individuals. Facilities can be community based or within another individual's home. They must abide by specific state regulations. Boarding homes are also called assisted living facilities, and some include nursing care but are not nursing facilities.
Time Based	Yes, only when counseling and/or coordination of care take more than 50% of total visit time.
Key Components	3/3—New Patient 2/3—Established Patient
Subcategories	*New Patient*—A patient who has not received any professional services (face-to-face) within the past three years from the physician or another physician of the same specialty who belongs to the same group practice. *Established Patient*—A patient who has received professional services (face-to-face) within the past three years from the physician or another physician of the same specialty who belongs to the same group practice.
Additional Points to Remember—Dos and Don'ts	✓ Do not report these codes when residents see physicians in the office. Instead, report the appropriate E/M code, such as Office or Outpatient Services or Preventive Care Services.

9—Domiciliary, Rest Home (e.g., Assisted Living Facility), or Home Care Plan Oversight Services (99339–99340)

Patient Status	Inter-Facility or Home, New or Established (codes do not specify new or established patients)
Location	Facility that provides domiciliary (home), rest home, boarding home (also called assisted living), or home care services
Description of Services	Supervision of a patient or resident at a supervised facility that provides room, board, and various types of non-medical assistance. Care plan oversight services include developing and revising care plans, reviewing status reports and results of diagnostic tests, and communicating with other providers, family, and caregivers involved in patient's care. The patient is not present for these services. Only one physician can report these services for a specific patient during the same month.
Time Based	Yes. Report one of two codes, per month: • 99339—15–29 minutes • 99340—30 minutes or more
Key Components	Not applicable
Subcategories	Not applicable
Additional Points to Remember—Dos and Don'ts	✓ Do not report these codes for care plan oversight for patients receiving recurrent care plan oversight for a home health agency, hospice, or nursing facility. Instead, report codes for Care Plan Oversight Services (99374–99380). ✓ Do not report these codes if the physician spends fewer than 15 minutes per month on care plan oversight services for a patient.

10—Home Services (99341–99350)

Patient Status	Home, New or Established (code ranges are separate for new and established patients)
Location	Home (private residence)
Description of Services	Examination and assessment of a patient in his own home. Home-bound patients have conditions that do not enable them to function independently. Home services, provided by a home health agency, are often alternatives to placement in an assisted living or nursing facility. Physicians who provide home E/M services often work for home health agencies, which also provide nursing care for home-bound patients.
Time Based	Yes, only when counseling and/or coordination of care take more than 50% of total visit time.
Subcategories	• *New Patient*—A patient who has not received any professional services (face-to-face) within the past three years from the physician or another physician of the same specialty who belongs to the same group practice. • *Established Patient*—A patient who has received professional services (face-to-face) within the past three years from the physician or another physician of the same specialty who belongs to the same group practice.
Key Components	3/3—New Patient 2/3—Established Patient
Additional Points to Remember—Dos and Don'ts	✓ Do not report Home Services codes when a home health agency or physician provides care plan oversight services. Instead, report codes 99374–99375 or 99339–99340. ✓ Do not report Home Services codes for patients who reside in a domiciliary, rest home, or assisted living home.

11—Prolonged Services (99354–99365)

Patient Status	Outpatient, Inpatient, New or Established (codes do not specify new or established patients; some codes are separate for Outpatient and Inpatient).
Location	Office or other outpatient facility, Inpatient hospital
Description of Services	Prolonged Services—When more than the usual E/M time is spent on face-to-face or non-face-to-face services. Codes apply to outpatients or inpatients. • Report these codes with a primary E/M code (any level) to show that the service lasted longer than the time listed in the primary E/M code descriptor. The primary E/M code must first follow the 50% rule before coding an additional prolonged services code. • Prolonged time does not have to be continuous. Physician Standby Services—Prolonged physician attendance *without* direct patient face-to-face contact.
Time Based	Yes—Report once per date of service. Codes are divided by • First hour • Each additional 30 minutes *Exception:* Physician Standby Service code is for each 30 minutes.
Key Components	Not applicable
Subcategories	***With Direct Face-to-Face Patient Contact:*** Report when the prolonged service is 30 minutes or more. The primary E/M service must have an average time in the code descriptor in order to assign a prolonged services code as an *additional* code (see Prolonged Services Example that follows this table). Codes are divided by office or other outpatient setting or inpatient setting. • It is acceptable to report a code for the *first hour* (99354, 99356) for the first 30 minutes to 1 hour 14 minutes. It is also acceptable to report a code for *each additional 30 minutes* (99355, 99357) for each additional 30 minutes beyond the first hour and for the *final* 15 to 30 minutes (see Total Duration of Prolonged Services table in the CPT manual listing codes and times). ***Without Direct Face-to-Face Patient Contact:*** Report when the prolonged service is 30 minutes or more, beyond the usual non-face-to-face time, including reporting the prolonged service on a different date than the primary service. The primary E/M service does not need to have an average time in the code descriptor. • Report the code for the first hour (99358) for the first 30 minutes to 1 hour 14 minutes, regardless of the place of service. Report the code for *each additional 30 minutes* (99359) for each additional 30 minutes beyond the first hour and for the *final* 15 to 30 minutes of service, regardless of the place of service. Prolonged activities include records review and telephone services. ***Physician Standby Services:*** Report when a physician provides standby services that another physician requested. Standby services are when the physician is available to assist with a patient's case if the patient develops complications (cardiac surgery, high-risk delivery). This service *excludes* face-to-face contact, and the physician cannot provide other patient care during standby. • Report the code for *each 30 minutes* of standby per day (99360). Report the *second and subsequent 30 minutes* with the same code only if there were an additional full 30 minutes of standby provided.
Additional Points to Remember— Dos and Don'ts	✓ Do not report prolonged services if the prolonged time is less than 30 minutes, which is included in the primary E/M service. ✓ Do not report standby services when the standby results in a procedure. Instead, report the code for the procedure.

Prolonged Services Example: Dr. Pena, a nephrologist, sees new patient Sue Li, age 62, for multiple conditions, including acute renal failure, uncontrolled diabetes, hypertension, and congestive heart failure. Dr. Pena documents that he spent one hour with the patient in counseling and coordinating additional care with other providers. He also documents a comprehensive history and exam and high medical decision-making. The total service lasted one hour, with 35 minutes spent in counseling and coordination of care. Dr. Pena also documents that he spent an additional half hour reviewing records and diagnostic tests after the patient's visit and communicating results to family members.

To code this case, turn to your CPT manual and perform the following steps:

Search the index for the main term *evaluation and management,* subterm *office and other outpatient,* which lists codes 99201–99215. You can also turn directly to the

Office and Other Outpatient category in the E/M section. Review the code ranges for a new patient—99201–99205. Code 99205 matches the comprehensive history and exam and high medical decision-making. Also, the time for code 99205 is 60 minutes. Use time as the sole determining factor for choosing the code, since counseling or coordinating care (35 minutes) took more than 50% of the total visit time. Dr. Pena also documents an additional half hour in activities that related to the patient's care, but the patient was not present.

Next, assign a prolonged services code for the additional half hour. Search the index for *prolonged services*. You will find code choices 99354–99357, 99360, and 99358–99359 for services without direct patient contact. Turn to codes 99358–99359 (without direct patient contact). Code 99358 is for the first hour, but you can still assign it for a half hour (see directions in the Total Duration of Prolonged Services table). The final code assignment is **99205** and **99358**.

12—Case Management Services (99363–99368)

Patient Status	Outpatient or Site Not Specified (Medical Team Conferences), New or Established (codes do not specify new or established patients)
Location	Office or other outpatient facility, Unspecified site (Medical Team Conferences)
Description of Services	Case management occurs when a physician or other healthcare professional manages a patient's care, including developing, coordinating, and supervising services. Anticoagulant Therapy—Report for the use of **anticoagulants** (blood thinners) to prevent and treat blot clots. Medical Team Conferences—Report for face-to-face conferences of at least three health care professionals (nonphysicians) of different specialties to develop, revise, coordinate, and implement services for a patient.
Time Based	Yes. Anticoagulant Therapy codes are divided by • first 90 days of therapy, including at least eight International Normalized Ratio (INR) measurements. An INR is a blood test that measures the effect of an anticoagulant drug. • each additional 90 days of therapy, including at least three INR measurements Medical Team Conferences are 30 minutes or more.
Key Components	Not applicable
Subcategories	*Anticoagulant Management:* Anticoagulant therapy treats **thromboembolic** (blood clot) disorders that are associated with atrial fibrillation, cerebrovascular accident, acute myocardial infarction, pulmonary embolism, and other heart valve disease. **Warfarin** is a common blood thinner (brand name Coumadin®). • Services include monitoring patients' responses to therapy, including complications; ordering and reviewing the INR; communicating with the patient; and adjusting the dosage. *Medical Team Conferences:* Report when physicians or other qualified healthcare professionals participate in meetings with at least three other caregivers (different specialties) to monitor and manage patients' needs. Each team member should have performed face-to-face patient evaluations or treatments in the previous 60 days. • Codes are separate depending on if there is face-to-face contact with patient and/or family and if the physician is present.
Additional Points to Remember—Dos and Don'ts	✓ Do not report Anticoagulant Management codes if the physician does not perform the specified minimum number of services.

anticoagulants (an-ti-ko-ag′ u-lənts)

thromboembolic (throm bo-em-bol′ik)

warfarin (wor′fər-in)

13—Care Plan Oversight Services (99374–99380)

Patient Status	Inter-Facility, Home, New or Established (codes do not specify new or established patients)
Location	Home Health Agency, Hospice, Nursing Facility
Description of Services	Care plan oversight is recurrent physician supervision of a patient receiving home health, hospice, or nursing facility services, which include developing and revising care plans, reviewing status reports and results of diagnostic tests, and communicating with other providers, family, and caregivers involved in patient's care.
	The patient is not present for these services.
	Only one physician can report these services for a specific patient during the same month.
	Codes are separated by care plan oversight for a home health agency (99374–99375), hospice (99377–99378), or nursing facility (99379–99380).
Time Based	Yes. Codes are divided by
	• 15–29 minutes
	• 30 minutes or more
Key Components	Not applicable
Subcategories	Not applicable
Additional Points to Remember—Dos and Don'ts	✓ Do not report Care Plan Oversight codes for patients who *do not* need recurrent supervision.
	✓ Do not report Care Plan Oversight codes when work is very low intensity or infrequent. Instead, this work is included in the pre- and postencounter work for other E/M codes for home, office/outpatient, nursing facility, or domiciliary care.

TAKE A BREAK

That was a lot of information to review! Let's complete some exercises to practice what you learned.

Exercise 19.12   E/M Categories 8–13

Part 1: Refer to the CPT guidelines, code descriptors, and the tables for categories 8–13 to answer the following questions.

1. For category Domiciliary, Rest Home (e.g., Boarding Home), or Custodial Care Services, what does the term "personal assistance" mean? _____

2. How many of the three key components must be met for code 99348? _____

3. During a prolonged service with face-to-face patient contact, should the provider separately report supplies used? _____ How do you know? _____

4. Why can't you separately report prolonged face-to-face services lasting less than 30 minutes? _____
_____

5. How should you report physician standby services when the time spent in standby ultimately leads to the physician performing a procedure for the patient? ___
_____

6. How should each member of the same specialty report his medical team conference services for the same patient, on the same day? _____

Part 2: Assign procedure code(s) to the following cases, referencing both the index and CPT sections. Refer to the CPT manual and the tables provided for specific information on each category.

1. Dr. Fletcher asks Dr. Beck to be on standby in case his services are needed for Rita Chambers, a 62-year-old patient in surgery at Williton. She is at risk for developing cardiac complications. Total standby time is 55 minutes, and Dr. Beck did not perform any procedures.

   Code(s): _____

2. Dr. Bates works for Williton Home Health. He reviews a care plan for Jimmy McDaniel, a 50-year-old, and discusses treatment with clinical and social treatment team members. His review lasts 30 minutes. The patient is not present.

   Code(s): _____

3. Dr. Hoffman visits new patient Ronald Newman, age 82, at home. Services include a comprehensive history, detailed exam, and moderate MDM.

   Code(s): _____

4. Eleanor Bush, age 85, is a new assisted living patient of Sebring Fields Assisted Living, whom Dr. Haynes

continued

TAKE A BREAK *continued*

evaluates. The service involved a detailed exam, comprehensive history, and high MDM.

Code(s): _____

5. Dr. Hoffman visits new patient Linda Parks, age 45, at home. Services include moderate MDM, detailed exam, and expanded problem-focused history.

Code(s): _____

6. Dr. Vaughn, of Tusca Hospice, reviews a care plan this month for Evan Rhodes, age 25, and spends 45 minutes reviewing the patient's records and discussing care with family members and other clinicians. The patient is not present.

Code(s): _____

14—Preventive Medicine Services (99381–99429)

Patient Status	Outpatient, New or Established (some codes specify new or established patients, while others combine new and established)
Location	Office or other outpatient facility
Description of Services	Preventive medicine consists of services to prevent illness in patients who do not have chief complaints. Examples of services are an annual exam, check-up, or a well-baby or well-child visit. Services involve an age-appropriate comprehensive history and exam for infants, children, or adults, as well as counseling, guidance, and risk factor reduction.
	• Some services are divided by new or established and the patient's age.
	• Report separate codes for services provided during a preventive visit, such as immunizations and screening tests.
Time Based	The following subcategories are based on time:
	• Preventive Medicine, Individual Counseling (15, 30, 45, or 60 minutes)
	• Behavior Change Interventions, Individual (3–10, more than 10, or 15–30 minutes)
	• Preventive Medicine, Group Counseling (30 or 60 minutes)
Key Components	Not applicable
Subcategories	**Counseling Risk Factor Reduction and Behavior Change Intervention:** These services should not already be included as part of another E/M service. A physician or other qualified health care professional can render these services which include the following types of services:
	Preventive Medicine, Individual Counseling: Report for counseling and risk factor reduction for an individual patient without an established illness. Services include diet and exercise recommendations, counseling for substance abuse, and information on preventing injuries.
	Behavior Change Interventions, Individual: Report for counseling an individual patient to change an *established behavior,* such as smoking, drinking alcohol, or overeating.
	Preventive Medicine, Group Counseling: Report for counseling and risk factor reduction for a group of patients without established illnesses. Services include diet and exercise recommendations, counseling for substance abuse, and information on preventing injuries.
	Other Preventive Medicine Services: Report for administration and interpretation of a health risk assessment consisting of a questionnaire, tests, and exam to determine a patient's risk for developing specific conditions. This category also includes a code for an unlisted preventive service.
Additional Points to Remember—Dos and Don'ts	✓ Do report a separate E/M code for Office or Other Outpatient Services (99201–99215) when the physician reviews a specific condition during a preventive service. The review must meet the criteria required in the E/M code descriptor in order to assign the code. Report the code for the preventive service, and report the code for the Office or Other Outpatient service by appending modifier -25 (separate E/M service) to the Office or Other Outpatient E/M service.

15—Non-Face-to-Face Physician Services (99441–99444)

Patient Status	Outpatient, Established
Location	Office or other outpatient facility, Other setting
Description of Services	Report telephone services and online services that the physician provides to an established patient, parent, or patient's guardian in response to a patient's phone call or online inquiry. Services may include discussing the patient's condition, treatment, and medications.
Time Based	Telephone services are based on increments of 5–10, 11–20, or 21–30 minutes. Online services are reported once per seven days for the same episode of care.
Key Components	Not applicable
Subcategories	***Telephone Services:*** Report for physician telephone services that *do not* relate to an E/M service of the past seven days. • Do not report for telephone services that are part of a surgical post-op period. • Do not report a telephone service that *leads to* a face-to-face E/M service in the next 24 hours or soonest appointment. The telephone service is considered part of the E/M service. ***On-Line Medical Evaluation:*** Report for physician online services that *do not* relate to an E/M service of the past seven days. Services include related phone calls, prescriptions, and lab orders. The physician must electronically store the evaluation and communication with the patient and/or family. • Do not report for online services that are part of a surgical post-op period. • Report once for the same episode of care during a seven-day period. • More than one physician can report these services for the same patient.
Additional Points to Remember—Dos and Don'ts	✓ Do not report Telephone Services codes for nonphysician qualified healthcare professionals. Instead, report codes 98966–98968 (Non-Face-to-Face Nonphysician Services).

16—Special Evaluation and Management Services (99450–99456)

Patient Status	Outpatient, New or Established (codes do not specify new or established patients)
Location	Office or other outpatient facility, Other setting
Description of Services	Basic Life and/or Disability Evaluation Services are for patients who want to enroll in a life and/or disability insurance policy, and the insurance company requires a medical evaluation before they will write the policy. Some physicians contract with insurance companies to provide these evaluations. In other cases, patients request the evaluation from their personal physicians.
	Work-Related or Medical Disability Evaluation Services are for patients who are injured at work or elsewhere and need a medical evaluation, which the workers' compensation or disability insurance typically requires. Either the treating physician or another physician performs these services.
	Do not report codes from this category if the physician actively manages a patient's condition during the encounter.
Time Based	No
Key Components	Not applicable
Subcategories	***Basic Life and/or Disability Evaluation Services:*** The code descriptor lists all services included with the exam, such as vital signs and medical history.
	Work-Related or Medical Disability Evaluation Services: The code descriptor lists all services included with the exam, such as a medical history and treatment plan. Physicians provide these services for two different situations:
	• Periodic evaluation by the physician *treating* the patient for a disability. Results guide the physician regarding future treatment decisions. Insurance companies may require a periodic evaluation in order to justify continuing care and reimbursement.
	• Insurance company-mandated evaluation from an *independent* physician whom the insurance company designates, not from the treating physician. This is called an *independent medical evaluation (IME)*. Some physicians contract with insurance companies to provide IMEs.
Additional Points to Remember—Dos and Don'ts	✓ Do separately report other E/M services or other procedures when the physician performs them with Special Evaluation and Management Services.
	✓ Do append modifier -32 when the insurance or another party mandates the evaluation.

17—Newborn Care Services (99460–99465)

Patient Status	Inpatient, other setting, New or Established (codes do not specify new or established patients)
Location	Hospital, Birthing Center, Other Setting
Description of Services	Report for E/M services for a normal newborn (birth to 28 days) in different settings. Services include maternal and/or fetal and newborn history, exam, ordering tests, treatment, discussions with family, and documentation.
	• Services do not apply to newborns with conditions requiring inpatient acute care, including critical or intensive care. See other E/M categories for these services.
	• Newborn care service codes are per day and divided by initial or subsequent services and admission and discharge on the same day for a hospital or birthing center.
	Other newborn services include
	• Delivery/Birthing Room Attendance and Resuscitation Services
Time Based	No
Key Components	Not applicable
Subcategories	**Delivery/Birthing Room Attendance and Resuscitation Services:**
	Attendance at delivery—Report for services for attending a delivery at the delivering physician's request and for stabilizing the newborn's condition.
	Delivery/birthing room resuscitation—Report for resuscitation (restore lung and heart functions), positive pressure ventilation (breathing assistance), and chest compressions. Report additional codes for procedures that physicians perform as a necessary part of the resuscitation, such as endotracheal intubation (inserting a tube in the trachea to assist breathing). Physicians must perform these procedures as a necessary component of the resuscitation.
	Report the two types of services listed *above* in addition to normal newborn services (99460–99463).
Additional Points to Remember—Dos and Don'ts	✓ Do report separate codes for procedures (54150—newborn circumcision) *in addition to* newborn services.
	✓ Do report codes for separate E/M services for critical or intensive care by the same physician on the same date *in addition to* newborn services. Append modifier -25 (separate E/M service) to the critical or intensive care E/M code.

18—Inpatient Neonatal Intensive Care Services and Pediatric and Neonatal Critical Care Services (99466–99480)

Patient Status	Outpatient, Inpatient, New or Established (codes do not specify new or established patients)
Location	Transport (en route to a hospital), Inpatient—Neonatal Intensive Care Unit (NICU), Pediatric Intensive Care Unit (PICU), or other critical care unit
Description of Services	Face-to-face hands-on transport care for a critically ill patient (24 months old or younger) with a life-threatening condition. Services are provided during an inter-facility transport (en route to a hospital). Do not separately report services normally included with critical care transport, such as blood pressure and pulse oximetry. (See CPT manual for complete list under Pediatric Critical Care Patient Transport.)
	Inpatient critical care for neonatal (28 days or younger), infant, or pediatric (29 days to five years old) critically ill patients with life-threatening conditions. Do not separately report services normally included with inpatient critical care. (See CPT manual for complete lists under Critical Care Services and Inpatient Neonatal and Pediatric Critical Care.)
	Intensive care services for neonates age 28 days or younger, including those of low birth weight (up to 2500 grams—5 lbs, 8 oz). Services are for patients who are *not critically ill* but require intensive observation and frequent interventions.
	Refer to extensive CPT guidelines for coding all of these services.
Time Based	Yes. Pediatric Critical Care Patient Transport includes • 99466—first 30 to 74 minutes (per day) • +99467—each additional 30 minutes (add-on code) (per day) Inpatient Neonatal and Pediatric Critical Care and Initial and Continuing Intensive Care Services are per day.
Key Components	Not applicable
Subcategories	*Pediatric Critical Care Patient Transport:* Do not report these codes when services are less than 30 minutes. Do not report these codes for services that other members of the transport team provide.
	Inpatient Neonatal and Pediatric Critical Care: Codes are divided by initial and subsequent and patient's age. Report these codes for a single physician once per day, per patient.
	Initial and Continuing Intensive Care Services: Codes are divided by initial and subsequent services. Subsequent services are divided by birth weight. Report these codes for a single physician once per day, per patient.
Additional Points to Remember—Dos and Don'ts	✓ Do not report critical care for critically injured children older than age five with codes for Inpatient Neonatal and Pediatric Critical Care. Instead, report codes from Critical Care Services (99291–99292).
	✓ Do not report critical care for outpatient services with codes for Inpatient Neonatal and Pediatric Critical Care. Instead, report codes from Critical Care Services (99291–99292).

19—Other Evaluation and Management Services (99499)

No table is provided for this category because it only contains one code for an unlisted E/M service.

TAKE A BREAK

Let's take a break and then review coding the remaining categories of E/M services.

Exercise 19.13 **E/M Categories 14–19**

Instructions: Assign procedure code(s) to the following cases, appending appropriate modifiers, and referencing both the index and CPT sections. Refer to the CPT manual and the tables provided for specific information on each category.

1. Yvette Bare sends an email to Dr. Flynn, a pediatrician, regarding her daughter Yvonne, age eight. She states in her email that Yvonne has chronic tonsillitis and requests a prescription refill for an antibiotic. Dr. Flynn saw Yvonne six weeks ago for the same problem, so he responds to Mrs. Bare's email and sends a prescription to her pharmacy.

   Code(s): _____

2. Dr. Hilburn, an occupational medicine specialist, sees Jonathan Sheldon, age 28, for a work-related disability evaluation that his workers' compensation insurance requires. (Dr. Hilburn conducts IMEs through a contract with the insurance, and they reimburse him for each evaluation that he performs.) Mr. Sheldon sustained a lumbar sprain while lifting a large box at his job for a package delivery company. Dr. Hilburn has been treating the patient since his injury occurred. He completes a medical history of Mr. Sheldon's lumbar strain, performs a physical examination, confirms the diagnosis of lumbar strain, assesses his capabilities and stability, calculates the degree of impairment, develops recommendations for treatment, and completes the documentation and report that the insurance requires.

   Code(s): _____

3. Brandi Gilmer, age 26, delivers baby boy, Brandon, vaginally after an occipital presentation. Brandon's Apgar scores are 8 and 10. The infant has no perinatal conditions or congenital anomalies. Dr. Flynn, a pediatrician, provides evaluation and management services for baby Brandon on the day of his birth. He performs a newborn history, conducts a newborn physical examination, orders diagnostic tests, meets with the family, and documents his work in the medical record.

   Code(s) for Dr. Flynn: _____

4. Dr. Wooten, an OB/GYN, delivers baby Miriam to Myra Board, age 23, at Middledale Community Hospital. Dr. Rios, a neonatal cardiologist, diagnoses baby Miriam in critical condition with tetralogy of Fallot. He wants to move her to Williton Medical Center, the closest major hospital, which is 100 miles away. He accompanies baby Miriam on the medical helicopter and provides 1 hour and 45 minutes of critical care services during the flight.

   Code(s): _____

5. Dr. Hoffman sees new patient Rosa Santiago, age 52, for an annual exam. He determines that she is perfectly healthy, and Rhonda, the medical assistant, schedules her for a return appointment next year.

   Code(s): _____

6. Terri Love, age 45, sees Dr. Hoffman for her regular annual check-up. During the exam, Ms. Love states that she "feels fine," but upon questioning, the patient admits to recently having cloudy urine. She provides a urine sample, and Dr. Hoffman diagnoses a urinary tract infection (UTI). He prescribes an antibiotic. Dr. Hoffman's services include an annual exam, as well as services that include a problem-focused history and exam and straightforward MDM for the UTI.

   Code(s): _____

CHAPTER REVIEW

Multiple Choice

Instructions: Circle one best answer to complete each statement.

1. NPPs who can assign some E/M codes include all of the following *except*
   a. physician assistant (PA).
   b. nurse practitioner (NP).
   c. certified nursing assistant (CNA).
   d. certified nurse midwife (CNM).

2. After a physician turns in an encounter form to office staff, you, as the coder audit the patient's documentation and
   a. compare it to the E/M level on the encounter form.

   b. change information the physician documented in the record to match the encounter form.

   c. change the code on the encounter form if it does not match the documentation.

   d. compare the documentation with the health history form to check documentation accuracy.

3. A(n) _____ is a patient who has not received any professional services within the past three years from the physician or another physician of the same specialty who belongs to the same group practice.
   a. new patient
   b. established patient
   c. inpatient
   d. outpatient

4. Which of the following is *not* a category of E/M service?
   a. Office or Other Outpatient Services
   b. Consultations
   c. Non-Face-to-Face Physician Services
   d. Adult Intensive Care Services

5. Which of the following is *not* one of the four types of medical decision-making?
   a. Straightforward
   b. Detailed
   c. Moderate
   d. High

6. _____ is when the physician reviews information about the patient's body systems by asking the patient a series of questions to identify past or current signs and/or symptoms.
   a. Chief complaint
   b. Examination
   c. Review of systems
   d. Medical decision-making

7. The level of risk of medical decision-making that includes chest X-ray, EKG, and urinalysis is
   a. minimal.
   b. low.
   c. moderate.
   d. high.

8. The history of present illness element that asks the patient to describe how her condition feels is
   a. severity.
   b. context.
   c. quality.
   d. duration.

9. The _____ is the type of history that includes constitutional symptoms:
   a. CC
   b. HPI
   c. ROS
   d. PFSH

10. The type of examination that includes a general multisystem exam is
   a. problem-focused.
   b. expanded problem-focused.
   c. detailed.
   d. comprehensive.

Chapter Assignments

Instructions: Assign CPT-4 procedure code(s) to the following cases, referencing both the index and CPT sections. Optional: For additional practice, assign ICD-9-CM diagnosis codes using both the Index and Tabular.

1. Sarah Benavidez, age 71, sees Dr. Lombard, a neurologist, in the office for follow up on peripheral autonomic neuropathy. She also has type II diabetes. Dr. Lombard conducts and documents a comprehensive examination and medical decision-making of high complexity.

   Diagnosis code(s): _____

   Procedure code(s): _____

2. Dr. Goldstein, a psychiatrist, sees Ralph Mccune, age 30, for the third time in the partial hospitalization program at Williton Medical Center. The patient suffers from chronic **schizoaffective** disorder with acute exacerbation. Dr. Goldstein performs and documents a problem-focused history, a problem-focused examination, and medical decision-making of low complexity.

   Diagnosis code(s): _____

   Procedure code(s): _____

3. Dr. Manfred, an oncologist, sees Loretta Embry, age 72, in Williton Medical Center's ED after she collapsed at home. He has been treating her for metastatic ovarian cancer, which has spread to multiple sites, and she recently began chemotherapy. Dr. Manfred conducts and documents a comprehensive history and examination, and he orders a number of lab tests. Medical decision-making is of high complexity as he reviews multiple lab reports and risk factors. Dr. Manfred diagnoses dehydration and hyponatremia due to chemotherapy. He begins IV hydration, but the patient does not stabilize, so he admits her as an inpatient.

   Diagnosis code(s): _____

   Procedure code(s): _____

4. Dr. Hoffman asks Dr. Grisham, an orthopedist, to see Albert Dominguez, age 33, in his office to evaluate a lump behind the knee. Dr. Grisham performs and documents a comprehensive history and exam, and medical decision-making of moderate complexity. He diagnoses osteochondroma and does not recommend surgery unless the lump causes a lot of pain. Dr. Grisham calls Dr. Hoffman with his findings and follows up with a written report.

   Diagnosis code(s): _____

   Procedure code(s): _____

5. Jeremy Morey, age 58, sees Dr. Hoffman for his routine annual preventive care physical. He also saw Dr. Hoffman last year for the same reason. Dr. Hoffman tells him that pure hypercholesterolemia (high cholesterol) appears to be under control and he finds no new problems.

   Diagnosis code(s): _____

   Procedure code(s): _____

6. Dr. Hoffman performs an annual nursing facility assessment for Tony Boutte, age 87, at Valley Nursing Facility. He performs and documents a detailed history, comprehensive examination, and medical decision-making of moderate complexity. He documents Mr. Boutte's diagnoses of benign hypertension with heart failure and **degenerative dementia**.

   Diagnosis code(s): _____

   Procedure code(s): _____

7. Dr. Mills, ED physician, admits Karese Jones, age 26, to Williton Medical Center for observation. The patient experienced chest pain and severe dizziness and drove herself to Williton. After further workup, physicians determine that she had a panic attack and discharge her from observation to home the same day. Observation care includes a comprehensive exam, moderate MDM, and a detailed history

   Diagnosis code(s): _____

   Procedure code(s): _____

8. Randolph Keller is an NF patient. Dr. Guzman, a psychologist, meets with clinical team members and Mrs. Keller, the patient's wife, about his treatment, progress, and prognosis. The patient suffers from senile dementia with acute confusion. The meeting is held at the NF, and it lasts 40 minutes. A physician is not present for the meeting. Assign the procedure code for Dr. Guzman's services.

   Diagnosis code(s): _____

   Procedure code(s): _____

9. On Tuesday, Heather Wolfe, age 22, arrives by ambulance at Williton's ED. Dr. Mills sees her and calls in Dr. Valdez, an orthopedic surgeon. Ms. Wolfe suffers from multiple closed pelvic fractures, which include disruption of the pelvic circle. Dr. Valdez orders tests and then admits the patient. The admission service includes moderate MDM, comprehensive history, and exam. The patient remains in the hospital on Wednesday, Thursday, Friday, and Saturday. Wednesday's services for Dr. Valdez include a detailed history and exam with moderate MDM; on Thursday, Friday, and Saturday they include a problem-focused history and exam and low MDM. Dr. Barber, the attending physician, discharges the patient on Sunday, after spending 45 minutes examining her and providing discharge instructions to her and her family. Assign E/M codes for each day of the patient's stay.

   Diagnosis code(s): _____

   Procedure code(s): _____

10. Dr. Mills, an ED physician at Williton, directs telemetry, cardiac resuscitation, and endotracheal intubation for an emergent patient's care over the phone with emergency management services (EMS) while the ambulance is on route to the hospital. The patient went into cardiac arrest in the ambulance.

    Diagnosis code(s): _____

    Procedure code(s): _____

schizoaffective (skit′so-ə-fek′tiv)—psychiatric condition in which a person demonstrates symptoms of both schizophrenia and mood disorders

degenerative dementia—severe loss of intellectual function with no discernible cause

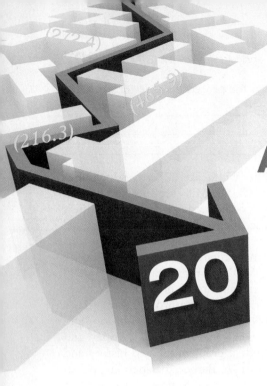

Anesthesia

Learning Objectives

After completing this chapter, you should be able to

- Spell and define the key terminology in this chapter.
- Define anesthesia and discuss its history.
- Describe the types of anesthesia providers.
- Explain the types of anesthesia.
- Discuss anesthesia complications and risks.
- Define the anesthesia code package.
- Assign anesthesia codes.
- Name the qualifying circumstances codes.
- Identify modifiers for anesthesia.
- Explain the unique features of anesthesia coding, billing, and reimbursement.

Key Terms

anesthesia
anesthesia code package
anesthesia time
base unit value

intraservice time
modifiers for anesthesia providers
physical status modifier
qualifying circumstances codes
time units

INTRODUCTION

At this stop on your coding journey, you will learn about anesthesia services and different anesthesia providers. You will also learn about various types of anesthesia that providers use, depending on the type of procedure that a patient receives. There are also specific anesthesia modifiers to append to anesthesia services, including modifiers that represent the patient's overall health and modifiers to identify the type of anesthesia provider involved in a service. You will have the opportunity to expand your coding knowledge and continue to practice the skills you already acquired for coding both procedures and diagnoses.

"We keep moving forward, opening new doors, and doing new things, because we're curious, and curiosity keeps leading us down new paths."—WALT DISNEY

ANESTHESIA

Anesthesia is a medical specialty involving administering anesthetic drugs to patients during diagnostic or therapeutic procedures, monitoring their conditions throughout the procedures (by checking heart rate, blood pressure, respiration, and organ functions), ensuring the patients' safety while they are under anesthesia, and providing care before and after the procedures. Anesthetic drugs cause partial or total sensation loss so that the patient can undergo a medical procedure without feeling pain. Anesthesia also prevents them from moving during procedures and can be combined with other drugs that relieve a patient's fears and anxiety about surgical procedures. A patient may or may not lose consciousness while under anesthesia, depending on the type of anesthesia given and the nature of the procedure. The anesthesia code range is 00100–01999, and you can find anesthesia codes in the second section of the CPT manual.

It is important to understand that simply locating an anesthesia code in the CPT manual is not all that is involved with coding anesthesia services. There are many different insurance regulations governing coding, billing, and reimbursement for anesthesia, which can be very complex. There is also a process for checking each anesthesia CPT code for its correlation to a specific procedure, using a crosswalk that the American Society of Anesthesiologists (ASA) created. Here are some other reasons that anesthesia coding is challenging:

- The ASA assigns base unit values (BUVs) to anesthesia codes and some modifiers, which represent the various complexity levels of anesthesia services. Insurances, including Medicare, use BUVs to determine reimbursement.

- Insurances may reimburse more if specific modifiers are present with the CPT code.

- Some anesthesia services do not require an anesthesia code but instead require a code that represents the actual procedure.

- Time units are required with anesthesia services and can differ among payers.

- Insurance coding requirements for reimbursement can differ depending on the payer and on each patient's specific situation and diagnoses.

So keep in mind that there are many different coding criteria to consider when coding for an anesthesia service that ultimately affect reimbursement, and you will learn more about them as you work through this chapter.

History of Anesthesia

We take anesthesia for granted today, knowing that physicians can deaden pain of surgery with anesthesia, but this was not always the case. In ancient times, physicians gave patients opiates, like poppy seeds, or herbs, like hemp and cannabis, to reduce pain or render a patient unconscious. Problems occurred because physicians could not often predict the quantity of anesthesia that a patient needed, so many patients either still had pain during a procedure or died from an overdose of an anesthetic drug. Physicians also hypnotized patients to eliminate pain before surgical procedures.

In the 1800s, physicians gave patients carbon dioxide, morphine, cocaine, chloroform, ether, or alcohol to deaden pain. You may have seen old westerns where the unfortunate patient only received a shot of whiskey and the opportunity to bite down on a bullet or strap of leather to eliminate the pain! The patient was also permitted to hold the whiskey bottle for ready access in case the effect of the whiskey wore off and he needed more. In 1846, William Morton held the first demonstration of ether used as anesthesia for a patient who had a neck tumor removed (■ FIGURE 20-1). Morton was a dentist who pioneered using ether, even though he was not the first person to discover it. Morton spent his life trying to market the use of ether, but in spite of his efforts, he died bankrupt.

The late 1800s brought advances in anesthesia administration as people learned **aseptic** techniques for sterilization to keep the patient and the operating environment germ-free. In the 1900s, there were additional advancements in anesthesia: the discovery of new anesthetic drugs and the use of **endotracheal intubation**, also called intubation. Intubation is when the physician inserts a flexible tube into the patient's mouth or nose,

aseptic (a-sep′tik)—free from infection; sterile

endotracheal intubation (end ō-tra′ke-əl in-too-ba′ shən)

Figure 20-1 ■ A daguerreotype (early photograph) believed to be a re-enactment of the first demonstration of ether anesthesia by Dr. William T. G. Morton at Massachusetts General Hospital on October 16, 1846.

Photo credit: © Everett Collection Inc./Alamy.

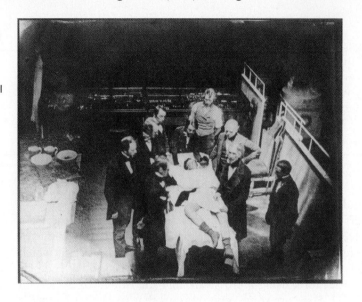

laryngoscope (lə-ring′gə-skōp)—an endoscope used to visually examine the larynx (voice box)

anesthetized (uh-nes′-thi-tahyz)

extubation (ek-stoo-bā′-shən)

through the vocal folds, into the pharynx (throat), and into the trachea (windpipe). The tube is called an endotracheal tube (ET) (■ Figure 20-2). A **laryngoscope** helps the physician to view internal structures in order to insert the ET. Clinicians can then administer anesthesia gases through the ET.

Intubation allows air to move in and out of the lungs while the patient is **anesthetized** (given anesthesia) during surgery. Intubation is also used for patients who need a mechanical ventilator during surgery. Removing the endotracheal tube after anesthesia administration is called **extubation**.

Anesthesia providers eliminate pain during patients' surgeries, and they can also help patients who do not need surgery but instead require anesthesia for pain control (called

Figure 20-2 ■ Endotracheal tube placement.

Photo credit: © Nucleus Medical Art, Inc./Alamy.

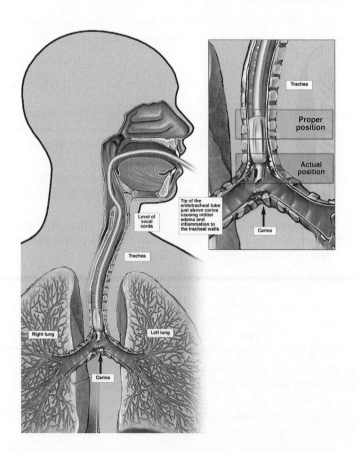

pain management) for conditions like cancer. Some anesthesia providers specialize in pain management to help patients live without constant pain. Other times, anesthesia providers oversee anesthesia for a patient's procedure and then administer postoperative pain management medications after surgery for pain control.

Keep in mind that when you are coding for this type of case, you should assign an anesthesia procedure code for the anesthesia services and a separate procedure code for the type of pain management, such as epidural anesthesia. Append modifier -59 (indicating a separate procedure) to the additional anesthesia pain management service.

ANESTHESIA PROVIDERS

Recall from Chapter 18 that an anesthesiologist is a physician who is trained in the specialty of anesthesia administration. An anesthesiologist is a medical doctor of anesthesia (MDA). MDAs can specialize in anesthesia for cases in pediatrics, obstetrics, cardiothoracic, neurosurgical, orthopedics, critical care, trauma, organ transplant, ambulatory, and pain management. They work on cases alone, with other MDAs, and can also supervise other anesthesia providers.

A certified registered nurse anesthetist (CRNA) is a registered nurse with advanced education and training in the field of anesthesia. CRNAs can work alone on cases, with other CRNAs, or MDAs can supervise their work. An MDA has more education and training than a CRNA and is licensed to practice medicine. CRNAs can work in hospitals and ambulatory surgery centers and may also work in surgery suites, physician offices, and pain management clinics. Both medical residents and nursing anesthetist students who train in anesthesia work under a physician's supervision until they have all necessary experience and are permitted to work independently.

An anesthesiologist assistant (AA) is a specialty physician assistant who assists the anesthesiologist and can also work alongside a CRNA. An anesthesia technician, certified anesthesia technician, and certified anesthesia technologist assist the anesthesiologist, AA, and CRNA. They also operate, maintain, and monitor equipment and oversee supplies.

Anesthesia providers are not surgeons. They perform functions related to anesthesia administration, while surgeons perform the actual procedures. However, there are occasions when surgeons also administer the patient's anesthesia, such as a procedure to remove a toenail or to perform a skin biopsy.

CMS requires that the following providers administer anesthesia in order to reimburse services:

- qualified anesthesiologist
- doctor of medicine or osteopathy (other than an anesthesiologist)
- dentist, oral surgeon, or podiatrist who is qualified to administer anesthesia under state law
- CRNA under the supervision of the operating surgeon or an anesthesiologist who is immediately available if needed (physically located in the same area)
- AA under the supervision of an anesthesiologist who is immediately available if needed (physically located in the same area)

TAKE A BREAK

Let's take a break and then review more about anesthesia and anesthesia providers.

Exercise 20.1   **Anesthesia, Anesthesia Providers**

Instructions: On the line preceding each statement, write T for True or F for False.

1. _____ The late 1800s brought advances in anesthesia administration as people learned aseptic techniques for sterilization to keep the patient and the operating environment germ-free.

2. _____ Intubation allows air to move in and out of the lungs while the patient is anesthetized during surgery.

continued

TAKE A BREAK *continued*

3. _____ An AA monitors equipment and oversees supplies.

4. _____ Anesthesia providers perform functions related to anesthesia administration, while surgeons perform the actual procedures.

5. _____ A CRNA is a registered nurse who specializes in anesthesia administration.

6. _____ AAs and CRNAs may administer anesthesia under the supervision of the operating surgeon or an anesthesiologist who is on call in another area of the facility.

TYPES OF ANESTHESIA

Anesthesia providers give patients anesthesia through various methods, including: intravenously, face mask, endotracheal tube, through the nose, or an injection directly into an anatomic site where surgery will occur. Patients receive specific types of anesthesia depending on the procedure the physician performs and whether the patient needs to be awake or asleep. Anesthesia can involve a combination of drugs, including drugs to relieve anxiety and fear and to create amnesia so that the patient does not remember the surgery. Types of anesthesia include general, moderate (conscious) sedation, local and regional anesthesia, nerve block, patient-controlled analgesia, and monitored anesthesia care (MAC).

General Anesthesia

General anesthesia, also called unconscious sedation, is a type of anesthesia which prevents patients from experiencing pain from major surgical procedures. The patient's entire body, including the brain, is anesthetized. The patient receives general anesthesia by breathing vapors through an endotracheal tube or mask or with a combination of IV sedation. The patient is unconscious, cannot communicate with the physician, and remembers nothing about the surgery. Patients under general anesthesia do not have the ability to breathe independently, and the recovery from general anesthesia is longer than any other type of anesthesia. General anesthesia also carries a greater risk of developing complications. General anesthetic drugs include propofol and sevoflurane. Here are some examples of procedures requiring general anesthesia:

- Major orthopedic procedures
- Various general surgeries
- Cardiac surgery
- Neurosurgery
- Pediatric surgery

The type of anesthesia administered depends on the type of procedure, the patient's physical condition and health history, and the potential for possible complications. The anesthesia provider obtains this information by reviewing the patient's medical information, typically during a preoperative or preanesthesia meeting with the patient.

Moderate (Conscious) Sedation

Moderate (conscious) sedation is when the patient loses partial consciousness but is not completely asleep. Patients under moderate sedation receive a combination of drugs to relieve pain and to help them relax. They can communicate with the physician and respond to verbal commands, can breathe independently, and have a shorter recovery time with fewer complications than with general anesthesia. Drugs used for conscious sedation include Demerol® and Versed®. Moderate sedation is also referred to as twilight sedation or twilight sleep. Patients receive moderate sedation for outpatient procedures (same-day surgeries) where they return home the same day. Examples of procedures where patients need moderate sedation include the following:

- Cataract surgery (some cataract surgeries include anesthetic drops instead of conscious sedation, or can include general anesthesia if the patient does not want to be awake during the procedure)
- Craniotomy that requires the patient to respond to the physician's commands
- Vasectomy
- Minor surgeries such as foot or fracture repairs
- Plastic or reconstructive surgery
- Dental reconstructive surgery or dental prosthetics
- **Endoscopy** (such as procedures to diagnose and treat stomach, colon, and bladder conditions)

endoscopy (en-dos'kə-pe)—viewing inside the body through a natural body opening or small incision with a long narrow instrument

Local and Regional Anesthesia

Local and regional anesthesia are types of anesthesia that prevent patients from experiencing pain in a specific body site; regional anesthesia affects a larger body area than local anesthesia. Under local and regional anesthesia, the patient remains awake and can communicate with the physician and also remembers circumstances of the procedure. Local anesthesia, also called conduction anesthesia, is sometimes provided in the form of a spray, solution, or ointment. Local and regional anesthetic drugs include Marcaine® and bupivacaine. Here are some examples of procedures requiring local or regional anesthesia:

- Skin or tissue biopsies
- Cesarean section childbirth
- Procedures performed on the arms, legs, hands, feet, urinary tract, or sexual organs
- Cosmetic surgery
- Dental procedures

Nerve Blocks

A nerve block is an anesthetic injected into or around a nerve to block pain, also called block anesthesia; nerve blocks are used therapeutically to control chronic pain or used during procedures. They can be in the form of local anesthesia, regional anesthesia, or analgesia (medicine that eliminates pain). Analgesia provides pain relief by blocking pain receptors in the peripheral and/or central nervous system, but the patient does not lose consciousness. Providers can create permanent nerve blocks for patients using

- alcohol or **phenol** (a solution that burns) to destroy nerve tissue
- cryoanalgesia to freeze nerves
- radiofrequency ablation, using heat to destroy nerves

phenol (fe'nol)

Drugs that are used for local nerve blocks include lidocaine and novacaine, and drugs that are used for regional nerve blocks include morphine and methadone. Types of nerve blocks include the following:

- *Epidural block*—Epidural anesthesia numbs nerves in the spinal cord, the lower half of the body, and is commonly used for pregnant patients in labor. It is also used for surgeries in the legs and pelvis. Using a needle, the anesthesia provider inserts a catheter (small tube) into the patient's back in the epidural space to deliver anesthesia and leaves the catheter in place in case the patient needs more anesthesia during the procedure (■ FIGURE 20-3).
- *Epidural blood patch*—An epidural blood patch is different from an epidural nerve block. It is a procedure that anesthesia providers perform to relieve headache pain that a lumbar puncture (spinal tap) or epidural anesthesia caused.

Figure 20-3 ■ A needle is injected posteriorly into the epidural (above the dura) space. The space contains spinal nerves, which travel up the spinal cord to the brain.

Photo credit: © Nucleus Medical Art, Inc./Alamy.

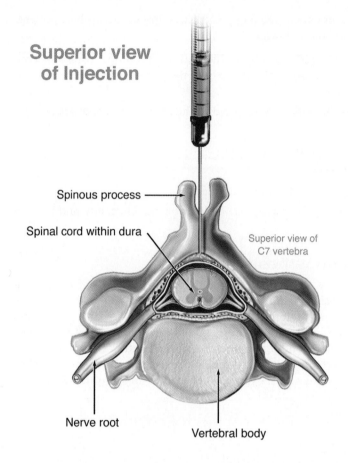

Superior view of Injection

Spinous process

Spinal cord within dura

Superior view of C7 vertebra

Nerve root

Vertebral body

Lumbar punctures involve puncturing the dura (membrane containing the spinal cord and brain) to collect cerebrospinal fluid (CSF) to diagnose meningitis, hydrocephalus, and intracranial hypertension or to administer chemotherapy medications. Patients can experience headaches from lumbar punctures because CSF leaks out of the puncture site, reducing intracranial pressure.

Epidural anesthesia involves injecting drugs into the epidural space to anesthetize nerves in the spinal cord. If the dura is punctured accidentally, it can cause a CSF leak, which can cause a postdural puncture headache.

To perform a blood patch, the anesthesia provider injects the patient's own blood into epidural space that is close to the original puncture site. The blood then forms a clot, which patches the leak.

An *epidural nerve block* involves injecting a corticosteroid into the epidural space to decrease pain from a herniated disk, spinal stenosis, or other disorders.

- *Spinal block*—Anesthesia is injected into the fluid that surrounds the spinal cord or cerebrospinal fluid (CSF); spinal blocks are used for urologic and genital procedures, as well as procedures on the lower body.

- *Peripheral nerve block*—Anesthesia is injected into the peripheral nerves in the patient's arm or leg for procedures on the arms and legs.

- *Axillary block*—Anesthesia is injected into the armpit for procedures on the hand, wrist, elbow, and forearm.

plexus (plek′səs)

- *Plexus block*—Anesthesia is injected into an area of a nerve plexus, or network of nerves, for procedures near the nerve network, such as the cardiac plexus or pelvic plexus.

supraclavicular (soo-prə-klə-vik′u-lər)

- *Supraclavicular block*—Anesthesia is injected above the clavicle (collarbone) for procedures on the wrist, hand, upper arm, and elbow.

- *Infraclavicular block*—Anesthesia is injected toward the **brachial** plexus (network of nerves) below the clavicle (collarbone) for procedures on the wrist, forearm, and elbow.
- *Interscalene block*—Anesthesia is injected into the neck for procedures on the shoulder and arm.
- *Bier block*—A Bier block is used for procedures on extremities or for pain management. First, a tourniquet is used on the upper arm or leg and is inflated. Anesthesia is injected into a vein in the arm or leg, anesthetizing nerve endings and peripheral nerves. The tourniquet prevents the block from traveling to other areas of the body.
- *Wrist block*—Anesthesia is injected near wrist nerves, such as the **median nerves** and **ulnar nerves** for procedures on the fingers and hand.
- *Saddle block or caudal block*—Anesthesia is injected into the lower spine for procedures on the legs or buttocks.
- *Intrapleural block*—Anesthesia is injected between the **parietal pleura** and **visceral pleura** for a thoracotomy or biopsy of the pleura.
- *Intraarticular block*—Anesthesia is injected into a joint for procedures on the joint.
- *Field block*—Anesthesia is injected into an area surrounding the procedure site.
- *Rescue block*—A postsurgical anesthesia injection keeps the patient comfortable and pain-free.

infraclavicular (in-frə-klə-vik′u-lər)

brachial (brā′-kē-əl)

interscalene (int′-ər-ska′-leen)

median nerves—nerves in the forearm

ulnar nerves (ul′nər)—nerves in the forearm and front and back of the hand

caudal (kaw′dəl)

intrapleural (in-trə-ploor′əl)

parietal pleura (pə-ri′ə-təl ploor′ə)—serous (smooth) membrane covering the chest wall

visceral pleura (vis′ər-əl ploor′ə)—serous (smooth) membrane covering the lungs

intraarticular (in-trə-är-tik′-yə-lər)

Patient-Controlled Analgesia

Patient-controlled analgesia (PCA) is pain medication that a patient administers, in response to the level of pain. A PCA pump is an electronically controlled analgesia pump that delivers pain medication intravenously. The patient pushes a button on a hand-held device to direct the pump to deliver the medication. The provider sets the limit on the maximum amount of medication that the pump can deliver to the patient during a specific time interval. PCA pumps help patients with postoperative pain control and also relieve pain for terminally ill cancer patients.

Monitored Anesthesia Care

Monitored anesthesia care (MAC) is a specific type of anesthesia service where an anesthesiologist or CRNA addresses any problems or **physiological** changes the patient may have while under various types of anesthesia. The anesthesia provider is also ready to address *potential* problems or changes that could occur during a diagnostic or therapeutic procedure, to ensure the patient's safety and the best health outcomes. MAC can include oxygen administration and patient monitoring using the same procedures the anesthesia provider employs in general or other types of anesthesia. MAC may involve a combination of anesthesia drugs and/or conversion to a different type of anesthesia during a procedure, such as converting from one type of anesthesia at the start of the procedure to general anesthesia later. Anesthesia providers determine the need for MAC by assessing the type of procedure for the patient, the patient's health status and medical history, risks of anesthesia to the patient, and the potential for converting the type of anesthesia during the procedure. Like other anesthesia services, MAC services include preoperative, intraoperative, and postoperative care of the patient.

physiological (fiz-e-o-loj′i-kəl)—pertaining to the physical functions of the body

Insurances that reimburse for MAC approve services if they are medically necessary based on the patient's condition, medical history, and patient information documented in the anesthesia record. They do not reimburse providers who provide MAC for *all* anesthesia cases. There are modifiers for MAC anesthesia that you should append to the anesthesia CPT code so the insurance will know that MAC anesthesia was provided. We will review these modifiers later in this chapter.

TAKE A BREAK

Good job! Let's take a break and then review more about types of anesthesia.

Exercise 20.2 Types of Anesthesia

Instructions: Match the term in the list to its description.

1. _____ An anesthesia provider may administer a combination of anesthesia drugs, such as intravenous anesthesia and nerve blocks.

2. _____ A type of anesthesia which prevents patients from experiencing pain from major surgical procedures.

3. _____ Anesthetic injected into or around a nerve to block pain.

4. _____ Anesthesia injected into an area of a nerve plexus.

5. _____ The patient loses partial consciousness but is not completely asleep.

6. _____ A procedure that anesthesia providers perform to relieve a patient's headache pain that a lumbar puncture or epidural anesthesia caused.

Bier block	moderate sedation	spinal block
epidural block	monitored anesthesia care (MAC)	local anesthesia
epidural blood patch	nerve block	patient-controlled analgesia (PCA)
general anesthesia	plexus block	

ANESTHESIA COMPLICATIONS AND RISKS

Although advances in anesthesia enable providers to eliminate patients' pain during many types of surgeries, anesthesia is not without risks. Patients with comorbidities are at a greater risk for developing complications from anesthesia than are normal, healthy patients. Risks also depend on the complexity of a procedure and the type of anesthesia administered. Side effects, risks, and complications during or after anesthesia can include any of the following:

nausea and vomiting	shakiness	seizures
disorientation	hallucinations	myocardial infarction
sleepiness	headache	pyrexia
confusion	problems urinating	irregular heart rhythm
chills	loose stools	difficulty breathing

- Sore throat after general anesthesia because of endotracheal tube placement
- Temporary or permanent loss of function or numbness in areas where nerve blocks were administered
- Allergic reactions to anesthesia drugs
- Death

Before the day of a patient's scheduled surgical procedure, the surgeon or another clinician will review information about the procedure and anesthesia administration. The patient will receive instructions to follow before surgery, such as avoiding food after a specific time because he needs to receive anesthesia on an empty stomach, or stopping certain medicines or herbal remedies within a specific amount of time before surgery.

Preoperative Anesthesia Services

Before or on the day of surgery, the anesthesia provider meets with the patient and/or family to review anesthesia complications and risks, called a preoperative service. The anesthesia provider also asks several questions to better understand the patient's overall health and any current medications the patient takes that may interfere with anesthesia.

The provider determines the type of anesthesia that the patient will need and documents the anesthesia evaluation on a preanesthesia evaluation form for the patient's medical record (■ FIGURE 20-4). Here are some examples of information that the anesthesia provider discusses with the patient and/or family prior to anesthesia administration:

- Current health status, such as current colds or influenza
- Presence of diseases, such as diabetes, hypertension, or renal problems
- Snoring problems, which may indicate breathing difficulty
- Psychiatric disorders, such as anxiety and depression (the patient's medications could interfere with anesthesia, or the patient may experience psychiatric problems upon awakening from anesthesia)
- Prescription and over-the-counter (OTC) medications, vitamin supplements, or herbal remedies or supplements, which could interfere with anesthesia
- Allergies to medications, foods, or latex (found in medical supplies and surgical gloves)
- Previous reactions to anesthesia
- Social history, including tobacco and alcohol use, and use of recreational drugs
- Types of anesthesia medications that will be used during the procedure
- Postoperative care
- Discussion with the patient and family of risks and benefits of anesthesia

Some surgeries are emergent when the patient is unconscious and cannot meet with the anesthesia provider, or the patient may be confused and cannot clearly communicate. In these cases, the provider will attempt to contact family members to obtain information about the patient, if possible.

Informed Consent

The anesthesia provider also obtains the patient's consent, or permission, to administer anesthesia on an informed consent form that the patient signs, showing that he understands the benefits and risks of anesthesia. The consent form is a legal document which shows that the patient was informed about the procedure, benefits, and risks; agreed to the procedure; and agreed to receive anesthesia. Anesthesia providers should ensure that they answer all of the patients' questions and allow adequate time to meet with patients so patients do not feel that the provider is rushing them into making a decision about receiving anesthesia. Because the patient signs a consent form, if he later develops a complication, then he cannot blame the provider if the complication were listed as one of the possible complications or risks of anesthesia. A family member may also sign a consent form if the patient is unable to sign because of his health condition. ■ FIGURE 20-5 shows an example of a consent form that a patient signs agreeing to undergo a procedure and receive anesthesia.

ANESTHESIA CODE PACKAGE

Recall that a surgical package includes preoperative, intraoperative, and postoperative care. The **anesthesia code package** includes the same services and is very similar to a surgical code package. The anesthesia CPT code includes preoperative and postoperative visits with the anesthesia provider and anesthesia administration before and during a surgical, diagnostic, therapeutic, or obstetrical procedure. The code package includes both induction of (start of) and emergence from (end of) anesthesia. You learned earlier in this chapter about preoperative visits between the anesthesia provider and the patient.

Preoperative care also includes placing monitoring devices on the patient and facilitating anesthesia administration with other equipment, such as an ET. Anesthesia *administration* begins when the anesthesia provider induces the patient, monitoring the patient's vital signs and reactions to anesthesia to ensure that the patient receives the correct amount of anesthesia and has no adverse reactions.

PRE-ANESTHESIA EVALUATION

AGE	SEX □ M □ F	HEIGHT in./cm.	WEIGHT lb./kg.	PRE-PROCEDURE VITAL SIGNS B/P P R T

PROPOSED PROCEDURE

PREVIOUS ANESTHESIA/OPERATIONS (*If none, check here* □)	CURRENT MEDICATIONS (*If none, check here* □)
FAMILY HISTORY OF ANESTHESIA COMPLICATIONS (*If none, check here* □)	ALLERGIES (*If NKDA, check here* □)

AIRWAY/TEETH/HEAD AND NECK	HISTORY FROM □ PARENT/GUARDIAN □ POOR HISTORIAN □ CHART □ SIGNIFICANT OTHER □ PATIENT

SYSTEM	WNL	COMMENTS	PERTINENT STUDY RESULTS
RESPIRATORY Asthma Pneumonia Bronchitis Productive cough COPD Recent cold Dyspnea SOB Orthopnea Tuberculosis	□	Tobacco Use: □ No □ Yes _____ Pack/Day for _____ Years	Chest X-ray Pulmonary Studies
CARDIOVASCULAR Angina MI Arrhythmia Murmur CHF MVP Exercise Tolerance Pacemaker Hypertension Rheumatic fever	□		EKG
HEPATO/GASTROINTESTINAL Bowel obstruction Jaundice Cirrhosis N&V Hepatitis Reflux/heartburn Histal hernia Ulcers	□	Ethanol Use: □ No □ Yes Frequency _____	
NEURO/MUSCULOSKELETAL Arthritis Paresthesia Back problems Syncope CVA/stroke Seizures DJD TIAs Headaches Weakness Loss of consciousness Neuromuscular disease Paralysis	□		
RENAL/ENDOCRINE Diabetes Renal failure/Dialysis Thyroid disease Urinary retention Urinary tract infection Weight loss/gain	□		
OTHER Anemia Bleeding tendencies Hemophilia Pregnancy Sickle cell trait Transfusion history			

PROBLEM LIST/DIAGNOSES	ASA PS 1 2 3 4 5 E	LAB STUDIES Hgb/Hc/CBC Electrolytes Urinalysis
PLANNED ANESTHESIA/SPECIAL MONITORS		OTHER
		POST-ANESTHESIA NOTE
PRE-ANESTHESIA MEDICATIONS ORDERED		
SIGNATURE OF EVALUATOR(S)		
		Signed Date Time

OPTIONAL FORM 517 BACK

Figure 20-4 ■ Pre-Anesthesia Evaluation Form.

Source: U.S. General Services Administration, http://www.gsa.gov.

MEDICAL RECORD	**REQUEST FOR ADMINISTRATION OF ANESTHESIA AND FOR PERFORMANCE OF OPERATIONS AND OTHER PROCEDURES**

A. IDENTIFICATION

1a. *(Check all applicable boxes)*		1b. DESCRIBE
OPERATION OR PROCEDURE	SEDATION	
ANESTHESIA	TRANSFUSION	

B. STATEMENT OF REQUEST

2. The nature and purpose of the operation or procedure, possible alternative methods of treatment, the risks involved, and the possibility of complications have been fully explained to me. I acknowledge that no guarantees have been made to me concerning the results of the operation or procedure. I understand the nature of the operation or procedure to be (describe operation or procedure in layman's language)

which is to be performed by or under the direction of Dr. _____

3. I request the performance of the above-named operation or procedure and of such additional operations or procedures as are found to be necessary or desirable, in the judgment of the professional staff of the below-named medical facility, during the course of the above-named operation or procedure.

4. I request the administration of such anesthesia as may be considered necessary or advisable in the judgment of the professional staff of the below-named medical facility.

5. Exceptions to surgery or anesthesia, if any are: _____
(If "none", so state)

6. I request the disposal by authorities of the below-named medical facility of any tissues or parts which it may be necessary to remove.

7. I understand that photographs and movies may be taken of this operation, and that they may be viewed by various personnel undergoing training or indoctrination at this or other facilities. I consent to the taking of such pictures and observation of the operation by authorized personnel, subject to the following conditions:

   a. The name of the patient and his/her family is not used to identify said pictures.

   b. Said pictures be used only for purposes for medical/dental study or research.

(Cross out any parts above which are not appropriate)

C. SIGNATURES
(Appropriate items in parts A and B must be completed before signing)

8. COUNSELING PHYSICIAN/DENTIST: I have counseled this patient as to the nature of the proposed procedure(s), attendant risks involved, and expected results, as described above. I have also discussed potential problems related to recuperation, possible results of non-treatment, and significant alternative therapies.

_____
(Signature of Counseling Physician/Dentist)

9. PATIENT: I understand the nature of the proposed procedure(s), attendant risks involved, and expected results, as described above, and hereby request such procedure(s) be performed.

_____ _____ _____
(Signature of Witness, excluding members of operating team) | *(Signature of Patient)* | *(Date and Time)*

10. SPONSOR OR GUARDIAN: (When patient is a minor or unable to give consent) _____
sponsor/guardian of _____ understand the nature of the proposed procedure(s), attendant risks involved, and expected results, as described above, and hereby request such procedure(s) be performed.

_____ _____ _____
(Signature of Witness, excluding members of operating team) | *(Signature of Sponsor/Legal Guardian)* | *(Date and Time)*

PATIENT'S IDENTIFICATION (For typed or written entries, give: Name -- last, first, middle; ID no. (SSN or other); hospital or medical facility)	REGISTER NO.	WARD NO.

REQUEST FOR ADMINISTRATION OF ANESTHESIA AND FOR PERFORMANCE OF OPERATIONS AND OTHER PROCEDURES

Medical Record

OPTIONAL FORM 522 (REV. 8/2003)
Prescribed by GSA/ICMR FMR (41 CFR) 102-194.30(i)

Figure 20-5 ■ Request for Administration of Anesthesia and for Performance of Operations and Other Procedures.

Source: U.S. General Services Administration, http://www.gsa.gov.

Intraoperative anesthesia care involves monitoring and managing the patient's physiological status during a procedure and ensuring the patient's safety. If a patient experiences complications to anesthesia, then the anesthesia provider must render appropriate care to the patient, including life-saving interventions, such as cardiopulmonary resuscitation, restoration of fluids and blood, and respiratory therapy.

The following services are *included* in the anesthesia code package:

- Blood administration
- Fluid administration
- Electrocardiogram (ECG), an electrical recording of heart functions
- Temperature
- Blood pressure
- **Oximetry,** also called pulse oximetry, a test to measure the amount or level of oxygen in the blood
- **Capnography,** a test to measure the amount or level of carbon dioxide in the blood
- Mass **spectrometry,** a test to measure the amount of gases and anesthetics the patient inhales and exhales

oximetry (ok-sim′ə-tre)

capnography (kap-nog′rə-fe)

spectrometry (spek-trom′ə-tre)

Postoperatively, the anesthesia provider reverses the effects of anesthesia so that the patient can awaken (called emergence) and return to *baseline functioning,* or a normal state of functioning. The patient is taken to a postoperative room or another area to recover from the surgical procedure and effects of anesthesia. For an outpatient hospital procedure, the patient can return home after the anesthesia provider and other clinicians, such as nurses, ensure that the patient has no negative effects or complications. For an inpatient procedure, the patient does not return home until the attending physician discharges him.

It is important to note that more than one anesthesia provider can be involved in a specific patient's case, with one provider overseeing preoperative care and another overseeing the intraoperative and postoperative care. Check individual payers' coding and billing requirements when there is more than one provider involved in a case because requirements differ among payers.

Unusual Forms of Patient Monitoring

Unusual forms of patient monitoring, such as the placement of specific catheters, are *excluded* from the anesthesia code package because the anesthesia provider must perform *additional work* beyond what is normally required for anesthesia administration. Catheter placements allow the anesthesia provider to measure specific parameters about a patient's condition. The type of catheter that the provider uses depends on the patient's situation, and not all patients receive catheters. You can code unusual forms of patient monitoring separately because they are

- not part of the anesthesia services
- not part of the total time the provider renders anesthesia services
- separate surgical procedures (some payers require you to append modifier -59 to indicate a distinct procedural service to codes for these procedures)

There are three types of catheter placements, which are considered unusual forms of patient monitoring. You should code and bill them separately from anesthesia services:

1. *Intra-arterial catheter (also called an A-line)*—This catheter is placed in an artery, usually on the inner wrist, but sometimes in an artery of the groin or foot or on the inner side of the elbow. The A-line allows the anesthesia provider to closely monitor blood pressure, draw blood for lab tests, and measure the amount of oxygen in the blood.

2. *Central venous catheter (CVC)*—Also called a central line or central venous line, this is a catheter placed into a large vein, such as the external or internal **jugular**

jugular (jug′u-l ər)

veins in the neck, the **subclavian** vein in the chest, or the **femoral** vein in the groin. Using the CVC, the anesthesia provider can administer fluids and medication, measure the amount of oxygen in the blood, and measure cardiovascular functions, like **central venous pressure (CVP)**. Many times, clinicians refer to the CVC as a CVP line because it measures CVP.

3. ***Swan-Ganz catheter***—The Swan-Ganz catheter is also placed into a large vein, like the internal jugular, subclavian, or femoral vein, and then passed through the heart into the pulmonary artery. The catheter has an inflatable balloon at its tip, and when it is inflated, the balloon allows the catheter to remain within a pulmonary blood vessel to measure pressure inside the heart. The anesthesia provider uses the Swan-Ganz catheter to monitor heart functions, sepsis, and effects of medications. Two cardiologists from Cedars-Sinai Medical Center in Los Angeles, California, invented it, Dr. Jeremy Swan and Dr. William Ganz.

You can locate codes for these services by first searching for the main term *catheterization* in the index and then the subterm for the body site where the provider places the catheter.

Epidural catheters and nerve blocks for postoperative pain control are other examples of services excluded from the anesthesia code package that you should code separately.

Throughout the time that the anesthesia provider renders care to the patient, the provider documents the time and other information on the patient's medical record of anesthesia (■ FIGURE 20-6).

The medical record of anesthesia includes details about the patient's anesthesia administration and monitoring from the beginning of a procedure to the time the patient is recovering postoperatively. The anesthesia provider documents intraoperative anesthesia services including administration and monitoring, drugs administered, techniques used, fluids or blood products given, vital signs, complications, and adverse reactions. The anesthesia provider also documents postanesthesia information in the patient's medical record. Refer to Figure 20-4 to review the preanesthesia evaluation form. The bottom right section contains space for postanesthesia notes.

It is important to note that when an anesthesiologist and another anesthesia provider, such as a CRNA, are both involved in a patient's anesthesia services, they must specifically document in the patient's record which provider performed specific services.

subclavian (səb-klā'-vē-ən)

femoral (fem'or-əl)

central venous pressure (ve'nəs)—blood pressure in a vein, which is measured in the right atrium

---

INTERESTING FACT: Patients Can Awaken from Anesthesia Too Soon

Once a patient is unconscious from anesthesia, the anesthesiologist monitors his medications and health status to keep him that way. In rare cases, though, something can go wrong. In one out of every 1,000 to 2,000 surgeries, patients gain anesthesia awareness when they should be unconscious. They may hear the doctors talking and remember it afterward. Worse yet, they may feel pain but be unable to move or tell the doctors.

"It's a real problem, although it's quite rare," says Dr. Alex Evers, an anesthesiologist at Washington University in St. Louis. "Anesthesia awareness can lead to posttraumatic stress disorder," a severe anxiety disorder that can arise after a terrifying ordeal.

Scientists developed strategies to identify and prevent anesthesia awareness. Small studies suggested

that brain monitors might help. But in 2008, Evers and his colleagues reported the results of the largest study to compare different techniques. Brain monitoring did no better than standard monitoring in preventing anesthesia awareness. Addiction to alcohol or drugs increases the risk for anesthesia awareness, but doctors cannot accurately predict who will be affected. A research team in Canada identified variations in a gene that may allow animals to form memories while they are under anesthesia. Ongoing studies are exploring whether this gene plays a role in anesthesia awareness in people.

(U.S. Department of Health and Human Services, National Institutes of Health, newsinhealth.nih.gov/issue/Apr2011/Feature1, accessed 4/25/11.)

AUTHORIZED FOR LOCAL REPRODUCTION

MEDICAL RECORD-ANESTHESIA

PROCEDURE

	ITEM	START	STOP
	Anesthesia		
	Procedure		

DATE	OR NO.	PAGE OF	SURGEON(S)

PRE-PROCEDURE
- ☐ Identified ☐ ID Band ☐ Questioning
- ☐ Chart Review   ☐ Permit Signed
- ☐ NPO Since _____
- Pre-anesthetic State: ☐ Calm
- ☐ Awake   ☐ Asleep
- ☐ Apprehensive   ☐ Confused
- ☐ Uncooperative   ☐ Unresponsive

PATIENT SAFETY
- ☐ Anes. Machine # _____ Checked
- ☐ Safety Belt On   ☐ Axillary Roll
- ☐ Arm Restraints   ☐ Arms Tucked
- ☐ Pressure points checked and padded
- ☐ Eye Care: ☐ Ointment ☐ Saline
- ☐ Taped   ☐ Pads   ☐ Goggles

MONITORS AND EQUIPMENT
- ☐ Steth ☐ Esoph ☐ Precord ☐ Other
- ☐ Non-Invasive B/P   ☐ Nerve Stimulator
- ☐ Continuous EKG   ☐ V Lead EKG
- ☐ Pulse Oximeter   ☐ Oxygen Analyzer
- ☐ End Tidal CO_2 ☐ Resp Gas Anlyzr
- ☐ Temp _____   ☐ EEG
- ☐ Warming Blanket   ☐ Fluid Warmer
- ☐ Airway Humidifier   ☐ _____
- ☐ NG/OG Tube   ☐ Foley Catheter
- ☐ Art Line _____
- ☐ CVP _____
- ☐ PA Line _____
- ☐ IV(s) _____
- ☐ _____

ANESTHETIC TECHNIQUES
- Method: ☐ General   ☐ Spinal
- ☐ Epidural ☐ Caudal   ☐ Brachial
- ☐ Bier Block ☐ Ankle Blk ☐ M.A.C.
- General: ☐ Pre-O_2 ☐ L.T.A.
- ☐ Rapid Sequence ☐ Cricoid Pressure
- ☐ Intravenous   ☐ Inhalation
- ☐ Intramuscular ☐ Rectal
- Regional: ☐ Position _____
- ☐ Prep _____ ☐ Local _____
- ☐ Needle _____
- ☐ Drug(s) _____
- ☐ Dose_____ ☐ Attempts x ____
- ☐ Site _____ ☐ Level _____
- ☐ Catheter _____ ☐ See Remarks

AIRWAY MANAGEMENT
- ☐ Intubation   ☐ Oral   ☐ Nasal
- ☐ Direct Vision ☐ Magill's ☐ Blind
- ☐ Diff. see Rmks ☐ Fiber Op ☐ Stylet
- ☐ Attempts x __ ☐ Blade _____
- ☐ Tube size __ ☐ Endobronchial
- ☐ Regular ☐ RAE ☐ Armored ☐ Laser
- ☐ Cuffed   ☐ Min. occ. pres. ☐ Air ☐ NS
- ☐ Uncuffed, leaks at _____ cm H_2O
- ☐ Secured at _____ ☐ ET CO_2 Present
- ☐ Breath Sounds _____
- ☐ Circuit: ☐ Circle ☐ Non-rebreaking
- ☐ Airway: ☐ Oral ☐ Nasal ☐ Natural
- ☐ Mask Case   ☐ Via Tracheostomy
- ☐ Nasal Cannula   ☐ Simple O_2 Mask

RECOVERY ROOM

Time	B/P	O_2 Sat.

☐ PACU	P	R	T
☐ ICU ☐ L&D			

- ☐ Awake ☐ Spont Resp ☐ Oral Airway
- ☐ Asleep ☐ Ventilator ☐ Nasal Airway
- ☐ Stable ☐ Extubated ☐ Face Shield O_2
- ☐ Unstable ☐ Intubated ☐ T-Piece O_2

CONTROLLED DRUGS

Drug	Used	Destroyed	Returned

Provider	Witness

TIME:

			TOTALS
☐ Hal ☐ Ent ☐ Iso (%)			
☐ N_2O ☐ Air (L/min)			
AGENTS Oxygen (L/min)			
( )			
( )			
( )			
( )			
( )			

FLUIDS

Urine (ml)			
EBL (ml)			
MONITORS EKG			
% O_2 Inspired (FIO₂)			
O_2 Saturation (SAO₂)			
End Tidal CO_2			
Temp: ☐ °C ☐ °F			

VITAL SIGNS

Baselin Values

200
180
160
140
120
B/P   100
80
P   60
40
20
R

VENT

Tidal Vol. (ml)			
Resp. Rate			
Peak Pres. (cm H_2O)			
PEEP (cm H_2O)			
Symbols for Remarks			
Position			

SYMBOLS
- X ANESTHESIA
- ⊙ OPERATION
- ∨∧ B/PCUFF PRESSURE
- ⊥T ARTERIAL LINE PRESSURE
- Δ MEAN ARTERIAL PRESSURE
- ● PULSE
- ○ SPONTANEOUS RESP
- ⊘ ASSISTED RESP
- ⊗ CONTROLLED RESP
- T TOURNIQUET

ANESTHESIA PROVIDER(S)

REMARKS

PATIENT'S IDENTIFICATION (For typed or written entries give: Name-last, first, middle: ID No. (SSN or other); hospital or medical facility.)

ANESTHESIA
Medical Record
OPTIONAL FORM 517 (7-95)
Prescribed by GSA/ICMR,1
FPMR (41 CFR) 101-11.203(b)(10)

Figure 20-6 ■ Medical Record—Anesthesia.

Source: U.S. General Services Administration, http://www.gsa.gov.

TAKE A BREAK

That was a lot of information to remember! Let's take a break and then review more about risks, complications, and the anesthesia code package.

Exercise 20.3 Anesthesia Complications and Risks, Anesthesia Code Package

Instructions: Fill in each blank with the best answer, choosing from the list of words and terms provided.

1. _____ is when the anesthesia provider obtains the patient's permission to administer anesthesia.

2. _____ measures the amount or level of carbon dioxide in the blood.

3. Postoperatively, the anesthesia provider reverses the effects of anesthesia so that the patient can awaken and return to _____, or normal state.

4. Using the _____, the anesthesia provider can administer fluids and medication, measure the amount

of oxygen in the blood, and measure cardiovascular functions.

5. Unusual forms of patient monitoring, such as the placement of specific _____, are excluded from the anesthesia code package.

6. _____ anesthesia care involves monitoring and managing the patient's physiological status during a procedure.

baseline functioning	informed consent	postoperative
capnography	intra-arterial	preoperative
catheters	intraoperative	spectrometry
central venous catheter	oximetry	Swan-Ganz catheter

ANESTHESIA CODES

You can find codes for various types of anesthesia by searching under the main term *anesthesia* in the index. Then search for the subterm for the anatomic site of the procedure (■ FIGURE 20-7) or search for the subterm showing the type of procedure (■ FIGURE 20-8). Turn to the index in your CPT manual to find the anesthesia code choices listed under *anesthesia*.

You can find codes in the Anesthesia section immediately following E/M codes. Just like the E/M section and other sections in the CPT manual, the Anesthesia section also has coding guidelines preceding the codes. Be sure to review the guidelines before assigning codes from the Anesthesia section.

Remember from earlier in this chapter that you learned that anesthesia coding also involves checking the ASA's crosswalk for correlation of a specific anesthesia code to a specific procedure. This step ensures that you choose the correct anesthesia code for the procedure performed. Providers can purchase the copyrighted crosswalk from the ASA, called the *CROSSWALK® Book, A Guide for Surgery/Anesthesia CPT® Codes*. The *CROSSWALK® Book* contains each CPT anesthesia code that describes anesthesia services for specific CPT procedure codes. The ASA determined which anesthesia services are appropriate for a given procedure. You will not use the ASA *CROSSWALK®* in this chapter. You will only code

Anesthesia
See Analgesia
Abbe-Estlander Procedure 00102
Abdomen
Abdominal Wall 00700, 00730, 00800-00802, 00820, 00836
Halsted Repair 00750-00756

Figure 20-7 ■ Index entry for anesthesia for an anatomic site, the abdominal wall.

Anesthesia
Prostatectomy
Perineal 00908
Radical 00865
Walsh Modified Radical 00865

Figure 20-8 ■ Index entry for anesthesia for a procedure, prostatectomy.

■ TABLE 20-1 **ANESTHESIA CODE RANGES**

Subsection—Anatomic Site/Type of Procedure	Code Range
Head	00100–00222
Neck	00300–00352
Thorax (Chest Wall and Shoulder Girdle)	00400–00474
Intrathoracic	00500–00580
Spine and Spinal Cord	00600–00670
Upper Abdomen	00700–00797
Lower Abdomen	00800–00882
Perineum	00902–00952
Pelvis (Except Hip)	01112–01190
Upper Leg (Except Knee)	01200–01274
Knee and **Popliteal** Area	01320–01444
Lower Leg (Below Knee, Includes Ankle and Foot)	01462–01522
Shoulder and Axilla	01610–01682
Upper Arm and Elbow	01710–01782
Forearm, Wrist, and Hand	01810–01860
Radiological Procedures (diagnostic or therapeutic)	01916–01936
Burn Excisions or Debridement	01951–01953
Obstetric	01958–01969
Other Procedures	01990–01999

perineum (per-ə-nē′-əm)—the tissue around the pelvic outlet, between the anus and genitalia

popliteal (päp-lə-tē′-əl)—pertaining to the area behind the knee

using the CPT manual so that you understand the basics about assigning anesthesia codes. But do not forget that if you have to code anesthesia services when you are working in the healthcare field, you will need to reference the crosswalk. (To learn more about the *CROSSWALK*® and other publications from the ASA, visit the ASA's website at http://asahq.org. You can also purchase the crosswalk from other publishers authorized to sell it.)

■ TABLE 20-1 lists anesthesia code ranges from the beginning of the Anesthesia section in the CPT manual. Subsections represent anatomic sites or types of procedures.

■ FIGURE 20-9 shows the Anesthesia section and the first subsection of the body site of *head*. Turn to the Anesthesia section in your CPT manual to review the various subsections and procedures that they contain.

Other subsections of anesthesia are arranged first by a category of procedures, such as radiological, obstetric, or other procedures. ■ FIGURE 20-10 shows the index entries for anesthesia for radiological procedures.

Do you remember learning earlier in the chapter that there can be more than one anesthesia provider administering anesthesia for a specific patient's case? For example, an anesthesiologist can oversee the case, while a CRNA assists. When there is more than one

Anesthesia

Head (00100-00222)

00100 Anesthesia for procedures on salivary glands, including biopsy

00102 Anesthesia for procedures involving plastic repair of cleft lip

00103 Anesthesia for reconstructive procedures of eyelid (eg, blepharoplasty, ptosis surgery)

00104 Anesthesia for electroconvulsive therapy

Figure 20-9 ■ Anesthesia subsection for procedures performed on the head.

Anesthesia

Radiological Procedures 01905-01922

Arterial

Therapeutic 01924-01926

Figure 20-10 ■ Index entry for anesthesia for radiological procedures.

> **Anesthesia**
>
> Sedation
>
> Moderate 99148-99150
>
> with Independent Observation 99143-99145

anesthesia provider for the same patient, assign an anesthesia procedure code for each provider and diagnosis code(s) so that each can bill the patient's insurance. Keep in mind that different insurances have different regulations for coding and billing anesthesia services when there are multiple providers for the same case, so it is best to check individual regulations for more information.

Moderate (Conscious) Sedation Codes

Searching for moderate (conscious) sedation codes is different from searching for many other types of anesthesia. Search under the main term, *anesthesia*, and subterm *sedation* (■ FIGURE 20-11). CPT includes codes for conscious sedation in the Medicine section (99143–99150), not in the Anesthesia section.

Recall that Appendix G in the CPT manual lists procedure codes for diagnostic and therapeutic services that include moderate sedation as an integral part of the procedure. Turn to Appendix G to review the codes listed. When you see procedure codes in CPT that have a ⊙ symbol before the code, it means that the procedure includes moderate sedation. When a physician performs a procedure listed in Appendix G and also administers conscious sedation, he *does not* report a separate code for the sedation, since it is included with the procedure. Instead, he reports only the code for the procedure.

However, there are unusual occasions when another physician administers conscious sedation for procedures listed in Appendix G. Refer to the following CPT guidelines from Appendix G to determine how to code moderate sedation for these situations:

1. When a physician performs a procedure in Appendix G in a facility setting (e.g., hospital, ambulatory surgery center, skilled nursing facility), and a second physician provides moderate sedation,
   - The first physician reports the procedure code.
   - The second physician reports a moderate sedation code from 99148–99150.

2. When a physician performs a procedure in Appendix G in a *nonfacility* setting (e.g., physician office, freestanding imaging center), and a second physician provides moderate sedation,
   - The first physician reports the procedure code.
   - The second physician *does not report* a moderate sedation code.

Intraservice time is included in moderate sedation codes. CPT guidelines state that intraservice time begins when the physician administers sedation, continues with face-to-face attendance to the patient, and ends when the physician no longer has personal contact with the patient. The physician's assessment of the patient before sedation and the patient's recovery time are both *excluded* from intraservice time.

Moderate sedation codes 99148–99150 are categorized by intraservice time and the patient's age (■ FIGURE 20-12).

99148	Moderate sedation services (other than those services described by codes 00100-01999), provided by a physician other than the health care professional performing the diagnostic or therapeutic service that the sedation supports; younger than 5 years of age, first 30 minutes intraservice time
99149	age 5 years or older, first 30 minutes intraservice time
+99150	each additional 15 minutes intraservice time (List separately in addition to code for primary service)

Figure 20-13 ■ Moderate sedation codes 99143–99145.

⊘**99143** Moderate sedation services (other than those services described by codes 00100-01999) provided by the same physician performing the diagnostic or therapeutic service that the sedation supports, requiring the presence of an independent trained observer to assist in the monitoring of the patient's level of consciousness and physiological status; under 5 years of age, first 30 minutes intraservice time

⊘**99144**   age 5 years or older, first 30 minutes intraservice time

+99145   each additional 15 minutes intraservice time (List separately in addition to code for primary service)

There are other occasions when an independent trained observer is present during a procedure to *assist* with monitoring the patient under moderate sedation. In these cases, the physician performing the procedure reports *both* the procedure code and the moderate sedation code (99143–99145). Codes 99143–99145 are also based on intraservice time and the patient's age (■ FIGURE 20-13).

According to CPT guidelines, moderate sedation includes the following services, which you should not code separately:

patency (pa′tən-se)

tympanotomy (tim-pə-nät′-ə-mē)

nephrectomy (ni-frek′-tə-mē)

arthroscopic (är-thrə-skäp′-ik)

- Assess the patient before sedation (excluded from intraservice time)
- Establish IV access and fluids to maintain **patency** (unobstructed), when performed
- Administer agent(s) for sedation
- Maintain sedation
- Monitor oxygen saturation, heart rate, and blood pressure
- Oversee recovery (excluded from intraservice time)

TAKE A BREAK

You are doing very well! Let's take a break and then practice coding anesthesia services.

Exercise 20.4   Anesthesia Codes

Instructions: Review each patient's case and then assign anesthesia procedure code(s) (CPT). *Do not* assign separate CPT codes for surgical procedures. Optional: For additional practice, assign the patient's diagnosis code(s) (ICD-9-CM).

1. Edward Rollins, a CRNA, meets with Mr. and Mrs. Batiste regarding their son, Jeremy, age 10. He is having a **tympanotomy** (incision into the tympanic membrane or eardrum) to treat chronic otitis media. Mr. Rollins oversees all anesthesia services for Jeremy's procedure.

   Diagnosis code(s): _____

   Procedure code(s): _____

2. Dr. Joyner, an anesthesiologist, meets with Christina Maxie, a 25-year-old, who is donating a kidney to her sister. Dr. Joyner oversees all preoperative, intraoperative, and postoperative services for Mrs. Maxie's **nephrectomy** (surgical removal of a kidney).

   Diagnosis code(s): _____

   Procedure code(s): _____

3. Judy Gifford, age 26, delivers her son via cesarean section due to cephalopelvic disproportion and obstructed labor. Dr. Joyner performs preoperative, intraoperative, and postoperative anesthesia services for the patient.

   Diagnosis code(s): _____

   Procedure code(s): _____

4. Edward Rollins, CRNA, is in charge of all anesthesia services today for Samuel Richmond, age 43. The patient undergoes a repair of an incarcerated unilateral inguinal hernia (incarcerated refers to an obstruction; a hernia is part of the abdomen or small intestine that bulges through the groin or scrotum).

   Diagnosis code(s): _____

   Procedure code(s): _____

TAKE A BREAK *continued*

5. Susan Fryer, age 62, has coronary artery disease (of native coronary artery) and has a scheduled cardiac catheterization. Dr. Joyner meets with the patient before the procedure and also handles all of her intraoperative and postoperative anesthesia care.

   Diagnosis code(s): _____

   Procedure code(s): _____

6. Dr. Joyner oversees all aspects of anesthesia care for an **arthroscopic** repair (repair by visualizing a joint with an arthroscope, a type of endoscope). The patient is Anthony Hornback, age 22. He suffers from a torn medial meniscus in the left knee.

   Diagnosis code(s): _____

   Procedure code(s): _____

POINTERS FROM THE PROS: Interview with a Coding Instructor

Terri Barbour is the Medical Faculty Team Leader/Instructor for a two-year college. She has 25 years of experience in the healthcare field and is a medical assistant, certified professional coder through the American Academy of Professional Coders, and a registered nurse. Ms. Barbour worked as a physician practice manager and as a healthcare consultant, which included chart auditing for evaluation and management services.

Why did you become interested in teaching?

For as long as I can remember, I have always wanted to become a teacher; however, I strongly believe that before teaching a skill, you have to master that skill. Although I do not consider myself a master of coding, I do have faith in my ability to take a difficult concept and explain it in an easier format.

How do you think having a nursing degree has helped you to teach coding?

In order to code correctly, you need to understand what you are coding. My nursing degree has enabled me to comprehend the physiological processes associated with diseases, as well as the procedures to treat diseases; with this, I can provide a more thorough explanation to my coding students so that they, in turn, can correctly assign the appropriate codes.

What advice would you like to give coding students who want to advance their careers beyond coding?

Do it! An education is something that no one can take away—it is yours for life! It will enable you to be independent and also develop a strong sense of self-pride. It is a long road, especially as an adult when you are already holding down a job, house, etc., but time has a way of passing anyway—make the most of it!

What advice would you like to give coding students to help them prepare to work successfully with various personality types?

The best advice I can possibly give is don't let someone else ruin your day! You will have the opportunity to meet many people, most of whom are wonderful, amazing people; however, there are always a select few who seem to enjoy making someone else feel inferior or less important. These people are not worth a second thought! Maintain your professionalism, continue your duties, and move on!

(Used by permission of Teresa Barbour.)

QUALIFYING CIRCUMSTANCES CODES

Many times, physicians administer anesthesia to patients whose cases are complex, including a patient who:

- is over age 70 or under age 1
- has total body hypothermia (low body temperature) or controlled hypotension (low blood pressure)
- suffers from emergent condition(s)

Patients who are very old (over age 70) or young (under age 1) have additional health risks that make anesthesia administration and monitoring more difficult. Patients' anesthesia cases may also be more complex because of total body hypothermia

Figure 20-14 ■ Qualifying circumstances codes.

> **Qualifying Circumstances for Anesthesia (99100-99140)**
> (For explanation of these services, see **Anesthesia Guidelines**)
>
> ✦**99100** Anesthesia for patient of extreme age, younger than 1 year and older than 70 (List separately in addition to code for primary anesthesia procedure)
>
> ✦**99116** Anesthesia complicated by utilization of total body hypothermia (List separately in addition to code for primary anesthesia procedure)
>
> ✦**99135** Anesthesia complicated by utilization of controlled hypotension (List separately in addition to code for primary anesthesia procedure)
>
> ✦**99140** Anesthesia complicated by emergency conditions (specify) (List separately in addition to code for primary anesthesia procedure)
>
> (An emergency is defined as existing when delay in treatment of the patient would lead to a significant increase in the threat to life or body part.)

or controlled hypotension. Total body hypothermia, which decreases oxygen demand, occurs when the anesthesia provider purposely lowers a patient's total body temperature during a procedure to reduce the amount of ischemic damage that could occur, as in a cardiac procedure.

Deliberate controlled hypotension occurs when the anesthesia provider lowers a patient's blood pressure to decrease blood loss from a procedure, such as during a total hip replacement. Patients may also suffer from emergent conditions that require more complex anesthesia care.

CPT contains four separate codes, called **qualifying circumstances codes**, that describe each of these four complex situations (■ FIGURE 20-14). Qualifying circumstances codes are located in the Medicine chapter of CPT, but the guidelines for assigning them are at the beginning of the Anesthesia chapter.

Notice that the qualifying circumstances codes are add-on codes. Recall that the ✦ symbol in front of a code means that the code is an add-on code, and you cannot report it alone.

extracapsular (eks-trə-kap′su-lər)—situated outside a capsule

Providers assign qualifying circumstances codes *in addition to* anesthesia codes. For example, if Mr. Robinson, an 82-year-old patient, has **extracapsular** surgery to remove a cataract and to insert an intraocular lens implant, you would assign the following codes for the anesthesia provider:

00142—Anesthesia for procedures on eye; lens surgery

99100—Anesthesia for patient of extreme age, younger than 1 year and older than 70

You can also assign more than one qualifying circumstance code to the same patient if necessary.

Note that you would *not* assign a code for the surgery. The *surgeon's* coder would assign the surgical code (66984—Extracapsular cataract removal with insertion of intraocular lens prosthesis).

Many insurances reimburse providers more for anesthesia care to patients with qualifying circumstances, but some insurances do not recognize the codes and will not pay for them. When more than one anesthesia provider administers anesthesia for the same patient, insurances typically only pay extra for qualifying circumstances to one provider, not to all of them. So only one provider, such as the supervising anesthesiologist, should report the qualifying circumstances code to the insurance. It is best to check individual payers' guidelines for specific information on coding and billing for qualifying circumstances.

Anesthesia
Special Circumstances
Emergency 99140
Extreme Age 99100
Hypotension 99135
Hypothermia 99116

Figure 20-15 ■ Index entry for qualifying circumstances codes.

You can locate codes for qualifying circumstances under the main term, *anesthesia*, and subterm *special circumstances* (■ FIGURE 20-15).

TAKE A BREAK

Good work! Let's take a break and then practice coding qualifying circumstances.

Exercise 20.5 Qualifying Circumstances Codes

Instructions: Review each patient's case and assign anesthesia procedure code(s) and qualifying circumstances code(s) (CPT). Do not assign procedure codes for surgical procedures. Optional: For additional practice, assign the patient's diagnosis code(s) (ICD-9-CM).

1. Dr. Joyner, an anesthesiologist, oversees the anesthesia case, including anesthesia administration, for Andrew Minor, age 70. The patient undergoes a repair of an abdominal aortic aneurysm (excessive dilation of a blood vessel). Dr. Nassar, the vascular surgeon, determines that the surgery is necessary to save the patient's life.

   Diagnosis code(s): _____

   Procedure code(s): _____

2. Edward Rollins, CRNA, oversees anesthesia care for Terrence Scruggs, a 9-month-old, for an **orchiopexy** due to an undescended left testicle.

   Diagnosis code(s): _____

   Procedure code(s): _____

3. Maggie Stinson, age 82, suffered a fracture of the femoral head (highest part of the femur—thigh bone). She undergoes a total hip arthroplasty to treat the condition. Dr. Joyner manages the case, including all intraoperative care.

   Diagnosis code(s): _____

   Procedure code(s): _____

4. Clarissa Anthony, a 3-month-old, has an atrial septal defect (congenital disorder where there is an abnormal opening in the walls of the atria). She needs to have open heart surgery to repair it, and Dr. Joyner oversees all aspects of the case.

   Diagnosis code(s): _____

   Procedure code(s): _____

5. Edward Rollins, CRNA, administers anesthesia for Kristin Rael, age 16, for emergency spinal decompression (to relieve pressure on the nerve roots and restore normal spacing between vertebrae). The patient suffers from **cauda equina** syndrome (compression of the spinal nerve roots located at the base of the spine). Mr. Rollins manages all aspects of anesthesia care for the patient.

   Diagnosis code(s): _____

   Procedure code(s): _____

6. Dr. Joyner administers anesthesia for Steven Lineberry, age 75, for coronary artery bypass graft (CABG) surgery using a pump oxygenator (also called a heart–lung machine, which performs the work of the lungs and heart in open heart surgery). The procedure includes induced hypothermia. The patient suffers from arteriosclerosis. Dr. Joyner oversees preoperative, intraoperative, and postoperative care.

   Diagnosis code(s): _____

   Procedure code(s): _____

MODIFIERS FOR ANESTHESIA

There are several HCPCS modifiers to assign for anesthesia, including modifiers that show the patient's overall health status, represent the type of anesthesia provider who rendered care, and represent MAC services. We will review each type of modifier next.

orchiopexy (r-kē-ō-pek′-sē)— to place an undescended testicle inside the scrotum

cauda equina (kaud′-ə-ē-kwī′-nə)

Physical Status Modifiers

A **physical status modifier** is a HCPCS modifier that describes the patient's overall health status at the time of anesthesia. Physical status modifiers start with the letter P, followed by the number 1 to 6, as follows:

- P1: A normal healthy patient
- P2: A patient with mild **systemic** disease (affecting the entire body) (certain types of anemia)
- P3: A patient with severe systemic disease (hypertension, diabetes)

systemic (sis-tem′ik)

moribund (mor'ĭ-bənd)

- P4: A patient with severe systemic disease that is a constant threat to life (respiratory failure, acute angina, traumatic injuries)
- P5: A **moribund** (dying) patient who is not expected to survive without the operation (life-threatening traumatic injuries, unconscious)
- P6: A declared brain-dead patient whose organs are being removed for donor purposes

The anesthesia provider, not the coder, documents a physical status modifier for every patient's case in the patient's medical record. Anesthesia providers may interpret the meanings of physical status modifiers differently. In other words, one provider may assign P3 for a disorder that another provider feels is better represented by P4. You, as the coder, should still review the medical documentation and the modifier assigned. If you have any questions, then you should query the anesthesia provider for additional clarification.

The physical status modifier helps to describe the level of difficulty of the patient's case, and you should append it to the anesthesia procedure code. Patients' cases that involve health problems that these modifiers represent are more complex to manage during anesthesia services. Providers can also charge a higher fee for an anesthesia service represented by a code that includes a physical status modifier of P3 to P5. Not all payers recognize physical status modifiers, but some insurances will pay more for cases with modifiers that represent a complex case, such as P3, P4, or P5. Insurances will not typically pay more for physical status modifiers P1, P2, or P6, since these modifiers do not indicate a more complex anesthesia case. Diagnosis codes reported for the patient's encounter should justify appending specific physical status modifiers to the anesthesia procedure code.

Modifiers for Anesthesia Providers and Monitored Anesthesia Care (MAC)

There are HCPCS modifiers representing the type of anesthesia provider who rendered anesthesia services (**modifiers for anesthesia providers**). Other HCPCS modifiers represent cases that include MAC. Append these modifiers to *anesthesia codes* for Medicare patients' services, and other payers also recognize the modifiers. It is best to check with an individual payer's guidelines to determine whether to append the modifiers.

Anesthesia provider modifiers and their definitions are as follows:

Physician Modifiers:

- **AA**—Anesthesia services performed personally by the anesthesiologist
- **AD**—Medical supervision by a physician; more than four concurrent (at the same time) anesthesia procedures
- **QK**—Medical direction of two, three, or four concurrent anesthesia procedures involving a qualified individual
- **QY**—Medical direction of one CRNA
- **GC**—Anesthesia services that a resident performed under the direction of a teaching physician. The teaching physician reports the GC modifier to show that he rendered the service.

Medical direction occurs when the anesthesiologist

- performs the pre-anesthesia evaluation and examination and develops the plan for anesthesia

induction (in-dək'-shən)

- personally administers various procedures, when appropriate, including the **induction** of and emergence from anesthesia
- oversees another anesthesia provider involved in anesthesia care
- frequently monitors anesthesia care of the patient
- is physically available to provide emergency care if needed
- provides postanesthesia care

CRNA Modifiers:

- **QX**—CRNA service; with medical direction by a physician
- **QZ**—CRNA service: without medical direction by a physician

Physician modifiers and CRNA modifiers help insurances to identify when anesthesia providers should receive full reimbursement for a service, such as when an anesthesiologist is working alone, or partial reimbursement for a service, such as when an anesthesiologist supervises a CRNA. When both an anesthesiologist and a CRNA work together on a patient's case, each provider can code and bill the anesthesia service, appending the appropriate modifier(s) to the anesthesia code. They report the same CPT code for anesthesia services and the same physical status modifier, but they report *different* modifiers to show who provided the service.

Monitored Anesthesia Care Modifiers:

- **G8**—MAC for deep complex, complicated, or markedly invasive surgical procedures
- **G9**—MAC for patient who has a history of a severe cardiopulmonary condition
- **QS**—MAC service. The QS modifier is for informational purposes.

Other Anesthesia Modifiers   Recall that there are also CPT modifiers specific to anesthesia services, which you learned in Chapter 18:

- **-23—Unusual anesthesia**
  Occasionally, because of unusual circumstances, a procedure which usually requires either *no anesthesia, local, or regional anesthesia,* must be done under *general anesthesia.* When this occurs, append modifier -23 to the procedure code *for the basic service of anesthesia,* not to the procedure code for the surgery.

- **-47—Anesthesia by surgeon**
  Recall that an anesthesiologist or CRNA administers anesthesia to a patient, while a surgeon performs the procedure. There are times when the surgeon performs the procedure *and* administers the anesthesia without an anesthesiologist or CRNA. An example is an obstetrician who administers regional anesthesia (such as an epidural to relieve pain) to a patient in labor.

  o Modifier -47 applies only to times when the surgeon performs the surgery and administers regional or general anesthesia. Modifier -47 does not include local anesthesia. When the surgeon performs surgery and administers regional or general anesthesia, assign a code for the procedure, assign the code for the procedure again, and append modifier -47 to show that the surgeon also administered the anesthesia. Assign two codes for the procedure so that the insurance will process the claim for the procedure itself, and for the anesthesia the surgeon administered during the procedure.

  o *Note:* Do not append modifier -47 to anesthesia procedure codes.

- **-73—Discontinued outpatient hospital/ambulatory surgery center (ASC) procedure prior to the administration of anesthesia**
  Modifier -73 represents a discontinued outpatient procedure *before* anesthesia administration. Append modifier -73 to the surgical procedure code to indicate that a surgical or diagnostic procedure requiring anesthesia was terminated due to extenuating circumstances that threatened the well-being of the patient, and after the patient had been prepared for the procedure and taken to the procedure room. Do not append modifier -73 when the patient elects to cancel a procedure.

- **-74—Discontinued outpatient hospital/ambulatory surgery center (ASC) procedure after administration of anesthesia**
  Modifier -74 represents a discontinued outpatient procedure *after* anesthesia administration (local, regional block, general). Append modifier -74 to the surgical or

diagnostic procedure code to indicate that a procedure requiring anesthesia was terminated *after the induction* of anesthesia, or after the physician started the procedure such as the incision made, intubation started, or endoscope inserted. Do not append modifier -74 when the patient elects to cancel a procedure.

TAKE A BREAK

Hang in there! You are making progress! Let's take a break and then practice assigning modifiers.

Exercise 20.6 Modifiers for Anesthesia

Instructions: Review the following cases for Medicare patients. Then assign anesthesia procedure code(s) and any qualifying circumstances code(s) (CPT).

Append a physical status modifier to the anesthesia code for each case.

Append HCPCS modifiers representing the anesthesia provider and/or MAC.

Append any applicable CPT modifiers.

Do not assign CPT codes for surgical procedures.

Optional: For additional practice, assign the patient's diagnosis code(s) (ICD-9-CM).

1. Edward Rollins, CRNA, administers anesthesia and oversees the case without medical direction for Eugene Gravitt, age 67, a normal healthy patient. Mr. Gravitt undergoes a corneal transplant due to corneal edema that occurred when he suffered substantial damage from a motor vehicle accident five years ago. Mr. Rollins administers general anesthesia to the patient, which is not normally required for the surgery. In the preoperative interview, the patient requested general anesthesia because he was anxious about remaining awake for the procedure.

   Diagnosis code(s): _____

   Procedure code(s): _____

2. Dr. Joyner, an anesthesiologist, supervises five anesthesia cases simultaneously, including one for Agnes Creek, age 79, for removal of a shoulder cast. Mrs. Creek suffered a fracture of the neck of the scapula (shoulder blade). She has uncontrolled type II diabetes. Assign code(s) for Dr. Joyner's services for Mrs. Creek.

   Diagnosis code(s): _____

   Procedure code(s): _____

3. Dr. Joyner supervises Edward Rollins on an anesthesia case for Antonio Hung, age 66, a normal healthy patient. The patient undergoes a transurethral resection of the prostate (TURP) (removal of part or all of the prostate gland). He suffers from benign prostatic hyperplasia (BPH) (enlarged prostate).

   Diagnosis code(s): _____

   Procedure code(s) for Dr. Joyner, anesthesiologist:

   _____

   Procedure code(s) for Mr. Rollins, CRNA:

   _____

4. Donald Maxie, age 28, is the recipient of a kidney transplant using a kidney that his sister donated. The patient has ESRD, which Dr. Joyner determines is a constant threat to life. Dr. Joyner administers anesthesia and oversees the patient's case. Edward Rollins provides assistance with the case.

   Diagnosis code(s): _____

   Procedure code(s) for Dr. Joyner, anesthesiologist:

   _____

   Procedure code(s) for Mr. Rollins, CRNA:

   _____

5. Edward Rollins administers moderate anesthesia care without medical direction for Josephine Carrasco, age 78. Ms. Carrasco is having a pacemaker inserted due to cardiac arrhythmia, which Mr. Rollins determines is a severe systemic condition.

   Diagnosis code(s): _____

   Procedure code(s): _____

6. Dr. Joyner directs Dr. Pleth, a medical resident, in administering anesthesia for Amelia Harden, age 74, for burn excision and debridement of the trunk involving 27% of total body surface area. The third-degree burns are the result of a house fire that occurred last week, and Dr. Joyner rates this as a severe systemic condition.

   Diagnosis code(s): _____

   Procedure code(s) for Dr. Joyner, anesthesiologist:

   _____

ANESTHESIA BILLING AND REIMBURSEMENT

Anesthesia has unique coding, billing, and reimbursement requirements, which involve units of time, base unit values, and a specific payment formula. Let's review these requirements next so that you have a better understanding of how to follow them.

Anesthesia Time

When providers bill anesthesia services to insurances, they list anesthesia time on the CMS-1500 form in block 24G, which represents *units* of time. **Anesthesia time** is the period of time when an anesthesia provider is present with the patient. It starts when the provider prepares the patient for anesthesia induction in the operating room or another area. It ends when the provider is no longer furnishing anesthesia services to the patient and when other clinicians, such as nurses, take over the patient's postoperative care. The anesthesia provider documents total anesthesia time in the patient's anesthesia medical record. Refer to Figure 20-6 (anesthesia medical record), where you can see blocks for the provider to list the anesthesia start and stop times in the top right corner of the record.

Medicare and many other payers compute **time units**, or time divided into increments of 15 minutes, meaning that each increment of 15 minutes equals one unit. Providers divide the *total anesthesia time* by 15 to calculate the number of units to report on the CMS-1500 form.

For example, if total anesthesia time was 30 minutes, then the provider would bill two units (two 15-minute increments) on the claim form. Providers can round up the time to the nearest decimal, when appropriate, such as rounding up 59 minutes of anesthesia to 60 minutes, or 4 units. Other payers compute time units in increments of 30 minutes or other intervals, such as the total minutes of a procedure, so it is best to check individual payers' policies to determine the amount of time that represents one unit. (Note that there are no time units associated with code 01996—*Daily hospital management of epidural or subarachnoid continuous drug administration.*)

Base Unit Value

For Medicare and many other payers, anesthesia services do not have relative value units (RVUs) like other services in the Medicare Physician Fee Schedule (MPFS). Recall that an RVU is a number assigned to each CPT or HCPCS code that represents the amount of physician work involved and expense incurred to provide the service, along with the cost of malpractice insurance.

Instead of RVUs, anesthesia codes are assigned **base unit values (BUVs)**, which is a number that represents the complexity level of the anesthesia, risk to the patient, and the anesthesia provider's skills needed to render services. The ASA assigns base unit values to anesthesia codes, qualifying circumstances codes, and physical status modifiers, updating base unit values yearly in a publication called the Relative Value Guide® (RVG).

Insurances also use the ASA's BUVs to calculate anesthesia payments. CMS publishes base unit values on their website, and you can refer to ▪ FIGURE 20-16 for examples of anesthesia procedures with different base unit values for Medicare.

The BUV assigned to an anesthesia code (00211) for a complex procedure is higher than the BUV assigned to an anesthesia code for a simpler procedure. In Figure 20-16, a craniotomy (cutting the skull) or **craniectomy** (removing part of the skull), requires a more complex level of anesthesia than a vasectomy (procedure for male sterilization), so the craniotomy or craniectomy has a base unit value of 10, while the vasectomy base unit value is only 3.

craniectomy (kray-ne-ek′tə-me)

Providers can charge for anesthesia services depending on the BUVs. For example, an anesthesia provider may charge $60 for each BUV. The charge for code 00211 (10 base units × $60) would be $600. The charge for code 00921 (3 base units × $60) would be $180.

00211	Anesthesia for intracranial procedures; craniotomy or craniectomy for evacuation of hematoma
Base unit value = 10	
00921	Anesthesia for procedures on male genitalia (including open urethral procedures); vasectomy, unilateral or bilateral
Base unit value = 3	

Figure 20-16 ▪ Comparison of base unit values for two different anesthesia codes from CMS.

Anesthesia Payment Formula

Payers also use base units to calculate payments. A common formula that many payers use to calculate anesthesia payments is as follows:

> ***Anesthesia payment*** = Base unit values (for anesthesia procedure codes) + Time units + Modifying units (BUVs for qualifying circumstances codes and physical status modifiers) × Conversion factor.

Note: Some payers may use this formula to calculate an allowable charge, rather than a payment. They will then pay a *portion or a percentage* of the allowable charge once they calculate it using the formula.

The formula may seem complex, but it is relatively simple to calculate the insurance payment. It is important that you understand the formula so that you realize when you assign anesthesia procedure codes, assign qualifying circumstances codes, and append physical status modifiers, they may have BUVs that will affect reimbursement. If you assign incorrect codes or modifiers, then it could affect reimbursement, and insurance could pay too little or too much. Let's review an anesthesia case from earlier in this chapter to determine how the patient's insurance calculates the anesthesia payment.

Example: Mr. Robinson, an 82-year-old patient, has extracapsular surgery to remove a cataract and to insert an intraocular lens implant. He receives conscious sedation for the procedure.

The total anesthesia time the anesthesiologist documents is 45 minutes. The Medicare patient is a normal, healthy patient, and the anesthesiologist assigns P1 as the patient's physical status modifier.

Codes and their base unit values are as follows:

- **00142—Anesthesia for procedures on eye; lens surgery**
  Base unit value = 4
- **99100—Anesthesia for patient of extreme age, younger than 1 year and older than 70**
  Base unit value = 1 (qualifying circumstances)
- **Anesthesia time is 45 minutes**
  Time units = 3 (15-minute increments)
- **Physical status modifier—P1**
  Base unit value = 0
- **Conversion factor = $19.79**

The *conversion factor* is a dollar amount each insurance assigns to one base unit value. It is based on the geographic location where the provider rendered anesthesia services. There are differences in costs associated with providing anesthesia services in different locations, such as a large city or a small rural town. It costs more to provide services in a large city because the cost of living is higher, than it costs to provide services in a small town, so the conversion factor changes by provider location. Let's say for this example that Medicare's conversion factor for the provider's location is $19.79.

The formula for calculating anesthesia payment for this example is as follows:

> Base unit values (for anesthesia code 00142) = 4 *plus*
>
> Time units = 3 *plus*
>
> Modifying units (base unit values for qualifying circumstances codes) = 1 *plus*
>
> Modifying units (base unit values for physical status modifiers) = 0 *multiplied by*

Conversion factor of $19.79:

$$4 + 3 + 1 + 0 = 8 \times \$19.79 = \$158.32 \text{ (payment from Medicare)}$$

■ TABLE 20-2 EXAMPLES OF MEDICARE'S 2011 CONVERSION FACTORS

Carrier Number	Locality Number	City/State	Anesthesia Conversion Factor
10102	0	Alabama	$19.88
831	1	Alaska	$28.85
3102	0	Arizona	$20.84
520	13	Arkansas	$19.79
1192	26	Anaheim/Santa Ana, CA	$21.95
1192	18	Los Angeles, CA	$21.77

(Department of Health and Human Services, Centers for Medicare and Medicaid Services.)

Refer to ■ TABLE 20-2 to review examples of Medicare's conversion factors for different geographic locations, using the 2011 *national* conversion factor of $21.05. Notice how the conversion factors change, depending on the location where the provider rendered anesthesia services. (For more information about Medicare's conversion factors and regulations on anesthesia coding, billing, and reimbursement, which frequently change, visit the Medicare website at www.cms.gov.)

The ASA's Relative Value Guide® also lists anesthesia codes where time units are appropriate to bill for anesthesia services. Providers should only bill *time* units in block 24G of the CMS-1500 form, not BUVs. Insurances already consider BUVs when calculating their payments. Adding BUVs to time units is considered fraudulent billing. Keep in mind that payers may use different formulas to calculate anesthesia payments, so check with individual payers' policies for specific information.

Many anesthesia software programs can convert total anesthesia time into the appropriate number of units, based on the specific payer's guidelines, and can also calculate expected anesthesia reimbursement, applying the payment calculation that each payer uses.

Coding and Billing Multiple Anesthesia Services

Providers also use the ASA's BUVs for anesthesia codes to determine how to assign codes for multiple procedures. When you are coding and billing for multiple anesthesia services for the same patient during the same encounter, follow these rules:

1. Assign only the most complex anesthesia procedure code with the highest BUV. *Note:* The primary procedure may *not* be the most complex anesthesia procedure.

WORKPLACE IQ

You are working as a coder for a busy anesthesiology practice with 10 anesthesiologists and 5 CRNAs. Today, your manager asks you to educate a new coder, Julie, on the anesthesia payment formula that many insurances use to calculate anesthesia payments. After you review the formula with Julie, she asks you why she needs to bother learning it, telling you, "I don't do billing. I'm a coder. Why do I need to know this when we have billers who handle insurance billing and collections?"

What would you do?

2. Add the anesthesia time for all procedures combined, and divide it by the time unit increment the payer uses, such as 15 minutes.

3. Bill the total dollar amount for all anesthesia services combined.

Medicare has specific guidelines for billing multiple anesthesia procedures, so check the Medicare website at http://www.cms.gov for more detailed information.

TAKE A BREAK

Way to go! Let's take a break and then review anesthesia billing and reimbursement.

Exercise 20.7 Anesthesia Billing and Reimbursement

Part 1—Theory

Instructions: Fill in each blank with the best answer.

1. Anesthesia time _____ when the provider is no longer furnishing anesthesia services to the patient and when other clinicians, such as nurses, take over the patient's postoperative care.

2. A common formula that many payers use to calculate anesthesia payments is as follows:

   Anesthesia payment = Base unit values + Time units + _____ × Conversion factor.

3. The _____ is a dollar amount each insurance assigns to one BUV, based on the geographic location where the provider rendered anesthesia services.

4. _____ is the period of time when an anesthesia provider is present with the patient.

5. Providers should only bill _____ on the CMS-1500 form and exclude BUVs for anesthesia codes, qualifying circumstances codes, or physical status modifiers, because insurances already allow for them in their payment calculations.

6. The ASA assigns _____ to anesthesia codes, qualifying circumstances codes, and physical status modifiers.

Part 2—Application

Instructions: Using the information provided for each patient's case, determine the anesthesia time and the amount that the insurance will pay for anesthesia services. Use the following anesthesia payment formula: Payment = base units + time units + modifying units × conversion factor. Calculate time in 15-minute increments. Record the time units, and then calculate the anesthesia payment.

1. Dr. Stuart repairs an open ankle fracture for Mr. Key, a 71-year-old patient. Dr. Joyner is the anesthesiologist for the procedure. The patient is a normal, healthy patient. Total anesthesia time is 60 minutes.

   Base units = Anesthesia code 01480 is 3 base units

   Time units = _____

   Modifying units = Qualifying circumstances code 99100 is 1 base unit

   Physical status modifier = P1 is 0 base units

   Conversion factor = $21.02

   Anesthesia payment from insurance = $ _____

2. Dr. Stuart excises a tumor from the humerus for Mrs. Donaldson, a 75-year-old patient. Dr. Joyner is the anesthesiologist for the procedure. The patient is a normal, healthy patient. Total anesthesia time is 44 minutes.

   Base units = Anesthesia code 01758 is 5 base units

   Time units = _____

   Modifying units = Qualifying circumstances code 99100 is 1 base unit

   Physical status modifier = P1 is 0 base units

   Conversion factor = $23.07

   Anesthesia payment from insurance = $ _____

3. Dr. Drimond performs an incisional hernia repair in the lower abdomen (■ FIGURE 20-17) for Mr. Horne, a 52-year-old patient. Dr. Joyner is the anesthesiologist for the procedure. The patient is a normal, healthy patient. Total anesthesia time is 90 minutes.

   Base units = Anesthesia code 00832 is 6 base units

   Time units = _____

   Modifying units = none

   Physical status modifier = P1 is 0 base units

   Conversion factor = $19.55

   Anesthesia payment from insurance = $ _____

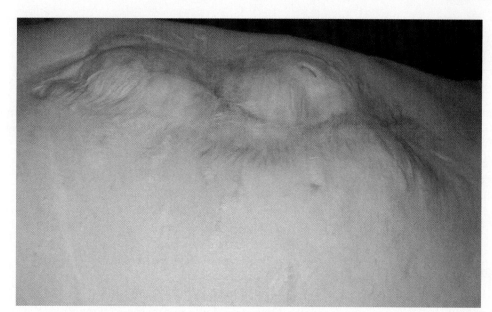

Figure 20-17 ■ Bulges in a patient's abdomen due to an incisional hernia.

Photo credit: Slaven/Custom Medical Stock.

DESTINATION: MEDICARE

This Medicare exercise will help you to find additional information about anesthesia billing and reimbursement. Follow the instructions listed next to access Chapter 12 of the Medicare Claims Processing Manual for Physicians/Nonphysician Practitioners:

1. Go to the website http://www.cms.gov.

2. At the top of the screen on the banner bar, choose *Regulations and Guidance.*

3. Under *Guidance,* choose *Manuals.*

4. On the left side of the screen, under *Manuals,* choose *Internet-Only Manuals (IOMs).*

5. Scroll down to *Publication 100-04 Medicare Claims Processing Manual,* and click *100-04.*

6. Scroll down to the list of Downloads, and choose *Chapter 12—Physicians/ Nonphysician Practitioners.*

Answer the following questions, using the search function (Ctrl + F) to find information that you need:

1. For anesthesia payment at the medically directed rate, a physician (anesthesiologist) can medically direct two, three, or four concurrent procedures involving qualified individuals. Who are the qualified individuals?

2. How many base units per procedure does Medicare allow when the anesthesiologist renders more than four procedures concurrently, or performs other services while directing concurrent procedures?

3. Which modifier should you append to the anesthesia code with the highest BUV when there are multiple bilateral surgeries performed?

4. What medical and surgical services will Medicare reimburse separately under the fee schedule when the anesthesiologist performs them in addition to anesthesia?

CHAPTER REVIEW

Multiple Choice

Instructions: Circle one best answer to complete each statement.

1. Which of the following anesthesia providers can provide anesthesia services as long as an anesthesiologist is immediately available if needed?
   a. CRNA
   b. Doctor of osteopathy
   c. Podiatrist
   d. All of the above

2. Moderate sedation may be used for what types of procedures?
   a. Skin biopsy, cesarean section
   b. Cataract, vasectomy, and endoscopy
   c. Open heart surgery
   d. Lumbar puncture

3. _____ block is anesthesia injected into the lower spine for procedures on the legs or buttocks.
   a. Caudal
   b. Epidural
   c. Peripheral nerve
   d. Spinal

4. Which of the following is *not* a side effect, risk, or complication during or after anesthesia?
   a. Disorientation
   b. Myocardial infarction
   c. Pyrexia
   d. Diabetes

5. Which of the following services is *not* included in the anesthesia code package?
   a. Oximetry
   b. A-line
   c. Blood administration
   d. Mass spectrometry

6. What is the main term that you should first search for in the index to locate anesthesia codes?
   a. The name of the procedure
   b. The word "anesthetize"
   c. The name of the anesthetic drug administered
   d. The word "anesthesia"

7. In the early history of anesthesia, patients experienced problems because
   a. anesthetic drugs caused all patients to have cardiac arrest.
   b. physicians were unwilling to administer anesthetic drugs.
   c. physicians could not often predict the quantity of anesthesia that a patient needed.
   d. physicians did not use anesthetic drugs until the 1920s.

8. In the 1900s, there were additional advancements in anesthesia with the use of
   a. nasogastric intubation.
   b. endotracheal intubation.
   c. Swan-Ganz catheters.
   d. epidural blood patches.

9. _____ is when the patient loses partial consciousness but is not completely asleep.
   a. General anesthesia
   b. Moderate (conscious) sedation
   c. Local anesthesia
   d. Regional anesthesia

10. The patient (or family member) signs a(n) _____, a legal document showing that he understands the benefits and risks of anesthesia.
    a. anesthesia consult
    b. informed consult
    c. preoperative consent
    d. informed consent

Coding Assignments

Instructions: Assign anesthesia procedure code(s) (CPT) to the following cases, referencing both the index and CPT sections.

- Append physical status modifiers and any applicable CPT modifiers.

- Assign applicable qualifying circumstances procedure codes.

- For Medicare patients only, also assign HCPCS modifiers representing the anesthesia provider and/or MAC.

- Do not assign CPT codes for surgical procedures, as you are coding for the anesthesiologist or the CRNA, not for the surgeon.

Optional: For additional practice, assign the patient's diagnosis code(s) (ICD-9-CM).

1. Dr. Joyner, an anesthesiologist, administers anesthesia and oversees all anesthesia services for Matthew Delk, age 13. The procedure at Williton Medical Center is an emergent tracheostomy to open the patient's trachea because it swelled shut. The obstructed trachea is due to **anaphylactic** shock, an allergic reaction in response to a **sulfonamide** (antibacterial drug) that Dr. Hoffman prescribed for **sinusitis** (sinus infection). The patient previously had no known allergies to sulfonamide. The patient will not survive without the procedure.

   Diagnosis code(s): _____

   Procedure code(s): _____

2. Dakota Bowen, a 3-week-old, needs open heart surgery with a pump oxygenator to repair an interatrial septal defect, also called an atrial septal defect. Dr. Joyner, who oversees anesthesia care for the case, determines that baby Dakota has a severe systemic disease that is a constant threat to life.

Diagnosis code(s): _____

Procedure code(s): _____

3. Dr. Joyner personally performs anesthesia services for Jenny Major, age 66, for a left-sided **radical mastectomy**, due to breast cancer. Ms. Major also has type II diabetes. Dr. Joyner determines that her overall health status is a P3 rating because of the breast cancer, a severe systemic disease. Mrs. Major has Medicare.

Diagnosis code(s): _____

Procedure code(s): _____

4. Edward Rollins, CRNA, oversees anesthesia care at Williton for Tony Felderini, age 71. Mr. Rollins works on the case alone. The procedure is laparoscopic placement of a gastric restrictive device for obesity (a weight loss procedure to decrease the amount of food intake). Mr. Rollins determines that the patient's health status qualifies him as having moderate systemic disease, due to obstructive sleep apnea and hypertension. The patient has Medicare.

Diagnosis code(s): _____

Procedure code(s): _____

5. Dr. Santos, an obstetric anesthesiologist, administers epidural anesthesia for Kristen Sproul, age 27, a normal healthy female. She delivers a healthy baby boy with no complications. Hint: an epidural is also **neuraxial** (relating to the central nervous system) labor anesthesia.

Diagnosis code(s): _____

Procedure code(s): _____

6. Kim Wong, CRNA, administers anesthesia for Scott Schuller, age 19, for removal of four impacted molars (wisdom teeth). Dr. Breneman, an oral surgeon, performs the surgery in his office. Mr. Schuller has type I diabetes, which is currently uncontrolled.

Diagnosis code(s): _____

Procedure code(s): _____

7. Santiago Delgado, age 68, has acute appendicitis. His surgeon, Dr. Gupta, performs an emergency appendectomy through the anterior abdominal wall. Dr. Joyner personally oversees the anesthesia case. Without surgery, the patient runs the risk of a life-threatening infection and will most likely not survive. Mr. Delgado has Medicare.

Diagnosis code(s): _____

Procedure code(s): _____

8. At Williton, Shauntell Wilson, age 21, undergoes a kidney transplant to treat ESRD. A team of surgeons perform the procedure and oversee her care. Dr. Joyner conducts the preoperative interview and meets with the patient and her parents. He performs preoperative, intraoperative, and postoperative anesthesia services. Tiffany Moss, CRNA, assists Dr. Joyner with the case, which he supervises. Modifier -P4 represents the patient's health status. Ms. Wilson has Medicare, which she qualifies for based on her disabling condition.

Procedure code(s) for Dr. Joyner, anesthesiologist:

_____

Procedure code(s) for Ms. Moss, CRNA:

_____

9. Elizabeth McGhee, age 32, is a normal healthy patient. At Williton, she undergoes posterior lumbar interbody fusion (PLIF) to reinforce intervertebral disc spaces. The patient suffers from **spondylolisthesis**, when the lumbar vertebra are displaced and cause painful compression of nerve roots. Tiffany Moss, CRNA, oversees anesthesia services for the patient's case and works without an anesthesiologist's supervision. Ms. Moss also administers a morphine epidural injection for postoperative pain management. (Code this service separately.) Ms. McGhee's insurance company, Delf Insurance, requires HCPCS modifiers that indicate the anesthesia provider.

Diagnosis code(s): _____

Procedure code(s): _____

10. Today at Williton, Dr. Nguyen performs a CABG procedure for Arthur Good, age 74, who has coronary arteriosclerosis. The procedure includes a pump oxygenator and induced hypothermia. Because of his history of cardiac procedures, Dr. Joyner provides MAC for this Medicare patient.

Diagnosis code(s): _____

Procedure code(s): _____

anaphylactic (an-ə-fə-lak′-tik)

sulfonamide (suhl-fon′-uh-mahyd)

sinusitis (sī-n(y)ə-sīt′-əs)

radical mastectomy—removal of the breast, pectoral muscles, axillary lymph nodes, and associated skin and subcutaneous tissue

neuraxial (noo-rak′se-əl)

spondylolisthesis (spän-də-lō-lis-′thē-səs)

SECTION SIX

Surgery Coding

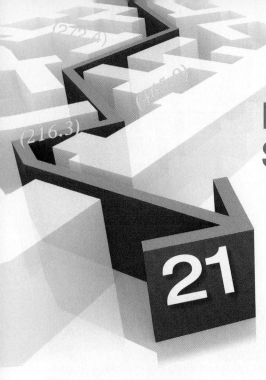

Introduction to Surgery Coding

21

Learning Objectives

After completing this chapter, you should be able to

- Spell and define the key terminology in this chapter.
- Name the body systems of the Surgery subsections.
- Identify section divisions of Surgery subsections.
- Discuss common suffixes used in medical terms of surgical procedures.
- Review common surgical procedures and their meanings.
- List the integral components of a procedure.
- Define the global surgical package under CPT and Medicare.
- Discuss Surgery section coding guidelines found at the beginning of the section.
- Identify where to find additional guidelines in the Surgery section.
- Explain the purpose of *CPT® Assistant* guidelines.
- Discuss procedures located in the General subsection of the Surgery section.

Key Terms

incidental to
global surgical package
materials supplied by the physician
operating microscope

separate procedure
special report
Surgery section guidelines
unlisted service or procedure

INTRODUCTION

At this stop on your coding journey, you will start in the Surgery section to learn about coding guidelines and instructions that provide you with helpful information about assigning many different surgery codes. You will practice reviewing the guidelines, including interpreting them for specific codes. Once you become familiar with where to find guidelines in the Surgery section of the CPT manual and learn how to interpret them, you will be better able to assign surgery codes for various specialties. Let's continue on your coding journey and take a new step toward another goal—coding surgeries!

"I have always been delighted at the prospect of a new day, a fresh try, one more start, with perhaps a bit of magic waiting somewhere behind the morning."

—JOSEPH PRIESTLEY

SURGERY SECTION (10021–69990)

The Surgery section is the largest section of codes in the CPT manual, and it is categorized by *subsections* of surgeries for specific body systems (■ TABLE 21-1), except for the operating microscope.

■ TABLE 21-1 **SURGERY SUBSECTIONS**

Subsection (Body System)	Code Range
General	10021–10022
Integumentary System	10040–19499
Musculoskeletal System	20005–29999
Respiratory System	30000–32999
Cardiovascular System	33010–37799
Hemic and **Lymphatic** Systems	38100–38999
Mediastinum and **Diaphragm**	39000–39599
Digestive System	40490–49999
Urinary System	50010–53899
Male Genital System	54000–55899
Female Genital System	56405–58999
Maternity Care and Delivery	59000–59899
Endocrine System	60000–60699
Nervous System	61000–64999
Eye and Ocular Adnexa	65091–68899
Auditory System	69000–69979
Operating Microscope	69990

hemic (he′mik)—pertaining to the blood

lymphatic (lim-′fat-ik)—pertaining to the lymphatic system, including lymph nodes and vessels

mediastinum (me-de-əs-ti′ nəm)—the space between the pleural sacs of the lungs, which contains all the organs and structure of the chest except the lungs

diaphragm (′dī-ə-fram)—structure separating the chest and abdominal cavity, composed of tissue and muscle

Keep in mind that when you code for a provider, you will not need to know how to code surgeries for every body system, unless you work as a coder for a multispecialty physician group or work in a hospital. Typically, when you work for a physician or group of physicians, you will code for their specialty, such as obstetrics and gynecology. You would then only need to know how to code procedures related to the female genital system, rather than other body systems, such as the digestive or nervous systems. However, this does not mean that a physician cannot perform procedures on more than one body system. This chapter covers general information about the Surgery section, and you will learn how to code procedures from each body system in subsequent chapters in order to adequately prepare you to work for any type of provider.

SURGERY SUBSECTIONS

Recall from Chapter 17 that each of the six CPT sections is further divided into additional classifications. In the Surgery section, additional classifications include the body system, anatomic site, and types of procedures. Here are the names of the individual section divisions:

- Subsection
- Subheading
- Category
- Subcategory

Turn to the beginning of the Surgery section in your CPT manual. Then refer to the example that follows to determine the subsection, subheading, and categories listed (■ FIGURE 21-1).

Before each subsection of the Surgery chapter, CPT has a table of contents with the name of the subsection, along with its corresponding subheadings, categories, and subcategories, and the page numbers where they are located. In the table of contents, there is an asterisk (*) following any subsection, subheading, category, and subcategory with coding instructions that you should review before assigning codes from the classification.

Figure 21-1 ■ Example of divisions of the Surgery section.

Surgery ◄Section
General ◄Subsection
Integumentary System ◄Subsection
Skin, Subcutaneous and Accessory Structures ◄Subheading
Incision and Drainage ◄Category
Debridement ◄Category
Paring or Cutting ◄Category

Skin Replacement Surgery and Skin Substitutes ◄Category
Surgical Preparation ◄Subcategory
Application of Skin Replacements and Skin Substitutes ◄Subcategory

SURGICAL PROCEDURES

It is important to understand that when you code any type of surgery or procedure, you should know what the procedure is and why the physician performed it. It is very helpful to know common procedures because physicians perform them across specialties. If you do not recognize a procedure, then you should search for the definition and not guess. Do not assume that you have chosen a correct code if you do not know anything about the procedure. There can be many different variations of the same procedure, so it is crucial to take the time to investigate and understand all of the information that the physician documents in the patient's record to ensure that you assign the correct code. A misunderstanding on your part can lead to incorrect code assignment and incorrect insurance reimbursement. *Always* research a procedure that you do not understand, and query the physician for clarification.

The first step in understanding a procedure is to define the term that describes it through knowledge of medical terminology. ■ TABLE 21-2 lists common suffixes that you will see at the end of medical terms for various procedures. You should become familiar with the definitions of the suffixes so that you can better define types of procedures.

In addition to knowing common prefixes to help you to better define medical terms, you also should become familiar with common procedures that physicians perform on various body systems across specialties (■ TABLE 21-3). You are already familiar with specific surgical procedures that you reviewed in previous chapters. You will see these

■ TABLE 21-2   COMMON SUFFIXES IN MEDICAL TERMS DESCRIBING PROCEDURES

Suffix	Meaning
-desis	To stabilize or fuse together (*Example*: arthrodesis—to fuse joints together)
-ectomy	Excision, or surgical removal (*Example*: appendectomy—surgical removal of the appendix)
-pexy	Surgical fixation (*Example:* hysteropexy—surgical fixation of the uterus to keep it from moving)
-plasty	Surgical repair (*Example:* dermatoplasty—a procedure to surgically repair skin with grafts)
-scopy	To visually examine (*Example:* colonoscopy—to examine the colon visually)
-stomy	To surgically create an opening (*Example*: tracheostomy—a procedure to create an opening in the trachea)
-tomy	Incision, or cutting into (*Example:* thoracotomy—an incision into the thorax, or chest)

■ **TABLE 21-3   COMMON SURGICAL PROCEDURES**

Procedure Name	Definition
ablation	Separating, detaching, or destroying
amputation	Removing a body part, such as a leg or arm
anastomosis	Joining two structures that are not normally joined together
biopsy	Removing skin, tissue, muscle, or bone to test for the presence of disease
closure	Closing an open wound with stitches, staples, or another mechanism
debridement	Cleaning out an area using various methods, such as scraping or fluids, to remove contaminated or necrotic tissue or tissue containing foreign bodies
decompression	Removing pressure
destruction	Reducing to tiny fragments or destroying, also called lysis
diagnostic (screening) endoscopy	Using an endoscope to diagnose a condition
dilation	Expanding or stretching an opening
drainage	Removing fluids
endoscopy	Viewing a body cavity using a long narrow hollow instrument that has a light and a camera
excision	Cutting out all or part of an organ or tissue
exploration	Examining an organ or structure to determine a diagnosis
graft	Attaching a piece of skin, fascia, muscle, or bone from one area of the body to another
incision	Cutting with a sharp instrument
incision and drainage	Cutting and draining
injection	Forcing a fluid or other substance into a cavity, tissue, or vessel
insertion	Putting something in place
laparotomy	Cutting into the abdominal cavity
ligation	Tying off using any substance, such as cotton, silk, or wire
lysis	Destruction
reconstruction	Restoring or reforming a part
removal	Taking out
repair	Restoring damaged or diseased tissues to normal function
resection	Removing part of a structure or organ
revision	Repairing or replacing work performed during a previous procedure
surgical (therapeutic) endoscopy	Using an endoscope to treat a condition; a surgical endoscopy always includes a diagnostic endoscopy
suture	Closing a wound with stitches
transplant, transplantation	Replacing an organ or tissue with organ or tissue from a donor

ablation (ab-la′shən)

debridement (di-brēd′-mənt)

dilation (dī-lā′-shən)

endoscopy (en-dos′kə-pe)

laparotomy (lap-ə-rot′ə-me)
ligation (li-ga′shən)
lysis (lī′-səs)

procedures, and procedures in Table 21-3, and others, throughout the Surgery section. To find codes for common surgical procedures, you can search under the name of the procedure in the index and then search for the anatomic site where the physician performed the procedure. Or you can search for the anatomic site, and then look for the name of the procedure.

TAKE A BREAK

Let's take a break and review suffixes and common surgeries.

Exercise 21.1   Surgery Section, Subsections, and Surgical Procedures

Instructions: Fill in each blank with the best answer. Refer to Tables 21-2 and 21-3 for assistance.

1. The suffix _____ means to surgically create an opening.

2. Surgical fixation is represented by the suffix _____.

3. _____ is the surgical procedure that involves removing fluids.

4. _____ is to examine an organ or structure to determine a diagnosis.

5. Cutting into the abdominal cavity is called _____.

6. _____ is to reduce to tiny fragments.

INTEGRAL COMPONENTS OF A PROCEDURE

It is important for you to fully understand every procedure that you code because you must ensure that you assign codes correctly and do not assign separate codes for integral parts of a procedure. In other words, there are certain activities that physicians perform which are naturally part of a procedure, and you should never code them separately. For example, an incision into a patient to perform surgery is an integral component of the surgery. It is understood that the physician must incise the patient to begin the surgery. Therefore, you should not code the incision separately. Other examples of activities which you should *not* code separately because they are integral to procedures, include:

- Preparing the patient for surgery, including shaving hair and cleaning the surgical site
- Draping the patient—covering the patient and surrounding area with a sterile barrier, such as a sheet, to separate sterile areas from nonsterile areas
- Positioning the patient for surgery, including elevating specific anatomic sites, such as a knee
- Exploring specific areas of the patient, including further investigation of an anatomic site
- Destroying, also called lysis, such as destroying lesions to allow the physician to complete a procedure
- Debriding, excising necrotic or contaminated tissue and removing foreign bodies (■ Figure 21-2)

Figure 21-2 ■ Debridement of a patient's face and shoulder. Debridement removes necrotic and infected tissue to facilitate wound healing.

Photo credit: CDC.

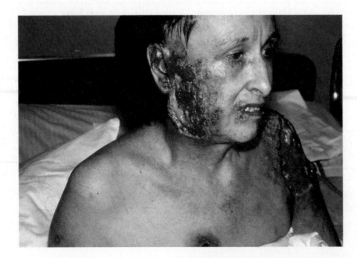

- Performing **lavage** (washing out)
- Achieving **hemostasis** (controlling or stopping the flow of blood)
- Performing any diagnostic procedure when the physician also performs a therapeutic procedure. (Example: a colonoscopy detects polyps (diagnostic colonoscopy), so the physician removes the polyps during the procedure (the diagnostic colonoscopy then becomes a surgical colonoscopy).) Only code the surgical colonoscopy; do not code separately for a diagnostic colonoscopy because the diagnostic colonoscopy is included with the surgical colonoscopy.
- Administering local and regional anesthesia (that the surgeon administers)
- Closing the incision after surgery
- Using a surgical tray of supplies during surgery, including a gown, mask, Betadine® (for cleaning the incision site), sponges, towels, and dressings (excluding surgical instruments)
- Using an **operating microscope**, a microscope that a physician uses to see small structures, such as in eye surgery (called microsurgery) (■ FIGURE 21-3). When a surgery requires an operating microscope, and the physician cannot perform the surgery without it, the microscope is an integral component of the procedure, and you cannot code it separately. (You can assign code 69990 for the operating microscope when it is *not* an integral component of a procedure.)

Always query the physician if you are not sure if an activity is an integral component of a procedure.

lavage (lah-vahzh′)

hemostasis (he-mo-sta′sis)

Surgical Trays

Let's review a little more about when you can code for surgical trays, since they are typically considered to be an integral component of a procedure that you do not normally code. Providers use different surgical trays for different procedures. The supplies in the tray are what the physician will need to have on hand to complete a specific procedure. Many insurances consider surgical trays to be **incidental to**, or part of, a procedure, and they do not allow you to code and bill for them separately. The insurance payment for the procedure *includes* supplies that the provider uses in the surgical tray. Medicare will not pay providers separately for surgical trays that physicians use during office procedures (see Medicare Claims Processing Manual, Chapter 12). Medicare may pay for other types of supplies, depending on the procedure.

Some payers may reimburse providers separately for surgical trays or may pay for trays and supplies which the physician uses that are *above and beyond* the supplies normally required for a procedure. For example, a physician may need more towels and sponges for a procedure on a patient who bleeds excessively. The provider bills the patient's insurance for the additional supplies using either CPT code 99070 or HCPCS

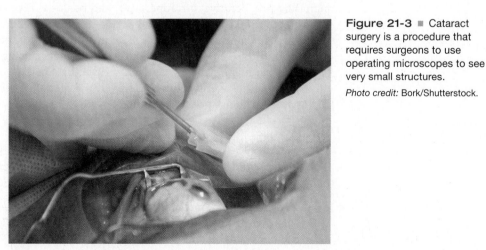

Figure 21-3 ■ Cataract surgery is a procedure that requires surgeons to use operating microscopes to see very small structures.

Photo credit: Bork/Shutterstock.

INTERESTING FACT: Diabetes Patients Commonly Experience Debridement

Patients with diabetes have an increased risk for developing foot sores, or ulcers. Foot ulcers, which are often painless, are the most common reason for hospital stays for people with diabetes. It may take weeks or even several months for foot ulcers to heal. Debridement is the process of a physician or nurse removing dead skin and tissue in order to better see a patient's foot ulcer. There are many ways to do this, including using a scalpel and special scissors. Here is a typical list of steps for debridement:

✔ The skin surrounding the wound is cleaned and disinfected.

✔ The wound is probed with a metal instrument to see how deep it is and to see if there is any foreign material or object in the ulcer.

✔ The doctor cuts away the dead tissue using a scalpel or special scissors, then washes out the ulcer.

✔ The sore may seem bigger and deeper after the doctor or nurse debrides it. The ulcer should be red or pink in color and look like fresh meat.

There are other ways to remove dead or infected tissue:

✔ Soak the foot in a whirlpool bath.

✔ Use a syringe and catheter (tube) to wash away dead tissue.

✔ Apply wet to dry dressings to the area to pull off dead tissue.

✔ Put special chemicals, called enzymes, on the ulcer. The enzymes dissolve dead tissue from the wound.

(U.S. Department of Health and Human Services, National Institutes of Health, www.nlm.nih.gov/medlineplus/ency/patientinstructions/000077.htm, accessed 4/21/11.)

code A4550, depending on which code the insurance requires. Code descriptions are as follows:

99070—Supplies and materials (except spectacles), provided by the physician over and above those usually included with the office visit or other services rendered (list drugs, trays, supplies, or materials provided)

A4550—Surgical trays

You can find CPT code 99070 in the index under the main term *supply*, subterm materials. Code A4550 is listed in the HCPCS Index under the main term surgical, subterm *tray*.

THE GLOBAL SURGICAL PACKAGE

In order to better understand when to assign codes for surgeries, it is also important to review the global surgical package. Recall from Chapter 18 that a **global surgical package** represents a group, or package, of services that all relate to a single surgery, including preoperative, intraoperative, and postoperative services. The insurance specifies a time frame, called the global period, during which the provider must render all of the services related to the surgery. The insurance will issue *one payment* to the provider to cover multiple services that the provider renders during the global period, instead of issuing individual payments for each service. Payers have different criteria for elements of a surgical package and time frames of the global period, so it is best to check with each payer for their specific guidelines.

CPT's Global Surgical Package

The Surgery guidelines at the beginning of the Surgery section in the CPT manual contain the CPT definition of a surgical package, which includes the following services:

- Local infiltration, metacarpal (long bones of the hand)/metatarsal (long bones of the foot)/digital block (anesthetic nerve block of the fingers) or topical anesthesia (excludes general anesthesia)

- Subsequent to the decision for surgery, conducting one related E/M encounter on the date immediately prior to or on the date of procedure (including history and physical)
- Immediate postoperative care, including dictating operative notes and talking with the family and other physicians
- Writing orders
- Evaluating the patient in the postanesthesia recovery area
- Typical postoperative follow-up care

Medicare's Global Surgical Package

Medicare providers render services that are related to the global surgical package in any setting, including hospitals, ambulatory surgery centers (ASCs), and physicians' offices. The following services are included in Medicare's global surgical package (Medicare Claims Processing Manual, Chapter 12, publication #100-04):

- Preoperative Visits—Preoperative visits occur *after the physician decides to operate*, beginning on the day *before surgery* for major procedures, and the day *of surgery* for minor procedures. Preoperative services include examination and workup to determine if the patient is healthy enough for surgery.
- Intra-operative Services—These services are normally a usual and necessary part of a surgical procedure. Intra-operative services include performing the surgical procedure.
- Complications Following Surgery—This includes all additional medical or surgical services required of the surgeon during the postoperative period of the surgery because of complications which *do not* require additional trips to the operating room (OR).
- Postoperative Visits—Follow-up visits *during the postoperative period* of the surgery that are related to recovery from the surgery. Follow-up services include wound checks and review of the overall health of the patient.
- Postsurgical Pain Management—The surgeon provides postsurgical pain management, including methods for reducing the patient's postsurgical pain.
- Supplies—Included in the patient's procedure and follow-up, except for supplies identified as exclusions by the insurance.
- Miscellaneous Services—Items such as dressing changes; local incisional care; removal of operative pack; removal of cutaneous sutures, staples, lines, wires, tubes, drains, casts, and splints; insertion, irrigation, and removal of urinary catheters, routine peripheral intravenous lines, and nasogastric and rectal tubes; and changes and removal of tracheostomy tubes.

Physicians who perform the patient's surgery and render all of the usual pre- and postoperative services code and bill Medicare and other payers for the global package with one CPT code *for the surgical procedure only*. Insurances do not allow providers to bill individual services with individual charges for visits or other services that are included in the global package. Instead, providers should report and submit code 99024 with *no charge* to the insurance to show that the service, such as a postoperative office visit, was related to the surgery and occurred within the postoperative period. The CPT index main term for code 99024 is *post-op visit*:

> **99024**—Postoperative follow-up visit, normally included in the surgical package, to indicate that an evaluation and management service was performed during a postoperative period for a reason(s) related to the original procedure

Medicare classifies surgeries as major, with a 90-day postoperative period, or minor, with a 10-day postoperative period. Some surgeries may also have a zero-day postoperative period (only the day of surgery). CMS publishes Medicare's number of global days for specific CPT codes in the Physician Fee Schedule Relative Value File, which you can access through the CMS website. ■ TABLE 21-4 lists examples of Medicare's global days for specific CPT codes:

ischial tuberosity (is′ke-əl too-bə-ros′ĭ-te)—a normal protrusion or bump that is part of the hip bone

trochanter (tro-kan′tər)—a normal protrusion or bump below the neck of the thigh bone

coccygectomy (kok-sĭ-jek′ tə-me)—surgical excision of the tailbone

subfascial (səb-fash′ əl)—below the tissue that surrounds a muscle

intramuscular (in-trə-mus′ ku-lər)—within a muscle

methylmethacrylate (meth-əl-mcth-ak′rə-lāt)—a substance used in making acrylic resin

arthrography (ahr-throg′ rə-fe)—taking an X-ray after injecting a dye that makes the structure visible

■ TABLE 21-4 **EXAMPLES OF MEDICARE'S GLOBAL DAYS FOR SPECIFIC CPT CODES**

CPT Code	Description	Global Days
27078	Radical resection of tumor; **ischial tuberosity** and greater **trochanter** of femur	90
27080	**Coccygectomy**, primary	90
27086	Removal of foreign body, pelvis or hip; subcutaneous tissue	10
27087	Removal of foreign body, pelvis or hip; deep (**subfascial** or **intramuscular**)	90
27090	Removal of hip prosthesis (separate procedure)	90
27091	Removal of hip prosthesis; complicated, including total hip prosthesis, **methylmethacrylate** with or without insertion of spacer	90
27093	Injection procedure for hip **arthrography**; without anesthesia	0

Source: Department of Health and Human Services, Centers for Medicare and Medicaid Services, 2011 National Physician Fee Schedule Relative Value File. CPT only © 2011. American Medical Association. All rights reserved.

Other payers may follow Medicare's global days for specific procedures, but it is best to check with individual payers so that you know what services are included in the global days and what services you should separately code.

Also remember that there are specific modifiers related to the global surgical package which give the insurance further information about procedures that are rendered during the global period. For example, remember that you appended modifier -79 to a procedure that is *unrelated* to the patient's initial surgery. Modifier -79 tells the insurance to pay the procedure separately because it had nothing to do with the surgery or its global period.

Services Excluded from Medicare's Global Surgical Package

Medicare carriers *do not include* the following services in the global surgical package payment, and Medicare may pay for these services separately:

- The surgeon's initial consultation or evaluation of the patient's condition to determine the need for surgery. Please note that this policy only applies to *major surgical procedures*. The initial evaluation is *always included* in the allowance *for a minor* surgical procedure.

- Services provided by *other physicians*, except when the surgeon and the other physician(s) agree on the transfer of care. This agreement may be in the form of a letter or an annotation in the discharge summary, hospital record, or ASC record.

- Visits *unrelated to the diagnosis for which the surgical procedure is performed*, unless the visits occur due to complications of the surgery.

- Treatment for the underlying condition, or an added course of treatment, which is *not part* of normal recovery from surgery.

- Diagnostic tests and procedures, including diagnostic radiological procedures

- Clearly distinct surgical procedures that are conducted during the postoperative period, which are *not* re-operations or treatment for complications. (A new postoperative period begins with the subsequent procedure that is unrelated to the initial procedure and its global period.)

- Treatment for postoperative complications, which *requires a return trip to the OR*.

- If a less extensive procedure fails, and a more extensive procedure is required, then Medicare pays the second procedure separately.

- For certain services performed in a physician's office, separate payment can no longer be made for a surgical tray (code A4550). However, splints and casting supplies are separately payable.

- **Immunosuppressive** therapy for organ transplants.

immunosuppressive (im-u-no-sə-pres′iv)—reducing the body's immune response

- Critical care services (codes 99291 and 99292) *unrelated to the surgery* where a seriously injured or burned patient is critically ill and requires the physician's constant attendance.

Many payers follow Medicare's guidelines for the surgical package, but it is always best to check with each payer for specific guidelines on the elements that they include in the surgical package.

TAKE A BREAK

Good job! Let's take a break and review more about integral components and the global surgical package.

Exercise 21.2   **Integral Components of a Procedure, the Global Surgical Package**

Instructions: On the line preceding each statement, write T for True or F for False.

1. _____ The CPT global surgical package includes, subsequent to the decision for surgery, one related Evaluation and Management (E/M) encounter on the date immediately prior to or on the date of the procedure.

2. _____ CPT's global surgical package includes any and all postoperative follow-up care.

3. _____ Medicare's global surgical package includes all additional medical or surgical services required of the surgeon during the postoperative period of the surgery, including complications which require additional trips to the OR.

4. _____ Intra-operative services are normally a usual and necessary part of a surgical procedure and include preoperative visits, the surgical procedure, and postsurgical pain management.

5. _____ Medicare's global surgical package does not include the surgeon's initial consultation or evaluation of the patient's condition to determine the need for surgery.

6. _____ Medicare's global surgical package excludes diagnostic tests and procedures, such as diagnostic radiological procedures.

DESTINATION: MEDICARE

This Medicare exercise will help you to review additional information about Medicare's global surgical package. Follow the instructions listed next to access Chapter 12 of the Medicare Claims Processing Manual for Physicians/Nonphysician Practitioners:

1. Go to the website http://www.cms.gov.
2. At the top of the screen on the banner bar, choose *Regulations and Guidance.*
3. Under Guidance, choose *Manuals.*
4. On the left side of the screen, under Manuals, choose *Internet-Only Manuals (IOMs).*
5. Scroll down to Publication #*100-04 Medicare Claims Processing Manual*, and click *100-04.*
6. Scroll down to the list of Downloads, and choose Chapter 12—*Physicians/ Nonphysician Practitioners.*

Answer the following questions, using the search function (Ctrl + F) to find information that you need:

1. In what settings will Medicare reimburse providers for performing services included in the global surgical package?
2. Will Medicare pay providers for a patient's visits that are unrelated to the diagnosis for which the physician performed the surgery?
3. Is an endoscopy suite considered to be an OR?
4. When should a provider begin counting the number of days for a major surgery?

SURGERY GUIDELINES

You already learned that each of the six sections in CPT include guidelines at the beginning of the section, in addition to guidelines that you will find *throughout* the section. Guidelines can also apply to subsections, subheadings, or categories of codes. It is important that you read and analyze coding guidelines that you find throughout the CPT manual because it can affect your final code assignments. The guidelines are meant to help you better understand how and why you should assign specific codes. Always keep in mind that individual payers may have their own coding guidelines that you will also have to follow, in addition to following CPT guidelines.

Let's start by reviewing the **Surgery section guidelines**, which are guidelines listed at the beginning of the Surgery section that will help you to code surgical procedures correctly. Then we will review additional instructions found throughout the Surgery section. Turn to your CPT manual and locate the Surgery section guidelines at the beginning of the Surgery section. They are divided into the following categories:

- Physicians' Services
- CPT Surgical Package Definition
- Follow-up Care for Diagnostic Procedures
- Follow-up Care for Therapeutic Surgical Procedures
- Materials Supplied by Physician
- Reporting More Than One Procedure/Service
- Separate Procedure
- Unlisted Service or Procedure
- Special Report
- Surgical Destruction

Let's review each of the categories next so that you can better understand them.

Physicians' Services

The Evaluation and Management Section (99201–99499) contains codes for physicians' services rendered in the office, home, or hospital, as well as consultations and other medical services. Assign codes for "Special Services and Reports" (99000–99091) from the Medicine section. They represent *adjunct services,* or services that a provider renders *in addition to* another service. Turn to the Special Services and Reports codes (99000–99091) as you review the examples of Special Services and Reports listed next:

- Handling and/or conveyance of a lab specimen from a physician's office to a laboratory (99000–99001)
- Postoperative follow-up visit included in the surgical package (99024)
- Hospital on-call services, office services provided in or out of the office during times when the office is normally closed, and emergency services provided in or out of the office (99026–99050)
- Supplies and materials (99070)
- Educational supplies, such as books and pamphlets (99071)
- Medical testimony, patient group education, special reports, patient transports, and analyzing and interpreting clinical and physiologic data (99075–99091)

CPT Surgical Package Definition

CPT lists elements of the surgical package that you should *not* code and bill separately, which you reviewed earlier in this chapter.

Follow-up Care for Diagnostic Procedures

arthroscopy (är-'thräs-kə-pē)—to visually examine a joint using an arthroscope

Follow-up care for diagnostic procedures (e.g., endoscopy, **arthroscopy**, injection procedures for radiography) only includes care that is related to *recovery from* the diagnostic

POINTERS FROM THE PROS: Interview with a Senior Consultant

John Elders has worked in healthcare for 43 years and is a Senior Consultant for a healthcare software and consulting services firm. He helps clients to verify correct CPT and HCPCS codes for their charge description master (CDM) line items and also provides assistance with ICD-9-CM code assignments.

What interests you the most about the job that you perform?

The diversity of the clients I deal with. Each conversation is a new experience.

What are the most challenging aspects of your job?

Staying on top of the Medicare regulations and coding guidelines.

Please give an example of a time when you educated a physician(s) about coding processes and the outcome.

I performed an audit for a physician who employed a physician's assistant (PA) who was incorrectly reporting E/M codes for services that were not documented or medically necessary. I discussed these with the physician, and he, in turn, discussed them with the PA. The physician agreed that he needed to be more involved in the training and education of his staff.

What advice would you like to give to coding students to help them prepare to work successfully in the healthcare field and to communicate with physicians?

Listen closely. Ask questions. Remember that Internet search engines are your best friends, and you should know how to use them well. Know your subject matter and where to find regulatory support for the advice you give.

(Used by permission of John R. Elders.)

procedure. Follow-up care *excludes* care of the patient's condition which warranted the diagnostic procedure. You can code and bill separately for services to care for the patient's condition.

Follow-up Care for Therapeutic Surgical Procedures

Follow-up care for therapeutic surgical procedures only includes care that is usually a *part of the surgical service.* You can code and bill separately for complications, exacerbations, recurrence, or the presence of other diseases or injuries requiring additional services.

Materials Supplied by Physician

Assign codes for **materials supplied by the physician** (sterile trays or drugs), *over and above* those usually included with the procedure(s). Assign code 99070 to drugs, trays, supplies, and materials provided, or assign a specific supply code that the insurance requests.

Reporting More Than One Procedure or Service

You may need to append one or more modifiers when a physician performs more than one procedure or service on the same date, same session, or during a postoperative period. Modifiers provide insurances with more information about the services or procedures so that they will consider the claim for payment. Refer to Appendix A in the CPT manual for modifier definitions. You also reviewed appending modifiers to multiple services in various situations in Chapter 18 of this text.

Separate Procedure

A **separate procedure** is often an integral component (part) of another major service or procedure, and these integral procedures are called *minor* procedures. You should not code minor procedures when they are integral components of a major procedure.

CPT lists minor procedures with the words "separate procedure" in the code descriptor. You should not assign codes for services that are designated as a "separate procedure" if they were an integral component of another total procedure. For example, refer to the

inguinofemoral (ing′gwĭ-no′-fem-or-əl)—groin and thigh region

lymphadenectomy (lim-fad-ə-nek′tə-me)

hypogastric (hī-pə-gas′-trik)—lowest region of the abdomen

obturator nodes (äb-t(y)ə-rāt′-ər)—lymph nodes in the abdominal/pelvic region

following three codes for an **inguinofemoral lymphadenectomy** (removal of one or more lymph nodes) or a pelvic lymphadenectomy:

38760   Inguinofemoral lymphadenectomy, superficial, including Cloquets node (separate procedure)

38765   Inguinofemoral lymphadenectomy, superficial, in continuity with pelvic lymphadenectomy, including external iliac, **hypogastric**, and **obturator nodes** (separate procedure)

38770   Pelvic lymphadenectomy, including external iliac, hypogastric, and obturator nodes (separate procedure)

Notice that each code descriptor for the lymphadenectomy contains the words *separate procedure*. This means that the three types of lymphadenectomies listed are *minor* procedures which are normally integral components of a major procedure. Therefore, you should *not* code them separately if they are *part of* a major procedure.

Be very careful when you are assigning codes with the words *separate procedure* as part of their descriptors. You should only assign separate procedure codes when the physician does *not* perform them as integral components of a major procedure. Whenever they are integral to a major procedure, you should only assign a code for the major procedure. Refer to code 54130 for an example:

54130   Amputation of penis, radical; with bilateral inguinofemoral lymphadenectomy

(For lymphadenectomy (separate procedure), see 38760–38770)

Notice that the descriptor for code 54130 *includes* lymphadenectomy because the lymphadenectomy is an integral part of the penis amputation, so you should not assign a separate code for a lymphadenectomy. However, if a physician performs an inguinofemoral or pelvic lymphadenectomy, and it is *not* an integral part of another procedure, then you *should assign* a code for the lymphadenectomy. The CPT note following the code descriptor gives you this information:

(For lymphadenectomy (separate procedure), see 38760–38770)

For example, a physician may diagnose a patient with bladder cancer and decide to perform a pelvic lymphadenectomy to determine if the bladder cancer has metastasized to the pelvic lymph nodes. The physician only performs the pelvic lymphadenectomy, and it is not an integral part of another procedure. In this case, you would assign a code for the pelvic lymphadenectomy because it was *not* an integral part of another procedure performed at the same time.

A physician may also perform a procedure designated in CPT as a *separate procedure* in *addition to unrelated* major or minor procedures that occur during the same encounter or episode of care. For these cases, assign a code to the *separate procedure*, and append modifier -59 to indicate that the procedure is *not* a component of another procedure but is a distinct, independent procedure. This may represent a different session, different procedure or surgery, different site or organ system, separate incision or excision, separate lesion, or separate injury (or area of injury in extensive injuries). You also reviewed how to append modifier -59 in Chapter 18 of this text.

Unlisted Service or Procedure

Recall from Chapter 17 that there are many unlisted procedure codes in CPT Category I that have very general descriptions, which are intended to cover a variety of services and procedures. They are called *unlisted* codes, and they represent an **unlisted service or procedure**. Report an unlisted code for a procedure or service for which there is no specific CPT code in either Category I or Category III. AMA designated many unlisted codes in the six sections of CPT that you can assign for reporting unlisted procedures. These include procedures that providers do not often perform, procedures that are experimental, or new procedures that do not yet have a specific Category I or Category III code. There are reporting guidelines associated with many unlisted procedures, and you should review and understand the guidelines before reporting the unlisted code.

Guidelines at the beginning of the Surgery section show all unlisted CPT codes within the Surgery section, arranged in numeric order. They include the following examples:

- **15999**—Unlisted procedure, excision pressure ulcer
- **17999**—Unlisted procedure, skin, mucous membrane and subcutaneous tissue
- **19499**—Unlisted procedure, breast

Unlisted codes appear throughout the Surgery section. They are arranged by anatomic site and/or type of procedure and appear at the end of specific subsections, subheadings, categories, and subcategories. Unlisted codes end in 98 or 99. You should only assign unlisted codes as a *last resort*, after checking for a more specific Category I or Category III code.

Because the descriptor for unlisted codes is so general, it is impossible to tell from the unlisted descriptor what service was provided because it only states "unlisted," along with a specific anatomic site or procedure type. Insurances require that you submit additional documentation, or a *special report*, with the insurance claim for an unlisted procedure to show what service or procedure the clinician actually provided and to establish medical necessity. Insurances may request the patient's medical documentation or a letter from the clinician explaining the procedure and why he performed it. Be aware that when you have to send additional information with claims, insurances typically take longer to process them because they spend more time reviewing the additional information the provider submitted.

Special Report

Also recall from Chapter 17 that for services that providers rarely perform, or services that are new or unusual, insurances may require a **special report**, including medical documentation or letters from clinicians to justify medical necessity of a procedure and provide greater detail about the procedure performed. Providers send special reports with claims for Category I unlisted codes and Category III codes. Special reports include the definition or description of the nature, extent, and need for the procedure, as well as the time, effort, and equipment used to provide the service.

Surgical Destruction

Surgical destruction is a part of a surgical procedure, so do not code different methods of destruction separately unless the destruction technique substantially alters the standard management of a problem or condition. Destruction, also called lysis, includes **electrosurgery**, **cryosurgery**, and **laser** and **chemical treatment**.

Now that you reviewed the various categories of guidelines that appear at the beginning of the Surgery section, we will next review additional guidelines that appear *throughout* the Surgery section.

electrosurgery (e-lek-tro-sur′jər-e)—surgical procedures performed using an instrument which conducts electrical current

cryosurgery (kri-o-sur′jər-e)—destroying tissue by using extreme cold

laser treatment—treatment with a light beam that is transformed into radiation and heat energy

chemical treatment—using a chemical to treat or destroy tissue

TAKE A BREAK

Give yourself a pat on the back! Let's take a break and review more about surgery guidelines.

Exercise 21.3 Surgery Guidelines

Instructions: Fill in each blank with the best answer.

1. Individual payers may have their own _____ that you will have to follow, in addition to following CPT guidelines.

2. Follow-up care for diagnostic procedures only includes care that is related to _____ the diagnostic procedure.

3. You should not assign codes for services designated as a _____ if they were an integral component of another procedure.

4. Insurances require that you submit additional documentation, or a _____, with the insurance

continued

TAKE A BREAK *continued*

claim for an unlisted procedure to show what service or procedure the clinician actually provided and to establish medical necessity.

5. If a physician performs an inguinofemoral or pelvic lymphadenectomy and it is not an integral part of another procedure, then you should assign a code for the _____.

6. Surgical _____ is a part of a surgical procedure, so do not code different methods of this separately unless the technique substantially alters the standard management of a problem or condition.

WORKPLACE IQ

You are working as a coder at Williton Medical Center in the Health Information Management Department. Today, your manager asks you to train Cindy, a new coder, on the definition of a surgical package. Your manager wants you to define the surgical package and then explain to Cindy how the surgical package relates to her job.

What would you do?

ADDITIONAL GUIDELINES IN THE SURGERY SECTION

Just as in all six sections in CPT, the Surgery section lists additional coding guidelines for you to follow before coding from various subsections, subheadings, categories, subcategories, and codes. Guidelines include instructions, notes, and coding tips to help you to assign the correct code, so be sure that you read and understand guidelines because they can affect your final code assignment.

When you review CPT's coding instructions in your coding manual, do not be afraid to highlight the notes in your manual or write any additional reminders to yourself. The CPT Professional Edition contains various blank pages, which you can use specifically for notes. If you have the electronic version of the Professional Edition of CPT, then you can type notes into the Notes tab and save them for future reference.

Review the following examples of various types and formats of coding guidelines and instructions that you will find in the CPT manual for 2011:

Example 1: Coding instructions for subsection Musculoskeletal System

Surgery

Musculoskeletal System

Cast and strapping procedures appear at the end of this section.

The services listed next include the application and removal of the first cast or traction device only. Subsequent replacement of cast and/or traction device may require an additional listing.

Definitions

The terms "closed treatment," "open treatment," and "percutaneous skeletal fixation" have been carefully chosen to accurately reflect current orthopaedic procedural treatments.

Closed treatment specifically means that the fracture site is not surgically opened (exposed to the external environment and directly visualized). This terminology is used to describe procedures that treat fractures by three methods: (1) without manipulation; (2) with manipulation; or (3) with or without traction.

Open treatment is used when the fractured bone is either: (1) surgically opened (exposed to the external environment) and the fracture (bone ends) visualized and internal fixation may be used; or (2) the fractured bone is opened remote from the fracture site in order to insert an **intramedullary** nail across the fracture site (the fracture site is not opened and visualized).

intramedullary (in-trə-med′u-lar-e)—within the bone marrow (material in a bone cavity), spinal cord, or medulla oblongata (a structure between the base of the brain and spinal cord)

Example 2: Coding instructions for subsection Musculoskeletal System, subheading Spine (Vertebral Column)

Surgery

Musculoskeletal System

Spine (Vertebral Column)

Cervical, thoracic, and lumbar spine.

Within the Spine section, bone grafting procedures are reported separately and in addition to arthrodesis. For bone grafts in other Musculoskeletal sections, see specific code(s) descriptor(s) and/or accompanying guidelines.

Example 3: Coding instructions for subsection Integumentary System, subheading Skin, Subcutaneous, and Accessory Structures, category Debridement

▶**Debridement**◀ (11000–11047)

▶Wound debridements (11042–11047) are reported by depth of tissue that is removed and by surface area of the wound. These services may be reported for injuries, infections, wounds and chronic ulcers. When performing debridement of a single wound, report depth using the deepest level of tissue removed. In multiple wounds, sum the surface area of those wounds that are at the same depth, but do not combine sums from different depths. For example: When bone is debrided from a 4 sq cm heel ulcer and from a 10 sq cm ischial ulcer, report the work with a single code, 11044. When subcutaneous tissue is debrided from a 16 sq cm dehisced abdominal wound and a 10 sq cm thigh wound, report the work with 11042 for the first 20 sq cm and 11045 for the second 6 sq cm. If all four wounds were debrided on the same day, use modifier 59 with 11042, 11045 and 11044.◀

In Example 3, did you notice the facing triangles enclosing the word Debridement and enclosing the coding instructions? Do you remember what they mean? Recall from Chapter 17 that facing triangles indicate that text for the descriptor is new or revised since last year, or there are new or revised instructions for assigning a code. Always be sure to read any coding instructions, especially because they may change from year to year.

Example 4: Coding tip for Application of Skin Replacements and Skin Substitutes

--------------*Coding Tip*---

Surface Area Requirement for Reporting

When square centimeters are indicated, this refers to 1 sq cm up to the stated amount.

Example 5: Coding Instructions for Codes 31287 and 31288

31287   Nasal/sinus endoscopy, surgical, with **sphenoidotomy**;

31288   with removal of tissue from the sphenoid sinus

▶(Do not report <u>31287</u>, <u>31288</u> in conjunction with <u>31297</u> when performed on the same sinus)◀

sphenoidotomy (sfe-noi-dot′ə-me)—making a surgical incision into the sphenoid sinus (in front of the ear)

Notice that the coding instructions in Example 5 are listed in parentheses. You will see instructions in parentheses that apply to one code or to several codes, including information about deleted codes. It is important to read the information in parentheses to ensure that you assign the correct code(s).

TAKE A BREAK

Good work! Let's take a break and review more surgery guidelines.

Exercise 21.4 Additional Guidelines in the Surgery Section

Instructions: Review coding instructions in the Surgery section as directed, and then answer each question.

1. According to the coding instructions for codes 41733–41747, what three activities are involved in a living donor **hepatectomy** (excision of the liver)? _____
_____

2. Review the coding instructions following code 52334. What code should you report for a **cystourethroscopy** with **fulguration** of congenital posterior **urethral** valves? _____

3. Review the coding instructions for subsection Nervous System, subheading Skull, **Meninges**, and Brain, and category Surgery of Skull Base. Which type of procedure should you report separately if the patient requires a **cranioplasty**? _____

4. Review the coding instructions for subsection Integumentary System, subheading Skin, Subcutaneous and Accessory Structures, category Excision—Malignant Lesions. What two types of closures of defects should you report separately? _____
_____

5. Review the coding instructions following code 22525. What codes can you report with code 22525? _____
_____

6. Review the coding instructions following code 37025. What codes should you report for transcatheter coronary stent placement? _____

CPT® ASSISTANT GUIDELINES

In addition to the coding guidelines and instructions that you will find throughout the Surgery section and the entire CPT manual, the AMA also offers additional coding guidelines to help you code accurately. Recall from Chapter 17 that AMA publishes a monthly newsletter called *CPT® Assistant*, which contains helpful information that clarifies how and when to assign specific codes. Providers purchase yearly subscriptions of *CPT® Assistant* from AMA. Also remember that the arrow symbol ➲ appears after many code descriptors in the CPT manual and includes a reference to a specific issue of *CPT® Assistant* or *CPT® Changes: An Insider's View*, an annual book with all of the coding changes for the current year. Review the following example of a *CPT® Assistant* reference for a code:

> **10040** Acne surgery (eg, **marsupialization**, opening or removal of multiple **milia**, **comedones**, cysts, pustules)
>
> ➲ *CPT Assistant* <u>Fall 1992:10</u>, <u>Feb 2008:8</u>

In the example of code 10040, the *CPT® Assistant* reference includes the newsletter issue and page number for you to review more about assigning code 10040. Providers can also purchase archives, or back issues, of *CPT® Assistant* if they need to reference older issues.

One of the features of the *CPT® Assistant* newsletter is a question-and-answer forum where providers submit coding questions that AMA coding experts answer. They then publish both the questions and answers so that other providers can also benefit from the information.

SURGERY: GENERAL SUBSECTION

Remember that the Surgery section contains many different subsections that represent procedures on different body systems and anatomic sites (Table 21-1). You will learn more about coding from various Surgery subsections in other chapters of this text. However, the first and smallest subsection of the surgery chapter is General, and since it only

hepatectomy (hep-ə-'tek-tə-mē)

cystourethroscopy (sis-tō-yu-'rē-thrə-skōp-ē)—to examine the bladder and urethra with an endoscope

fulguration (ful-gu-ra'sh ən)—destroying tissue using an electrical current

urethral (u-re'thrəl)—pertaining to the urethra, tube that carries urine from the urinary bladder to outside the body

meninges (mə-nin'jēz)—the three membranes that surround the brain and spinal cord

cranioplasty (kra'ne-ō-plas-te)—surgical repair of the skull

marsupialization (mahr-soo-pe-əl-i-za'shən)—creating a pouch

milia (mil'e-ə)—clusters of tiny cysts often found in the eyelids, cheeks, and forehead

comedones (ko'mə-do'nēz)—blackheads

includes two codes, let's review them in this chapter. The two codes and corresponding coding instructions in parentheses are as follows:

10021   Fine needle aspiration; without imaging guidance

10022   with imaging guidance

(For placement of percutaneous localization clip during breast biopsy, use <u>19295</u>)

(For radiological supervision and interpretation, see <u>76942</u>, <u>77002</u>, <u>77012</u>, <u>77021</u>)

▶(For percutaneous needle biopsy other than fine needle aspiration, see <u>20206</u> for muscle, <u>32400</u> for pleura, <u>32405</u> for lung or mediastinum, <u>42400</u> for salivary gland, <u>47000</u> for liver, <u>48102</u> for pancreas, <u>49180</u> for abdominal or retroperitoneal mass, <u>50200</u> for kidney, <u>54500</u> for testis, <u>54800</u> for epididymis, <u>60100</u> for thyroid, <u>62267</u> for nucleus pulposus, intervertebral disc, or paravertebral tissue, <u>62269</u> for spinal cord)◀

(For evaluation of fine needle aspirate, see <u>88172</u>, <u>88173</u>)

Fine-needle aspiration, also called a needle aspiration biopsy, is when a physician inserts a fine, or thin, hollow needle under the skin to take a sample of cells. The needle is attached to a syringe that extracts cells, which are contained in fluid or blood. The physician rotates the needle within layers of cells to remove an adequate specimen. The cells from the sample are then placed on a glass slide and stained, and a pathologist reviews them under a microscope to determine whether any malignancy exists.

Note that code 10022 includes imaging guidance with fine-needle aspiration, which is when the physician uses imaging, such as ultrasound, to see the needle and determine where to move it. A physician may also use other imaging, including fluoroscopy, MRI, and CT.

Also note that the coding instructions in parentheses direct you to assign other codes for

- placement of percutaneous localization clip during breast biopsy—when the physician leaves a metal clip in the patient to mark the biopsy site in case he needs to remove more tissue from the same site in the future
- radiological supervision and interpretation of the needle aspiration
- percutaneous needle biopsy

Note that there are different types of needle biopsies, including a *percutaneous needle biopsy*, when a physician uses a needle bigger than a fine needle to obtain a *single* biopsy (■ FIGURE 21-4).

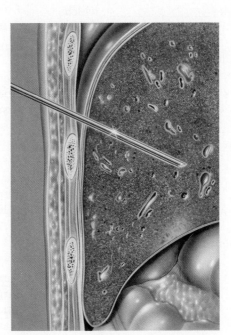

Figure 21-4 ■ Illustration of a percutaneous needle biopsy of the liver to diagnose liver cirrhosis and hepatitis, involving intercostal penetration between the rib bones (spongy ovals at left) to reach the liver (at center, brown). Part of the digestive tract can be seen at lower right.

Credit: John Bavosi/Photo Researchers, Inc.

A *percutaneous core needle biopsy* is when a physician uses a larger needle to take *several* tissue samples for biopsy, removing a separate sample with each needle insertion.

Be sure to carefully review the medical documentation to determine if the physician performed a fine-needle aspiration, percutaneous needle biopsy, or percutaneous core needle biopsy, and always query the physician if you are unsure.

TAKE A BREAK

Great job! Let's take a break and review more about the General subsection of Surgery.

Exercise 21.5   Surgery: General Subsection

Instructions: Fill in each blank with the best answer.

1. Fine-needle aspiration, also called a needle _____, is when a physician inserts a fine, or thin, hollow needle under the skin to take a sample of cells.

2. Code 10022 includes _____ with fine-needle aspiration.

3. A percutaneous _____ needle biopsy is when a physician uses a larger needle to take several tissue samples for biopsy, removing a separate sample with each needle insertion.

CHAPTER REVIEW

Multiple Choice

Instructions: Circle one best answer to complete each statement.

1. The medical terminology suffix that means excision or surgical removal is
   a. –ectomy.
   b. –stomy.
   c. –tomy.
   d. –plasty.

2. CMS publishes Medicare's number of global days for specific CPT codes in the _____, which you can access through the CMS website.
   a. CPT Appendix A
   b. Physician Fee Schedule Relative Value File
   c. Medicare Claims Processing Manual
   d. Medicare Global Surgical Package

3. You should *not* assign separate codes for services designated as a(n) _____ if they were an integral component of another procedure.
   a. separate procedure
   b. global procedure
   c. adjunct service
   d. unlisted service

4. A(n) _____ means to attach a piece of skin, fascia, muscle, or bone from one area of the body to another
   a. anastomosis
   b. closure
   c. lysis
   d. graft

5. You can find coding guidelines in all of the following locations except
   a. CPT Assistant.
   b. sections.
   c. index.
   d. subsections.

6. The _____ subsection appears first in the Surgery section and contains two codes.
   a. Debridement
   b. Integumentary System
   c. General
   d. Incision and Drainage

7. Some payers may reimburse providers separately for _____ which the physician uses that are *above and beyond* supplies normally required for a procedure.
   a. surgical scissors
   b. surgical sponges
   c. surgical trays
   d. surgical prep

8. Turn to the Respiratory System subsection under Surgery. What is the second subheading listed?
   a. Excision
   b. Accessory Sinuses
   c. Larynx
   d. Nose

9. Turn to the Cardiovascular System subsection under Surgery. Code 36100 is listed under Intra-Arterial-Intra-Aortic, which is a
   a. subheading.
   b. category.

c. subcategory.

d. subclassification.

10. Turn to the Nervous System subsection under Surgery. Code 63700 is listed under Repair, which is a
    a. subheading.
    b. category.
    c. subcategory.
    d. subclassification.

Coding Assignments

Instructions: Assign procedure code(s) (CPT) to the following surgery cases, which represent procedures that you reviewed in Table 21-3. You can locate a procedure in the index by searching for the type of the procedure or searching for the body site and then the type of procedure. Optional: For additional practice, assign the patient's diagnosis code(s) (ICD-9-CM).

1. Dr. Wong, a proctologist (a physician who diagnoses and treats disorders of the anus, rectum, and colon), performs destruction of an anal lesion using cryosurgery. The patient is Margaret Head, age 70, and she undergoes the procedure in the surgical suite of Dr. Wong's practice.

   Diagnosis code(s): _____

   Procedure code(s): _____

2. Arthur Conrad, age 63, suffers from an embolism of the pulmonary artery. Today at Williton Medical Center, Dr. Kinney, a cardiopulmonary surgeon (a specialist in heart and lungs), excises the embolism (embolectomy) without using cardiopulmonary bypass.

   Diagnosis code(s): _____

   Procedure code(s): _____

3. At Williton, Dr. Cleveland, a general surgeon, performs an exploration of the mediastinum, **transthoracic** approach (through the thorax, or chest) for a biopsy. He sends the biopsy to pathology for interpretation. The patient is David Wynn, age 42. The pathology report reveals a malignant **thymoma** (tumor of the thymus gland).

   Diagnosis code(s): _____

   Procedure code(s): _____

4. Kelly Stanton, age 34, suffers from adhesions (abnormally joined tissue) of the ureter due to ovarian vein syndrome (obstruction of the tube that carries urine from the kidney to the urinary bladder by enlarged veins in the ovary). Dr. Rosales, an OB/GYN, performs lysis of the adhesions at Williton.

   Diagnosis code(s): _____

   Procedure code(s): _____

5. Lisa Holden, age 30, is an established patient who sees Dr. Hoffman for a painful red lump on her neck. Dr. Hoffman diagnoses a sebaceous cyst (swollen hair follicle) and incises and drains it. He does not perform any other services during the encounter.

   Diagnosis code(s): _____

   Procedure code(s): _____

6. Dr. Choo, an ophthalmologist, performs a revision of a previous **blepharoplasty** (repair of eyelid) of the upper eyelid for Nancy Compton, age 62. He performs the surgery at Williton and diagnoses the patient with mechanical ptosis resulting from the first surgery.

   Diagnosis code(s): _____

   Procedure code(s): _____

7. Mary Craft, age 60, has a colonoscopy (endoscopy to visually examine the colon) today at Williton, as a recommended diagnostic screening for colon cancer. Dr. Cote, a gastroenterologist, performs the procedure. He finds no evidence of growths or any disorders.

   Diagnosis code(s): _____

   Procedure code(s): _____

8. Jonisha Smith, age 22, had a mammogram which revealed suspicious lesions in the left breast. Today at Williton, Dr. Rosales performs a percutaneous needle core biopsy for two lesions in the lower inner quadrant. He uses CT imaging guidance for the needle placements (radiological supervision and interpretation). The pathologist's report reveals carcinoma, stage I.

   Diagnosis code(s): _____

   Procedure code(s): _____

9. Jeffrey Riggs, age 50, is one of Dr. Hoffman's established patients. Mr. Riggs has diabetes type II, uncontrolled, and also suffers from peripheral arterial disease. He develops necrosis and gangrene in his right great toe, and Dr. Hoffman refers him to Dr. Frye, a vascular surgeon. Dr. Frye determines that he will have to amputate the patient's toe (interphalangeal joint), and he performs the surgery today at Williton.

   Diagnosis code(s): _____

   Procedure code(s): _____

10. Dr. Choo, an ophthalmologist, sees Valerie Berger, age 28, for complaints of right eye pain, redness, and discharge. Dr. Choo examines her eye using a slit lamp and finds a torn piece of contact lens on her cornea, which he removes.

    Diagnosis code(s): _____

    Procedure code(s): _____

transthoracic (trans-thə-ras′ik)

thymoma (thi-mo′mə)

blepharoplasty (blef′ə-ro-plas-te)

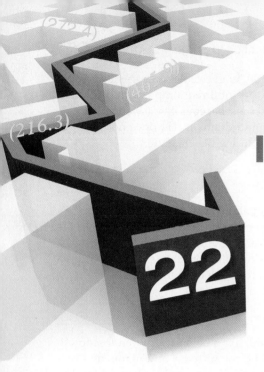

Integumentary System

Learning Objectives

After completing this chapter, you should be able to

- Spell and define the key terminology in this chapter.
- Describe the subsection Surgery—Integumentary system.
- Discuss how to code from the subheading Skin, Subcutaneous, and Accessory Structures.
- Define lesions.
- Explain how to use the codes in the category Excision—lesions—benign and malignant.
- Identify how to use the codes in the subheading Nails.
- Define how to use the codes in the subheading Pilonidal Cyst.
- Describe how to use the codes in the subheading Introduction.
- Explain how to use the codes in the subheading Repair.
- Discuss how to use the codes in the subheading Destruction.
- Identify how to use the codes in the subheading Breast.

Key Terms

complex repair
fine needle aspiration
flap

intermediate repair
simple repair
skin graft

INTRODUCTION

You have reached a very interesting stop on your journey—coding procedures of the integumentary system. You will learn about many different types of procedures that physicians perform, including lesion excisions and wound repairs. CPT includes several coding instructions for specific integumentary procedures, and it is important to review and understand them before assigning codes from the categories. This stop may be a little uncomfortable, but, you will gain confidence by the new information that you learn and apply. Let's continue to move onward to the integumentary system!

"March on. Do not tarry. To go forward is to move toward perfection. March on, and fear not the thorns, or the sharp stones on life's path."—KAHLIL GIBRAN

SURGERY—INTEGUMENTARY SYSTEM (10040–19499)

integumentary (in-teg-yə-ment'-ə-rē)

The **integumentary** system is a subsection of the Surgery section, or chapter. Recall from Chapter 10 that the integumentary system consists of the skin, nails, hair, hair follicles, and related glands. (See Figures 10-26 and 10-27.) The skin is the largest body organ and protects the body from harmful organisms, regulates body temperature, and produces Vitamin D, which helps bones to grow. The skin consists of three layers:

- Epidermis (upper layer of skin)
- Dermis (middle layer of skin)
- Subcutaneous fascia (deepest layer of skin made of fatty tissue)

Integumentary literally means pertaining to (-ary) a covering or skin (integument/o). Dermatology is the study of (-ology) the skin (dermat/o). A dermatologist is a physician who specializes in the diagnosis, treatment, and prevention of skin disorders. But a dermatologist is not the only physician who can perform integumentary system procedures; many other types of physicians can also render services listed in the integumentary subsection, including plastic surgeons (physicians who specialize in correcting disorders involving the skin and underlying structures.)

The integumentary subsection is divided into numerous subheadings organized by body site (nails) or type of procedure (repair), and then further divided into categories of procedures (incision, biopsy) (see ■ TABLE 22-1), as well as subcategories of procedures. The integumentary subsection also includes breast procedures, such as breast reconstruction surgery.

■ TABLE 22-1   **INTEGUMENTARY SYSTEM SUBHEADINGS AND CATEGORIES**

Subheadings and Categories	Code Range
INTEGUMENTARY SYSTEM	**10040–19499**
Skin, Subcutaneous, and Accessory Structures	**10040–11646**
Incision and Drainage	*10040–10180*
Debridement	*11000–11047*
Paring or Cutting	*11055–11057*
Biopsy	*11100–11101*
Removal of Skin Tags	*11200–11201*
Shaving of Epidermal or Dermal Lesions	*11300–11313*
Excision—Benign Lesions	*11400–11471*
Excision—Malignant Lesions	*11600–11646*
Nails	**11719–11765**
Pilonidal Cyst	**11770–11772**
Introduction	**11900–11983**
Repair (Closure)	**12001–16036**
Repair—Simple	*12001–12021*
Repair—Intermediate	*12031–12057*
Repair—Complex	*13100–13160*
Adjacent Tissue Transfer or Rearrangement	*14000–14350*
Skin Replacement Surgery and Skin Substitutes	*15002–15431*
Flaps (Skin and/or Deep Tissues)	*15570–15738*
Other Flaps and Grafts	*15740–15776*
Other Procedures	*15780–15879*
Pressure Ulcers (Decubitus Ulcers)	*15920–15999*
Burns, Local Treatment	*16000–16036*
Destruction	**17000–17999**
Destruction, Benign or Premalignant Lesions	*17000–17250*
Destruction, Malignant Lesions, Any Method	*17260–17286*
Mohs Micrographic Surgery	*17311–17315*
Other Procedures	*17340–17999*
Breast	**19000–19499**
Incision	*19000–19030*
Excision	*19100–19272*
Introduction	*19290–19298*
Mastectomy Procedures	*19300–19307*
Repair and/or Reconstruction	*19316–19396*
Other Procedures	*19499*

SKIN, SUBCUTANEOUS, AND ACCESSORY STRUCTURES (10040–11646)

sebaceous (si-bā′-shəs)—
secreting fatty material
(sebum)

The subheading Skin, Subcutaneous, and Accessory Structures (hair, nails, sweat glands, and **sebaceous** glands) contains eight different categories of codes, depending on the type of procedure that the physician performs (Table 22-1). Common procedures for the categories include incision and drainage (I & D), debridement, biopsy, and excision, all of which you first learned about in Chapter 21. Let's review how to assign codes for procedures in each category, and then practice coding.

Incision and Drainage (10040–10180)

Incision and drainage, also called I & D, is when the physician has to drain fluid, such as pus or blood, from a lesion or mass to allow it to heal. Examples of types of lesions and masses include

- *abscess*—collection of pus (■ FIGURE 22-1)
- *bulla*—fluid-filled blister
- *cyst*—sac of fluid
- *hematoma*—collection of blood
- *seroma*—collection of serum (clear fluid)

The physician must anesthetize the area to drain before puncturing it with a needle (called a puncture aspiration) or cutting it with a scalpel to drain the fluid. The physician then performs one or more of the following activities:

- packs the wound with gauze or another absorbent material
- allows the wound to continue to drain on its own but does not pack it
- inserts a drain, or wick, which is a strip of gauze or tube that helps with continued drainage outside of the wound

The physician may also perform a biopsy of the fluid to determine if there is an infection that needs treatment.

Review the I & D codes for code ranges 10040–10180 for a better understanding of the types of procedures listed in this category, which CPT arranges according to the patient's condition. You should also become familiar with additional terms listed in the code descriptors, which you can find in ■ TABLE 22-2.

When you reviewed the I & D codes, did you notice that CPT categorizes some of them according to whether the procedure was single or multiple, and simple or complicated? Unfortunately, CPT does not define these terms, and providers may interpret them differently. Typical definitions include:

- *single I & D*—The physician incises and drains a single area, as opposed to draining *multiple* areas (multiple I & D).

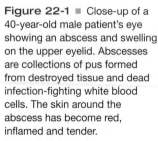

Figure 22-1 ■ Close-up of a 40-year-old male patient's eye showing an abscess and swelling on the upper eyelid. Abscesses are collections of pus formed from destroyed tissue and dead infection-fighting white blood cells. The skin around the abscess has become red, inflamed and tender.

Photo credit: DR P. MARAZZI/ SCIENCE PHOTO LIBRARY.

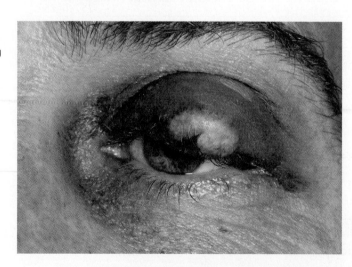

■ TABLE 22-2   COMMON TERMS FOR INCISION AND DRAINAGE CODES

Term	Definition
aspiration (as-pə-rā′-shən)	using suction to remove fluid
carbuncle (kahr′bəng-kəl)	an infection of subcutaneous tissue which includes pus and dying tissue, usually caused by *Staphylococcus aureus* bacteria
cutaneous (kyu̇-tā′-nē-əs)	pertaining to the skin
furuncle (fu′rung-kəl)	a localized swelling and inflammation of a hair follicle and adjacent tissue, with a hard central core and pus, usually caused by a bacterial infection
hidradenitis (hi-drad-ən-īt′-əs)	inflammation of a sweat gland
paronychia (par-o-nik′e-ə) (■ FIGURE 22-2)	inflammation of tissues surrounding the nail
pilonidal cyst (pī-lə-nīd′-əl)	a cyst containing hair
suppurative (sup′u-ra-tiv)	containing pus

- *simple I & D*—The physician drains an area and then allows it to continue to drain on its own.
- *complicated I & D*—The physician places a drain in the wound or packs the wound for continued drainage and requests that the patient return for follow-up care. A complicated case may also involve infection or the drainage of a large area.

Always carefully review the patient's record before you assign codes, and query the physician if you are not certain if an I & D is single, multiple, simple, or complicated.

For I & D procedures of the skin, you can locate codes in the index under the main term *incision and drainage,* and then search for the subterm of the name of the mass that the physician drains (cyst, bulla, abscess) and subterm *skin.* You can also search for the main term *incision and drainage* and subterm *skin.*

Note that a physician can perform I & D on any anatomic site, not just the skin, and you can find these codes in other subsections of the Surgery chapter. For example, a physician might drain **bursa** from the elbow, which has nothing to do with the skin. In this case, you would search the index for the main term *incision and drainage,* subterm *bursa,* and subterm *elbow* to find the code to cross reference (23931). Be very careful when you are coding I & D procedures so that you do not incorrectly assign codes for skin and related structures as the body site if the patient's procedure involved another area. Also investigate whether the I & D is an integral component of another procedure. If it is, then you should not code it separately.

bursa (bur′sə)—a sac of fluid between a tendon and a bone

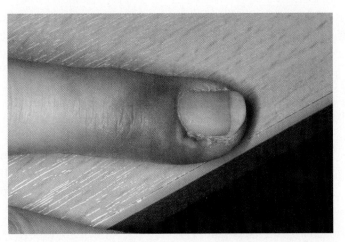

Figure 22-2 ■ Acute paronychia. Close-up of a nail bed of a finger with paronychia, inflammation and infection of the tissues surrounding the fingernails.

Photo credit: Hercules Robinson/ Alamy.

Refer to the following example to learn more about coding an I & D procedure of the skin.

Example: Mr. Rudy, age 36, sees Dr. Hoffman because of a painful lump on his left upper arm. Dr. Hoffman notes that the patient's skin is warm, red, and swollen. He determines that Mr. Rudy has an abscess, so he incises the skin with a scalpel and drains the pus.

To code this case, search the index for the main term *incision and drainage*, subterm *abscess*, and subterm *skin*, which then directs you to cross-reference codes 10060–10061 (■ FIGURE 22-3).

Since there was no information supporting a complicated or multiple procedure, you should assign code **10060** for a simple procedure (single abscess). The patient's diagnosis code is **682.3** (main term *abscess* and subterm *arm*).

10060	Incision and drainage of abscess (eg, carbuncle, suppurative hidradenitis, cutaneous or subcutaneous abscess, cyst, furuncle, or paronychia); simple or single
10061	complicated or multiple

Figure 22-3 ■ Codes 10060 and 10061.

Debridement (11000–11047)

Recall from Chapter 21 that debridement involves excising necrotic tissue or foreign bodies from wounds. Codes under the Debridement category cover debridement of tissue from wounds of the skin, subcutaneous tissue, fascia, muscle, and bone. (*Note:* To code debridement of *burns,* refer to category Burns, Local Treatment—codes 16000–16036.)

Before debridement, the physician assesses the depth of the wound by probing it with an instrument. He then disinfects the area around the wound. The physician removes tissue that is necrotic (dead tissue that may be infected), contaminated, or devitalized (with reduced blood flow and oxygen) and also removes any foreign bodies (Figure 21-2). Wounds may be the result of infections, chronic ulcers, burns, or other injuries.

Physicians debride wounds to remove tissue that will not regenerate and heal and to remove anything else that stops wound healing, such as a build-up of pus. The physician debrides a wound until he removes all contaminated tissue and only healthy tissue remains. Debridement also includes irrigating (cleaning) the wound with water, saline, or another solution. Physicians may also biopsy tissue that was debrided in order to identify any infection or other condition. Without debridement, a wound can become more severe or infected and may cause additional problems for a patient, including continuous spread of infection throughout the body, amputation of an infected body part, or death.

Physicians may perform one type of debridement or a combination of debridement procedures for a patient's wound. Here are some examples of debridement types:

- *Mechanical debridement*—The physician places a saline dressing on the wound until it dries, and he then removes the dressing, along with the necrotic tissue that adhered to the dressing. This process can be painful and removes the patient's healthy tissue with necrotic tissue. Mechanical debridement may also involve irrigation and using a whirlpool.

autolytic (aw-to-lit′ik)
- *Autolytic debridement*—The physician dresses the wound to keep it moist. The body's own cells then debride necrotic tissue but do not destroy healthy tissue. The patient also experiences little pain.

- *Sharp or surgical debridement*—The physician anesthetizes the area to debride and uses a scalpel, laser, or other surgical instrument to remove necrotic tissue.

- *Chemical or enzymatic debridement*—The physician places a solution or gel into the wound to remove necrotic tissue, however, this procedure can also damage healthy tissue.

Do not assign a debridement code if the debridement is an *integral component* of another procedure that the physician performs. You may code debridement separately from another procedure performed at the same session if the debridement is *above and beyond* what is normally required for the procedure.

Review the Debridement codes for code ranges 11000–11047 for a better understanding of the types of procedures listed in this category, which CPT arranges according to the patient's:

- **condition**—such as eczema (a skin inflammation characterized by lesions, crusting, and fluid discharge) or fracture
- **anatomic site**—such as skin, subcutaneous tissue, muscle, fascia, bone, external genitalia, perineum, or abdominal wall
- **total amount of debrided tissue**—for example, 10% of body surface area, each additional 10% of body surface, first 20 square cm or less, or each additional 20 square cm

Refer to code 11008—*Removal of prosthetic material or mesh, abdominal wall for infection* to better understand its meaning. Code 11008 is an add-on code, which you should only report *in addition to* another procedure. This code descriptor means that the physician removed prosthetic material or mesh, which a surgeon first applied during a patient's abdominal wall surgery. Physicians use prosthetic material and mesh to reinforce a weak area and hold it in place; for example, a physician applies mesh after a hernia repair. Assign code 11008 when the material or mesh causes infection, and the physician removes it.

Did you notice the coding instructions listed before the Debridement category? The instructions state that you should report the depth of debridement for a *single* wound according to the *deepest level* of tissue removed. When you are coding debridement for *multiple* wounds, add the surface area of wounds that are the same depth. (***Note:*** Do not combine areas if multiple wounds were debrided at different depths.) Refer to the following example to learn more about coding debridement for multiple wounds.

Example: Dr. Daniels, an emergency physician at Williton Medical Center, sees Mr. Miller, a 58-year-old. Mr. Miller has two deep ulcers, a heel ulcer (4 sq cm) and a hip ulcer (10 sq cm). Dr. Daniels performs bone debridement for both ulcers.

The CPT coding instructions allow you to *add the ulcer sizes together*, since both involved bone debridement of the same depth, for a total of 14 sq cm. Search the index for the main term *debridement* and subterm *bone*, which directs you to codes 11044 and 11047 (■ Figure 22-4).

The total area Dr. Daniels debrides is 14 sq cm, so assign code **11044** because it represents the "first 20 sq cm or less." The patient's diagnosis codes are **707.07** (main term *ulcer* and subterm *heel*) and **707.8** (main term *ulcer* and subterm *hip*).

11044	Debridement, bone (includes epidermis, dermis, subcutaneous tissue, muscle and/or fascia, if performed); first 20 sq cm or less
11047	each additional 20 sq cm, or part thereof (List separately in addition to code for primary procedure)

Figure 22-4 ■ Codes 11044 and 11047.

INTERESTING FACT: Maggots Help Heal Wounds

Physicians can also debride wounds using a method that has been around for centuries: fly maggots. Sterile fly larvae (maggots) debride wounds that are unresponsive to conventional debridement techniques. Maggots secrete an enzyme that breaks down necrotic tissue, which they then ingest. Clinicians apply maggots to the patient's wound and cover it with a dressing. Within a few days, the maggots have eaten enough and are full, and they are removed and replaced with a new colony. Maggot therapy treats various wounds including pressure ulcers, chronic ulcers, and burns.

LESIONS

The next six categories all involve procedures to remove or biopsy lesions:

- Paring or Cutting
- Biopsy
- Removal of Skin Tags
- Shaving of Epidermal or Dermal Lesions
- Excising Benign Lesions
- Excising Malignant Lesions

nevi (nevus) (ne′vi, nē′-vəs)

corn—thick, hard epidermis typically found on the toe joints or between the toes, which friction causes

callus (′kal-əs)—thick, hard skin typically found on the soles of the feet, palms of the hands, and the knees, which friction causes

Lesions are abnormal growths or masses and are also called tumors, **nevi** (singular is **nevus**), moles, scars, sores, or ulcers. Lesions form when tissue is damaged from age, cancer, burns, disease, infection, or injury. Physicians remove malignant lesions to stop an invading cancer from spreading. They may also remove benign lesions such as warts, moles, or skin tags (small flaps of skin) to improve the patient's appearance or to eliminate pain or pressure (as with a **corn** or **callus**).

Primary skin lesions (■ FIGURE 22-5) appear at the start of disease or infection (acne, warts), may be congenital (birthmark), or may be the result of reactions to environmental factors (chemicals) or radiation (exposure to the sun). *Secondary skin lesions*

Macule, Patch

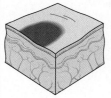

Flat, nonpalpable change in skin color. Macules are smaller than 1 cm, with a circumscribed border, and patches are larger than 1 cm and may have an irregular border.

Examples Macules: freckles, measles, and petechiae. Patches: Mongolian spots, port-wine stains, vitiligo, and chloasma.

Papule, Plaque

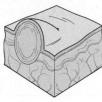

Elevated, solid, palpable mass with circumscribed border. Papules are smaller than 0.5 cm; plaques are groups of papules that form lesions larger than 0.5 cm.

Examples Papules: elevated moles, warts, and lichen planus. Plaques: psoriasis, actinic keratosis, and also lichen planus.

Nodule, Tumor

Elevated, solid, hard or soft palpable mass extending deeper into the dermis than a papule. Nodules have circumscribed borders and are 0.5 to 2 cm; tumors may have irregular borders and are larger than 2 cm.

Examples Nodules: small lipoma, squamous cell carcinoma, fibroma, and intradermal nevi. Tumors: large lipoma, carcinoma, and hemangioma.

Vesicle, Bulla

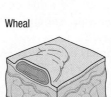

Elevated, fluid-filled, round or oval shaped, palpable mass with thin, translucent walls and circumscribed borders. Vesicles are smaller than 0.5 cm; bullae are larger than 0.5 cm.

Examples Vesicles: herpes simplex/zoster, early chickenpox, poison ivy, and small burn blisters. Bullae: contact dermatitis, friction blisters, and large burn blisters.

Wheal

Elevated, often reddish area with irregular border caused by diffuse fluid in tissues rather than free fluid in a cavity, as in vesicles. Size varies.

Examples Insect bites and hives (extensive wheals).

Pustule

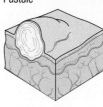

Elevated, pus-filled vesicle or bulla with circumscribed border. Size varies.

Examples Acne, impetigo, and carbuncles (large boils).

Cyst

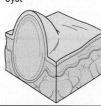

Elevated, encapsulated, fluid-filled or semisolid mass originating in the subcutaneous tissue or dermis, usually 1 cm or larger.

Examples Varieties include sebaceous cysts and epidermoid cysts.

Figure 22-5 ■ Primary skin lesions.

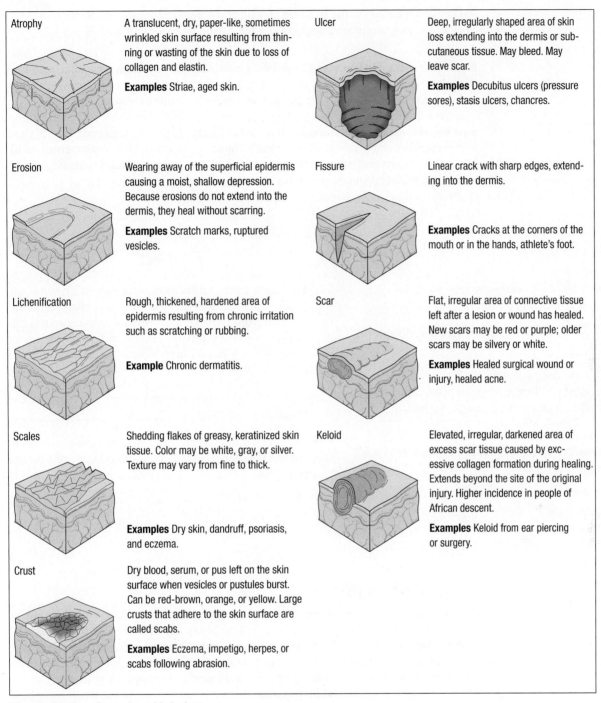

Atrophy

A translucent, dry, paper-like, sometimes wrinkled skin surface resulting from thinning or wasting of the skin due to loss of collagen and elastin.

Examples Striae, aged skin.

Erosion

Wearing away of the superficial epidermis causing a moist, shallow depression. Because erosions do not extend into the dermis, they heal without scarring.

Examples Scratch marks, ruptured vesicles.

Lichenification

Rough, thickened, hardened area of epidermis resulting from chronic irritation such as scratching or rubbing.

Example Chronic dermatitis.

Scales

Shedding flakes of greasy, keratinized skin tissue. Color may be white, gray, or silver. Texture may vary from fine to thick.

Examples Dry skin, dandruff, psoriasis, and eczema.

Crust

Dry blood, serum, or pus left on the skin surface when vesicles or pustules burst. Can be red-brown, orange, or yellow. Large crusts that adhere to the skin surface are called scabs.

Examples Eczema, impetigo, herpes, or scabs following abrasion.

Ulcer

Deep, irregularly shaped area of skin loss extending into the dermis or subcutaneous tissue. May bleed. May leave scar.

Examples Decubitus ulcers (pressure sores), stasis ulcers, chancres.

Fissure

Linear crack with sharp edges, extending into the dermis.

Examples Cracks at the corners of the mouth or in the hands, athlete's foot.

Scar

Flat, irregular area of connective tissue left after a lesion or wound has healed. New scars may be red or purple; older scars may be silvery or white.

Examples Healed surgical wound or injury, healed acne.

Keloid

Elevated, irregular, darkened area of excess scar tissue caused by excessive collagen formation during healing. Extends beyond the site of the original injury. Higher incidence in people of African descent.

Examples Keloid from ear piercing or surgery.

Figure 22-6 ■ Secondary skin lesions.

(■ FIGURE 22-6) form from primary skin lesions, appear as a disease progresses, or happen when a patient causes them by scratching, scraping, pulling, or picking.

Paring or Cutting (11055–11057)

Paring involves cutting a thin slice or surface from the lesion using a blade or **curet** (also **curette**), a sharp-edged spoon-shaped instrument, to remove a lesion, such as a corn or callus. Cutting involves cutting out the entire lesion or part of it. Lesion removal eliminates the pressure, pain, or friction that the lesion causes. Review the three codes under this category, which include the medical term hyperkeratotic. **Hyperkeratotic** means excessive growth of the horny layer of the skin, the outer layer of the epidermis.

curet, curette (ku-ret′)

hyperkeratotic (hi-per-ker-ə-tot′-ik)

Assign codes based on the number of lesions the physician removes. Refer to the following example to learn more about coding for paring or cutting of lesions.

> **Example:** Mrs. Knapp sees Dr. Avery, a podiatrist (a physician specializing in foot disorders) because of a callus on her great toe that is causing painful pressure while walking. Dr. Avery assesses the patient and pares the callus to reduce its size.
>
> Search the index for the main term *paring*, subterm *skin lesion*, and subterm *benign hyperkeratotic*, which directs you to codes 11055–11057. Assign code **11055**, since it represents a *single lesion*. The patient's diagnosis code is **700** (main term *callus*). Note: You cannot find paring and cutting procedures under the main term *cutting*; you must search under *paring*.

TAKE A BREAK

Wow! That was a lot of information to remember! Let's take a break and practice coding skin procedures.

Exercise 22.1 **Incision and Drainage, Debridement, Paring, or Cutting**

Instructions: Review the patient's case and assign codes for the procedure(s) appending a modifier when appropriate. Optional: For additional practice, assign the patient's diagnosis code(s) (ICD-9-CM).

1. Dr. Hoffman performs a puncture aspiration of a soft tissue hematoma on Janet Truax's left leg.

   Diagnosis code(s): _____

   Procedure code(s): _____

2. Dr. Stark, a general surgeon, sees Robert Thomas, age 46, for chronic infection and necrosis of the abdominal wall from internal dehiscence (opening apart) following a hernia repair. He debrides 30 sq cm of subcutaneous tissue, muscle, and fascia and removes the mesh prosthesis.

   Diagnosis code(s): _____

   Procedure code(s): _____

3. Dr. Avery, a podiatrist, sees Lucinda Rosha, age 62, to cut out two corns on her left foot and one corn on her right foot.

   Diagnosis code(s): _____

   Procedure code(s): _____

Biopsy (11100–11101)

A biopsy is when the physician removes tissue and cells from a lesion of the skin or mucous membranes to send to a pathologist. The physician may remove one or several lesions from the same patient during the same encounter. The pathologist views the tissue sample microscopically to determine the cell structure of the tissue (histology) and presence of disease (pathology), including whether the sample is malignant or benign.

Do not assign a code for the biopsy until the pathologist reviews the tissue sample so that you can appropriately code the patient's diagnosis. Physicians remove entire lesions or parts of them to test for the following skin cancers:

- basal cell carcinoma
- melanoma
- squamous cell carcinoma

If the pathologist finds that part of a lesion is cancerous, then the physician will remove the entire lesion and may test the patient for further evidence of metastasis to other body sites, such as the lymph nodes. With some lesions, like skin tags, physicians remove them but do not send them to the pathologist to review because they are inherently benign, and no disease is present.

Before a biopsy, physicians anesthetize the area of the lesion removal or may provide other types of anesthesia (local or general) to the patient, depending on how extensive the procedure is. They may perform biopsies in their offices or in the hospital. Physicians use different methods to remove lesions based on the size and type of lesion:

- *Curette biopsy*—using a curette to scrape away the lesion's surface
- *Excisional biopsy*—cutting out the *entire* lesion and surrounding area, called margins; Physicians excise margins (healthy tissue) to send to the pathologist so that he can compare the tissue structure of the lesion to the tissue structure of the healthy tissue.
- **Fine needle aspiration**—inserting a fine, or thin, hollow needle under the skin to take a sample of cells
- *Incisional biopsy*—cutting out a *part* of the lesion because it is too large to remove all of it
- *Punch biopsy*—using a punch instrument (rounded knife) to remove a core from the subcutaneous layer of the lesion's center (■ Figure 22-7). This procedure is the same as an incisional biopsy, but the shape of the tissue sample is round. This method is used when the physician suspects melanoma and squamous cell carcinoma. *Note:* Removal of an entire lesion using a punch may not involve a biopsy, so be sure to read the medical documentation carefully.
- *Shave biopsy*—shaving off the top of the lesion with a small scalpel. This procedure is used when the physician suspects basal cell carcinoma, and is also called scoop or scallop biopsy.

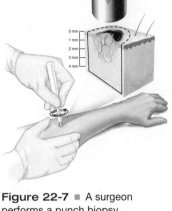

Figure 22-7 ■ A surgeon performs a punch biopsy.

After removing part or all of the lesion, the physician achieves hemostasis of the wound using various methods. Depending on the lesion size and depth, the physician may need to suture the wound closed. There are three types of wound closures: *simple, intermediate, and complex*. A simple closure involves closing the epidermis or dermis, or superficial layer of the skin. When the physician uses simple closure to repair the wound, you should *not* assign a separate code for the lesion excision. Simple closure is included in the lesion excision code. However, if wound closure is more involved, such as with intermediate or complex closure, then assign a separate code for wound closure. You will learn more about wound repairs and closures later in this chapter.

Review the two codes available for skin biopsies. Note that code 11101 is an add-on code for each additional lesion after the first lesion removed. It is not necessary to append modifier -51 to code 11101 because the code descriptor already defines *additional* lesions.

Did you notice that there are also coding instructions for this category? The instructions state that if a physician excises an *entire lesion* for a biopsy, then you should only code the *lesion excision* because the biopsy is *bundled* into the lesion excision code. You will learn more about lesion excisions later in this chapter. Refer to the following example to learn more about coding biopsies of lesions.

> **Example:** Mr. Frederick, a 54-year-old, sees Dr. Dillard, a dermatologist, in the office for removal of four lesions from his back to be sent for biopsy. Dr. Dillard performs shave biopsies for each lesion and sends samples to the pathologist at Williton Medical Center. The pathology report is positive for basal cell carcinoma.
>
> To code this case, search the index for the main term *biopsy* and subterm *skin lesion*, which directs you to codes 11100–11101. Assign code **11100** for the first lesion, and assign **11101 × 3** for the next three lesions (you can also report the codes as 11101, 11101, 11101). *Note:* If you perform the billing, you would also report the number of lesions in block 24-G of the CM-1500 form. (Refer to Figure 1-1.) The patient's diagnosis code is **173.5** (main term *neoplasm*, subterm *skin*, and subterm *back, malignant primary*).

Removing Skin Tags (11200–11201)

An **acrochordon**, or skin tag, is a small, benign flap of skin which may have a **peduncle** (stalk) (■ Figure 22-8). Many times, skin tags appear and increase in number as a person ages. They are most often found on the neck, upper chest, eyelids, axillae, and groin.

acrochordon (ak-rə-kȯr′-dän)

peduncle (pə-dung′kəl)

Figure 22-8 ■ Skin tag on the perianal skin of a 42-year-old male patient.

Photo credit: Dr. P. Marazzi/Photo Researchers, Inc.

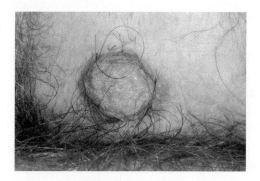

Physicians remove skin tags that bleed, itch, cause pain, are inflamed, or cause friction or rubbing (for example, a skin tag on the neck may rub against the shirt collar). The physician may also remove skin tags for cosmetic reasons to improve a patient's appearance, but insurances typically deny reimbursement for cosmetic procedures.

Methods of removing skin tags include the following:

- *Cryotherapy*—freeze skin tags with liquid nitrogen
- *Chemical destruction*—destroy skin tags using chemical agents
- *Electrosurgical destruction*—destroy skin tags with a spark of electrical current
- *Excision*—excise skin tags using scissors or another sharp instrument
- *Ligature strangulation, or ligation*—tie off the skin tag at its base with thread, eliminating blood flow to the skin tag; it eventually dies and falls off.

fibrocutaneous (fi-bro kyù-tā′-nē-əs)

Review the two codes available for removing skin tags. The word **fibrocutaneous** in the code descriptor means a fibrous skin tumor or growth. Notice that you should assign code 11200 for *up to 15 lesions* and add-on code 11201 for *each additional 10 lesions*. Did you see the coding instructions for this category? The instructions state that the codes include **electrocauterization** of the wound and also include local anesthesia.

electrocauterization (e-lek-tro-kaw-tər-ĭ-za′ shən)—destroying tissue with a hot instrument

Additional points to note are that just as with skin biopsies of lesions, skin tag removal includes simple closure of the wound. If the physician performs a more involved wound repair, such as intermediate or complex, then assign a separate code for the closure.

Refer to the following example to learn more about coding removal of skin tags.

Example: Mrs. David, a 65-year-old, sees Dr. Dillard, a dermatologist, in the office for removal of seven skin tags from her neck. The patient tells Dr. Dillard that she wants the skin tags removed because they are ugly.

Search the index for the main term *removal* and subterm *skin tags*, which directs you to codes 11200–11201. Assign code **11200** because the code represents up to 15 lesions. The patient's diagnosis code is **701.9** (main term *tag* and subterm *skin*).

Shaving of Epidermal or Dermal Lesions (11300–11313)

Shaving is when the physician uses a sharp instrument to remove an epidermal or dermal lesion, without a full-thickness excision (excision of the epidermis, dermis, and subcutaneous tissue). Codes in this category include local anesthesia and chemical or electrocauterization of the wound. Keep in mind that if the physician uses electrocautery to remove the entire lesion, then do not assign a code for shaving. Instead, assign a code for destruction of a lesion (codes 17000–17250). Shaving does not require suture closure of the wound.

Review the codes for this category. Notice that CPT arranges the codes by the anatomic site of the lesion and the lesion's diameter.

Calculating Total Lesion Size   Recall that when the physician excises a lesion, he also removes healthy tissue surrounding the lesion, called *margins*. In order to calculate the entire size of an excised lesion, you need to add the lesion size (the physician reports this in centimeter-cm) to its margins, and there are always two margins (■ FIGURE 22-9). Calculate the margin size using the most narrow part that the physician excises.

Example: excision, malignant lesion of the back, 1.0 cm, Code 11606

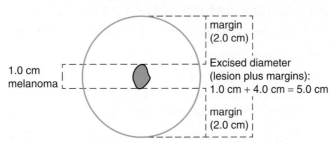

Figure 22-9 ■ Excision of a 5.0-cm lesion.

Source: From *CPT® manual,* March 2011. Reprinted by permission of American Medical Association.

For example, a physician documents that he excises a 3.0 cm lesion with 1.0 cm margins. The total lesion size is 5.0 cm (3.0 + 1.0 + 1.0). For other lesions, the physician may also document:

- *Total lesion excision was 7.0 cm.* This means that the physician already added the margins to the lesion, and you do not have to add them.

- *A lesion excised was 4.0 cm with 1.0-cm margins.* The margin size was 1.0 cm for each margin. Add 4.0 (lesion) + 1.0 (first margin) + 1.0 (second margin) = 6.0 cm.

You should code the size of the lesion with margins *before* the physician sends the lesion and margins to pathology because the size of it will shrink. Append modifier -51 (multiple procedures) to each lesion after the first lesion excised for the same patient during the same session. Recall from Chapter 18 that when you are reporting multiple procedures, you should report the most complex (highest charge) procedure first because the insurance reduces payment on subsequent procedures. An exception to appending modifier -51 is if the lesion code includes more than one lesion. Simple closure is included in lesion removals.

Refer to the following example to learn more about coding for shaving of a lesion.

Example: Mrs. Coaler, a 43-year-old, sees Dr. Dillard in the office for shaving a 1.7-cm benign lesion with margins from her back.

Search the index for the main term *shaving* and subterm *skin lesion*, which directs you to codes 11300–11313. Assign code **11302** because the code represents lesion removal from the trunk and a size of 1.7 cm. The patient's diagnosis code is **216.5** (main term *neoplasm*, subterm *skin*, and subterm *trunk, benign*).

TAKE A BREAK

Good work! Let's take a break and practice coding more skin procedures.

Exercise 22.2 **Biopsy, Removal of Skin Tags, Shaving of Epidermal or Dermal Lesions**

Instructions: Review the patient's case and assign codes for the procedure(s) appending a modifier when appropriate. Optional: For additional practice, assign the patient's diagnosis code(s) (ICD-9-CM).

1. Dr. Dillard, a dermatologist, performs punch biopsies for Melvin Pepper, age 43, on two lesions on his back and one on his arm. The pathology report is positive for melanoma on all three lesions.

Diagnosis code(s): _____

Procedure code(s): _____

2. Dr. Dillard removes 20 skin tags from Betty Salsa's back and abdomen.

Diagnosis code(s): _____

Procedure code(s): _____

3. Ruby Tunica, age 31, sees Dr. Dillard for shaving of epidermal lesions. He removes a 0.5-cm lesion from her right eyelid, a 0.6-cm lesion from her left eyelid, and a 1.0-cm lesion from her left cheek.

Diagnosis code(s): _____

Procedure code(s): _____

Excision—Lesions—Benign (11400–11471) and Malignant (11600–11646)

CPT classifies the skin lesion excision codes by three criteria:

- Benign or malignant
- Total excised diameter
- Anatomic site where lesion was removed (excluding eyelids—code these lesion removals from the Surgery subsection *Eye and Ocular Adnexa*)

Turn to the codes in these categories in your CPT manual. You will see that there are coding instructions for *both* benign lesions and malignant lesions. Lesion excision codes for both benign and malignant lesions include local anesthesia, full-thickness (through the dermis) lesion removal, and simple (nonlayered) closure. Report intermediate or complex closure separately.

Remember to assign the code for the lesion excision *after* reviewing the pathology report to determine if the lesion is malignant or benign. Then determine from the physician's documentation the total size of the lesion excision, including margins. The physician measures the lesion and margins before he excises the lesion. Also, report each lesion excision separately. You cannot combine sizes of excised lesions and assign one code.

Note that the benign lesions include codes for excising skin and subcutaneous tissue for patients with hidradenitis for abscess removal, based on the location of the abscess, such as inguinal.

Refer to the following example for coding a lesion excision.

Example: Mr. Alexander sees Dr. Dillard to have a 5.0-cm lesion with 1.0-cm margins excised from his face. The pathologist's report reveals that the lesion is melanoma.

Search the index for the main term *excision*, subterm *skin*, subterm *lesion*, and subterm *malignant*, which refers you to codes 11600–11646. Assign code **11646** because it represents a lesion on the face and a total size over 4.0 cm. The patient's diagnosis code is **173.3** (main term *neoplasm*, subterm *skin*, and subterm *face*, *malignant primary*).

NAILS (11719–11765)

This subheading includes procedures for both fingernails and toenails. It is important to append HCPCS modifiers to these procedure codes to indicate the specific fingernail or toenail involved (■ TABLE 22-3).

Refer to the codes in the Nails subheading and review the diagram of the fingernail (Figure 10-27). Codes cover the following procedures:

nondystrophic (non-dis-trō′-fik)

- Trimming of **nondystrophic** (normal) nails
- Debridement of 1–5 nails

onychocryptosis (än-i-kō-krip-tō′-səs)

- Avulsion—forceful tearing of the nail plate to treat **onychocryptosis** (ingrown toenail), perform a biopsy, or treat an infection (single nail, and each additional nail—*Note:* Modifier -51 does not apply.)
- Evacuation of hematoma
- Excision of nail and nail matrix
- Biopsy of nail
- Repair of nail bed
- Reconstruction of nail bed
- Wedge (partial) excision of skin and nail fold (for ingrown toenail)

■ TABLE 22-3   **HCPCS MODIFIERS FOR FINGERS AND TOES**

Modifier	Definition
FA	Left hand, thumb
F1	Left hand, second digit
F2	Left hand, third digit
F3	Left hand, fourth digit
F4	Left hand, fifth digit
F5	Right hand, thumb
F6	Right hand, second digit
F7	Right hand, third digit
F8	Right hand, fourth digit
F9	Right hand, fifth digit
TA	Left foot, great toe
T1	Left foot, second digit
T2	Left foot, third digit
T3	Left foot, fourth digit
T4	Left foot, fifth digit
T5	Right foot, great toe
T6	Right foot, second digit
T7	Right foot, third digit
T8	Right foot, fourth digit
T9	Right foot, fifth digit

Refer to the following example to code a nail procedure.

Example: Mr. Hamilton, age 46, dropped a heavy box on his right great toenail, which developed a bruise and a hematoma. Dr. Hoffman drains the hematoma.

Search for the main term *evacuation*, subterm *hematoma*, and subterm *subungual*, which leads you to code 11740. Do you need a modifier for the right great toe? If you answered yes, then you are correct! Append modifier -T5 to the CPT code, **11740-T5**. The patient's diagnosis is **703.8** (main term *hemorrhage* and subterm *nail (subungual)*).

PILONIDAL CYST (11770–11772)

Recall from Table 22-2 that a pilonidal cyst contains hair. It is located in the **sacrococcygeal** (tailbone) area, the cleft of the buttocks. Ingrown hairs, dead skin cells, and dirt cause pilonidal cysts. They appear as pits or pimples and can become infected, forming an abscess. A *pilonidal sinus* is the opening from which the pilonidal cyst drains. Turn to the Pilonidal Cyst subheading in your CPT manual. Notice that codes include a pilonidal cyst or sinus excision, which includes simple (single layer closure), extensive (layered closure), or complicated (layered closure that may require skin flaps).

sacrococcygeal (sā-krō-käk-sij′(-ē)-əl)

Refer to the following example to code a pilonidal cyst excision.

Example: Dr. Hoffman sees Mrs. Harrison, a 35-year-old established patient, because of pain in her tailbone when she walks or sits. Dr. Hoffman diagnoses her with a pilonidal cyst, excises it, and performs a single-layer closure.

Search the index for the main term *excision*, subterm *cyst*, and subterm *pilonidal*, which lists codes 11770–11772. Assign code **11770**, which represents a simple excision. The patient's diagnosis code is **685.1** (main term *cyst*, subterm *pilonidal*).

INTRODUCTION (11900–11983)

The Introduction subheading includes codes for many different types of services that involve introducing a substance or object into the body. Review the following services and their definitions to become more familiar with them:

keloids (kē′-loids)—thick scars resulting from excessive growth of tissue

psoriasis (sə-rī′-ə-səs)—a chronic skin disease with red patches covered with white scales

hypertrophic (hī-per-trō′-fik)—related to excessive growth or enlargement

areola (ə-rē′-ə-lə)—small space within tissue; or, a round colored section of tissue

alopecia (al-ə-pē′-sh(ē-)ə)—lack of hair or loss of hair

- *Intralesional injection (11900–11901)*—The physician injects a drug, such as a corticosteroid, into a skin lesion to treat **keloids, psoriasis, hypertrophic** scars, cystic acne, and eczema. Note that code 11900 includes *up to seven lesions*, and code 11901 is for *more than seven lesions*. It is important to choose *only one code* per patient. It is *incorrect* to report *both codes* for the *same patient* during the same encounter. To assign these codes, search for the main term *injection*, subterm *intralesional*, and subterm *skin*.

- *Tattooing, also called medical tattooing (11920–11922)*—The physician injects a colored pigment into the skin to hide a discoloration which disease, a congenital deformity, injury, or trauma cause. Medical tattooing is also used to tattoo an **areola** and nipple after breast reconstruction and to tattoo eyebrows and eyelashes for patients with hair loss from cancer or **alopecia**. Notice that CPT arranges the codes by the total area of skin tattooed. Code 11922 is an *add-on code* that represents *each additional 20.0 sq cm or part thereof*. To assign these codes, search for the main term *tattoo* and subterm *skin*.

- *Subcutaneous injection of filling material (11950–11954)*—The physician injects collagen or other injectable filler, such as silicone, into the patient's skin to diminish the appearance of wrinkles. This is a cosmetic procedure, which insurances typically do not reimburse. The codes are categorized by the amount of filler material the patient receives. To assign these codes, search for the main term *collagen injection*, or search for the main term *silicone* and subterm *contouring injections*.

- *Tissue expanders—insertion, replacement, and removal (11960–11971)*—The physician inserts an inflatable tissue expander under the skin so it stretches and expands over time, and the patient's body will grow extra skin (■ FIGURE 22-10). The physician will use the new skin to replace skin on areas of the body where skin was lost from burns, trauma, or injury. To assign these codes, search for the main term *tissue* and subterm *expander*.

- *Implantable contraceptive capsules—insertion, removal, and removal with reinsertion (11975–11977)*—The physician implants a contraceptive, such as Norplant®, Jadelle®, or Implanon®, under the skin on the upper arm. The capsule remains there for several years until the physician removes it. Patients seen for contraceptive encounters typically have a diagnosis from category V25—*Encounter for contraceptive management*. Also assign a HCPCS code for the drug implanted, such as J7307—*Etonogestrel (contraceptive) implant system, including implant and supplies*.

  Be careful to choose the correct code from this category, depending on the specific circumstances of the patient's encounter, including insertion, removal, or removal with reinsertion. To assign these codes, search for the main term *implantation* or main term *removal* and subterm *contraceptive capsules*.

- *Subcutaneous hormone pellet implantation (11980)*—also called hormone replacement therapy. The physician inserts a hormone pellet about the size of a grain of rice under the skin of the lateral buttocks to replace hormones the patient loses

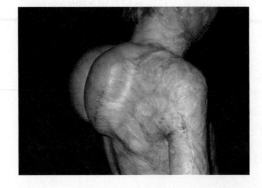

Figure 22-10 ■ Inflated tissue expanders in the back of a 12-year-old boy who had extensive scarring after third-degree burns.

Photo credit: Dr. P. Marazzi/Photo Researchers, Inc.

due to age or disease. The pellet secretes estradiol and/or testosterone. Both women and men may receive hormone replacement therapy. The patient's body absorbs the pellet, so patients need to receive implants at regular intervals to maintain the correct level of hormone(s) in their systems. To assign these codes, search for the main term *implantation* and subterm *hormone pellet*.

- ***Nonbiodegradable drug implant—insertion, removal, and removal with reinsertion (11981–11983)***—The physician implants a drug under the patient's skin to deliver drugs to treat certain disorders, such as **central precocious puberty (CPP)** in children. Assign a HCPCS code (J-code) that represents the type of drug implanted.

central precocious (pri-ˈkō-shəs) puberty (CPP)— early onset of puberty

Be sure to carefully choose the correct code from this category, since there are three choices, based on: insertion, removal, or removal with reinsertion. To assign these codes, search for the main term *implantation*, subterm *drug delivery device* or the main term *removal*, and subterm *drug delivery implant*.

Refer to the following example to code an introduction.

Example: Mrs. Taylor sees Dr. Allen, a gynecologist, for a contraceptive implant. This is the first time that the patient receives an implant.

Search the index for the main term *implantation* and subterm *contraceptive capsules*, which lists codes 11975 and 11977. Assign code **11975**, which represents insertion of the capsules. The patient's diagnosis code is **V25.5** (main term *admission*, subterm *for*, subterm *insertion (of)*, and subterm *subdermal implantable contraceptive*).

TAKE A BREAK

Way to go! You are doing great learning about many new procedures! Let's take a break and practice coding more skin procedures.

Exercise 22.3 Excision of Benign and Malignant Lesions, Nails, Pilonidal Cyst, Introduction

Instructions: Review the patient's case and assign codes for the procedure(s), appending a modifier when appropriate. Optional: For additional practice, assign the patient's diagnosis code(s) (ICD-9-CM).

1. Dr. Dillard, a dermatologist, excises two lesions from Raymond Sapp's back, one lesion from his arm, and one lesion from his hand. The pathology report is positive for melanoma (malignant) of all four lesions. The back lesions are 1.5 cm and 2.1 cm including margins. The arm lesion is 0.5 cm including margins. The hand lesion is .04 cm including margins.

   Diagnosis code(s): _____

   Procedure code(s): _____

2. Dr. Avery, a podiatrist, sees Ronald Clintone, age 22, for an ingrown toenail of the right great toe and performs a wedge excision of the skin of the nail fold.

   Diagnosis code(s): _____

   Procedure code(s): _____

3. Dr. Hoffman sees Maggie Shorner, age 40, to remove a pilonidal cyst which requires a layered closure.

   Diagnosis code(s): _____

   Procedure code(s): _____

4. Dr. Dillard sees Joseph Bernham, age 36, to inject corticosteroid into nine keloid scars.

   Diagnosis code(s): _____

   Procedure code(s): _____

5. Dr. Hoffman removes a lesion from the left arm of Betty Graves, age 73. The lesion size is 2.0 cm with 1.0 margins. He sends the lesion to Williton Medical Center's pathologist who confirms melanoma.

   Diagnosis code(s): _____

   Procedure code(s): _____

6. Dr. Dillard sees Marcy Didier, age 14, to remove three skin lesions: 1.0 cm with 0.5 cm margins from the cheek, 2.0 cm with 1.0 cm margins from the neck, and 3.0 cm with 0.5 cm margins from the forehead. The lesions are benign.

   Diagnosis code(s): _____

   Procedure code(s): _____

continued

TAKE A BREAK *continued*

7. Dr. Dillard removes a lesion from the skin of the back for Ralph Rhoades, age 63. The lesion measures 5.0 cm with 2.0 cm margins. The pathology report reveals melanoma.

   Diagnosis code(s): _____

   Procedure code(s): _____

8. Dr. Dillard sees Sarah Boch, age 30, for a lesion on her back. He excises a lesion of 3.0 cm plus 1.0-cm margins. The pathology report states that the lesion is benign.

   Diagnosis code(s): _____

   Procedure code(s): _____

9. Wanda Mase, age 44, visits Dr. Dillard for an implant of estradiol pellets under the skin following a bilateral **hysterosalpingoopherectomy** (removal of uterus, fallopian tubes, and ovaries).

   Diagnosis code(s): _____

   Procedure code(s): _____

10. Nancy Buckley, age 55, sees Dr. Dillard for breast reconstruction following a left breast mastectomy to tattoo the areola on the left breast. He tattoos a total area of 15 sq cm.

    Diagnosis code(s): _____

    Procedure code(s): _____

---

hysterosalpingoopherec-tomy (his-ter-ō-sal-pin-gō-ō-ə-fə-ʹrek-tə-mē)

REPAIR (CLOSURE) (12001–16036)

There are many different types of procedures under this subheading, including the following categories:

- Simple, intermediate, and complex wound repairs
- Adjacent tissue transfer or rearrangement
- Skin replacement surgery and skin substitutes
- Flaps (skin and/or deep tissues)
- Other flaps and grafts and other procedures
- Pressure ulcers
- Local treatment of burns

You will learn about procedures listed under each category in the following sections.

Repairs—Simple (12001–12021), Intermediate (12031–12057), Complex (13100–13160)

Turn to the codes for these categories in your CPT manual. These codes are for repairing three types of wounds, depending on how far the wound penetrates the layers of the skin: simple, intermediate, and complex. Refer to Figure 10-26 to review the skin anatomy while you study the coding guidelines in this section. When you review the codes from these categories, notice that there are many coding instructions for you to review before assigning codes. You will review information in the coding instructions but will start by defining each type of repair:

scar revision—repairing or modifying the appearance of a scar

undermining—condition when area of the wound under the skin is larger than the skin opening

retention sutures—heavy sutures placed deep within the muscles and fascia of the abdominal wall

- **Simple repair** *(12001–12021)*—repair of a superficial wound, which primarily involves the epidermis, dermis, or subcutaneous tissues with simple one-layer closure (closing one layer of skin). A simple repair includes local anesthesia and chemical or electrocauterization to close the wound.

- **Intermediate repair** *(12031–12057)*—repair of a wound that involves the epidermis, dermis, and subcutaneous tissues, with layered closure (closing more than one layer) of subcutaneous tissue and superficial (nonmuscle) fascia. Intermediate repair also includes single-layer closure of heavily contaminated wounds.

- **Complex repair** *(13100–13160)*—repair of a wound that requires more than a layered closure, such as **scar revision**, debridement, extensive **undermining**, stents, or **retention sutures**. Codes include debridement of complicated lacerations or avulsions.

12001	**Simple repair** of superficial wounds of **scalp, neck, axillae, external genitalia, trunk and/or extremities** (including hands and cfeet); 2.5 cm or less

Figure 22-11 ▪ Code 12001.

All of the codes listed under each type of repair are arranged according to three criteria:

1. type of repair (simple, intermediate, or complex)
2. anatomic site repaired
3. total length of repair (reported in centimeter-cm)

Review the codes listed under *Repair—Simple* to become familiar with the code choices. Notice that there are codes which list all of the anatomic sites applicable to that code, such as code 12001, which includes scalp, neck, axillae, external genitalia, trunk, and/or extremities (including hands and feet) (▪ FIGURE 22-11). This does not mean that the physician must repair *all* of the sites in order for you to assign the code. However, if the physician repairs one or more of the sites, you can assign the code.

An important point to remember when you are coding multiple wound repairs for the same patient during the same session is that you can *add together the length of the same type of repairs* (such as simple) and assign *one code*, as long as the code descriptor includes all of the body sites repaired.

For example, a patient's wound repairs include three simple repairs: a 1.0-cm wound on the neck, a 2.0-cm wound on the trunk, and a 3.0-cm wound on the right hand. Because all of the repairs were simple (same type), and all of the anatomic sites are listed in the same code descriptor (12001), you can add the lengths together and assign one code. The total length of all three repairs is 6.0 cm, which represents code 12002 (2.6 cm to 7.5 cm).

However, if the repairs are *different types,* such as a simple repair and a complex repair, then you cannot add the lengths. You also cannot add the lengths if the repairs are the same type but from different anatomic sites that do not share the same code descriptor.

For example, if a patient had a 1.0-cm simple repair of the trunk and a 2.0-cm intermediate repair of the right arm, you could not add the lengths of the repairs because they are not the same type. Also, if a patient had a 1.0-cm simple repair of the trunk and a 2.0-cm simple repair of the face, you could not add the lengths of the repairs because the anatomic sites do not share the same code descriptor, even though the repairs are the same type. A simple trunk repair is listed in code 12001, while a simple face repair is listed in code 12011.

It is important to understand that physicians typically document wound repairs by describing the procedures, such as "simple closure was performed" or "layered closure of the wound." Do not expect that all medical documentation will clearly state that the patient had a simple, intermediate, or complex repair. Always query the physician if you are unsure.

Additional information listed in the coding instructions for the Repair (Closure) subheading include some of the following points. Be sure to review the coding instructions carefully before you assign codes.

1. Wound closure includes sutures, staples, or **tissue adhesives**, alone or in combination with each other or **adhesive strips**.
2. If the physician only uses adhesive strips for the repair, then do not assign a code for the repair. Instead, assign an E/M code to report the service.
3. When you are coding multiple wound repairs for the same patient during the same encounter, report the most complex repair first, followed by the other repairs, and append modifier -51.

Refer to the following example to code a repair.

tissue adhesives—a liquid glue applied to a wound to hold the edges together during healing

adhesive strips—sticky-backed pieces of fabric or synthetic material

Example: Mr. Ramirez, a 38-year-old patient, arrives at Williton Medical Center's ED, where Dr. Daniels repairs four wounds that the patient suffered while cutting tree branches in his backyard: a 15.5-cm wound repair of the face with one-layer closure, a 25.5-cm layered closure of the subcutaneous tissue of the left forearm, and a 10-cm one-layer closure of the right external ear. Do not assign an E code to this case.

Search the index for the main term *repair* subterm *skin*, and subterm *wound*, which lists codes for the three types of repairs. Turn to the code ranges and review the coding instructions to determine each type of repair based on the physician's documentation. Assign the following procedure codes:

12036 (intermediate repair of the arm) and

12017-51 (simple repair of the face and ear)

Assign the following diagnosis codes:

873.40 (main term *wound, open* and subterm *face*)

881.0 (main term *wound, open*, subterm *arm*, and subterm *forearm*)

872.00 (main term *wound, open*, subterm *ear*, and subterm *external*)

Adjacent Tissue Transfer or Rearrangement (14000–14350)

Codes in this category include an excision and/or repair by adjacent tissue transfer or rearrangement. An adjacent tissue transfer (rearrangement) is when a physician transfers or transplants a section of skin or skin and tissue (flap) from one part of the patient's body to a site that is adjacent to it (beside it) (■ FIGURE 22-12).

Tissue transfers help to repair scars and wounds, which could result after lesion removal. In an adjacent tissue transfer, part of the skin transferred remains connected to its original site to maintain the blood supply when it is attached to the new site. Adjacent tissue transfers *include* lesion excisions, so you should not report them separately.

Review the codes in this category. Notice that CPT arranges them by *anatomic* site and the *size of the defect*. The size of the defect (measured in square centimeters) is the length of the tissue transfer for the **recipient site**, the site that needs to be repaired. The **donor site** is the site where the physician removes skin and tissue to repair the defect at the recipient site.

Adjacent tissue transfers include simple repair, so do not report it separately. However, if the physician performs intermediate or complex repair, you can report the repair separately from the tissue transfer.

If the physician has to place skin grafts (skin and tissue) on both the primary defect (recipient site) and secondary defect (donor site), then you must add the lengths of both repairs and assign one code. Refer to coding instructions for this category for more information before you assign codes.

Adjacent tissue transfer or rearrangement includes the following types:

- **Z-plasty**—a tissue transfer involving placement of triangle-shaped skin flaps to repair a defect that a scar causes and to eliminate increased tension from the scar. The physician incises the scar in the shape of the letter Z.

- **W-plasty**—a tissue transfer where the physician incises wound edges (such as a scar) in the shape of the letter W, creating triangular skin flaps.

- **V–Y plasty**—a tissue transfer where the physician incises wound edges in the shape of the letter V, and after suturing the transfer into place, it takes the shape of the letter Y.

WORKPLACE IQ

You are working as a medical coder for Brandyburg Urgent Care Center. A new coder, Jane Lynn, brings you a patient's chart and asks for your help coding the procedures that Dr. Stevens performed. She says that she coded the procedures but would like you to code them, also, so that she can verify her answers. Jane Lynn said she especially wants you to check her conversions from inches to centimeters (1 inch = 2.54 cm). Dr. Stevens performed the following procedures and documented measurements in inches: Layered closure of the left leg, 1.7 in.; one-layer closure of the neck, 1.2 in.; debridement and undermining of the left leg, 2.2 in.; one-layer closure of the left arm, .75 in.; and layered closure of the neck, 3.4 in.

What would you do?

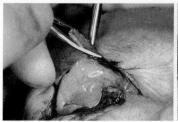 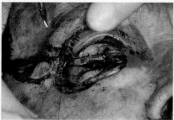 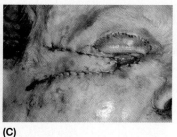

(A)   (B)   (C)

Figure 22-12 ■ (A) A skin flap is taken from a patient's upper eyelid to repair a defect from an excision of basal cell carcinoma on the lower eyelid. (B) The skin flap is transplanted to the lower eyelid. (C) The skin flap is sutured into place.

Photo credits: (A-C) Dr. P. Marazzi / Photo Researchers, Inc.

- *Rotation flap*—a flap of skin and subcutaneous tissue attached at its base; The physician rotates the flap to cover a defect.

- *Random island flap*—a flap with its own blood supply intact.

- *Advancement flap*—a flap placed perpendicular to a defect.

Refer to the following example to code a tissue transfer or rearrangement.

Example: Mr. Kelly, a 68-year-old, sees Dr. James, plastic surgeon, for a W-plasty repair of a 28.5-sq cm **cicatrix** (scar) on his neck, which was causing tightness.

Search the index for the main term *tissue*, subterm *transfer*, subterm *adjacent*, and subterm *skin*, which lists codes 14000–14350. Assign code **14041**, which represents an adjacent tissue transfer of the neck, total size 10.1 sq cm to 30.0 sq cm. The patient's diagnosis code is **709.2** (main term *scar, scarring*).

cicatrix ('sik-ə-triks)—a scar made up of fibrous tissue, resulting from a skin wound

Skin Replacement Surgery and Skin Substitutes (15002–15431)

Skin replacement and skin substitutes include skin grafts and other materials to repair defects and replace skin. This category of codes includes surgical preparation or creation of a recipient site for a graft, flap, skin replacement, or skin substitute (15002–15005), which involves cleaning the site and ensuring that the surface is appropriate for repair of the defect.

POINTERS FROM THE PROS: Interview with a Medical Receptionist

Dara Morris works as a Medical Receptionist for an urgent care center where she greets and checks in patients, verifies insurance, answers the phone, schedules outpatient testing, and dispenses medication, and "makes sure their visit can, at the very least, start off as a pleasant experience." She also assists the billing specialist with verifying procedure and diagnosis codes on encounter forms.

What are the most challenging aspects of your job?

The most challenging aspect of my job would be dealing with or handling all of the different personalities that you may come across in a day. Some days all of the patients are as nice as can be, but other days it does not matter, you just cannot seem to please them no matter what you say or do.

Describe the frequency and types of communication that you have with physicians and/or employees of other departments, organizations, or providers.

Every day there are numerous times I have to talk to doctors or coworkers, whether it is on the phone,

through our software messaging system, or face-to-face. Communication between all staff is a big key factor to making a patient's visit go as smoothly and efficiently as possible.

What advice can you give to new coders to help them to communicate effectively with physicians, since physicians can sometimes be intimidating?

Never take anything personally. Some doctors are nicer than others, and some are more down-to-earth than others. A lot of doctors do not realize the tone of voice or attitude they use when speaking to you, especially when they are busy. At the end of the day, just know that you did your job to the best of your ability.

What advice would you like to give to coding students about working with different personalities?

Empathize with the patients. Most patients are sick and/or injured and are not in the best of spirits because of this. Make them feel welcome and comfortable in the office.

(Used by permission of Dan Morris.)

■ **TABLE 22-4   PROCEDURES INVOLVING SKIN REPLACEMENT SURGERY AND SKIN SUBSTITUTES**

Procedure	Definition
acellular (ā-selʹ-yə-lər) *dermal allograft*	a skin substitute made from the basement membrane of skin from a donor or cadaver (excluding the epidermis cells), to help prevent rejection
acellular xenograft (zenʹ-ə-graft) *implant*	material obtained from a nonhuman species, such as a pig, that is placed under the skin to reconstruct a soft tissue defect
allograft (alʹ-ə-graft)	a tissue graft from another member of the same species, such as human to human
autograft	a tissue graft from another site from the same person
full-thickness skin graft (FTSG)	a skin graft consisting of the epidermis and the full depth of the dermis
permanent graft	an autograft that is intended to be a long term replacement for the original skin
pinch graft	a skin graft which is a combination of a full-thickness graft at the center and a partial thickness of the epidermis only around the edges
split-thickness skin graft (STSG)	a skin graft consisting of the epidermis and a portion of dermis, or a mucosal graft consisting of only a partial thickness of mucosa
temporary graft	a skin graft, usually an allograft or xenograft, that is intended to be temporary, usually until the patient regrows enough skin to obtain an autograft
tissue-cultured allogenic (al-ō-jə-nēʹ-ik) *skin substitute*	taking a graft from a human and then growing new cells on it before grafting it into the recipient site
tissue-cultured autograft	taking a graft from the same person and then growing new cells on it before grafting it into the recipient site
xenograft (also called heterograft)	a skin graft from a nonhuman species, such as a pig

Do not report codes 15002–15005 for surgical preparation and debridement of a wound left to heal by *secondary intention,* a wound without surgical closure that heals on its own. Instead, report wound management or debridement codes. *Primary intention* is a wound that heals after surgical closure.

A **skin graft** is when the physician takes skin from one area of the body (donor site) and transfers it to a wound (recipient site). The skin from the donor site is completely removed from its connecting blood supply before the physician transfers it to the recipient site. A **flap** is similar to a graft, but it involves transferring skin with its blood supply intact, or the physician removes the skin and blood vessels and *connects them* to the recipient site. Flaps can also involve subcutaneous tissue, muscle, fascia, and bone.

Review the codes within this category and you will find many subcategories of codes for various types of procedures (■ TABLE 22-4). You should become familiar with these procedures to better understand how to assign codes for them.

Be sure to read the coding instructions listed before any subcategories to ensure that you fully understand how and when to assign codes from the subcategory. Search for the main term *skin* to find skin replacement and skin substitutes. You will need to look for subterms that describe the specific procedure. You can also search for the name of the procedure and the subterm *skin* or search under the main term *skin graft and flap.*

Many of the codes within this category specify the size of the skin replacement and skin substitutes, which is measured in square centimeters, or percentage of body area affected. If the physician documents the size in inches, then convert inches to centimeters: 1 inch = 2.54 centimeters.

Refer to the following example to code a skin replacement surgery/skin substitute.

dystrophic epidermolysis (dis-trōʹ-fik ep-ə-dər-mälʹ-ə-səs)

Example: Thad Butler, a seven-year-old, undergoes surgery to repair a defect on his left arm from recessive **dystrophic epidermolysis** bullosa (RDEB) (an inherited disease that causes skin blisters and scars). Dr. James places an acellular dermal allograft measuring 22 sq cm on the patient's arm.

To code this case, search the index for the main term *skin graft and flap*, subterm *allograft*, and subterm *acellular dermal*, which lists codes 15330–15336. Assign code **15330**, which represents the arm, first 100 sq cm or less. The patient's diagnosis code is **757.39** (main term *epidermolysis* and subterm *bullosa*).

TAKE A BREAK

Hang in there! You are doing great! Let's take a break and practice coding more skin procedures.

Exercise 22.4 Repairs—Simple, Intermediate, and Complex, Adjacent Tissue Transfer or Rearrangement, Skin Replacement Surgery and Skin Substitutes

Instructions: Review the patient's case and assign codes for the procedure(s), appending a modifier when appropriate. Optional: For additional practice, assign the patient's diagnosis code(s) (ICD-9-CM).

1. Sherry Carr, age 16, arrives at Williton's ED after a crash that occurred when she was driving an off-road vehicle in the woods. Dr. Mills, the ED physician, repairs a 7.0-cm wound on the neck with a one-layer closure, a 2.5-cm wound on the face with a simple closure, and a 10.2-cm wound on the right forearm with complex closure with debridement.

   Diagnosis code(s): _____

   Procedure code(s): _____

2. Dr. Ferguson, a dermatologist, repairs a wound on the left hip for Brandon Dugger, age 39. He performs a rotation flap repair in which the donor site is 4.5 cm × 2.5 cm and the recipient site is 2.0 cm × 1.5 cm. (Hint: Calculate the area of both sites and add them together to obtain the total size of the defect.)

   Diagnosis code(s): _____

   Procedure code(s): _____

3. Dr. James, a plastic surgeon, performs temporary wound repair for Ralph Frith, age four. He uses an acellular dermal replacement on the right thigh, measuring 2% of the patient's body area.

   Diagnosis code(s): _____

   Procedure code(s): _____

Flaps (Skin and/or Deep Tissues) (15570–15738) and Other Flaps and Grafts (15740–15776)

When you review the codes under *Flaps (Skin and/or Deep Tissue)*, note the coding instructions, which include assigning a separate code when the physician must repair a donor site with a skin graft or local flap. Coding instructions also note that the areas listed in code descriptors pertain to the *recipient site*, not the donor site. CPT divides codes in this category by the *type of flap* and the *location of the recipient site*.

Note that under the category *Other Flaps and Grafts*, there are additional coding instructions regarding cutaneous flaps and neurovascular pedicle procedures. CPT arranges codes in this category by the *type of flap*.

Review the following definitions (■ TABLE 22-5), which will help you to better understand codes in both categories.

Refer to the following example to code a flap.

Example: Mr. Brooks, a 45-year-old, sees Dr. James, a plastic surgeon, to reconstruct part of his nose, which was previously excised due to melanoma. Dr. James removes a 7.3-cm flap from the patient's forehead, cutting into the fascia, leaving the blood supply intact. He uses **electrocoagulation** for hemostasis and rotates the flap to fit the size of the defect.

electrocoagulation (e-lek-trō-kō-ag-yə-lā′-shən)—stopping bleeding using a heated instrument

Search the index for the main term *skin graft and flap* and subterm *fasciocutaneous*, which lists codes 15731–15738. Assign code **15731**, which represents a forehead flap. The patient's diagnosis code is **173.30** (main term *neoplasm*, subterm *skin*, and subterm *nose, malignant primary*).

■ TABLE 22-5   **PROCEDURES WITHIN FLAP CATEGORIES**

Procedure	Definition
delayed flap	a flap with blood vessels intact; the physician may wait several days before detaching it and attaching it to the recipient site, to ensure that it has the proper amount of blood supply
free flap	a flap removed from the donor site with blood vessels attached, which the physician then reattaches to the recipient site
island pedicle flap	a flap that is still connected to blood vessels, arteries, and veins, through a base, or stem, called a pedicle
neurovascular pedicle flap	a flap that is still connected to nerves, arteries, and veins through a base, or stem, called a pedicle
pedicle flap	a flap that is still connected to its blood supply through a pedicle
punch graft	a procedure when physician uses a small tool to remove scarred skin (such as in acne) and then places a graft onto the area removed
tubed flap	a procedure when physician sutures the flap's sides together, forming the shape of a tube (used, among other purposes, to replace breasts removed during mastectomies)

Other Procedures (15780–15879)

Other Procedures is a category that contains a variety of procedures, including many that are cosmetic. CPT arranges the codes by procedure and anatomic site, if appropriate. It is important to become familiar with the types of procedures in this category to better understand how to assign the codes (■ TABLE 22-6).

Review the remaining codes listed in this category to become more familiar with them. Refer to the following example to code other procedures.

Example: Dr. Fitzpatrick, an ophthalmologist, performs blepharoplasty on both of Mrs. Marshall's upper eyelids. The patient has ptosis, and she feels that it makes her look much older than she really is.

Search the index for the main term *blepharoplasty*, which lists codes 15820–15823. Assign code **15822-50** (bilateral). The patient's diagnosis code is **374.30** (main term *ptosis* and subterm *eyelid*).

■ TABLE 22-6   **OTHER PROCEDURES**

Procedure	Definition	Reason for Procedure
abrasion (ə-brā′-zhən)	an area of skin where the cells have been rubbed or scraped away	remove lesions, such as warts; remove skin damaged by sun
cervicoplasty (sur-vī-kō-plas′te)	plastic surgery on the neck	cosmetic, to tighten the skin on the neck
chemical peel	using a caustic or acidic chemical to remove skin cells	remove wrinkles
dermabrasion (dər-mə-brā′-zhən)	using fine sandpaper or wire brushes to scrape away skin cells	remove acne scars, other scars, and tattoos
lipectomy (lī-pek′tə-me)	removal of a small area of fatty tissue	cosmetic; also to restore body function lost due to carrying excess fat
rhytidectomy (rit′ĭ-dek′tə-me)	plastic surgery to eliminate wrinkles from the face; also called a face lift	cosmetic, to tighten the skin on the face

Pressure Ulcers (Decubitus Ulcers) (15920–15999)

Recall from Chapter 4 that a pressure ulcer, also called a bedsore, pressure sore, or decubitus ulcer, develops due to lack of blood supply to a specific area of the body. It is most common on the buttocks of patients who are bedridden or in a wheelchair due to lack of movement. These patients cannot move much on their own, or have no one to help them move, so pressure ulcers develop. Pressure ulcers are classified into four stages according to their severity:

- Stage I—skin redness, hardness, and warmth, with itching and/or pain (Figure 4-50)
- Stage II—skin loss of the first or second layer of the skin (epidermis and dermis); appears as a blister or an abrasion (Figure 4-51)
- Stage III—skin loss of both layers of the skin, along with loss of deeper subcutaneous tissue (under the skin); appears as a crater in the skin (Figure 4-52)
- Stage IV—most destructive stage with skin loss of epidermis, dermis, subcutaneous tissue; damage to the muscles, bones, and additional body structures; could cause necrosis (death of tissue) (Figure 4-53)

Physicians treat a pressure ulcer by excising the ulcer and then suturing it closed. The procedure may also involve preparing the site of the ulcer for a flap or graft. Review the codes in this category to become familiar with their descriptors. Notice that CPT arranges the codes by the *anatomic site of the ulcer* (e.g., coccygeal, sacral—pertaining to bones at the base of the spine), *reasons for the excision*, and *additional procedures* the physician performs with the ulcer excision (e.g., flap, coccyectomy—removal of the coccyx, ostectomy—removal of all or part of a bone).

Refer to the following example to code pressure ulcers.

Example: Dr. Alston treats Mr. Cruz, an 82-year-old nursing home resident, for a Stage IV sacral pressure ulcer. He excises the ulcer, performs an ostectomy (to remove bone), and places a muscle flap on the defect.

Search the index for the main term *ostectomy*, subterm *pressure ulcer*, and subterm *sacral*, which lists codes 15933, 15935, and 15937. Assign code **15937**, which includes the preparation for the muscle flap and the ostectomy. Did you read the coding instructions listed directly below code 15937? They instruct you to assign an *additional code* for the muscle flap. Assign code **15734** for the muscle flap (main term *skin graft and flap* and subterm *muscle*). The patient's diagnosis codes are **707.03** (main term *ulcer*, subterm *pressure*, and subterm *sacrum*) and **707.24** (main term *ulcer*, subterm *pressure*, subterm *stage*, and subterm *IV (healing)*).

myocutaneous (mī-ō-kyŭ-tā′-nē-əs)

TAKE A BREAK

Good work! Let's take a break and practice coding more procedures.

Exercise 22.5 Flaps (Skin and/or Deep Tissues), Other Flaps and Grafts, Other Procedures, Pressure Ulcers (Decubitus Ulcers)

Instructions: Review the patient's case and assign codes for the procedure(s), appending a modifier when appropriate. Optional: For additional practice, assign the patient's diagnosis code(s) (ICD-9-CM).

1. Lydia Amerson, age 41, sees Dr. James, a plastic surgeon, for repair of a complicated wound of her cheek where a malignant tumor had previously been removed from her jaw. Dr. James performs a **myocutaneous** (muscles and skin) flap repair.

   Diagnosis code(s): _____

   Procedure code(s): _____

2. Dr. Lombard, a neurologist, treats Lois Melanson, age 35, for facial nerve paralysis from Bell's palsy. He

continued

TAKE A BREAK *continued*

performs a bilateral free fascia graft in order to restore facial nerve function.

Diagnosis code(s): _____

Procedure code(s): _____

3. Dr. James treats Brian Oakes, age 87, for an **ischial** pressure ulcer (hip bone), stage III. He excises the

ulcer and closes it with sutures. (Hint: Immediate surgical closure of a wound is called primary suture.)

Diagnosis code(s): _____

Procedure code(s): _____

---

ischial (is′-kə-əl)

Burns, Local Treatment (16000–16036)

Local treatment means that the physician cleans and debrides the burn, applies topical antimicrobial cream to fight infection, and applies dressings. Codes in this category describe both initial and subsequent burn treatment and specify total body surface area (TBSA) treated.

Recall from Chapter 8 that TBSA is the percentage burned out of the total area of the entire body, using the "rule of nines." The rule of nines divides the body into sections, with each section representing a percentage of TBSA, and divisible by 9. (Refer to Figure 8-21.) Also recall that burns are classified as first, second, or third degree.

Note that code 16020 represents dressings and/or debridement of partial thickness burns for a small, medium, or large burn. The physician performs the procedure as initial or subsequent because many times, patients with burns need multiple debridements and dressing changes as the burn heals. Refer to the definitions listed here to help you better understand small, medium, and large burns represented in code descriptors:

- *Small burn*—less than 5% TBSA
- *Medium burn*—5%–10% TBSA, whole face or whole extremity
- *Large burn*—more than 10% TBSA, more than one extremity

escharotomy (es-kə-rot′ə-me)

Code 16035 and add-on code 16036 are for an **escharotomy**. An eschar is dry, dead skin or a scab that develops after a burn. An escharotomy is when the physician incises the eschar to alleviate tension it creates on any tissue surrounding the burn.

Refer to the following example to code burns.

Example: Dr. James, a plastic surgeon, sees Jason Murray, a 12-year-old, for the second time to debride and apply dressing to a second-degree burn on his upper left arm, involving 4% of TBSA.

Search the index for the main term *debridement*, subterm *burns*, which lists codes 01951–01953 and 16020–16030. Assign code **16020**, which represents a small partial-thickness burn. The patient's diagnosis codes are **943.23** (main term *burn*, subterm *arm*, subterm *upper*, and subterm *second-degree*) and **948.00** (main term *burn*, subterm *extent*, and subterm *less than 10 percent*).

TAKE A BREAK

Way to go! Let's take a break and practice coding burns and procedures from additional categories.

Optional: For additional practice, assign the patient's diagnosis code(s) (ICD-9-CM).

Exercise 22.6 Burns, Local Treatment

Instructions: Review the patient's case and assign codes for the procedure(s), appending a modifier when appropriate.

1. Dr. James, a plastic surgeon, treats Jeanette Mallon, age 26, for multiple first- and second-degree burns on

TAKE A BREAK *continued*

both lower legs. He debrides the burns and applies dressings. He documents that he treated 36% of TBSA, with 16% for first-degree burns and 20% for second-degree burns.

Diagnosis code(s): _____

Procedure code(s): _____

2. Dr. James dresses and debrides a small partial thickness second-degree burn involving the right forearm (less than 5% TBSA) for Janie Pack, age 76.

Diagnosis code(s): _____

Procedure code(s): _____

3. Dr. James treats Gary Leary, age 31, for second-degree burns to his upper arms. He debrides blisters and skin and applies a skin substitute. Dr. James documents that he treated 9% of TBSA.

Diagnosis code(s): _____

Procedure code(s): _____

DESTRUCTION (17000–17999)

The Destruction subheading contains the following types of procedures:

- Destruction of benign, premalignant, or malignant lesions
- Mohs micrographic surgery
- Cryotherapy
- Chemical exfoliation
- Electrolysis

You will learn more about these procedures in the following sections.

Destruction Benign or Premalignant Lesions (17000–17250) and Malignant Lesions, Any Method (17260–17286)

Lesion destruction is not the same as lesion excision. Lesion excision involves excising part or all of a lesion, which the physician sends to a pathologist to determine if it is benign or malignant. Lesion destruction involves destroying the entire lesion, which the physician cannot send to pathology because there is nothing left. Methods of destruction include laser surgery, electrosurgery, cryosurgery, chemosurgery (using chemicals), and surgical curettement.

Review the codes in these categories, which CPT arranges by the number of lesions destroyed; if the lesion is benign, premalignant, or malignant; the anatomic site of the lesion; and its diameter.

Refer to the following example to code a lesion destruction.

Example: Dr. James uses cryosurgery to destroy two malignant lesions for Mr. Ortiz, a 63-year-old patient. The lesions are on his face, and the first lesion is 1.7 cm, and the second lesion is 0.8 cm.

Search the index for the main term *destruction*, subterm *lesion*, subterm *skin*, and subterm *malignant*, which lists codes 17260–17286 and 96567. Assign codes **17262** (1.7-cm lesion) and **17261-51** (0.8-cm lesion). The patient's diagnosis code is **173.3** (main term *neoplasm*, subterm *skin*, and subterm *face, malignant primary*).

Mohs Micrographic Surgery (17311–17315) and Other Procedures (17340–17999)

Dr. Frederic E. Mohs invented Mohs micrographic surgery, also called chemosurgery, for treating skin cancer, such as basal cell carcinoma and squamous cell carcinoma. Mohs surgery involves the surgeon removing a cancerous lesion while minimizing the amount of healthy tissue removed (margins). The surgeon performs the procedure and also acts as the pathologist.

He excises the lesion in layers, dividing the specimen into pieces. Each piece of the specimen is called a *tissue block*. The surgeon uses a microscope for histological examination of each tissue block until he no longer finds evidence of malignancy in any specimen removed. Mohs surgery is very successful at removing all malignant tissue and eliminating cancer recurrence.

CPT arranges codes for Mohs surgery according to

- anatomic site

- involvement of muscle, cartilage, bone, tendon, major nerves, or vessels

- first stage (removal of the first layer)

- additional stage (removal of subsequent layers)

- total number of tissue blocks

If the surgeon repairs a defect with a flap or graft, then code it separately. It is important to review the coding guidelines for this category before assigning the codes.

The category **Other Procedures** (17340–17999) lists four additional procedures, including

- cryotherapy

- chemical exfoliation for acne

- **electrolysis epilation**

- unlisted procedure

Refer to the following example to code Mohs micrographic surgery.

electrolysis epilation (e-lek-trol′ə-sis ep-ə-lā′-shən)—removing hair by the root using an electrical current

mastotomy (ma-′stät-ə-mē)

partial mastectomy (ma-stek′-tə-mē)—removal of only enough breast tissue to ensure that the margins of the specimen are free of malignant cells, also called lumpectomy or tylectomy

simple complete mastectomy—removal of only the breast tissue, nipple, and a small portion of the overlying skin, also called simple mastectomy and total mastectomy

subcutaneous mastectomy—excision of breast tissue but not the overlying skin, nipple, and areola, making it possible for the breast form to be reconstructed

radical mastectomy—removal of the breast, pectoral muscles, axillary lymph nodes, and associated skin and subcutaneous tissue

modified radical mastectomy—simple mastectomy plus removal of axillary lymph nodes but not the pectoral muscles

mastopexy (mas′-tō-pek-sē)

mammoplasty (mam′-ō-plast-ē)

> **Example:** Mrs. Webb sees Dr. Ferguson, a dermatologist, for Mohs micrographic surgery to remove squamous cell carcinoma from her back. He performs the surgery in two stages, using five tissue blocks for the first stage and three tissue blocks for the second stage.
>
> Search the index for the main term *Mohs micrographic surgery,* which lists codes 17311–17315. Assign code **17313** (first stage, up to five tissue blocks) and **17314** (each additional stage, up to five tissue blocks). *Note*: Code 17314 is an add-on code, so do not append modifier -51. The patient's diagnosis code is **173.5** (main term *neoplasm*, subterm *skin*, and subterm *back, malignant primary*).

BREAST (19000–19499)

The subheading Breast includes many different categories of breast procedures. Turn to the categories within this subheading to review the procedures, and refer to ■ TABLE 22-7 for a summary of categories and the procedures listed in each. Refer to Figure 10-23 to review a diagram of the mammary glands.

Refer to the following example to code a breast procedure.

> **Example:** Dr. Wooten, a gynecologist, performs a percutaneous needle core breast biopsy for Ms. Tucker. He sends the specimen from the lesion to the pathologist, and the pathology report reveals that the specimen is benign.
>
> Search the index for the main term *biopsy* and subterm *breast*, which lists codes 19100–19103. Assign code **19100**, which represents the procedure *without* imaging guidance. The patient's diagnosis code is **216.5** (main term *neoplasm*, subterm skin, and subterm *breast, benign*).

■ TABLE 22-7   **BREAST CATEGORIES AND PROCEDURES**

Category Name	Code Range	Procedures Included
Incision	19000–19030	• Puncture aspiration of cyst
		• **Mastotomy** *(surgical removal of all or part of the breast)* with exploration or drainage of an abscess
		• Injection procedure for ductogram or galactogram *(image of breast ducts)*
Excision	19100–19272	• Breast biopsy
		• Ablation of a fibroadenoma *(benign breast growth)*
		• Nipple exploration *(to investigate abnormal nipple discharge)*
		• Excisions of cysts, fibroadenoma, tumors, fistulas *(abnormal duct)*
Introduction	19290–19298	• Preoperative placement of needle localization wire or metallic localization clip *(clip placed at surgical site to easily identify it)*
		• Placement of radiotherapy catheter *(to deliver radiation after partial mastectomy)*
Mastectomy Procedures	19300–19307	• **Partial mastectomy** *(also called lumpectomy, tylectomy)*
		• **Simple complete mastectomy**
		• **Subcutaneous mastectomy**
		• **Radical mastectomy**
		• **Modified radical mastectomy**
Repair and/or Reconstruction	19316–19396	• **Mastopexy** *(lift breast or change its shape)*
		• **Mammoplasty** *(enlarge breast size, called mammoplasty augmentation, or reduce breast size, called reduction mammoplasty)*
		• Removal of implant
		• Insertion of prosthesis
		• Nipple/areola reconstruction
		• Breast reconstruction
Other Procedures Affecting the Breast	19499	• Unlisted procedure, breast

TAKE A BREAK

Give yourself a pat on the back! You are progressing well! Let's take a break and practice coding more skin procedures.

Exercise 22.7 Destruction of Benign or Premalignant Lesions and Malignant Lesions, Any Method, Mohs Micrographic Surgery, Other Procedures, Breast

Instructions: Review the patient's case and assign codes for the procedure(s), appending a modifier when appropriate. Optional: For additional practice, assign the patient's diagnosis code(s) (ICD-9-CM).

1. Dr. Ferguson, a dermatologist, uses surgical curettement to destroy 15 premalignant actinic keratoses (skin growths) for Eugene Whaley, age 39.

   Diagnosis code(s): _____

   Procedure code(s): _____

2. Kenneth Sacco, age 68, sees Dr. Ferguson for Mohs micrographic surgery to remove basal cell carcinoma from his face. Dr. Ferguson performs the surgery in three stages, using six tissue blocks for the first stage, three tissue blocks for the second stage, and two tissue blocks for the third stage.

   Diagnosis code(s): _____

   Procedure code(s): _____

3. Dr. Wooten, OB/GYN, performs open excision of two breast lesions from the outer quadrant of the lower left breast for Debbie Abeyta, age 43. Dr. Wooten identified the locations preoperatively with a radiological marker. The pathology report indicated that the lesions were benign.

   Diagnosis code(s): _____

   Procedure code(s): _____

continued

TAKE A BREAK *continued*

4. Dr. Ferguson treats John Herman, age 47, for chemo-surgical destruction of 10 benign lesions on his right upper arm.

   Diagnosis code(s):_____

   Procedure code(s):_____

5. Daniel McClain, age 53, sees Dr. Ferguson for electrosurgical destruction of malignant skin lesions: one lesion on the right eyelid 0.3 cm in diameter, two lesions on the left eyelid 0.3 cm in diameter and 0.4 cm in diameter, one lesion on the nose 1.0 cm in diameter, and one malignant lesion in the mucous membrane of the mouth (cheek) 0.5 cm in diameter.

   Diagnosis code(s):_____

   Procedure code(s):_____

6. Dr. Wooten treats Betsy Wasserman, age 35, for cryosurgical ablation of a *fibroadenoma* of the upper outer quadrant of her left breast (benign tumor made of fibrous and glandular tissue). Dr. Wooten uses ultrasound guidance to perform the procedure.

   Diagnosis code(s):_____

   Procedure code(s):_____

7. Dr. Ferguson treats Kelly Withers, age 23, for malignant lesions on the skin of her face and neck. He performs laser surgery to destroy three lesions on the neck of 0.3 cm diameter, 0.4 cm diameter, and 0.5 cm diameter and one lesion on the face of 0.6 cm diameter.

   Diagnosis code(s):_____

   Procedure code(s):_____

8. Antoinette Svoboda, age 32, sees Dr. Ferguson for Mohs micrographic surgery to remove squamous cell carcinoma from her right arm and hand. Dr. Ferguson performs the surgery on the arm in one stage, using three tissue blocks. He performs the surgery on the hand in two stages, using three tissue blocks for the first stage and two tissue blocks for the second stage.

   Diagnosis code(s):_____

   Procedure code(s):_____

9. Matthew O'Reilly, age 16, sees Dr. Ferguson for chemical **exfoliation** (peeling off layers of skin) for acne, using acne paste.

   Diagnosis code(s):_____

   Procedure code(s):_____

exfoliation (eks-fō-lē-ā′-shən)

DESTINATION: MEDICARE

This Medicare exercise will help you to find additional information about the National Correct Coding Initiative (NCCI). Recall from Chapter 15 that CMS developed the National Correct Coding Initiative (NCCI) to identify procedure codes that providers should not report together. NCCI edits are rules incorporated into a computer software program that automatically flag procedures that are incompatible. The purpose of NCCI edits is to prevent improper Medicare payments when providers report incorrect code combinations. Follow the instructions listed next to access Chapter 5 of the Medicare Contractor Beneficiary and Provider Communications Manual:

1. Go to the website http://www.cms.gov.
2. At the top of the screen on the banner bar, choose *Regulations and Guidance.*
3. Under Guidance, choose *Manuals.*
4. On the left side of the screen, under Manuals, choose *Internet-Only Manuals (IOMs).*
5. Scroll down to Publication # *100-09 Medicare Contractor Beneficiary and Provider Communications Manual,* and click *100-09.*
6. Scroll down to the list of Downloads, and choose *Chapter 5—Correct Coding Initiative,* which is listed as com109c05.

Answer the following questions, using the search function (Ctrl + F) to find information that you need:

1. Can a physician perform both an excision of a malignant lesion of the arm and destruction of the same lesion during the same session?

2. During the same encounter, can you report both a fine needle aspiration and a breast lesion excision after preoperative placement of a radiologic marker? Why or why not?

CHAPTER REVIEW

Multiple Choice

Instructions: Circle the best answer to complete each statement.

1. Physicians debride wounds to
   a. perform a biopsy of the fluid to determine if there is an infection.
   b. stop an invading cancer from spreading.
   c. remove tissue that will not regenerate and heal.
   d. inject a drug, such as a corticosteroid, into a skin lesion to treat keloids, psoriasis, hypertrophic scars, cystic acne, and eczema.

2. CPT classifies the skin lesion excision codes by all of the following criteria *except*
   a. malignant or benign.
   b. epidermis, dermis, or subcutaneous.
   c. total excised diameter.
   d. anatomic site where lesion was removed.

3. When the physician documents *Lesion excised was 3.0 cm with 1.0 cm margins*, what is the total size of the lesion you should code?
   a. 1.0
   b. 3.0
   c. 4.0
   d. 5.0

4. Methods of removing skin tags include all of the following *except*
   a. cryotherapy.
   b. chemical destruction.
   c. ligation.
   d. shaving.

5. Code debridement as a separate procedure *except* when
   a. the physician performs debridement of complicated lacerations or avulsions.
   b. there is prolonged cleansing because of gross contamination.
   c. the physician removes substantial amounts of devitalized or contaminated tissue.
   d. the physician debrides the wound without closing it immediately.

6. Which of the following structures is *not* included with procedure codes under the subsection Integumentary System?
   a. Eyes
   b. Nails
   c. Breasts
   d. Hair

7. The layers of the skin are
   a. epidermis, dermis, and hair follicles.
   b. epidermis, dermis, and subcutaneous fascia.
   c. integumentary, epidermis, and dermis.
   d. integumentary, epidermis, and hair follicles.

8. An abscess is a(n)
   a. sac of fluid.
   b. collection of pus.
   c. fluid-filled blister.
   d. collection of serum (clear fluid).

9. An elevated, often reddish area with an irregular border caused by diffuse fluid in tissues rather than free fluid in a cavity is called a
   a. vesicle.
   b. plaque.
   c. cyst.
   d. wheal.

10. CPT classifies the skin lesion excision codes by all of the following criteria *except*
    a. whether it is malignant or benign.
    b. total excised diameter.
    c. the anatomic site where lesion was removed.
    d. the length of the repair where the lesion was removed.

Coding Assignments

Instructions: Assign procedure code(s) to the following cases, appending a modifier when appropriate. Optional: For additional practice, assign the patient's diagnosis code(s) (ICD-9-CM).

1. Dr. Ferguson, a dermatologist, performs puncture aspiration of an abscess on the left thigh for Kay Wakefield, age 64.

   Diagnosis code(s): _____

   Procedure code(s): _____

2. Dr. Ferguson treats Margaret Ramer, age 46. He uses electrosurgery to destroy two skin lesions on the face, one of 0.5 cm diameter and one of 1.2 cm diameter; and one lesion on the ear of 0.8 cm diameter. He also excises one skin lesion from scalp which is 1.9 cm in diameter *plus* 1.0 cm margins. The pathology report confirms basal cell carcinoma for the scalp lesion. The other lesions were benign.

   Diagnosis code(s): _____

   Procedure code(s): _____

3. Leonard Coulter, age 83, sees Dr. Ariss, a podiatrist, to have his toenails trimmed. Mr. Coulter has type II diabetes with peripheral neuropathy and has had problems with ingrown and infected toenails in the past.

   Diagnosis code(s): _____

   Procedure code(s): _____

4. Dr. Ferguson treats Nicholas Patch, age 51, for 10 benign anal **papillae** (small nipple-like lesions). He destroys the lesions using laser surgery.

   Diagnosis code(s): _____

   Procedure code(s): _____

5. Dr. Mills, Williton's ED physician, repairs a 6-cm laceration above the eyebrow for Juan Boyette, age eight, using a one-layer closure.

   Diagnosis code(s): _____

   Procedure code(s): _____

6. Dr. Faulkner, surgical oncologist, performs a radical mastectomy for Heidi Mulvey, age 46, who has breast cancer with metastasis. He removes the pectoral muscles as well as the axillary and internal mammary lymph nodes.

   Diagnosis code(s): _____

   Procedure code(s): _____

   papillae (pə-pil′ə)

7. An ambulance transports Rhonda Britt, age 26, to Williton's ED, where Dr. Daniels examines her. Ms. Britt suffered multiple lacerations from a motor vehicle accident where she was a passenger in her friend's car. Dr. Daniels repairs the lacerations and orders further testing for other injuries. Lacerations include a one-layer closure of the face (5.5 cm), one-layer closure of the nape of the neck (4.0 cm), layered closure of the face (20.3 cm), and layered closure of the face involving superficial fascia (15.2 cm).

   Diagnosis code(s): _____

   Procedure code(s): _____

8. Dr. Jarvis, a general surgeon at Williton, excises a stage III sacral pressure ulcer for Gary Levi, age 66. The procedure includes skin flap closure and ostectomy.

   Diagnosis code(s): _____

   Procedure code(s): _____

9. Susan Michael, age 45, is an established patient who sees Dr. Hoffman for an annual check-up. During the exam, she asks Dr. Hoffman to remove several skin tags from her neck and chest. He excises 9 skin tags from the left side of her neck, 7 from the right, and 12 from her chest. Dr. Hoffman does not perform separate E/M services in addition to the patient's check-up, and he determines that Ms. Michaels is otherwise healthy.

   Diagnosis code(s): _____

   Procedure code(s): _____

10. Dr. Hoffman sees established patient Margaret Miller, age 60, for a physical. During the exam, he finds two lesions on her left shoulder, which he removes and sends to Williton's pathology department. Lesions measure 3.2 cm and 4.5 cm. The pathology report indicates that the lesions are benign. Dr. Hoffman does not perform separate E/M services in addition to the patient's physical, and he determines that the patient is healthy.

    Diagnosis code(s): _____

    Procedure code(s): _____

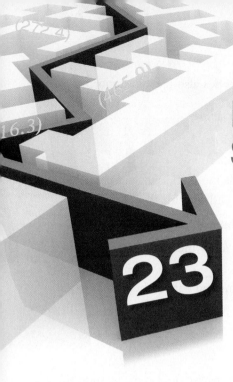

Musculoskeletal System

23

Learning Objectives

After completing this chapter, you should be able to

- Spell and define the key terminology in this chapter.
- Describe and apply the guidelines for coding procedures on the musculoskeletal system.
- Describe coding procedures in the General subheading.
- Discuss how to code procedures from additional subheadings.
- Demonstrate how to code spine procedures.
- Demonstrate how to code for the application of casts and strapping.
- Define how to code endoscopy/arthroscopy procedures.

Key Terms

arthrodesis
external fixation
musculoskeletal system
replantation
skeletal traction

skull traction
spinal instrumentation
spinal osteotomy
spinal vertebrae
wound exploration

INTRODUCTION

You have reached another amazing stop on your journey—coding procedures of the musculoskeletal system! You will learn about many different types of procedures that physicians perform, including fracture repairs, joint replacements, excision of neoplasms, and procedures to cut bones apart or fuse them together. CPT includes several coding instructions for specific musculoskeletal procedures, and it is important to review and understand them before assigning codes from the categories. This stop may be a little overwhelming at first because the musculoskeletal system contains so many parts and there are various types of procedures, but you will gain confidence as you learn and apply the new information. Let's continue to move onward and learn how to code procedures for the musculoskeletal system!

"By persisting in your path, though you forfeit the little, you gain the great."—
RALPH WALDO EMERSON

MUSCULOSKELETAL SYSTEM (20005–29999)

The Musculoskeletal System is the second subsection of the Surgery section. Recall from Chapter 10 that the **musculoskeletal system** consists of the muscles and bones. The skeletal system is made up of bones and joints that hold the body together and enclose and protect organs and structures (Figure 10-31). Bones also play an important role in creating blood cells.

The skeletal system classifies bones according to shape:

- Long bones (long and narrow, such as arms and legs)
- Short bones (cube-shaped, such as wrists and ankles)
- Flat bones (thin and either curved or flat, such as the skull, ribs, and breastbone)
- Irregular bones (odd-shaped, such as hip bones and vertebrae).

The muscular system (Figure 10-32) contains three types of muscles:

striated (strī′- āt-əd)

- Skeletal (**striated**) muscles attach to bones and allow the body to move.
- Cardiac muscles form the walls of the heart.

visceral (vis′-ə-rəl)

- Smooth (**visceral**) muscles line the body's organs and enable them to function.

Connective tissue joins structures throughout the body for structure and support:

tendons (ten′-dəns)

- **Tendons** connect muscles to bones.

ligaments (lig′-ə-mənts)

- **Ligaments** connect bones to other bones.

Remember from Chapter 10 that an orthopedic specialist, or orthopedic surgeon, diagnoses, treats, and prevents musculoskeletal system disorders. Orthopedic literally means pertaining to (-ic) straight (orth/o) foot (ped/o). Depending on the severity of the diagnosis and procedure, other types of physicians may also diagnose and treat musculoskeletal system disorders, such as physicians working in an ED, an urgent care clinic, or a family practice.

Musculoskeletal Subheadings and Categories

The Musculoskeletal subsection is divided into 16 subheadings organized by body site (e.g., head, neck) or procedure (e.g., casts, endoscopy) (■ TABLE 23-1), except for the *General* subheading. There are over 100 categories pertaining to the musculoskeletal system, so they have not been included in Table 23-1. Turn to your CPT manual to review the Musculoskeletal System subheadings and categories.

■ TABLE 23-1   **MUSCULOSKELETAL SYSTEM SUBHEADINGS**

Subsection, Subheadings	Code Range
MUSCULOSKELETAL SYSTEM	**20005–29999**
General	20005–20999
Head	21010–21499
Neck (Soft Tissues) and Thorax	21501–21899
Back and Flank	21920–21936
Spine (Vertebral Column)	22010–22899
Abdomen	22900–22999
Shoulder	23000–23929
Humerus (Upper Arm) and Elbow	23930–24999
Forearm and Wrist	25000–25999
Hand and Fingers	26010–26989
Pelvis and Hip Joint	26990–27299
Femur (Thigh Region) and Knee Joint	27301–27599
Leg (Tibia and Fibula) and Ankle Joint	27600–27899
Foot and Toes	28001–28899
Application of Casts and Strapping	29000–29799
Endoscopy/Arthroscopy	29800–29999

CPT divides musculoskeletal system codes into various subheadings that represent body sites, with some exceptions. The subheadings share many of the same types of procedures, including:

- *Incision* to drain abscesses from subcutaneous, fascial, and subfascial tissue and bones; relieve pressure on joints, fascia, or other structures; remove a foreign body
- *Excision* to remove tumors (malignant or benign), cysts, and all or part of tendons, other soft tissue, or bones; or to obtain a biopsy
- *Introduction or Removal* to inject a dye or contrast medium for arthrography studies (joint X-rays)
- *Repair, Revision, and/or Reconstruction* to shorten, lengthen, or replace tendons and bones; to reform or reshape tissue and bones damaged by disease or injury
- *Fracture and/or Dislocation* to treat fractures and joint dislocations using open or closed methods, manipulation, or internal fixation
- *Manipulation* to manipulate a joint to reposition it, performed under general anesthesia
- **Arthrodesis** to fuse or stabilize joints
- *Amputation* to remove all or part of a limb
- *Other Procedures* unlisted procedures not elsewhere described within the category.

You can locate these procedures in the index by searching for the type of procedure (incision), the anatomic site involved (femur), or the condition (wound). You learned about fractures, dislocations, and open wounds as diagnoses in Chapter 8. In this chapter, you will learn about procedures to treat these conditions. It will be very helpful to refer to Chapter 8 Tables and Figures to refresh your memory while working through this chapter:

- Table 8-2—Fracture Types and Definitions
- Table 8-3—Types of Open Wounds
- Figure 8-11—Comminuted fracture
- Figure 8-12—Greenstick fracture
- Figure 8-14—Closed ankle dislocation
- Figure 8-16—Avulsion of a forearm draped for surgery

Also refer to ■ FIGURE 23-1, which shows diagrams of many different types of fractures.

Musculoskeletal Terminology

Turn to the beginning of the Musculoskeletal subsection in your CPT manual. Notice that CPT provides many common terms and their definitions in the coding guidelines. These apply to codes in all subheadings. ■ TABLE 23-2 outlines these terms that you will find in the guidelines in bold print, along with other terms, so that you can become familiar with them. It is also a good idea to keep your medical references handy, such as a medical dictionary and anatomy or physiology reference, when you code musculoskeletal procedures because you will need to identify specific bones and parts of bones, as well as muscles, tendons, and ligaments.

Let's learn more about the details of each of the 16 subheadings (Table 23-1) and how to assign codes for specific procedures.

GENERAL (20005–20999)

The subheading General contains seven categories of common codes that do not relate to a specific anatomical site. It has the following categories:

- Incision
- Wound Exploration—Trauma (e.g., Penetrating Gunshot, Stab Wound)
- Excision
- Introduction or Removal

Figure 23-1 ■ Classification of fractures by direction of fracture.

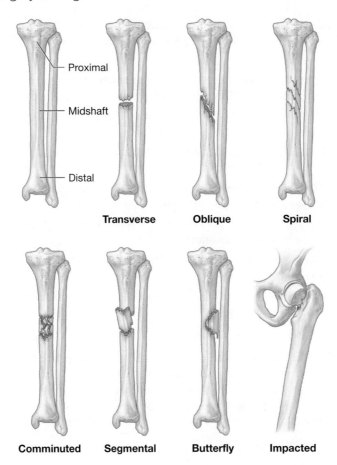

Proximal

Midshaft

Distal

Transverse   **Oblique**   **Spiral**

Comminuted   **Segmental**   **Butterfly**   **Impacted**

tendon sheaths—membrane layers surrounding a tendon

■ TABLE 23-2   **COMMON MUSCULOSKELETAL SYSTEM TERMS**

Term	Definition
digital (finger and toes) subfascial tumors	tumors involving the tendons, **tendon sheaths**, or joints of the digit
dislocation	joint injury that is not a fracture
epiphysis (i-'pif-ə-səs)	round end of a long bone (■ FIGURE 23-2)
excision	removal without removing a significant amount of surrounding normal tissue
fascial or subfascial soft tissue tumors	tumors confined to the tissue within or below the deep fascia, but not involving the bone; often intramuscular
head	the rounded top portion of a long bone
neck	the portion of a long bone just below the head
osteoplasty (os'te-o-plas-te)	surgical repair of a bone
process	an enlargement or protrusion from a bone
radical resection	the removal of a tumor with wide margins of normal tissue, including simple or intermediate repair; usually used for malignant or aggressive benign tumors
shaft	the long straight portion of a long bone
subcutaneous soft tissue tumors	tumors confined to subcutaneous tissue below the skin but above the deep fascia, usually benign
vertebroplasty (vur'tə-bro-plas-te)	surgical repair of a vertebra

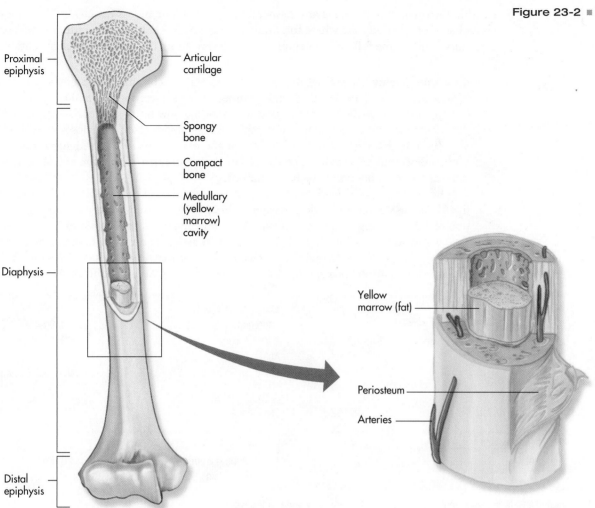

Figure 23-2 ■ Epiphysis.

- Replantation
- Grafts (or Implants)
- Other Procedures

You can locate codes for these procedures in the index by searching for the type of procedure, such as incision and drainage or replantation, and then the body site, or start your search with the body site and then search for the type of procedure.

Incision (20005)

The incision category contains one code for incision and drainage of a soft tissue abscess, subfascial (soft tissue below the deep fascia). You learned in Chapter 22 that an abscess is a collection of pus, which an infection can cause. Remember that an incision and drainage (I & D) of the skin's layers is a procedure that you can find under the Integumentary subsection. An incision under the Musculoskeletal system subsection is to drain a deeper abscess located *below* the layers of the skin. The I & D may also involve debridement, as well as a course of antibiotics to treat the underlying infection.

Wound Exploration (20100–20103)

Codes in the Wound Exploration category describe the work that surgeons perform on penetrating wounds resulting from trauma such as a gunshot or stab. You should review the CPT coding guidelines for wound explorations before assigning codes.

Wound exploration is when surgeons explore a wound and often enlarge or dissect it in order to determine the wound depth or to remove a foreign body, such as a bullet; to debride the area; and to repair any tissue, fascia, muscle, or blood vessels. CPT divides codes based on the body site where the wound occurs: neck, chest, abdomen/flank/back, or extremity. Refer to the following example to learn more about coding a wound exploration.

> **Example:** Jeremy Ladwig, age 19, arrives at Williton's ED by ambulance after sustaining a gunshot wound to his left thigh in a hunting accident involving a rifle. Dr. Stuart, an orthopedic surgeon, dissects the wound to determine how far the bullet has penetrated, debrides the wound, removes the bullet, repairs minor blood vessels, and closes the wound.
>
> To code this case, search the index for the main term *wound* and subterms *exploration*, *penetrating*, *extremity*, or search for the main term *exploration* and subterms *extremity*, *penetrating wound* (■ FIGURE 23-3).
>
> Both search paths lead you to code 20103, which you should cross-reference to the Musculoskeletal subsection. Assign code **20103** because it describes the exploration of a penetrating wound on an extremity. The diagnosis code is **890.0** (main term *wound* and subterms *leg*, *thigh*). You should also assign E codes to describe how the injury occurred: **E985.2** (main term *shooting* and subterm *rifle*), **E008.9** (main term *activity* and subterm *other sports*), **E000.8** (main term *status* and subterm *recreation*).

Wound		**Exploration**	
Closure		Abdomen	49000-49002
Debridement		Adrenal Gland	60540-60545
Dehiscence		Anal	
		Ankle	27610, 27620
Exploration			
Penetrating		**...**	
Abdomen/Flank/Back	20102	Esophagus	
Chest	20101	Endoscopy	43200
Extremity	20103	Extremity	
Neck	20100	Penetrating Wound	20103
		Finger Joint	26075-26080

Figure 23-3 ■ Index entry options for exploration of a penetrating wound.

Be very careful when assigning codes for a wound exploration to ensure that you choose the code from the correct section in CPT. In other words, if the wound exploration includes a simple, intermediate, or complex repair without any wound enlargement, assign a code from the Integumentary System subsection. If the wound exploration involves an organ, such as the stomach, then assign a code for wound exploration and repair of the stomach, not for wound exploration of the musculoskeletal system.

Do not use codes in the Wound Exploration category when a surgeon performs a thoracotomy or laparotomy in order to repair a major structure or major blood vessel related to a penetrating wound. Instead, use the appropriate code for a **thoracotomy** (an incision into the chest for procedures inside the chest, such as the heart) or for a **laparotomy** (an incision into the abdomen for procedures in the abdominal area).

thoracotomy
(thōr-ə-'kät-ə-mē)

laparotomy (lap-ə-rät'-ə-mē)

Excision (20150–20251)

Most of the codes in the excision category are for bone or muscle biopsies. As you already learned, physicians perform biopsies to obtain samples of skin, tissues, muscle, fascia, or bone to diagnose various conditions. These procedures are *not* to excise tumors. Biopsies may involve different types of anesthesia, depending on the type of biopsy. They also may require sutures to close the wound, but suturing is not always necessary. Procedures in the Excision category include

- *Excision of epiphyseal bar (20150)*—removal of part of a bone to allow it to grow.
- *Biopsy muscle—superficial or deep muscle (20200–20205)*—procedure to remove a muscle sample from a superficial muscle (below the skin's surface) or deep muscle (below the fascia).

- *Biopsy muscle—percutaneous needle (20206)*—procedure to diagnose diseases such as muscular dystrophy (weakened muscles); it involves inserting a needle into a muscle to obtain one or more tissue samples to send to pathology.
- *Biopsy bone, trocar (hollow needle) or needle—superficial or deep (20220–20225)*—procedure includes the use of a large needle and may also include a smaller one to extract bone tissue; codes are divided based on the type of bone.
- *Biopsy bone, open—superficial or deep (20240–20245)*—procedure to open bone tissue with an incision; codes are divided based on the type of bone.
- *Biopsy vertebral body, open—thoracic, lumbar or cervical (20250–20251)*—procedure to extract muscle tissue from the vertebra.

Did you notice that there are CPT guidelines following some of the codes in the Excision category? One of the guidelines directs you to assign a separate code for imaging guidance. Remember that imaging guidance is when the physician uses imaging, such as ultrasound, to watch a procedure from the inside of the body, such as the movement of a needle during a biopsy, to determine where to move it. A physician may also use other imaging, including fluoroscopy, MRI, and CT.

Introduction or Removal (20500–20697)

Refer to ■ TABLE 23-3 to review procedures and their definitions included in the Introduction or Removal category. You can locate codes in the index by searching for the name of the procedure or the anatomic site of the procedure. Turn to the codes in this category to review them while you read more about them in this section.

fistula (fis′-tyu-lə)
aponeurosis (ap-ə-n(y)-rō′-səs)
interstitial (int-ər-stish′-əl)
brachytherapy (brak′ē-thār′ă-pē)

■ TABLE 23-3 PROCEDURES IN INTRODUCTION OR REMOVAL

Procedure	Description
Injection of sinus tract (20500–20501)	You learned in Chapter 22 that a sinus tract is the opening where a cyst (or abscess) drains, which is also called a **fistula**. The physician injects an antibiotic or other substance into the fistula to treat or sterilize it to promote healing. The procedure may include imaging guidance.
Removal of foreign body (20520–20525)	Removal of a foreign body from a muscle or tendon sheath (membrane surrounding a tendon allowing it to move).
Therapeutic injection, carpal tunnel (20526)	Also called a carpal tunnel injection or a median nerve injection, the injection of a corticosteroid (medication to reduce swelling) for carpal tunnel syndrome (CTS).
Injection(s), single tendon sheath, ligament, aponeurosis (membrane of connective tissue), or tendon (20550–20551)	Injection with steroids or anesthetics to treat inflammation and pain. Report an injection code once for each injection (modifier -51 multiple procedures will not apply), and report steroids with J codes (from HCPCS).
Injection(s), single or multiple trigger points (20552–20553)	Injection with steroids or anesthetics into soft tissue to treat specific areas that cause pain (trigger points). Report an injection code once for each injection (modifier -51 multiple procedures will not apply), and report steroids with J codes (HCPCS).
Placement of needles or catheters for interstitial (inside tissue) radioelement application (20555)	Radioelement application is also called **brachytherapy** which involves placing a radioelement (radiation) into a malignant tumor using capsules, ribbons, or seeds. To apply the radiation, the physician inserts a needle and threads a catheter through it, which delivers the radioelement. Coding guidelines direct you to assign separate codes for imaging guidance for the needle and catheter placement and for radioelement application.
Arthrocentesis, aspiration, and/or injection (20600–20610)	Aspiration of a small joint or bursa (fluid-filled sac that helps movement of bones, tendons, and muscles), also called joint aspiration, or collecting synovial fluid from a joint with a needle and syringe to diagnose disorders like infections or to alleviate pain. Codes are divided by the type of joint or bursa involved in the procedure. You should separately report imaging guidance used during the procedure.
Aspiration and/or injection (20612–20615)	Aspiration of a ganglion cyst (fluid-filled cyst in tendons and joints, typically in the wrist) or bone cyst (fluid-filled cyst in the bone) to aspirate (remove) fluid or inject medication. Report procedure for multiple ganglion cysts by appending modifier -59 (separate procedure) to subsequent procedures.

Figure 23-4 ■ Skeletal traction in a patient with the leg suspended by strings to treat bones broken in a car accident.

Photo credit: B.S.I.P./Custom Medical Stock.

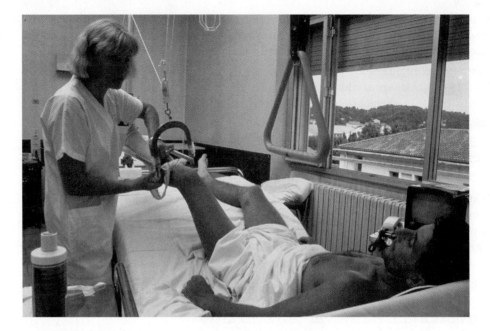

Other procedures in the Introduction or Removal category include insertion, application, removal, or adjustment of hardware that secures broken bones into place, including

- Wire or pin with application of skeletal traction
- Cranial tongs, caliper, or stereotactic frame
- Halo—cranial, pelvic, or femoral
- Implant, superficial—buried wire, pin, or rod
- External fixation systems

Skeletal traction (pulling) involves placing pins and/or wires through broken bones, which are then exposed to the outside of the body. Stirrups, ropes, pulleys, and weights are attached to the pins and wires to secure bones in place until they heal (■ FIGURE 23-4).

Skull traction involves applying cranial tongs or calipers to the head to treat cervical spine factures and dislocations. Physicians place pins in the skull that are attached to ropes and weights on the outside, which secure the spine into place. A stereotactic frame is also attached to the head with pins. Many times, it is used during stereotactic radiosurgery, or radiation therapy, to secure the head and direct radiation to a specific area.

A cranial, pelvic, or femoral halo is a type of external fixation, a device to help stabilize a fracture or dislocation to promote healing (■ FIGURE 23-5).

In **external fixation**, the surgeon drills several holes through a bone and inserts wires or pins through the holes with the ends extending outside the skin. Then the surgeon attaches the ends to clamps and rods called the frame. The frame helps to align the bone during healing, and the physician can easily adjust the frame to realign the bone at any time. The CPT manual Professional Edition includes many external fixation diagrams within the Introduction or Removal category to help you better understand the procedures. The various types of frames include

- *Uniplane frame*—one surface, extending to one side of the limb or bone
- *Multiplane frame*—More than one surface, extending to at least two sides of the limb or bone
- *Halo frame*—Surrounding the bone entirely and used on the cranium (to stabilize the cervical spine), pelvis, or femur

Codes describe applying, removing, and adjusting various types of frames. Some codes include *both* the application and removal, while others describe only the applica-

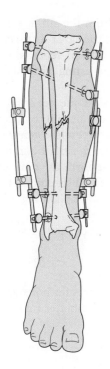

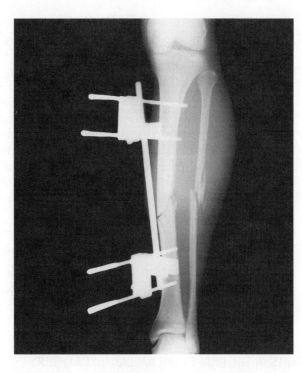

Figure 23-5 ■ External fixation device used to treat a fracture of the tibia and fibula.

Photo credit: SPL / Photo Researchers, Inc.

tion or only the removal, so read the details of the code carefully before final code assignment. Note that code 20665 represents removal of tongs or halo that *another physician* first applied.

Replantation (20802–20838)

A **replantation** is when the physician reattaches an amputated arm, forearm, hand, digit (finger or toe), thumb, or foot. Amputations occur from many different types of injuries at work (such as machinery accidents), in the home (such as accidents involving power tools and equipment), or from motor vehicle accidents. Physicians cannot reattach all amputated body parts, especially if the injury is severe enough to complete destroy tissues, muscles, and bones, like a severe crushing injury or avulsion. Replantations can also involve microsurgery, when physicians visualize nerves and vessels of smaller body parts, such as fingers.

Temperature plays a significant role in whether a physician can reattach an amputated part. The tissues in the amputated part can necrotize in several hours if they are left at room temperature, which makes reattachment unsuccessful. But if the tissue is kept at a temperature just above freezing, the amputated part can last much longer.

Take a look at the codes under the Replantation category. Did you notice that each of them includes coding guidelines? The guidelines state that if a patient has an incomplete amputation (the part has not been completely detached from the rest of the body), then you should assign a code for a *repair*, not a replantation, because a replantation attaches an entire body part, not a partial body part. These repairs may be done on bones, ligaments, tendons, nerves, or blood vessels. There are additional coding guidelines for these procedures that you should carefully review before final code assignment.

Grafts (or Implants) (20900–20938)

You learned about skin grafts in Chapter 22, including allografts (from a member of the same species, including cadavers) and autografts (from the same person, also called autologous). In this category for the musculoskeletal system, grafts include *harvesting* (obtaining) grafts of bone, cartilage, fascia lata (deep fascia in the thigh), tendon, tissue, and grafts for spine surgery. There are separate codes elsewhere in CPT for the *placement* of the graft, called the repair.

For example, a physician harvests a bone graft from the rib to place on a patient's nose. You can code for *both* the harvesting of bone from the rib and also code for the repair of the nose (graft placement), since the procedures involved separate incision sites. But sometimes the code descriptor for the repair *includes* harvesting, and then you should only report the code for the repair.

Surgeons perform grafts when an injured or diseased site needs an implant to complete the healing process. For example, bone grafts help healing by providing a surface where new bone can form. A tendon graft can help to rebuild a tendon damaged from injury. Physicians may harvest grafts and implant them during the initial encounter. Or they may repair an injury during one encounter and perform the graft and implant days or weeks later. This may be because the injured or diseased site did not heal as expected and needs a graft to heal completely. Physicians may also implant a graft to the same site more than once if the first attempt fails.

Refer to ■ TABLE 23-4 for more information about codes for harvesting grafts.

Other Procedures (20950–20999)

The Other Procedures category includes various procedures for bone grafts and implants and methods to heal fractures. Refer to ■ TABLE 23-5 for a better understanding of these procedures.

osteogenesis (äs-tē-ə-jen′-ə-səs)

costochondral (kos-to-kon′drəl)

gastrocnemius (gas-tro-ne′me-əs)—calf muscle

paratenon (par ə-ten′on)—loose connective tissue from the tendon compartment

■ TABLE 23-4 **TYPES OF GRAFTS IN THE GRAFTS (OR IMPLANTS) CATEGORY**

Type of Graft	Code(s)	Harvesting Site(s)	Purpose	Examples
Bone	20900–20902	Iliac crest (hip), femur, tibia, or any other bone	**Osteogenesis** (growth of new bone), stability	• Stimulate new bone growth in a fractured tibia (Codes are divided by grafts that are minor or small, major or large.)
Cartilage	20910–20912	Ribs (**costochondral**), nasal septum	Reconstruction	• Reconstruct areas of the face, such as the nose (Codes are divided by costochondral or nasal septum.)
Fascia lata	20920–20922	Side of mid-upper thigh or calf (**gastrocnemius**)	Soft tissue repair	• Repair skin defects, severe acne scars, and wrinkles, and treat facial paralysis (Codes are divided by use of a stripper, a cutting instrument, to remove fascia lata or use of other instruments in a complex removal of fascia lata.)
Tendon	20924	Palmaris (along the wrist), toe extensor (in the toe), plantaris (back of lower leg)	Repair another tendon	• Reconstruct the anterior cruciate ligament (in the knee)
Tissue	20926	**Paratenon**, fat, dermis	Augmentation, reconstruction	• Reconstruct a breast or augment a breast
Spine	20930–20938	Ribs, spine	Spinal fusion (join) vertebra to stop movement between them	• Repair fractures • Reduce pain • Provide stability to treat spinal disorders (Codes are divided by allografts, frozen cadaver bone, and autografts, patient's own bone. Grafts can be morselized, from several pieces, or structural, from one piece, and may be obtained through a separate incision or the same incision as the repair. Separately report the primary repair for placement of the graft, unless the repair includes harvesting.)

■ TABLE 23-5   **OTHER PROCEDURES CATEGORY**

Procedure	Definition
Monitoring of interstitial fluid pressure (includes insertion of device) to detect muscle compartment syndrome (20950)	• Patients who have fracture repairs of an extremity sometimes experience bleeding or swelling in the area of the fracture, called the compartment. This bleeding or swelling can then cause a build-up of interstitial fluid, which compresses muscles, nerves, and blood vessels. Left untreated, the condition results in necrosis of tissue. • Physicians monitor interstitial fluid pressure with a device, by inserting various types of catheters into the compartment, that sense pressure and send results to some type of monitor. When there is too much interstitial fluid, the physician performs a fasciotomy (incising fascia) to relieve it.
Bone graft with microvascular anastomosis (20955–20962)	• This procedure includes both harvesting a bone graft and implanting it, which includes attaching the bone, vessels, and nerves using microsurgery. Remember that physicians use an operating microscope for microsurgery. The use of the microscope is *included* in these codes, so do not report it separately. • CPT divides bone graft codes by the site of the bone graft (fibula, **metatarsal**), not by the site of the implant.
Free osteocutaneous flap with microvascular anastomosis (20969–20973)	• This procedure includes both harvesting a bone and soft tissue graft, with the blood supply intact (flap), and implanting it by attaching the bone, tissue, and vessels using microsurgery. The use of the microscope is *included* in these codes, so do not report it separately. • CPT divides these codes by the site of the bone and tissue graft (iliac crest, metatarsal), not by the site of the implant.
Electrical stimulation to aid bone healing (20974–20975) **Low intensity ultrasound stimulation to aid bone healing (20979)**	• When bone encounters injury, it undergoes a unique process of self-regeneration to form new bone to heal itself. But in 5%–10% of patients this process is disrupted, which leads to delayed bone healing or nonunions. • Electrical stimulation involves administering an electrical current to fractured bones to help them heal faster. This can include implanting electrodes on the bone (invasive procedure) and removing them after healing, or placing electrodes on the skin at the fracture site (noninvasive procedure). • Ultrasound involves administering sound waves to fractured bones.
Ablation, bone tumor(s) radiofrequency, percutaneous, including computed tomographic (CT) guidance (20982)	• An electrode needle is inserted into a tumor to deliver radiofrequency (electrical current) to ablate a tumor with heat. CT guidance first determines the tumor's location.
Computer-assisted surgical navigational procedure for musculoskeletal procedures; imageless (20985)	• Computer-assisted navigation (CAN) equipment involves different methods to perform procedures by allowing physicians to locate specific areas. CAN may use images (such as CT scans) or may be imageless, instead using infrared probes for navigation.
Unlisted procedure (20999)	• For any procedures not covered by codes under the General subheading.

metatarsal (met ə-tahr′səl)—bones between the phalanges of the toes and the ankle (tarsus)

INTERESTING FACT: Purring Cats May Heal Fractures

Some researchers believe that cats can heal their own fractures faster by the sound frequency of their purrs. There has been various research on reasons cats purr, and no one seems to really know why. But there has also been evidence through research that cats with fractures and other injuries heal faster than dogs with the same injuries, and the difference has been attributed to purring. (Von Muggenthaler, 2001; Whitney & Mehlhaff, 1987)

TAKE A BREAK

Wow! That was a lot of information to cover! Good job! Let's take a break and then review more about the musculoskeletal system and coding procedures from the General subheading.

Exercise 23.1   Musculoskeletal System, General

Part 1—Theory

Instructions: Fill in the blank with the best answer.

1. A _____ bone is thin, such as the skull, ribs, and breastbone.

2. To shorten, lengthen, or replace tendons and bones or reform or reshape tissue and bones damaged by disease or injury is called _____.

3. _____ involves using skeletal pins plus an attaching device for temporary or definitive treatment of an acute or chronic bone deformity.

4. The portion of a long bone just below the head is called the _____.

5. _____ is the procedure to remove a muscle sample from a superficial (below the skin's surface) muscle or deep muscle (below the fascia).

6. Treating specific areas that cause pain using steroids or anesthetics in soft tissue is called _____.

Part 2—Coding

Instructions: Review the patient's case, and assign procedure code(s), appending a modifier when appropriate. Optional: For additional practice, assign the patient's diagnosis code(s) (ICD-9-CM).

1. Dr. Stuart, an orthopedic surgeon, treats Jason Freedman, age 5, today at Williton. The patient has osteogenesis imperfecta (a genetic bone disorder in which the body produces poor quality or insufficient collagen). The surgeon applies a cranial halo with eight pins in order to stabilize the cervical spine.

   Diagnosis code(s): _____

   Procedure code(s): _____

2. Mary Sui, age 63, needs several dental implants (replacement teeth) due to loss of some of her upper teeth (a condition called partial **endentulism**) and loss of part of her maxilla (upper jaw) from sleep-related

bruxism (teeth clenching). Today at Williton, Dr. Stuart performs a bone graft of the hip to transfer to her maxilla. After several months, new bone will grow, and Ms. Sui will undergo dental implant surgery.

   Diagnosis code(s): _____

   Procedure code(s): _____

3. At Williton, Dr. Stuart implants electrodes in the femur for Susan Queeny, age 49, to heal a nonunion of the fractured femur.

   Diagnosis code(s): _____

   Procedure code(s): _____

4. An ambulance transports Richard Radonculus, age 25, to Williton after a car accident when the car he was driving collided with two other vehicles. Two fingers on his right hand (index finger and middle finger) were completely amputated during the crash. Dr. Daniels, an ED physician, examines the patient and calls Dr. Bamm, an orthopedic surgeon. Dr. Bamm determines that the patient needs to have immediate surgery to completely reattach both fingers, and he performs the surgery, including distal tip to sublimis tendon insertion. Code for Dr. Bamm's service(s).

   Diagnosis code(s): _____

   Procedure code(s): _____

5. Hans Rich, age 52, sees Dr. Stuart in his office for a lump on his wrist. Dr. Stuart diagnoses the patient with a ganglion cyst and aspirates it.

   Diagnosis code(s): _____

   Procedure code(s): _____

6. At Williton, Dr. Stuart adjusts an external fixation system, including replacing the hardware, for Arthur Deco, age 33. The patient suffered multiple tibial fractures that require external fixation to heal properly. The patient requires anesthesia to perform the procedure. Code for Dr. Stuart's services.

   Diagnosis code(s): _____

   Procedure code(s): _____

endentulism   bruxism
(ē-den′tyū-liz-əm)   (brək′-siz-əm)

POINTERS FROM THE PROS: Interview with a Chiropractor

Dr. Bryan Mock is a Doctor of Chiropractic (D.C.) and is trained in chiropractic medicine, a specialty branch of medicine focused on healing spinal and nervous system disorders using medical and holistic (physical, emotional, social, nutritional, and spiritual) methods to treat patients. Dr. Mock sold his chiropractic and physical rehabilitation practice and now teaches medical courses full time.

What interested you the most about being a chiropractor?

My role as a chiropractor and business owner was unique. I would see the patients, create the documentation, and work with my coding/billing employees to ensure the work was submitted correctly (to insurances). I would say I enjoyed patient interactions the most and working with insurance and coding issues the least.

What were the most challenging aspects of your job?

In regards to billing and coding, the most challenging aspect was catching improperly bundled codes. An example of this would be 97012 and 97110, which (insurances) bundled together incorrectly and paid for 97110 (when a patient had both services). Another aspect was watching that (insurances) reimbursed at the proper

level, (including) being paid for an exam at 99212 when we submitted 99213 with supporting documentation. I was truly surprised at the frequency of these occurrences. Obviously, a lot of my time was spent in working with my coder to ensure proper coding and payments.

What was your role in determining the correct diagnosis and procedure codes for patients' services?

I was the one documenting the diagnoses. Our office used diagnoses that were musculoskeletal or neurofunctional in nature. My coder (assigned the) usual sets of ICD-9 codes, and I would only review the special diagnoses.

Describe any challenges that your office faced regarding medical documentation correlating to correct diagnosis and procedure codes:

At times, it appeared that different insurance companies needed different types of documentation to support the same codes. We (would send) identical codes and documentation to two different insurance companies. One would automatically bundle (codes) and downcode, and the other would pay according to what we submitted.

(Used by permission of Dr. Bryan Mock.)

Additional Musculoskeletal Subheadings

Now that you learned about coding procedures in the General subheading, let's review procedures in additional subheadings for the Musculoskeletal subsection. Turn to the Musculoskeletal subsection in your CPT manual to review procedures under additional subheadings, such as Head, Neck (Soft Tissues) and Thorax, Back, and Flank. Did you notice that most of the subheadings represent body sites? As you learned earlier in this chapter, the subheadings for body sites share many of the same types of procedures, like incision, excision, and introduction. CPT arranges the procedures first by body site (under a subheading, such as head), and then by the type of procedure and then by a more specific site, such as a particular bone of the face. You can find procedures in the index by searching for the body site (head, thorax), and then the type of procedure, or search for the type of procedure (incision and drainage, introduction), and then by the body site.

Did you also notice how many procedures there are in the additional subheadings? Hundreds of them! There are too many for us to review in this chapter! So instead, we will only review some of the procedures, which you will see in ■ TABLE 23-6. When you review information in Table 23-6 for a specific subheading, you should also turn to your CPT manual to read through some of the other procedures under the subheading. In addition, you will find it very helpful to refer to Figure 10-31, which is the skeletal system, and to additional figures referenced in Table 23-6.

There are three subheadings for musculoskeletal procedures that we will discuss separately from Table 23-6 because they can be a little confusing, and it is important that you fully understand them, including Spine (Vertebral Column), Application of Casts and Strapping, and Endoscopy/Arthroscopy.

Let's review the information in Table 23-6 and the corresponding figures, and then walk through the coding examples listed after the table.

■ **TABLE 23-6 ADDITIONAL SUBHEADINGS IN THE MUSCULOSKELETAL SYSTEM SUBSECTION**

Subheadings and Code Ranges	Anatomic Sites	Examples of Procedures
Head (21010–21499) (■ Figure 23-6)	skull, soft tissue of face and scalp, jaw bones, facial bones, and **temporomandibular** joint (TMJ)	Head prosthesis (21076–21089)—The physician designs and prepares a prosthesis for patients with oral or facial deformities, including loss of bone and tissues from tumor excision, or injuries such as burns.
Neck (Soft Tissues) and Thorax (21501– 21899)	soft tissues of the neck and soft tissue and bones of the thorax, including the ribs	**Costotransversectomy** (21610)—Partial rib excision with excision of the vertebral transverse process (located at the sides of vertebra that attach to spinal muscles) to treat various disorders, including thoracic tumors.
Back and Flank (21920–21936)	soft tissues of the back and flank	Excision, tumor, soft tissue of back or flank (side of the body between the ribs and hip) (21930–21933)
Abdomen (22900–22999)	soft tissue of abdominal wall	Radical resection (removal) of tumor (e.g., malignant neoplasm), soft tissue of abdominal wall (22904–22905)—Physicians perform this procedure to remove tumors, including desmoid tumors (benign fibrous neoplasms), which are more common in women than men.
Shoulder (23000–23929)	clavicle (collar bone), scapula (shoulder blade), head and neck of the **humerus** (upper arm), **sternoclavicular** joint (between the breast bone and clavicle), **acromioclavicular (AC)** joint (at the outside end of the clavicle, between the collar bone and shoulder blade), and shoulder (**glenohumeral**) joint	**Scapulopexy** (23400)—Attaching the scapula to the rib cage using metal wires without arthrodesis. The procedure treats paralysis, Sprengel's deformity (one shoulder blade is higher than the other), and facioscapulohumeral muscular dystrophy (weakened muscles affecting the face, scapula, and upper arms).
Humerus (Upper Arm) and Elbow (23930–24999)	shaft of the humerus, the head and neck of the radius (outside of forearm), the olecranon process (the outer bump of the elbow), and the elbow joint	**Tenotomy** (24310, 24357–23459)—procedure that involves cutting a tendon, removing inflamed tissue, and/or repairing tears, for conditions such as severe cases of epicondylitis. Surgeons usually perform the repair with an open procedure or a combination of an open and arthroscopic procedure (visualizing a joint with an arthroscope, or endoscope).
		Lateral **epicondylitis** (tennis elbow) is an overuse injury from repeated hand and wrist movements that damage the tendons. Tendons surround the muscles of the forearm, wrist, and hand where they attach to the humerus at the elbow joint. Tendon damage causes pain or soreness around the outside of the elbow and makes it difficult or impossible for patients to rotate the forearm or flex the wrist. Many activities besides tennis can cause tendon injury, even something as simple as turning a screwdriver on a constant basis.
Forearm and Wrist (25000–25999)	soft tissues, tendons, muscles, bones, and joints of the forearm and wrist, shaft of the radius, the head, neck, and shaft of the ulna (inside of forearm), and carpal (wrist) bones and joints	Injection procedure for wrist arthrography (25246)—The patient receives an injection of contrast agent (substance that enhances the radiographic image) for arthrography, imaging that can show injuries to the wrist joint and ligaments.
		Separately report code 73115 for radiological supervision and interpretation (S & I) for this procedure.
Hand and Fingers (26010–26989)	soft tissue, tendon, and bones of the hand and fingers	Repair, revision, and/or reconstruction (26340–26596)—To treat various types of hand injuries involving soft tissues, tendons, ligaments, nerves, muscles, arteries, veins, and bones.
		The hand, not including the wrist, consists of 19 bones and also contains numerous other structures, which makes treatment complex. Hand injuries, which account for nearly 10% of emergency department visits, include lacerations (the most common hand injuries), contusions, fractures, and infections (the least common hand injuries).
Pelvis and Hip Joint (26990–27299)	soft tissue and bone of the pelvis and hip region, the ilium (largest pelvic bone) and adjoining bones, and head and neck of the femur (thigh bone)	**Arthroplasty** (partial or total hip replacement) (27125–27138)—Total hip replacement is one of the most important surgical advances of the last century, first performed in 1960, with over 193,000 total hip replacements performed in the U.S. each year. Patients receive hip or other joint replacements when a joint is damaged by disease, such as arthritis; an acute injury, such as a fracture; or an overuse injury, such as running or jumping.

continued

■ TABLE 23-6 *continued*

Subheadings and Code Ranges	Anatomic Sites	Examples of Procedures
		The hip joint consists of two main bones: the femoral head, which is the round ball on the top of the femur, and **acetabulum**, which is the socket it fits into. Ligaments connect the ball to the socket and provide stability to the joint. Cartilage covers the surface of the ball and socket and provides a smooth durable cover to cushion the ends of the bones. Synovial membrane covers all remaining surfaces of the hip joint and it releases a small amount of fluid to lubricates and minimize friction in the hip joint. When these parts wear out from age, overuse, or injury, the mobility of the hip decreases and pain increases. In total hip arthroplasty (■ FIGURE 23-7), the surgeon replaces both the ball (femoral head) and socket with artificial components. In **hemiarthroplasty**, the surgeon replaces only the femoral head but not the socket. The replacement parts may be made of titanium, stainless steel, ceramic, or polyethylene (plastic) or other similar material, based on the needs of each patient.
Femur (Thigh Region) and Knee Joint (27301–27599)	soft tissue and bone of the thigh, shaft of the femur, knee joint, and tibial plateau (below knee joint)	Repair, Revision, and/or Reconstruction (27380–27499)—To treat diseases, disorders, and injuries. Common injuries to the knee involve tearing the tendons and ligaments. If you are a sports fan, you have probably heard of athletes who suffer a torn anterior **cruciate** ligament (ACL) (one of four knee ligaments), which requires a reconstruction or repair. ACL injuries happen when an outside force (such as a tackle) injures the knee or the knee turns sharply during quick movements. To reconstruct the ACL, surgeons replace the ligament with a graft, usually an autograft, such as the patellar (knee) tendon or one of the hamstring (behind the knee) tendons. Surgeons repair the ACL when the patient has an **avulsion** fracture (when the ligament and a piece of the bone separate from the rest of the bone). In this case, they reattach the bone fragment on the end of the ACL to the bone. Surgeons may perform ACL reconstruction and repair with an open procedure or arthroscopically.
Leg (Tibia and Fibula) and Ankle Joint (27600–27899)	soft tissues of the lower leg and ankle, **tibia** (largest bone in lower leg), **fibula** (second largest bone in lower leg), and ankle joint	Arthrodesis (27870–27871)—Fusing joints together so that they no longer move to treat chronic pain from arthritis, infections, disease, or fractures that do not heal correctly.
Foot and Toes (28001–28899)	soft tissues and bones of the foot and toes, and nails	Repair, Revision, and/or Reconstruction (28200–28360)—A common procedure of the foot is a **hallux valgus** (bunion) repair (28289–28299). A bunion is a condition in which the big toe points toward the second toe, causing a bump on the inside edge of the big toe (■ FIGURE 23-8). Hallux refers to the big toe and valgus refers to the abnormal angle of the toe. Patients may experience pain and red, calloused skin at this site. Women have bunions more often than men, often as a result of poor fitting high-heeled shoes or being flat-footed. Wearing wide-toed shoes can help correct a bunion. The foot can experience many different types of structural problems with a bunion, so surgeons use a variety of procedures to correct bunion deformities. Refer to your CPT manual to review various bunion procedures and diagrams of how orthopedic surgeons and podiatrists (physicians who diagnose and treat foot disorders) perform them. Some hallux valgus procedures include implants to replace bone and/or wires to help stabilize the joint. Many procedure names are eponyms, which you will find in the index under *bunion repair* (e.g., Mitchell procedure, Lapidus-type procedure). You can also search the index for the main terms **ostectomy** (surgical removal of a bone or part of a bone) or **exostectomy** (surgical removal of bone bump) to locate the codes for bunion repair.

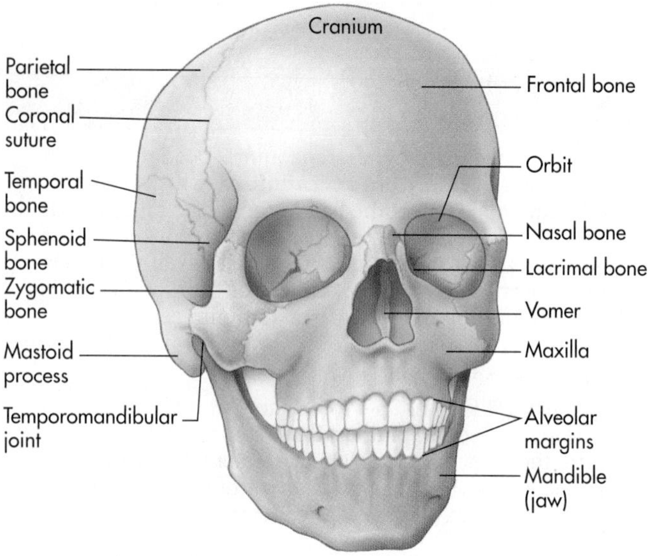
Cranium
Parietal bone
Coronal suture
Temporal bone
Sphenoid bone
Zygomatic bone
Mastoid process
Temporomandibular joint
Frontal bone
Orbit
Nasal bone
Lacrimal bone
Vomer
Maxilla
Alveolar margins
Mandible (jaw)

Figure 23-6 ■ Bones of the skull.

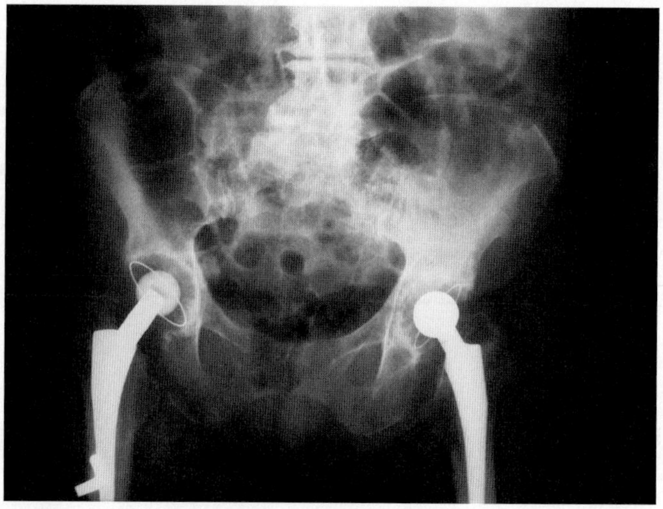

Figure 23-7 ■ Pelvic X-ray of a total hip arthroplasty.
Photo credit: monika3steps/Shutterstock.

temporomandibular (tem pə-ro-mən-dib′u-lər)—joint of the jaw, joining the head to the lower jaw bone (mandible)

costotransversectomy (kŏs′-tō-tran(t)s-vər-sek-tə-mē)

scapulopexy (skap-yə-lō-pek′-sē)

humerus (hu′mər-əs)

sternoclavicular (stur-no-klə-vik′u-lər)

acromioclavicular (ə-krō-mē-ō-klə-′vik-yə-lər)

glenohumeral (gle-no-hu′mər-əl)

tenotomy (ten - ot′ - ə-mē)

epicondylitis (ep-ĭ-kon-də-li′tis)

arthroplasty (är′-thrə-plas-tē)

acetabulum (as-ĕ-tab′yū-lŭm)

hemiarthroplasty (hem e-ahr′thro-plas te)

cruciate (krü′-shē- āt)

avulsion (ə-vul′-shən)

tibia (tib′e-ə)

fibula (fib′-u-lə)

hallux valgus (hal′əks-val′gəs)

ostectomy (os-tek′tə-me)

exostectomy (eks-os-tek′tə-me)

Refer to the following examples for coding procedures from additional subheadings in the Musculoskeletal System subsection. If you like, you can try coding these examples on your own and then read the explanation of how to assign the codes after you finish each case.

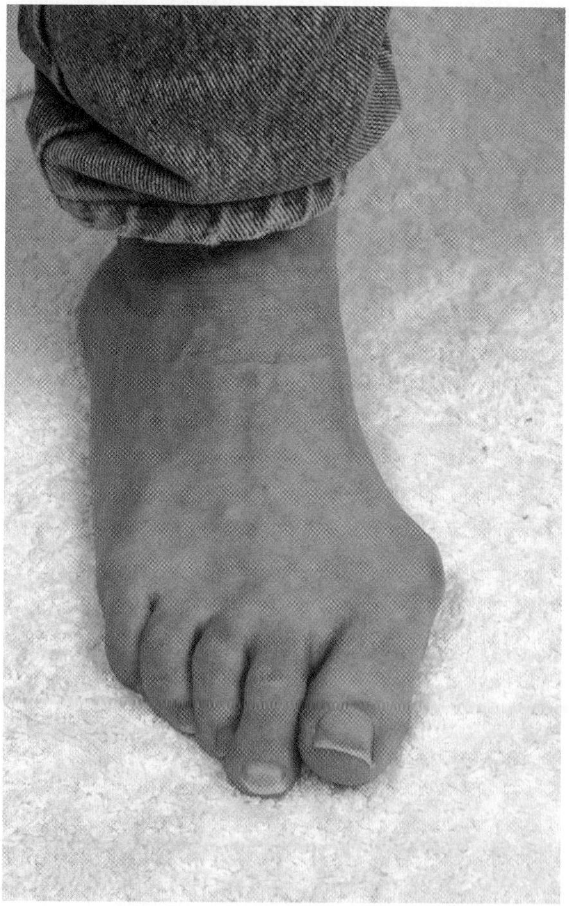

Figure 23-8 ■ A bunion of the right foot.
Photo credit: Bubbles Photolibrary/Alamy.

Example 1—Procedure of the head: Dr. Breneman, an oral surgeon, sees Kaitlin Coughlin, age 23, at Williton for a **keratinizing and calcifying odontogenic cyst (KCOC)** (a benign neoplasm with cystlike tendencies) of the mandible (lower jawbone). Dr. Breneman excises it and performs an **intraoral osteotomy** (cutting into the bone from the inside of the mouth).

To code this case, search the index for the main term *mandible*, subterm *cyst*, and subterm *excision*, which directs you to cross reference codes 21040 and 21046–21047. The excision requires an intraoral osteotomy, so assign code **21047**. The diagnosis code is **213.1** (main term *neoplasm*, subterm *mandible*, and subterm *benign*).

keratinizing and calcifying odontogenic cyst (KCOC) (ker′ a-tin-z-ing kal′-sə-fī-ng o-don′to-jen′ik)

intraoral osteotomy (os-te-ot′ə-me)

Example 2—Procedure of the thorax: Dr. Carver, an orthopedic surgeon, sees Joshua Oppegard, age 20, at Williton for a rib fracture which he suffered during football practice. Dr. Carver provides closed treatment to two ribs and prescribes pain medication.

To code this case, search the index for the main term *rib*, subterm *fracture*, and subterm *closed treatment*, which leads you to code 21800. Notice that code 21800 is for *each* rib, so assign **21800 x 2**. The diagnosis code is **807.02** (main term *fracture*, subterm *rib*). Do not assign E codes to this case.

Example 3—Procedure of the clavicle: Jorge Trujillo, age 21, sees Dr. Gould, an orthopedic surgeon, for a left shoulder dislocation that occurred when he fell on his outstretched arm while playing soccer. After several months of conservative care, the injury has not healed. Dr. Gould determines that the ligaments are severely torn and recommends surgical repair to hold the clavicle in place. Today at Williton, he reconstructs the acromioclavicular joint with open repair including a fascial graft.

To code this case, search the index for the main term *clavicle*, subterm *dislocation*, subterm *acromioclavicular joint*, and subterm *open treatment*. The index directs you to cross reference the code range 23550–23552. Assign code **23552-LT** for an open treatment with fascial graft (left side). Notice that the code description includes obtaining the graft, so you do not need to assign an additional code. The diagnosis code is **831.04** (main term *dislocation* and subterm *acromioclavicular*). There is a difference between an open *injury* and an open *surgical procedure*. Mr. Trujillo's *injury* is closed because Dr. Gould did not state that the bone pierced the skin. However, Dr. Gould performed an *open treatment* because he made a full-length incision to access the injured site.

Example 4—Procedure of the hip: Dr. Stuart, an orthopedic surgeon, performs a total right hip arthroplasty at Williton for Madeline McGinnon, age 81, who has severe osteoarthritis of the hip. He uses a metal head on a polyethylene socket.

To code this case, search the index for main term *hip* and subterm *arthroplasty*, which directs you to cross reference codes 27130–27132. Assign code **27130-RT** because it describes the full procedure on the right side, rather than a conversion or revision. The diagnosis code is **719.5** (main term *osteoarthrosis* and subterms *localized*, *primary*, *pelvic region and thigh*).

TAKE A BREAK

Wow! That was a lot to remember! Let's take a break and then review more about coding from additional musculoskeletal system subheadings.

Exercise 23.2 Additional Musculoskeletal Subheadings

Part 1—Theory

Instructions: Fill in the blank with the best answer.

1. Attaching the scapula to the rib cage using metal wires without arthrodesis is called a(n) _____.

2. _____ is an overuse injury from repeated hand and wrist movements that damage the tendons.

3. A(n) _____ is a partial rib excision with excision of the vertebral transverse process (located at the sides of vertebra that attach to spinal muscles) to treat various disorders, including thoracic tumors.

4. _____ means to treat various types of hand injuries involving soft tissues, tendons, ligaments, nerves, muscles, arteries, veins, and bones.

5. The hip joint consists of two main bones: the femoral head, which is the round ball on the top of the femur, and the _____, the socket into which it fits.

6. _____ means to fuse joints together so that they no longer move, in order to treat chronic pain from arthritis, infections, disease, or fractures that do not heal correctly.

Part 2—Coding

Instructions: Review the patient's case, and assign procedure code(s), appending a modifier when appropriate. Optional: For additional practice, assign the patient's diagnosis code(s) (ICD-9-CM).

1. Dr. Breneman, an oral surgeon, performs a bone graft of the mandible (lower jaw) for Kaitlin Coughlin, age 23, to repair an area where he previously removed a cyst.

   Diagnosis code(s): _____

   Procedure code(s): _____

2. Dr. Stuart, an orthopedic surgeon, treats Dan Shain, age 38, for a dislocated right shoulder. He performs closed treatment with manipulation (moving the dislocation back into normal position).

   Diagnosis code(s): _____

   Procedure code(s): _____

3. Dr. Gould, an orthopedic surgeon, performs a tenotomy for Jolene Heyman, age 35, due to lateral epicondylitis in the left elbow. He debrides excess soft tissue and bone and then repairs the tendon using an open approach.

   Diagnosis code(s): _____

   Procedure code(s): _____

4. Pedro Fiala, age 48, has a deep abscess on the left elbow due to *Staphylococcus aureus*. Dr. Stuart treats him in the office, making an incision and draining the **exudate** (fluid). He prescribes antibiotics to treat the infection.

   Diagnosis code(s): _____

   Procedure code(s): _____

5. Today at Williton, Dr. Carver, an orthopedic surgeon, performs a complete arthrodesis of the left wrist for Helena Aycock, age 52. The patient suffers from chronic pain that has not responded to other treatments. Dr. Carver does not perform bone grafting.

   Diagnosis code(s): _____

   Procedure code(s): _____

6. Keisha Darrington, age 23, has surgery today at Williton because she jammed her right thumb in a dresser drawer, resulting in a fracture. Dr. Stuart manipulates both thumb joints under anesthesia and restores the thumb to normal function.

   Diagnosis code(s): _____

   Procedure code(s): _____

exudate (eks'u-dāt)

SPINE (VERTEBRAL COLUMN) (22010–22899)

Before you can begin assigning codes for procedures involving the spinal column, it is important for you to understand the anatomy of the spine. The spinal (vertebral) column runs from the neck to the tailbone, beginning at the brainstem (■ FIGURE 23-9), and contains the spinal cord and the nerves attached to it.

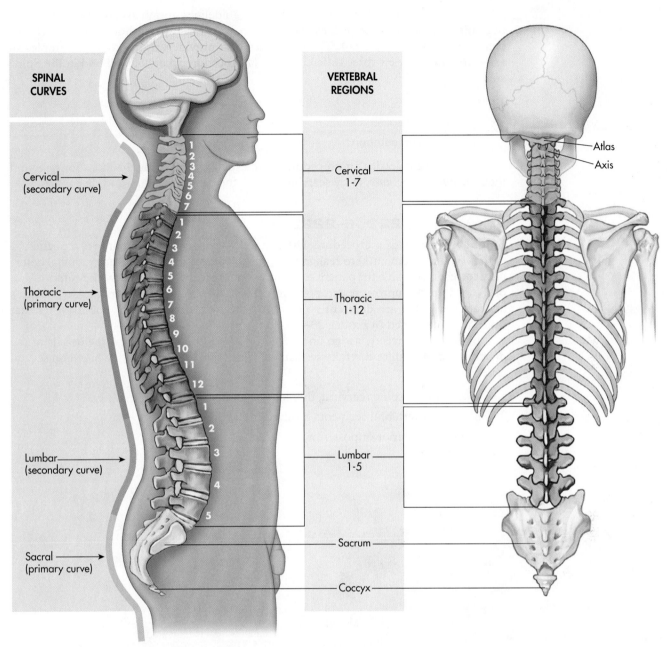

SPINAL CURVES

Cervical (secondary curve)

Thoracic (primary curve)

Lumbar (secondary curve)

Sacral (primary curve)

VERTEBRAL REGIONS

Cervical 1-7

Thoracic 1-12

Lumbar 1-5

Sacrum

Coccyx

Atlas

Axis

Figure 23-9 ■ The spinal column.

The **spinal vertebrae**, or bones of the spine, are located in five separate areas. Each bone is numbered according to its location. Notice in Figure 23-9 how the vertebrae are identified by their location: cervical (neck), thoracic (upper back), lumbar (lower back), sacral (bones formed together near the tailbone), and coccygeal (bones formed together that make up the tailbone). Vertebrae are identified by a letter, representing the first letter of the vertebrae location—**C**ervical, **T**horacic, **L**umbar—and a number, identifying an individual vertebra, listed in ascending order as the vertebrae move down the spine (cervical—C1–C7, C1 is called the atlas and C2 is called the axis; thoracic—T1–T12; lumbar—L1–L5). These letters and numbers identify the vertebrae involved in procedures, and physicians include them in their documentation. CPT divides spinal procedure codes by the spinal location (e.g., cervical, thoracic, lumbar), the surgical approach (e.g., anterior, posterior), and the number of **vertebral** segments (the vertebrae) or *inter-spaces* (compartments, or spaces, between vertebrae which contain a fleshy tissue called the intervertebral disc) involved in the procedure.

vertebral (vər-te′brəl)

The Spine subheading contains extensive guidelines and instructional notes at the beginning and throughout each category, which as you know, you should carefully review before final code assignment. The guidelines also provide various coding examples to assist you. Let's review three different types of procedures that you will find in the Spine subheading:

- Osteotomy
- Arthrodesis
- Spinal instrumentation

You can locate codes for procedures of the spine by searching the index for *spine* and then the *type of procedure*, or by searching under the *type of procedure* and then *spine*..

Osteotomy (22206–22226)

Spinal osteotomy is a procedure where the physician incises and removes a portion(s) of the vertebral segment(s) to realign the spine to correct a spinal deformity. Spinal deformity corrections enable the patient to resume a more erect posture, relieve the compression of the abdomen, improve respiration through the diaphragm, and improve the patient's appearance. There are different types of osteotomies, depending on the disorder that needs to be corrected (■ FIGURE 23-10).

In order to correctly assign an osteotomy procedure code, review the details of the documented procedure carefully so that you can assign the correct code based on several criteria:

- section of the spine (cervical, thoracic, or lumbar)
- number of vertebral segments involved in the procedure
- approach (anterior or posterior)

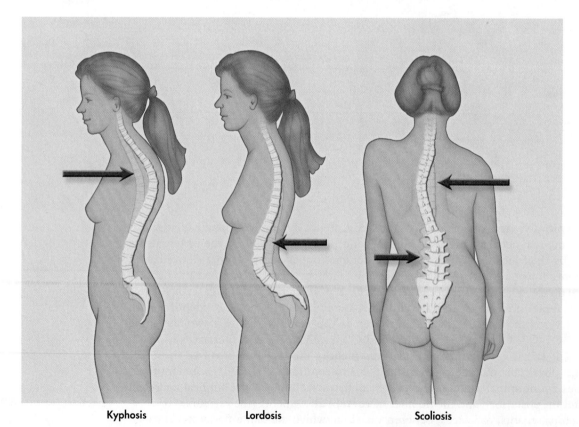

Kyphosis   Lordosis   Scoliosis

Figure 23-10 ■ Disorders of the spinal column.

- number of columns, including
  - anterior (anterior half of the vertebral body)
  - middle (posterior half of the *vertebral body*—main portion of a vertebrae that contains the spinal cord—and the *pedicle*—back of the vertebral body)
  - posterior

    articular facets—located at the back of vertebrae, joining them together
    lamina—top, or roof, of the spinal canal
    spinous process—projections of vertebrae where ligaments and muscles attach

Note that there are many coding guidelines for the Osteotomy category that you should read before final code assignments.

Arthrodesis (22532–22819)

Arthrodesis is the surgical fusion of a joint so that it no longer moves. Physicians perform arthrodesis to relieve pain or provide support in a diseased or injured joint. Spinal arthrodesis fuses together two or more vertebrae and can include bone grafts. Physicians also perform arthrodesis on other joints, including the ankle, wrist, knee, shoulder, and hip. Although arthrodesis may seem like a drastic step to take, patients who choose arthrodesis usually have little motion left in joints, have adapted to living without motion, and are suffering from chronic pain, such as with arthritis. As procedures for artificial joint replacements and implants improve, more patients are able to receive joint replacements instead of arthrodesis.

arthrodesis (ahr-thrō-de′sis)

Physicians may perform arthrodesis as the only procedure or together with another procedure, such as osteotomy, fracture care, vertebral **corpectomy**, or **laminectomy**. In these cases, report the primary procedure code first, then report the code for arthrodesis, and append modifier -51. Carefully review coding guidelines and instructional notes throughout the Arthrodesis category to learn when you need to append a modifier and when to assign additional codes for other procedures. CPT divides codes by the surgical approach, section of the spine, and the number of vertebrae treated.

corpectomy (kor-pek′tə-me)—surgical removal of a vertebra

laminectomy (lam-ĭ-nek′tə-me)—surgical removal of the posterior (back) arch of a vertebra

Spinal Instrumentation (22840–22865)

Orthopedic surgeons use **spinal instrumentation**, also called fixation, to assist in stabilizing the vertebrae of the spine. In spinal instrumentation, surgeons attach metal rods, screws, and pins to the vertebrae to align two or more vertebral segments. Surgeons attach the rods to each end of the span of vertebrae being stabilized. They may or may not also attach them to the vertebrae between the ends.

- Segmental instrumentation occurs when the surgeon places fixation rods at each end of the section begin treated and also attaches the section to at least one vertebra in the middle of the span.

- Nonsegmental instrumentation occurs when the surgeon places fixation devices at each end of section being treated and nowhere else.

Many of the codes in the Spinal Instrumentation category are add-on codes that you assign in addition to the primary procedure, so you should carefully review the instructions after each add-on code to ensure correct code assignment.

APPLICATION OF CASTS AND STRAPPING (29000–29799)

It is important to understand that applying casts and straps is related to fracture care, as well as care for other types of injuries. Did you notice that many of the other subheadings in the Musculoskeletal System subsection include a category for Fracture and/or Dislocation? These categories include codes for treating fractures and dislocations. Let's review common terms associated with treatment of fractures, including casting and strapping

■ TABLE 23-7   **TERMS USED WITH TREATMENT OF FRACTURES AND DISLOCATIONS**

Term	Definition
Open Fracture	break in a bone that punctures the skin
Closed Fracture	break in a bone that does not puncture the skin
Dislocation	movement of one or more bones at a joint from its usual place
Strain	bodily injury from excessive tension, effort, or use
Sprain	a sudden or violent twist or wrench of a joint causing the stretching or tearing of connective tissue and often rupturing of blood vessels
Open Treatment (Reduction)	the realignment of a fractured or dislocated body part back to its normal position when the injury pierces the skin
Closed Treatment (Reduction)	the realignment of a fractured or dislocated body part back to its normal position when the injury does not pierce the skin (can include manipulation)
Internal Fixation	treatment of an injury by attaching bones together with pins, rods, plates, or screws, which are not visible on the outside of the body (can include internal fixation)
External Fixation	treatment of an injury by attaching bones together with pins, rods, plates, or screws, which are attached to another device that is placed on the outside of the body (can include internal fixation)
Manipulation (Reduction)	application of manual force (pull, bend) to reduce or restore a fracture or dislocation to its normal alignment
Percutaneous Skeletal Fixation	fixation (e.g., pins, screws) is applied to the fracture site, and the physician uses imaging to visualize the procedure
Skeletal Traction	application of a pulling force to a limb through a wire, pin, screw, or clamp that is attached to bone
Skin Traction	application of a force (weights) to a limb using felt or strapping applied directly to the skin only
Cast	a rigid casing used to prevent movement of a diseased or broken body part, made of plaster or fiberglass
Strap	taping a body area to stabilize it using strips or pieces of overlapping adhesive plaster
Splint	a rigid device used to prevent motion of a joint or of the ends of a fractured bone, made of cloth, wood, plastic, or metal; static splints allow for complete movement, and dynamic splints allow for partial movement

(■ TABLE 23-7), and then we will review more about assigning the codes under the Application of Casts and Strapping category. You should already be familiar with some of these terms, which you learned previously.

The subheading Application of Casts and Strapping has the following categories and code ranges:

- Body and Upper Extremity (29000–29280)
- Lower Extremity (29305–29590)
- Removal or Repair (29700–29750)
- Other Procedures (unlisted procedure) (29799)

Each of the first two categories is further divided into subcategories for the specific service: casts, splints, or strapping (any age). The third category is further divided by the type of procedure. This subheading includes guidelines. Here are some of the most important points:

- The codes for treating a fracture or dislocation include applying the first cast, splint, or strap. A physician who applies the initial cast, strap, or splint and *also* assumes all of the follow-up care *cannot* report the application of casts and strapping codes as an initial service. Instead, the physician reports the code for treating the fracture as the initial service because it includes applying the cast, strap, or splint. Note that the physician can separately report the application of a new cast, strap, or splint for the patient for the same injury by reporting the code with modifier -58 (staged procedure). Physicians or hospitals (if service is in the ED or hospital) may also report HCPCS Q codes for supplies (casting, strapping, splinting) or CPT code 99070 (supplies).

- Codes for applying casts and strapping also include follow-up services to remove them.

- Report codes for cast removal only when the physician who removes the cast is different from the physician who applied it. For example, the ED physician applies the cast, but an orthopedic surgeon removes it eight weeks later. The orthopedic surgeon would report the code for the cast removal.

Coding regulations for casts, splints, and straps can vary among payers, including Medicare. Be sure to check individual payer guidelines for specific information. You can locate codes for treatment of fractures and dislocations in the index under various main terms, depending on the type of procedure, such as *fracture, dislocation, cast, strapping,* or *splint,* or search under the body site, like *femur, tibia,* or *fibula,* and then by the diagnosis (fracture).

Example: Dr. Gould, an orthopedic surgeon, removes a full arm cast from the left arm of Curtis Rothman, age 17. Dr. Daniels, one of Williton's ED physicians, previously applied the cast when he saw the patient in the ED.

To code this case, search the index for the main term *cast* and subterm *removal,* which directs you to cross reference codes 29700–29715. Assign code **29705-LT** because it describes removal of a full arm cast (left arm). The diagnosis code is **V54.89** (main term *removal* and subterm *cast*).

DESTINATION: MEDICARE

In this Medicare exercise, you will learn more about osteoporosis and Medicare reimbursement for bone mass measurements. Follow the instructions listed next to access *Overview Bone Mass Measurement:*

1. Go to the website http://www.cms.gov.
2. At the top of the screen on the banner bar, choose *Outreach and Education.*
3. Under Medicare Learning Network (MLN), choose *MLN Products.*
4. Under MLN Products, choose *MLN Catalog of Products.*
5. Scroll down to Downloads, and choose *MLN Catalog of Products.*
6. Go to page 16 and click on the brochure *Bone Mass Measurements.*

Answer the following questions:

1. What is the purpose of measuring bone mass?
2. How many women and men over age 50 will have an osteoporosis-related fracture in their lifetime?
3. How frequently will Medicare pay for bone mass measurements?
4. What is another name for bone mass measurement?

TAKE A BREAK

Great job! You are progressing very well! Let's take a break and then review more about coding for procedures on the spine and casts and strapping.

Exercise 23.3 Spine (Vertebral Column), Application of Casts and Strapping

Part 1—Theory

Instructions: Fill in the blank with the best answer.

1. _____ and _____ identify the vertebrae involved in procedures, and physicians include them in their documentation.

2. _____ is the surgical fusion of a joint so that it no longer moves.

3. _____ are compartments, or spaces, between vertebrae, which contain a fleshy tissue called the intervertebral disc.

4. Closed treatment (reduction) is the realignment of a(n) _____ back to its normal position when the injury does not pierce the skin.

5. In spinal instrumentation, surgeons attach _____ to the vertebrae to align two or more vertebral segments.

6. _____ is a procedure where the physician incises and removes a portion(s) of the vertebral segment(s) to realign the spine to correct a spinal deformity.

Part 2—Coding

Instructions: Review the patient's case, and assign procedure code(s), appending a modifier when appropriate. Optional: For additional practice, assign the patient's diagnosis code(s) (ICD-9-CM).

1. Dr. Gould, an orthopedic surgeon, treats Kristin Senter, age 10 months, for a congenital clubfoot (an anomaly, which can be congenital or acquired, where the foot turns toward the ankle, also called **talipes equinovarus**). Dr. Gould stretches the left leg and applies a long leg clubfoot cast.

   Diagnosis code(s): _____

   Procedure code(s): _____

2. Today in the office, Dr. Gould removes a long arm cast (full arm) from the right arm for Leroy Battaglia, age 12, that another physician applied while Leroy was at summer camp. Leroy suffered a radius fracture.

   Diagnosis code(s): _____

   Procedure code(s): _____

3. Dr. Carver, an orthopedic surgeon, applies a *walking cast*, or *total contact cast* (a short leg cast with a plastic sole that allows the patient to walk on it rather than using crutches) to the left leg for Bernard Lankford, age 67. Mr. Lankford has diabetic ulcers on his foot and leg from diabetic neuropathy, and the cast will help to protect his foot.

   Diagnosis code(s): _____

   Procedure code(s): _____

4. Michelle Rawson, age 13, arrives at Williton's ED with her mother. She fell from playground equipment earlier in the day. Dr. Mills examines her and orders X-rays. He diagnoses her with a displaced fracture of the right radius and ulna. He manipulates the fracture and applies a *short arm cast* (a cast that extends from the elbow to the finger). He refers her to Dr. Gould for follow-up care and cast removal.

   Dr. Mills' diagnosis code(s): _____

   Procedure code(s): _____

5. Today at Williton, Dr. Reilly, an orthopedic spinal surgeon, treats Clyde Henninger, age 65, for pain in the thoracic spine due to degenerated and protruding discs at T9–T10 and T10–T11. He prepares two interspaces and performs an arthrodesis on both spaces using an **anterolateral** approach (front and to the side).

   Diagnosis code(s): _____

   Procedure code(s): _____

6. Today at Williton, Dr. Reilly treats Rachelle Strock, age 42, for chronic lower back pain due to degenerative disc disease at the L4–L5 level. She has not responded adequately to physical therapy, exercise, and other conservative (nonsurgical) treatment. Dr. Reilly performs an arthroplasty to remove the entire disc and uses an anterior approach.

   Diagnosis code(s): _____

   Procedure code(s): _____

talipes equinovarus
(tal′-ə-pēz ek-wi-nō-var′-əs)

anterolateral
(an-ter- ō lat′-ə-rəl)

ENDOSCOPY/ARTHROSCOPY (29800–29999)

Do you remember that an endoscopy is the visual examination of a body cavity or organ with a long, narrow, hollow viewing instrument with a light, mirror, and a camera? Arthroscopy is endoscopy of a joint. Physicians perform arthroscopy for diagnostic and surgical purposes. Diagnostic endoscopy/arthroscopy includes a biopsy if the physician needs to perform it, but there is not always a need for a biopsy during an endoscopy. Surgical endoscopy/arthroscopy always includes a diagnostic endoscopy/arthroscopy. Append modifier -51 to the subsequent procedure when the physician performs an arthroscopy with an **arthrotomy** (incision of a joint). Remember that when you report multiple procedures, you should always list the procedure with the highest charge first because it represents the most complex procedure. The insurance will reduce payment for subsequent procedures with modifier -51 appended.

arthrotomy (är-thrät′-ə-mē)

Surgeons perform surgical endoscopies/arthroscopies for many reasons:

- Remove tissue or a foreign body, release or decompress a tendon or ligament
- Debride damaged tissue or bone, or repair injured or diseased tissue, such as a tear
- Treat a fracture, apply transplants or grafts, or drain and irrigate an infection
- Perform arthrodesis or dissect adhesions

Orthopedic surgeons use an arthroscope (an endoscope used for joints) to examine the interior of a joint and perform surgery whenever possible. Surgeons can perform arthroscopic procedures on any joint and most commonly perform them on the knee, shoulder, wrist, and spine. Surgeons use arthroscopic surgery to correct a variety of problems, including to remove floating cartilage, repair torn surface cartilage, trim damaged cartilage, or reconstruct ligaments.

To perform arthroscopy, a surgeon makes two small incisions, called portals, over the *surgical field* (area of surgery). He inserts the arthroscope through one portal and the surgical instruments through the other portal. A camera on the end of the arthroscope transmits an image of a joint to a video monitor, so the surgeon can direct the procedure. Arthroscopy has a faster recovery time than an open procedure where the surgeon uses larger incisions because arthroscopy incisions are smaller. In addition, with arthroscopy, anesthesiologists are often able to use local or regional anesthesia, rather than general anesthesia, and this fact also contributes to the patient's faster recovery time.

When you review patients' medical records, identify whether physicians performed procedures using an open approach or arthroscopically because the codes are located under different subheadings in the CPT manual. Open procedures for the Musculoskeletal System subsection appear under the subheading for the anatomical region where the physician performs the procedure. Arthroscopic procedures for *all* musculoskeletal anatomical sites appear under the subheading *Endoscopy/Arthroscopy*. CPT further divides arthroscopic codes by body site, but there are no separate categories for body sites. Diagnostic procedures are separate from surgical procedures. Remember that a surgical endoscopy always includes a diagnostic endoscopy, so you should never separately code for a diagnostic endoscopy.

Also note that many arthroscopic procedures include the phrase *separate procedure* following the code descriptor. Do you remember what this means? If you said that modifier -59 helps the insurance to know that the provider performed a separate procedure from other procedures that would normally be bundled together under one code, then you are correct! In other words, if you read the medical documentation and find that the arthroscopy is part of a major procedure that the physician performs, then you cannot separately report the arthroscopy. If you do, it is considered *unbundling,* which is incorrect coding!

It is also important to note a few other points when coding arthroscopies:

1. If a surgeon performs an arthroscopy in an attempt to treat a specific condition but cannot do so successfully, he may then convert the procedure to an open procedure. When this happens, you should only report the code for the open procedure.
2. The knee has three compartments, medial, lateral, and patellofemoral. When you are coding for knee arthroscopies, be sure to carefully review not only the code

descriptors but the coding guidelines in the CPT manual and in CPT Assistant®. This is because for certain types of arthroscopies you should report a separate arthroscopy code for each compartment visualized, and for other arthroscopies you should report *one code* regardless of how many compartments were involved. Wrists have six separate compartments, but you should not assign separate arthroscopy codes for each compartment visualized.

3. Some arthroscopic codes contain the phrase *arthroscopically aided* in the code descriptor, which indicates that the physician performed part of the procedure as an *open procedure*. You should still assign the code for the arthroscopic procedure.

To locate codes in the index for an arthroscopy, search for the main term *arthroscopy* and subterm *diagnostic* or *surgical*, then the subterm for the anatomical site involved. Refer to the following example to learn more about coding arthroscopic procedures.

bucket handle tear—tear in the semilunar cartilage, along the middle portion of the meniscus

meniscus (mə-nis′kəs)—a crescent-shaped structure of dense fibrous tissue found in some of the joints

meniscectomy (men-i-sek′-tə-mē)

labrum (lā′-brəm)

fibrocartilage (fi-bro-kahr′tĭ-ləj)—cartilage composed of thick fiber-like strands

Example: Dr. Carver, an orthopedic surgeon, performs a diagnostic arthroscopy on the left knee for William Booker, age 27, due to pain and swelling. X-rays are negative for a patellar fracture. The procedure reveals a **bucket handle tear** of the lateral **meniscus**, which Dr. Carver repairs. He shaves the meniscus and then repairs the tear.

Turn to your CPT manual to code this case. Remember that a surgical arthroscopy always includes diagnostic arthroscopy, so you will not need to assign a separate code for the diagnostic procedure. Search the index for main term *arthroscopy*, subterm *surgical*, and subterm *knee*, which directs you to cross reference codes 29871–29889. Assign code **29882-LT** because it includes a **meniscectomy** (surgical removal of the meniscus) for either medial or lateral, but not both, and it also identifies a meniscus repair for either medial or lateral, but not both. The diagnosis code is **836.1** (main term *tear* and subterms *meniscus, lateral, bucket handle*).

TAKE A BREAK

That was a lot of information to remember! Good work! Let's take a break and practice coding endoscopies/arthroscopies.

| Exercise 23.4 | **Endoscopy/Arthroscopy** |

Instructions: Review the patient's case and then assign codes for the procedure(s), appending a modifier when appropriate. Optional: For additional practice, assign the patient's diagnosis code(s) (ICD-9-CM).

1. Today at Williton, Dr. Carver, an orthopedic surgeon, repairs a torn right rotator cuff (four muscles surrounding the humerus that help the arm to move) for Mario Decastro, age 20. Dr. Carver performs the procedure arthroscopically.

   Diagnosis code(s): _____

   Procedure code(s): _____

2. At Williton, Dr. Breneman, an oral surgeon, performs a surgical arthroscopy of the temporomandibular joint for Miguel Taplin, age 31, to correct a TMJ disorder

(pain, lack of movement, and tenderness in the joint, which has various causes, including injuries).

   Diagnosis code(s): _____

   Procedure code(s): _____

3. Zachary Branstetter, age 24, suffers from a torn **labrum** (a rim of **fibrocartilage** around the acetabulum). Dr. Carver repairs it arthroscopically at Williton and also debrides cartilage during the procedure.

   Diagnosis code(s): _____

   Procedure code(s): _____

4. Dr. Gould, an orthopedic surgeon, performs an arthroscopically aided open repair of the right posterior cruciate ligament (one of four ligaments of the knee) for Jeannie Martino, age 26, to treat an avulsion.

   Diagnosis code(s): _____

   Procedure code(s): _____

WORKPLACE IQ

You are working as a new coder for Dr. Gould, an orthopedic surgeon. Although you practiced coding musculoskeletal system procedures in coding class, you have never coded them for a physician. However, Kathy, the office manager, said that another coder will happily train you. Today, you are reviewing medical documentation to become more familiar with the types of procedures that Dr. Gould performs. You find the terms *interspace* and *segment* and vaguely remember what they mean, but you're not sure how they apply to specific codes.

What would you do?

CHAPTER REVIEW

Multiple Choice

Instructions: Circle one best answer to complete each statement.

1. A(n) _____ is a joint injury that is not a fracture.
   a. excision
   b. dislocation
   c. reduction
   d. fixation

2. The _____ is an enlargement or protrusion from a bone.
   a. head
   b. neck
   c. shaft
   d. process

3. _____ tumors are confined to the tissue within or below the deep fascia, but do not involve the bone.
   a. Fascial
   b. Subcutaneous
   c. Percutaneous
   d. Closed

4. Select codes for musculoskeletal tumor excision and resection based on the tumor
   a. size and location.
   b. behavior, malignant or benign.
   c. cause.
   d. pathology report.

5. Report codes for cast removal only when the physician who removes the cast is
   a. the same as the physician who applied it.
   b. the same as the physician who provided all the follow-up care.
   c. different from the physician who applied it.
   d. the emergency department physician.

6. Diagnostic endoscopy/arthroscopy includes
   a. surgical endoscopy/arthroscopy.
   b. removal of a foreign body.
   c. a biopsy.
   d. incision and drainage.

7. _____ is when surgeons enlarge a wound or dissect it in order to determine the wound depth or to remove a foreign body.
   a. Wound debridement
   b. Wound suturing
   c. Wound incision
   d. Wound exploration

8. _____ is a procedure where the physician incises and removes a portion(s) of the vertebral segment(s) to realign the spine to correct a spinal deformity.
   a. Spinal instrumentation
   b. Spinal osteotomy
   c. Arthrodesis
   d. Osteotomy instrumentation

9. Radioelement application is also called _____ and involves placing a radioelement (radiation) into a malignant tumor using capsules, ribbons, or seeds.
   a. radiotherapy
   b. immunotherapy
   c. brachytherapy
   d. chemotherapy

10. The spinal vertebrae, or bones of the spine, are located in _____ separate areas.
    a. four
    b. five
    c. six
    d. seven

Coding Assignments

Instructions: Assign procedure code(s) to the following cases. Optional: For additional practice, assign the patient's diagnosis code(s) (ICD-9-CM).

1. The radiology department asks Dr. Gould, an orthopedic surgeon, to inject contrast medium as part of an elbow arthrography. The patient is Brent Rosinski, age 29, and the purpose of the procedure is to determine the cause of pain in the joint of the right elbow. Code for Dr. Gould's services.

   Diagnosis code(s): _____

   Procedure code(s): _____

2. Today at Williton, Dr. Reilly, an orthopedic spinal surgeon, treats Isabelle Berns, age 33, for fractures of vertebrae L3 and L4. He performs a percutaneous vertebroplasty (osteoplasty, repair of the vertebrae) where he injects bone cement bilaterally into both vertebrae to help stabilize them.

   Diagnosis code(s): _____

   Procedure code(s): _____

3. Dr. Stuart, an orthopedic surgeon, treats Debora Navarrette, age 52, at Williton. She suffers from thoracic outlet syndrome (compression of blood vessels or nerve fibers between the neck and the axilla). He excises a portion of the third rib on the right side.

   Diagnosis code(s): _____

   Procedure code(s): _____

4. Tom Moxley, age 14, suffers from **pectus excavatum**, a congenital deformity of the anterior chest wall, in which several ribs and the sternum grow abnormally. Dr. Carver, an orthopedic surgeon, treats the patient today at Williton. He performs a minimally invasive Nuss procedure with a thoracoscopy that involves placing a steel bar into the chest to correct the deformity while the bones solidify.

   Diagnosis code(s): _____

   Procedure code(s): _____

5. Dr. Gould treats Dena Bryand, age 48, for chronic disabling pain in the right ankle joint that has not responded to conservative care. He performs an arthroscopic arthrodesis of the ankle.

   Diagnosis code(s): _____

   Procedure code(s): _____

6. Dr. Burns, Williton's ED physician, treats Rick Borrero, age 33, for a closed Colles fracture (radius) that the patient sustained when he fell off a horse he was riding. Dr. Burns performs a closed reduction and applies a *gauntlet cast* (a cast from the lower forearm to the hand) to the right hand and wrist. He refers Mr. Borrero to Dr. Stuart, an orthopedic surgeon, for follow-up care and cast removal. Assign codes for Dr. Burns' services.

   Diagnosis code(s): _____

   Procedure code(s): _____

7. Dean Pinette, age 31, arrives at Williton's ED with his wife after he cut off the middle finger of his left hand with a table saw. Dr. Mills examines the patient, and Mr. Pinette's wife gives the detached finger, which she has wrapped in a wet towel, to Dr. Mills. Dr. Mills calls Dr. Kellison, the orthopedic hand surgeon on call. Dr. Kellison determines that he needs to immediately perform surgery. He successfully performs a replantation (reattachment) of the finger. After the patient recovers, Dr. Kellison counsels him on power tool safety.

   Diagnosis code(s): _____

   Procedure code(s): _____

8. Dr. Stark, a general surgeon, treats Gwen Oleson, age 46, for an abdominal wall tumor. Dr. Starks excises a tumor from the intramuscular tissue. The tumor measures 4.0 cm in diameter. The pathology report states that the tumor is benign.

   Diagnosis code(s): _____

   Procedure code(s): _____

9. Dr. Carver treats Jay Roane, age 57, for chronic obstructive sleep apnea today at Williton. He performs a **hyoid myotomy** with suspension (HMS), in which he moves forward the horseshoe-shaped bone in the neck where the tongue muscles attach. This procedure will stabilize the airway space behind the back of the tongue.

   Diagnosis code(s): _____

   Procedure code(s): _____

10. Dr. Gould performs a radical resection to remove a tumor from the **latissimus dorsi** (back muscle) for Ruby Oslund, age 71. The tumor measures 5.0 cm. The pathology report later states that it is a **leiomyosarcoma** (malignant tumor of smooth muscle).

    Diagnosis code(s): _____

    Procedure code(s): _____

pectus excavatum
(pek-təs ek-skə-vāt-əm)

hyoid myotomy
(hi′oid-mi-ot′ə-me)

latissimus dorsi
(lə-tis′ī-məs dor′si)

leiomyosarcoma
(le-o-mi-o-sahr-ko′mə)

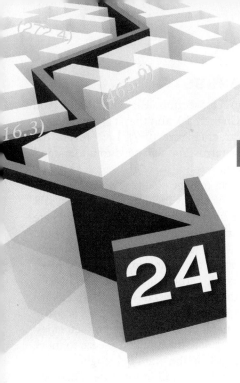

Respiratory System

Learning Objectives

After completing this chapter, you should be able to

- Spell and define the key terminology in this chapter.
- Describe the subsection Surgery—Respiratory system.
- Discuss how to code from the subheading Nose.
- Identify how to use the codes in the subheading Accessory Sinuses.
- Explain how to code from the subheading Larynx.
- Define how to use the codes in the subheading Trachea and Bronchi.
- Describe how to code in the subheading Lungs and Pleura.

Key Terms

accessory sinuses
cardiopulmonary bypass (heart–lung machine)
direct laryngoscopy
heart–lung transplant
indirect laryngoscopy

lower respiratory system
lung transplant
ultrasound
upper respiratory system
vocal cords

INTRODUCTION

You have reached the next stop on your journey—coding procedures of the respiratory system. Remember that the respiratory system allows the body to inhale oxygen and distribute it throughout the bloodstream to cells in the body in order to sustain life. You will learn about many different types of procedures that physicians perform, including *laryngoscopy* (to visually examine the larynx with an endoscope) and *bronchoscopy* (to visually examine the bronchi with an endoscope). Remember that an endoscopy is a procedure where the physician views the inside of the patient's body using a lighted, flexible tube with an attached lens. The CPT manual includes several coding instructions for the Respiratory subsection, including guidelines for specific categories, including endoscopies, and guidelines for individual codes. As always, it is important to review and understand guidelines before assigning codes. This stop may be a little tricky at first, but you will gain self-confidence by completing the practice exercises and applying the new information presented in this chapter. So, let's get started with the respiratory system, taking time to learn about new procedures and how to code them!

"The greatest things ever done on Earth have been done little by little."
—WILLIAM JENNINGS BRYAN

CPT-4 codes in this chapter are from the CPT-4 2012 code set. CPT is a registered trademark of the American Medical Association.

ICD-9-CM codes in this chapter are from the ICD-9-CM 2012 code set from the Department of Health and Human Services, Centers for Disease Control and Prevention.

RESPIRATORY SYSTEM (30000–32999)

The Respiratory System is a subsection of the Surgery section. Remember that you learned information about the respiratory system in Chapter 10, and that it is divided into an upper airway (Figure 10-6) and lower respiratory tract (Figure 10-7). Let's review the respiratory system and how it functions and learn new terms. You will need to understand the respiratory system anatomy before you code procedures.

Both the upper airway and the lower respiratory tract may be collectively referred to as the respiratory system. The **upper respiratory system** or airway includes the nose, **larynx** (voice box), and **pharynx** (throat). The pharynx contains three pairs of tonsils, which are lymphoid tissues. The **lower respiratory system** or tract contains the lungs, bronchi and bronchioles (branches of tubes that carry oxygen), and alveoli (air sacs at the ends of bronchioles). The diaphragm is a muscular membrane separating the abdominal cavity from the thoracic cavity, helping the body to inhale oxygen and exhale carbon dioxide (Figure 10-8).

The nose inhales oxygen (air) into the body with the help of the chest muscles, abdominal muscles, and diaphragm. The *nasal cavity* is the area inside the nose that detects smell, and the *nasal septum* is the thin wall that separates the nasal cavity into right and left sides. The nose also contains sensory nerves, some of which regulate the reflex to sneeze to move foreign bodies out of the respiratory system. Other nerves help the brain to recognize smell.

Nasal turbinates, or **conchae**, are spongy bones inside the wall of the nose. There are three different pairs of turbinates on each side of the nose: inferior (the largest), middle, and superior turbinates (the smallest) (■ FIGURE 24-1). **Mucosa** is the mucous membrane that covers the turbinates, which helps to warm the air that you breathe.

The *sinus cavity* contains air-filled chambers, or spaces, called *paranasal sinuses,* inside the skull and face bones. The *sinus membrane* lines the sinuses and produces mucus, which prevents bacteria, dirt, and dust in the air from entering the body. It also moistens the air and warms it. *Cilia* are small hairs that line the sinus membrane and move mucus from the sinus cavity to the nasal cavity. There are four pair of paranasal sinuses, also called **accessory sinuses** (■ FIGURE 24-2), which have both a left and right side: the *frontal sinuses* (located over the eyes), *maxillary sinuses* (located under the eyes), **ethmoid sinuses** (located between the eyes and nose), and **sphenoid sinuses** (located at the center of the base of the skull, at the back of the nose).

Air passes from the nose and sinuses into the **nasopharynx**, passes through the **oropharynx**, and continues into the larynx through the **epiglottis**. The epiglottis is a flap of skin which opens to allow air into the larynx and closes when swallowing to prevent

---

larynx (lar′-i ŋ(k)s)

pharynx (far′-iŋ(k)s)

conchae (käŋ′- kē)

mucosa (myü-kō′-zə)

ethmoid (eth′-moid)

sphenoid (sfee′-noid)

nasopharynx (ney-zoh-far′-ingks)—the first division of the pharynx, the area of the throat joining to the nasal cavity

oropharynx (ohr-oh-far′-ingks)—the second division of the pharynx, the area of the throat joining to the mouth

epiglottis (ep-i-glot′-is)

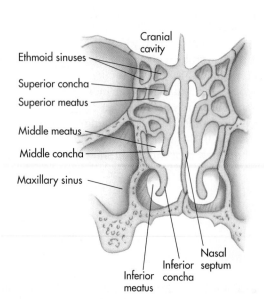

Figure 24-1 ■ Positions of the entrance to the ethmoid and maxillary sinuses.

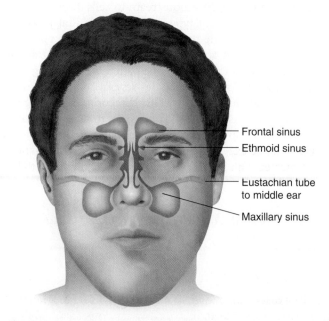

Figure 24-2 ■ Paranasal sinuses.

food and liquid from entering the trachea. When the epiglottis is closed, food and liquid enter the *esophagus*, a tube that carries it from the pharynx to the stomach. The larynx contains ligaments and soft tissue folds (**vocal cords**) that produce sound when air passes through them, which produces speech. The larynx also cleans and moistens the air before passing it into the trachea (windpipe).

The *trachea* is a tube which passes air into the chest cavity. The end of the trachea divides into two bronchi, and each bronchus leads to a lung. Each main bronchus divides into small **bronchi**. The bronchi further divide into smaller **bronchioles**. These small, branching tubes carry air to and from the **alveoli**. The *alveoli* are thin-walled sacs in which the exchange of oxygen and carbon dioxide takes place. The *lungs* are upside-down, cone-shaped organs, which are divided into *lobes*. The right lung is divided into three lobes, and the left lung is divided into two lobes. Each lobe receives air from its own bronchus. Most of the lung tissue is made up of *capillaries* and alveoli. The lungs are covered with a protective lining called the *pleura*.

bronchi (brong′-kahy)—a branch that comes off the trachea

bronchioles (brong′-kee-ohls)

alveoli (al-vē′-ə-lī)

Respiratory disorders occur when the lungs and organs of the respiratory system do not function properly because of a congenital condition; underlying disease, such as cancer; infection, such as sinusitis; or trauma. Other respiratory conditions that physicians treat include pleural effusion (fluid in the pleura), benign neoplasms, and presence of foreign bodies.

CPT divides the Respiratory subsection into five subheadings by body site (e.g., nose, lungs) and then into categories of types of procedures (e.g., incision, endoscopy) (■ TABLE 24-1). Turn to the codes in the subsection to become more familiar with them as you review Table 24-1.

Recall that otorhinolaryngologists and otolaryngologists specialize in preventing, diagnosing, and treating ear, nose, and throat disorders and are also referred to as ENT (ear, nose, throat) specialists. It is important to note that other types of physicians may also perform procedures listed in the Respiratory section, depending on the patient's case, like primary care physicians, pulmonologists, thoracic surgeons, or ED physicians. Depending on the procedure, the patient may also need to have general anesthesia or local anesthesia for the procedure.

You can locate codes in the index for respiratory system procedures by searching for either the body site (nose), and then the type or procedure (incision, removal, polypectomy), or by the type of procedure and then the body site. Let's review respiratory terms with an exercise, then look at some examples of codes in each of the subheadings to learn more about them and then practice coding.

TAKE A BREAK

Let's take a break and then review terms of the respiratory system.

Exercise 24.1   Respiratory System

Instructions: Fill in each blank with the best answer.

1. The _____ is the thin wall that separates the nasal cavity into right and left sides.

2. The sinus cavity contains air-filled chambers, or spaces, called _____.

3. The _____ lines the sinuses and produces mucus.

4. The _____ is a flap of skin which opens to allow air into the _____ and closes when swallowing.

5. The end of the trachea divides into two _____, and each _____ leads to a _____.

6. The right lung is divided into _____ lobes, and the left lung is divided into _____ lobes.

NOSE (30000–30999)

The subheading Nose contains seven different categories of codes, depending on the type of procedure that the physician performs (Table 24-1). Common procedures in this category include incision, excision, and repair. You can find procedures in this subheading by

■ TABLE 24-1   **RESPIRATORY SYSTEM SUBSECTION, SUBHEADINGS, AND CATEGORIES**

Subsection, Subheadings, and Categories	Code Range
RESPIRATORY SYSTEM	**30000–32999**
Nose	**30000–30999**
Incision	*30000–30020*
Excision	*30100–30160*
Introduction	*30200–30220*
Removal of Foreign Body	*30300–30320*
Repair	*30400–30630*
Destruction	*30801–30802*
Other Procedures	*30901–30999*
Accessory Sinuses	**31000–31299**
Incision	*31000–31090*
Excision	*31200–31230*
Endoscopy	*31231–31297*
Other Procedures	*31299*
Larynx	**31300–31599**
Excision	*31300–31420*
Introduction	*31500–31502*
Endoscopy	*31505–31579*
Repair	*31580–31590*
Destruction	*31595*
Other Procedures	*31599*
Trachea and Bronchi	**31600–31899**
Incision	*31600–31614*
Endoscopy	*31615–31656*
Introduction	*31715–31730*
Excision, Repair	*31750–31830*
Other Procedures	*31899*
Lungs and Pleura	**32035–32999**
Incision	*32035–32225*
Excision	*32310–32405*
Removal	*32420–32540*
Introduction and Removal	*32550–32553*
Destruction	*32560–32562*
Endoscopy	*32601–32665*
Repair	*32800–32820*
Lung Transplantation	*32850–32856*
Surgical Collapse Therapy; Thoracoplasty	*32900–32960*
Other Procedures	*32997–32999*

searching the index for the *type of procedure* or for the *body site (nose, turbinate)*, and then the *type of procedure (excision, incision)*. So let's take a look at the procedures in each category and learn why physicians perform them, and then practice coding. Turn to each category of codes in your CPT manual as you read more about them.

Incision (30000–30020)

Both procedures in the Incision category are for the drainage of an abscess or hematoma from the nose (*internal approach*—from inside the nose) or from the nasal septum. Notice that the CPT guidelines direct you to codes 10060 or 10140 for draining an abscess or hematoma using an *external approach* (from outside the nose). Coding guidelines for draining an abscess or hematoma from the nasal septum direct you to other codes when the physician performs a lateral **rhinotomy** (incision into the nose).

rhinotomy (rī-nät′-ə-mē)

Excision (30100–30160)

CPT arranges procedures in the Excision category by type (e.g., biopsy, excision, resection), condition (e.g., nasal polyp, dermoid cyst), and body site (e.g., intranasal, inferior turbinate). Examples of procedures in this category are

- *Biopsy, intranasal (inside the nose) (30100)*—Recall that a biopsy is when a physician removes tissues or cells to examine them or send them to a pathologist for testing to determine whether any condition or disease is present.

- *Excision of nasal polyp(s)—simple or extensive (30110–30115)*—A *nasal polyp* is a growth from the mucous membrane inside the nose, which infection, allergies, or asthma can cause. Patients with nasal polyps may have difficulty breathing through their noses and experience a decreased sense of smell. CPT defines a *simple excision* as a procedure performed in an office setting and an *extensive excision* as a procedure requiring facilities available in a hospital setting. CPT also directs you to append modifier -50 for a bilateral excision.

- *Excision or destruction of an intranasal lesion (30117–30118)*—This surgery may take an internal or external approach.

- *Excision or surgical planing of skin of nose for* **rhinophyma** *(30120)* (thick skin due to sebaceous gland infection, which occurs in patients with **rosacea**, a condition with erythema and papules)—The physician removes the thickened skin in layers, which includes dermabrasion.

rhinophyma (rī-nō-fī′-mə)
rosacea (rō-zā′-shē- ə)

- *Excision of inferior turbinate, partial or complete (turbinectomy) (30130), and Submucous resection of inferior turbinate—partial or complete (30140)*—A physician may need to excise all or part of the mucosa and bone of the inferior turbinate (30130) or resect the inferior turbinate due to hypertrophy from allergies or infection.

  - In order for you to report the code for a submucous resection (30140), the physician must document that he incised the mucosa over the turbinate, elevated the mucosa, and then removed the bone underneath *without* removing the mucosa. Note that there are several CPT guidelines for these two procedures that direct you to other codes, when the physician performs different or additional procedures.

- *Rhinectomy—partial or total—* A **rhinectomy** is the surgical excision of the nose, most commonly performed to remove neoplasms, such as carcinoma.

rhinectomy (rī-nek′- tə-mē)

Review the following example for coding a procedure performed on the nose. You can try coding this case on your own and checking the answer listed next, or code along with the steps listed.

Example: At Williton Medical Center, Dr. Rosa, an otorhinolaryngologist, performs a complete inferior turbinectomy (right and left inferior turbinate) for Judy Brown, a 53-year-old patient, suffering from turbinate hypertrophy.

To locate the code for this procedure, search the index for the main term *turbinate* and subterm *excision*, and you will then see the code range 30130–30140. Cross-reference the codes in the Respiratory System subsection, and you will find that code **30130** describes the procedure, which is the correct code to assign. The patient's diagnosis code is **478.0** (*hypertrophy, turbinate*).

Introduction (30200–30220)

The Introduction category contains codes for three procedures:

- *Injection into turbinate(s), therapeutic (30200)*—A physician can inject drugs, such as corticosteroids, into the turbinates to treat allergic rhinitis and other infections.

- *Displacement therapy (Proetz type) (30210)*—A method of irrigating blocked sinuses (due to **ethmoditis** or allergies) with a saline solution that is then suctioned out.

- *Insertion, nasal septal prosthesis (button) (30220)*—A physician inserts a silicone nasal septal prosthesis, called a button, to repair a nasal septum perforation. Perforations can be the result of infection, trauma, or previous surgery. Patients with perforations may have epistaxis, rhinorrhea, pain, and breathing difficulty. The button is not intended to be permanent and does not replace surgery but it is helpful for patients who cannot medically withstand surgery.

ethmoditis (eth-moy-dīt'-əs)—inflammation of the ethmoid bone

Removal of Foreign Body (30300–30320)

As you can imagine, foreign bodies in the nose are most commonly seen in children who insert a variety of objects into their noses, including food and toys. Patients suffering from psychiatric conditions may also insert objects into their noses. Many times, a patient does not have any symptoms, but a parent or caregiver sees the patient insert an object into his nose and brings him to the healthcare provider for treatment. Patients often experience symptoms when an object remains in the nose for an extended time, including rhinorrhea, epistaxis, pain, and sneezing.

The Removal of Foreign Body category contains three codes for removal of an intranasal foreign body, depending on whether the procedure is:

- *office type (30300)*—The physician removes the foreign body in an office, outpatient clinic, urgent care center, or the emergency department.

- *requiring general anesthesia (30310)*—The patient needs general anesthesia in order for the physician to remove the foreign body.

- *by lateral rhinotomy (30320)*—The physician needs to incise the nose from the inner eyebrow to the **nasolabial fold** in order to remove the foreign body.

nasolabial fold (na-so-la'be-il)—the crease that runs from the bottom of each nostril to the corner of the mouth

TAKE A BREAK

That was a lot of information to cover! Let's take a break, review more about procedures related to the nose, and then practice coding.

Exercise 24.2 Incision, Excision, Introduction, Removal of Foreign Body

Part 1—Theory

Instructions: Fill in the blank with the best answer.

1. CPT guidelines direct you to codes _____or _____ for draining an abscess or hematoma using an external approach.

2. For excision of a nasal polyp, CPT defines a _____ excision as a procedure performed in an office setting and an _____ excision as a procedure requiring facilities available in a hospital setting.

3. A _____ is the surgical excision of the nose, most commonly performed to remove neoplasms, such as carcinoma.

4. A method of irrigating blocked sinuses with a saline solution that is then suctioned out is called _____.

5. A physician inserts a silicone nasal septal prosthesis, called a _____, to repair a nasal septum perforation.

6. Foreign bodies in the nose are most commonly seen in _____ and in _____ patients who insert a variety of objects into their noses, including food and toys.

Part 2—Coding

Instructions: Review each patient's case, then assign codes for the procedure(s), appending a modifier when

TAKE A BREAK *continued*

appropriate. Optional: For additional practice, assign the patient's diagnosis code(s) (ICD-9-CM).

1. Jane White, a 52-year-old, presents to Williton Medical Center's ED with complaints of nasal pain, edema, and purulent (pus) discharge. Dr. Daniels, the ED physician, assesses the patient and orders a CT scan and lab work. The tests reveal a nasal septum abscess, which *Staphylococcus aureus* caused. Dr. Daniels performs an incision and drainage (I & D) of the abscess.

   Diagnosis code(s):_____

   Procedure code(s): _____

2. Dr. Rosa, an otorhinolaryngologist, performs an extensive nasal polypectomy at Williton Medical Center for Eugene Collor, a 62-year-old who suffers from nasal polyps.

   Diagnosis code(s):_____

   Procedure code(s): _____

3. Dr. Rosa repairs a nasal septum perforation at Williton for Lou Carroll, a 63-year-old. Dr. Rosa uses a nasal septal button on the defect.

   Diagnosis code(s):_____

   Procedure code(s): _____

4. While playing marbles with her friends, Miranda Tubbs, age 4, pushes a small marble up her right nostril and cannot retrieve it. Later that day, Mrs. Tubbs witnesses Miranda pressing her nose and picking at it. When questioned, Miranda says the marble fell up her nose. Mrs. Tubbs takes her to Williton's ED, where Dr. Daniels examines her nose and uses a pair of forceps to remove the marble. She is awake and alert during the procedure.

   Diagnosis code(s):_____

   Procedure code(s): _____

5. Kelsi Lawson, age 12, sees Dr. Rosa in his clinic with complaints of pain and edema of her nose. Dr. Rosa sends her to a separate area of the clinic for magnetic resonance imaging (MRI), a radiology test to view the patient's nasal structures. The MRI reveals a lesion of the nasal septum. Dr. Rosa performs a simple excision and finds that it is a dermoid cyst.

   Diagnosis code(s):_____

   Procedure code(s): _____

6. Dr. Rosa performs a corticosteroid injection into the inferior turbinates for Jenn Femer, age 26, to treat allergic rhinitis.

   Diagnosis code(s):_____

   Procedure code(s): _____

Repair (30400–30630)

CPT arranges codes in the Repair category by the type of procedure. The first eight codes in the Repair category are for **rhinoplasty**, which is the surgical repair of the nose. A rhinoplasty is commonly referred to as a "nose job." Physicians perform rhinoplasties for patients who want their noses to look better or for patients who have suffered trauma to the nose; have a congenital deformity, such as a **cleft lip** or **cleft palate**; or have had carcinoma removed, which left the nose deformed. A physician can perform a *closed* rhinoplasty, where the incisions are intranasal, or an *open* rhinoplasty, where the incisions are also intranasal, but the physician incises the nose externally on the **columella** to gain better access to internal structures.

A rhinoplasty may be primary or secondary. A *primary* rhinoplasty is the initial procedure, and a *secondary* rhinoplasty, which is typically more complex, is performed when the:

- primary rhinoplasty was unsuccessful.
- patient experiences trauma to the nose following the initial procedure.
- patient is dissatisfied with the outcome of the initial procedure.

A secondary rhinoplasty may involve grafts of cartilage (usually from the ear), bone, or tissue to reconstruct the nose. It may also involve repairing the nasal septum if part of it was removed during the primary procedure. CPT categorizes secondary rhinoplasties by the following types of revisions:

- *minor revision (30430)*—small amount of nasal tip work
- *intermediate revision (30435)*—bony work with osteotomies (incisions into bones)
- *major revision (30450)*—nasal tip work and osteotomies

rhinoplasty (rī′-nō-plas-tē)

cleft lip—a congenital anomaly where the lip does not completely form, resulting in a cleft

cleft palate—a congenital anomaly causing a fissure to form in the roof of the mouth because the maxilla is not fully formed

columella (kăl-ə-mel′-ə)—the lower portion of the nasal septum

septoplasty (sep′-tə-plas-tē)

rhinoseptoplasty(rī′-nō-sep-tə-plas-tē)

synechia (si-nēk′-ē-ə)

Did you notice the CPT coding note that appears before the codes in the Repair category? It directs you to assign additional codes when the physician obtains tissues for a graft.

The Repair category also includes the procedure for a **septoplasty**, with or without cartilage scoring (incising), contouring, or replacement with graft. A septoplasty is the surgical repair of the nasal septum, which a patient may need because of a deviated, or displaced, nasal septum.

A patient may also undergo a **rhinoseptoplasty**, which is the surgical repair of the nose and nasal septum, to repair structures to correct breathing disorders, repair damage caused by trauma, or to reshape the nose for cosmetic reasons.

Additional procedures in the Repair category include

- *Lysis of intranasal synechia (adhesion) (30560)*
- *Repair of a fistula or nasal septal perforation (30580)*
- *Septal or other intranasal dermatoplasty (30620)*

Other terms located in code descriptors with which you should be familiar are located in ■ Table 24-2.

■ **TABLE 24-2**   **TERMS IN THE REPAIR CATEGORY**

Term	Definition
Bony pyramid	Inside surface of the nasal bone
Lateral and alar cartilages (■ FIGURE 24-3)	Cartilage at the tip of the nose and just above the tip
Oromaxillary *fistula*	Abnormal opening between the roof of the mouth and the maxillary sinus
Oronasal *fistula*	Abnormal opening between the mouth and the nasal cavity
Spreader grafting	Synthetic or cartilage graft between the nasal septum and wall of the nose to improve breathing

alar (ā′-lər)

oromaxillary (ohr-oh-mak′-sə-ler-ē)

oronasal (ohr-oh - nā′-zəl)

Destruction (30801–30802)

The Destruction category contains two codes for the ablation of mucosa of the inferior nasal turbinates, unilateral or bilateral, using any method. Physicians can ablate turbinate soft tissue to reduce its size to improve breathing in snoring disorders and obstructive sleep apnea. Radiofrequency is a common method of soft tissue ablation and involves a needle electrode that destroys tissue using heat from an electrical current.

Codes for ablations are based on the depth of the ablation, including:

- *superficial (30801)*—involving the surface of the mucosa, or
- *intramural (submucosal) (30802)*—involving ablation deeper into the mucosa

Other Procedures (30901–30999)

The Other Procedures category contains eight codes, including an unlisted procedure of the nose. The first four procedures are to control a nasal hemorrhage (epistaxis), which patients experience for various reasons, including trauma, surgery, infection, allergy, foreign bodies, medications, nasal sprays, bleeding disorders, or aggressive nose blowing or nose picking. Control of a nasal hemorrhage is either:

- *Anterior* (front of the nose from the nasal septum), the most common situation—An anterior procedure can be *simple* (limited cautery and/or packing) (30901) or *complex*

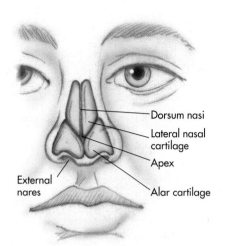

Figure 24-3 ■ Nasal cartilages and external structure.

Dorsum nasi

Lateral nasal cartilage

Apex

External nares

Alar cartilage

(extensive cautery and/or packing) (30903). CPT notes direct you to report modifier -50 when the procedure is bilateral.

- **Posterior** (back of the nose)—A posterior procedure can be *initial* (30905) or *subsequent* (30906).

Additional services in the Other Procedures category include

- **Ligation arteries, ethmoidal or internal maxillary artery** (facial artery that extends to the upper jaw), **transantral** (across the antrum—an air-filled cavity of the maxilla, the upper jaw) **(30915–30920)**— a procedure for treating posterior epistaxis when cautery or packing fails

- **Fracture nasal inferior turbinate(s), therapeutic (30930)**—a procedure to relocate a turbinate that causes an obstruction.

TAKE A BREAK

Congratulations! You are doing great! Let's take a break and review more about the nose, then practice coding more nose procedures.

| Exercise 24.3 | **Repair, Destruction, Other Procedures** |

Part 1—Theory

Instructions: Fill in the blank with the best answer.

1. A _____ is commonly referred to as a "nose job."

2. Surgical repair of the nasal septum is called _____.

3. A patient may undergo a _____, which is the surgical repair of the nose and nasal septum to repair structures to correct breathing disorders.

4. An abnormal opening between the roof of the mouth and the maxillary sinus is called an _____.

5. _____ is a synthetic or cartilage graft between the nasal septum and wall of the nose to improve breathing.

6. A procedure for treating posterior epistaxis when cautery or packing fails is called _____ of arteries.

Part 2—Coding

Instructions: Review each patient's case, then assign codes for the procedure(s), appending a modifier when appropriate. Optional: For additional practice, assign the patient's diagnosis code(s) (ICD-9-CM).

1. Dr. Rosa, an otorhinolaryngologist, performs a septoplasty at Williton on Jason Snyder, a 17-year-old, to repair a deviated nasal septum, which happened from a blow to his nose while he was playing high school football. He experienced epistaxis and difficulty breathing when Dr. Rosa diagnosed his condition.

   Diagnosis code(s):_____

   Procedure code(s): _____

2. Dr. Rosa performs a bilateral soft tissue ablation of the intramural inferior turbinates for Karen Hart, a 41-year-old, to treat inferior turbinate hypertrophy.

   Diagnosis code(s):_____

   Procedure code(s): _____

continued

TAKE A BREAK *continued*

3. Joe Greenwald, age 28, arrives at Williton's ED for uncontrolled bilateral epistaxis. Dr. Daniels examines the patient and determines that the bleeding is anterior. Workup reveals that the patient suffers from sinusitis. Dr. Daniels performs limited cautery and packing of the nasal hemorrhage to treat the patient.

Diagnosis code(s):_____

Procedure code(s): _____

4. Maria Vasquez, age 32, sees Dr. Rosa because she is unhappy with the appearance of her nose. She states, "I have a bump on it that I can't stand and would like it removed. I also hate the tip of it because it looks pointy." Dr. Rosa and the patient view computer images of her "new" nose as it would appear if he performed surgery. Ms. Vasquez opts for surgery, and today at Williton, Dr. Rosa performs a primary rhinoplasty and elevates the nasal tip.

Diagnosis code(s):_____

Procedure code(s): _____

5. After her surgery and healing, Ms. Vasquez sees Dr. Rosa again because she states that she is still unhappy with the tip of her nose. She states that even though her nose now looks the way it appeared on the computer image, she still feels self-conscious about it. Dr. Rosa agrees to perform a secondary rhinoplasty to revise the nasal tip further but advises the patient that she must have realistic expectations of the outcome and he will not perform further surgeries. Code for the second surgery that Dr. Rosa performs today at Williton for a revision of the tip of the patient's nose.

Diagnosis code(s):_____

Procedure code(s): _____

6. Dakota Chapman, age 2, has a congenital obstruction of the nasolacrimal duct (which transports tears from the lacrimal sac to the nasal cavity). Dr. Kumar, an otolaryngologist specializing in pediatric cases, fractures the turbinates bilaterally and then repositions them. The surgery is successful.

Diagnosis code(s):_____

Procedure code(s): _____

ACCESSORY SINUSES (31000–31299)

The Accessory Sinuses subheading contains four categories that cover the types of procedures that the physician performs, including incision, excision, endoscopy, and other procedures (which contains only one code for an unlisted procedure of the accessory sinuses). Let's review more about how to assign codes for procedures in the first three categories and then practice coding. You can locate codes for accessory sinuses in the index by searching for the *body site* (sinus) or *type of procedure* (sinusoscopy). Turn to the codes in each category as you read more about them in the following sections.

Incision (31000–31090)

CPT divides the codes in the Incision category by:

lavage (luh- vahzh′)— washing, irrigation

- *Type of procedure*—**lavage**, sinusotomy
- *Location of procedure*—maxillary, frontal, sphenoid
- *Additional procedures performed*—removal of polyps, biopsy, osteoplastic flap
- *Approach of procedure*—intranasal, transorbital

Review the following Incision category procedures and their definitions to become more familiar with them:

ostium (äs′-tē-əm)

- *Lavage by cannulation; maxillary sinus (antrum puncture or natural ostium)* **(31000–31002)**—The physician irrigates the maxillary or sphenoid sinus by puncturing the antrum or creating an **ostium** (opening) to remove infected mucus that will not improve with antibiotics. Causes of the infection may include chronic sinusitis, a tooth infection that spread to the sinus, or trauma.

- *Sinusotomy* **(31020–31032, 31050–31090)**—A sinusotomy is an incision into the sinus to drain fluid build-up from sinusitis, remove an **osteoma** (benign neoplasm of the bone) or **mucocele**, or treat other conditions causing a sinus obstruction. There are different types of sinusotomies, depending on the patient's condition. It is important to be familiar with terms listed in code descriptors so that you can fully understand procedures and assign accurate codes. Here are some examples of terms listed in code descriptors for sinusotomies:

  - *Caldwell-Luc procedure* **(31030–31032)** —A procedure where the physician incises the patient's gum and bone to create an opening to the maxillary sinus to improve drainage for chronic sinusitis; remove **antrochoanal** (in the maxillary sinus) polyps, cysts, or lesions; and treat other conditions involving facial bones and sinuses.
  - *Trephine operation* **(31070)**—In this procedure, the physician uses a trephine to access the frontal sinus.

  Note that there are CPT coding guidelines throughout procedures in the Incision category, so be sure to review them before final code assignment. Also keep in mind that procedures in the Incision category do not involve an endoscope. If the physician performs a nasal or sinus endoscopy, then you will need to assign a code from the Endoscopy category (31231–31297). You will review these codes later in this chapter.

osteoma (äs-tē-ō′-mə)

mucocele (myü′-kə-sēl)— a sac of mucus

antrochoanal (an-trō-cha′-nəl)

Excision (31200-31230)

There are five codes in the Excision category, including variations of two procedures, ethmoidectomy and maxillectomy. An **ethmoidectomy** occurs when a physician opens the ethmoid sinus cavity to improve drainage of the ethmoid sinus and correct sinusitis or remove an obstruction. Note that there are three types of ethmoidectomy:

ethmoidectomy (eth-moi-dek′-tə-mē)

- Intranasal, anterior (31200)—The physician accesses the front (anterior) of the ethmoid sinus cavity and the procedure is done from the inside.
- Intranasal, total (31201)—The physician accesses both the front (anterior) and back (posterior) of the ethmoid sinus cavity and is done from the inside.
- Extranasal, total (31205)—The physician accesses the ethmoid sinus through the nasal dorsum (ridge of the nose) and medial canthus (corner of the eye where the upper and lower lids meet).

A **maxillectomy** is when a physician removes part or all of the maxilla (upper jaw bone), most commonly to remove a malignant neoplasm (31225-31230). The patient may then need a prosthetic to replace the missing bone. There are two types of maxillectomy:

maxillectomy (mak-sə-lek′-tə-mē)

- Without orbital exenteration (removal of an organ)—The physician does not remove the eyeball and surrounding tissue.
- With orbital exenteration (en bloc—all together)—The physician removes the eyeball and surrounding tissue.

CPT notes direct you to other codes when the physician only performs orbital exenteration without the maxillectomy or when the procedure involves skin grafts.

Codes in the Excision category do not include an endoscope.

Endoscopy (31231-31297)

Remember that there are two types of endoscopies, a *diagnostic* endoscopy, where the physician views the body structures through a fiberoptic flexible tube with a magnifier (endoscope) inserted into a body cavity or area, such as the nostrils, and a *surgical* endoscopy, where the physician views the body structures with an endoscope *and* also performs a procedure (to remove polyps, obtain a biopsy, or enlarge the sinuses). *Functional endoscopic sinus surgery* (FESS) describes procedures that physicians use to diagnose and treat nasal or sinus conditions by using an endoscope to view structures. Physicians also use CT scans of the sinus to help diagnose various conditions.

Remember that when the physician performs a surgical endoscopy, you only assign one code (surgical endoscopy) because the diagnostic endoscopy is already included. There are numerous CPT coding guidelines in the Endoscopy category that you should review before final code assignment. Notice that the guidelines in the beginning of the category alert you that a surgical sinus endoscopy includes a sinusotomy (if appropriate) and a diagnostic endoscopy.

The guidelines also state that a diagnostic evaluation (endoscopy) uses an endoscope to view the following areas:

meatus (mee-ey'-tuhs)

- nasal cavity
- middle and superior **meatus** (opening in the nasal cavity)
- turbinates
- spheno-ethmoid recess (opening of the sphenoidal sinus)

Assign only one CPT code for a diagnostic endoscopy, since the physician examines all of the areas listed. Do not report multiple codes for an endoscopy of each area.

The Endoscopy category includes two types of diagnostic endoscopies (31231–31235):

- Nasal endoscopy

sinusoscopy (sī-nus-os′kō-pē)—endoscopic exam of the sinus

- Nasal/sinus endoscopy—can include a maxillary or sphenoid **sinusoscopy**

A physician can perform a nasal or nasal/sinus diagnostic endoscopy in the office to determine the severity of a patient's infection or the cause of an obstruction.

Nasal/sinus surgical endoscopies (31237–31297) include a diagnostic endoscopy and may also include a biopsy, polypectomy, debridement, or control of nasal hemorrhage. Keep in mind that endoscopy procedures can be unilateral—affecting either the right or left side—or bilateral, affecting *both* the left and right sides. For example, code 31276 represents a surgical nasal/sinus endoscopy with *frontal sinus* exploration. If the physician performs the procedure on *both* the left frontal sinus and the right frontal sinus, then you should append modifier -50 to 31276 to show that the procedure is bilateral.

TAKE A BREAK

Good job! Let's take a break and review the accessory sinuses and then practice coding procedures.

Exercise 24.4 **Accessory Sinuses**

Part 1—Theory

Instructions: Fill in the blank with the best answer.

1. Name the four criteria that CPT uses to divides codes in the Incision category: 1)_____, 2) _____, 3)_____, 4)_____.

2. A _____ is an incision into the sinus to drain fluid build-up from sinusitis.

3. A procedure where the physician incises the patient's gum and bone to create an opening to the maxillary sinus to improve drainage for chronic sinusitis is called a _____ procedure.

4. In this procedure, the physician uses a trephine to access the frontal sinus: _____

5. In this type of ethmoidectomy, the physician accesses the ethmoid sinus through the nasal dorsum and medial canthus: _____

6. A _____ is a procedure where a physician removes part or all of the maxilla, most commonly to remove a malignant neoplasm.

Part 2—Coding

Instructions: Review each patient's case, then assign codes for the procedure(s), appending a modifier when appropriate. Optional: Assign the patient's diagnosis code(s) (ICD-9-CM).

1. At Williton Medical Center, Dr. Rosa, an ENT, irrigates the maxillary sinuses for James Cunningham, age 52, to treat chronic sinusitis.

   Diagnosis code(s): _____

   Procedure code(s):_____

2. Today at Williton, Dr. Rosa performs an intranasal total ethmoidectomy (excision of anterior and posterior ethmoid sinus cells, which form a honeycomb-shaped cavity) to drain mucus. The patient is Nora Williams, age 52, who suffers from chronic sinus infections.

   Diagnosis code(s): _____

   Procedure code(s):_____

TAKE A BREAK *continued*

3. Dr. Rosa performs an endoscopic **antrostomy** (a procedure to open the maxillary sinus) to drain fluid due to maxillary sinusitis for Norma Fields, age 63.

   Diagnosis code(s): _____

   Procedure code(s): _____

4. Jake Bradley, a 28-year-old, sees Dr. Rosa for a left transorbital frontal sinusotomy (a procedure to open the sinus) to treat acute frontal sinusitis.

   Diagnosis code(s): _____

   Procedure code(s): _____

5. In his office, Dr. Rosa performs a bilateral nasal endoscopy for Lavelle Armstrong, age 33, because he has severe nasal congestion and facial pain. Dr. Rosa finds nasal polyps and excises them.

   Diagnosis code(s): _____

   Procedure code(s): _____

6. Dr. Rosa performs a bilateral diagnostic nasal endoscopy in his office for Gerald Grame, age 46. He diagnoses the patient with acute sinusitis and prescribes an antibiotic.

   Diagnosis code(s): _____

   Procedure code(s): _____

antrostomy (an-träs′-tə-mē)

LARYNX (31300–31599)

The subheading Larynx contains six different categories that cover the types of procedures that the physician performs on the larynx (voice box). The larynx plays a role in breathing and swallowing and creates an airway to the lungs. It is made up of bones and muscles. The larynx contains two pair of mucous membranes, the upper and lower vocal cords, or vocal folds. The lower pair are called *true vocal cords* and vibrate when the lungs exhale air to create speech and singing. The upper pair are called *false vocal cords* and do not produce sound. During swallowing, the vocal cords prevent food from entering the trachea and lungs.

CPT lists the following six categories in the Larynx subheading:

1. Excision
2. Introduction
3. Endoscopy
4. Repair
5. Destruction
6. Other Procedures—contains one code for an unlisted procedure of the larynx.

You will next learn more about procedures in the first five categories. Turn to the codes in each category as you read more about them in the following sections.

Excision (31300–31420)

The Excision category contains 14 codes for six different procedures. CPT categorizes the procedures by type (e.g., laryngotomy, laryngectomy), which other procedures were performed at the same time, and the approach (e.g., horizontal, anterovertical). Review the following procedures from the Excision category to learn more about how and why physicians perform them:

- **Laryngotomy** (31300–31320)—A laryngotomy is an incision into the larynx to remove a tumor or **laryngocele**, an air or liquid sac in the larynx that may be congenital or acquired. The laryngotomy may also be diagnostic, where the physician examines the laryngeal structures to diagnose a condition.

  laryngotomy (lar-ən-gät′-ə-mē)
  laryngocele (lə-riŋ′-gə-sēl)

  - A physician may also perform a laryngotomy as a life-saving measure for a patient whose larynx is obstructed by trauma.
  - A **thyrotomy**, or **laryngofissure** (31300), is an incision through the larynx and thyroid cartilage.

    thyrotomy (thī-rät′-ə-mē)
    laryngofissure (lə-riŋ′-gō-fish-ər)

  - A **cordectomy** (31300) is the surgical removal of a vocal cord.

    cordectomy (kor-dek′-tə-mē)

laryngectomy
(lə-riŋ-jek′-tə-mē)

- **Laryngectomy** (31360–31368)—A laryngectomy is the partial or total surgical excision of the larynx, most commonly to remove laryngeal cancer when chemotherapy and/or radiation are unsuccessful. A physician may also perform a laryngectomy following trauma to the larynx.

  - In a *total* laryngectomy, the physician removes the entire larynx. The procedure may also include a radical neck dissection (removal of lymphatic tissue and the internal jugular vein, covered in more detail in Chapter 26). After a total laryngectomy, the patient can no longer breathe through his mouth, so the physician creates a **stoma** (round opening, or mouth) in the patient's neck and attaches the stoma to the trachea. The patient breathes through the stoma.

stoma (stō′-mə)

aryepiglottic
(ar-ē-ep-ə-glät′-ik)

  - A *subtotal supraglottic* laryngectomy (SSL) involves removing structures of the supraglottic larynx, including the epiglottis, false vocal cords, **aryepiglottic** folds (located at the larynx entrance), and part of the thyroid cartilage.

hemilaryngectomy
(hem-i-lə-riŋ-jek′-tə-mē)

  - A *partial* laryngectomy, also called a **hemilaryngectomy** (31370–31382), is when the physician removes the right or left half of the larynx, but the patient is still able to breathe, swallow, and speak after the procedure. CPT arranges partial laryngectomies by the body sites resected (e.g., horizontal, laterovertical), so be sure to carefully read medical documentation to ensure that you assign the correct code.

pharyngolaryngectomy
(fə-riŋ′-gō-lar-ən-jek-tə-mē)

- **Pharyngolaryngectomy** (31390–31395)—A procedure to excise the larynx and pharynx, most commonly to treat malignant neoplasms, but physicians can also perform the procedure to treat traumatic injuries or other conditions. Depending on the extent of cancer metastasis, the physician may also remove a section of the patient's esophagus, thyroid gland, and parathyroid glands.

  - After a pharyngolaryngectomy, patients may need additional procedures to reconstruct the areas of the neck that the physician removed, including skin grafts and grafts from the intestine to replace excised esophageal structures.

  - As with a total laryngectomy, the patient will have a stoma in the neck. A pharyngolaryngectomy may also include a radical neck dissection (a procedure to excise lymphatic tissue, veins, and nerves), with or without reconstruction.

arytenoidectomy
(ar-ə-tē-noi-dek′-tə-mē)
arytenoidopexy
(ar-ət-ə-noid′-ə-pek-sē)

- **Arytenoidectomy** *or* **arytenoidopexy**, external approach (31400)—Procedures to excise, or perform surgical fixation, of the arytenoid cartilage or muscle. The arytenoid muscle is made up of fibers between arytenoid cartilage, which is attached to the vocal cords, allowing them to move. Physicians perform the procedure externally (without using an endoscope) or endoscopically (code 31560) for patients with bilateral vocal cord paralysis (BVCP) or any conditions that inhibit vocal cord movement, such as infection, malignant neoplasms, injury from previous surgery, or injury after intubation.

epiglottidectomy
(ep-ə-glät-əd-ek′-tə-mē)
glossectomy (gläs-ek′-tə-mē)

- **Epiglottidectomy** (31420)—A procedure to excise part or all of the epiglottis to treat obstructive sleep apnea, malignant neoplasm, or other conditions. Physicians may also perform a **glossectomy** (an excision of part or all of the tongue) at the same time if they are treating metastatic cancer.

Introduction (31500–31502)

The Introduction category contains two codes:

- *Intubation, endotracheal, emergency procedure (31500)*—Recall that intubation is a procedure where the physician inserts a flexible tube into the patient's mouth and down into the trachea. The tube is called an endotracheal tube (ET) (Figure 20-2), and is attached to a ventilator that provides oxygen to the patient, called *artificial respiration*. An ET helps the patient breathe during a surgical procedure with general anesthesia, or in cases when the patient suffers from an *emergent condition*, such as trauma or disease, and cannot breathe independently. **Extubation** is the process of removing the ET from the patient's throat.

extubation (ek-stü-bā′-shən)

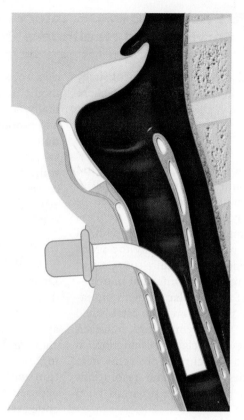

FIGURE 24-4 ■ Tracheotomy tube placement.
Source: Blamb/Shutterstock.com.

- **Tracheotomy** *tube change prior to establishment of fistula tract (31502)*—A tracheotomy is an incision through the neck into the trachea to place a breathing tube, called a tracheotomy tube, which enables the patient to breathe through the tube when he cannot breathe unassisted (■ FIGURE 24-4).

  tracheotomy (trā-kē-ät′-ə-mē)

  - Physicians perform tracheotomies to clear the airway prior to throat surgery, as patients may experience postsurgical edema that makes it difficult or impossible for them to breathe until the edema subsides.

  - Physicians may also perform a tracheotomy emergently for patients who are unable to breathe due to traumatic injury, edema, or hematoma, or who have obstructive sleep apnea or malignant neoplasms.

  - The tracheotomy tube remains in the patient's throat as long as the patient requires it to breathe. Clinicians must periodically change the tube because it can become occluded with mucus.

  - The physician may also create a fistula tract for placing a tracheotomy tube if there is not enough room to insert it otherwise.

  - Do not confuse a tracheotomy with a **tracheostomy**, the creation of an opening, or stoma, in the trachea for a tracheostomy tube. A tracheostomy is a different procedure and is typically more permanent than a tracheotomy. You will learn more about tracheostomies later in this text.

    tracheostomy (trā-kē-äst′-ə-mē)

Endoscopy (31505–31579)

In a **laryngoscopy**, a physician diagnoses and/or treats conditions of the larynx. It may include using an laryngoscope or other instrument to view structures of the larynx, including the glottis and vocal folds. Laryngoscopy is the only procedure in the Endoscopy category. A physician may perform a larygoscopy to remove foreign bodies or diagnose swallowing, breathing, and bleeding disorders; voice problems; or throat pain.

laryngoscopy (lar-ən-gäs′-kə-pē)

POINTERS FROM THE PROS: Interview with a Director of Patient Financial Services and Healthcare Consultant

You first read advice from Trish Zubritzky in Chapter 14. She has additional information to share with you.

As the director of patient financial services, describe the types and frequency of your interactions with coding staff.

(It) was a daily occurrence, both of an informal and formal nature. Daily communication was essential to managing my facility's claims production. If a particular problem with a physician or system process occurred, a formal meeting might be called with all necessary participants to review and rectify the problem quickly. But I'd say most of the daily contact and problem resolution was more of an informal nature—one-on-one discussions of a particular problem or reason a claim(s) was being held beyond the established system hold days. Formal monthly meetings, however, were critical in managing clean claims production on an ongoing basis. Patterns or recurrent problems were addressed with all parties involved and resolutions sought to eliminate and prevent the situation from occurring again.

As a healthcare consultant, describe how you educated clients and whom you educated.

General instruction was sometimes necessary to better familiarize hospital and office staff with CPT/HCPCS coding and governmental regulations. This general overview was designed to eliminate any staff misconceptions as well as improve understanding they might already have. Training occurred both informally, as we discussed their departmental processes and problems, as well as formally in classroom instruction with a set agenda and training material. Facility-specific education sessions were also often done to train clients on their newly designed workflow processes and restructured charge methodologies. These education sessions were conducted with front-line staff, supervisors, management and physicians.

What advice can you give to individuals working in billing and collections who want to transition to coding?

Do it! Your experience with billing and collections will definitely help you. You already understand the impact of compliant and noncompliant coding. You've probably researched more than one denied or rejected claim and found it was because of a coding (or charging) inaccuracy of some sort. Your subsequent interaction with coding staff to rectify these claims has exposed you to the expanse of codes and intricacies of code assignment. The biggest obstacle you might face may be some of the advanced medical terminology utilized and depth of anatomy you need to know, but I found that was easily overcome by hard work. And hard work is something I know all dedicated billing and collection staff understand fully and can do!

(Used by permission of Patricia Zubritzky.)

CPT arranges codes by the type of laryngoscopy that the physician performs (e.g., indirect, direct), along with other procedures that the physician performs during the same encounter (e.g., biopsy, removal of foreign body, reconstruction). The type of laryngoscopy also depends on the type of laryngoscope that the physician uses.

In an **indirect laryngoscopy,** the physician holds a mirror in the back of the patient's throat and shines a light into the throat (attached to the physician's headpiece) to view laryngeal structures. The physician performs the procedure in his office, and the patient is not under anesthesia during the procedure. In a **direct laryngoscopy,** the patient is anesthetized with local or general anesthesia, and the physician looks directly at the larynx through a laryngoscope, inserting it into the mouth or nose to see the larynx.

Laryngoscopies can be either diagnostic or surgical. Remember that a surgical laryngoscopy always includes a diagnostic laryngoscopy, so you should never separately report a diagnostic laryngoscopy in addition to a surgical one.

Notice that the first five procedures in the Endoscopy category are for different types of *indirect* laryngoscopies:

- diagnostic
- with biopsy
- with removal of foreign body
- with removal of lesion

- with vocal cord injection (injection of material, such as collagen, to improve conditions like vocal cord paralysis, restore weakened muscles, improve the voice, and enable the patient to successfully swallow liquids)

Review the following example for coding a laryngoscopy.

Example: Mrs. Weaver brings her son Edward, age 2, to Williton's ED because he is gagging and his voice is hoarse. Dr. Daniels, the ED physician, examines the patient and calls in Dr. Greene, an otolaryngologist, who recommends a laryngoscopy. The patient receives anesthesia, and Dr. Greene performs a direct laryngoscopy, discovers a thumbtack stuck in the patient's vocal folds, and removes it. The patient recovers from the procedure without any complications.

To locate a code for this procedure, search the index for the main term *laryngoscopy* and subterm *direct*, which leads you to 31515–31571. Cross-reference the codes in the Respiratory System subsection, and you will find that code **31530** includes removal of a foreign body, which is the correct code to assign. The patient's diagnosis code is **933.1** (*foreign body, entering through orifice, larynx*).

Repair (31580–31590)

The Repair category includes five codes for different types of a **laryngoplasty** (surgical repair of the larynx), including a laryngoplasty

laryngoplasty
(lǝ-riŋ´-gǝ-plas-tē)

- *for laryngeal web, 2-stage, with keel insertion and removal*—A laryngeal web is a congenital disorder where a webbed membrane spreads between the vocal folds, causing stridor (high-pitched wheezing), hoarseness, or **aphonia** (no voice). To treat a laryngeal web, the physician divides the web and then inserts a keel stent in the vocal folds to stop the web from forming again. The two-stage procedure includes both the insertion and subsequent removal of the stent.

aphonia (ā-fō´-nē-ǝ)

- *for laryngeal stenosis, with graft or core mold, including tracheotomy*— Laryngeal stenosis, which can be congenital or acquired, is narrowing of the larynx. Acquired laryngeal stenosis is typically due to intubation or trauma. Physicians can remove tissue or scars that cause stenosis and perform grafting or construct a stent mold to repair the defect.

- *with open reduction of fracture*—The physician repairs a laryngeal fracture.

- *cricoid split.* The physician incises cricoid cartilage (ring-shaped cartilage at the larynx base) to open the airway. The procedure treats subglottic (below the glottis) stenosis, a disorder that can be congenital or acquired.

- *not otherwise specified (for burns, reconstruction after partial laryngectomy)*

The last procedure in the Repair category is for ***Laryngeal reinnervation by neuromuscular pedicle.*** Physicians perform it to treat laryngeal **dystonia**, a neuromuscular disorder, which causes the patient to speak in a whispered or strained voice, or to treat vocal fold paralysis. The physician utilizes a neuromuscular pedicle to reinnervate (restore nerves) to the affected area and restore the patient's voice.

dystonia (dis-tō´-nē-ǝ)

Destruction (31595)

There is only one code in the Destruction category for ***Section recurrent laryngeal nerve, therapeutic (separate procedure), unilateral.*** The recurrent laryngeal nerve is part of the **vagus** nerve, a cranial nerve that creates movement in the larynx. (You will learn more about cranial nerves in Chapter 30). The physician sections (incises) the recurrent laryngeal nerve to treat disorders like spastic **dysphonia**, a neurological condition, which causes the patient to have a strained, low-pitched voice.

vagus (vā´-gǝs)

dysphonia (dis-fō´-nē-ǝ)

TAKE A BREAK

Wow! That was a lot of area to cover! Let's take a break and review the larynx and then practice coding procedures.

Exercise 24.5 Larynx

Part 1—Theory

Instructions: Fill in the blank with the best answer.

1. A _____ is a life-saving measure for a patient whose larynx is obstructed by trauma.

2. A procedure to excise the larynx and pharynx, most commonly to treat malignant neoplasms, is called a(n) _____.

3. A _____ is an incision through the neck into the trachea to place a breathing tube, called a _____.

4. In an _____ the physician holds a mirror in the back of the patient's throat and shines a light into the throat to view laryngeal structures.

5. A _____ is a congenital disorder where a webbed membrane spreads between the vocal folds, causing stridor, hoarseness, or aphonia.

6. _____, which can be congenital or acquired, is narrowing of the larynx.

Part 2—Coding

Instructions: Review each patient's case, then assign codes for the procedure(s), appending a modifier to the procedure when appropriate. Optional: For additional practice, assign the patient's diagnosis code(s) (ICD-9-CM).

1. Dr. Kelly, a pediatric ENT, performs an arytenoidectomy using an external approach at Williton Medical Center for Nathan Wheeler, age 11. The patient has suffered from aphonia for several years, which his physicians hoped would resolve. Because it did not, his parents opted for surgery. Dr. Kelly diagnoses the patient with partial BVCP of idiopathic etiology (unknown cause).

   Diagnosis code(s): _____

   Procedure code(s): _____

2. An ambulance transports Ralph Elliot, age 58, to Williton Medical Center's ED because he cannot breathe. Mr. Elliot was involved in a motor vehicle accident where he was the passenger in a car his wife was driving. They rear-ended a pick-up truck on the highway, and Mr. Elliot was ejected from the vehicle. Dr. Mills, the ED physician, immediately assesses the patient, along with the trauma team, and determines that he has acute respiratory failure. He intubates the patient, places him on a ventilator, and proceeds with further workup.

   Diagnosis code(s): _____

   Procedure code(s): _____

3. Today at Williton, Dr. Rosa performs a total laryngectomy with radical neck dissection for Mario Garzinini, age 62, a lifelong smoker who has been diagnosed with squamous cell carcinoma of the larynx metastasized to the skeletal muscles.

   Diagnosis code(s): _____

   Procedure code(s): _____

4. Gene Alvarez, age 47, has obstructive sleep apnea and is also obese. Today at Williton, Dr. Rosa performs a planned tracheostomy to treat the sleep apnea.

   Code(s) _____

5. Dr. Hoffman refers Jerome Burton, age 54, to Dr. Rosa. Dr. Rosa sees Mr. Burton in his office and the patient states, "I can't stop coughing and always feel that there is a lump in my throat." Dr. Rosa examines the patient and also notes that his voice is hoarse. He schedules a direct laryngoscopy today at Williton, where he excises a tumor and strips the vocal cords. The pathology report confirms carcinoma of the larynx. Code for today's procedure at Williton.

   Diagnosis code(s): _____

   Procedure code(s): _____

6. Mr. Peters brings his daughter, Sally, age 3, to Williton's ED because she continues to grab her throat and complain that she feels like "someone's choking me." After examining the patient, Dr. Mills calls Dr. Kelly, who subsequently performs a direct diagnostic laryngoscopy and then removes a dime from the laryngeal folds. Sally recovers from the procedure without complications.

   Diagnosis code(s): _____

   Procedure code(s): _____

TRACHEA AND BRONCHI (31600–31899)

The Trachea and Bronchi subheading contains five different categories of codes based on the types of procedure that the physician performs on the trachea or bronchi, including:

1. Incision
2. Endoscopy

3. Introduction

4. Excision, Repair

5. Other Procedures—contains one code for an unlisted procedure of the trachea or bronchi

You will next learn how to assign codes for procedures in the first four categories. Refer to the definitions of trachea and bronchi in the beginning of this chapter, along with anatomy diagrams, if you need to better understand them. You can locate codes for trachea and bronchi procedures by searching the index for *trachea* or *bronchi* and then the *type of procedure*, or begin your search with the *type of procedure*. Turn to the codes in each category as you read more about them in the following sections.

Incision (31600–31614)

The Incision category includes five codes for three types of tracheostomy, a procedure to create an opening (stoma) in the trachea to insert a tracheostomy tube (also called a trach tube) to enable the patient to breathe. The tracheostomy tube may connect to a ventilator to provide artificial respiration. A tracheostomy can be temporary or permanent. Physicians perform tracheostomies for patients who have an obstructed airway (due to foreign body, trauma, or edema), respiratory failure, or to suction excessive mucus built up in the airway. An emergency medical technician (EMT) or paramedic may also perform a life-saving tracheostomy on a trauma patient whose injuries have damaged the patient's airway.

There are three types of tracheostomies:

1. **Planned** (31600, 31601)—tracheostomy that the physician performs for patients (including those who are younger than two years old) who are unable to breathe on their own due to diseases. Some of the conditions that can interfere with breathing are CHF, cystic fibrosis (an inherited condition where thick mucus forms in the lungs, eventually causing death from respiratory failure; the disease also affects other organs, but many patients affected by it can live into their 30s, 40s, or 50s) and emphysema. The patient may have been previously intubated and connected to a ventilator but may have experienced problems with intubation, such as laryngotracheal stenosis, infection, and edema. The physician can then extubate the patient, perform a tracheostomy, and connect the patient's trach tube to a ventilator.

   Did you notice that the code descriptor for a planned tracheostomy includes *separate procedure*? This means that if the physician performs another procedure at the same time as the tracheostomy, you should only code the tracheostomy if it is distinct and separate from the other procedure. For example, if the physician performs a procedure involving the trachea or a body site near it and also performs a tracheostomy, then you *should not* assign a separate code for the tracheostomy because it is a *related* procedure.

   However, if the physician performs another procedure on a completely different body site, such as the abdomen, then you should separately code the tracheostomy. Do you remember which modifier you should append to the tracheostomy code when it is a separate procedure? If you guessed modifier -59, then you are correct! Appending modifier -59 will ensure that the payer will understand that the tracheostomy was a separate procedure, and the insurance should separately pay it.

2. **Emergency procedure** (31603, 31605)—tracheostomy that the physician performs to save a patient's life, due to conditions like respiratory failure, foreign body occlusion, or traumatic injury. Notice that there are two types of emergency tracheostomy: *transtracheal* (across the trachea) and *cricothyroid membrane* (also called a **crycothyrotomy**). The transtracheal is the most common type because a crycothyrotomy can injure the patient and cause possible permanent vocal cord injury.

   crycothyrotomy
   (cri-co-thy-rot′-o-mē)

3. **Fenestration procedure with skin flaps** (also called inferior tracheal flaps or Bjork flaps)—tracheostomy where the physician removes part of the tracheal cartilage, creating flaps, which he sutures to the skin to ensure the stoma remains open. This procedure is common for patients who require a permanent stoma, such as those with sleep apnea.

Payers have different global periods for tracheostomy procedures, so be sure to check individual payer guidelines for more specific information.

The Incision category also includes three additional procedures:

alaryngeal (ā-lä·rin′je·əl)—without a larynx

prosthesis (präs-thē′-səs)

- *Construction of tracheoesophageal fistula to insert an **alaryngeal** speech prosthesis*—A **prosthesis** is an artificial device that replaces a missing part. The physician creates a fistula between the trachea and esophagus and inserts a speech prosthesis for a patient who had a total laryngectomy. The prosthesis enables the patient to speak again.

- *Tracheal puncture with aspiration and/or injection*—The physician punctures the trachea with a needle and inserts a catheter to aspirate a fluid sample for lab testing or can inject a medication to treat a specific condition, such as a malignancy.

- *Tracheostoma revision*—The physician reconstructs a stoma that developed scar tissue or stenosis. The procedure can be simple or complex, depending on whether the procedure involves a rotation flap.

Endoscopy (31615–31656)

The Endoscopy category includes three different procedures:

tracheobronchoscopy (tra-cheo-brong-käs′kah-pe)

- **Tracheobronchoscopy** (31615)—The physician inserts an endoscope through an established tracheostomy incision to view the trachea and bronchi. The procedure helps to diagnose reasons for tracheal stenosis, including benign or malignant neoplasms.

- *Endobronchial ultrasound (EBUS)* (31620, an add-on code)—This procedure is done to diagnose diseases like lung cancer or disorders or infections that cause lymph nodes in the chest to become enlarged. The procedure involves using an ultrasound catheter probe to image body structures.

bronchoscopy (brän-käs′-kə-pē)

- *Bronchoscopy* (31622–31656)—This procedure is discussed next.

Bronchoscopy is the process of inserting a bronchoscope (endoscope) into the mouth or nose. The physician, who is typically a thoracic surgeon or pulmonologist, can view the larynx, trachea, lungs, and bronchi (■ FIGURE 24-5). Through an aspirating needle attached to the bronchoscope, the physician may obtain tissue samples from various body sites, called *transbronchial needle aspiration*. An ultrasound probe, or processor, is also attached to the bronchoscope and can send ultrasound waves into specific body areas.

Ultrasound is a radiology imaging method for viewing various structures, including internal organs, muscles, joints, and tendons, using sound waves. The physician sees the images on a screen. You probably know that pregnant women have ultrasound tests to determine fetal development and discover disorders. If the physician finds an abnormality on the ultrasound image, then she will take a tissue or fluid sample biopsy from the body site and send it to a pathologist for testing.

hemoptysis (hi-mäp′-tə-səs)

lumen (lü′-mən)

There are two types of bronchoscope: rigid and flexible. The physician uses a rigid bronchoscope during medical emergencies, when patients have **hemoptysis** (coughing and spitting up blood). A *rigid* bronchoscope has a larger channel, or **lumen**, which allows the physician to suction excess blood and utilize additional instruments, such as electrocautery, to achieve hemostasis. The *flexible* bronchoscope is the most commonly used, with a thinner and longer lumen. Physicians still use it for suctioning or for other purposes.

The majority of procedures in the Endoscopy category are for bronchoscopy. Notice the CPT guidelines at the beginning of the Endoscopy category, which state that you should code the endoscopy for each body site the physician examines. The guidelines also remind you that a surgical endoscopy always includes a diagnostic endoscopy when the same physician performs both procedures. In addition, it is important to note that many bronchoscopy codes include fluoroscopy when the physician performs it, so you should not separately code for fluoroscopy.

Review the bronchoscopy code descriptors (31622–31656), and note that bronchoscopies can include many different types of procedures, like brushing—placing a brush at the end of a bronchoscope to collect cells for pathology testing (31623), placing catheters to deliver radiation treatment (31643), injecting contrast (dye) for a radiology

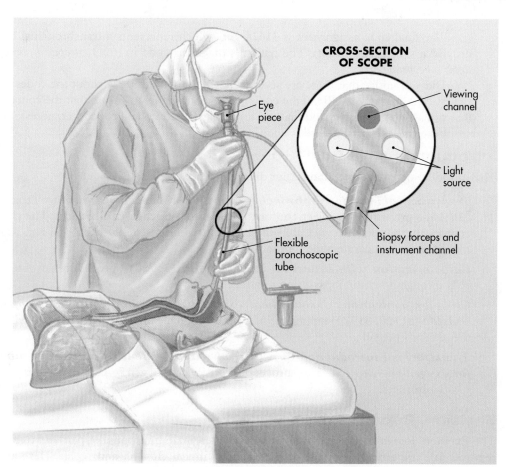

Figure 24-5 ■ A physician uses a bronchoscope during a bronchoscopy.

procedure (31656—assign the radiology procedure code separately), and performing lung biopsy (31628)—read the operative report closely to determine exactly where the physician took a biopsy to ensure correct code assignment. You can also query the physician if you are unsure after reading the documentation.

Review the following example for coding a bronchoscopy with biopsy.

Example: Dr. Lightner, a pulmonologist at Williton Medical Center, performs a bronchoscopy with a transbronchial lung biopsy of the right upper lobe for Mr. Sims, age 53, for a lung mass. Dr. Lightner sends the biopsy to the pathology department, and the pathologist determines that the patient has lung carcinoma.

To locate a code for this procedure, search the index for *endoscopy*, subterm *bronchi*, and subterm *biopsy*, and you will find two code ranges: 31625–31629 and 31632–31633. Cross-reference the codes in the Respiratory System subsection, and you will find that

- Code 31625 includes a *bronchial or endobronchial biopsy*, but Dr. Lightner performed a *transbronchial* biopsy.

- Code 31626 includes *placement of fiducial markers*, which was *not* part of the procedure.

- Code 31627 includes *computer-assisted, image-guided navigation*, which was *not* documented.

- Code 31628 includes a *transbronchial biopsy* of a *single lobe*. This code looks promising.

- Code 31629 is also a *transbronchial biopsy* code, *but* it represents a biopsy *by needle aspiration*, which was *not* part of the procedure.

- Codes 31632 and 31633 are add-on codes for *each additional lobe* biopsied, including by needle aspiration. If Dr. Lightner biopsied more than one lobe, then you would report one of these codes.

The final code assignment is **31628-RT**, which represents a transbronchial biopsy of a single lobe (right). The patient's diagnosis code is **162.3** (*neoplasm, lung, upper lobe, primary*).

Did you notice that there are several CPT coding notes throughout the codes in the Endoscopy category? Read the coding notes thoroughly to ensure that the code(s) that you assign are correct and that you also assign an additional code when necessary.

Introduction (31715-31730)

The Introduction category contains four different procedures:

- *Transtracheal injection for bronchography* (X-ray of the lower respiratory tract) (31715)—procedure to inject contrast dye into the trachea and bronchi. The dye enables the physician to see abnormal structures more clearly on the X-ray. You should assign a separate code for the X-ray.
- *Catheterization with bronchial brush biopsy* (31717)—procedure to obtain cells through a brush biopsy using a catheter.
- *Catheter aspiration; nasotracheal or tracheobronchial with fiberscope, bedside* (31720, 31725)—drainage of fluid through a catheter can be performed at the patient's bedside.
- *Transtracheal introduction of needle wire dilator/stent or indwelling tube for oxygen therapy* (31730)—procedure to delivery oxygen to patients with respiratory disorders.

Excision, Repair (31750–31830)

The Excision, Repair category contains several codes, including wound repair and tumor removal. You are already familiar with excision, surgical closure, and repair. Here are examples of some of them:

tracheoplasty
(trā′-kē-ə-plas-tē)

- **Tracheoplasty**—surgical repair of the trachea to treat disorders like tracheal stenosis or airway collapse. The surgeon may use materials such as mesh to strengthen areas of the trachea that have been weakened by disease or incised to correct stenosis.

bronchoplasty
(bräη′-kə-plas-tē)

- **Bronchoplasty**—surgical repair of the bronchus to close a bronchial fistula or remove a bronchial lesion.
- *Excision of tracheal tumor or carcinoma*
- *Surgical closure of tracheostomy or fistula*
- *Repair of tracheostomy scar*

TAKE A BREAK

Nice work! Let's take a break to review the trachea and bronchi and then practice coding procedures.

Exercise 24.6   **Trachea and Bronchi**

Part 1—Theory

Instructions: Fill in the blank with the best answer. Refer to your CPT manual when necessary.

1. What codes are available to report a tracheostomy that the physician performs to save a patient's life, due to conditions like respiratory failure? _____

2. When a patient has a total laryngectomy, the physician creates a _____ between the trachea and esophagus and inserts a speech prosthesis.

3. What codes are you permitted to report first, before reporting add-on code 31620?

4. A _____ is when the physician reconstructs a stoma that developed scar tissue or stenosis.

5. Should you ever report a radiology code in addition to code 31715? If so, which code(s)?

6. What are the two types of bronchoscopies?

Part 2—Coding

Instructions: Review the patient's case and then assign the appropriate procedure code(s), appending a modifier when appropriate. Optional: Assign the patient's diagnosis code(s) (ICD-9-CM).

TAKE A BREAK *continued*

1. Joseph McCoy, age 58, had a tracheostomy tube placed previously due to acute respiratory arrest. His respiratory status has improved over the last year and he no longer needs the tracheostomy. Today at Williton, Dr. Rosa, an ENT, closes the tracheostomy without plastic repair.

   Diagnosis code(s): _____

   Procedure code(s): _____

2. Kathy Fernandez, age 38, has a chronic cough and chest pain. Today at Williton, Dr. Rosa performs a bronchoscopy with endobronchial biopsies of the right upper and lower lobes. The pathology report shows acute bronchitis.

   Diagnosis code(s): _____

   Procedure code(s): _____

3. Nelson Sims, age 32, arrives at Williton Medical Center by ambulance after a motor vehicle accident on Highway 9. Mr. Sims' car, which he was driving, crossed over the center line and hit another car head-on. The trauma team assesses the patient, who experiences hemoptysis, and Dr. Johnston, a pulmonologist, inserts a rigid bronchoscope and then suctions blood from the patient's lungs.

   Diagnosis code(s): _____

   Procedure code(s): _____

4. Lyn Wong, age 63, had a total laryngectomy for laryngeal squamous cell carcinoma. Today at Williton, Dr. Rosa constructs a tracheoesophageal fistula to place an alaryngeal speech prosthesis. Code for today's procedure.

   Diagnosis code(s): _____

   Procedure code(s): _____

5. In Williton's ED, Dr. Rosa performs an emergency transtracheal tracheostomy for Eduardo Mendoza, age 72, who suffers from respiratory failure.

   Diagnosis code(s): _____

   Procedure code(s): _____

6. Dr. Rosa reconstructs a tracheostoma for Harvey Hanson, age 68. His stoma has extensive scarring, which Dr. Rosa removes. The procedure involves a rotation flap.

   Diagnosis code(s): _____

   Procedure code(s): _____

LUNGS AND PLEURA (32035–32999)

The Lungs and Pleura subheading contains 10 different categories of codes based on the type of procedure that the physician performs, including incision, excision, removal, introduction, destruction, endoscopy, repair, transplantation, surgical collapse therapy, and other procedures. You can locate codes for the lungs and pleura by searching the index for the body site and then the type of procedure, or start your search with the type of procedure. Turn to the codes in the Lungs and Pleura subheading as we discuss them in ■ TABLE 24-3 so that you can become more familiar with them.

Lung Transplantation (32850–32856)

CPT includes codes for **lung transplants**, where the physician removes a diseased lung from a patient and replaces it with a donor lung from a cadaver (called an allograft). Clinicians carefully screen donor lungs to ensure that they are healthy enough to be used for a transplant. Let's review more about the interesting process of lung transplants before we look at the available procedure codes.

WORKPLACE IQ

You are working in Dr. Lightner's office as a coding auditor. One of your job duties is to investigate insurance claim denials involving incorrect codes. Today, you review an insurance denial for a claim where code 31628 was reported four times to indicate that Dr. Lightner performed four lung biopsies. The patient had insurance coverage for this procedure, but you need to determine why the insurance did not pay.

What would you do?

■ **TABLE 24-3   EXAMPLES OF PROCEDURES IN THE LUNGS AND PLEURA SUBHEADING**

Category	Procedure	Description
Incision	*Thoracostomy* (thōr-ə-'käs-tə-mē)	A chest tube or intercostal catheter is inserted into the pleural space to remove a pleural effusion, **empyema** (pus in the pleural space), or pneumothorax (air or gas in the pleural space).
	Thoracotomy (thōr-ə-'kät-ə-mē)	An incision is made into the pleural space to perform procedures on the heart and lungs, including removing neoplasms and foreign bodies and performing a biopsy.
Excision	*Pleurectomy, parietal* (plu-'rek-tə-mē)	The parietal pleura is excised to treat pleural effusion, traumatic injuries, and pleural **mesothelioma** (carcinoma, typically caused by exposure to asbestos).
	Biopsy, lung	A biopsy is done to remove tissue from the lung for pathological exam. The physician may use a bronchoscope or a needle (to remove the tissue using imaging guidance), perform an open biopsy (incision into the lungs to remove tissue), or use a thoracoscope (endoscope in the thoracic cavity).
Removal	*Pneumocentesis* (n(y)ü-mə-sen-'tē-səs)	The physician punctures the lung to withdraw fluid from the lung, which may have built up due to a traumatic injury.
	Thoracentesis (thō-rə-sen-'tē-səs)	Also called thoracocentesis or pleural tap, this procedure withdraws air or fluid from the pleural space in the thorax. The air or fluid may have built up due to conditions such as cancer, pneumonia, pneumothorax (air or gas in the pleural space), hemothorax (blood in the pleural space) or CHF. The procedure may involve inserting a chest tube for draining or using suction.
	Pneumonectomy (n(y)ü-mə-'nek-tə-mē)	This is excision of a lung, typically to remove a malignant neoplasm. (A lobectomy is removal of a lobe of the lung, and a wedge resection is removal of a lung segment.)
Introduction and Removal	Insertion of indwelling tunneled pleural catheter with cuff	A catheter is inserted into the pleural space for removing fluid, with a cuff to hold it in position.
Destruction	Installation of agent for *pleurodesis* (plu-'räd-ə-səs)	The physician inserts a substance, such as providone iodine, into the pleural space to reduce fluid accumulation from pleural effusion.
Endoscopy	*Thoracoscopy, diagnostic* (thōr-ə-'käs-kə-pē)	The physician performs an endoscopy of the thorax and pleural cavity to view the chest and lungs and diagnose conditions like carcinoma or empyema.
Repair	Repair lung hernia through chest wall	Repair of a hernia of the lung, which is a rare condition.
Lung Transplantation	Lung transplant, single or double	All or part of a lung is replaced with a healthy donor lung. We will review additional information about lung transplants in the next section.
Surgical Collapse Therapy; Thoracoplasty	*Thoracoplasty* ('thōr-ə-kō-plas-tē)	The thorax is repaired to treat conditions like scoliosis (abnormal curvature of the spine), which can cause a hump to form in the thoracic vertebra, or to treat thoracic empyema.
	Pneumonolysis (n(y)ü-mə-'näl-ə-səs)	This procedure is done to collapse diseased cavities of the lungs to allow the lung to heal faster. It was a former treatment for tuberculosis.
Other Procedures	Total lung lavage	To wash out, or irrigate, protein deposits from the lung, which disorders like pulmonary alveolar proteinosis (PAP) can cause.

empyema (em-pī- ē'-mə)

mesothelioma (mēz -ə-thē-lē- ō'-mə)

Lung transplants are for patients who are likely to die from lung disease within one to two years. Their conditions are so severe that other treatments, such as medicines or breathing devices, no longer work. Lung transplants are a last resort treatment for people who have no other options for treatment of severe disease, such as

- *COPD*—the most common reason why adult patients need lung transplants. COPD is a progressive disease which exacerbates over time and makes it difficult for patients to breathe.

- *Idiopathic pulmonary fibrosis (IPF)*—a condition where tissue deep in the lungs becomes thick and stiff, or scarred, over time.

- *Cystic fibrosis (CF)*—the most common reason why children need lung transplants.

- *Alpha-1 antitrypsin deficiency (AAT deficiency)*—a condition that raises a patient's risk for developing certain types of lung disease, especially if the patient smokes.

- *Pulmonary hypertension (PH)*—a condition of increased pressure in the pulmonary arteries, which carry blood from the heart to the lungs to pick up oxygen.

A lung transplant can improve a person's quality of life, and for patients with certain lung disorders, transplants also may help them live longer than they would without surgery.

Lung transplants are not very common because of the small number of donor organs available. About 1,800 lung transplants were done in the United States in 2010. More donor lungs would mean a larger number of suitable lungs available for transplant. Most patients who undergo lung transplants are between ages 18 and 65, but younger or older patients may also have lung transplants.

Before a lung transplant, each patient must undergo a careful screening process that clinicians oversee to make sure that the patient is a good candidate for a lung transplant. If he is, the patient is then placed on a waiting list to wait until a lung(s) becomes available. Patients must also be healthy enough to undergo lung transplant surgery. Lung transplants are done in medical centers (large hospitals) where the staff has a lot of organ transplant experience. Patients who need a lung transplant must apply to the medical center's transplant program. Transplant teams at the medical center manage all parts of the center's transplant program. A transplant team may include the following members:

- thoracic surgeon

- pulmonologist

- cardiologist

- immunologist (a physician who specializes in immune system disorders)

- respiratory technician (a physician who renders care to patients with breathing and lung disorders)

- transplant coordinator (a healthcare professional who schedules the patient's lung transplant surgery).

Other team members may include a social worker, psychiatrist, financial coordinator (to determine the total costs and methods of payment), and other specialists and medical personnel, such as a nutritionist and nurses.

Patients who are accepted into a medical center's transplant program are then placed on the Organ Procurement and Transplantation Network (OPTN) national waiting list. The OPTN manages the nationwide organ-sharing process and maintains the waiting lists for all organ donations. The number of people on the lung transplant waiting list changes often. About half of the people on the list receive a lung in any given year. The transplant team works with patients to ensure that they will be ready for the transplant and remain as healthy as possible until a donor lung becomes available.

Some patients only need one lung during a transplant and undergo a *single-lung transplant*. Other patients receive two lungs and undergo a *double-lung transplant*. Patients with severe heart and lung disorders receive both a heart and lung(s), which is called a **heart–lung transplant**. A rare kind of lung transplant is a *living donor lobar lung transplant*. For this surgery, a healthy adult donates a segment, or lobe, of one lung to another person. This type of transplant usually is done in children.

The OPTN matches donor lungs to recipients (receivers) based on need. The OPTN considers the severity of a patient's disease, how quickly it exacerbates, and whether the transplant will improve the recipient's chances of survival, and if so by how much. Organs are matched for blood type and the size of the donor lung and the recipient. If the OPTN and the medical center think that they have a good match for a patient, the transplant team asks the patient to arrive at the medical center as quickly as possible. Donor lungs last about six hours once removed from the cadaver and must be transplanted into the recipient within that time.

Patients who receive lung transplants are under general anesthesia, on a ventilator, and typically on a cardiopulmonary bypass (heart-lung machine), where a machine performs the work of the lungs and heart to allow the surgeon to perform procedures in a bloodless surgical field (area of surgery) and so that the heart does not move during surgery. The surgeon incises the chest and then incises the main airway to the diseased lung and the blood vessels connecting the lung to the heart. The surgeon removes the diseased lung(s), places the donor lung(s) into the chest, and connects the main airway of the donor lung to the patient's airway, along with connecting blood vessels to the heart (■ FIGURE 24-6). A single-lung transplant usually takes 4–8 hours to complete; a double-lung transplant takes 6–12 hours.

Lung transplants have serious risks. The patient's body may reject the new lung (which is most common during the first six months after surgery), or the patient may develop infections. The short- and long-term complications of a lung transplant can be

Figure 24-6 ■ (A) The airway and blood vessels between a recipient's diseased right lung and heart are cut. The inset image shows the location of the lungs and heart in the body. (B) A healthy donor lung is stitched to the recipient's blood vessels and airway.

Source: National Institutes of Health, National Heart, Lung, and Blood Institute: http://www.nhlbi.nih.gov/health/health-topics/topics/lungtxp/.

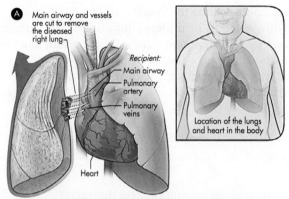

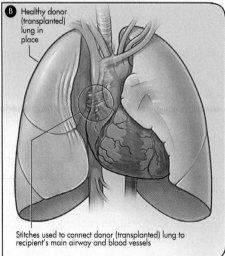

In recent years, short-term survival after lung transplantation has improved. Recent data on single-lung transplants show that

✔ About 78% of patients survive the first year.

✔ About 63% of patients survive three years.

✔ About 51% of patients survive five years.

Survival rates for double-lung transplants are slightly better. Recent data show that the median survival for single-lung recipients is 4.6 years. The median survival for double-lung recipients is 6.6 years (National Institutes of Health, National Heart, Lung, and Blood Institute).

life-threatening. The first year after the transplant is the most critical because it is when the risk of complications is highest.

The patient's immune system will regard the new lung as a foreign object and will create antibodies (proteins) to fight against the new lung. This reaction may cause the patient's body to reject the new organ. To prevent this from happening, the patient takes immunosuppressive drugs to suppress the functions of the immune system. But because the immune system is suppressed, the patient is more likely to develop infections. In addition, long-term use of immunosuppressive drugs can cause diabetes, kidney damage, osteoporosis (thinning of the bones) and increases the patient's risk of developing cancer.

Turn to the codes under the category Lung Transplantation in the Lungs and Pleura subheading. Let's briefly review procedures in this category:

- *Donor pneumonectomy from cadaver donor (32850)*— harvesting a lung(s) from a cadaver and preserving it with cold solution until it is transplanted

- *Lung transplant, single or double (32851–32854)* (may involve **cardiopulmonary bypass**)— transplanting the cadaver lung(s) into the recipient

- *Backbench preparation of cadaver donor lung allograft, unilateral or bilateral (32855–32856)*—preparing the donor lung(s) for transplant, including preparing connected arteries and veins for transplant

When patients receive a heart-lung transplant, assign a code from the Cardiovascular subsection, category Heart/Lung Transplantation.

TAKE A BREAK

Great job! You reviewed procedures in the last subheading of the Respiratory System section and covered a lot of ground! You have done very well! Let's take a break to review the lungs and pleura and then practice coding procedures.

Exercise 24.7   Lungs and Pleura

Part 1—Theory

Instructions: Fill in the blank with the best answer.

1. A _____ is when the physician incises the pleural space to perform procedures on the heart and lungs, including removing neoplasms and foreign bodies and performing a biopsy.

2. _____ is when the physician punctures the lung to withdraw fluid, which may have built up due to a traumatic injury.

3. When the physician inserts a substance, such as providone iodine, into the pleural space to reduce fluid accumulation from pleural effusion, the procedure is called _____.

4. _____ is when the physician collapses a diseased cavity of the lung to allow the lung to heal faster. It was a former treatment for tuberculosis.

5. The most common reason why adult patients need lung transplants is _____.

continued

TAKE A BREAK *continued*

6. The most common reason why children need lung transplants is _____.

Part 2—Coding

Instructions: Review the patient's case and then assign the appropriate procedure code(s), appending a modifier when appropriate. Optional: Assign the patient's diagnosis code(s) (ICD-9-CM).

1. At Williton Medical Center, Dr. Lightner, a pulmonologist, performs a thoracostomy with open flap drainage for Brenda Byrd, age 58, to treat an empyema resulting from pneumonia.

   Diagnosis code(s): _____

   Procedure code(s): _____

2. Judy Hopkins, age 63, is a lifelong cigarette smoker. Six years ago, she was diagnosed with breast cancer and had a right breast mastectomy. Since then, she has not had any problems, until recently. She has experienced hemoptysis, loss of appetite, and shortness of breath. In his office, Dr. Lightner examines Mrs. Hopkins and decides to perform a thoracotomy with biopsy of the right and left lungs. He sends tissue samples to the pathology department at Williton for testing. After Dr. Lightner reviews the pathologist's report, he concludes that the patient has lung cancer, which started in the right breast.

   Diagnosis code(s): _____

   Procedure code(s): _____

3. Jamar Jones, age 25, works for Overfield Moving Company. Today, he and his crew moved the contents of a large home, including a grand piano. Unfortunately, the men lost their grip on the piano, and it turned sideways and fell on Mr. Jones, crushing his chest. City Ambulance Service transported him to Williton where Dr. Holt, a pulmonologist, performed a pleural tap to treat a hemothorax. The piano was unharmed.

   Diagnosis code(s): _____

   Procedure code(s): _____

4. Today at Williton, Bruce Watts, age 60, undergoes a lobectomy of the upper lobe of the right lung to treat small cell carcinoma.

   Diagnosis code(s): _____

   Procedure code(s): _____

5. Debbie Mendez, the transplant coordinator at Williton, calls Amy Moriani, age 22, who suffers from cystic fibrosis. She is on OPTN's lung transplant waiting list for a double-lung transplant. Debbie asks Ms. Moriani to come to Williton right away. New lungs are available for her and on the way, and the transplant team will be waiting to transplant them. The cadaver donor is an 18-year-old man who died in a motor vehicle accident. The team performs the transplant, which includes the heart–lung machine, donor pneumonectomy, and backbench preparation of the cadaver donor lung allograft. After surgery, the team sends Ms. Moriani to the intensive care unit (ICU) to recover.

   Diagnosis code(s): _____

   Procedure code(s): _____

6. At Williton, Dr. Lightner inserts a chest tube to drain pleural fluid for Harvey Norris, age 80, to treat an acute pneumothorax.

   Diagnosis code(s): _____

   Procedure code(s): _____

DESTINATION: MEDICARE

In this exercise, your Medicare destination is a computer-based training module called *Medicare Fraud & Abuse: Prevention, Detection, and Reporting*. Follow the instructions listed next to access this training module.

1. Go to the website http://www.cms.gov.
2. At the top of screen on the banner bar, choose *Outreach & Education*.
3. Scroll down to Medicare Learning Network (MLN), and choose *MLN Products*.
4. Scroll down to Related Links, and choose *Web-Based Training (WBT) Courses*.
5. You will then see a list of web-based training courses. Click on *Medicare Fraud & Abuse: Prevention, Detection, and Reporting*.

6. If you never accessed the MLN's computer-based training, then you will have to register as a new user. Registration is free and takes a few minutes registered, you will only need your login and password each time you access the computer-based MLN. After registering, click *Web-Based Training Courses*, and click *Medicare Fraud & Abuse: Prevention, Detection, and Reporting* again.

7. On the next screen, click the radio button for *No credits* or *Continuing Education Units (CEU).* (CMS grants 1 CEU to coders certified through the American Academy of Professional Coders, AAPC, for scoring 70% or higher on the posttest.) Then click *Take Course.* You will take both a pretest and posttest so that you can monitor how well you learned the material.

CHAPTER REVIEW

Multiple Choice

Instructions: Circle one best answer to complete each statement.

1. Accessory sinuses cavities include all of the following *except*
   a. maxillary.
   b. ethmoid.
   c. frontal.
   d. nasal.

2. The purpose of the respiratory system is to
   a. bring oxygen to the body.
   b. remove carbon dioxide from the body.
   c. bring carbon dioxide to the body and remove oxygen from the body.
   d. bring oxygen to the body and remove carbon dioxide from the body.

3. Nasal turbinates are _____ inside the wall of the nose.
   a. soft tissues
   b. spongy bones
   c. muscular tissues
   d. fascia

4. Cilia are _____ that line the sinus membrane and move mucus from the sinus cavity to the nasal cavity.
   a. mucous membranes
   b. bony prominences
   c. small hairs
   d. soft tissues

5. A rhinectomy is the surgical _____ of the _____.
   a. excision, nose
   b. incision, nose
   c. removal, nose
   d. excision, sinus

6. Patients with foreign bodies in their noses are most likely
   a. disabled.
   b. elderly.
   c. children.
   d. male.

7. The medical term for a "nose job" is a(n)
   a. sinusotomy.
   b. rhinoplasty.
   c. septoplasty.
   d. rhinoseptoplasty.

8. The two types of bronchoscopy are
   a. mobile and immobile.
   b. hard and soft.
   c. rigid and flexible.
   d. static and dynamic.

9. An X-ray of the lower respiratory tract is called a(n):
   a. bronchography.
   b. thoracography.
   c. pleurography.
   d. septography.

10. Excision of the parietal pleura to treat pleural effusion, traumatic injuries, and pleural mesothelioma (carcinoma, typically caused by exposure to asbestos) is called a(n):
    a. pneumonectomy.
    b. thoracotomy.
    c. pleurectomy.
    d. parietalectomy.

Coding Assignments

Instructions: Review the patient's case and then assign the appropriate procedure code(s), appending a modifier when appropriate. Optional: Assign the patient's diagnosis code(s) (ICD-9-CM).

1. Dr. Lightner, a pulmonologist, performs a laryngotomy to remove a malignant neoplasm from the larynx for Ray Green, age 63.

   Diagnosis code(s):_____

   Procedure code(s): _____

2. Ellen Rahnor, age 57, has a sinus endoscopy at Williton, where Dr. Lightner removes several nasal polyps.

   Diagnosis code(s):_____

   Procedure code(s): _____

3. Dr. Mills, Williton's ED physician, performs emergency endotracheal intubation on George Reynolds, age 68. The patient suffers from COPD.

   Diagnosis code(s):_____

   Procedure code(s): _____

4. Dr. Lightner performs an indirect laryngoscopy with biopsy of tissue for Ruth Mayfield, age 78. The pathology report reveals a benign neoplasm of the larynx.

   Diagnosis code(s):_____

   Procedure code(s): _____

5. Mandy Carothers, age 32, has a pleural effusion. On Monday, Dr. Lightner inserts providone iodine to reduce the fluid accumulation. This is the first treatment.

   Diagnosis code(s):_____

   Procedure code(s): _____

6. On Tuesday, Dr. Lightner performs two more treatments for Mandy Carothers to reduce fluid accumulation.

   Diagnosis code(s):_____

   Procedure code(s): _____

7. Dr. Lightner performs thoracentesis for Greg Manzierre, age 52, to treat a pneumothorax.

   Diagnosis code(s):_____

   Procedure code(s): _____

8. Today at Williton, Dr. Lightner excises the parietal pleura to treat a pleural effusion for Margaret Jones, age 57.

   Diagnosis code(s):_____

   Procedure code(s): _____

9. Dr. Lightner performs pneumocentesis to remove fluid build-up in the lung for Macey Newman, age 19, who suffers from CF.

   Diagnosis code(s):_____

   Procedure code(s): _____

10. Williton's transplant team performs a single lung transplant for Sally Gartner, age 54, who suffers from COPD. The patient is on the heart–lung machine during the procedure. Other procedures include the donor pneumonectomy and backbench preparation of the cadaver donor lung allograft. The patient recovers in the ICU.

    Diagnosis code(s):_____

    Procedure code(s): _____

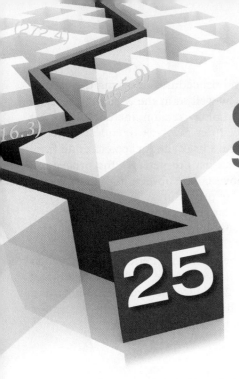

Cardiovascular System

Learning Objectives

After completing this chapter, you should be able to

- Spell and define the key terminology in this chapter.
- Describe procedures found in the Cardiovascular subsection.
- Discuss heart and pericardium procedures, and explain how to code them.
- Define various procedures of the arteries and veins and how to code them.

25

Key Terms

cardiac valves
cardiovascular system
coronary artery bypass graft (CABG)

great vessels
pacemaker
patient-activated event recorder

INTRODUCTION

Do you remember learning about the anatomy of the heart in Chapter 11 when we reviewed the circulatory system (Figure 11-1)? You also learned how arteries and veins function (Figures 11-2, 11-3), as well as about diseases and disorders of the heart, arteries, and veins. In this chapter, you will learn even more and will have the opportunity to apply your knowledge to coding many different types of procedures. These procedures can often be complex and difficult to understand. So take your time and go slowly, referring to information and diagrams in Chapter 11 to help you. You can also consult your medical references and perform Internet searches to find out more about how and why physicians perform specific procedures. The road in this chapter may wind a little more than in other chapters, but just hold on because you can do it! Let's travel this journey together so that you can continue to build your coding skills by successfully learning about procedures of the heart, arteries, and veins!

"Formulate and stamp indelibly on your mind a mental picture of yourself as succeeding. Hold this picture tenaciously. Never permit it to fade."
—NORMAN VINCENT PEALE

CARDIOVASCULAR SYSTEM (33010–37799)

The **cardiovascular system** includes the heart and blood vessels. In the CPT manual, there are only two subheadings in the Cardiovascular subsection of Surgery: Heart and Pericardium and Arteries and Veins. The **pericardium** is a sac surrounding the heart, made up of an outer layer called the parietal pericardium, and an inner layer called the visceral pericardium. Pericardial fluid lies between the inner and outer layers of the pericardium.

pericardium
(per-ə-kärd′-ē-əm)

An important point to note is that you will find procedures involving the cardio-vascular system in the Cardiovascular subsection, as well as in the Medicine section, including specific tests on the heart, and in the Radiology section, including imaging procedures of the heart. Some cardiovascular procedures involve two codes: one code from the Cardiovascular subsection for the procedure itself, and a second code from the Radiology section for imaging that the physician uses to perform the procedure. There are many CPT notes throughout the Cardiovascular subsection to alert you to assign separate radiology codes with cardiovascular procedures. In this chapter, we will concentrate on procedures of the Cardiovascular subsection, and we will review additional procedures in chapters covering the Radiology section and the Medicine section.

There are numerous procedures listed under the Heart and Pericardium as well as the Arteries and Veins subheadings, including numerous categories and subcategories of procedures and extensive CPT guidelines. ■ TABLE 25-1 lists the two subheadings and their categories. Let's begin by reviewing some of the procedures under the Heart and Pericardium subheading, and then we will move on to Arteries and Veins.

HEART AND PERICARDIUM (33010–33999)

The Heart and Pericardium subheading includes 29 categories of procedures, but as you have probably guessed, we will not have time to review procedures in all of the categories. Instead, let's look at *some* of the categories and discuss the types of procedures that you will find, and then you can practice coding.

CPT arranges codes in the Heart and Pericardium subheading by the *location* of the procedure and the *type* of procedure. To locate codes for these procedures in the index, search for the *body site* and then the *type of procedure,* or begin your search with the *type of procedure.* Turn to the codes in your CPT manual as we discuss them, starting with the first category, Pericardium.

■ TABLE 25-1   **CARDIOVASCULAR SYSTEM SUBHEADINGS AND CATEGORIES**

Cardiovascular System	33010–37799
Heart and Pericardium	**33010–33999**
Pericardium	33010–33050
Cardiac Tumor	33120–33130
Transmyocardial Revascularization	33140–33141
Pacemaker or Pacing Cardioverter-Defibrillator	33202–33249
Electrophysiologic Operative Procedures	33250–33266
Patient-Activated Event Recorder	33282–33284
Wounds of the Heart and Great Vessels	33300–33335
Cardiac Valves	33400–33478
Other Valvular Procedures	33496
Coronary Artery Anomalies	33500–33507
Endoscopy	33508
Venous Grafting Only for Coronary Artery Bypass	33510–33516
Combined Arterial Venous Grafting for Coronary Bypass	33517–33530
Arterial Grafting for Coronary Artery Bypass	33533–33518
Coronary Endarterectomy	33572
Single Ventricle and Other Complex Cardiac Anomalies	33600–33622

continued

■ **TABLE 25-1** *continued*

Cardiovascular System	33010–37799
Septal Defect	33641–33697
Sinus of Valsalva	33702–33722
Venous Anomalies	33724–33732
Shunting Procedures	33735–33768
Transposition of the Great Vessels	33770–33783
Truncus Arteriosus	33786–33788
Aortic Anomalies	33800–33853
Thoracic Aortic Aneurysm	33860–33877
Endovascular Repair of Descending Thoracic Aorta	33880–33891
Pulmonary Artery	33910–33926
Heart/Lung Transplantation	33930–33945
Cardiac Assist	33960–33983
Other Procedures	33999
Arteries and Veins	**34001–37799**
Embolectomy/Thrombectomy	34001–34490
Venous Reconstruction	34501–34530
Endovascular Repair of Abdominal Aortic Aneurysm	34800–34834
Endovascular Repair of Iliac Aneurysm	34900
Direct Repair of Aneurysm or Excision (Partial or Total) and Graft Insertion for Aneurysm, Pseudoaneurysm, Ruptured Aneurysm, and Associated Occlusive Disease	35001–35152
Repair **Arteriovenous** Fistula	35180–35190
Repair Blood Vessel Other Than for Fistula, With or Without Patch Angioplasty	35201–35286
Thromboendarterectomy	35301–35390
Angioscopy	35400
Transluminal Angioplasty	35450–35476
Bypass Graft	35500–35671
Composite Grafts	35581–35583
Adjuvant Techniques	35585–35586
Arterial Transposition	35691–35697
Excision, Exploration, Repair, Revision	35700–35907
Vascular Injection Procedures	36000–36598
Arterial	36600–36660
Intraosseous	36680
Hemodialysis Access, Intervascular Cannulation for Extracorporeal Circulation, or Shunt Insertion	36800–36870
Portal Decompression Procedures	37140–37183
Transcatheter Procedures	37184–37216
Endovascular Revascularization	37220–37235
Intravascular Ultrasound Services	37250–37251
Endoscopy	37500–37501
Ligation	37565–37785
Other Procedures	37788–37799

arteriovenous (är-tir-ē-ō-vē′-nəs)—pertaining to an artery and a vein

Pericardium (33010–33050)

pericardiocentesis
(per-ə-kärd-ē-ō-sen-tē′-səs)

The Pericardium category contains eight procedure codes. **Pericardiocentesis**, is the first procedure in the category, which involves removing excess fluid from the pericardium by aspirating it with a needle, wire, and catheter. The procedure includes imaging to perform the procedure, such as ultrasound. CPT notes alert you to report radiological procedures separately using a code from the Radiology section.

effusion (i-fyü′-zhən)

There is always a small amount of fluid in the pericardium for lubricating the structures of the heart. A pericardiocentesis can be *diagnostic* to test the fluid for a definitive diagnosis about a specific disorder or disease, such as cancer metastasis or an infection. The procedure can also be *therapeutic* to eliminate the excess fluid (called an **effusion**) which is visible on an X-ray or cardiac ultrasound. The excess fluid can prevent the heart from functioning normally, so the physician has to remove it. In some cases, the patient's case is emergent, such as with a cardiac **tamponade**, a disorder that prevents the heart from pumping blood properly, which **pericarditis** (inflammation of the pericardium), trauma, or hypothyroidism can cause. Pericardiocentesis can be *initial* (first time performed) or *subsequent* (performed after the initial procedure).

tamponade (tam-pə-nād′)
pericarditis (per-ə-kär-dīt′-əs)

Other procedures in the Pericardium category include

pericardiostomy
(per-ə-kärd-ē-äs′-tə-mē)

pericardiotomy
(per-ə-kärd-ē-ät′-ə-mē)

pericardiectomy
(pĕr-ĭ-kär-dē-ĕk′tə′-mē)

- **Pericardiostomy** and **pericardiotomy**—procedures to insert a catheter to drain pericardial effusions or remove a foreign body
- **Pericardiectomy**—removal of the pericardium because other disorders caused it to become too thick
- Creation of pericardial window—procedure to drain a pericardial effusion
- Excision of a pericardial cyst, tumor, or foreign body

Cardiac Tumor (33120–33130)

The Cardiac Tumor category contains only two procedures for treating cardiac tumors, including excising an intracardiac tumor (inside the layers of the heart) and resecting an external cardiac tumor (on the outer aspect of the heart). Physicians diagnose cardiac tumors through imaging, such as a CT, MRI, or echocardiogram (cardiac ultrasound). Removing a cardiac tumor can involve an *invasive* procedure (involving larger surgical incisions) or a *minimally invasive* procedure using endoscopy (involving smaller surgical incisions).

myxomas (mik-sō′-məs)
rhabdomyomas
(rab-dō-mī-ō′-məs)
lipomas (li-pō′-məs)

Most cardiac tumors are benign, including a **myxomas**, which can form in the heart chambers, and a **rhabodomyomas**, a benign muscle tumor. **Lipomas** (tumors of fat) and fibromas (tumors of fibers and connective tissue) are other types of benign cardiac tumors. In addition, cardiac sarcoma is a rare form of a malignant cardiac neoplasm.

Transmyocardial Revascularization (33140–33141)

Transmyocardial revascularization (TMR) is a laser procedure to increase blood flow in the coronary arteries. Physicians perform this procedure when other methods to treat ischemia (restricted blood flow) or chronic chest pain have failed, and the only other alternative is a heart transplant. During TMR, the physician uses a laser to create several openings in the heart muscle that allow blood to flow. The physician can perform TMR along with other cardiac procedures during the same operative session.

Pacemaker or Pacing Cardioverter-Defibrillator (33202–33249)

cardioverter-defibrillators
(kärd-ē-ō-vərt′-ər dē-fib′-rə-lāt-ərs)

Pacemakers and implantable **cardioverter-defibrillators** (ICDs), are small devices with a battery-operated pulse generator connected to leads (wires). Electrodes are attached to the leads, which are then attached to the heart. Physicians implant pacemakers and ICDs in a skin pocket (in the chest or abdomen) to help control abnormal heart rhythms.

epicardium (ep′i-kär′dē-um)

Physicians place leads directly on the **epicardium** (outer layer of the heart) through an open incision (**thoracotomy**), with endoscopy (called **thoracoscopy**), or transvenously (through a vein and then into the right atrium or right ventricle).

A pacemaker or ICD monitors heart rhythm and sends electrical pulses or shocks (during an emergent situation), to prompt the heart to beat at a normal rate. These devices are for patients with arrhythmias, disorders of heart rhythm including tachycardia (rapid heartbeat) and bradycardia (slow heartbeat). During an arrhythmia, the heart may not be able to pump enough blood to the body, which may cause fatigue, shortness of breath, or fainting. Severe arrhythmias can damage the body's vital organs and may even cause loss of consciousness or death.

A pacemaker monitors and helps control heartbeat. The electrodes detect the heart's electrical activity and send data through the wires to the computer in the pulse generator. If the heart rhythm is abnormal, the computer will direct the generator to send electrical pulses to the heart. The pulses then travel through the wires to reach the heart. Newer pacemakers can also monitor blood temperature, breathing, and other factors and adjust heart rate to respond to different levels of physical activity. A pacemaker also records the heart's electrical activity and rhythm. The physician analyzes the recordings to adjust a patient's pacemaker so that it functions well.

Pacemakers have one to three wires that are each placed in different chambers of the heart:

- The wires in a single-chamber pacemaker usually carry pulses between the right ventricle (the lower right chamber) and the pulse generator (using one lead).

- The wires in a dual-chamber pacemaker carry pulses between the right atrium (the upper right chamber) and the right ventricle and the pulse generator. The pulses help coordinate the timing of these two chambers' contractions (using two leads).

- The wires in a biventricular pacemaker carry pulses between an atrium and both ventricles and the generator. The pulses help coordinate electrical signaling between the two ventricles (using three leads). This type of pacemaker is also called a *cardiac resynchronization therapy* (CRT) device.

Patients with pacemakers have to avoid close or prolonged contact with electrical devices or devices that have strong magnetic fields, such as cell phones, portable media players, microwave ovens, high-tension wires, metal detectors, industrial welders, and electrical generators. These devices can disrupt the electrical signaling of the pacemaker and stop it from working properly.

Pacemakers can be temporary or permanent. Temporary pacemakers are used to treat temporary heartbeat problems, such as a slow heartbeat caused by a heart attack, heart surgery, or an overdose of medicine. Temporary pacemakers are also used during emergencies. They're used until a permanent pacemaker can be implanted or until the temporary condition subsides. Permanent pacemakers are used to control long-term heart rhythm problems.

Pacemaker batteries last between 5 and 15 years (with an average of 7 years), depending on how active the pacemaker is. Physicians replace both the pulse generator and the battery before the battery starts to run down. Replacing the generator and battery is less-involved than the original surgery to implant the pacemaker. Eventually, the pacemaker's wires may also need to be replaced. Report two separate codes for a removal of a pulse generator and insertion of a new one.

An ICD sends electrical pulses and shocks to the ventricles of the heart, called **defibrillation**. An ICD helps treat more serious heart disorders, such as cardiac arrest. An ICD can deliver low-energy electrical pulses (for less serious heart disorders) or high-energy electrical pulses (for more serious heart disorders), while a pacemaker can only deliver low-energy electrical pulses (■ FIGURE 25-1). Some ICDs can perform functions of a pacemaker, too (National Institutes of Health).

CPT arranges codes for pacemakers and cardioverter defibrillators by the

- type of procedure (e.g., insertion, repositioning, repair)

- equipment involved (e.g., electrodes, pacemaker, cardioverter-defibrillator)

- location (e.g., atrial, ventricular)

thoracotomy
(thōr-ə-kät′-ə-mē)

thoracoscopy
(thōr-ə-käs′-kə-pē)

defibrillation
(dē-fib-rə-lā′-shən)

Figure 25-1 ■ The location and general size of an ICD (A) and pacemaker (B) in the upper chest. The wires with electrodes on the ends are inserted into the heart through a vein in the upper chest.

Source: National Heart, Lung, and Blood Institute; National Institutes of Health; U.S. Department of Health and Human Services.

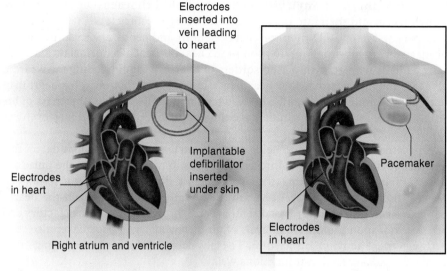

When the physician uses imaging to perform the procedure, be sure to assign a separate code from the Radiology section of the CPT manual.

The Pacemaker or Pacing Cardioverter-Defibrillator category includes many different procedure codes and extensive CPT coding guidelines at the beginning of the category and throughout various procedures, so be sure to review the guidelines before final code assignment. You can locate codes in the index by searching for the *type of procedure* (repair), *equipment* (pacemaker), or *anatomic site* (heart).

Electrophysiologic Operative Procedures (33250–33256)

supraventricular dysrhythmias (sü-pra-ven-trik′-yə-lər dis-rith′-mē-əs)

electrophysiologic (i-lek-trō-fiz-ē-ä-lä′-jik)

This category contains codes for procedures to treat **supraventricular dysrhythmias**, abnormalities of heart rhythm caused by electrical impulses originating from the sinoatrial (SA) node (located in the right atrium, which generates electrical impulses of the heart) and atria. **Electrophysiologic** *operative procedures* include ablating tissue and reconstructing areas of the heart to eliminate dysrhythmias, and the physician may use endoscopy to ablate tissue and reconstruct the atria.

Other electrophysiology procedures involve monitoring the heart's electrical activity through wire electrodes placed in the heart, and you can find codes for these procedures in the Medicine section of the CPT manual.

Patient-Activated Event Recorder (33282–33284)

This category contains only two procedure codes, one for implanting a **patient-activated event recorder** (also called a loop recorder), and the other for removing it. Event recorders are medical devices that record the heart's electrical activity, but they are not implanted into the patient's body like a pacemaker or ICD. Physicians most often use these monitors to diagnose arrhythmias. Event monitors are also used to detect *silent myocardial ischemia* when not enough oxygen-rich blood reaches the heart muscle. "Silent" means that there are no symptoms.

An event monitor reports information similar to an EKG. An EKG is a simple test that detects and records the heart's electrical activity but may not diagnose all heart disorders. But an event monitor can measure the heart's electrical activity over a longer period of time.

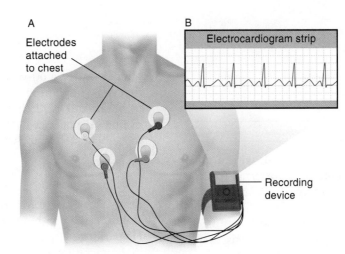

A
Electrodes
attached
to chest

B
Electrocardiogram strip

Recording
device

Figure 25-2 ■ (A) An event monitor attached to a patient. (B) An electrocardiogram strip, which maps the data from the event monitor.

Source: National Institutes of Health; U.S. Department of Health and Human Services.

The event monitor is a small, portable device. The patient can wear it while performing normal daily activities or while asleep. Some people have heart rhythm problems that only occur during certain activities, such as sleep or physical exertion. Using an event monitor increases the chances of recording these electrical abnormalities. Most event monitors have wires that connect the device to sensors. The sensors are stuck to the patient's chest using sticky patches (■ Figure 25-2).

Event monitors only record the heart's electrical activity when symptoms occur. For many event monitors, the patient needs to start the monitor when he feels symptoms. Some event monitors start automatically if they detect abnormal heart rhythms (National Institutes of Health).

TAKE A BREAK

Wow! That was a lot of information to cover! Let's take a break and then review more about the heart and pericardium and then practice coding procedures.

Exercise 25.1   Heart and Pericardium

Part 1—Theory

Instructions: Fill in the blank with the best answer.

1. _____ involves removing excess fluid from the pericardium by aspirating it with a needle, wire, and catheter.

2. _____ is a laser procedure to increase blood flow in the coronary arteries.

3. Physicians implant _____ and _____ in a skin pocket (in the chest or abdomen) to help control abnormal heart rhythms.

4. Pacemakers have one to three _____ that are each placed in different chambers of the heart.

5. _____ are abnormalities of heart rhythm caused by electrical impulses originating from the sinoatrial (SA) node and atria.

6. _____ operative procedures include ablating tissue and reconstructing areas of the heart to eliminate dysrhythmias, and the physician may use endoscopy to ablate tissue and reconstruct the atria.

Part 2—Coding

Instructions: Review each patient's case, and then assign codes for the procedure(s), appending a modifier to the procedure when appropriate. Optional: Assign the patient's diagnosis code(s) (ICD-9-CM).

1. Connie Viteri, age 53, is taken to the operating room at Williton Medical Center to have a tumor removed from her heart. During the surgery Dr. Michalek, a cardiovascular surgeon, places Mrs. Viteri on cardiopulmonary bypass during the resection of the heart tumor.

   Diagnosis code(s): _____

   Procedure code(s): _____

2. Dr. Michalek sees Cody Broker, age 56, at the Ambulatory Center at Williton Medical Center to implant a continuous loop cardiac event recorder into the subcutaneous tissue of the chest to investigate arrhythmia.

   Diagnosis code(s): _____

   Procedure code(s): _____

3. Adam Kochan, a 38-year-old, presents to Williton Medical Center with atrial fibrillation. Dr. Michalek

continued

TAKE A BREAK *continued*

performs an endoscopic operative ablation and reconstruction of the atria.

Diagnosis code(s): _____

Procedure code(s): _____

4. Dr. Michalek sees Julie Sizer, age 24, with a chief complaint of sharp, intermittent retrosternal (behind the sternum or breast bone) pain that is reduced by sitting up or leaning forward. Chest films reveal **pulmonary edema** with acute pericardial effusion. Dr. Michalek performs a pericardiocentesis in the Ambulatory Surgery Department at Williton.

Diagnosis code(s): _____

Procedure code(s): _____

5. Janice Whitely, a 60-year-old female, has a pacemaker that was implanted two years ago for ventricular tachycardia. Dr. Michalek replaces the dual-chamber pacing cardioverter-defibrillator pulse generator from the subcutaneous pocket in her chest.

Diagnosis code(s): _____

Procedure code(s): _____

6. Dr. Michalek sees Mr. Burns, a 52-year-old man, in Williton's ED with angina and myocardial ischemia. He performs a transmyocardial laser revascularization by thoracotomy to restore the flow of blood and oxygen to the heart.

Diagnosis code(s): _____

Procedure code(s): _____

---

pulmonary edema (pul-mə-ner′-ē i-dē′-mə)—edema of the lungs, usually due to mitral stenosis or left ventricular failure

cardiotomy (kärd-ē-ät′-ə-mē)

Wounds of the Heart and Great Vessels (33300–33335)

This category includes codes for repair of a cardiac wound, exploratory **cardiotomy** (incision into the heart), which is used to remove a foreign body, thrombus, or neoplasm, and graft insertion of the aorta or great vessels. The **great vessels** are the superior vena cava, inferior vena cava, pulmonary artery, and aorta.

Turn to the procedures listed in this category. Did you notice that physicians can perform them with or without shunt bypass or cardiopulmonary bypass? In a *shunt bypass*, physicians use a coronary shunt to divert blood flow during heart surgery to maintain a bloodless surgical field (area being operated on). *Cardiopulmonary bypass* is a method to keep a patient alive during heart surgery, using a heart–lung machine that performs functions of the heart and lungs, "bypassing" both organs during a patient's heart surgery. The heart–lung machine allows the physician to operate on the heart when it is not beating; if the heart continued to beat, it would make specific procedures difficult, if not impossible, to perform. A heart–lung machine can also sustain life for patients with cardiac failure who are waiting for a heart transplant.

INTERESTING FACT: Many Women Do Not Know Signs of a Heart Attack

The U.S. Department of Health and Human Services' Office on Women's Health funded a study, which indicated that 57% of Latina women, 40% of African American women, and 32% of Caucasian women had three or more risk factors for having a heart attack. Surprisingly, only 60% of these women were aware of the symptoms of a heart attack and of the need to call 9-1-1 if having symptoms, including

✔ Chest pain, discomfort, pressure, or squeezing

✔ Shortness of breath

✔ Nausea

✔ Light-headedness or sudden dizziness

✔ Unusual upper body pain or discomfort in one or both arms, back, shoulder, neck, jaw, or upper part of the stomach

✔ Unusual fatigue

✔ Breaking out in a cold sweat

(U.S. Department of Health and Human Services, www.hhs.gov/ash/news/20120206.html)

Cardiac Valves (33400–33478)

This category includes procedures on the valves of the heart. The valves open and close in response to blood flowing through the atria and ventricles. **Cardiac valves** include

- *Mitral valve* and *triscuspid valve*, called atrioventricular (AV) valves, which are located between the atria and ventricles
- *Aortic valve* and *pulmonary valve*, called semilunar (SL) valves, located in the arteries away from the heart

  Let's discuss a few of the procedures that you will find in this category:

- **Valvotomy** (incision into a valve) is done to correct disorders that prevent the heart valve from correctly opening and closing.

- **Valvuloplasty** (valve repair) is done to open a valve which is occluded or **stenotic** (stiff), which prevents adequate blood flow.

- ***Replacement of a valve***—Physicians replace heart valves due to aortic stenosis (narrow valve) or aortic insufficiency (weakened valve that cannot close). Some replacement valves include

  - *Homograft valve*—heart valve from a human cadaver
  - *Animal valve*—heart valve from a pig (porcine) or cow (bovine)
  - *Mechanical valve*—prosthetic valve made of metal and/or polyester; mechanical valves may cause the patient's blood to clot, which can be life-threatening. Patients with mechanical valves must take anticoagulant medications (called blood thinners) throughout their lives to prevent blood clots.

valvotomy (val-vät′-ə-mē)

valvuloplasty (val-vyə-lō-plas′-tē)

stenotic (stə-nät′-ik)

Other Valvular Procedures (33496), Coronary Artery Anomalies (33500–33507), Endoscopy (33508)

These three categories include various procedures, such as

- ***Repair of a dysfunctional prosthetic valve*** (*Other Valvular Procedures*)
- ***Repair of coronary arteriovenous or arteriocardiac chamber fistula; repair of coronary artery anomalies, involving ligation or graft;*** these procedures also include **endarterectomy** (excision of plaque from an artery); or **angioplasty** (to open or widen a narrow artery); and may also include the use of cardiopulmonary bypass during the procedure (*Coronary Artery Anomalies*)
- ***Surgical endoscopy to harvest veins for coronary artery bypass***, an add-on procedure. We will discuss coronary artery bypass in the next section (*Endoscopy*).

endarterectomy (en-därt-ə-rek′-tə-mē)
angioplasty (an-jē-ə-plas′-tē)

Coronary Bypass—Venous Grafting (33510–33516), Arterial-Venous Grafting (33517–33530), Arterial Grafting (33533–33548)

A **coronary artery bypass graft (CABG)** (pronounced "cabbage") is a procedure for improving blood flow to the heart. You first learned about this procedure in Chapter 11. Physicians perform it for patients with severe coronary artery disease (CAD). CAD is the #1 killer of both men and women in the United States. CAD occurs if plaque builds up in the coronary arteries (called **atherosclerosis**).

Coronary arteries supply oxygen-rich blood to the heart. **Plaque** is made up of fat, cholesterol, calcium, and other substances found in the blood. Plaque can cause stenosis or occlusion of the coronary arteries and reduce blood flow to the heart muscle (ischemia). Plaque buildup also makes it more likely that blood clots will form in the coronary arteries. Blood clots can partially or completely occlude blood flow. CAD can cause angina, shortness of breath, or an MI.

CABG is one treatment for CAD. During CABG, a physician connects, or grafts, a healthy artery or vein taken from elsewhere in the body, like the leg, arm, or chest, to the

atherosclerosis (ath-ə-rō-sklə-rō′-səs)
plaque (plak)

Figure 25-3 ■ Coronary artery bypass grafting: (A) The location of the heart. (B) How physicians attach vein and artery bypass grafts to the heart.

Source: National Institutes of Health; U.S. Department of Health and Human Services.

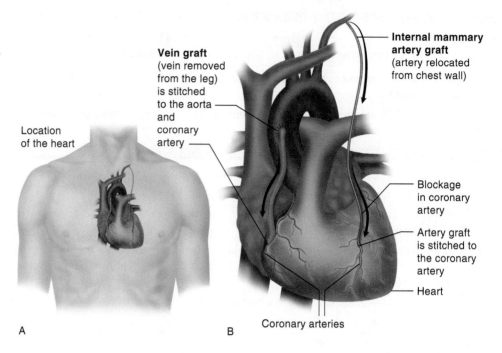

Vein graft
(vein removed
from the leg)
is stitched
to the aorta
and
coronary
artery

Internal mammary
artery graft
(artery relocated
from chest wall)

Location
of the heart

Blockage
in coronary
artery

Artery graft
is stitched to
the coronary
artery

Heart

A

B

Coronary arteries

sternotomy (stər-nät′-ə-mē)

occluded coronary artery. The grafted artery or vein *bypasses* (goes around) the blocked portion of the coronary artery because the physician attaches one end of it to the aorta and the other to the occluded or diseased coronary artery, past the occluded area. This surgery creates a new passage, and oxygen-rich blood is routed *around the blockage* to the heart muscle (■ FIGURE 25-3).

CABG can be minimally invasive, involving an endoscope and robotic surgery that the surgeon directs, or it can be invasive, involving a **sternotomy** (incision into the sternum) to open the chest to perform the surgery using a heart–lung machine to sustain the patient during the procedure. The procedure may involve a large incision or smaller incision (called a keyhole procedure) into the chest, depending on the patient's condition and type of procedure needed.

The principle of a CABG procedure is similar to a highway bypass. Did you ever drive or ride on a bypass highway, or bypass road, that was designed to avoid a congested road with a lot of traffic? Bypass highways are designed specifically as *new routes* of travel where none existed before. CABG works the same way, creating an artery or vein "highway bypass," a new route for blood to travel where none ever existed.

CABG is the most common type of heart surgery in the U.S., and cardiothoracic surgeons perform it. Research has shown that results of CABG surgery are excellent. Following CABG, 85% of patients have significantly reduced symptoms of CAD, less risk of future MIs, and a decreased chance of dying within 10 years (National Institutes of Health). However, patients who have had CABG still need to be vigilant about their health because the grafts can also occlude in the future.

Physicians do not always treat CAD with CABG. Many people who have CAD can be treated other ways, such as with lifestyle changes, medicines, or angioplasty. During angioplasty, the surgeon places a small mesh tube, called a stent, in an artery to help keep it open by pushing plaque against the artery walls (see Figure 11-17).

CABG or angioplasty with stent placement may be options for patients with severe occlusions in the coronary arteries, especially if their hearts are already weak. But when angioplasty is not an option, CABG is considered more effective than other types of treatment. Goals of CABG include

- Improving the patient's quality of life by decreasing angina and other CAD symptoms
- Allowing the patient to resume a more active lifestyle
- Improving heart functions, especially if the heart sustained damage from an MI

- Lowering the risk of an MI, especially for patients with other health problems, such as diabetes
- Improving the patient's survival rate

Just because a patient has CABG surgery does not mean that he will never need to have it again. For example, a grafted artery may eventually become occluded or diseased. Patients may be able to prevent this situation by taking prescribed medicines to reduce plaque formation and making lifestyle changes that the physician recommends. It is important to note that many patients may not be candidates for heart surgery, including CABG and angioplasty, and they are instead treated with medicines and other measures.

Turn to the codes for coronary bypass procedures in your CPT manual, starting with code 33510. Notice that there are three separate categories of codes for coronary bypass procedures and numerous CPT guidelines for assigning the codes. You should thoroughly review not only the CPT guidelines but also the code descriptors to ensure that you completely understand the procedures. Let's review the three categories next, along with a few summary points of the CPT guidelines.

- *Venous Grafting Only for Coronary Artery Bypass* (33510–33516)—Assign these codes to report CABG procedures using venous grafts only.
  - Do not report these codes for CABG procedures using arterial grafts and venous grafts during the same procedure (see 33517–33523 and 33533–33536).
  - Procuring (taking) the saphenous vein graft is included in these codes, so you should not separately report it.
  - Separately report harvesting of an upper extremity vein (35500) or femoropopliteal vein (femoral vein connecting to the popliteal vein, located in the groin) segment (35572) in addition to the bypass procedure.
- *Combined Arterial–Venous Grafting for Coronary Bypass* (33517–33530, **all add-on codes**)—Assign these codes for CABG procedures using venous grafts and arterial grafts during the same procedure.
- *Arterial Grafting for Coronary Artery Bypass* (33533–33536)—Assign these codes for CABG procedures using arterial grafts only or a combination of an arterial–venous graft.

In order to correctly code for coronary bypass procedures, you need to know if the physician performed the procedure using veins only, arteries only, or a combination of both. Since there are different code ranges in three separate categories, depending on the type of grafts, you need to be sure that you assign codes from the correct category.

You also need to know the *total number* of grafts that the physician performs. To count the number of bypass grafts, review the medical documentation to determine how many **anastomoses** (vessels joined) the physician performed to attach the healthy vein or artery to the diseased coronary artery. You may have heard people refer to coronary artery bypass as "heart bypass" or "triple bypass surgery" or "quadruple bypass." These terms, triple (3) and quadruple (4), refer to the number of bypass grafts involved in the surgery.

Refer to the following example to better understand how to code a coronary bypass procedure.

anastomoses
(ă-nas-tō-mō′-sez′)

Example: Nathan Simms, age 65, suffers from CAD. He experiences chronic angina and also had an acute MI. Today at Williton Medical Center, Dr. Swamy, a cardiothoracic surgeon, performs a triple bypass for three coronary vessels: left anterior descending (LAD), right coronary artery (RCA), and left coronary artery (LCA). He performs the bypass using multiple segments from the saphenous vein. The procedure involves a sternotomy, and the patient recovers in the ICU after the procedure.

To code this case, let's first determine whether the procedure involved vein grafts only, arterial grafts only, or a combination of both. The documentation states that Dr. Swamy used segments from the *saphenous vein*. The documentation does not include the use of any other vessels for the grafts. So, the procedure involved *only vein* grafts.

Search the index for the type of procedure, *bypass graft*, subterm *coronary artery*, and subterm *venous graft*, which leads you to the code range of 33510–33516.

Next, turn to the category in your CPT manual that represents vein grafts, *Venous Grafting Only for Coronary Artery Bypass* (33510–33516). Take a look at the codes in the category. Did you notice that CPT arranges them by the *total number of grafts* involved in the procedure? The documentation includes vein grafts of *three* coronary vessels, LAD, RCA, and LCA. Code **33512** represents CABG using three venous grafts, which is the final code assignment.

Should you also report a code for procuring the saphenous vein, since it represents additional work that the physician performed before performing the bypass? If you said no, then you are correct! Remember that the CPT guidelines alert you that procuring the saphenous vein is *already included* in the procedure for the bypass graft, so you should not code it separately.

TAKE A BREAK

Good job! Let's Take A Break and review more about the heart and pericardium and then practice coding procedures.

Exercise 25.2   Heart and Pericardium

Part 1—Theory

Instructions: Fill in the blank with the best answer.

1. The _____ are the superior vena cava, inferior vena cava, pulmonary artery, and aorta.

2. A(n) _____ is a heart valve from a human cadaver.

3. _____ is the #1 killer of both men and women in the United States.

4. _____ is made up of fat, cholesterol, calcium, and other substances found in the blood.

5. During _____, a physician connects, or grafts, a healthy artery or vein taken from elsewhere in the body, like the leg, arm, or chest, to the occluded coronary artery.

6. In order to correctly code for _____ bypass procedures, you need to know if the physician performed the procedure using _____ only, _____ only, or a combination of both.

Part 2—Coding

Instructions: Review each patient's case, and then assign codes for the procedure(s), appending a modifier to the procedure when appropriate. Optional: Assign the patient's diagnosis code(s) (ICD-9-CM).

1. Melanie Haverty, age 34, has a history of mitral valve prolapse (heart disorder in which one or both mitral valve flaps in the heart do not close completely, usually producing either a click or murmur). Dr. Michalek, a cardiovascular surgeon, sees her at his office. At Williton, he subsequently performs a replacement of the mitral valve after placing the patient on cardiopulmonary bypass. Code for the procedure at Williton.

    Diagnosis code(s): _____

    Procedure code(s): _____

2. Bing Markovich, age 87, has a history of repair of his heart valve four years ago. He now presents to Williton for scheduled surgery on a malfunctioning artificial prosthetic valve. In the operating room, Dr. Michalek places the patient on cardiopulmonary bypass and repairs the leakage around the valve.

    Diagnosis code(s): _____

    Procedure code(s): _____

3. Dr. Dillard, a cardiovascular surgeon, repairs a fistula of the arteriocardiac chamber (opening between the coronary arterial system and a chamber of the heart) on Goldie Hillario, a 73-year-old female. Dr. Dillard does not use cardiopulmonary bypass during this procedure. After the procedure, Miss Hillario is admitted to the ICU to recover.

    Diagnosis code(s): _____

    Procedure code(s): _____

4. Lisa Minichew, age 42, sees Dr. Mills, the ED physician at Williton, after she suffers an acute anterior wall MI. Dr. Mills calls in Dr. Dillard, who performs a cardiac catheterization (inserts a catheter into the heart to examine it). Dr. Dillard then performs a double CABG using venous grafts for coronary artery disease. To obtain the venous grafts, Dr. Dillard performs a video-assisted harvesting of the saphenous vein.

    Diagnosis code(s): _____

    Procedure code(s): _____

TAKE A BREAK *continued*

5. Dr. Pille, a resident in the cardiovascular program at Williton, is the assistant surgeon to Dr. Dillard, who performs five venous grafts in a CABG on Jenny Aune, age 63. The patient's diagnosis is coronary artery disease. Code for Dr. Pille's services.

Diagnosis code(s): _____

Procedure code(s): _____

6. Dr. Dillard admits Cal Tuff, age 64, to Williton with a diagnosis of arteriosclerotic heart disease. Dr. Dillard performs a CABG using two coronary arterial grafts and three venous grafts.

Diagnosis code(s): _____

Procedure code(s): _____

Additional Categories

Of the 29 total categories listed under the Heart and Pericardium subheading, we already reviewed procedures in 14 of them. There are 15 additional categories left, which you can review in your CPT manual. They include procedures for repairs, shunts, grafts, **embolectomy** (removal of an embolus), and endarterectomy to treat disorders like arteriosclerosis, stenosis, fistula, and aneurysm. Let's discuss some of the categories and types of procedures that you will find so that you can be more familiar with them, and then practice coding:

embolectomy
(em-bə-lek′-tə-mē)

- *Coronary Endarterectomy* (33572)—The excision of plaque in an artery. Physicians perform a coronary endarterectomy (add-on code) along with a CABG.

- *Single Ventricle and Other Complex Cardiac Anomalies* (33600–33619)— These procedures include repair, closure, and anastomosis to treat various cardiac anomalies, such as closure of an atrial septal defect, a disorder of the interatrial septum, which divides the atria.

- *Septal Defect* (33641–33697)—This category includes repairs and closures of septal defects (defects in the ventricular septum, which divides the left and right ventricles), including those that involve the atria and ventricles.

- *Heart/Lung Transplantation* (33930–33945)—This category includes procedures for both heart transplants and heart/lung transplants, along with backbench work that the physician performs to prepare the heart or heart and lung for transplantation. You already learned about lung transplants in Chapter 24 and that patients may need both new lungs and a new heart, which the transplant team can transplant at the same time. In order to be eligible to receive a heart transplant, a patient must have a heart disorder so severe that all other treatments have failed, and the patient will not survive without the transplant. These conditions include **cardiomyopathy** (weak heart muscle), congestive heart failure, or abnormalities in the heart's pumping ability.

cardiomyopathy
(kärd-ē-ō-mī-äp′-ə-thē)

  - Like patients who need lung transplants, patients who qualify for heart transplants are on a waiting list that the Organ Procurement and Transplantation Network (OPTN) oversees. Donor hearts should be from cadavers who are younger than 65 years and who have little or no heart disease or chest trauma and no exposure to HIV or hepatitis. Donor hearts can survive without blood circulation for up to four hours.

  - The patient also works with an interdisciplinary transplant team at a transplant center, which includes a cardiologist, cardiovascular surgeon, and transplant coordinator, to name a few.

  - About 3,000 people in the United States are on the waiting list for a heart transplant on any given day. About 2,000 donor hearts are available each year. Wait times vary from days to several months and depend on a recipient's blood type and condition.

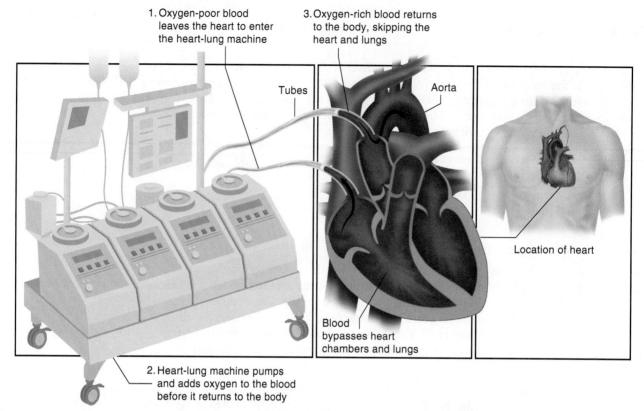

1. Oxygen-poor blood leaves the heart to enter the heart-lung machine

3. Oxygen-rich blood returns to the body, skipping the heart and lungs

Tubes

Aorta

Location of heart

Blood bypasses heart chambers and lungs

2. Heart-lung machine pumps and adds oxygen to the blood before it returns to the body

Figure 25-4 ■ How a heart–lung bypass machine works during surgery.
Source: National Institutes of Health; U.S. Department of Health and Human Services.

- Time spent on the waiting list plays a part in who receives a donor heart. For example, if two patients have equal need, the one who has been waiting longer will likely get the first available donor heart.

- At some heart transplant centers, patients carry a pager so the center can contact them at any time. Patients are asked to tell the transplant center staff if they are going out of town. They often need to be prepared to arrive at the hospital within two hours of being notified about a donor heart.

- Surgeons use open-heart surgery to perform heart transplants. The surgeon makes a large incision into the patient's chest to open the rib cage and operates on the heart, using cardiopulmonary bypass (■ FIGURE 25-4).

POINTERS FROM THE PROS: Interview with a Coding Expert

You first read advice from Danielle Taimuty, MA, CPC, CEMC, in Chapter 6. She has additional pointers to share with you.

Describe the skills that you feel a coder needs to have to be successful:

Analytical skills, problem solving, organization, confidence speaking and teaching physicians, and patience.

What advice can you give coding students to help them to prepare to work with many types of personalities?

Always keep an open mind and try to put yourself in the other person's shoes.

What qualities do you look for in an employee when determining if you should promote them?

The main characteristics I look for are the desire to help others and the willingness to go the extra mile for our clients.

(Used by permission of Danielle Taimuty.)

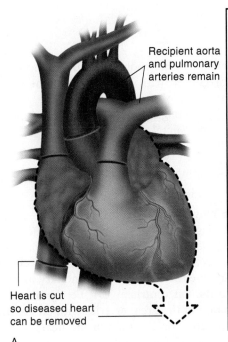

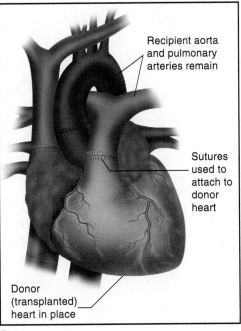

Recipient aorta and pulmonary arteries remain

Heart is cut so diseased heart can be removed

A

Recipient aorta and pulmonary arteries remain

Sutures used to attach to donor heart

Donor (transplanted) heart in place

B

Figure 25-5 ■ (A) A diseased heart is cut for removal. (B) The healthy donor heart is sutured to the recipient's arteries and veins.
Source: National Institutes of Health; U.S. Department of Health and Human Services.

transesophageal echocardiography (TEE) (trans-i-säf-ə-jē′-əl ek-ō-kärd-ē-äg′-rə-fē)—alternative way to perform an echocardiogram by inserting a probe into the esophagus to use ultrasound waves to obtain clear images of the heart

bicuspid aortic valve (bī-kəs′-pəd ā-ort′-ik)—defect of the aortic valve that results in the formation of two leaflets or cusps instead of the normal three

regurgitation (rē-gər-jə-tā′-shən)—failure of the cusps (leaflets) of the heart valve to come together tightly when closing, allowing blood to leak back into the heart

aneurysmal dilatation (an-yə-riz′-məl dil-ə-tā′-shən)—weakening that results in a bulge in the blood vessel wall

sinus of Valsalva (sahy′-nuhs val-sal′-vuh)—any of the pouches of the aorta and the pulmonary artery opposite the flaps of the semilunar valves (which permit blood to be forced into the arteries and prevent backflow of blood from the arteries into the ventricles); blood returning to the heart flows into the sinuses of Valsalva, closing the valves

- The surgeon removes the patient's diseased heart and sutures the healthy donor heart into place. The patient's aorta and pulmonary arteries are not replaced as part of the surgery (■ FIGURE 25-5).

- Heart transplant surgery usually takes about four hours. Patients often spend the first days after surgery in the ICU of the hospital. The amount of time a heart transplant recipient spends in the hospital varies. Recovery often involves one to two weeks in the hospital and three months during which the transplant team at the heart transplant center continues to monitor the patient.

- Just like a lung transplant, the patient's body will regard the new heart as a foreign object, and the patient will need to take immunosuppressive drugs to suppress the immune system and stop it from rejecting the new heart.

- About 88% of patients survive the first year after transplant surgery, and 75% survive for five years. The 10-year survival rate is about 56% (National Institutes of Health).

TAKE A BREAK

Nice work! Let's Take A Break and then practice coding more procedures. This exercise will give you experience coding procedures that we did not cover in our discussion. Be sure to consult your medical references if you need additional information.

Exercise 25.3   **Heart and Pericardium**

Instructions: Review each patient's case and then assign codes for the procedure(s), appending a modifier to the procedure when appropriate. Optional: For additional practice, assign the patient's diagnosis code(s).

1. Amy Marmo is a 2-day-old infant in the neonatal intensive care unit (NICU) at Williton Medical Center. She has cyanosis and hypotension. Echocardiog-

raphy shows hypoplastic left heart syndrome (left side of the heart does not develop completely). Dr. Ferrigno, a pediatric cardiovascular surgeon, applies right and left pulmonary artery bands (hybrid approach stage 1) to reduce the blood flow through the pulmonary artery.

Diagnosis code(s): _____

Procedure code(s): _____

2. Katy Demyan, a 3-week-old baby in the NICU at Williton, has a diagnosis of tetralogy of Fallot. Dr. Ferrigno performs a tetralogy of Fallot procedure, the

continued

TAKE A BREAK *continued*

closure of a ventricular septal defect with a pulmonary graft valve attached.

Diagnosis code(s): _____

Procedure code(s): _____

3. Giu Ta is a 39-year-old male who presents to Williton's ED with congestive heart failure. **Transesophageal echocardiography (TEE)** demonstrates a **bicuspid aortic valve** with severe **regurgitation** and **aneurysmal dilatation** of the noncoronary **sinus of Valsalva**. Dr. Dillard performs a repair of the fistula of the sinus of Valsalva, using cardiopulmonary bypass.

Diagnosis code(s): _____

Procedure code(s): _____

4. Lance Knauf is 16 years old and has a congenital condition, **Scimitar syndrome**. At Williton, Dr. Dillard repairs the isolated partial anomalous venous return.

Diagnosis code(s): _____

Procedure code(s): _____

5. Erik Portalis is a newborn male in Williton's NICU who is diagnosed with **truncus arteriosus**, a congenital anomaly of the branching of the pulmonary arteries. Dr. Ferrigno performs a surgical closure of the ventricular septal defect with a patch (also known as Rastelli type operation).

Diagnosis code(s): _____

Procedure code(s): _____

6. Saundra Yingst is a 1-month-old infant whom Dr. Ferrigno diagnoses with transposition of the aorta and pulmonary artery (the "great" arteries are reversed in their origins from the heart, with the aorta connected to the right ventricle and the pulmonary artery connected to the left ventricle). Dr. Ferrigno repairs the transposition of the great arteries with an atrial baffle procedure, creating a tunnel in the heart to redirect the flow of blood. He uses cardiopulmonary bypass.

Diagnosis code(s): _____

Procedure code(s): _____

Scimitar syndrome (sim′-i-ter)—congenital heart defect involving abnormal pulmonary veins

truncus arteriosus (trəŋ′-kəs är-tir-ē-ō′-səs)—the part of the embryonic arterial system which develops into the ascending aorta and the pulmonary trunk

thrombectomy (thrəm-bek′-tə-mē)

infrarenal (in-frə-rēn′-əl)

ARTERIES AND VEINS (34001–37799)

Arteries and Veins, the second subheading in the Cardiovascular subsection, contains 26 categories, as you saw earlier in the chapter in Table 25-1. Turn to this subheading in your CPT manual to become familiar with the categories and procedures listed. CPT categorizes the procedures mostly by the type of procedure but sometimes by the body site. To locate procedures in the index, search for the body site or the *type of procedure*.

Physicians perform procedures listed in this subheading on arteries and veins throughout the body, other than the coronary vessels. Examples of procedures in the Arteries and Veins subheading include excision of an embolus or thrombus, repair of an aneurysm or fistula, removal of plaque from an artery, grafting a vein for bypass, insertion of a catheter into a vessel to inject contrast dye for imaging or inject medication, and creation of an arteriovenous (AV) fistula for hemodialysis access (a graft under the skin, typically in the forearm, to begin hemodialysis).

As you can see from reviewing the procedures in the Arteries and Veins subheading, there are hundreds of procedures! Just as with the Heart and Pericardium subheading, we also will not review all of the procedures in the Arteries and Veins subheading. But we will focus on some of them so that you can become familiar with how physicians perform them and why. Let's get started by reviewing procedures in ■ TABLE 25-2, and you can also follow along in your CPT manual by turning to each of the categories as we discuss them. Also be sure to refer to the diagrams for arteries (Figure 11-2) and veins (Figure 11-3) so that you have a better understanding of their anatomy.

WORKPLACE IQ

You are working as a coder for Dr. Newton, a cardiovascular surgeon. Today, you are training a new coder, Julie, to assign codes for various procedures involving pacemakers. Julie says that she is very confused and does not know what a pacemaker looks like or what procedures to follow for coding pacemakers.

What would you do?

■ TABLE 25-2   **ARTERIES AND VEINS CATEGORIES OR PROCEDURES**

Category or Procedure	Description
Embolectomy/ Thrombectomy (34001–34490)	An embolus, or embolism, can cause an occlusion of a blood vessel—artery or vein. It is composed of bacteria, plaque, liquid, or even gas. An *embolectomy* is the excision of an embolus to remove the occlusion from the blood vessel, which can be done with or without using a catheter.
	A thrombus is a blood clot that can also occlude a blood vessel. A **thrombectomy** is the excision of the clot using a catheter with a balloon tip that is inflated to dilate the vessel and eliminate the clot. A thrombectomy may also include injecting a medication into the blood vessel, which will aspirate the clot.
Endovascular Repair of Abdominal Aortic Aneurysm (34800–34834)	An abdominal aortic aneurysm (AAA) occurs when the abdominal aorta abnormally dilates and bulges. It is caused by a weakening of vessel walls. Most AAAs are **infrarenal**, meaning below the kidneys.
	Endovascular repair includes the use of catheters for stent placement. The stent is placed to reinforce the vessel walls so that they do not bulge. You should separately report codes for fluoroscopic guidance (live X-ray) that the physician uses to view the procedure as he performs it.
	Notice that there are several CPT guidelines for this procedure, which you will need to carefully review before final code assignment.
Angioscopy (35400)	In angioscopy, the physician views the inside of a blood vessel using an angioscope, an endoscope to examine a vessel (angi/o). The angioscope can transmit the image of the vessel to a monitor, using fluoroscopy. The physician can then diagnose various disorders, such as an embolus, lesion, or plaque.
Transluminal Angioplasty (35450–35476)	*Transluminal* means across (trans) the lumen (inside of a vessel). A transluminal angioplasty is a procedure to widen a blood vessel that is occluded from atherosclerosis, using a catheter with a balloon on a guidewire. Once the catheter is inside the vessel, the physician inflates the balloon to dilate the vessel and then removes the balloon. The physician may also insert a stent to keep the vessel open.
	The procedure can be open (using an incision) or percutaneous (using a puncture in the skin). Note that if a physician performs transluminal angioplasty with another procedure, you should append modifier -51 (multiple procedures) or -52 (reduced services) to the transluminal angioplasty code.
	Separately report radiology imaging used for the procedure with a code from the Radiology section.
Bypass Graft (35500–35671)	You already learned about CABG earlier in this chapter. The principle of a bypass graft for veins is the same: treating an occluded vessel by creating a new road for blood to travel, using a healthy vein from the patient or using synthetic material. The new road *bypasses* the area of the vessel that is occluded, allowing blood to flow freely.
	The procedure treats patients with arterial stenosis, lesions, atherosclerosis, or peripheral vascular occlusive disease.
	Take a look at the some of the code choices for a bypass vein graft, starting with code 35501. Notice that the code descriptors specifically name the vessels involved in the procedure.
	Also notice that there are several CPT guidelines at the beginning of the Bypass Graft category to assist you with assigning bypass graft codes, including the fact that codes 35501–35587 already include procurement of (obtaining) the saphenous vein graft, so you should not report a separate code for it. Be sure to read the guidelines carefully before final code assignment.
Composite Grafts (35681–35683)	A composite graft incorporates synthetic material into a graft procedure. The codes for composite grafts are all *add-on codes* that you should report *in addition* to the code for the primary graft procedure.
	There are also CPT guidelines to direct you on correctly assigning these codes.
Vascular Injection Procedures (36000–36598)	Vascular injection procedures involve injecting contrast dye for radiological imaging or injecting medication into blood vessels.
	Notice that some of the codes for vascular injection procedures describe *selective catheter placement*, which means that the physician treats a specific vessel using a catheter but needs to enter another vessel, and then move through one or more additional vessels, to reach the vessel that needs treatment. Vessels connect to one another through *branches* (Figures 11-2, 11-3). These branches are categorized in groups, called first-, second-, or third-order vessels.

continued

■ TABLE 25-2   *continued*

Category or Procedure	Description
	The CPT code that you choose for selective catheter placement depends on how far the physician advances the catheter and the specific order of vessels involved. This is why you will see first-order, second-order, and third-order branches mentioned in the code descriptors for selective catheter placement. A *vascular family* is a group of vessels composed of first-, second-, and third-order branches and branches beyond the third order.
	Turn to Appendix L in your CPT manual. Appendix L lists the various vascular families of the body and the order of the branches to help you better understand the names of the vessels and the order they represent.
	Nonselective catheter placement occurs when the physician performs a procedure using a catheter and places it into one vessel without advancing it any further.
Intraosseous (36680)	Intraosseous literally means in (inter) the bone (osseous). There is one code in this category for placement of a needle for intraosseous infusion. Many times, this procedure is performed emergently to administer fluids and medication directly into the bone marrow in patients who either cannot receive fluids intravenously or need them faster than the intravenous route can deliver.
Transluminal Atherectomy (37225–37233)	An **atherectomy** is a procedure to excise (-ectomy) plaque (ather/o, or atheroma) that occludes a blood vessel, using an extraction catheter, which has rotating blades for cutting and a grinder for breaking up the plaque. The plaque can be vacuumed out of the blood vessel, gathered by the catheter, or left in the form of miniscule fragments in the bloodstream for the body to absorb and excrete.
	Did you notice that the CPT notes for a transluminal atherectomy are the same as they are for a transluminal angioplasty? So if a physician performs a transluminal atherectomy with another procedure, you should append modifier -51 (multiple procedures) or -52 (reduced services) to the transluminal atherectomy code. You should also separately report radiology imaging used for the procedure with a code from the Radiology section.
Endoscopy (37500–37501)	This procedure is *surgical vascular endoscopy for ligation of perforator veins. Perforator veins* join the two sets of veins in the body: superficial veins (near the skin) and deep veins. The perforator veins have valves that help blood to flow to the heart. But if the valves do not work properly, blood can flow backward, away from the heart, enlarging the superficial veins. This causes the veins to become varicose (enlarged, twisted). This condition is called venous insufficiency, or varicose veins, which is more common in the legs (■ FIGURE 25-6).
	The physician may **ligate** a vein (tie it off) and then remove it, using an open procedure without an endoscope. There are many other codes for vein ligation that do not involve an endoscope. Take a look at some of them under the Ligation category.

TAKE A BREAK

Way to go! You finished reviewing procedures in the Cardiovascular System! Let's Take A Break and then review more about the procedures and then practice coding them.

Exercise 25.4 Arteries and Veins

Part 1—Theory

Instructions: Fill in the blank with the best answer.

1. A(n) _____ is the excision of an embolus to remove the occlusion from the blood vessel.

2. A(n) _____ occurs when the abdominal aorta abnormally dilates and bulges.

3. Using _____, the physician can diagnose various disorders, such as an embolus, lesion, or plaque.

4. A(n) _____ angioplasty is a procedure to widen a blood vessel that is occluded from atherosclerosis, using a catheter with a balloon on a guidewire.

5. The procedure that incorporates synthetic material into a graft procedure is called a(n) _____.

6. A(n) _____ is a procedure to excise plaque that occludes a blood vessel, using an extraction catheter, which has rotating blades.

Part 2—Coding

Instructions: Review each patient's case, and then assign codes for the procedure(s), appending a modifier to the procedure when appropriate. Optional: For additional practice, assign the patient's diagnosis code(s) (ICD-9-CM).

1. Fannie Fail, a 54-year-old, presents to the office with a blood clot in her right leg. Dr. Dillard, a cardiovascular surgeon, performs a thrombectomy of the femoral artery using a leg incision. The vascular return is reestablished and Ms. Fail recovers nicely.

TAKE A BREAK *continued*

Diagnosis code(s): _____

Procedure code(s): _____

2. Gina Fava, a 35-year-old, is a hairstylist and is on her feet most of her day. She has pain and swelling in both legs and Dr. Dillard diagnoses severe varicose veins. At Williton, he performs a femoral vein valvuloplasty on both legs.

Diagnosis code(s): _____

Procedure code(s): _____

3. Herbert Ringler, an 89-year-old, has an AAA. Today at Williton, Dr. Michalek, a cardiovascular surgeon, repairs the AAA with a modified bifurcated prosthesis.

Diagnosis code(s): _____

Procedure code(s): _____

4. Anthony Scheiffer, a 64-year-old, presents to Williton's ED with acute onset of abdominal pain of 24 hours' duration. He reports to Dr. Mills, the ED physician, that the pain is mainly in the lower quadrants and flanks (between the rib and hip). Dr. Mills examines the patient and orders further workup. An ultrasound scan of the abdomen reveals a 6-cm aneurysm of the right common iliac artery (main artery in the pelvis).

Dr. Mills consults Dr. Michalek, a cardiovascular surgeon, who performs an emergency endovascular repair of the iliac artery aneurysm using a stent.

Diagnosis code(s): _____

Procedure code(s): _____

5. Jacob Winick, age 25, sustained a shrapnel injury of his left leg during a previous injury sustained during the Iraq war. This injury resulted in an arteriovenous fistula (abnormal connection or passageway between an artery and a vein). Today at Williton, Dr. Dillard repairs the fistula.

Diagnosis code(s): _____

Procedure code(s): _____

6. Dr. Michalek diagnoses Maria Disla, age 65, with plaque in the lining of the **axillary** artery (large blood vessel that transports oxygenated blood to the thorax, axilla, and upper extremity). Today at Williton, Dr. Michalek performs a **thromboendarterectomy** of the axillary artery.

Diagnosis code(s): _____

Procedure code(s): _____

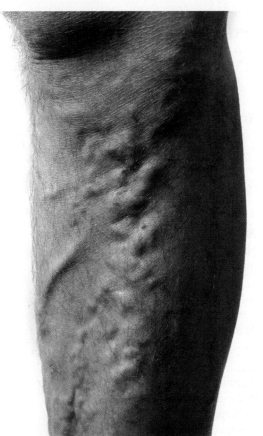

Figure 25-6 ■ Varicose veins on a male patient's leg.

Photo credit: Audie/Shutterstock.

atherectomy
(ath-ə-rek′-tə-mē)

ligate (lī′-gāt)

axillary (′ak-sə-ler-ē)

thromboendarterectomy
(thräm-bō-en-där-tə-rek′-tə-mē)—excision of a thrombus from an artery

DESTINATION: MEDICARE

This Medicare exercise will help you to learn more about cardiac pacemakers. Follow the instructions listed to access one of the MLN products on cardiac pacemaker guidelines.

1. Go to the website http://www.cms.gov.
2. At the top of the screen on the banner bar, choose *Outreach & Education*.
3. Under the *Medicare Learning Network*, click *MLN Products*.
4. Under *MLN Products*, click *MLN Catalog of Products*.
5. Scroll down to *Downloads*, and choose *MLN Catalog of Products*.
6. Press the Ctrl key and the F key at the same time to access the search function.
7. Type "pacemaker" into the search field. Then click on the fact sheet called *Cardiac Pacemakers: Complying with Documentation and Coverage Requirements.* Answer the questions listed next.

1. Name one of the four covered indications for a dual-chamber pacemaker:

   _____

2. Does Medicare consider cardiac pacing acceptable for sinus node dysfunction? _____

3. Does Medicare cover a dual-chamber pacemaker for patients with frequent or persistent supraventricular tachycardias? _____

tracheomalacia
(trā-kē-ə-mə-lā′-sh(ē-)ə)

pseudoaneurysm
(süd′-ō-an-yə-riz-əm)—
a vascular abnormality of the
aorta resembling an aneurysm

CHAPTER REVIEW

Multiple Choice

Instructions: Circle one best answer to complete each statement.

1. The _____ is a sac surrounding the heart.
   a. endocardium
   b. intracardium
   c. epicardium
   d. pericardium

2. Where can you find codes for cardiovascular procedures in the CPT manual?
   a. Evaluation and Management section, Cardiovascular subsection, and Medicine section
   b. Cardiovascular subsection, Medicine section, Radiology section
   c. Evaluation and Management section, Cardiovascular subsection, and Radiology section
   d. Cardiovascular subsection, Pathology and Laboratory section, and Medicine section

3. Physicians diagnose cardiac tumors through
   a. radiologic imaging.
   b. needle core biopsies.
   c. open heart procedures.
   d. angioplasty.

4. _____ is a laser procedure to increase blood flow in the coronary arteries.

   a. Transmyocardial infarction (TI)
   b. Aortic revascularization (AR)
   c. Transmyocardial revascularization (TMR)
   d. Angioplastic transmyocardial revascularization (ATR)

5. According to CPT guidelines, a _____ system includes a pulse generator and one electrode inserted in either the atrium or ventricle.
   a. dual-chamber pacemaker
   b. single-chamber pacemaker
   c. pacing cardioverter-defibrillator
   d. implantable cardioverter-defibrillator

6. According to CPT guidelines, codes for electrophysiologic operative procedures describe the surgical treatment of
   a. supraventricular dysrhythmias.
   b. superventricular dysrhythmias.
   c. atrioventricular dysrhythmias.
   d. arteriovenous dysrhythmias.

7. A patient-activated event recorder is called a(n) _____ recorder.
   a. electrical
   b. monitor
   c. loop
   d. arrhythmic

8. The procedure for allowing a machine to perform the work of the heart and lungs to maintain a bloodless surgical field is called
   a. pulmonary bypass.
   b. cardiovascular bypass.
   c. pulmonocardiac bypass.
   d. cardiopulmonary bypass.

9. The mitral valve and triscuspid valve are called _____ valves.
   a. atrioventricular
   b. ventriculoatrial
   c. semilunar
   d. semiventricular

10. A condition of a weak heart muscle is called
    a. tetralogy of Fallot.
    b. cardiac tamponade.
    c. cardiomyopathy.
    d. cardiac insufficiency.

Coding Assignments

Instructions: Review each patient's case and then assign codes for the procedure(s), appending a modifier when appropriate. Optional: Assign the patient's diagnosis code(s) (ICD-9-CM).

1. Agnes Hartt, age 84, has COPD and **tracheomalacia** (degeneration of the elastic and connective tissue of the trachea). Today at Williton, Dr. Michalek, a cardiovascular surgeon, performs an aortopexy (procedure to stabilize the trachea).

   Diagnosis code(s): _____

   Procedure code(s): _____

2. Doug Harvard, a 48-year-old, sees Dr. Michalek for a previously diagnosed thoracic aortic aneurysm. After performing an evaluation in the office, Dr. Michalek sends Mr. Harvard to Williton where he repairs the ascending aorta with a graft, using cardiopulmonary bypass.

   Diagnosis code(s): _____

   Procedure code(s): _____

3. Betty Manz, age 82, presents to Dr. Michalek's office with a **pseudoaneurysm** of the descending thoracic aorta. She is asymptomatic; however, Dr. Michalek arranges for surgery at Williton and subsequently repairs the pseudoaneurysm with an endoprosthesis (internal artificial device or material).

   Diagnosis code(s): _____

   Procedure code(s): _____

4. Mr. Tague had gastric bypass surgery two weeks ago. At his follow-up visit with Dr. Dillard, a cardiovascular surgeon, he complains of shortness of breath and chest pain. Dr. Dillard examines the patient and orders a chest X-ray and echocardiogram. After testing is completed, Dr. Dillard diagnoses Mr. Tague with a pulmonary artery embolism and tells the patient that he will need surgery. Dr. Dillard subsequently performs an embolectomy without cardiopulmonary bypass. Mr. Tague recovers from the surgery without any problems.

   Diagnosis code(s): _____

   Procedure code(s): _____

5. Andrew Toothman is a 5-year-old male who has cystic fibrosis and primary cardiomyopathy He is on the transplant list at Williton Medical Center for both a heart and lungs. Finally, a heart and lungs arrive, and Andrew's parents take him to Williton where Dr. Ferrigno, a pediatric cardiovascular surgeon, and the transplant team perform a heart–lung transplant.

   Diagnosis code(s): _____

   Procedure code(s): _____

6. Today at Williton, Dr. Michalek inserts a left ventricular assist device (mechanical pump to perform functions of the heart) into the left ventricle for Rob Rexroat, age 54. Mr. Rexroat suffers from advanced congestive heart failure and is in the ICU awaiting a heart transplant.

   Diagnosis code(s): _____

   Procedure code(s): _____

7. Glenda Fout, age 80, sees Dr. Dillard at Williton for an angioscopy of the right femoral artery for peripheral vascular disease.

   Diagnosis code(s): _____

   Procedure code(s): _____

8. Nancy Niemiec, age 78, has an atherosclerotic obstruction of the renal artery (artery that supplies the kidneys with blood) which causes renal stenosis. Dr. Michalek performs an angioplasty of the renal artery (called percutaneous transluminal renal angioplasty, PTRA) at Williton.

   Diagnosis code(s): _____

   Procedure code(s): _____

9. Betsy Karn, age 73, sees Dr. Michalek at Williton. She suffers from an occluded femoral artery. Dr. Michalek performs a left femoropopliteal bypass graft, using a vein.

   Diagnosis code(s): _____

   Procedure code(s): _____

10. Vladimir Vlacek, age 71, suffers from leg pain and edema. Dr. Dillard examines the patient and orders further workup. He then diagnoses Mr. Vlacek with an obstructed femoral artery. At Williton, Dr. Dillard performs a bypass graft of the right femoropopliteal artery with Gore-Tex (synthetic graft) using a portion of the saphenous vein.

    Diagnosis code(s): _____

    Procedure code(s): _____

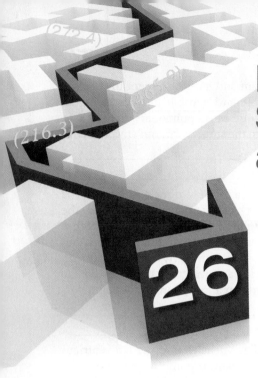

Hemic and Lymphatic Systems, Mediastinum, and Diaphragm

26

Learning Objectives

After completing this chapter, you should be able to

- Spell and define the key terminology in this chapter.
- Describe the functions and structure of the hemic and lymphatic systems.
- Identify various spleen, bone marrow, and lymphatic disorders.
- List procedures that physicians perform on the spleen.
- Explain procedures under the General subheading, including bone marrow transplants.
- Discuss procedures of the lymph nodes and lymphatic channels.
- Explain the structure and function of the mediastinum and diaphragm.
- Describe procedures of the mediastinum and diaphragm.

Key Terms

bone marrow
diaphragm
hemic

lymphatic system
mediastinum
spleen

INTRODUCTION

Your journey has brought you to learning about procedures of the hemic and lymphatic systems, mediastinum, and diaphragm, subsections of the Surgery chapter. You will learn about the function of the spleen, bone marrow procedures, and procedures involving the lymph nodes. You will continue to apply skills you have already learned to code these new procedures.

"Bear in mind, if you are going to amount to anything, that your success does not depend upon the brilliance and the impetuosity with which you take hold, but upon the everlasting and sanctified bull doggedness with which you hang on after you have taken hold."—Dr. A. B. Meldrum

HEMIC AND LYMPHATIC SYSTEMS (38100–38999)

The subsection Hemic and Lymphatic Systems contains codes that represent procedures related to the bone marrow, blood, the lymph nodes, and lymphatic channels (vessels that transport lymph to the bloodstream) (■ Table 26-1).

■ TABLE 26-1   **PROCEDURES LISTED UNDER HEMIC AND LYMPHATIC SYSTEMS**

Subsection, Subheading, and Categories	Code Range
HEMIC AND LYMPHATIC SYSTEMS	**38100–38999**
Spleen	**38100–38200**
Excision	*38100–38102*
Repair	*38115*
Laparoscopy	*38120–38129*
Introduction	*38200*
General	**38204–38242**
Bone Marrow or Stem Cell Services/Procedures	*38204–38242*
Lymph Nodes and Lymphatic Channels	**38300–38999**
Incision	*38300–38382*
Excision	*38500–38555*
Limited Lymphadenectomy for Staging	*38562–38564*
Laparoscopy	*38570–38589*
Radical Lymphadenectomy (Radical Resection of Lymph Nodes)	*38700–38780*
Introduction	*38790–38794*
Other Procedures	*38900–38999*

Hemic literally means pertaining to (-ic) the blood (hem/o). Recall from Chapter 9 that blood has many important functions in the body to maintain homeostasis, including delivering nutrients, eliminating wastes, transporting oxygen and hormones, and fighting infections. The body performs these functions by using erythrocytes, red blood cells (RBCs); leukocytes, white blood cells (WBCs); and thrombocytes, platelets (which help blood to clot). Blood is made up of cells, platelets, and plasma (Figure 9-16). A hematologist is a physician who diagnoses and treats blood disorders.

Bone marrow is soft, spongy tissue inside bones. The body produces RBCs, WBCs, and platelets in bone marrow. Stem cells are cells in the bone marrow, which can grow to become other types of cells, a process called *differentiation*. Stem cells help the body to repair damaged tissue.

Bone marrow can be red or yellow (■ FIGURE 26-1). The red marrow produces blood cells and platelets, and the yellow marrow is made up of fat cells. An infant's bone marrow is completely red, but as the body ages, the bone marrow becomes yellow.

Lymphology is the study of (-ology) the lymph (lymph/o), or the study of the lymphatic system. The **lymphatic system** consists of vessels, nodes, ducts, and organs and moves lymph, a clear fluid containing protein, throughout the body (■ FIGURE 26-2). Blood that moves throughout the circulatory system contains plasma (the liquid part of the blood). Some of the plasma escapes from the capillaries, and the lymphatic system then transports it and eventually returns it to the blood. The lymphatic system produces lymphocytes (cells that are found in the lymph, lymphoid tissues, and blood), which produce antibodies to defend the body against disease, bacteria, and viruses.

The lymphatic system is made up of lymph capillaries, which transport lymph to lymphatic vessels and into lymph nodes (also called lymph glands) that filter bacteria by producing lymphocytes. The network of lymph capillaries runs throughout the body. Lymph nodes (■ FIGURE 26-3) are bean-shaped and can be found especially in the groin, neck, chest, collar bone, inner thigh, and axillae.

When an infection invades the body, lymph nodes can swell as large as an olive because they produce lymphocytes to fight the infection. You may have heard the term "swollen glands," which means a person's lymph nodes are swollen because they are fighting an infection. Lymph nodes may also enlarge because of an invading tumor. The

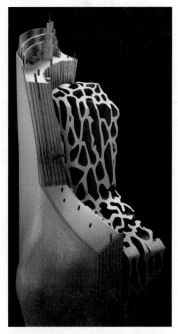

Figure 26-1 ■ Internal structure of a bone showing bone marrow.

Photo credit: © MedicalRF.com/Alamy.

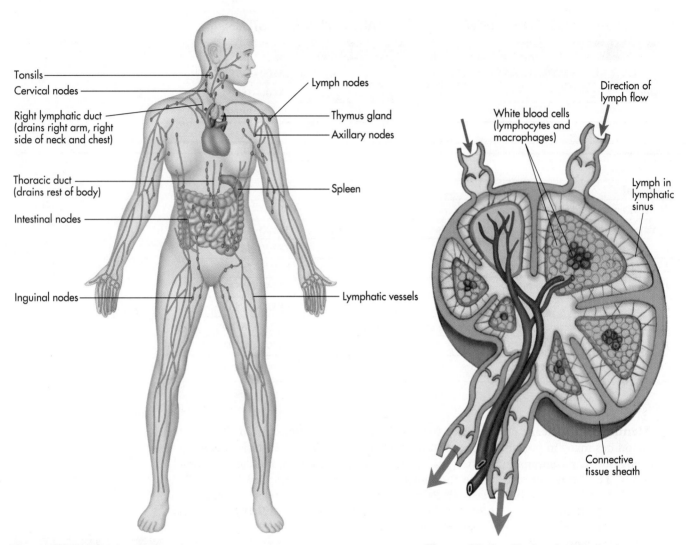

Figure 26-2 ■ The lymphatic system.

Figure 26-3 ■ The lymph node structure.

lymphatic system is part of the body's immune system, or defense against invading organisms, the skin being the first line of defense. Depending on the patient's condition and severity of illness, diagnosing and treating disorders of the lymphatic system may involve an immunologist (a physician who specializes in the immune system), an oncologist (a physician who specializes in cancer treatment), or other types of physicians.

The **spleen** is an organ of the lymphatic system (Figure 26-2) and is located in the upper left quadrant of the abdomen. The spleen produces lymphocytes, creates and stores RBCs, and filters blood by destroying old RBCs.

It is important to know about the types of conditions that a patient may have so that you will better understand how to assign codes for procedures in the Hemic and Lymphatic Systems subsection. Here are some spleen, bone marrow, and lymphatic disorders:

- Anemia—a condition where bone marrow cannot create RBCs
- **Cystic hygroma** (also called **lymphagioma**)—abnormal lymph vessel; congenital neck mass, formed from lymphatic tissue
- Leukemia—cancer of the blood where cells develop and grow abnormally
- **Lymph node abscess**—abscess formed within a lymph node
- **Lymphadenitis**—inflammation of lymph node(s)

cystic hygroma
(sis′ tik hi-gro′ ma)

lymphagioma
(lim-fan-jē-ō′-mə)

lymph node abscess
(limf nōd ab′ ses)

lymphadenitis
(lim-fad′ en ī tis)

- Lymphedema—swelling of the lymph node or lymphatic system, due to blockage caused by an underlying disease or disorder
- **Lymphoma**—tumor of a lymphoid cell (relating to lymph or lymph tissue)
- **Myeloproliferative** diseases—a group of conditions where the body produces too many bone marrow cells
- **Splenomegaly**—enlarged spleen caused by infection, cancer, anemia, blood clot, or cyst; enlargement causes storage of RBCs and platelets and diminishes their numbers throughout the body; an enlarged spleen can rupture

lymphoma (lim fo′ mah)

myeloproliferative
(mī ĕ-lō-pro-lif′ er-ah-tiv)

splenomegaly
(sple nō meg′ ah-le)

Spleen (38100–38200)

Codes listed under the subheading *Spleen* describe procedures that physicians perform on the spleen, such as excision (**splenectomy**) and repair (**splenorrhaphy**). Even though the spleen plays an important role in the body's immune system, an adult's body can function without it, but people without spleens are more susceptible to infections than people with spleens. A child without a spleen is much more susceptible to infections because a child's body has not developed other immune responses yet, as an adult's body has.

splenectomy (spl-nek′tah me)

splenorrhaphy
(sple-nor′ ah-fe)

Physicians perform splenectomies when the spleen is ruptured due to trauma (medical emergency), when there is cancer in the spleen, or when the patient suffers from hypersplenism, an overactive and possibly enlarged spleen, which other disorders, such as lymphoma, can cause.

Notice that codes 38100 and 38101 for splenectomy list "separate procedure" as part of the code descriptors. Remember from Chapter 21 that some procedures and services are integral components (parts) of another major service or procedure, and these integral procedures are called *minor* procedures. You should not separately code minor procedures (separate procedures) when they are integral components of a major procedure.

A splenorrhaphy is necessary when the patient's spleen is ruptured by trauma, such as from injuries in a motor vehicle or sports accident. Underlying infections can also cause the spleen to enlarge and increase the chances of a splenic rupture.

Splenoportography is an X-ray where the patient receives a contrast injection to view the splenic vein and the portal vein (the large vein connected to the digestive system, spleen, pancreas, liver, and gall bladder). Physicians can view occlusions in both veins, and the procedure is especially important before a patient receives a liver transplant. Assign the code for splenoportography from the Radiology section of CPT.

splenoportography
(spleen ō por′ tŏ grah-fe)

Turn to the categories within the *Spleen* subheading to review the procedures, which CPT arranges by type of procedure, and refer to ■ TABLE 26-2 for a summary of categories and the procedures listed in each.

To find codes for procedures of the spleen, search the index for the main term *spleen* and then the subterm for the *type of procedure*, or search for the *type of procedure*, which may also include the subterm *spleen*. Refer to the following example to code a procedure involving the spleen.

■ TABLE 26-2　**CATEGORIES AND PROCEDURES UNDER SPLEEN**

Category Name	Code Range	Procedures Included
Excision	38100–38102	Splenectomy, total or partial—excision of the spleen
Repair	38115	Splenorrhaphy—repair of ruptured spleen, with or without partial splenectomy
Laparoscopy	38120–38129	• Splenectomy—performed by laparoscopy (a surgical procedure that includes diagnostic laparoscopy, using a laparoscope)
		• Unlisted laparoscopy procedure, spleen
Introduction	38200	Injection procedure for splenoportography

Example: Dr. Simpson, an internist (physician who specializes in internal medicine) at Williton Medical Center, performs a total splenectomy for Ralph Porter, age 36, whose spleen ruptured from injuries he suffered in a car accident where he was the driver. Dr. Simpson documents splenic rupture with **parenchymal** fragmentation.

Search the index for the main term *splenectomy* and subterm *total*, which lists code 38100. Assign code **38100**, which represents a total splenectomy. The patient's diagnosis code is **865.04** (main term *laceration*, subterm *spleen*, subterm *with*, and subterm *disruption of parenchyma*) and **E819.0** (main term *accident* and subterm *motor vehicle*).

parenchymal (păr-ĕn′kĭ-măl)—essential part of an organ, such as tissue that is essential to providing its unique function

TAKE A BREAK

That was a good bit of information to cover! Let's take a break, review more about the hemic and lymphatic systems, and practice coding spleen procedures.

Exercise 26.1   Hemic and Lymphatic Systems, Spleen

Part 1—Theory

Instructions: Fill in the blank with the best answer.

1. _____ are cells in the bone marrow, which can grow to become other types of cells, a process called _____.

2. The _____ consists of vessels, nodes, ducts, and organs that move lymph throughout the body.

3. These are bean-shaped and can be found especially in the groin, neck, chest, collar bone, inner thigh, and axillae: _____

4. Cancer of the blood where cells develop and grow abnormally is called _____.

5. A radiology procedure where the patient receives a contrast injection to view the splenic vein and the portal vein is called _____.

6. Physicians perform a _____ when the spleen is ruptured due to trauma (medical emergency) or when there is cancer in the spleen.

Part 2—Coding

Instructions: Review the patient's case and then assign codes for the procedure(s), appending a modifier when appropriate. Optional: For additional practice, assign the patient's diagnosis code(s) (ICD-9-CM).

1. John Timothy, age 46, was driving his car on U.S. Highway 422 when he collided with a truck. He suffered multiple injuries. Dr. Mills, an ED physician at Williton Medical Center, examines the patient. He performs a detailed history, comprehensive exam, and medical decision making of high complexity. Dr. Mills diagnoses the patient with a concussion with a 15 minute loss of consciousness, fractured radius of the distal end, and traumatic ruptured spleen. Dr. Mills consults with Dr. Nelson, a general surgeon, who determines that he can repair the spleen, rather than remove it, and he performs surgery. Code for Dr. Mills' services and Dr. Nelson's procedure.

   Diagnosis code(s): _____

   Dr. Mills' procedure code(s): _____

   Dr. Nelson's procedure code(s): _____

2. Julie Raymond, age 28, was in a motorcycle accident, where she was the passenger, and the motorcycle hit a car. An ambulance transports her to Williton's ED. Ms. Raymond suffers from severe abdominal pain. Dr. Mills examines her and orders further workup. Dr. Mills performs an expanded problem focused history, comprehensive exam, and medical decision making of high complexity. He determines that she has a lacerated spleen and consults with Dr. Nelson, who determines that the patient needs immediate surgery. Dr. Nelson admits her to Williton and performs a laparoscopic splenectomy. Code for Dr. Mills' services and Dr. Nelson's procedure.

   Diagnosis code(s): _____

   Dr. Mills' procedure code(s): _____

   Dr. Nelson's procedure code(s): _____

3. Simone Gonzales, age 26, was driving the motorcycle, and Ms. Raymond was her passenger. Ms. Gonzales also lacerated her spleen during the accident and was taken immediately to the operating room for a total splenectomy. Unlike Ms. Raymond, Ms. Gonzales had to have an open procedure, as her injuries were too severe for laparoscopic removal.

   Diagnosis code(s): _____

   Procedure code(s): _____

TAKE A BREAK *continued*

4. Millicent Lavage, age 72, arrives at Williton's ED because of edema of her left side. Dr. Mills examines her and orders radiology testing. A CT scan reveals a splenic mass, which Dr. Nelson biopsies. The pathology report indicates a benign splenic neoplasm. Dr. Nelson then performs a partial splenectomy to treat the patient's condition.

Diagnosis code(s): _____

Procedure code(s): _____

5. Dr. Nelson performs a partial splenectomy for Marcus Lieberman, age 35, due to a rupture in a section of his spleen.

Diagnosis code(s): _____

Procedure code(s): _____

6. After his surgery, Mr. Lieberman has an episode of postoperative bleeding, with dehiscence of an internal suture, which results in a return to the operating room (OR) for Dr. Nelson to perform an additional repair of the spleen.

Diagnosis code(s): _____

Procedure code(s): _____

General (38204–38242)—Bone Marrow or Stem Cell Services/Procedures

Procedures under the General subheading include the category Bone Marrow or Stem Cell Services/Procedures, which involve steps to preserve, prepare, and purify bone marrow/stem cells prior to transplantation or reinfusion. CPT guidelines state that providers are only permitted to report one code per day, regardless of the total number of bone marrow or stem cells involved in a procedure.

A *bone marrow transplant* is when a physician transplants healthy bone marrow into a patient with abnormal or diseased bone marrow from leukemia, lymphoma, multiple myeloma, immunodeficiency disorders, or aplastic anemia. The transplant is needed to replace defective stem cells. The process of transplantation is similar to a blood transfusion. The patient remains awake during the procedure, which takes about an hour to perform.

POINTERS FROM THE PROS: Interview with a Medical Instructor

Peter Viola is a medical instructor for a postsecondary school where he teaches medical coding, health insurance, medical terminology, anatomy and physiology, and medical law and ethics to students who are pursuing Associate in Science degrees in Medical Assisting or Medical Office Administration. Mr. Viola spent over 25 years in management and oversaw health information management departments, including coding, transcription, correspondence, and storage of patient medical records. He holds a Masters degree in Business Administration and is a Registered Health Information Administrator (RHIA) through the American Health Information Management Association (AHIMA).

Why did you become interested in teaching?

I wanted to make a difference in my field of study. I could achieve this goal by instructing and molding future individuals who would be working in health care.

Please give an example of a time when you educated a physician(s) on processes of coding or any other procedures, and the outcome:

I developed a managed care billing/coding/documentation process that validated the codes assigned vs. the physician's actual documentation. I also provided group and individual orientation and instruction in appropriate assignment of codes, along with appropriate physician documentation.

What advice would you like to give to coding students to help them prepare to work successfully with various personality types?

Make sure they take psychology and management courses. Also, participate in personality profiling surveys to learn about different personalities and the proper techniques to effectively deal with them.

(Used by permission of Peter Viola.)

Before the transplant, the patient receives chemotherapy or radiation, which destroys defective stem cells before transplanted cells are introduced. The patient can receive one of the following types of bone marrow transplants:

autologous (aw-tol′ o-gus)

- **Autologous** *transplant*—The patient provides stem cells, and the physician removes and destroys abnormal cells before returning bone marrow to the patient.

allogenic (al-o-jĕ-ne′-ik)

- **Allogenic** *transplant*—A donor provides stem cells. The donor must be a good genetic match to the patient and must have the same blood type. Many times, the donor is the patient's sister, brother, parent, or other relative. Donors can also be people not related to the patient who choose to donate stem cells for any transplant, and their stem cells become part of a bone marrow registry of available donors. The patient is then matched to a donor in the registry.

- *Umbilical cord transplant*—Stem cells come from the umbilical cord of an infant after birth. These stem cells undergo testing and are then frozen (cryopreservation) until it is time to transplant them into a patient.

apheresis (af-er-ē′-sis)

A *bone marrow harvest* is when the physician collects bone marrow from a donor's hip bone using a needle and syringe. The physician can also remove specific cells, including T cells (white blood cells), or deplete them from donated bone marrow (**apheresis**) to eliminate the risk of the recipient's body rejecting the donor cells, called *graft-versus-host disease (GVHD)*.

Physicians perform a *bone marrow aspiration*, also called bone marrow sampling, which is removing bone marrow fluid for diagnosis or to collect stem cells for a transplant. A *bone marrow biopsy* is the removal of bone and marrow, typically from the hip bone. The aspiration or biopsy, both performed using a needle, helps the physician to diagnose bone marrow disorders, such as leukemia, myeloproliferative disorders (abnormal growth of platelets and blood cells in bone marrow), anemia, and cancers. An aspiration or biopsy can also help the physician evaluate if a bone marrow transplant was successful.

Turn to the categories within the General subheading to review the procedures, and refer to ■ TABLE 26-3 for a summary of categories and the procedures listed in each. CPT arranges the codes by type of procedure and whether cells, platelets, or plasma were involved in the procedure. To locate codes in the index, search under the body site (stem cell) and then the type of procedure, or search for the type of procedure (harvesting) and then the body site.

Refer to the following example to code a procedure involving bone marrow/stem cells.

hematopoietic progenitor cell (he-ma-t-poy-et′ik prŏg-ĕn′-ĭ-tŏr)—stem cells in the umbilical cord and bone marrow

Example: Dr. Hicks, an oncologist specializing in bone marrow disorders, performs a bone marrow biopsy for Ms. Hunt, a 26-year-old, due to an abnormal CBC. The biopsy is positive for lymphoma.

Search the index for the main term *biopsy* and subterm *bone marrow*, which lists code 38221. Assign code **38221**, which represents the bone marrow biopsy. The patient's diagnosis code is **202.80** (main term *lymphoma*).

■ **TABLE 26-3** **CATEGORY AND PROCEDURES UNDER GENERAL**

Category Name	Code Range	Procedures Included
Bone Marrow or Stem Cell Services/ Procedures	38204–38242	• Management of recipient **hematopoietic progenitor cell** donor search and cell acquisition • Blood-derived hematopoietic progenitor cell harvesting for transplantation, allogenic or autologous • Transplant preparation of hematopoietic progenitor cells, including cryopreservation, thawing, and specific cell depletion • Bone marrow aspiration or biopsy • Bone marrow harvesting for transplantation • Bone marrow or blood-derived peripheral stem cell transplantation, allogenic or autologous

TAKE A BREAK

Let's take a break, review more about the General subheading, and practice coding bone marrow/stem cell procedures.

Exercise 26.2   General; Bone Marrow or Stem Cell Services/Procedures

Part 1—Theory

Instructions: Fill in the blank with the best answer.

1. Before a _____, the patient receives chemotherapy or radiation, which destroys defective stem cells before transplanted cells are introduced.

2. In this type of transplant, stem cells come from the umbilical cord of an infant after birth: _____

3. In this type of transplant, a donor provides stem cells. The donor must be a good genetic match to the patient and must have the same blood type. _____

4. In this type of transplant, the patient provides stem cells, and the physician removes and destroys abnormal cells before returning bone marrow to the patient: _____

5. A _____ is when the physician collects bone marrow from a donor's hip bone using a needle and syringe.

6. Physicians perform a _____, also called bone marrow sampling, which is removing bone marrow fluid for diagnosis or to collect stem cells for a transplant.

Part 2—Coding

Instructions: Review the patient's case and then assign codes for the procedure(s), appending a modifier when appropriate. Optional: For additional practice, assign the patient's diagnosis code(s) (ICD-9-CM).

1. Collin Cortez, an 18-year-old high school senior, sees Dr. Hoffman with complaints of fever, fatigue, and a stiff neck. Dr. Hoffman orders blood tests, and the results later show an elevated WBC count. Dr. Hoffman refers the patient to Dr. Klootwyk, an oncologist, to perform a bone marrow aspiration from the sternum at Williton Medical Center to determine the cause of the patient's symptoms. Code for Dr. Klootwyk's services.

Diagnosis code(s): _____

Procedure code(s): _____

2. Trina Timpkin, age 12, needs a bone marrow transplant. Her mother, Julia Timpkin, age 46, volunteers to be tested to determine if she is a histological match, and she is. Today at Williton, Dr. Klootwyk performs bone marrow harvesting for Mrs. Timpkin so that she can donate bone marrow cells to her daughter.

Diagnosis code(s): _____

Procedure code(s): _____

3. Mrs. McCormick, age 49, had bone marrow harvesting prior to receiving chemotherapy for non-Hodgkin's lymphoma (any of a large group of cancers of lymphocytes and WBCs). The disease involves lymph nodes of multiple sites. Today at Williton, Dr. Klootwyk transplants Mrs. McCormick's own bone marrow.

Diagnosis code(s): _____

Procedure code(s): _____

4. Unfortunately, after surgery, Dr. Klootwyk determines that Mrs. McCormick's transplantation was not successful. Clinicians find a donor for Mrs. McCormick, and today, Dr. Klootwyk performs a second bone marrow transplant using donor bone marrow cells.

Diagnosis code(s): _____

Procedure code(s): _____

5. Dr. Klootwyk determines that Collin Cortez's bone aspiration smears were inadequate, and she could not accurately diagnose his condition. She schedules him for a second procedure, a bone marrow biopsy of the iliac bone, which she performs today at Williton.

Diagnosis code(s): _____

Procedure code(s): _____

6. Dr. Willis, an oncologist, prepares hematopoietic progenitor cells for transplant for Daniel Miles, age 32, who has Hodgkin's disease involving multiple lymph nodes. Procedures include cryopreservation and storage, thawing without washing, and specific T-cell (lymphocyte) depletion within harvest.

Diagnosis code(s): _____

Procedure code(s): _____

DESTINATION: MEDICARE

This Medicare exercise will help you to find additional information about procedures that you should not report together under the NCCI. Follow the instructions listed to access Chapter 5 of the Medicare Contractor Beneficiary and Provider Communications Manual:

1. Go to the website http://www.cms.gov.
2. At the top of the screen on the banner bar, choose *Regulations and Guidance*.
3. Under *Guidance*, choose *Manuals*.
4. On the left side of the screen, under *Manuals*, choose *Internet-Only Manuals (IOMs)*.
5. Scroll down to Publication # *100-03 Medicare National Coverage Determinations (NCD) Manual*, and click *100-03*.
6. Scroll down to the list of Downloads, and choose *Chapter 1—Coverage Determinations, Part 2*.

Answer the following questions, using the search function (Ctrl + F) to find information that you need.

1. Under what condition will Medicare pay for treatment for patients with Myelodysplastic Syndromes (MDS)?
2. Is treatment using Erythropoiesis Stimulating Agents (ESAs) covered for cancer patients who have anemia due to bone marrow fibrosis?
3. Does Medicare cover autologous stem cell transplantation (AuSCT) for patients who have acute leukemia in remission if they have a high probability of relapse?

LYMPH NODES AND LYMPHATIC CHANNELS (38300–38999)

Turn to the categories within the Lymph Nodes and Lymphatic Channels subheading to review the procedures, and refer to ■ TABLE 26-4 to review common terms you will find in procedure code descriptors for lymph nodes and lymphatic channels. You can find codes for procedures in this subheading by searching the index for the body site (lymph node)

■ TABLE 26-4 COMMON TERMS FOR LYMPH NODES AND LYMPHATIC CHANNELS PROCEDURES

Term	Definition
Biopsy	Diagnose diseases, including lymphoma; determine if chemotherapy or radiation effectively treated cancer
Cannulation (of thoracic duct) (kan-yə-lā′-shən)	Insertion of a tube (cannulation) into the thoracic duct to collect lymph to determine disorders of lymph flow
Lymphadenectomy (lim-fad-ən-ek′-tə-mē)	• Removal of a lymph node, most commonly because of cancer; many cancers metastasize to the lymph nodes, and the physician removes the lymph nodes to prevent cancer from spreading throughout the body. • Removal can also determine the stage, or extent, of the cancer (0, I–IV). • Limited lymphadenectomy—removal of lymph nodes • Radical lymphadenectomy—removal of lymph nodes and nearby structures
Lymphangiography (lim-fan-jē-äg′-rə-fē)	Radiology procedure where contrast medium is injected into the patient to visualize lymph nodes and lymph circulation to diagnose diseases, such as cancer
Lymphangiotomy (lim-fan-jē-ät′-ə-mē)	Incision into a vessel of the lymphatic system
Sentinel lymph node (sent′-ən-əl)	The first lymph node, or group of lymph nodes, to which primary cancer metastasizes. The physician removes the sentinel node and sends it to pathology for examination. If there is no evidence of cancer in the sentinel lymph node(s), it is unlikely that cancer has metastasized anywhere else in the body.

■ **TABLE 26-5 PROCEDURES OF THE LYMPH NODES AND LYMPHATIC CHANNELS**

Category Name	Code Range	Procedures Included
Incision	38300–38382	• Drainage of lymph node abscess—simple or extensive • Lymphangiotomy • Suture and/or ligation of thoracic duct—cervical, thoracic, or abdominal approach
Excision	38500–38555	• Biopsy or excision of lymph node (open, superficial); needle, superficial; deep; or internal • Dissection, deep jugular nodes • Excision of cystic hygroma—may include deep neurovascular dissection
Limited Lymphadenectomy for Staging	38562–38564	• Limited lymphadenectomy for staging (separate procedure)—pelvic or retroperitoneal, to determine the stage of cancer ***Note:*** Do not code this procedure separately if it is an integral component of another service.
Laparoscopy	38570–38589	• Laparoscopy, with lymph node biopsy or lymphadenectomy ***Note:*** A surgical laparoscopy always includes a diagnostic laparoscopy. • Unlisted laparoscopy procedure
Radical Lymphadenectomy (Radical Resection of Lymph Nodes)	38700–38780	• Lymphadenectomy—based on lymph node location (e.g., **suprahyoid**, cervical, axillary)
Introduction	38790–38794	• Injection procedure for lymphagiography This is a radiology procedure where radiology technician injects contrast into the lymphatic channel and visualizes the lymphatic system and lymph nodes on X-rays to help diagnose **lymphadema** (swelling and fluid retention) and lymphoma. • Injection procedure to identify sentinel node The physician injects a radioactive tracer (chemical that radiation can visualize) and blue dye into a tumor to find lymph nodes to remove to determine cancer metastasis. The *hot node* contains the radioactive tracer, and the *blue node* contains the blue dye. The physician then removes the lymph nodes, and a pathologist determines if they contain cancer. ***Note:*** This procedure is bundled into a lymphadenectomy. Do not report it separately if it is performed with a lymphadenectomy. • Cannulation of thoracic duct
Other Procedures	38900–38999	• Intraoperative identification (e.g., mapping) of sentinel lymph node The physician performs this procedure to determine the extent of cancer metastasis to the lymphatic system. It is an add-on code, and physicians perform mapping with a lymph node biopsy or dissection, or with a lymphadenectomy. • Unlisted procedure, hemic or lymphatic system

and then the type of procedure, or search for the type of procedure (biopsy) and then the body site.

■ TABLE 26-5 shows a summary of the categories listed under the subheading Lymph Nodes and Lymphatic Channels.

To better understand a lymphadenectomy of the neck (also called neck dissection), including radical and modified radical neck dissections, it is important to know more about the six lymph node regions of the neck (■ FIGURE 26-4).

The six regions of lymph nodes of the neck are as follows:

- I: submental (below the chin) and **submandibular** (below the mandible) triangles
- II: upper third jugular (neck) nodes
- III: middle third jugular nodes

suprahyoid (sū-prā-hī′-oyd)—lymph nodes and other anatomical structures located above the hyoid bone, the bone supporting the tongue

lymphadema (lim(p)-fi-′dē-mə)

submandibular (sub man-dib′ u-lar)

Figure 26-4 ■ Lymph nodes found in the neck.

Source: Tinydevil/Shutterstock.

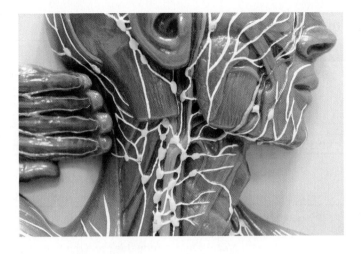

spinal accessory nerve (spīn′-ăl ăc- sĕs′-ŏr-ē)— eleventh cranial nerve, classified as a motor nerve

sternocleidomastoid muscle (stŭrn-nō-klī-dō-măs′-toyd)— muscle supplied by the spinal accessory nerve, which bows and rotates the head

- IV: lower jugular nodes
- V: posterior triangle group of lymph nodes
- VI: lymph nodes around the neck's midline

A *radical (complete) neck dissection* (code 38720) is when the physician excises lymphatic tissue from the first five regions, including the internal jugular vein (IJV) located in the neck, **spinal accessory nerve (SAN)**, and **sternocleidomastoid muscle (SCM)**. A *modified radical neck dissection* (code 38724) is when the physician removes tissue in the first five regions but preserves the IJV, SAN, and SCM.

Refer to the following example to code a procedure involving the lymph nodes.

Example: Dr. Boyd, an oncologist, performs a limited lymphadenectomy for staging for Mr. Morales, age 57, who has melanoma.

Search the index for the main term *lymphadenectomy*, subterm *limited, for staging*, and subterm *pelvic*, which lists code 38562. Assign code **38562**, which represents the procedure. The patient's diagnosis code is **172.9** (main term *melanoma*).

TAKE A BREAK

Let's take a break and review more about the lymphatic system and then code procedures.

Exercise 26.3   Lymph Nodes and Lymphatic Channels

Part 1—Theory

Instructions: Fill in the blank with the best answer.

1. Insertion of a tube into the thoracic duct to collect lymph to determine disorders of lymph flow is called _____.

2. A(n) _____ is the removal of a lymph node, most commonly because of cancer.

3. _____ is region II of the lymph nodes.

4. The _____ is the first lymph node, or group of lymph nodes, to which primary cancer metastasizes.

5. The _____ node contains the radioactive tracer, and the _____ node contains the blue dye.

6. Incision into a vessel of the lymphatic system is called _____.

Part 2—Coding

Instructions: Review the patient's case and then assign codes for the procedure(s), appending a modifier when appropriate. Optional: For additional practice, assign the patient's diagnosis code(s) (ICD-9-CM).

1. Dr. Kavanaugh, a general surgeon, performs a special laparoscopic procedure of the lymphatic system for Mrs. Beight, age 53, at Williton Medical Center. The patient has lymphoma involving lymph nodes of the axilla. There is no CPT code that accurately describes the procedure. Dr. Kavanaugh prepares a special report for the insurance that outlines the procedure and why she performed it. The billing

TAKE A BREAK *continued*

specialist will include this special report with the CMS-1500 claim form.

Diagnosis code(s): _____

Procedure code(s): _____

2. Mr. Danko, age 57, presents to Williton Medical Center, where Dr. White, a general surgeon, performs a complete axillary lymphadenectomy after sentinel node visualization reveals metastasis of his lung cancer (middle lobe).

Diagnosis code(s): _____

Procedure code(s): _____

3. Mrs. Kerr, age 60, has a radical mastectomy today at Williton Medical Center. The patient suffers from breast cancer. Dr. Burch, an oncologist, performs an open lymph node biopsy of the deep axillary nodes during the same operative session as the mastectomy. The mastectomy includes removal of pectoral muscles and axillary lymph nodes. The cancer metastasized to the axillary lymph nodes. Code for both the mastectomy and the biopsy.

Diagnosis code(s): _____

Procedure code(s): _____

4. Dr. Lumley, a general surgeon, performs a procedure where he removes lymphatic tissue in the first five regions plus the IJV (including the SAN and the SCM) for Mrs. Neish, age 82, who suffers from lymphoma involving lymph nodes of multiple sites.

Diagnosis code(s): _____

Procedure code(s): _____

5. Dr. Layko, a general surgeon, performs an I & D of a cervical lymph node abscess for Irma England, age 66, at Williton Medical Center. Dr. Layko determines that the abscess is deeper and more complex than he previously diagnosed. In the operative report, he describes the procedure as "extensive."

Diagnosis code(s): _____

Procedure code(s): _____

6. Ron Spielvogel, age 62, suffers from prostate cancer. Today at Williton, Dr. Ford, an oncology surgeon, performs a limited pelvic lymphadenectomy for staging.

Diagnosis code(s): _____

Procedure code(s): _____

MEDIASTINUM AND DIAPHRAGM (39000–39599)

The **mediastinum** is located in the thorax and is surrounded by connective tissue (■ FIGURE 26-5). It separates the lungs and contains the esophagus, heart, and superior and inferior vena cava and aorta. Conditions affecting the mediastinum include tumors and infections (mediastinitis).

The **diaphragm** is a muscle that is involved in respiration. It is shaped like half of a dome and is located between the thoracic and abdominal cavities. It contracts and flattens during inhalation and relaxes during exhalation. Diaphragm disorders include hiatal hernia (which occurs when part of the stomach protrudes through the diaphragm), other diaphragmatic hernias, paralyzed **phrenic nerve** , and **eventration** (a congenital anomaly with poor muscle development).

The Mediastinum and Diaphragm subsection contains two subheadings, Mediastinum and Diaphragm (■ TABLE 26-6).

Turn to the categories within these subheadings to review the procedures, and refer to ■ TABLE 26-7 for more information.

Refer to the following example to code a procedure involving the mediastinum.

phrenic nerve (frĕn′-ĭc)— sensory and motor nerve that conveys signals to the pleura, pericardium (sac that contains the heart), and diaphragm

eventration (ē-ven-trā′-shən)

Example: Dr. Kennedy, a thoracic surgeon, excises a mediastinal cystic teratoma (dermoid cyst) for Ms. Gordon, a 28-year-old patient.

Search the index for the main term *mediastinum,* subterm *cyst,* and subterm *excision,* which lists codes 32662, 39200. Assign code **39200**, which represents the excision. The documentation does not state that Dr. Kennedy used thoracoscopy, so do not assign 32662. The patient's diagnosis code is **748.8** (main term *cyst* and subterm *mediastinum*).

Figure 26-5 ■ Structures of the thoracic cavity.

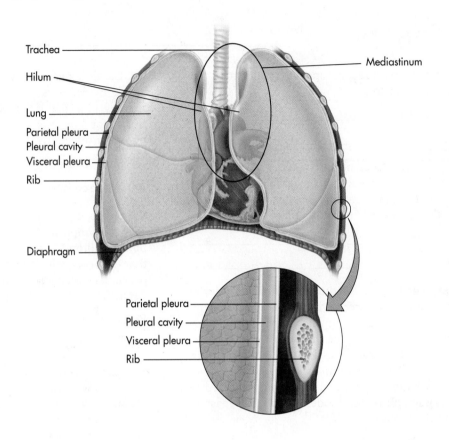

mediastinostomy
(me de-ah sti′ nos tō me)

imbrication (im′brĭ kā′ shun)

nephrectomy (nĕ frek′ to-me)

Subsection, Subheadings, and Categories	Code Range
■ TABLE 26-6 PROCEDURES LISTED UNDER MEDIASTINUM AND DIAPHRAGM	
MEDIASTINUM AND DIAPHRAGM	**39000–39599**
Mediastinum	**39000–39499**
Incision	*39000–39010*
Excision	*39200–39220*
Endoscopy	*39400*
Other Procedures	*39499*
Diaphragm	**39501–39599**
Repair	*39501–39561*
Other Procedures	*39599*

INTERESTING FACT: Dermoid Cysts Have Hair and Teeth

A dermoid cyst occurs while a fetus is developing and happens because certain cells do not form normally but still contain structures that are common to normal cells. Dermoid cysts can actually have sweat glands, teeth, hair, and nerves. Dermoid cysts can also rupture and cause cancer. They are found in the ovaries and on the face, back, and spinal cord. They also rarely occur in the brain, sinuses, and mediastinum.

■ **TABLE 26-7   PROCEDURES OF THE MEDIASTINUM AND DIAPHRAGM**

Subheading: Mediastinum

Category Name	Code Range	Procedures Included
Incision	39000–39010	**Mediastinostomy** (incision into the mediastinum), cervical (neck) or transthoracic (across the chest) approach *Note:* This procedure is performed for drainage, exploration, or foreign body removal. It can also include a median sternotomy (incision into the sternum).
Excision	39200–39220	Excision of mediastinal cyst or tumor
Endoscopy	39400	Mediastinoscopy with or without biopsy Endoscopy of the mediastinum, typically for biopsies or staging lung cancer. The physician incises the neck above the sternum in order to insert the mediastinoscope (endoscope).
Other Procedures	39499	Unlisted procedure, mediastinum

Subheading: Diaphragm

Category Name	Code Range	Procedures Included
Repair	39501–39561	• Repair of laceration of hernia or of neonatal diaphragmatic hernia • **Imbrication** (repair) of the diaphragm for eventration The patient has a condition where the diaphragm is relaxed and not shaped like a dome, leading to paralysis. The patient's condition can be congenital or acquired. • Resection, diaphragm, with simple or complex repair Commonly performed after excising invading cancer, also performed after a **nephrectomy** (surgical removal of a kidney).
Other Procedures	39599	Unlisted procedure, diaphragm

TAKE A BREAK

Let's take a break and review more about the mediastinum and diaphragm and practice coding procedures.

Exercise 26.4   Mediastinum and Diaphragm

Part 1—Theory

Instructions: Fill in the blank with the best answer.

1. The _____ separates the lungs and contains the esophagus, heart, and superior and inferior vena cava and aorta.

2. The _____ is a muscle that is involved in respiration. It is shaped like half of a dome.

3. Endoscopy of the mediastinum is typically performed for biopsies or for staging _____ cancer.

4. A _____ is a procedure performed for drainage, exploration, or foreign body removal.

5. Endoscopy of the mediastinum is called _____.

6. _____ is an infection of the mediastinum.

Part 2—Coding

Instructions: Review the patient's case and then assign codes for the procedure(s), appending a modifier when appropriate. Optional: For additional practice, assign the patient's diagnosis code(s) (ICD-9-CM).

1. Judy Peters, age 65, presents to Williton Medical Center for an excision of a mediastinal tumor. Dr. Fauzzi, a cardiothoracic surgeon, performs a substernal mediastinectomy. The pathology report shows the tumor is benign.

   Diagnosis code(s): _____

   Procedure code(s): _____

2. A car hit Ebbie Laughtner, age 70, while she was walking several dogs in the park. An ambulance transports her to Williton's ED, where Dr. Mills, the ED physician, diagnoses her with an acute traumatic diaphragmatic hernia. Dr. Fauzzi repairs the hernia.

   Diagnosis code(s): _____

   Procedure code(s): _____

continued

TAKE A BREAK *continued*

3. A falling piece of debris during a tornado struck Jackie Miller, age 22, as she was running for cover. A helicopter transports her to Williton's ED, and Dr. Mills examines her. He observes that the debris, a piece of metal, is embedded in the mediastinum, creating an open wound, necessitating emergency surgery. Dr. Fauzzi, a cardiothoracic surgeon, performs the surgery to remove the debris but determines that a cervical approach is contraindicated due to the patient's long-term tracheostomy status.

Diagnosis code(s): _____

Procedure code(s): _____

4. Mr. Williams, age 60, arrives at Williton's ED by ambulance after experiencing a crushing injury to the chest when a malfunctioning car rack collapsed on top of him in a garage at work. Dr. Mills examines the patient and determines that he needs to have immediate surgery.

Dr. Nelson, a general surgeon, performs a laceration repair of the diaphragm.

Diagnosis code(s): _____

Procedure code(s): _____

5. Dorothy Love, age 50, presents to Williton Medical Center for the excision of an anterior mediastinal dermoid cyst. Dr. Nelson performs the procedure.

Diagnosis code(s): _____

Procedure code(s): _____

6. Dr. Nelson performs a diaphragmatic hernia repair via a transabdominal approach for Carrie Parent, age 49, at Williton Medical Center. The hernia is chronic.

Diagnosis code(s): _____

Procedure code(s): _____

WORKPLACE IQ

You are working as a coder for Dr. Kennedy, a thoracic surgeon. Today, one of the billing specialists, Sandy, asks you to investigate denials for two patients. The claims for their services are old; in fact, Sandy submitted them before the previous coder, Ruth, retired. Sandy tells you that she thinks it may not be too late to appeal the denied claims if they contained incorrect procedure codes. Sandy asks you to verify the accuracy of two codes: 39520 and 39531.

What would you do?

CHAPTER REVIEW

Multiple Choice

Instructions: Circle one best answer to complete each statement.

1. The subsection Hemic and Lymphatic Systems contains codes for procedures for
   a. the mediastinum and diaphragm.
   b. imbrication and eventration.
   c. laparoscopic paraesophageal hernia repair.
   d. repair of a ruptured spleen.

2. The role that the blood plays in maintaining homeostasis includes
   a. delivering nutrients.
   b. keeping the body hydrated.
   c. eliminating wastes.
   d. a and c.

3. Bone marrow contains which types of blood cells?
   a. Lymph
   b. Red and white blood cells and platelets
   c. Yellow marrow
   d. Splenic

4. "Swollen glands" refers to
   a. enlarged lymph nodes due to production of lymphocytes to fight infection.
   b. cystic hygroma.
   c. GVHD.
   d. edema of the lymph system.

5. When the body produces too many bone marrow cells, the condition is referred to as
   a. splenomegaly.
   b. myeloproliferative disease.
   c. hypoxia.
   d. osteomyelitis.

6. An incision into the mediastinum would be described as
   a. mediastinotomy.
   b. mediastinectomy.
   c. eventration.
   d. mediastinoscopy.

7. The _____ consists of vessels, nodes, ducts, and organs and moves lymph, a clear fluid containing protein, throughout the body.
   a. mediastinum
   b. diaphragm
   c. lymphatic system
   d. splenic system

8. A(n) _____ is necessary when the patient's spleen is ruptured by trauma, such as from injuries in a motor vehicle or sports accident. Underlying infections can also cause the spleen to enlarge and increase the chances of a splenic rupture.
   a. splenomegaly
   b. splenorrhaphy
   c. splenoportography
   d. splenectomy

9. A radiology procedure where the patient receives a contrast injection to view the splenic vein and the portal vein is called a
   a. splenomegaly.
   b. splenorrhaphy.
   c. splenoportography.
   d. splenectomy.

10. Insertion of a tube into the thoracic duct to collect lymph to determine disorders of lymph flow is called
    a. limited lymphadenectomy for staging (pelvic or retroperitoneal).
    b. injection procedure for lymphagiography.
    c. cannulation.
    d. lymphadenectomy.

Coding Assignments

Instructions: Assign procedure code(s) to the following cases, appending a modifier when appropriate. Optional: For additional practice, assign the patient's diagnosis code(s) (ICD-9-CM).

1. A car hit Adrian Manderly, age 47, while he rode his bicycle to work. An ambulance transports him to Williton's ED. Dr. Burns, an ED physician, examines the patient and orders further workup. He diagnoses the patient with an acute, traumatic, diaphragmatic hernia, which Dr. Nelson, a general surgeon, subsequently repairs.

Diagnosis code(s): _____

Procedure code(s): _____

2. Arnold Quinn, age 67, wants to donate bone marrow. Yesterday, Dr. Niles, a specialist in oncology and hematology, harvested bone marrow from the patient to use cells for a child with whom he is a histological match.

Diagnosis code(s): _____

Procedure code(s): _____

3. Dr. Willis, an oncologist, prepares hematopoietic progenitor cells with T-cell depletion for transplant into Julie Rock, age 54. The patient suffers from acute lymphocytic lymphoma (increased number of WBCs in the lymph nodes).

Diagnosis code(s): _____

Procedure code(s): _____

4. Tyra Dawson, age 22, arrives at Williton's ED by helicopter. She was one of the passengers in a friend's plane when it crashed in a field. Dr. Mills, the ED physician, examines the patient and orders additional tests. He diagnoses her with a ruptured spleen due to trauma. Dr. Nelson performs the repair.

Diagnosis code(s): _____

Procedure code(s): _____

5. Greg Frommer, age 56, is a candidate for a liver transplant. Dr. Nelson performs the injection procedure for splenoportography and the S & I at Williton Medical Center to assess the competency of the splenic and portal veins. The patient's diagnosis is portal vein hypertension (hypertension in the portal vein, carries blood from the digestive system to the liver) with bleeding esophageal **varices** (dilated veins in the lower esophagus).

Diagnosis code(s): _____

Procedure code(s): _____

6. Mr. Gomez, age 40, presents to Williton Medical Center for surgery. He suffers from a mediastinal cyst. Dr. Nelson performs a mediastinoscopy and excises the cyst.

Diagnosis code(s): _____

Procedure code(s): _____

7. Dr. Willis performs a bone marrow aspiration for Sissy Mullen, age 2, today at Williton. The pathologist's

report later reveals that the patient has acute monocytic leukemia (cancer of the WBCs in bone marrow).

Diagnosis code(s): _____

Procedure code(s): _____

8. Janie Douglas, age 46, has a bone marrow biopsy at Williton. Dr. Willis performs the procedure, and the pathology report later reveals that the patient suffers from multiple myeloma (cancer of plasma cells).

Diagnosis code(s): _____

Procedure code(s): _____

varices ('var-ə-sēz)

teratoma (ter-ə-'tō-mə)

9. Dr. Willis performs an open biopsy of deep axillary lymph nodes today at Williton for Albert Pollard, age 61, who suffers from prostate cancer. The pathology report is negative for metastasis to the lymph nodes.

Diagnosis code(s): _____

Procedure code(s): _____

10. Dr. Nelson performs a mediastinotomy at Williton to remove a benign **teratoma** (tumor) for Joseph Cooley, age 50.

Diagnosis code(s): _____

Procedure code(s): _____

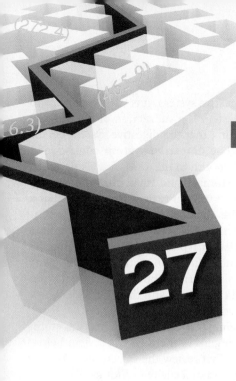

Digestive System

Learning Objectives

After completing this chapter, you should be able to

- Spell and define the key terminology in this chapter.
- Describe the digestive system anatomy.
- Discuss how to code from the subheading Lips.
- Identify how to use the codes in the subheading Vestibule of Mouth.
- Explain how to code from the subheading Tongue and Floor of Mouth.
- Define how to use the codes in the subheading Dentoalveolar Structures.
- Describe how to code in the subheading Palate and Uvula.
- Discuss how to use the codes in the subheading Salivary Gland and Ducts.
- Identify how to code in the subheading Pharynx, Adenoids, Tonsils, and Esophagus.
- Describe how to code in the subheadings Stomach, Intestines, Meckel's Diverticulum, and the Mesentery.
- Explain how to use the codes in the subheadings Appendix, Rectum, and Anus.
- Discuss how to code in the subheadings Liver, Biliary Tract, and Pancreas.
- Define how to use the codes in the subheading Abdomen, Peritoneum and Omentum.

Key Term

digestive system

INTRODUCTION

Get ready to really practice your pronunciation skills in this chapter! There are many new medical terms that we will discuss for the digestive system, and several of them can be challenging to pronounce. In this chapter, you will learn how to code several types of procedures that involve the mouth, stomach, intestines, and other structures, which we will discuss first when we review the digestive system anatomy. Be sure to consult your medical references to review procedures that we do not discuss or if you want to learn more about the procedures we cover in this chapter. Let's continue moving along on your coding journey!

"If you are facing a new challenge or being asked to do something that you have never done before, don't be afraid to step out. You have more capability than you think you do, but you will never see it unless you place a demand on yourself for more."—JOYCE MEYER

DIGESTIVE SYSTEM ANATOMY

Before you can accurately code procedures of the digestive system, it is very important to understand more about its anatomy. The digestive system is a subsection of the Surgery section, that you learned about in Chapter 10 including that the digestive system begins at the mouth and ends at the anus (Figure 10-11). The **digestive system** consists of a tube, called the **alimentary** tract, that runs from the mouth to the anus. You also learned that gastroenterology literally means the study of the stomach and small intestine, but the digestive system includes many other structures, which we will review. Remember that a gastroenterologist is a physician who specializes in the diagnosis, treatment, and prevention of digestive system disorders. A general surgeon may also perform procedures on the digestive system. A general surgeon specializes in different types of surgery, including the abdominal organs, thyroid, and skin. A plastic surgeon repairs various structures involving the digestive system, such as the lips and mouth. You also learned about the different types of dental specialties and physicians in Chapter 10 (Table 10-1), and these providers perform procedures related to the teeth and associated structures.

The digestive system is also called the gastrointestinal (GI) system, which means stomach and intestines. It is important to understand the organs of the digestive system before you begin coding digestive system procedures. So let's first review the structures of the GI system and their functions, beginning with the mouth and oral cavity (■ FIGURE 27-1).

alimentary (al-ə-ment′-ə-rē)

Mouth and Oral Cavity

The mouth is at the beginning of the digestive system and is where the process of digestion starts.

- The *labia*, or lips, surround the mouth and are the opening of the *oral cavity*, which includes a roof, made up of the *hard and soft palates*; sides, which are the *cheeks*; and a floor, composed of the *tongue*.

- The *lingual* **frenulum**, also called a **frenum**, is a thin stringy membrane under the tongue; there is also a frenulum under the top lip.

- The *vestibule* of the mouth consists of the mucosal and submucosal tissues that line the lips and cheeks.

- The tongue moves food around the mouth, and the teeth chew the food.

frenulum (fren′-yə-ləm)
frenum (frē′-nəm)

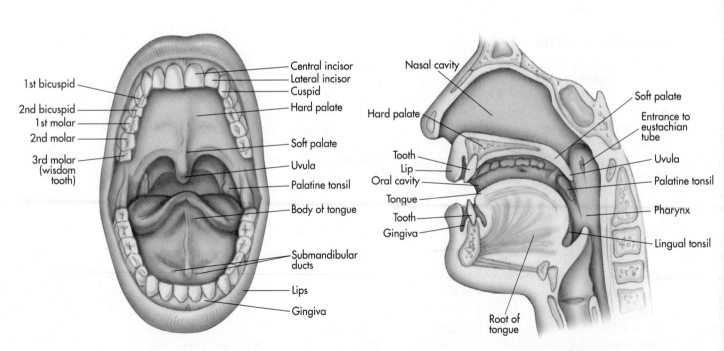

Figure 27-1 ■ The mouth and oral cavity.

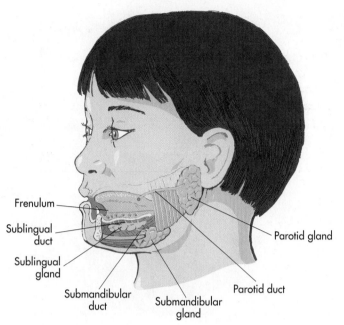

Figure 27-2 ■ The salivary glands.

Frenulum

Sublingual duct

Sublingual gland

Submandibular duct

Submandibular gland

Parotid duct

Parotid gland

- **Dentoalveolar** structures are the teeth and bones that hold the teeth. **Mastication** is the process of chewing, combining food with saliva, to form a **bolus** (ball), which is swallowed and moved through the pharynx (throat). You also learned about the pharynx in Chapter 10.

- The **gingiva**, or gums, is the mucosal tissue that lines the maxilla (upper jawbone) and mandible (lower jawbone) inside the mouth.

- There are three pair of major salivary glands: **parotid**, sublingual, and **submandibular** (■ FIGURE 27-2). There are also smaller, minor salivary glands found throughout the mouth and associated structures. Salivary glands are considered *accessory* (additional) *organs* of the digestive system and produce saliva during mastication.

- The **uvula** divides the oral cavity and the pharynx; it is the tissue that hangs from the center of the back of the mouth.

- The **palatine** tonsils are tissues at the back and sides of the throat that contain white blood cells that help to fight infection. You can actually see the palatine tonsils on either side of the uvula if you open your mouth wide enough and look into a mirror.

- **Adenoids**, or pharyngeal tonsils, which you cannot see, are also made up of infection-fighting (lymph) tissue and are located behind the nasal cavity.

dentoalveolar (dent-ō-al-vē′-ə-lər)

mastication (mas-tə-kā′-shun)

bolus (bō′-ləs)

gingiva (jin′-jə-və)

submandibular gland (səb-man-dib′-yə-lər)—one of a pair of salivary glands located below the lower jaw

parotid gland (pə-rät′-əd)—one of a pair of salivary glands located on the side of the face in front of the ear

uvula (yü′-vyə-lə)

palatine (pal′-ə-tīn)

adenoids (ad′-ən-oids)

Pharynx and Esophagus

The pharynx consists of the **nasopharynx** (which functions as part of the respiratory system and is located behind the nose), **oropharynx** (located at the back of the oral cavity), and **laryngopharynx** (the lowest part of the pharynx, also called the hypopharynx). The **esophagus**, a muscular tube, moves the bolus from the pharynx to the stomach. The opening to the esophagus, which is called the **pharyngoesophageal sphincter**, allows the bolus to enter. **Peristalsis** is the process when the muscles of the esophagus contract to move the bolus to the stomach.

nasopharynx (nā′-zō -far-iŋ(k)s)

oropharynx (or′- ō- far-iŋ(k)s)

laryngopharynx (lə-riŋ′-gə-far-iŋ(k)s)

esophagus (i-säf′-ə-gəs)

pharyngoesophageal sphincter (fə-riŋ′-gō-i-säf-ə-jē-əl sfiŋ(k)′-tər)

peristalsis (per-ə-stol′-səs)

chyme (kīm)

rugae (rü′-gə)

Stomach

After food reaches the stomach, it is called **chyme**, a thick liquid of partially digested food. The stomach uses its muscles to digest food, secreting enzymes and gastric acid. It absorbs some of the nutrients in the food it digests. The stomach moves chyme into the small intestine to continue the digestive processes. **Rugae** are folds inside the stomach that allow it to expand in size.

Figure 27-3 ■ The small intestine.

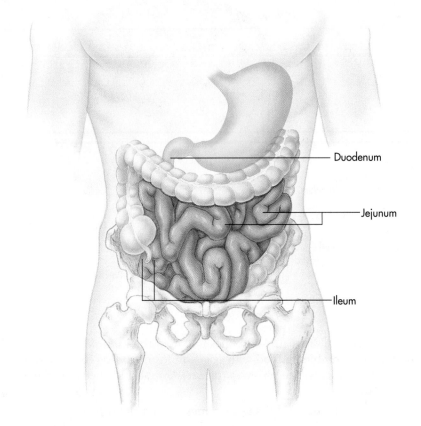

Duodenum

Jejunum

Ileum

The stomach has four parts (Figure 10-15):

* *Cardiac region*—the top of the stomach
* *Fundus*—holds food as it enters the stomach; above the body of the stomach
* *Body*—largest part of the stomach; lies toward the top and middle
* *Pyloric region*—where the stomach actually digests food; the pyloric sphincter is where food moves on to the small intestine

Small Intestine

The small intestine is a tube just over 20 feet long that absorbs most of the nutrients from food, including vitamins, sugar, and water. It contains digestive enzymes and also incorporates pancreas secretions (pancreatic juices) and liver secretions (bile) into the digestive process. The small intestine consists of three areas (■ FIGURE 27-3):

duodenum (d(y)ü-ə'-dē-nəm)

jejunum (ji-jü'-nəm)

ileum (il'-ē-əm)

villi (vil'ī)

* **Duodenum**—top, where food enters from the stomach
* **Jejunum**—middle
* **Ileum**—end

The walls of the small intestine contain protrusions called **villi**, which contain capillaries. The villi absorb glycerol (sugar) and fatty acids, and the capillaries absorb amino acids (which build protein and are an important part of nutrition) and sugars, sending them to the liver where they then move throughout the rest of the body.

Large Intestine

The large intestine, which is about five feet long, also absorbs water and vitamins and creates feces, which are transported out of the body through the anus (■ FIGURE 27-4). The large intestine has three parts, the cecum, colon, and rectum:

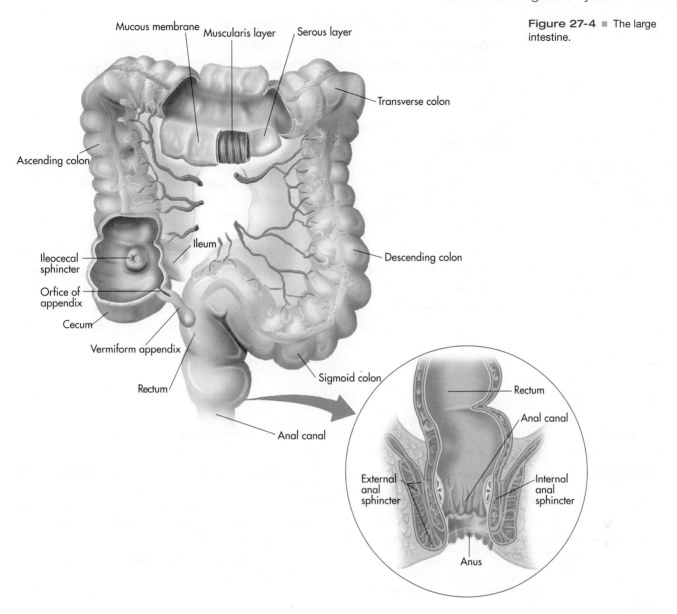

Figure 27-4 ■ The large intestine.

- **Cecum**—area where undigested food enters; the appendix is attached to it.

  cecum (sē′-kəm)

- *Appendix*—also called the vermiform (like a worm) appendix; contains muscle and lymphatic tissue that produces antibodies

- *Colon*—area that makes up the rest of the large intestine, divided into four regions: ascending, transverse, descending, and sigmoid (portion closest to anus and rectum)

- *Rectum*—feces move from the colon into the rectum, into the anal canal, and out the anus; the internal anal sphincter (through involuntary muscle contractions) and external anal sphincter (through voluntary muscle contractions) allow the feces to move out of the anus.

Accessory Organs

Accessory organs are also part of the digestive system but are not part of the alimentary tract. They include (see Figure 10-11):

- *Salivary glands*—produce saliva needed during mastication

- *Liver*—cleanses the body of toxins and filters red blood cells, producing the pigment **bilirubin**, which is excreted in feces

  bilirubin (bil-i-rü′-bən)

- *Biliary tract*—transports bile from the liver to the duodenum
- *Gallbladder*—stores bile that the liver produces
- *Pancreas*—secretes digestive enzymes that the small intestine uses for digestion

Additional Terms

There are some more terms that you need to know before you can code procedures of the digestive system:

peritoneum (per-ət-ən-ē′-əm)
parietal (pə-rī′-ət-əl)
viscera (vĭs′ər-ə)
visceral (vi′-sə-rəl)

- **Peritoneum**—two layers of membrane that line the abdominal cavity (the outer layer is attached to the abdominal wall and is called the **parietal** peritoneum). The peritoneum also covers the abdominal organs (called **viscera**) (the inner layer is called the **visceral** peritoneum). The area between the two layers is called the peritoneal cavity.

omentum (ō-ment ′-əm)
mesentery (mez′-ən-ter-ē)

- **Omentum**—a fold of the peritoneum that joins the stomach to the abdominal viscera
- **Mesentery**—folds of the peritoneum that join the abdominal organs to the abdominal wall
- *Upper GI*—consists of the esophagus, stomach, and the first part of the duodenum
- *Lower GI*—consists of the large intestine, including the colon and rectum

TAKE A BREAK

Wow! That was a lot of information to cover! Good job! Let's take a break and then review more about the digestive system.

Exercise 27.1   Digestive System

Instructions: Fill in the blank with the best answer.

1. _____ are also called pharyngeal tonsils, which are made up of infection-fighting (lymph) tissue, and are located behind the nasal cavity.

2. The opening to the _____ is called the _____ sphincter, which allows the bolus to enter.

3. Once food reaches the stomach, it is called _____, a thick liquid of partially digested food.

4. The _____ is the area of the large intestine where undigested food enters.

5. The _____ cleanses the body of toxins and filters red blood cells, producing the pigment _____.

6. A fold of the peritoneum that joins the stomach to the abdominal viscera is called the _____.

DIGESTIVE SYSTEM PROCEDURES (40490–49999)

CPT divides the Digestive System subsection into 18 different subheadings organized by body site (lips, vestibule of mouth, esophagus) (■ TABLE 27-1).

   Turn to the codes in the Digestive System subsection to review the types of procedures listed. Did you notice that many of the categories include the same procedures? CPT arranges categories by specific types of procedures. The following procedures are common to various categories in subheadings (we defined them in previous chapters):

- Destruction
- Endoscopy
- Excision
- Incision
- Introduction
- Laparoscopy

- Manipulation
- Repair
- Suture

■ TABLE 27-1   **DIGESTIVE SYSTEM SUBHEADINGS**

Subsection and Subheadings	Code Range
Digestive System	**40490–49999**
Lips	40490–40799
Vestibule of Mouth	40800–40899
Tongue and Floor of Mouth	41000–41599
Dentoalveolar Structures	41800–41899
Palate and Uvula	42000–42299
Salivary Gland and Ducts	42300–42699
Pharynx, Adenoids, and Tonsils	42700–42999
Esophagus	43020–43499
Stomach	43500–43999
Intestines (Except Rectum)	44005–44799
Meckel's Diverticulum and the Mesentery	44800–44899
Appendix	44900–44979
Rectum	45000–45999
Anus	46020–46999
Liver	47000–47399
Biliary Tract	47400–47999
Pancreas	48000–48999
Abdomen, Peritoneum, and Omentum	49000–49999

Examples of procedures from this list include excision of a lesion or tumor, including for a biopsy; incision to remove a foreign body or to drain an abscess, cyst, or hematoma; and repair of a laceration. There are other procedures not in this list, which we will review later in this chapter. As you can imagine, there are numerous procedures for the Digestive System subsection, and we will not be able to review all of them in this chapter. But we will discuss some of them, and it is important for you to use your medical references for procedures that we do not discuss so that you can become familiar with them.

Let's get started by reviewing procedures in the first three subheadings and then practice coding. Be sure to refer to the anatomy descriptions and diagrams at the beginning of this chapter for assistance with understanding procedures in each subheading that we review.

LIPS (40490–40799), VESTIBULE OF MOUTH (40800–40899), TONGUE AND FLOOR OF MOUTH (41000–41599)

Turn to the subheadings Lips, Vestibule of Mouth (passage between the inside and outside of the mouth), and Tongue and Floor of Mouth in your CPT manual. Codes in these subheadings include categories of procedures for excisions for biopsies, incisions to drain cysts and hematomas, and repairs of lacerations. Let's review some of the procedures listed in each subheading in ■ TABLE 27-2. To locate codes in these subheadings, search the index for the *body site* and then *type of procedure*, or start your search with the *type of procedure*. Turn to the codes in your CPT manual as we discuss them.

■ TABLE 27-2   **PROCEDURES OF THE LIPS, VESTIBULE OF MOUTH, AND TONGUE AND FLOOR OF MOUTH**

Subheading	Category and Code Range	Example(s) of Procedure	Description
Lips	**Excision (40490–40530)**	**Vermilionectomy** (lip shave), with mucosal advancement (40500)	A vermilionectomy, also called a lip shave, is excising a lesion from the **vermilion** border, the border around the lips where they meet the skin. The lesion may be from **actinic cheilitis** (precancerous condition that UV radiation exposure causes, such as from the sun) or from squamous cell carcinoma. The physician uses a mucosal (mucous membrane that lines the inside of the lips) advancement flap to repair the defect.
		Excision of lip; transverse wedge excision with primary closure (40510)	Excises part of the lip due to a neoplasm or to reduce the size of the lips for cosmetic reasons. A *transverse wedge excision* removes mucosa and submucosa (connective tissue supporting mucosa).
		Resection of lip, more than one-fourth without reconstruction (40530)	Removal of part of the lip due to a neoplasm or defect.
	Repair (40650–40761)	Repair (**cheiloplasty**) (40650–40654)	Surgical repair of a lip defect or to decrease or increase the size of the lips.
		Plastic repair of cleft lip/nasal deformity; primary or secondary, partial or complete, unilateral or bilateral (40700–40761)	A cleft lip/nasal deformity is when the upper lip and nose do not form completely, which is a congenital anomaly (■ FIGURE 27-5). Many times, the physician performs more than one surgery to completely repair the defect, which can be unilateral or bilateral.
Vestibule of Mouth	**Repair (40830–40845)**	**Vestibuloplasty** (40840–40845)	This procedure heightens the alveolar ridge by reducing the size of muscles attached to the jaw, to prepare the patient for dentures. The **alveolar** ridge is the area of bone that contains the teeth in the upper and lower jaws.
Tongue and Floor of Mouth	**Incision (41000–41019)**	Incision of lingual frenum (**frenotomy**) (41010)	Procedure performed on infants, incising a lingual frenulum that is too short, which makes it difficult for an infant to feed properly. The procedure is quick and is done without anesthesia.
	Excision (41100–41155)	Excision of lingual frenum (**frenectomy**) (41115)	Procedure to remove a frenulum that interferes with the growth of baby teeth, the fitting of dentures, or speech.
		Glossectomy, Hemiglossectomy (41120–41155)	Procedure to excise the tongue due to a malignant neoplasm. A hemiglossectomy is excision of only one side of the tongue.
	Other Procedures (41500–41599)	Suture of tongue to lip for **micrognathia** (Douglas type procedure) (41510)	Micrognathia is when the jaw or chin is abnormally small. It is a congenital anomaly that can cause problems with breathing, feeding, or growth of teeth. This procedure involves suturing the tongue to the lower lip.

vermilionectomy
(vər-mil-yən-ek′-tə-mē)
vermilion (vər-mil′-yən)
actinic cheilitis
(ak-tin′-ık kī-lıt′-əs)
cheiloplasty (kī′-lō-plas-tē)
vestibuloplasty
(ve-stib′-yə-lō-plas-tē)
alveolar (al-vē′-ə-lər)
frenotomy (frə-nə′-tə-mē)
frenectomy (frə-nek′-tə-mē)
glossectomy
(glah-tĕk′tə-mē)
hemiglossectomy
(hem-i-glah-sek-tĕk′tə-mē)
micrognathia
(mī-krō-nā′-thē-ə)

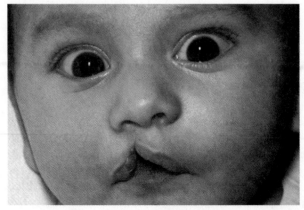

Figure 27-5 ■ An infant with a cleft lip.

Photo credit: NMSB / Custom Medical Stock.

TAKE A BREAK

Good work! Let's take a break and then practice coding procedures.

Exercise 27.2 Lips, Vestibule of Mouth, and Tongue and Floor of Mouth

Part 1—Theory

Instructions: Fill in the blank with the best answer.

1. A _____ is a surgical repair of a lip defect or to decrease or increase the size of the lips.

2. A _____ deformity is when the upper lip and nose do not form completely, which is a congenital anomaly.

3. This procedure heightens the alveolar ridge by reducing the size of muscles attached to the jaw, to prepare the patient for dentures. _____

4. This procedure is also called a lip shave, and includes excising a lesion from the vermilion border. _____

5. A _____ is a procedure to remove a frenulum that interferes with the growth of baby teeth, the fitting of dentures, or speech.

6. The condition where the jaw or chin is abnormally small is called _____.

Part 2—Coding

Instructions: Review each patient's case and then assign codes for the procedure(s), appending a modifier when appropriate. Optional: For additional practice, assign the patient's diagnosis code(s) (ICD-9-CM).

1. Dr. Medina, an oral maxillofacial surgeon, specializes in treating disorders of the mouth, jaws, face, and adjoining sites. Today at Williton Medical Center, he treats John Brewer, age 57, who has carcinoma of the mouth and neck, which metastasized from the lower jaw bone. Dr. Medina performs *commando* surgery to remove the patient's tongue, resect the floor of the mouth, and remove part of the jaw and neck.

   Diagnosis code(s) _____

   Procedure code(s): _____

2. At Williton, Dr. Medina performs a complete, primary repair (one-stage procedure) of a bilateral cleft lip and nasal deformity for Joseph Silva, a three-month-old child.

   Diagnosis code(s) _____

   Procedure code(s): _____

3. Dr. Bowman, a plastic surgeon, performs a lip excision for Maggie Fowler, age 32. The procedure includes a transverse wedge excision. The patient wants the surgery to reduce the size of her lips.

   Diagnosis code(s) _____

   Procedure code(s): _____

4. At Williton, Dr. Bowman performs a lip shave for Peter Fleming, age 62, which includes a lesion removal. The patient's diagnosis is actinic cheilitis.

   Diagnosis code(s) _____

   Procedure code(s): _____

5. Dr. Vargas, an oncologist, performs a biopsy of the upper lip for Omar Holland, age 57, due to a nonhealing lesion of the lip. The pathology report confirms squamous cell carcinoma.

   Diagnosis code(s) _____

   Procedure code(s): _____

6. George Byrd, age 48, arrives at Williton's ED with complaints of severe mouth pain. Dr. Mills, the ED physician, examines him and orders X-rays. The patient has an abscess on the floor of his mouth. Dr. Mills performs a lingual incision and drainage (I & D).

   Diagnosis code(s) _____

   Procedure code(s): _____

DENTOALVEOLAR STRUCTURES (41000–41899), PALATE AND UVULA (42000–42299), SALIVARY GLAND AND DUCTS (42300–42699)

The next three subheadings, Dentoalveolar Structures, Palate and Uvula, and Salivary Gland and Ducts, contain categories of procedures for incisions to drain abscesses, cysts, and hematomas; excisions of tissue for biopsies; and other procedures, such as closure of a fistula or placement of mucosal grafts. CPT arranges codes in these three subheadings by the body site and type of procedure. Turn to the codes in these subheadings to become more familiar with the types of procedures included.

An important point about insurance reimbursement for dentoalveolar procedures is that medical insurance reimburses for some of the procedures, and dental insurance reimburses for other procedures. Dental insurance covers procedures of the teeth and associ-

gingivectomy
(jin-jə-vek′-tə-mē)
gingivitis (jin-jə-vīt′-əs)
operculectomy
(ō-pər-kyə-lek′-tə-mē)
operculum (ō-pər′-kyə-ləm)

pericoronal (per-ə-kor′-ən-əl)
uvulectomy
(yü-vyə-lek′-tə-mē)
palatopharyngoplasty
(pal′-ət-ō-fə-riŋ-gō-plas-tē)
palatoplasty (pal′-ət-ə-plas-tē)
sialolithotomy
(sī-ə-lō-li-thät′-ə-mē)
sialolith (sī-al′-ə-lith)
sialolithiasis
(sī-ə-lō-li-thī′-ə-səs)
sialography (sī-ə-läg′-rə-fē)
Sjögren (shœ′-gren)

ated structures that different dental providers perform, and billing specialists submit claims on a special dental insurance claim form from the American Dental Association (ADA). The form captures specific information about the types of teeth involved in procedures and requires D-codes (HCPCS dental codes) for various procedures. But procedures that we may think of as dental because the teeth are involved may not be paid by dental insurance. Instead, medical insurance reimburses for these procedures. Not all dental insurance or medical insurance reimburses for the same dental procedures, so it is best to check with individual payers on their coverage.

To locate codes for these three subheadings, search the index for the *body site* (except for dentoalveolar, which you will not find in the index) and then the *type of procedure*, or start your search with the *type of procedure*. Let's review some of the procedures in the three subheadings in ■ TABLE 27-3 and then practice coding them. Turn to the codes in your CPT manual as we discuss them.

TAKE A BREAK

Nice job! Let's take a break and then practice coding more procedures.

Exercise 27.3 Dentoalveolar Structures, Palate and Uvula, and Salivary Gland and Ducts

Part 1—Theory

Instructions: Fill in the blank with the best answer.

1. Surgical excision of the uvula to treat snoring disorders or OSA is called _____.

2. A _____ is a procedure to remove gingival tissue that is infected with bacteria.

3. Surgical excision of tissue from the palate and oropharynx to treat OSA and/or snoring disorders is called _____.

4. A _____ is a procedure to remove a sialolith, a condition called _____.

5. This X-ray can detect the calculus in the salivary glands: _____.

6. A _____ repairs a cleft palate, and the physician may also repair the lip and nasal structures at the same time if they are also affected by clefts.

Part 2—Coding

Instructions: Review each patient's case, and then assign codes for the procedure(s), appending a modifier when appropriate. Optional: For additional practice, assign the patient's diagnosis code(s) (ICD-9-CM).

1. Mary Jensen, age 58, sees Dr. Medina, an oral maxillofacial surgeon, in Williton's dental clinic to remove a sialolith of the submandibular salivary gland, which he found on exam and X-ray at a previous appointment. The patient's chart documentation states that the procedure is complicated.

   Diagnosis code(s)_____

   Procedure code(s): _____

2. Today at Williton's outpatient clinic, Dr. May, an otolaryngologist, performs a needle biopsy of a tumor in the parotid gland. The patient is Jason Douglas, age 28. The pathology report reveals a pleomorphic adenoma (benign neoplasm).

   Diagnosis code(s)_____

   Procedure code(s): _____

3. Dr. May injects contrast for sialography of the submandibular salivary gland for Glenn Hopkins, age 62. He also performs the X-ray and discovers multiple sialoliths. He will schedule the patient for surgery to remove them.

   Diagnosis code(s)_____

   Procedure code(s): _____

4. Six-month-old Mandy Carlson has an incomplete unilateral cleft palate and cleft lip. Today at Williton's Cleft Palate Center, Dr. Medina repairs both conditions, with closure of the alveolar ridge involving soft tissue.

   Diagnosis code(s)_____

   Procedure code(s): _____

5. At the dental clinic, Dr. Soto, a periodontist, performs an operculectomy for Susie Herrara, age 23, to treat a periodontal infection in one of her wisdom teeth.

   Diagnosis code(s)_____

   Procedure code(s): _____

6. George Wade, age 57, has acute gingivitis in all four quadrants of his mouth. Dr. Soto performs a gingivectomy involving all quadrants to treat the patient's condition.

   Diagnosis code(s)_____

   Procedure code(s): _____

■ **TABLE 27-3   PROCEDURES OF DENTOALVEOLAR STRUCTURES, PALATE AND UVULA, AND SALIVARY GLAND AND DUCTS**

Subheading	Category and Code Range	Example(s) of Procedure	Description
Dentoalveolar Structures	*Excision, Destruction (41820–41850)*	**Gingivectomy,** excision gingiva, each quadrant (41820)	Procedure to remove gingival tissue that is infected with bacteria, called **gingivitis** (a gum infection), which causes inflammation and causes plaque to form along the gums. Brushing and flossing will not remove the plaque, so a periodontist or oral surgeon removes the plaque from the gums and then places a substance along the gums to help them to heal.
			• Note that the code descriptor is for each quadrant. The mouth is divided into four quadrants, based on dividing the maxilla and mandible in half: left maxillary (upper) quadrant, right maxillary (upper) quadrant, left mandibular (lower) quadrant, right mandibular (lower) quadrant. Report the procedure code for each quadrant involved.
		Operculectomy, excision pericoronal tissues (41821)	An **operculum** is a piece of **pericoronal** tissue (surrounding the crown, or top and sides of the tooth) that forms over a tooth. It can become infected, and an operculectomy is a procedure to remove the operculum.
Palate and Uvula	*Excision, Destruction (42100–42160)*	**Uvulectomy,** excision of uvula (42140)	Surgical excision of the uvula to treat snoring disorders or obstructive sleep apnea (OSA) to eliminate the uvula from obstructing the patient's airway.
		Palatopharyngo-plasty (42145)	Surgical excision of tissue from the palate and oropharynx to treat OSA and/or snoring disorders.
	Repair (42180–42281)	**Palatoplasty** for cleft palate (involving hard palate and/or soft palate) (42200–42225)	A cleft palate is a congenital anomaly where the roof of the mouth (hard palate) is incomplete and separated into two bones instead of being joined as one. The soft palate, the tissue that covers the hard palate, also has a cleft. The uvula is also split into two parts. The patient may also have a cleft lip, and nasal structures can also be involved.
			• A palatoplasty repairs a cleft palate and the physician may also repair the lip and nasal structures at the same time if they are also affected by clefts.
Salivary Gland and Ducts	*Incision (42300–42340)*	**Sialolithotomy** (42330–42340)	Procedure to remove a **sialolith**—a calculus, or stone, in the salivary glands—a condition called **sialolithiasis.** The calculus forms a lump and/or edema. An infection may also accompany the calculi. The physician can detect the calculus through an exam and an X-ray of the salivary gland (**sialography**).
			• CPT divides codes for this procedure by the type of salivary gland involved and whether the procedure is extraoral (outside the mouth) or intraoral (inside the mouth).
	Excision (42400–42450)	Biopsy of salivary gland, needle or incisional (42400–42405)	Procedure to excise tissue with a needle or through an incision to test for cancer in a tumor of the salivary gland or to test for **Sjögren** syndrome, an autoimmune condition where the salivary glands no longer function.
			• Note that CPT alerts you that if the physician uses imaging guidance for the procedure, then you should also report a radiology code for the imaging procedure from the Radiology section of CPT. You will learn more about radiology coding in Chapter 32.
	Other Procedures (42550–42699)	Injection procedure for sialography (42550)	Procedure to inject contrast into the salivary ducts of a gland to better view its structures on an X-ray (sialography). You should separately report the X-ray procedure (70390) from the Radiology section of CPT.
			• A sialography can help diagnose conditions such as a sialolith.
		Closure of salivary fistula (42600)	Procedure to close a salivary fistula, an abnormal passage between a salivary gland or duct and associated structures inside the mouth, such as the cheek. A salivary fistula can be caused by a congenital anomaly, an infection, or wound dehiscence at the surgical site after removal of the parotid gland.

POINTERS FROM THE PROS: Interview with a Medical Assistant

Jessica Chimile works as a medical assistant for a heart and vascular center where she performs a variety of duties, including preparing charts, rooming patients, updating medications, and performing diagnosis and procedure coding.

What are the most challenging aspects of your job?

As a recent graduate, I have found that one of the most challenging aspects is not knowing office procedures and responsibilities. When I've never been faced with certain situations, it is challenging to figure out exactly what should be done or said. I've also found going over medications with patients to be somewhat of a challenge. With so many drugs that come in generic form, it's challenging to learn different names and usages.

What advice can you give to new coders to help them communicate effectively with physicians?

Be confident when speaking to them. Make small talk to learn their personalities and interests. They all handle the stressful situations differently; you just have to learn

how to interact with them in a calming manner. It's vital for a business that a coder can effectively communicate with the physician to ensure that the proper CPT and ICD-9 codes are selected for correct reimbursement.

What advice would you like to give to coding students to help them prepare to work successfully in the field?

Learn as much as you can about everything you can, and especially about the procedures and diagnoses you will be coding, which will make you more effective at performing your job. Accept everyone for who they are. We all come from different backgrounds and have different experiences, but it is very important to remain professional and put your differences aside. It creates a very bad environment when even just two people are incapable of acting professionally together.

What personal motto do you live by?

Make the best out of every situation. Life can get stressful, but a simple smile can be enough to lighten up a hard day.

(Used by permission of Jessica Chemele.)

tonsillectomy
(tän(t)-sə-lek′-tə-mē)

adenoidectomy
(ad-ən-oi-dek′-tə-mē)

pharyngoplasty
(fə-riŋ′-gō-plas-tē)

pharyngostomy
(far-iŋ-gäs′-tə-mē)

nasopharyngeal
(nā-zō-fə-rin-j(ē-)′əl)

angiofibroma
(an-jē-ə fī-brō′-mə)

esophagectomy
(i-säf-ə-jek′-tə-mē)

esophagoscopy
(i-säf-ə-gäs′-kə-pē)

esophagogastroduodenoscopy (EGD) (eh-sə -fah-gō -gas-trō -doo- ə-den-ə′-ska-pē)

PHARYNX, ADENOIDS, AND TONSILS (42700–42999), ESOPHAGUS (43020–43499)

The subheadings of Pharynx, Adenoids, Tonsils, and Esophagus include procedures that you reviewed in other subheadings in the Digestive System subsection. Categories of procedures include an incision and drainage of an abscess, incision to remove a foreign body, biopsy, repair of a laceration, and excision of a lesion. The Esophagus subheading also includes procedures for endoscopy, laparoscopy, and manipulation. Both subheadings include categories for Other Procedures, which contain a variety of unique procedures.

CPT arranges codes in these subheadings by the type and location of the procedure, whether it was primary or secondary or simple or complicated, the type of approach, and other procedures performed along with the primary procedure. To locate codes for these two subheadings, search the index for the *body site* and then the *type of procedure*, or start your search with the *type of procedure*. Now, let's review some of the procedures in the two subheadings in ■ TABLE 27-4 and then practice coding them. Turn to the codes in your CPT manual as we discuss them.

TAKE A BREAK

You are doing great! Let's take a break and then practice coding more procedures.

> **Exercise 27.4** Pharynx, Adenoids, and Tonsils, Esophagus

Part 1—Theory

Instructions: Fill in the blank with the best answer.

1. The procedure to remove part of the esophagus to treat esophageal cancer by removing tumors is called a(n) _____.

2. A _____ is a procedure where the physician inserts a laparoscope into a small incision (about 1 cm) in the patient's abdomen or pelvis for diagnostic or surgical reasons.

TAKE A BREAK *continued*

3. Surgical repair of the pharynx to close any defects or change the size of the nasopharyngeal orifice is called a(n) _____ .

4. Endoscopic _____ is a procedure where the physician inserts a flexible endoscope into the patient's mouth, through the esophagus, into the stomach and pylorus, and into the duodenum.

5. Two of the most common procedures in the Digestive System subsection are _____ and _____ .

6. A _____ is a procedure to create an opening (fistula) through the neck and into the throat for the insertion of a feeding tube.

Part 2—Coding

Instructions: Review each patient's case, and then assign codes for the procedure(s), appending a modifier when appropriate. Optional: For additional practice, assign the patient's diagnosis code(s) (ICD-9-CM).

1. Justin Terry, age 12, experiences chronic tonsillitis and adenoiditis. Dr. May, an otolaryngologist, has prescribed antibiotics many times for the patient, but the infections continue to return. Today at Williton, Dr. May performs a primary tonsillectomy and adenoidectomy for Justin.

   Diagnosis code(s)_____

   Procedure code(s): _____

2. Three days after Justin Terry's surgery, he experiences postoperative nasopharyngeal bleeding, and his mother drives him to Williton's outpatient clinic for treatment. Dr. May controls the bleeding with both posterior and anterior nasal packs. (Hint: This service is within the global surgical period for the initial procedure.)

   Diagnosis code(s)_____

   Procedure code(s): _____

3. Today at Williton, Dr. May performs a near-total esophagectomy for Reginald Walters, age 68, to treat squamous cell carcinoma. Dr. May also performs a thoracotomy with a **pharyngogastostomy** (restructure of the pathway from the throat to the stomach after esophagectomy).

   Diagnosis code(s)_____

   Procedure code(s): _____

4. Dr. May performs an esophagoscopy for Barney Caldwell, age 67, including brushing to collect specimens for pathology testing. The pathologist's report reveals esophageal cancer of the distal third of the esophagus.

   Diagnosis code(s)_____

   Procedure code(s): _____

5. Lee Woo, age 57, has consistent stomach pain, which has not resolved in several weeks. Today at Williton, Dr. Gupta, a gastroenterologist, performs a diagnostic EGD and finds a peptic ulcer (also called a GI ulcer).

   Diagnosis code(s)_____

   Procedure code(s): _____

6. Dr. Gupta performs an ERCP for Josie Barker, age 58, and finds calculi of the biliary ducts, which he removes.

   Diagnosis code(s)_____

   Procedure code(s): _____

■ TABLE 27-4 **PROCEDURES OF THE PHARYNX, ADENOIDS, TONSILS, AND ESOPHAGUS**

Subheading	Category and Code Range	Example(s) of Procedure	Description
Pharynx, Adenoids, Tonsils	*Excision, Destruction (42800–42894)*	**Tonsillectomy, adenoidectomy** (42820–42836)	Two of the most common procedures in the Digestive System subsection are tonsillectomy and adenoidectomy. • Physicians perform a *tonsillectomy* when the patient suffers from recurring infections, such as chronic tonsillitis from streptococcal bacteria, that continue to return even with the use of antibiotics. Other reasons for a tonsillectomy include hyperplasia (excessive cell production) of the tonsils that causes airway obstruction and abscess of the tonsils. • Physicians perform an *adenoidectomy* for patients with chronic adenoiditis (recurring infection of the adenoids), chronic otitis media, chronic sinusitis, and hyperplasia of the adenoids, which also causes nasal airway obstruction.

continued

■ **TABLE 27-4** *continued*

Subheading	Category and Code Range	Example(s) of Procedure	Description
			• Both a tonsillectomy and adenoidectomy can involve excision with surgical instruments, by laser, or with radiofrequency ablation (heat from an electrical current).
			• Many times, physicians perform a tonsillectomy *with* an adenoidectomy. Take a look at the codes for these two procedures (42820–42836). CPT arranges codes by the individual procedure performed, or by the *combined* procedure (tonsillectomy *with* adenoidectomy), along with the patient's age (younger than 12, age 12 and over). Choose the code carefully based on these criteria.
			• CPT also categorizes codes by primary or secondary. A tonsillectomy or adenoidectomy can be a *primary* procedure (first time performed) or a *secondary* procedure (second time performed because the tonsils or adenoids originally removed grew back). CPT has *two different codes* for a primary or secondary *adenoidectomy* but has *only one* code for a *tonsillectomy* that can be either primary or secondary. Keep in mind that in order to determine if a procedure is secondary, you will need to review current and past medical documentation and may also need to query the physician.
			• Insurances typically require preauthorization before they will reimburse a tonsillectomy and/or adenoidectomy. They may also require supporting medical documentation. The medical documentation must clearly state reasons for the procedure and indicate that the procedure is being performed as a last resort and all other treatment interventions have failed, such as antibiotic treatment for recurring infections.
	Repair (42900–42953)	**Pharyngoplasty** (42950)	Surgical repair of the pharynx to close any defects or change the size of the nasopharyngeal orifice. The procedure treats speech disorders due to cleft palate or other conditions, and also treats OSA.
	Other Procedures (42955–42999)	**Pharyngostomy** (42955)	Procedure to create an opening (fistula) through the neck and into the throat for the insertion of a feeding tube. You learned about feeding tubes (enteral nutrition therapy) in Chapter 10, where patients typically receive tube feeding through a nasogastric (NG) tube. Sometimes, the patient cannot withstand an NG tube, which makes a pharyngostomy necessary.
			• Physicians may also perform a pharyngostomy for insertion of an endotracheal tube for ventilator-assisted breathing when the patient cannot withstand the insertion of the tube through the mouth and down the trachea.
		Control of **nasopharyngeal** hemorrhage (42960–42972)	*Nasopharyngeal* means pertaining to the nasopharynx. Notice in the CPT manual that there are three codes for this procedure, depending on whether it is simple or complicated, requires hospitalization, or has secondary surgical intervention.
			• The procedure is to stop bleeding (hemorrhage) from the nasopharynx (nose, posterior nasal cavity) after an adenoidectomy or bleeding that another condition causes, such as a nasopharyngeal **angiofibroma** (benign tumor behind the nasal cavity).
			• The procedure involves packing the nasopharynx (posterior) to control the bleeding, which may include balloon packs (balloons filled with saline solution) inserted into the nasopharynx. It may also include anterior packing or cautery (burning) to stop the bleeding.
Esophagus	*Excision (43100–43135)*	**Esophagectomy** (43107–43124)	Procedure to remove part of the esophagus to treat esophageal cancer by removing tumors (adenocarcinoma, squamous cell carcinoma) or to treat Barrett's esophagus (chronic acid reflux that travels from the stomach to the esophagus, which damages it). The physician must also rebuild the esophagus with portions of the small intestine or colon.
			Risk factors for developing esophageal cancer include
			• Being male
			• Being over age 65
			• Having Barrett's esophagus

■ TABLE 27-4 *continued*

Subheading	Category and Code Range	Example(s) of Procedure	Description
			• Having gastroesophageal reflux disease (GERD)
			• Long-term tobacco use and alcohol abuse
			CPT divides esophagectomy codes by whether the physician also performed a thoracotomy, and if the procedure were total or near total, or partial.
	Endoscopy (43200–43273)	**Esophagoscopy** (43200–43232)	Procedure performed under conscious sedation (included in the codes) where the physician inserts an endoscope through the patient's mouth, into the pharynx, and then into the esophagus for *diagnostic* or *therapeutic* purposes. As you learned previously, a *flexible* endoscope is equipped with a camera, light, and magnification to display images of internal structures on a monitor for the physician to review during the procedure. Physicians may also perform esophagoscopies with a *rigid* endoscope but it does not magnify internal structures.
			• Review the codes for esophagoscopy, beginning with 43200, which is for a *diagnostic* esophagoscopy to view the esophagus and diagnose various disorders, such as GERD. The procedure may also include collecting specimens for testing. Notice that the remaining codes (43201–43232) are *surgical* esophagoscopies that include performing additional procedures, such as biopsies, removal of foreign bodies, removal of tumors or polyps, and control of bleeding. Remember that a surgical endoscopy also includes a diagnostic endoscopy, so you should only assign one code for the surgical endoscopy.
			• Notice that for some of the procedures, there are CPT notes directing you to assign an additional radiology code when the physician uses imaging guidance during the procedure.
			• Esophagoscopy may also involve examining other body sites, including the stomach and intestines, which we will review next. You can locate codes for endoscopies by searching the index for *endoscopy* and then the body site(s) examined.
		Esophago-gastroduo-denoscopy (EGD) (43235–43259)	Esophagogastroduodenoscopy is not a procedure that you can pronounce quickly! For a good reason, in the healthcare field, it is simply called an EGD or an upper GI endoscopy. Code 43235 represents a diagnostic EGD, which may involve collecting specimens for testing.
			• An EGD involves inserting a flexible endoscope through the patient's mouth, pharynx, esophagus, stomach, and either the duodenum and/or jejunum. It is done for *diagnostic* reasons—to identify GI disorders, such as infections, ulcers, or neoplasms—or for *therapeutic* purposes—to perform biopsies, drain cysts, remove or ablate tumors or polyps, remove foreign bodies, or control bleeding (43236–43259).
		Endoscopic retrograde cholangio-pancreato-graphy (ERCP) (43260–43272)	Endoscopic retrograde cholangiopancreatography (ERCP), is a procedure where the physician inserts a flexible endoscope into the patient's mouth, through the esophagus, into the stomach and **pylorus** (the opening from the stomach to the duodenum), and into the duodenum. The physician injects a contrast agent and uses fluoroscopy to view the **hepatobiliary** system: the *pancreatic duct* (which transports pancreatic digestive enzymes into the duodenum), the *hepatic ducts* (which carry bile from the liver to the common bile duct), the *common bile duct* (the junction of the left and right hepatic ducts that transports bile to the duodenum), the *duodenal papilla* (the openings in the duodenum), and the *gallbladder*.
			The procedure can be diagnostic, which may include collecting specimens for testing (43260) or surgical (43261–43272). A surgical ERCP may also include biopsies, removal of calculi, removal of foreign bodies, and ablation of tumors or polyps.

continued

■ **TABLE 27-4** *continued*

Subheading	Category and Code Range	Example(s) of Procedure	Description
			• CPT code descriptors may include the specific body site involved (e.g., pancreatic duct, common bile duct). Also notice that all ERCP codes include conscious sedation (indicated by a bull's eye symbol before the code). There are also coding notes directing you to report imaging separately with codes from the Radiology section.
			• ERCP can diagnose and/or treat neoplasms, polyps, calculi, and chronic pancreatitis.
Laparoscopy (43279–43289)		Laparoscopy, surgical (43279–43283)	Remember that a laparoscopy is a procedure where the physician inserts a laparoscope (a thin, rigid tube with a light and video camera or device for digital imaging) into a small incision (about 1 cm) in the patient's abdomen or pelvis for diagnostic or surgical reasons. Laparoscopy eliminates the need for a large incision. The video camera transfers images of intra-abdominal structures to a monitor, which the physician views to perform the procedure. If the physician performs a surgical laparoscopy, then she inserts tubes, called ports, into other small incisions in the abdomen. She can then insert surgical instruments into the ports to perform surgery.
			• Laparoscopy involves fluoroscopic guidance to assist the physician with viewing intra-abdominal structures and performing procedures, such as hernia repair.
			• Just like an endoscopy, a surgical laparoscopy always includes a diagnostic laparoscopy.
			• Code 49320 from the Abdomen, Perineum, and Omentum subheading represents a *diagnostic* laparoscopy. Codes 43279–43283 represent *surgical* laparoscopies that involve the esophagus.

endoscopic retrograde cholangiopancreatography (ERCP) (en-də-skäp′-ik re′-trə-grād kə-lan-jē-ə-paŋ-krē-ə-täg′-rə-fē)
pylorus (pī-lōr′-əs)
hepatobiliary (hep-ət-ō-bil′-ē-er-ē)
pyloromyotomy (pī-lōr-ō-mī-ät′-ə-mē)
gastrectomy (ga-strek′-tə-mē)
gastroenterostomy (gas-trō- ent-ə-räs′-tə-mē)
enterolysis (en-ter-ol′-ī-sis)
colostomy (kə-läs′-tə-mē)

STOMACH (43500–43999), INTESTINES (EXCEPT RECTUM) (44005–44799), MECKEL'S DIVERTICULUM AND THE MESENTERY (44800–44899)

These three subheadings contain many types of procedures listed in categories that will sound familiar to you: incision, excision, laparoscopy, introduction, repair, and endoscopy. Each subheading also has a category for Other Procedures. CPT arranges codes in these subheadings by the type of procedure, location of the procedure, additional procedures performed, and whether the procedure is diagnostic or surgical.

To locate codes for these three subheadings, search the index for the *body site* and then the *type of procedure*, or start your search with the *type of procedure*. Let's review some of the procedures in the three subheadings in ■ TABLE 27-5 and then practice coding them. Turn to the codes in your CPT manual as we discuss them so that you can become familiar with them.

TAKE A BREAK

Way to go! Good work! Let's take a break and then practice coding more procedures.

Exercise 27.5 Stomach, Intestines (Except Rectum), Meckel'S Diverticulum and the Mesentery

Part 1—Theory

Instructions: Fill in the blank with the best answer.

1. According to the National Institutes of Health, _____ is a pandemic health problem (affecting large populations) in both developed and developing countries.

2. The _____ connects the yolk sac to an embryo.

3. A _____ is a procedure to create a stoma in the abdominal wall where the large intestine and colon can eliminate waste into a pouch.

4. Excision of part or all of the stomach, most commonly to treat stomach cancer, is called a(n)_____.

5. This procedure involves freeing an intestinal adhesion. _____

6. _____ is a congenital anomaly, which causes an abnormal pouch to form in the ileum.

TAKE A BREAK *continued*

Part 2–Coding

Instructions: Review each patient's case, and then assign codes for the procedure(s), appending a modifier when appropriate. Optional: For additional practice, assign the patient's diagnosis code(s) (ICD-9-CM).

1. At Williton Medical Center, Dr. Chew, a gastroenterologist specializing in pediatric cases, performs a pyloromyotomy for five-week-old Thurston Page, who suffers from infantile hypertrophic pyloric stenosis.

   Diagnosis code(s)_____

   Procedure code(s): _____

2. Dr. Gupta, a gastroenterologist, performs a laparoscopic gastric bypass and Roux-en-Y gastroenterostomy (100 cm) for Bridgett Munoz, age 42, who is morbidly obese. Her body mass index is 43.

   Diagnosis code(s)_____

   Procedure code(s): _____

3. Felix Leonard, age 63, has adenocarcinoma of the stomach. Today at Williton, Dr. Mullins, an oncologist, performs a total gastrectomy with esophagoenterostomy.

   Diagnosis code(s)_____

   Procedure code(s): _____

4. Dr. Gupta performs a laparoscopic enterolysis at Williton for Alvin Walsh, age 54, who suffers from intestinal adhesions from a past surgery.

   Diagnosis code(s)_____

   Procedure code(s): _____

5. Edna Sharp, age 82, has colon carcinoma. Today, Dr. Gupta performs a colostomy, which will be permanent.

   Diagnosis code(s)_____

   Procedure code(s): _____

6. Dr. Chew treats Radonna Jones, age 3, for Meckel's diverticulum, which he excises. The surgery is successful.

   Diagnosis code(s)_____

   Procedure code(s): _____

■ TABLE 27-5   **PROCEDURES OF THE STOMACH, INTESTINES, AND MECKEL'S DIVERTICULUM AND THE MESENTERY**

Subheading	Category and Code Range	Example(s) of Procedure	Description
Stomach	**Incision (43500–43520)**	**Pyloromyotomy** (43520)	Incision into the pylorus to treat pyloric stenosis, where the pylorus abnormally narrows and prevents food from traveling properly from the stomach to the small intestines. Infants may suffer from this condition, resulting in the inability to correctly digest food, which may result in projectile vomiting.
	Excision (43605–43641)	**Gastrectomy,** total or partial (43620–43634)	Excision of part or all of the stomach, most commonly to treat stomach cancer (such as adenocarcinoma), gastric ulcers, or a perforation in the wall of the stomach. The physician can perform the procedure using a laparoscope.
			• For a partial gastrectomy, the physician removes part of the stomach and then attaches the rest to a portion of the small intestine (duodenum, jejunum).
			• For a total gastrectomy, the physician removes the entire stomach and creates a new stomach by joining the esophagus to the small intestine. Patients with a total gastrectomy consume food frequently, in small amounts, to enable their bodies to appropriately digest it, since it travels directly to the small intestine.
	Other Procedures (43800–43999)	Laparoscopy, surgical, gastric restrictive procedure; with gastric bypass and Roux-en-Y **gastroenterostomy** (43846)	Procedure to decrease stomach size for patients who are morbidly obese (body mass index of more than 40) so that they are unable to consume large amounts of food at once. They also feel full faster. According to the National Institutes of Health, obesity is a pandemic health problem (affecting large populations) in both developed and developing countries.
			• Although this procedure involves laparoscopy, physicians can also perform it without a laparoscope.

continued

■ **TABLE 27-5** *continued*

Subheading	Category and Code Range	Example(s) of Procedure	Description
			• The physician performs a gastroenterostomy, portioning off a small stomach pouch from the existing stomach and joining it directly to the jejunum. The pouch then bypasses the remaining area of the stomach, which will not be used, and bypasses the duodenum. This reduces the number of calories that the body can absorb. The anastomosis is shaped like the letter Y.
			• This procedure can also treat other conditions, like carcinoma, and conditions that cause obesity or that obesity caused. Patients with diabetes or hypertension may also have this procedure.
			• You will see the terms *Roux-en-Y* and *gastric bypass* to describe other types of procedures for treating morbid obesity and other conditions. *Bariatric surgery* is a general term referring to several types of weight loss procedures.
Intestines (Except Rectum)	*Laparoscopy (44180–44238)*	Laparoscopy, surgical, **enterolysis** (freeing of intestinal adhesion) (44180)	Procedure to separate intestinal adhesions, resulting from scar tissue that a previous surgery or other condition caused. Patients with intestinal adhesions suffer from abdominal pain, nausea, vomiting, and diarrhea.
			• The physician uses a laparoscope to view the surgery and inserts surgical instruments through ports to excise scar tissue.
			• Note that CPT considers enterolysis to be a separate procedure. When the physician performs enterolysis with another unrelated procedure, you should append modifier -59 to the code for enterolysis. Modifier -59 alerts the insurance that it is separate and distinct from another unrelated procedure the physician performs during the same surgical session.
	Enterostomy— External Fistulization of Intestines (44186–44188)	**Colostomy** or skin-level **cecostomy** (44320–44322)	A colostomy is a procedure to create a stoma (opening) in the abdominal wall where the large intestine and colon can eliminate waste (feces) into a pouch (also called a bag), which is then emptied (■ FIGURE 27-6). Patients may also eliminate waste by using a catheter that transports waste into a sleeve.
			• Patients need this procedure when the physician excises part of the colon to treat carcinoma, the patient has had colon surgery, or the patient has another condition, such as an obstructed colon or carcinoma. Sometimes the colostomy is permanent, and other times, it can be reversed, depending on the patient's condition.
			• Colostomy "bags" have a stigma attached to them, and many patients refuse to have colostomy surgery because they do not want to use a bag that may leak or have a bad odor. But the bag is secured to the patient and is designed so that it does not leak feces or odor. However, if the seal from the bag onto the skin breaks, or the bag becomes full of waste and is not emptied, it can dislodge from the body, spilling its contents.
			• A cecostomy is a procedure to create a stoma in the abdomen at the location of the cecum. A catheter is inserted into the stoma to deliver an enema (a solution causing quick defecation) so the patient can empty the colon through the anus. This procedure treats fecal incontinence (inability to control the bowels) because regular enemas help the patient to maintain a schedule for evacuation, rather than evacuating accidentally and without warning.
Meckel's Diverticulum and the Mesentery	*Excision (44800–44820)*	Excision of Meckel's **diverticulum** (**diverticulectomy**) or **omphalomesenteric** duct (44800)	Procedure to excise *Meckel's diverticulum*, also called *diverticulum of Meckel*. It is a congenital anomaly, which causes an abnormal pouch to form in the ileum. Symptoms include rectal bleeding, abdominal pain, and bloody stools.
			• The *omphalomesenteric duct* connects the yolk sac to an embryo. The yolk sac is attached to an embryo and aids in the embryo's development during early pregnancy. It disappears during the seventh week of gestation. In rare cases, part of it remains in the small intestine, which is called Meckel's diverticulum.

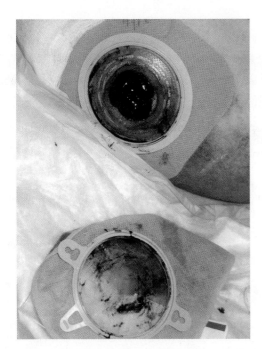

Figure 27-6 ■ A patient with a colostomy for perforated diverticulitis. Surgery was performed to feed a portion of the colon wall through the abdominal wall, bypassing the diseased region. The gut contents are collected in a stoma bag for disposal.

Photo credit: B. Slaven / Custom Medical Stock.

cecostomy (sē-käs′-tə-mē)
diverticulum
(dī-vər-tik′-yə-ləm)
diverticulectomy
(dī-vər-tik-yə-lek′-tə-mē)
omphalomesenteric
(äm(p)-fə-lō-mez-ən-ter′-ik)
appendiceal (ə-pen-də-sē′-əl)—
pertaining to the appendix
appendicitis (ə-pen-də-sīt′-əs)
appendectomy
(ap-ən-dek′-tə-mē)
proctectomy
(präk-tek′-tə-mē)
abdominoperineal (ab-däm-ə-nō-per-ə-nē′-əl)—pertaining
to the abdomen and the
perineum
proctosigmoidoscopy
(proc-tō-sig-moid-däs′-kə-pē)
sigmoidoscopy
(sig-moid-däs′-kə-pē)
sigmoidoscope
(sig-moid′-ə-skōp)
colonoscopy
(kō-lə-näs′-kə-pē)
anorectal (ā-nō-rek′-təl)—
pertaining to the anus and
rectum
hemorrhoids
(hem′-(ə-)-roids)
anoscope (ā′-nə-skōp)
proctosigmoidoscope
(proc-tō-sig-moid′-ə-skōp)
hemorrhoidectomy
(hem-ə-roi-dek′-tə-mē)
condyloma (kän-də-lō′-mə)
papilloma (pap-ə-lō′-mə)
molluscum contagiosum
(mə-ləs′-kəm kən-tā-jē-ō′-səm)
herpetic vesicle
(hər-pet′-ik ves′-i-kəl)

APPENDIX (44900–44979), RECTUM (45000–45999), ANUS (46020–46999)

You have made it far through this chapter, and you have done well! But we have additional subheadings to review before you finish, so hang in there! Take a look at the subheadings in your CPT manual for Appendix, Rectum, and Anus and the categories of codes listed for each. Did you notice that several of the categories are already familiar to you? They are many of the same categories that you reviewed earlier in the chapter, including incision, excision, laparoscopy, destruction, endoscopy, manipulation, introduction, and repair.

CPT arranges codes in these subheadings by the types of procedures performed and body sites involved. As with several other subheadings, to find codes for these three subheadings, search the index for the *body site* and then the *type of procedure*, or start your search with the *type of procedure*. Let's review some of these interesting procedures in ■ TABLE 27-6 and then practice coding them. You can follow along by reviewing the procedures in your CPT manual as we discuss them.

■ TABLE 27-6 **PROCEDURES OF THE APPENDIX, RECTUM, AND ANUS**

Subheading	Category and Code Range	Example(s) of Procedure	Description
Appendix	*Incision (44900–44901)*	Incision and drainage of **appendiceal** abscess, open or percutaneous (44900–44901)	Procedure to incise and drain an abscess of the appendix that appendicitis can cause. **Appendicitis** is a bacterial infection of the appendix causing inflammation and edema. If left untreated, the appendix can rupture and the infection can spread to other body sites, which is a life-threatening condition. • The incision and drainage (I & D) can be an open procedure, with an incision to access the abdominal structures and appendix, or percutaneous, introducing a catheter into the abdomen to drain the abscess. • Note that CPT directs you to assign a separate code for imaging during the procedure from the Radiology section.
	Excision (44950–44960)	**Appendectomy** (44950–44960)	Excision of the appendix because it is infected and/or ruptured. Appendicitis can lead to a potentially emergent condition if it is left untreated. Many times, physicians can treat appendicitis with antibiotics rather than surgery. • Symptoms of appendicitis include severe, sharp pain in the lower right abdomen, nausea, vomiting, fever, and constipation.

continued

■ TABLE 27-6 *continued*

Subheading	Category and Code Range	Example(s) of Procedure	Description
			• An appendectomy can be an invasive (open) procedure (44950–44960) or a minimally invasive laparoscopic procedure (44970).
			• In laparoscopic surgery, once the physician inserts the laparoscope into the abdomen, she inflates the abdomen with carbon dioxide to enlarge it so that there is enough space to perform the procedure.
			• In an open appendectomy, the physician must incise the abdominal wall and peritoneum to reach the appendix. The physician ligates the base of the appendix and then excises it, turning the stump that is left inward toward the cecum (■ FIGURE 27-7).
			• Did you notice the CPT note after code 44950 for an appendectomy? It states that when the physician performs an incidental appendectomy, you should not typically report a separate code. An *incidental appendectomy* is one that the physician performs for younger patients (less than 35 years old) during another intra-abdominal procedure, such as an abdominal hysterectomy (excision of the uterus). The physician removes the appendix not because it is infected or ruptured, but because removing it will prevent future problems.
Rectum	***Excision (45100–45172)***	**Proctectomy,** partial or complete (45110–45123)	A proctectomy is an excision or resection of the rectum, typically to treat carcinoma.
			• Notice that there are several different codes for proctectomies (45110–45123). CPT categorizes them by the type of procedure (e.g., partial, complete) and other procedures performed with the proctectomy, such as an **abdominoperineal** resection. This procedure involves removing the lower rectum and all or part of the anal sphincter (an opening that can constrict and relax).
			• A proctectomy can also be laparoscopic (45395–45397).
	Endoscopy (45300–45392)	**Proctosigmoidoscopy** (45300–45327)	Endoscopic procedure to examine the sigmoid colon, rectum, and anal structures for patients with changes in bowel habits, abdominal pain, pus in the stool, melena, or family history of carcinoma in these body sites. A proctosigmoidoscopy (45300–45327) can diagnose neoplasms, polyps, and other conditions. The physician may also perform other procedures with a proctosigmoidoscopy, such as a biopsy of a lesion or removal of a foreign body (surgical proctosigmoidoscopy, which includes a diagnostic proctosigmoidoscopy).
		Sigmoidoscopy (45330–45345)	Endoscopic procedure (45330–45345) using a **sigmoidoscope** to examine the rectum, sigmoid colon, and part of the descending colon for patients with symptoms of abdominal pain, changes in bowel habits, and rectal bleeding.
			This procedure is a screening exam for colorectal cancer, and the American Cancer Society recommends it every five years for patients 50 and over if they do not receive any other type of test for colorectal cancer, such as a sigmoidoscopy or other procedures. The test not only detects neoplasms but can also diagnose other conditions, like inflammatory bowel disease (inflammation of the colon and small intestine). The physician can also perform a biopsy of a lesion or remove polyps during the procedure (surgical sigmoidoscopy, which includes a diagnostic sigmoidoscopy). You can review the many variations of a sigmoidoscopy in your CPT manual.
			• Many payers will reimburse for a sigmoidoscopy every four to five years beginning at age 50. Medicare reimburses providers for the procedure every four years for patients 50 or older. You should report a HCPCS code when billing a screening sigmoidoscopy to Medicare. You will learn more about assigning HCPCS codes in Chapter 35.

■ **TABLE 27-6** *continued*

Subheading	Category and Code Range	Example(s) of Procedure	Description
		Colonoscopy (45355–45392)	Endoscopic procedure (45355–45392) to view the rectum and entire colon using a colonoscope (■ FIGURE 27-8). It helps the physician to diagnose neoplasms, ulcers, and polyps. During a colonoscopy, the physician may also perform a biopsy of a lesion, excise polyps, or control bleeding (surgical colonoscopy, which includes a diagnostic colonoscopy). CPT arranges colonoscopies by the type of procedure performed.
			• A colonoscopy is a screening exam for colorectal cancer. The American Cancer Society recommends a colonoscopy every 10 years for patients age 50 and older, if they do not have a sigmoidoscopy every 5 years.
			• Insurance reimbursement for a screening colonoscopy varies by payer. Medicare covers the procedure every 10 years as a screening test if the patient is not at high risk for developing colorectal cancer, but not within 4 years of having had a screening flexible sigmoidoscopy. Medicare covers the procedure every 2 years for patients who are at high risk for developing colorectal cancer. There is no minimum age requirement to reimburse for a colonoscopy. Colonoscopy is generally recommended as a follow-up test if anything unusual is found during one of the other screening tests. Medicare covers follow-up colonoscopy. You should also report a HCPCS code to Medicare when billing for a screening colonoscopy.
	Other Procedures (45990–45999)	**Anorectal** exam, surgical, requiring anesthesia, diagnostic (45990)	Exam of the anus and rectum, performed under anesthesia, to diagnose various conditions, such as an anal fissure (tear), fistula, lesion, or **hemorrhoids.**
			• The physician uses an endoscope, called an **anoscope**, to view the rectum and anus, and a rigid **proctosigmoidoscope** to view the sigmoid colon and rectum.
			• The CPT notes alert you that a surgical anorectal exam also includes an external perineal exam, digital rectal exam, and pelvic exam.
Anus	*Excision (46200–46320)*	**Fissurectomy**, including **sphincterotomy**, when performed (46200)	A fissure is a tear or a split. An anal fissure occurs in the anal canal and happens because of excessive straining during defecation, hard stools which are difficult to pass, inflammatory bowel disease, or other conditions.
			• Fissures can be extremely painful and bleed. If the fissure is not severe, many times the patient can use anal creams or suppositories to heal the fissure. In more serious cases, the physician performs a fissurectomy to close the fissure with sutures or electrocautery.
			• Physicians may also perform a sphincterotomy with a fissurectomy, which is incising the anal sphincter to eliminate pressure from the anal fissure and allow healing to take place.
		Hemorrhoidectomy (46221, 46945–46946, 46250–46262)	Hemorrhoids, also called piles, are rectal or anal veins that are swollen. Hemorrhoids in the anal canal are internal hemorrhoids, and hemorrhoids surrounding the anus are external hemorrhoids, also called thrombosed hemorrhoids (■ FIGURE 27-9). The *dentate line* is the area that divides the anus and rectum; internal hemorrhoids are above the dentate line, and external hemorrhoids are below the dentate line.
			A hemorrhoidectomy is a procedure to remove hemorrhoids.
			• Symptoms of hemorrhoids include pain, itching, and bleeding during defecation. Causes of hemorrhoids include increased pressure on the rectal and anal blood vessels, which happens during straining when defecating, sitting for prolonged periods, or during pregnancy in the second and third trimesters due to increased pressure to the pelvis.

continued

■ TABLE 27-6 *continued*

Subheading	Category and Code Range	Example(s) of Procedure	Description
			• Take a look at the hemorrhoid codes in your CPT manual (46221, 46945, 46250–46262). Did you notice that CPT arranges the codes by the type of hemorrhoid and method of removal? One of these methods includes rubber band ligation (46221), when the physician applies a rubber band tightly to the hemorrhoid to eliminate its blood supply until it falls off.
			• Also notice that CPT classifies hemorrhoidectomies by the number of columns or groups removed. A column refers to the shape of the hemorrhoid.
			• A physician can also treat hemorrhoids with destruction by thermal energy, such as cautery (46930).
	Destruction (46900–46942)	Destruction of lesion(s), anus, simple or extensive (46900–46924)	There are several codes for lesion destruction of the anus (46900–46924). Notice that the code descriptors list examples of the various types of lesions, which are defined here: • **condyloma**—also called a venereal wart or genital wart, which the human papilloma virus (HPV) causes • **papilloma**—benign tumor, such as a wart • **molluscum contagiosum**—virus affecting the epithelial layer of skin, causing lesions • **herpetic vesicle**—blister containing fluid that herpes simplex virus 1 (HSV-1) and herpes simplex virus 2 (HSV-2) cause You should already be familiar with many of the destruction methods listed in code descriptors because you learned them in Chapter 22 when you studied procedures of the integumentary system. Be careful, though, because destruction of anal lesions is not considered destruction of a skin lesion, so you should not assign codes from the Integumentary System subsection. • CPT categorizes lesion destructions as simple or extensive but does not define either of these terms. You may interpret simple to mean one lesion and extensive to mean multiple lesions; you may also query the physician for clarification.

Figure 27-7 ■ A physician performs an appendectomy by ligating the base of the appendix.

Photo credit: studio_chki/Shutterstock.

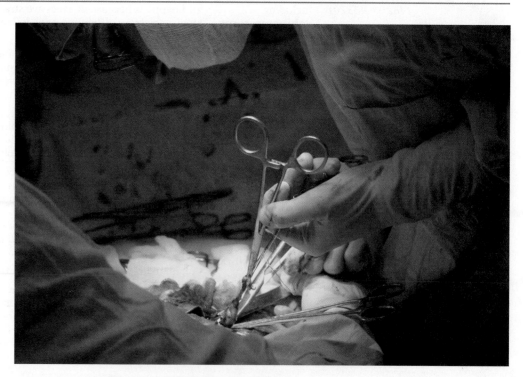

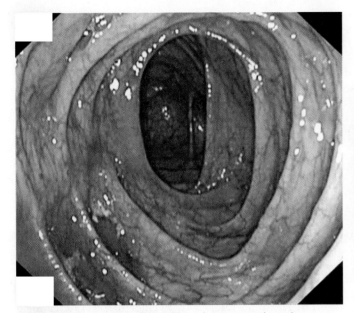

Figure 27-8 ■ Image of a healthy colon as seen through a colonoscope, during a colonoscopy.

Photo credit: Science Photo Library / Custom Medical Stock.

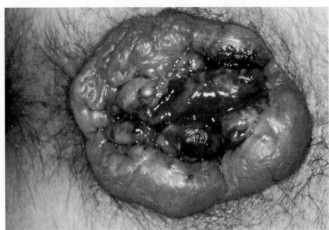

Figure 27-9 ■ Thrombosed external anal hemorrhoid (pile).

Photo credit: NMSB / Custom Medical Stock.

INTERESTING FACTS: Patients Can Swallow Their Own Colonoscopies

Instead of having a colonoscopy, patients can swallow a "camera pill," complete with a battery and a camera which takes thousands of pictures of the colon and rectum. The camera sends the images to a device that the patient wears. Several hours after swallowing the pill, the patient's physician reviews the images from the device. If the physician finds any disorders, such as colon polyps, the patient will still need to have a surgical colonoscopy to correct the problem. The patient passes the camera pill in the stool, and the pill is not used again. Research has shown that the camera pill cannot measure up to an actual colonoscopy, which detects more disorders. Many physicians do not believe that the camera pill will ever completely replace colonoscopies.

TAKE A BREAK

Great job! That was a lot of information to absorb! Let's take a break and then practice coding procedures.

Exercise 27.6 Appendix, Rectum, Anus

Part 1—Theory

Instructions: Fill in the blank with the best answer.

1. Symptoms of _____ include severe, sharp pain in the lower right abdomen; nausea; vomiting; fever; and constipation.

2. The _____ is the area that divides the anus and rectum.

3. A(n) _____ is an excision or resection of the rectum, typically to treat carcinoma.

4. A bacterial infection of the appendix that causes inflammation and edema is called _____.

5. An endoscopic procedure to examine the sigmoid colon, rectum, and anal structures for patients with changes in bowel habits, abdominal pain, pus in the stool, and melena is called a(n) _____.

6. Refer to the CPT guidelines listed under the subheading Rectum and the category Endoscopy to answer this question. If a patient is scheduled for a total colonoscopy, but the physician cannot complete the procedure due to unforeseen circumstances, what modifier should you append to the CPT code for the colonoscopy? _____

continued

TAKE A BREAK *continued*

Part 2—Coding

Instructions: Review each patient's case, and then assign codes for the procedure(s), appending a modifier when appropriate. Optional: For additional practice, assign the patient's diagnosis code(s) (ICD-9-CM).

1. Ben Griffith, age 19, arrives at Williton Medical Center's ED by ambulance. He has extreme abdominal pain, nausea, and vomiting. Dr. Mills, the ED physician, examines Mr. Griffith and orders further workup. He determines that the patient has appendicitis and a ruptured appendix with an abscess. Dr. Mills calls in Dr. Gupta, a gastroenterologist, who performs an emergent open appendectomy.

   Diagnosis code(s)_____

   Procedure code(s): _____

2. At Williton, Dr. Warner, an oncologist, performs a complete proctectomy with abdominoperineal resection for Ron Burgess, age 62, who suffers from rectal cancer. Dr. Warner also performs a colostomy for the patient.

   Diagnosis code(s)_____

   Procedure code(s): _____

3. Dr. Gupta performs a flexible screening sigmoidoscopy for Geraldine Tate, age 70. He finds no evidence of disease or disorders.

   Diagnosis code(s)_____

   Procedure code(s): _____

4. Terrence Garner, age 57, has a history of colon polyps. He sees Dr. Gupta at Williton for a screening colonoscopy. Dr. Gupta discovers several colon polyps and removes them with bipolar cautery. He sends the specimens to the pathology department for testing, and the pathologist determines that they are precancerous.

   Diagnosis code(s)_____

   Procedure code(s): _____

5. Gus Farmer, age 51, is one of Dr. Hoffman's established patients. He sees Dr. Hoffman with complaints of chronic anal pain and reports that when he has a bowel movement "it feels like I'm being sliced with pieces of glass, but I don't know exactly where it's coming from." Dr. Hoffman examines the patient and tells him that he has a severe anal fissure, or tear. He describes its location to the patient, stating, "If your anus were a clock, the fissure would be at 6 o'clock." Dr. Hoffman refers Mr. Farmer to Dr. Gupta for a fissurectomy. Dr. Hoffman's office manager, Chris, schedules the patient for an evaluation with Dr. Gupta. Dr. Hoffman's service includes an expanded problem-focused exam and medical decision-making of low complexity. Later that week, Dr. Gupta sees Mr. Farmer and performs a comprehensive history and exam with moderate medical decision-making. The same day at Williton, he performs a fissurectomy for Mr. Farmer. Code for Dr. Hoffman's services and for Dr. Gupta's services.

   Diagnosis code(s)_____

   Dr. Hoffman's procedure code(s): _____

   Dr. Gupta's procedure code(s): _____

6. In his clinic, Dr. Gupta evaluates Maggie Reynolds and determines that she has a deep anal fissure and that she needs a fissurectomy and most likely a sphincterectomy. Today at Williton, he performs both procedures for the patient.

   Diagnosis code(s)_____

   Procedure code(s): _____

DESTINATION: MEDICARE

This Medicare exercise will help you to learn more about bariatric surgery procedures. Follow the instructions listed next to access Medicare's National Coverage Determinations Manual:

1. Go to the website http://www.cms.gov.
2. At the top of the screen on the banner bar, choose *Regulations and Guidance*.
3. Under *Guidance*, choose *Manuals*.
4. On the left side of the screen, under Manuals, choose *Internet-Only Manuals (IOMs)*.

5. Scroll down to Publication #*100-03 Medicare National Coverage Determinations (NCD) Manual,* and click *100-03.*

6. Scroll down to the list of Downloads, and choose *Chapter 1—Coverage Determinations Part 2.*

Answer the following questions, using the search function (Ctrl + F) to find information that you need:

1. What are the two general types of bariatric surgery procedures?

2. In which specific type of bariatric surgery does the physician staple the upper part of the stomach?

3. In order for Medicare to cover certain bariatric procedures, what three criteria does the Medicare beneficiary have to meet?

4. Does Medicare cover an open and laparoscopic sleeve gastrectomy?

LIVER (47000–47399), BILIARY TRACT (47400–47999), PANCREAS (48000–48999)

Turn to your CPT manual and look at procedures in the next three subheadings in the Digestive System subsection: Liver, Biliary Tract (including gallbladder), and Pancreas. Did you notice the same types of procedures that you have seen throughout the Digestive System subsection, including incision, excision, repair, and laparoscopy? Notice that many procedures of the liver begin with the combining form *hepat/o*, meaning liver, such as **hepatotomy** (incision into the liver) and **hepatectomy** (excision of the liver). Gallbladder procedures begin with the combining form *cholecyst/o*, meaning gallbladder, like **cholecystectomy** (excision of the gallbladder) and **cholecystotomy** (incision into the gallbladder). The combining form *chol/e* means bile.

CPT arranges codes in these subheadings by the types of procedures performed and body sites involved, and you can find codes in the index by searching for the *body site* and then the *type of procedure.* Note that you will not find *biliary tract* in the index, so you should instead begin your search with *bile duct* or *gallbladder.* You can also find procedures by first searching for the *type of procedure.* Let's review procedures for these three subheadings in ■ TABLE 27-7, as you follow along in your CPT manual.

hepatotomy (hep-ə-tät′-ə-mē)
hepatectomy (hep-ə-tek′-tə-mē)
cholecystectomy (kō-lə-sis-tek′-tə-mē)
cholecystotomy (kō-lə-sis-tät′-ə-mē)

TAKE A BREAK

Nice work! Let's take a break and then practice coding more procedures.

Exercise 27.7 Liver, Biliary Tract, Pancreas

Part 1—Theory

Instructions: Fill in the blank with the best answer.

1. Excision of all or part of the pancreas is called a(n) _____.

2. A(n) _____ is when a physician uses a needle that is larger than a fine needle to obtain a single biopsy.

3. This procedure treats cysts that require continuous drainage and cannot be completely excised because that would destroy nearby structures. _____

4. Excision of the gallbladder, most typically to treat calculi, or gallstones, is called a(n) _____.

5. A(n) _____ is the removal of a liver from a cadaver or living donor and preservation to prepare it for transplantation.

6. A liver _____ means that a liver of the same species is transplanted into the patient.

Part 2—Coding

Instructions: Review each patient's case, and then assign codes for the procedure(s), appending a modifier when appropriate. Optional: For additional practice, assign the patient's diagnosis code(s) (ICD-9-CM).

1. Lindsay Mann, age 5, has biliary atresia and has been on a liver transplant waiting list. Finally, there is a living donor match for Lindsay. Today at Williton Medical Center, a transplant team oversees the patient's liver transplant surgery. Dr. Snidd, a gastroenterolo-

continued

TAKE A BREAK *continued*

gist and hepatologist (physician who specializes in diagnosing and treating liver disorders), works as a member of a surgical team, along with Dr. Cross, a pediatric gastroenterologist and hepatologist. They perform a hepatectomy on the living donor, Janice Wills, age 22, removing the left lateral segment. They also perform backbench reconstruction with two venous anastomoses and two arterial anastomoses and transplant the liver segment into Lindsay. The transplant is orthotropic (the donor liver is placed in the same location as the original liver). Assign code(s) to each patient's case for both physicians.

Ms. Wills' encounter:

Diagnosis code(s)_____

Dr. Snidd's procedure code(s): _____

Dr. Cross's procedure code(s): _____

Lindsay Mann's encounter:

Diagnosis code(s)_____

Dr. Snidd's procedure code(s): _____

Dr. Cross's procedure code(s): _____

2. At Williton, Dr. Gupta, a gastroenterologist, performs a biliary endoscopy for Margaret Thornton, age 52. He finds calculi in the bile duct and removes them during the procedure.

Diagnosis code(s)_____

Procedure code(s): _____

3. Dr. Gupta performs a laparoscopic cholecystectomy to treat gallstones for Gail Vega, age 56.

Diagnosis code(s)_____

Procedure code(s): _____

4. John Glover, age 60, undergoes a distal, near-total pancreatectomy today at Williton to treat carcinoma of the body of the pancreas. Dr. Gupta performs the Child-type procedure.

Diagnosis code(s)_____

Procedure code(s): _____

5. Ralph Harmon, age 37, has a pancreatic cyst, and Dr. Gupta performs a marsupialization to treat it.

Diagnosis code(s)_____

Procedure code(s): _____

6. Dr. Gupta injects contrast for a percutaneous cholangiography (an X-ray of the liver and bile ducts) and also performs the radiological procedure for Harold Robbins, age 48. Dr. Gupta finds what appear to be several lesions in the bile ducts. He will schedule the patient for further workup.

Diagnosis code(s)_____

Procedure code(s): _____

■ TABLE 27-7 **PROCEDURES OF THE LIVER, BILIARY TRACT, AND PANCREAS**

Subheading	Category and Code Range	Example(s) of Procedure	Description
Liver	*Incision (47000–47015)*	Biopsy of liver, needle; percutaneous (47000–47001)	You first learned about a percutaneous needle biopsy in Chapter 21. A percutaneous needle biopsy is when a physician uses a needle that is larger than a fine needle to obtain a single biopsy. A physician performs a percutaneous needle biopsy of the liver (47000) to test for liver disease, infections, and neoplasms, and to determine the reasons that a patient's body rejects a liver transplant. A physician may also excise part of the liver (wedge) for a biopsy (47100). • Note that CPT directs you to assign a separate radiology code if the physician uses imaging guidance to perform the biopsy.
	Liver Transplantation (47133–47147)	• Cadaver donor or living donor hepatectomy (47133, 47140–47142) • Backbench work (47143–47147)	We discussed heart transplants in Chapter 25, and the procedure code descriptors for a liver transplant are very similar. It is important to remember that there are different CPT codes for each procedure that physicians perform to complete the liver transplant: • A *hepatectomy* is the removal of a liver from a cadaver or living donor and preserving it to prepare it for transplantation.

■ TABLE 27-7 *continued*

Subheading	Category and Code Range	Example(s) of Procedure	Description
		• Recipient liver **allotransplantation** (47135–47136)	• *Backbench work* includes the physician's work to remove soft tissues surrounding the donor liver to prepare attached veins and arteries for transplantation and may include a cholecystectomy.
			• A liver allotransplantation means a liver of the same species is transplanted into the patient. When the donor is living, the physician removes part of the donor's liver, which later regenerates to its original size, and transplants the portion into the recipient. Once transplanted, the portion of the donor liver also regenerates into a normal-sized liver within the recipient.
			Infants and children may need liver transplants due to biliary **atresia** (an abnormal condition of the bile ducts that causes bile to remain in the liver).
			Adults need liver transplants due to viral hepatitis A or B and chronic hepatitis C (infections affecting the liver), liver damage from chronic alcoholism (alcoholic **cirrhosis**), and malignant neoplasms.
			Just like heart transplant candidates, patients who need liver transplants remain on a waiting list until a suitable liver is available, and the donor's blood type must match the recipient's blood type. Many patients die each year while waiting for a liver that never becomes available.
Biliary Tract	*Endoscopy (47550–47556)*	**Biliary** endoscopy (47550–47556)	Endoscopy of the biliary duct to diagnose conditions such as calculi, perform a biopsy, collect specimens for testing, or dilate a biliary duct stricture (narrowing).
			• Note that CPT lists an add-on code for biliary endoscopy (47550) if the physician performs it as an intraoperative procedure along with a primary procedure. Code 47552 represents a percutaneous biliary endoscopy.
			• CPT notes direct you to specific radiology codes if the physician uses imaging guidance for the procedure.
	Excision (47600–47715)	Cholecystectomy (47600–47620)	Excision of the gallbladder, most typically to treat calculi, or gallstones. Physicians may perform it with other procedures (47605–47620) or perform it laparoscopically (47562–47570), which may also involve other procedures.
Pancreas	*Excision (48100–48160)*	**Pancreatectomy** (48140–48160)	Excision of all or part of the pancreas to remove neoplasms (malignant or benign) or to treat pancreatitis (infection of the pancreas).
	Repair (48500–48548)	**Marsupialization** of pancreatic cyst (48500)	Incision into a cyst and suturing it open so that the cyst continues to drain. The procedure treats cysts that require continuous drainage and cannot be completely excised because that would destroy nearby structures.

ABDOMEN, PERITONEUM, AND OMENTUM (49000–49999)

You made it! This is the last subheading in the Digestive System subsection! Let's work through this last subheading together and then you can code more exercises. The Abdomen, Peritoneum, and Omentum subheading contains seven different categories of codes, which CPT categorizes by the type of procedure. You can find codes for procedures in the index by searching for the *body site* and then the *type of procedure* or starting your search with the *type of procedure*. Now, let's review some of the categories, along with examples of procedures, in ■ TABLE 27-8. Turn to the codes in your CPT manual to follow along with the table.

allotransplantation
(al-ō- tran(t)s-plan-tā′-shən)
atresia (ə-trē′-zhə)
cirrhosis (sə-rō′-səs)
biliary (bil′-ē-er-ē)—
pertaining to bile, the bile duct, or the gallbladder
pancreatectomy
(paŋ-krē-ə-tek′-tə-mē)
marsupialization
(mär-sü-pē-ə-li-zā′-shən)

■ TABLE 27-8 **PROCEDURES OF THE ABDOMEN, PERITONEUM, AND OMENTUM**

Subheading	Category and Code Range	Example(s) of Procedure	Description
Abdomen, Peritoneum, Omentum	**Incision (49000–49081)**	Exploratory laparotomy (49000)	Incision into the abdomen to explore internal abdominal structures, including the digestive tract, to diagnose a condition causing specific symptoms, such as abdominal pain; to diagnose the cause of a tumor or growth; or to identify a **volvulus** (bowel obstruction from twisted intestines). The physician examines organs such as the stomach, intestines, gallbladder, kidneys, liver, and pancreas. The physician may remove tissue for biopsies or perform other procedures during the laparotomy if the source of the problem is found, such as performing a laceration repair, achieving hemostasis, or draining an abscess.
		Drainage of abscess (49020–49061)	You first learned about draining an abscess of the skin in Chapter 22, and you also learned that an abscess can occur anywhere in or on the body. This procedure involves draining an abscess by an open or percutaneous approach from the following areas: • Peritoneal—pertaining to the peritoneum • Subdiaphragmatic or subphrenic—below the diaphragm • Retroperitoneal—behind the peritoneum The procedure used to drain an extraperitoneal **lymphocele** (collection of lymphatic fluid) is represented by code 49062.
	Introduction, Revision, Removal (49400–49465)	Insertion of peritoneal–venous shunt (49425)	A shunt is a device that includes a catheter (tube) that transports fluid from one area of the body to another. The procedure of inserting a peritoneal–venous shunt involves transporting excess peritoneal fluid (a condition called **ascites**) from the peritoneal cavity to the subclavian or jugular vein. Liver disease and cancer may cause the patient to have ascites.
		Insertion of gastrostomy tube under fluoroscopic guidance (49440)	Enteral nutrition therapy, also called tube feeding, provides a patient with nutrients through a tube in the nose (nasogastric, NG tube), stomach (gastrostomy, G tube), or small intestine (jejunostomy, J tube). • Gastrostomy means to create an opening (-ostomy) in the stomach (gastr/o). • A physician inserts a G tube percutaneously to reach the abdominal wall and then enter the stomach. • Patients may need tube feeding for different reasons, such as congenital anomalies or neurological problems involving the digestive system, which prevent a patient from normally digesting food, or swallowing disorders, including those resulting from a stroke or trauma.
	Repair (49491–49659)	Repair, hernia (49491–49566, 49570–49590)	You learned about various types of hernias in Chapter 10 (Table 10-2). A hernia occurs when part of an organ or tissue protrudes outside of the area that normally contains it, creating an opening and bulge. A hernia can be congenital or acquired. • CPT categorizes the hernia repair codes by the type of hernia involved in the procedure. Some codes specify if the hernia is initial (first time repaired) or recurrent (previously repaired), and the patient's age. • Notice that the CPT manual includes the terms **hernioplasty** (hernia repair), **herniorrhaphy** (hernia suture), and **herniotomy** (hernia incision) at the beginning of the repair category. A physician may employ one or all three types of procedures to repair a hernia. Hernia repair can also be laparoscopic (49650–49659).
	Other Procedures (49904–49999)	**Omental** flap (49904–49906)	An omental flap is when the physician harvests part of the omentum (■ FIGURE 27-10) to reconstruct other body sites, such as the chest wall or abdomen. The omental flap contains blood vessels that the physician can connect to other vessels when placing the flap. Notice that there are three codes for the omental flap (49904–49906), depending on whether the flap is extra-abdominal, is intra-abdominal, or will involve microvascular anastomosis. Be sure to review the CPT notes listed for each code before final code assignment.

Abdominal organs with greater omentum

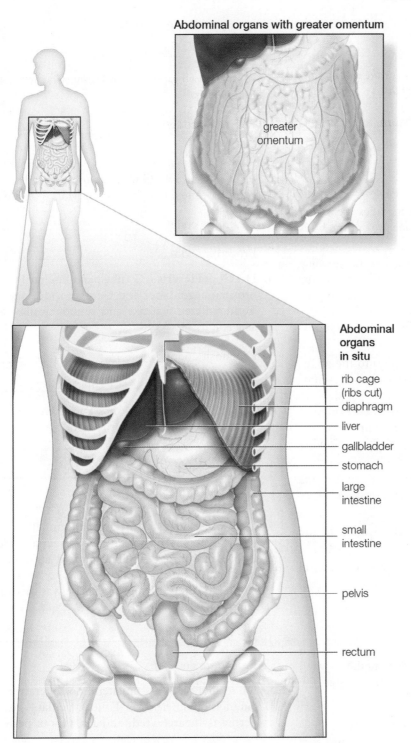

greater
omentum

Abdominal
organs
in situ

- rib cage
  (ribs cut)
- diaphragm

- liver

- gallbladder

- stomach

- large
  intestine

- small
  intestine

- pelvis

- rectum

Figure 27-10 ■ The human abdominal cavity, with the digestive organs covered by the omentum.
Source: © Universal Images Group Limited / Alamy

volvulus (′väl-vyə-ləs)

lymphocele (lim(p)′-fə-sēl)

ascites (ə-sīt′-ēz)

hernioplasty
(hər′-nē-ə-plast-ē)

herniorrhaphy
(hər-nē-or′-ə-fē)

herniotomy (hər-nē-ät′-ə-mē)

omental (ō-ment′-əl)

TAKE A BREAK

Wow! You made it through the chapter! Let's take a break and then review procedures and practice coding them.

Exercise 27.8   Abdomen, Peritoneum, and Omentum (49000–49999)

Part 1—Theory

Instructions: Fill in the blank with the best answer.

1. A _____ is a device that includes a catheter (tube) that transports fluid from one area of the body to another.

2. Enteral nutrition therapy, also called tube feeding, provides a patient with nutrients through a tube in the nose, called a nasogastric, or _____ tube; a tube in the stomach, called a gastrostomy, or _____ tube; or a tube in the small intestine, called a jejunostomy, or _____ tube.

3. A(n) _____ is an incision into the abdomen to explore internal abdominal structures, including the digestive tract.

    Turn to the subheading Abdomen, Peritoneum, and Omentum and the category Repair to review the CPT guidelines and answer the following questions:

4. For hernia repairs other than incisional, what code should you report for the use of mesh or other prosthesis? _____

5. Do hernia repair codes include debridement of the abdominal wall? _____

6. Are hernia repair codes for unilateral or bilateral procedures? _____

Part 2—Coding

Instructions: Review each patient's case, and then assign codes for the procedure(s), appending a modifier when appropriate. Optional: For additional practice, assign the patient's diagnosis code(s) (ICD-9-CM).

1. Newton Manning, age 48, suffers from severe generalized abdominal pain, nausea, and vomiting, and sees Dr. Gupta, a gastroenterologist, for an exam. Dr. Gupta orders several imaging studies but finds no cause for the pain. Today at Williton, Dr. Gupta performs an exploratory laparotomy and removes tissue from the stomach for biopsy, which he sends to the pathologist for analysis.

    Diagnosis code(s)_____

    Procedure code(s): _____

2. At Williton, Dr. Gupta laparoscopically drains an extraperitoneal lymphocele for Mary Higgins, age 52.

    Diagnosis code(s)_____

    Procedure code(s): _____

3. Dr. Gupta inserts a G tube percutaneously under fluoroscopic guidance for George Todd, age 82. Mr. Todd suffered a stroke and cannot swallow any food as a result.

    Diagnosis code(s)_____

    Procedure code(s): _____

4. Ronald Ingram, age 64, has a unilateral incarcerated inguinal hernia, which Dr. Gupta repairs for the second time.

    Diagnosis code(s)_____

    Procedure code(s): _____

5. Dr. Gupta harvests an extra-abdominal omental flap and transfers it to the chest wall to repair a defect for Bob Cannon, age 38. The patient suffered a chest wall injury during a motorcycle accident on State Route 50 when the motorcycle he was driving hit the guard rail.

    Diagnosis code(s)_____

    Procedure code(s): _____

6. Dr. Gupta repairs a unilateral postoperative abdominal incisional hernia for Timothy Jenkins, age 47. The hernia is incarcerated, and Dr. Gupta performs the procedure laparoscopically.

    Diagnosis code(s)_____

    Procedure code(s): _____

WORKPLACE IQ

You are working as a medical assistant for Dr. Gupta, a gastroenterologist. Today, Mr. Jenkins, age 52, calls to schedule a colonoscopy. You complete a preregistration for him in the computer system, and you ask for his insurance information. He provides the information and tells you, "My insurance should pay the whole thing, and I don't pay. It's part of the Affordable Care Act." You tell Mr. Jenkins that you still need to verify his coverage and benefits with his insurance plan. You schedule his procedure and end the call a little confused because you are not sure what questions to ask the insurance when you verify coverage because you have never heard of the Affordable Care Act.

What would you do?

CHAPTER REVIEW

Multiple Choice

Instructions: Circle one best answer to complete each statement.

1. The American Cancer Society recommends a colonoscopy every 10 years for patients who are ___ years old and older.
   a. 40
   b. 45
   c. 50
   d. 55

2. The _____ divides the oral cavity and the pharynx; it is the tissue that hangs from the center of the back of the mouth.
   a. lingual frenulum
   b. uvula
   c. gingiva
   d. adenoids

3. Folds inside of the stomach that allow it to expand in size are called
   a. fundus.
   b. chyme.
   c. rugae.
   d. bolus.

4. The _____ is the top of the small intestine, where food enters from the stomach, the _____ is the middle, and the _____ is the end.
   a. duodenum, ileum, jejunum
   b. jejunum, ileum, duodenum
   c. duodenum, jejunum, ileum
   d. ileum, jejunum, duodenum

5. The _____ transports bile from the liver to the duodenum.
   a. biliary tract
   b. gallbladder
   c. pancreas
   d. salivary glands

6. The two layers of membrane that line the abdominal cavity are called the _____. The outer layer is called the _____, and the inner layer is called the _____.
   a. omentum, parietal omentum, visceral omentum
   b. perineum, mesenteric perineum, omental perineum
   c. perineum, parietal perineum, visceral perineum
   d. peritoneum, parietal peritoneum, visceral peritoneum

7. Two of the most common procedures in the digestive system are
   a. biopsy and incision.
   b. tonsillectomy and adenoidectomy.
   c. pharyngoplasty and esophagectomy.
   d. EGD and ERCP.

8. A procedure to remove a sialolith from the salivary glands is called a(n)
   a. sialithotomy.
   b. sialolithectomy.
   c. sialolithotomy.
   d. sialolithoplasty.

9. A procedure to create a stoma in the abdominal wall where the large intestine and colon can eliminate waste into a pouch is called a(n)
   a. colostomy.
   b. colectomy.
   c. colotomy.
   d. colpostomy.

10. During an organ transplant, the physician's work to remove soft tissues surrounding the donor organ to prepare attached veins and arteries for transplantation is called
    a. backend work.
    b. backdoor work.
    c. backroom work.
    d. backbench work.

Coding Assignments

Instructions: Review each patient's case, and then assign codes for the procedure(s), appending a modifier when appropriate. Optional: For additional practice, assign the patient's diagnosis code(s) (ICD-9-CM).

1. MRI studies show that Melvin Blair, age 67, has a tumor of the posterior one-third of the tongue. At Williton, Dr. Ortega, an oncologist, removes the tumor and sends it to the pathologist, who confirms that it is carcinoma.

   Diagnosis code(s)_____

   Procedure code(s): _____

2. Freddy Jones, an eight-month-old, undergoes surgery today at Williton. Dr. May, an otolaryngologist, repairs his incomplete unilateral cleft palate and cleft lip. The procedure involves closure of the alveolar ridge involving soft tissue.

   Diagnosis code(s)_____

   Procedure code(s): _____

3. Jonathan Walton, age 18, has chronic tonsillitis. Today at Williton, Dr. May performs a tonsillectomy.

   Diagnosis code(s)_____

   Procedure code(s): _____

4. Johanna Rowe, age 20, is one of Dr. Hoffman's established patients. Ms. Rowe tells Dr. Hoffman that she experiences frequent nervousness, anxiety, and nausea with an urge to vomit, but she never does. She tells Dr. Hoffman, "My stomach is always growling, whether I'm hungry or just ate, and every time I eat, my stomach is almost instantly upset." Dr. Hoffman conducts an expanded problem-focused history and exam. He refers the patient to Dr. Gupta, a gastroenterologist, for a consultation to rule out any digestive disorders. Code for Dr. Hoffman's services.

   Diagnosis code(s)_____

   Procedure code(s): _____

5. Dr. Gupta sees Johanna Rowe for a consultation in his office. She reports the same symptoms that she described to Dr. Hoffman. She tells him that the symptoms began around the time that she changed jobs and divorced her husband. Dr. Gupta conducts a detailed history, comprehensive exam, and moderate medical decision-making. He determines that the patient needs an EGD in order to diagnose her problem. He dictates a report to send to Dr. Hoffman with the results of the consultation.

   Diagnosis code(s)_____

   Procedure code(s): _____

6. Today at Williton, Dr. Gupta conducts a diagnostic EGD for Johanna Rowe and finds no problems with her digestive tract. He later discusses his findings with the patient, and after further discussion regarding her personal problems that led to her symptoms, he suggests she receive psychological counseling. Then he calls Dr. Hoffman to tell him the results and suggests referring the patient to Dr. Francis, a psychologist, for a psychological evaluation because of her complaints of anxiety and nervousness. Dr. Hoffman agrees and will discuss the issue with the patient, and his office manager will coordinate the referral.

   Diagnosis code(s)_____

   Procedure code(s): _____

7. Jenny Maldonado, age 1 year, will not eat. Her mother takes her to Williton's ED, and Dr. Mills, the ED physician, examines her and orders X-rays. X-rays reveal that there is a penny lodged in the patient's esophagus. Dr. Mills discusses the case with Dr. May, who determines that the patient will need an esophagoscopy to remove the penny. He performs the surgery, which is successful.

   Diagnosis code(s)_____

   Procedure code(s): _____

8. Today at Williton, Dr. Gupta performs surgery for Eleanor Hodges, age 80, who has colon cancer. He removes part of her colon with an anastomosis.

   Diagnosis code(s)_____

   Procedure code(s): _____

9. Rhonda Yates, age 25, arrives at Williton's ED. Her mother drove her to the hospital because she could not drive herself due to severe abdominal pain, nausea, and vomiting. Dr. Burns, the ED physician, examines Ms. Yates and orders further workup. He diagnoses the patient with a ruptured appendix with appendicitis. Dr. Gupta subsequently performs an emergent open appendectomy.

   Diagnosis code(s)_____

   Procedure code(s): _____

10. Dr. Gupta performs a screening flexible colonoscopy for Bryan Webster, age 55. There is no evidence of disease or disorders.

    Diagnosis code(s)_____

    Procedure code(s): _____

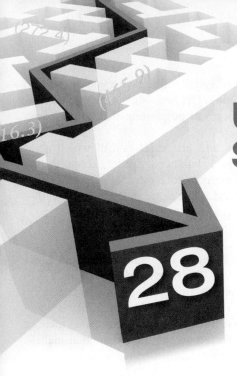

Urinary and Male Genital Systems

Learning Objectives

After completing this chapter, you should be able to
- Spell and define the key terminology in this chapter.
- Describe the anatomy of the urinary system and how it functions.
- Discuss urinary system procedures and how to code them.
- Explain the structure and functions of the male genital system.
- Define male genital system procedures and how to code them.

28

Key Terms

male genital system

renal hilum
urinary system

INTRODUCTION

You are doing very well traveling through many procedural coding stops along your coding journey! So far, you reviewed 11 chapters involving CPT coding for many different specialties. This stop on your journey takes you through procedures of the urinary and male genital systems. We journeyed through these systems a little in Chapter 10, when you learned about disorders of the genitourinary system, a system that includes the urinary system and the male and female reproductive systems. In Chapter 10, you also learned about urologists and nephrologists, and in this chapter, you will review procedures that they perform.

In this chapter, you will learn how to code urinary and male genital system procedures, starting with the urinary system. We still have a long way to go before finishing all chapters related to procedure coding, so let's continue on with this new destination where you can learn even more.

"The woods are lovely, dark, and deep, but I have promises to keep, and miles to go before I sleep, and miles to go before I sleep."—ROBERT FROST, "STOPPING BY WOODS ON A SNOWY EVENING"

URINARY SYSTEM ANATOMY

Before you can practice coding procedures of the urinary system, it is important for you to understand more about its anatomy. The **urinary system** produces and excretes urine, and it consists of two kidneys, two ureters, the bladder, sphincter muscles, and the urethra. Let's discuss these organs and structures and learn why they are important.

The body takes nutrients from food and uses them to maintain all bodily functions, including use of energy and self-repair. After your body has taken what it needs from food, it leaves waste products behind in the blood and in the bowel. We already reviewed the bowel in Chapter 27 when we discussed the digestive system. The urinary system produces urine to eliminate waste products and to maintain the body's electrolyte balance. **Electrolytes** are chemicals in the blood, such as sodium or potassium, that help organs and cells to function properly.

electrolytes (i-lek′-trə-līts)

The urinary system works with the lungs, skin, and intestines—all of which also excrete wastes—to keep electrolytes and water in the body balanced. Adults excrete about 1½ quarts of urine each day. The amount depends on many factors, especially the amounts of fluid and food a person consumes and how much fluid is lost through sweat and breathing. Certain types of medications can also affect the amount of urine excreted.

The urinary system removes waste called *urea* from the blood. Urea is produced when the body breaks down foods containing protein, such as meat and poultry, and certain vegetables. The bloodstream carries urea to the kidneys. The *kidneys* are two bean-shaped organs about the size of your fists (Figure 10-20). They are near the middle of the back, just below the rib cage. Although the body has two kidneys, it is able to function with only one if the other is lost to disease or injury. The external part of a kidney is covered with a membrane of connective tissue called the *renal capsule*. (The word *renal* means pertaining to the kidney.) The **renal hilum** is the indented part of the kidney that makes it look like a bean. The *renal artery* enters the kidney at the hilum.

The kidney has three layers (■ FIGURE 28-1):

- outer layer—*renal cortex*, which filters the blood
- middle layer—*renal medulla*, filtered blood flows through the renal medulla; it contains renal pyramids made up of tubules to collect urine
- inner layer—*renal pelvis*, which acts as a funnel to collect urine from the renal pyramids; it is made up of **major calyces** (cups) and **minor calyces**

The kidneys remove urea from the blood through tiny filtering tubules called *nephrons*. Each nephron is divided into two parts, the *renal corpuscle* and *renal tubule* (tube). Blood enters the renal corpuscle through the *glomerulus*, a ball formed of capillaries. The glomerulus has two layers of membranes called the *glomerular capsule*. Filtered blood, called *glomerular filtrate*, flows from the glomerular capsule into the various parts of the renal tubule, beginning with the *proximal tubule* (first part), then into the *nephron loop* and its two segments, the *descending loop* and *ascending loop*, then to the *distal tubule*. The filtrate then flows to collecting ducts, which connect to the minor **calyces** and then the

calyces (kā′-lə-sēz)

Figure 28-1 ■ Anatomy of the kidney.

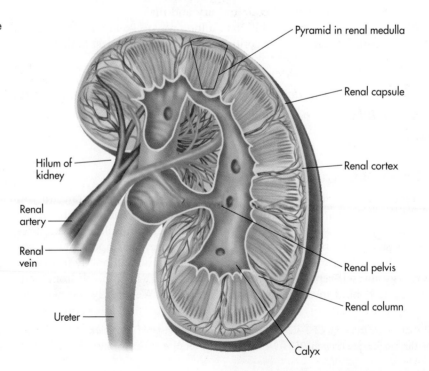

Figure 28-2 ■ The urinary bladder.

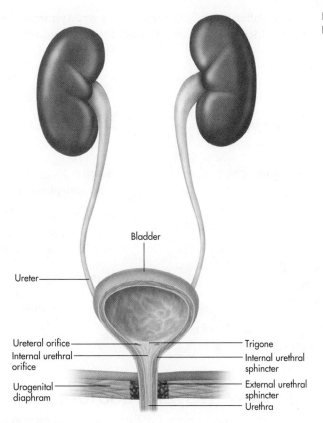

Bladder

Ureter

Ureteral orifice

Internal urethral orifice

Urogenital diaphram

Trigone

Internal urethral sphincter

External urethral sphincter

Urethra

major calyces (tubes of the renal pelvis). The filtrate, now called urine, flows into the major calyces, which form the *renal pelvis.*

The urine then travels from the kidneys into two thin tubes, called **ureters**, to the bladder. The ureters are about 8 to 10 inches long. Muscles in the ureter walls constantly tighten and relax to force urine downward away from the kidneys. The ureters empty small amounts of urine into the bladder about every 10 to 15 seconds.

The *bladder* is a hollow muscular organ shaped like a balloon (■ FIGURE 28-2). It sits in the pelvis, held in place by ligaments attached to other organs and pelvic bones. It is made up of several layers of muscle and connective tissue covers it. The bladder stores urine and swells and stretches into a round shape when it is full. It can hold up to 16 ounces (2 cups) of urine comfortably for 2 to 5 hours. A full bladder sends a message to the spinal cord and then the brain to trigger emptying, or voiding, called urination. Urine in the bladder empties into the *urethra,* a muscular tube, and then leaves the body.

Circular muscles called *sphincters* close tightly like a rubber band around the opening of the bladder into the urethra. When you urinate, the brain signals the bladder muscles to tighten, squeezing urine out of the bladder. At the same time, the brain signals the sphincter muscles to relax. As these muscles relax, urine exits the bladder through the urethra. When all the signals occur in the correct order, normal urination occurs.

Aging, illness, and injury can cause disorders of the urinary system. Aging changes the kidneys' structure, causing them to lose some of their ability to remove wastes from the blood. The muscles in the ureters, bladder, and urethra tend to lose some of their strength. Urinary tract infections (UTIs) occur if the bladder muscles do not tighten enough to empty the bladder completely, allowing urine to remain in the bladder. A decrease in strength of muscles of the sphincters and the pelvis can also cause incontinence, the unwanted leakage of urine. Illness or injury can also prevent the kidneys from filtering the blood completely or block the passage of urine.

Physicians diagnose urinary system conditions using different methods, including a **urinalysis,** a laboratory test for the presence of abnormal substances, such as protein or bacteria (signifying an infection) in the urine. You will learn more about the urinalysis in Chapter 33.

ureters (yur′-ət-ərs)

urinalysis (yur-ə-nal′-ə-səs)

urodynamic (yur-ə-dī-nam′-ik)

Another diagnostic method is a **urodynamic** test, which evaluates urine stored in the bladder and the flow of urine from the bladder through the urethra.

TAKE A BREAK

That was a lot of information to cover! Let's take a break and then review more about the urinary system.

Exercise 28.1   Urinary System Anatomy

Instructions: Fill in the blank with the best answer.

1. Adults excrete about _____ quarts of urine each day.

2. _____ is produced when the body breaks down foods containing protein, such as meat and poultry, and certain vegetables.

3. The kidney has three layers: the outer layer is called the _____, the middle layer is called the _____, and the inner layer is called the _____.

4. Each _____ is divided into two parts, the renal corpuscle and renal tubule.

5. Muscles in the _____ walls constantly tighten and relax to force urine downward away from the kidneys.

6. Circular muscles called _____ close tightly like a rubber band around the opening of the bladder into the urethra.

URINARY SYSTEM (50010–53899)

The Urinary System in the CPT manual is a subsection of the Surgery section. There are four subheadings in the Urinary System subsection, organized by *body site* (kidney, ureter, bladder, and urethra) and then *type of procedure* (■ TABLE 28-1). Many of the subheadings contain the same types of procedures, such as incision, excision, repair, laparoscopy, and endoscopy.

Turn to your CPT manual to page through procedures of the urinary system. Did you notice how many there are? We will not have time to review all of them in this chapter, so we will instead review some of them for various subheadings and categories. Be sure to refer back to the anatomy diagrams in this chapter and in Chapter 10, along with our discussion of the urinary system anatomy, as you read about procedures. As always, you can rely on your medical references and the Internet for more information about procedures we review and about new procedures that you find while working through the CPT manual. Let's get started then with the first subheading in the Urinary System subsection for the kidney.

Kidney (50010–50593)

Turn to the subheading Kidney in your CPT manual. Codes in this subheading include categories of procedures for excisions for biopsies, incisions to drain abscesses or remove kidney stones, repairs of a kidney wound or injury, and ablation of a renal cyst.

Many kidney procedures are unilateral, so you will need to append modifier -50 (for a bilateral procedure) to the code if the physician performs the procedure on *both* kidneys. Let's review some of the procedures listed in the Kidney categories in ■ TABLE 28-2. To locate codes for these procedures, search the index for the *body site* (kidney) and then *type of procedure* (e.g., biopsy, endoscopy) or *condition* (e.g., abscess, cyst), or start your search with the *type of procedure*. You can follow along in your CPT manual as we discuss the procedures.

Refer to the following example to learn more about coding procedures for the kidney.

Example: Shaun Spencer, age 52, has a malignant neoplasm of the kidney. Today at Williton Medical Center, Dr. Pigeon, a nephrologist, performs a nephrectomy by open approach, which includes a partial **ureterectomy** (excision of the ureter) and

ureterectomy (yur-ət-ər-ek′-tə-mē)

resection of a rib. The patient had previous surgery on the same kidney to treat another neoplasm.

You can try coding this case on your own and then review the following steps, or you can follow along and code with the steps listed. Search the index for the main term *nephrectomy* and subterm *with ureters,* which lists codes 50220–50236, 50546, and 50548. Assign code **50225,** since it describes all of the elements of the procedure, including previous surgery on the same kidney. The patient's diagnosis code is **189.0** (neoplasm, kidney, malignant, primary).

■ TABLE 28-1   **URINARY SYSTEM SUBHEADINGS AND CATEGORIES**

Subsection, Subheadings, and Categories	Code Range
Urinary System	**50010–53899**
Kidney	**50010–50593**
Incision	*50010–50135*
Excision	*50200–50290*
Renal Transplantation	*50300–50380*
Introduction	*50382–50398*
Repair	*50400–50540*
Laparoscopy	*50541–50549*
Endoscopy	*50551–50580*
Other Procedures	*50590–50593*
Ureter	**50600–50980**
Incision	*50600–50630*
Excision	*50650–50660*
Introduction	*50684–50690*
Repair	*50700–50940*
Laparoscopy	*50945–50949*
Endoscopy	*50951–50980*
Bladder	**51020–52700**
Incision	*51020–51080*
Removal	*51100–51102*
Excision	*51500–51597*
Introduction	*51600–51720*
Urodynamics	*51725–51798*
Repair	*51800–51980*
Laparoscopy	*51990–51999*
Endoscopy-Cystoscopy, Urethroscopy, Cystourethroscopy	*52000–52010*
Transurethral Surgery	*52204–52355*
Vesical Neck and Prostate	*52400–52700*
Urethra	**53000–53899**
Incision	*53000–53085*
Excision	*53200–53275*
Repair	*53400–53520*
Manipulation	*53600–53665*
Other Procedures	*53850–53899*

perirenal (per-i-rēn′-əl)

nephrostomy (ni-fräs′-tə-mē)

nephrotomy (ni-frät′-ə-mē)

nephrolithotomy (nef-rō-li-thät′-ə-mē)

pyelotomy (pī-(ə-)lät′-ə-mē)

nephrectomy (ni-frek′-tə-mē)

transurethral (trans-yu-rē′-thrəl)

pyeloplasty (pī′-(ə-)lə-plas-tē)

ureteropelvic (yu-rēt-ə-rō-pel′-vik)

calycoplasty (kā′lī-kō-plās′tē)

nephrorrhaphy (nef-ror′-ə-fē)

pyelostomy (pī-(ə-)läs′-tə-mē)

lithotripsy (lith′-ə-trip-sē)

extracorporeal (eks-tra-kor-pōr-ē′-əl)

■ TABLE 28-2   **PROCEDURES OF THE KIDNEY**

Category	Procedure(s)	Description
Incision (50010–50135)	Renal exploration, not necessitating other specific procedures (50010)	Procedure to examine renal structures, including for patients who suffer from hematuria or from external trauma, like a gunshot or knife wound. Physicians perform exploration by incising the abdomen to examine internal structures, including vessels. Physicians may also order renal imaging, such as a CT scan, to assess the patient's condition before performing renal exploration. • Often with blunt trauma kidney injuries, the laceration may cause a hematoma but does not damage blood vessels in the kidney. The hematoma may not spread because of the enclosed space surrounding the kidney. • Notice the CPT note directing you to digestive system codes if the exploration is retroperitoneal (behind the peritoneum).
	Drainage of perirenal or renal abscess, open or percutaneous (50020, 50021)	Procedure to drain fluid from a perirenal or renal abscess. A **perirenal** abscess *surrounds* a kidney and can involve both kidneys, and a renal abscess is *in* the kidney. An infection in the body or in the urinary tract (urinary tract infection - UTI) can cause an abscess. Ultrasounds and CT scans can show a perirenal or renal abscess. • The procedure can be performed through an open incision or may be percutaneous, using a catheter inserted through the skin and imaging to guide the procedure. • Symptoms of a perirenal or renal abscess include abdominal pain, fever, weight loss, dysuria, and hematuria. Many physicians successfully treat patients with these abscesses with antibiotics, rather than drainage.
	Nephrostomy, nephrotomy with drainage (50040)	Nephr/o is a combining form that means kidney. A nephrostomy is creating an opening in the kidney, and a nephrotomy is incising the kidney. • A nephrostomy involves percutaneous catheter insertion into the kidney in order to drain the urine into a bag that is placed outside the patient's body. The physician uses imaging to guide the procedure. • One of the reasons that the procedure is needed is because the patient has a ureter occlusion, like a kidney stone, that prevents urine from leaving the kidneys and flowing to the bladder. A renal ultrasound and other radiology tests can detect a ureter occlusion. • Urine that remains too long in the kidneys can cause kidney damage or infection. • Other reasons for a nephrostomy include ureter occlusion by a neoplasm or a tear in the ureter that allows urine to leak. It may also be performed as a diagnostic procedure to determine functions of the kidneys. • A nephrotomy involves incising the kidney to remove an obstruction.
	Nephrotomy, with exploration (50045)	An incision into the kidney to explore structures to diagnose causes of a hemorrhage or to diagnose neoplasms. • CPT notes alert you to review the renal endoscopy codes if the physician uses renal endoscopy to perform the nephrotomy.

■ **TABLE 28-2** *continued*

Category	Procedure(s)	Description
	Nephrolithotomy, removal of calculus (50060)	You learned that nephr/o means kidney. Lith/o is a combining form that means a stone, or calculus. A nephrolithotomy is a procedure to incise the kidney to remove a kidney stone, or calculus.
		• The kidneys form kidney stones, which are solid crystals of calcium, uric acid, and other substances (■ FIGURE 28-3).
		• Many stones are asymptomatic and very small, and an individual can "pass" them during urination. Other times, kidney stones grow in the kidneys and cause pain in the abdomen, sides, flank (between the ribs and hip), and groin. They may also move from the kidney to bladder or to the ureter, blocking the flow of urine.
	Pyelotomy (50120–50135)	Pyel/o is a combining form that means renal pelvis. A pyelotomy is an incision into the renal pelvis to:
		• Explore the renal pelvis to diagnose disorders
		• Drain urine from the renal pelvis
		• Remove a calculus or calculi
		The CPT note under code 50120 directs you to renal endoscopy codes if the physician performs renal endoscopy with the pyelotomy.
Excision (50200–50290)	**Nephrectomy** (50220–50240)	Procedure to partially or totally remove a kidney due to a neoplasm or to treat end-stage hydronephrosis, a condition that can severely damage the kidneys.
		• A nephrectomy may also include partial or total ureter excision or removal of lymph nodes.
		• A radical nephrectomy can also be done laparoscopically (50546).
	Ablation, open, 1 or more renal mass lesion(s), cryosurgical (50250)	Ablation by cryosurgery involves delivering a coolant at subfreezing temperatures through tubes or probes. Cryosurgery will cause tissue to die and slough off (fall off). The physician needs to perform the procedure on each individual lesion, but one CPT code represents one or more lesions. The procedure also includes ultrasound guidance and monitoring when performed.
Renal Transplantation (50300–50380)	• Cadaver donor or living donor nephrectomy • Backbench work • Recipient renal allotransplantation (50300–50380)	We discussed heart transplants in Chapter 25 and liver transplants in Chapter 27, and the procedures for a kidney transplant are very similar. It is important to remember that there are different CPT codes for each procedure that physicians perform to complete the kidney transplant:
		• A *nephrectomy* is the removal of a kidney from a cadaver or living donor and preservation to prepare it for transplantation. (50300, 50320)
		• *Backbench work* includes the physician's work to dissect and remove fat and prepare attached ureters, veins and arteries for transplantation (50323–50329).
		• A *renal allotransplantation* means a kidney of the same species is transplanted into the patient (50360). For a living donor, the physician removes *one* kidney from the donor and transplants it into the recipient. A cadaver donor has *two* kidneys that may be transplanted. The patient's diseased kidneys are not removed during the transplant to reduce the possibility of complications of the surgery.
		• Patients need kidney transplants due to chronic kidney disease or end-stage renal disease (ESRD), which you first learned about in Chapter 2. Other conditions can cause ESRD, such as hypertension and diabetes.

continued

■ **TABLE 28-2** *continued*

Category	Procedure(s)	Description
		• Just like heart and liver transplant candidates, patients who need kidney transplants remain on a waiting list until a suitable kidney is available. Many times, a patient's relative or friend will agree to donate a kidney.
		• Many insurances for patients who need a kidney transplant will also cover the living donor's expenses to donate a kidney. It is best to check with individual plans regarding specific coverage.
Introduction (50382–50398)	Removal of internally dwelling ureteral stent, via percutaneous approach, including radiological supervision and interpretation (50384)	Procedure to remove a temporary ureteral stent. The physician places the stent, a tube in the ureter, to allow the flow of urine, which is obstructed. A kidney stone may cause the occlusion. A temporary stent is needed until the physician performs a permanent procedure to treat the patient's condition. A ureteral stent can also be permanent, in the case of an inoperable neoplasm that obstructs urine flow.
		The percutaneous approach to remove the temporary stent is through the skin. The physician uses imaging to guide the procedure. He uses a catheter, needle, and guidewire to locate the stent and then remove it, usually with a snare (grabbing device) or forceps.
		CPT notes alert you to append modifier -50 for a bilateral procedure, and to assign a separate code for ureteral stent removal by **transurethral** (across the urethra) approach.
Repair (50400–50540)	**Pyeloplasty** (50400, 50405)	Repair of the renal pelvis to treat a **ureteropelvic** junction obstruction by excising it. The ureteropelvic junction is the connection between the renal pelvis and ureter.
		CPT categorizes a pyeloplasty as *simple* or *complicated*. It is complicated if it involves a congenital kidney abnormality, a secondary pyeloplasty, solitary kidney, or **calycoplasty** (repair of the calycx).
	Nephrorrhaphy, suture of kidney wound or injury (50500)	Procedure to repair a laceration after an injury from an object, like a knife or a bullet.
Laparoscopy (50541–50549)	Laparoscopy, surgical (50541–50545)	Procedure to ablate renal cysts or a renal lesion, or to perform a nephrectomy or pyeloplasty. A surgical laparoscopy always includes a diagnostic laparoscopy, so you should not separately report a diagnostic laparoscopy.
Endoscopy (50551–50580)	Renal endoscopy (50551–50580)	Endoscopy through an established nephrostomy, **pyelostomy** (opening in the renal pelvis), nephrotomy, or pyelotomy to perform various procedures, including a biopsy, ureteral catheterization, removal of foreign body or calculus, or fulguration (use of electrical current to destroy tissue) to treat a tumor.
		CPT directs you to report code 99070 for using supplies during the procedure. Remember that you can also report supplies with an appropriate HCPCS code, which you will review in Chapter 35.
Other Procedures (50590–50593)	**Lithotripsy, extracorporeal** shockwave (50590)	Extracorporeal shock wave lithotripsy (ESWL) is a procedure to treat kidney stones with a lithotriptor, equipment that aims shock waves, or pulsating sound waves, at the kidney stone to break it into pieces.
		The physician places a cushion filled with water at the kidneys and uses imaging, such as fluoroscopy, to locate the stone(s). The physician begins by operating the lithotriptor at a low level and gradually increases its intensity. The patient receives sedation or local anesthesia during the procedure.

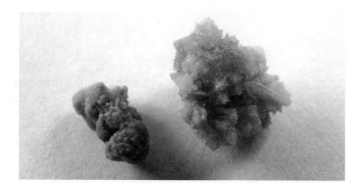

Figure 28-3 ■ Kidney stones.

Photo credit: remik44992/ Shutterstock.

TAKE A BREAK

Good job! Let's take a break and then review more about the kidneys.

Exercise 28.2   Kidneys

Part 1—Theory

Instructions: Fill in the blank with the best answer.

1. The repair of the renal pelvis to treat a ureteropelvic junction obstruction by excising it is called a(n) _____.

2. A(n) _____ is a procedure to partially or totally remove a kidney due to a neoplasm or to treat end-stage hydronephrosis.

3. Extracorporeal shock wave _____ is a procedure to treat kidney stones with equipment that aims shock waves, or pulsating sound waves, at the kidney stone to break it into pieces.

4. A(n) _____ involves percutaneous catheter insertion into the kidney in order to drain the urine into a bag that is placed outside the patient's body.

5. A procedure to ablate renal cysts or a renal lesion, or to perform a nephrectomy or pyeloplasty, is called _____.

6. _____ is a procedure to examine renal structures, including for patients who suffer from hematuria or from external trauma, like a gunshot or knife wound.

Part 2—Coding

Instructions: Review each patient's case, and then assign codes for the procedure(s), appending a modifier when appropriate. Optional: For additional practice, assign the patient's diagnosis code(s) (ICD-9-CM).

1. Ralph Hampton, age 45, has a renal pelvis abscess. At Williton, Dr. Suzuki, a urologist, inserts a needle percutaneously via translumbar (through the lower spine) approach and then advances it under fluoroscopic guidance into the abscess to drain it.

   Diagnosis code(s): _____

   Procedure code(s): _____

2. Rodney Jones, age 28, has ESRD, and his sister, Jan Jones, agrees to donate a kidney for a transplant. Today at Williton, the transplant team prepares for both surgeries. Dr. Pigeon, a nephrologist, performs the donor nephrectomy for Ms. Jones, the backbench standard preparation, and the renal allotransplantation for Mr. Jones. Dr. Pigeon does not remove Mr. Jones' own kidneys. Dr. Punjabi works with Dr. Pigeon and the rest of the transplant team on all three procedures.

   Code for Dr. Pigeon for Ms. Jones' surgery:

   Diagnosis code(s): _____

   Procedure code(s): _____

   Code for Dr. Pigeon for Mr. Jones' surgery:

   Diagnosis code(s): _____

   Procedure code(s): _____

   Code for Dr. Punjabi for Ms. Jones' surgery:

   Diagnosis code(s): _____

   Procedure code(s): _____

   Code for Dr. Punjabi for Mr. Jones' surgery:

   Diagnosis code(s): _____

   Procedure code(s): _____

3. Len Renson, age 19, suffered a kidney laceration from an automobile accident while driving to work on State Route 51. He collided with another vehicle which was traveling in the opposite direction. An ambulance

continued

TAKE A BREAK *continued*

transports Mr. Renson to Williton, where Dr. Pigeon repairs a large laceration during emergency surgery.

Diagnosis code(s): _____

Procedure code(s): _____

4. Macy Tobias, age 56, has renal calculi. They are causing her a great deal of pain, so Dr. Suzuki advises treatment with shock wave lithotripsy, which he performs today at Williton. The procedure is successful.

Diagnosis code(s): _____

Procedure code(s): _____

5. Today at Williton, Dr. Pigeon and Dr. Punjabi work on another kidney transplant case with the transplant team. They remove both kidneys from a **cadaveric** donor (a cadaver). After preparing the kidneys on the back table by removing **perinephric** (surrounding the kidneys) fat and preparing the veins, arteries, and ureters, they transplant the kidneys into Mandy

Quinn, age 37. The physicians also remove the patient's kidneys prior to the transplant. The patient has ESRD and renal abscesses from an infection that Staphylococcus aureus caused.

Code for Dr. Pigeon for all procedures:

Diagnosis code(s): _____

Procedure code(s): _____

Code for Dr. Punjabi for all procedures:

Diagnosis code(s): _____

Procedure code(s): _____

6. Ian Stone, age 45, has a calculus in his kidney. Dr. Punjabi performs a renal endoscopy through a nephrotomy. He removes the stone.

Diagnosis code(s): _____

Procedure code(s): _____

cadaveric (kə-dav′-(ə-)rik)

perinephric (per-ə-nef′-rik)

ureterotomy (yur-ət-ər-ät′-ə-mē)

ureterolithotomy (yu-rēt-ə-rō-li-thät′-ə-mē)

uretography (ure-tog′rah-fe)

ureteropyelography (yu-rēt-ə-rō-pī-ə-läg′-rə-fē)

ureterostomy (yur-ət-ər-äs′-tə-mē)

ileal conduit (il′-ē-əl kon′doo-it)

manometric (man-ə-me′-trik)

ureteroplasty (yu-rēt′-ə-rə-plas-tē)

ureterocystostomy (yu-ret-ə-rō-sis-tos′-tah-me)

urography (yu-räg′-rə-fē)

Ureter (50600–50980)

The Ureter subheading contains categories for incision, excision, introduction, repair, laparoscopy, and endoscopy.

Turn to the subheading Ureter in your CPT manual to review the types of procedures listed. Note that some of the ureter procedures are for a single ureter, such as code 50780, and you have to append modifier -50 (bilateral procedure) if the physician performs the procedure on both ureters. Let's review some of the procedures listed in the Ureter categories in ■ TABLE 28-3. To locate codes for these procedures, search the index for the *body site* (ureter) and then *type of procedure* (destruction, endoscopy), or start your search with the *type of procedure*. You can follow along in your CPT manual as we discuss the procedures.

Refer to the following example to learn more about coding procedures for the ureter.

Example: Dr. Suzuki, a urologist, performs a ureterography for Manny Thank, age 40. Dr. Suzuki previously examined the patient and found that his penis was red and swollen. Dr. Suzuki injects contrast through a ureteral catheter and uses imaging guidance, performing the radiological supervision and interpretation (S & I). He diagnoses the patient with a ureteral stricture.

You can try coding this case on your own and then review the following steps, or you can follow along and code with the steps listed. You will assign two procedure codes for this case, one for the injection of contrast, and the other for the imaging.

For the first code for the injection, search the index for main term *ureter*, subterm *injection*, and subterm *radiologic*, which directs you to codes 50684, 50690. Assign code **50684**, since it represents an injection procedure for ureterography.

For the second code for the radiological imaging, notice that a CPT note for code 50684 directs you to a radiology code of 74425 for the radiological supervision and interpretation. Refer to this code in the Radiology section, and you will find that it represents a **urography**, which is a radiologic exam of the urinary tract, including the ureter. Assign code **74425** as an additional code. The patient's diagnosis code is **593.3** (stricture, ureter).

■ TABLE 28-3   **PROCEDURES OF THE URETER**

Category	Procedure(s)	Description
Incision (50600–50630)	**Ureterotomy** (50600–50605)	Incision into the ureter for exploration to determine the cause of an occlusion, and for drainage or to insert an indwelling stent to treat stenosis and improve urine flow that stenosis causes. Stenosis can occur from scarring that develops after the patient suffers from an infection or injury. Ureteral stenosis causes obstructed flow of urine, which many times causes pain. • Notice the CPT note under code 50600 instructing you to assign an additional code if the physician performs ureteral endoscopy during the procedure.
	Ureterolithotomy (50610–50630)	An incision into a ureter to remove a calculus, or stone. There are three code choices for this procedure, and the code that you choose depends on the location of the incision: upper, middle, or lower third of the ureter. • There are several CPT notes for these codes directing you to review other codes for additional or other procedures performed.
Excision (50650–50660)	Ureterectomy (50650, 50660)	Excision of the ureter, most commonly to remove a malignant neoplasm. • When the physician removes a small portion of the bladder (bladder cuff) with the ureter, report code 50650. Code 50650 includes the "separate procedure" designation. CMS does not allow additional payment for the procedure when the physician performs it with other procedures in an anatomically related area. • Code 50660 represents a total ureterectomy of an ectopic ureter (abnormal condition where the ureter stops at the urethra or vagina instead of the bladder). The procedure includes a combination of approaches.
Introduction (50684-50690)	Introduction procedures (50684–50690)	Introduction procedures for injecting contrast, including for a **uretography** (image of the ureter) and **ureteropyelography** (image of the ureter and renal pelvis). The physician performs the procedure through an opening in the ureter (**ureterostomy**) or through an indwelling ureteral catheter. These images help the physician to diagnose various conditions. • Injection procedures also include visualizing an **ileal conduit** (channel). An ileal conduit is part of a procedure to create a new bladder from part of the bowel when the physician removes the patient's bladder. The physician joins the ureters to the ileum, the small intestine. • For injection procedures (50684, 50690), report radiological supervision and interpretation separately. • Introduction procedures also include changing a ureterostomy tube (stent) and **manometric** studies, tests that measure the pressure of liquid flowing through the ureters using fluid introduced through a ureterostomy or indwelling ureteral catheter.
Repair (50700–50940)	**Ureteroplasty** (50700)	Repair of the ureter to treat a ureteral stricture (narrowing) The procedure may include excision of the portion of the ureter with the stricture, then anastomosis of the ends that were not removed, or the procedure may include grafting tissue from the bladder to enlarge the stricture.

continued

■ **TABLE 28-3** *continued*

Category	Procedure(s)	Description
Laparoscopy (50945–50949)	Surgical laparoscopy (50945–50948)	Physicians may perform surgical laparoscopy for different reasons, including urethrolithotomy or **ureterocystostomy**, a procedure to resect the ureter to the bladder due to necrosis or disease.
		• Remember that surgical laparoscopy *always* includes diagnostic laparoscopy, so you should not separately report diagnostic laparoscopy.
		• Medicare guidelines state that if a physician converts a laparoscopic procedure to an open procedure, you may only code and bill the open procedure. Other insurances will reimburse for the partial laparoscopic procedure and the open procedure if you assign the laparoscopy code and append modifier -52 (reduced services) or -53 (discontinued procedure), and also report the code for the open procedure.
		• It is important to note that when the physician converts a laparoscopic procedure to an open procedure, you should assign a secondary diagnosis code of V64.41—*Laparoscopic surgical procedure converted to open procedure.*
Endoscopy (50951–50980)	Endoscopy through established ureterostomy or through ureterotomy (50951–50980)	Physicians perform ureteral endoscopies for various reasons, including to insert a catheter, perform a biopsy, or remove a foreign body.

TAKE A BREAK

Good work! You are doing great! Let's take a break and then review more about the ureter.

Exercise 28.3 **URETERS**

Part 1—Theory

Instructions: Fill in the blank with the best answer.

1. A(n) _____ is an image of the ureter and renal pelvis.

2. Another word for channel is _____.

3. An incision into the ureter for exploration to determine the cause of an occlusion is called a(n) _____.

4. A procedure to resect the ureter to the bladder due to necrosis or disease is called a(n) _____.

5. A(n) _____ is an excision of the ureter, most commonly to remove a malignant neoplasm.

6. An image of the ureter is called a(n) _____.

Part 2—Coding

Instructions: Review each patient's case, and then assign codes for the procedure(s), appending a modifier when appropriate. Optional: For additional practice, assign the patient's diagnosis code(s) (ICD-9-CM).

1. Dr. Suzuki determines that Avery Cool, age 29, has a calculus stuck in his right ureter. Today at Williton, he removes the stone by cutting into the lower third of the ureter to remove it.

   Diagnosis code(s): _____

   Procedure code(s): _____

2. Dr. Suzuki performs a ureteral endoscopy through a ureterotomy for Lamar Jones, age 59. He finds a tumor in the left ureter and removes it for a biopsy, which he sends to pathology. The pathologist determines that the tumor is benign.

   Diagnosis code(s): _____

   Procedure code(s): _____

TAKE A BREAK *continued*

3. Jerome Miller, age 65, is a Medicare patient who arrives at Williton for a surgical laparoscopy to remove a calculus from his right ureter. Dr. Suzuki performs the laparoscopy but determines that he needs to convert it to an open procedure to gain sufficient access to the calculus, which is larger than he anticipated. He excises the calculus from the middle third of the ureter.

Diagnosis code(s): _____

Procedure code(s): _____

4. Peter Homer, age 46, had bladder cancer, and Dr. Suzuki removed the bladder and created a new one from the bowel. Today at Williton, Dr. Suzuki performs an injection procedure to view the ileal conduit. He also performs the S & I of the radiology test.

Diagnosis code(s): _____

Procedure code(s): _____

5. Harry Snow, age 58, needs his ureterostomy tube changed, which Dr. Suzuki placed to allow urine to drain outside the body. Mr. Snow had cancer of the urinary bladder. Dr. Suzuki changes the tube each month and performs the procedure at Williton.

Diagnosis code(s): _____

Procedure code(s): _____

6. Jonathon Kreeson, age 40, has ureteral transitional cell carcinoma. Dr. Suzuki performs surgery to remove his left ureter, including bladder cuff (part of the bladder).

Diagnosis code(s): _____

Procedure code(s): _____

POINTERS FROM THE PROS: Interview with an Office Assistant

Angela Tomko works for a cardiology practice where she codes diagnoses and procedures, bills insurances and patients, transcribes office visits and surgeries, schedules appointments and tests, refills prescriptions, and answers phones.

What are the most challenging aspects of your job?

Getting all of the work completed in a timely manner.

What advice would you like to give to coding students about working with different personalities?

Be thick-skinned, though it can be frustrating, especially if you work with a difficult individual.

What advice would you like to give to coding students to help them prepare to work successfully in the healthcare field?

Always be prepared, and be positive about what you are doing.

What personal motto do you live by?

Do everything to the best of your ability.

(Used by permission of Angela Tomko.)

Bladder (51020–52700)

The Bladder (Figure 28-2) subheading contains categories that will sound familiar to you: incision, removal, excision, and introduction. There are also categories that are unfamiliar, such as urodynamics, which we will discuss later in this section. Turn to the Bladder subheading in your CPT manual, and you can follow along in your manual as we discuss bladder procedures in ■ TABLE 28-4. To locate codes for bladder procedures, search the index for the *body site* (bladder) and then *type of procedure* (destruction, excision) or *condition* (abscess, diverticulum), or start your search with the *type of procedure*.

cystotomy (sis-tät′-ə-mē)

cystostomy (sis-täs′-tə-mē)

cystolithotomy (sis-tō-lith-ät′-ə-mē)

cystectomy (sis-tek′-tə-mē)

ureterocele (yu-rēt′-ə-rə-sēl)

cystometrogram (sis-tə-me′-trə-gram)

cystoplasty (sis′-tə-plas-tē)

cystourethroplasty (sis-tō-yu-rē′-thrə-plas-tē)

■ TABLE 28-4   **PROCEDURES OF THE BLADDER**

Category	Procedure(s)	Description
Incision (51020–51080)	**Cystotomy, cystostomy, cystolithotomy** (51020–51045, 51050, 51065)	Cyst/o is a combining form that means bladder. A *cystotomy* is an incision into the bladder, and a *cystostomy* is creating an opening in the bladder. A *cystolithotomy* is incising a calculus of the bladder. The physician performs these procedures for various reasons, including cryosurgical lesion destruction, calculus removal, and inserting a catheter or stent.
Removal (51100–51102)	Aspiration of bladder (51100–51102)	Physicians can aspirate a patient's bladder to obtain a urine sample to test it for infection. Many times, bladder aspiration of urine is done for pediatric patients who cannot urinate using a clean catch method (collecting urine in a sterile cup). It is also performed for patients who are unable to urinate because certain conditions prevent it. • The physician can aspirate the bladder using a needle, a trocar (a long surgical tubelike instrument with a pointed end and hollow center), or a catheter, including a suprapubic catheter (inserted through the abdominal wall).
Excision (51500–51597)	Cystotomy, **cystectomy** (51520–51596)	A *cystotomy* involves excising a diverticulum, tumor, or **ureterocele** (cystic pouch in the ureter), and can involve removing the bladder neck (vesical neck). A *cystectomy* is the partial or complete excision of the bladder, most commonly to treat bladder cancer. A cystectomy may also involve other procedures, including removing surrounding lymph nodes.
	Pelvic exenteration (51597)	Radical procedure to treat vesical, prostatic (pertaining to the prostate gland) or urethral (pertaining to the urethra) malignancy. The physician excises the bladder, urethra, ureters, lymph nodes, prostate/vagina, uterus, colon and rectum. The procedure may also include a hysterectomy and resecting the rectum and colon.
Urodynamics (51725–51798)	Urodynamic tests (51725–51792)	Urodynamic tests measure how well the bladder, sphincters, and urethra store and release urine. Most urodynamic tests focus on the bladder's ability to hold urine and empty steadily and completely. Urodynamic tests measure the contraction of the bladder muscle as it fills and empties. A physician may recommend urodynamic tests if symptoms indicate disorders of the lower urinary tract. Lower urinary tract symptoms (LUTS) include: • urine leakage • frequent and/or painful urination • sudden, strong urge to urinate • difficulty starting a urine stream or emptying the bladder completely • recurrent UTIs Urodynamic tests range from simple visual observation to precise measurements using sophisticated instruments. For simple observation, a physician measures the length of time it takes a patient to produce a urinary stream, the volume of urine produced, and the ability or inability to stop the urine flow in midstream. • For precise measurements, imaging equipment takes pictures of the bladder filling and emptying, pressure monitors record the pressures inside the bladder, and sensors record muscle and nerve activity. The physician determines the type of urodynamic test the patient needs based on the health history, physical exam, and LUTS. The urodynamic test results help diagnose the cause and nature of a lower urinary tract problem. • One example of a urodynamic test is a **cystometrogram** (51725–51729) (■ FIGURE 28-4). A cystometrogram measures how much urine the bladder can hold, how much pressure builds up inside the bladder as it stores urine, and how full it is when the urge to urinate begins. A catheter is used to empty the bladder completely. Then a special, smaller catheter is placed in the bladder. This catheter has a pressure-measuring device called a manometer. Another catheter may be placed in the rectum or vagina to record pressure there.

■ TABLE 28-4   *continued*

Category	Procedure(s)	Description
		• Once the bladder is emptied completely, it is filled slowly with warm water. During this time, the patient is asked to describe how the bladder feels and indicate when the need to urinate arises. When the urge to urinate occurs, the volume of water and the bladder pressure are recorded. The patient may be asked to cough or strain during this procedure to see if the bladder pressure changes. A cystometric test can also identify involuntary bladder contractions. Cystometric tests are performed in a physician's office, clinic, or hospital with local anesthesia.
		Did you review the CPT guidelines at the beginning of the Urodynamics category? They alert you to append modifier -51 for multiple urodynamic tests performed for the same patient during the same session. Guidelines also state that a physician should either perform the urodynamic test or supervise it. Append modifier -26 to the urodynamic test codes when the physician only interprets test results or operates equipment.
Repair (51800–51980)	Repair procedures (51800–51980)	Take a look at the codes for bladder repairs. Did you notice that there are many different types of repairs? The type of repair depends on the patient's specific disorder that the physician needs to treat. Let's review the following types of repairs:
		• **Cystoplasty** *(bladder repair)*, **cystourethroplasty** *(repair of bladder and urethra)*, *plastic operation on bladder and/or vesical neck* (51800)—Repair of an obstruction in the bladder neck or urethra, with or without wedge resection of posterior vesical neck.
		• *Cystourethroplasty with unilateral or bilateral* **urethroneocystostomy**— Repair of a defect in the bladder and urethra, with reimplantation of one or both of the ureters into the bladder (ureteroneocystostomy)
		• *Anterior* **vesicourethropexy** *(to support the bladder neck and urethra)*— Older women frequently suffer from incontinence. Stress incontinence is the term used for leakage of urine during exercise, coughing, sneezing, laughing, or lifting. The Marshall-Marchetti-Krantz procedure is a type of surgery to treat incontinence. This procedure is also called a bladder lift. (51840—simple repair, or primary repair, 51841—complicated, or secondary repair).
		• **Cystorrhaphy**, suture of bladder wound—Repair of an injury or rupture to the bladder, simple or complicated (51860–51865).
		• *Cutaneous* **vesicostomy**—Temporary surgical procedure to create an opening in the lower abdomen (**umbilicus**), which allows urine to continuously drain from the bladder so that it will not remain in the kidneys (51980). The surgeon turns the edge of the bladder inside out and then sews it to the skin of the abdomen. It is a small incision and the opening is called a stoma. This procedure is usually performed on small children. They typically do not need an external drainage bag because they wear diapers. But they may need a temporary catheter.
Transurethral Surgery (52204–52355)	**Cystourethroscopy** (52204–52315, 52320–52355)	Transurethral means across the urethra. Notice that there are two subcategories under the Transurethral Surgery category, Urethra and Bladder and Ureter and Pelvis. Did you also notice that the majority of procedures in both subcategories are for a cystourethroscopy? A *cystourethroscopy* involves inserting an endoscope into the urethra and bladder to view internal structures and diagnose different conditions. A cystourethroscopy is used to perform various types of procedures, such as a biopsy and fulguration of the bladder neck or bladder tumors.
		• Physicians perform this procedure for patients with difficulty urinating, hematuria, UTIs, neoplasms, lower abdominal pain, or bladder stones.
		• The procedure can take up to 40 minutes to perform, and the patient must urinate before the procedure to ensure that the bladder is as empty as possible. The physician inserts a cystoscope into the urethra and then the bladder, takes a urine sample for testing, and introduces water into the bladder, inflating it, which enables the physician to adequately view the interior of the bladder. The physician may then take a biopsy, excise a neoplasm, or remove calculi from the bladder or urethra.

continued

■ **TABLE 28-4** *continued*

Category	Procedure(s)	Description
		There are several CPT guidelines for the Transurethral Surgery category, so be sure to read them carefully before final code assignment.
Vesical Neck and Prostate (52400–52700)	Transurethral resection of prostate (52601)	The *prostate gland* is an exocrine gland in the male reproductive system (■ FIGURE 28-5). It secretes fluid that combines with semen and the prostate gland's muscles contract to release the fluid during ejaculation.
		• A transurethral resection of the prostate (TURP) is a procedure that typically treats benign prostatic hypertrophy (BPH) (enlarged prostate). Many men develop BPH as they age, and the condition places pressure on the urethra. Patients urinate frequently but pass very small amounts of urine. TURP involves inserting an endoscope into the penis. The endoscope contains a wire loop to excise tissue from the prostate to remove the obstruction.

urethroneocystostomy
(u-re-thro-neo-sis-tos′tah-me)

vesicourethropexy (ves-i- kō-yu-rē-thrə pek′-se)

cystorrhaphy (sis-tär′-ə-fē)

vesicostomy (ves-i-käs′-tə-mē)

umbilicus (əm-bil′-i-kəs)

cystourethroscopy (sis-tō-yu-rē-thrə′-skə-pē)

Figure 28-4 ■ A cystometrogram showing the location of the catheter insertion.

Source: National Heart, Lung, and Blood Institute; National Institutes of Health; U.S. Department of Health and Human Services.

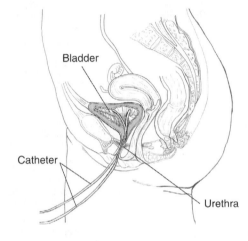

Figure 28-5 ■ The male reproductive anatomy.

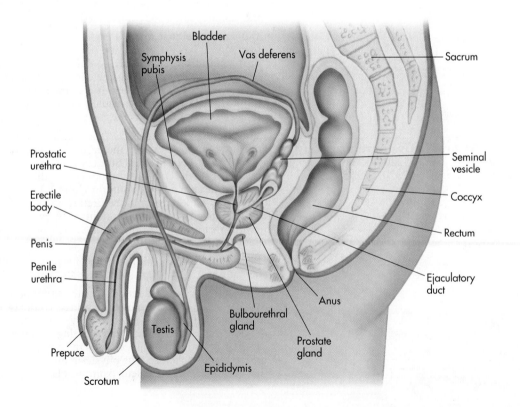

INTERESTING FACTS: Smoking Is the Cause of Most Bladder Cancer

In 2012, about 56,000 men and 18,000 women will be diagnosed with bladder cancer in the United States. Most will be over 70 years old. More than 9 of 10 Americans with bladder cancer have a type called transitional cell cancer (TCC). TCC begins in the cells on the surface of the inner lining of the bladder. Bladder cancer cells can spread through the blood vessels to the liver, lungs, bones, lymph vessels, and lymph nodes. Studies have found the following risk factors for bladder cancer:

✔ *Smoking:* Smoking causes most of the cases of bladder cancer. People who smoke for many years have a higher risk than nonsmokers or those who smoke for a short time.

✔ *Chemicals in the workplace:* Workers in the dye, rubber, chemical, metal, textile, and leather industries may be at risk of bladder cancer. Also at risk are hairdressers, machinists, printers, painters, and truck drivers.

✔ *Personal history of bladder cancer:* People who have had bladder cancer have an increased risk of getting the disease again.

✔ *Certain cancer treatments:* People with cancer who have been treated with certain drugs (such as cyclophosphamide) may be at increased risk of bladder cancer. Also, people who have had radiation therapy to the abdomen or pelvis may be at increased risk.

✔ *Arsenic:* Arsenic is a poison that increases the risk of bladder cancer. In some areas of the world, arsenic may be found at high levels in drinking water. However, the United States has safety measures limiting the arsenic level in public drinking water.

✔ *Family history of bladder cancer:* People with family members who have bladder cancer have a slightly increased risk of the disease.

(*What You Need To Know about Bladder Cancer* booklet, National Cancer Institute, National Institutes of Health, www.cancer.gov)

TAKE A BREAK

That was a lot of information to cover! Let's take a break and then review more about the bladder.

Exercise 28.4 Bladder

Part 1—Theory

Instructions: Fill in the blank with the best answer.

1. A(n) _____ is the partial or complete excision of the bladder, most commonly to treat bladder cancer.

2. A(n) _____ is a procedure that typically treats benign prostatic hypertrophy (BPH) (enlarged prostate).

3. Repair of a defect in the bladder and urethra, with reimplantation of one or both of the ureters into the bladder, is called a(n) _____.

4. _____ tests measure how well the bladder, sphincters, and urethra store and release urine.

5. A(n) _____ involves inserting an endoscope into the urethra and bladder to view internal structures and diagnose different conditions.

6. A(n) _____ involves excising a diverticulum, tumor, or ureterocele.

Part 2—Coding

Instructions: Review each patient's case, and then assign codes for the procedure(s), appending a modifier when appropriate. Optional: For additional practice, assign the patient's diagnosis code(s) (ICD-9-CM).

1. At Williton Medical Center, Dr. Suzuki, a urologist, performs a procedure for Johnny Blink, age 62, who has kidney stones in his bladder. Dr. Suzuki incises the bladder to remove the calculi with a basket, which he inserts in an endoscope and uses to retrieve the calculi. He also uses ultrasound fragmentation to destroy the calculi.

   Diagnosis code(s): _____

   Procedure code(s): _____

2. Mac Gold, age 72, suffers from urinary incontinence. He is an established patient of Dr. Hoffman, his primary care physician. Dr. Hoffman conducts an expanded problem-focused history and exam and advises Mr. Gold that he is referring him to see Dr. Suzuki for an evaluation.

   Diagnosis code(s): _____

   Procedure code(s): _____

continued

TAKE A BREAK *continued*

3. On Tuesday, Mr. Gold sees Dr. Suzuki for the first time in his office regarding urinary incontinence. Dr. Suzuki conducts a comprehensive history and exam with moderate medical decision-making. He determines that Mr. Gold will need further testing, and he discusses this option with the patient. Mr. Gold agrees to the testing. On Friday, at Williton, Dr. Suzuki measures postvoiding residual urine by ultrasound. The test, called a postvoid residual (PVR) test, measures the amount of urine left in the bladder after the patient urinates. After the procedure, Dr. Suzuki determines that the patient will need surgery to treat the incontinence. Code for services on Tuesday and Friday.

Tuesday:

Diagnosis code(s): _____

Procedure code(s): _____

Friday:

Diagnosis code(s): _____

Procedure code(s): _____

4. Janie Smith drives her husband, Tom, to Williton's ED because he cannot urinate. Dr. Mills, the ED physician, examines the patient and inserts a catheter into Mr. Smith's bladder (straight catheterization), which provides relief. Dr. Mills calls Dr. Suzuki to ask him to further evaluate the patient.

Diagnosis code(s): _____

Procedure code(s): _____

5. Whitey Smithson, age 69, has bladder cancer of **contiguous** sites of the bladder (adjacent to), which has metastasized to the colon and rectum. Today at Williton, a team of surgeons, including Dr. Suzuki, treats the patient's condition by performing a complete bladder removal; an **enterocystoplasty**, which anastomoses the intestine to reconstruct the bladder; and an open total **colectomy** (excision of all or part of the colon) with a complete proctectomy. Code for the patient's procedures for Dr. Suzuki working as part of the surgical team.

Diagnosis code(s): _____

Procedure code(s): _____

6. Albert Rock, age 68, has BPH with urinary obstruction and LUTS. He is having increased difficulty with urination. Dr. Hoffman refers him to Dr. Suzuki for an evaluation. Dr. Suzuki determines that the patient needs a complete TURP. He performs the procedure today at Williton and controls postoperative bleeding.

Diagnosis code(s): _____

Procedure code(s): _____

contiguous (kən-tig′-yə-wəs)

enterocystoplasty (en-tä-rō-sis′to-plas′te)

colectomy (kə-lek′-tə-mē)

Urethra (53000–53899)

There are not many procedures listed under the Urethra subheading, as compared to other subheadings of the Urinary System subsection. Categories of the Urethra subheading include incision, excision, repair, manipulation, and other procedures. Turn to the subheading Urethra in your CPT manual. Let's review some of the procedures listed in the categories. To locate codes for these procedures, search the index for the *body site* (urethra) and then *type of procedure* (biopsy, dilation) or *condition* (lesion, polyp), or start your search with the *type of procedure*. You can follow along in your CPT manual as we discuss the procedures. Be sure to consult your medical references to review procedures that we do not discuss or to find more information about procedures we review.

Take a look at the following procedures from the Urethra subheading, which you will find under different categories:

urethrotomy (yur-ə-thrät′-ə-mē)

urethrostomy (yr-ə-thräs′-tə-mē)

- **Urethrotomy** (incision into the urethra), **urethrostomy**, *external* (creating an opening in the urethra) (53000–53010)—A *urethrotomy* involves incising the urethra to relieve tension from a urethral stricture. A *urethrostomy* involves creating an opening in the urethra to treat an obstruction.

meatotomy (mē′ə-tŏt′ə′-mē)

- **Meatotomy**, *cutting of meatus (separate procedure); except infant, infant* (53020–53025)—Meatal stenosis is an abnormal narrowing of the urethral meatus, the external opening of the urethra. A meatotomy is a procedure to incise the meatus to treat stenosis. CPT divides codes by whether or not the patient is an infant.

urethroplasty (yu-rē′-thrə-plas-tē)

- **Urethroplasty** (53400–53431)—Repair of the urethra to treat an injury or defect in the urethral walls. The procedure could involve anastomosis or grafting.

- *Sling operation for correction of male urinary incontinence* (53440)—Procedure to treat stress urinary incontinence by creating a sling from material, which supports the urethra and helps the urethral sphincter to close properly and avoid urine leakage.

- *Dilation of urethral stricture by passage of sound or urethral dilator, male; initial or subsequent* (53600–53601)—Procedure to dilate a urethral stricture using sounds, or a metal urethral dilators, in the urethra. Physicians may use more than one size dilator throughout a procedure until they successfully dilate the urethra. Urethral dilation dates back to the 6th century B.C. The goal of urethral dilation is to increase the size of the urethra, but it can be a painful procedure with bleeding as one of the side effects, indicating a torn urethra. Injury to the rectum can also occur.

- *Transurethral destruction of prostate tissue; by microwave thermotherapy (TUMT)* (53850)—is often used as an alternative to TURP and treats BPH. The physician inserts a catheter into the bladder to insert a microwave antenna into the prostate. The microwaves destroy hyperplastic tissue of the prostate.

TAKE A BREAK

Nice work! You have finished reviewing all subheadings in the Urinary System subsection! Let's take a break and then review more about the urethra before moving on to the Male Genital System subsection.

Exercise 28.5 Urethra

Part 1—Theory

Instructions: Fill in the blank with the best answer.

1. The external opening of the urethra is called the _____.

2. A urethrotomy involves incising the _____ to relieve tension from a urethral stricture.

3. A urethroplasty is a repair of the urethra to treat an injury or defect in the _____.

4. During TUMT, the physician inserts a catheter into the bladder to insert a _____ into the prostate to destroy hyperplastic tissue.

5. A(n) _____ involves creating an opening in the urethra to treat an obstruction.

6. A sling operation is a procedure to treat _____ by creating a sling which supports the urethra and helps the urethral sphincter to close properly and avoid urine leakage.

Part 2—Coding

Instructions: Review each patient's case, and then assign codes for the procedure(s), appending a modifier when appropriate. Optional: For additional practice, assign the patient's diagnosis code(s) (ICD-9-CM).

1. Lou Lucky, age 45, has BPH with urinary obstruction. Today at Williton, Dr. Suzuki, a urologist, performs TUMT to relieve his symptoms.

   Diagnosis code(s): _____

   Procedure code(s): _____

2. Tom Young, age 34, has had difficulty voiding urine, due to scar tissue in his urethra. In his office, Dr. Suzuki dilates the urethra using dilators of increasing sizes.

   Diagnosis code(s): _____

   Procedure code(s): _____

3. George Good, age 49, has polyps in his urethra. Today at Williton, Dr. Suzuki excises polyps of the distal urethra.

   Diagnosis code(s): _____

   Procedure code(s): _____

4. Terrell Poling, who is three days old, has an incomplete opening of the urethral meatus. At Williton, Dr. Thomas, a urologist specializing in treating pediatric conditions, performs a meatotomy to correct the problem.

   Diagnosis code(s): _____

   Procedure code(s): _____

5. At Williton, Dr. Suzuki performs a closure of a urethral fistula for Marco Theos, age 61.

   Diagnosis code(s): _____

   Procedure code(s): _____

6. Today at Williton, Dr. Suzuki performs a sling operation for Bill Woyie, age 69, who has urinary incontinence.

   Diagnosis code(s): _____

   Procedure code(s): _____

WORKPLACE IQ

You work as the lead coder for Dr. Suzuki. Your manager, Cheryl, asks you to audit a group of insurance claims, which the billing specialist, Debbie, electronically billed to insurances. The insurances already processed the claims. The claims involve records that Tiffany, a coding specialist, coded for procedures. Cheryl asks you to verify that the codes reported on the CMS-1500 forms were correctly assigned to procedures documented in the patient's medical records. Cheryl instructs you to compile a report of your findings and include any recommendations for improvement. Your findings include missing modifiers that should have been appended to procedure codes. These include modifier -51 for multiple procedures and -LT, -RT, and -50 for unilateral or bilateral procedures. You now have to recommend improvements.

What would you do?

MALE GENITAL SYSTEM ANATOMY

You first learned about the male genital system in Chapter 10 (Figure 10-21). In this chapter, you will learn more about the structures and organs of the male genital system and how they function so that you will be better able to code procedures. Let's get started!

The **male genital system** contains organs and structures that are responsible for human reproduction and also includes structures for urination. Primary external genitalia are the *testes*, also called testicles or gonads, two glands suspended in the *scrotum* (sac), hanging on the left and right sides of the penis. The singular form of testes is testis. The serous membrane covering the testes is called the **tunica vaginalis**. The testes can produce sperm because the temperature inside the testes is cooler than the rest of the body. Sperm cannot be produced in normal body temperature.

tunica vaginalis (t(y)ü′-ni-kə vaj-ə-nā′-ləs)

Secondary external genitalia is the *penis,* which delivers sperm to the female. The penis also contains the urethra, which, as you already learned, transports urine outside the body. It also transports sperm outside the body. The portion of the penis attached to the body is the *root,* and the rest of the penis is called the *shaft.* At birth, the penis has a piece of skin at its tip called *foreskin* or **prepuce.** The tip of the penis is called the *glans penis.* **Circumcision** is a procedure to excise the foreskin from the penis, typically in infancy, which is done primarily for hygienic purposes. Not all cultures believe that circumcision is necessary.

prepuce (prē′-pyüs)

circumcision (sər-kəm-sizh′-ən)

The **epididymis** is a duct at the back and top of each testis where sperm mature. The **vas deferens** is a tube that transports sperm, connecting to the **seminal vesicle**, and forming the **ejaculatory duct**. The ejaculatory duct runs through the prostate gland and transports sperm into the urethra. The *spermatic cord* is a tube of blood vessels, which the vas deferens runs through. You already learned that the prostate gland is an exocrine gland. It is made of muscle and tissue surrounding the urethra.

epididymis (ep-ə-did′-ə-məs)

vas deferens (vas def′-ə-rənz)

seminal vesicle (sem′-ən-əl ves′-i-kəl)

An *erection* occurs when a male is aroused sexually, causing blood to fill in the **corpus cavernosum**, a pair of regions of spongy tissue inside the penis. *Ejaculation* occurs when muscle contractions cause semen to be ejected from the urethra. During sexual intercourse, ejaculation propels sperm into the vagina, which then travel to the uterus.

ejaculatory duct (i-jak′-yə-lə-tōr-ē)

corpus cavernosum (kor′-pəs kav-ər-nō′-səm)

urologist (yu-räl′-ə-jəst)

You already learned that a **urologist** prevents, diagnoses, and treats urinary system disorders, and a urologist also prevents, diagnoses, and treats male genital system conditions.

TAKE A BREAK

Great job! Let's take a break and then review more about the male genital system.

Exercise 28.6   Male Genital System Anatomy

Instructions: Fill in the blank with the best answer.

1. The portion of the penis attached to the body is the _____, and the rest of the penis is called the _____.

TAKE A BREAK *continued*

2. Primary external genitalia include the _____, also called testicles or gonads.

3. _____ is a procedure to excise the foreskin from the penis, which is done primarily for hygienic purposes, normally in infancy.

4. The _____ is a tube that transports sperm, connecting to the _____, and forming the _____ duct.

5. The serous membrane covering the testes is called the _____.

6. The _____ is a tube of blood vessels, which the vas deferens runs through.

MALE GENITAL SYSTEM (54000–55899)

The Male Genital System in the CPT manual is a subsection of the Surgery section. There are nine subheadings in the Male Genital System subsection, organized by *body site*, such as penis, testis, and spermatic cord, and then *type of procedure* (■ TABLE 28-5). Many of the subheadings contain the same types of procedures, such as incision, excision, and repair.

Notice that there are two additional subsections listed after the Male Genital System subsection: *Reproductive System Procedures*, which contains one procedure (55920) to treat

■ TABLE 28-5   MALE GENITAL SYSTEM SUBHEADINGS AND CATEGORIES

Subsection, Subheadings, and Categories	Code Range	Subsection, Subheadings, and Categories	Code Range
Male Genital System	**54000–55899**	**Scrotum**	**55100–55180**
Penis	**54000–54450**	*Incision*	*55100–55120*
Incision	*54000–54015*	*Excision*	*55150*
Destruction	*54050–54065*	*Repair*	*55175–55180*
Excision	*54100–54164*	**Vas Deferens**	**55200–55450**
Introduction	*54200–54250*	*Incision*	*55200*
Repair	*54300–54440*	*Excision*	*55250*
Manipulation	*54450*	*Introduction*	*55300*
Testis	**54500–54699**	*Repair*	*55400*
Excision	*54500–54535*	*Suture*	*55450*
Exploration	*54550–54560*	**Spermatic Cord**	**55500–55559**
Repair	*54600–54680*	*Excision*	*55500–55540*
Laparoscopy	*54690–54699*	*Laparoscopy*	*55550–55559*
Epididymis	**54700–54901**	**Seminal Vesicles**	**55600–55680**
Incision	*54700*	*Incision*	*55600–55605*
Excision	*54800–54861*	*Excision*	*55650–55680*
Exploration	*54865*	**Prostate**	**55700–55899**
Repair	*54900–54901*	*Incision*	*55700–55725*
Tunica Vaginalis	**55000–55060**	*Excision*	*55801–55865*
Incision	*55000*	*Laparoscopy*	*55866*
Excision	*55040–55041*	Other Procedures	*55870–55899*
Repair	*55060*		

extraparenchymal
(eks-tra-pə-reŋ′-kə-məl)

tunica albuginea
(t(y)ü′-ni-kə al-b(y)ə-jin′-ē-ə)

cryptorchidism
(krip-tor′-kid-izm)

orchiopexy (or′-kē-ō-pek-sē)

epididymovasostomy (ep-ə
-did-ə-mō-vas-äs′-tə-mē)

varicocele (var′-i-kō-sēl)

vesiculectomy
(vĕ-sik′u-lek′tah-me)

prostatectomy
(präs-tə-tek′-tə-mē)

a malignant neoplasm of the pelvic organs or genitalia with radioactivity, and *Intersex Surgery* (55970–55980), which contains procedures to correct congenital genital anomalies or injuries.

Procedures of the Male Genital System

Turn to your CPT manual to review the procedures of the male genital system. Did you notice that there are not very many procedures? We will review some of these procedures from different subheadings and categories, all combined into one table for easy reference. Be sure to refer back to Figure 10-21 as you read about procedures and then code them so that you have a good understanding of the male anatomy. You can also consult your medical references and the Internet for more information about procedures we review and about new procedures that you find while working through the CPT manual. To locate codes for male genital system procedures, search the index for the *body site* (e.g., penis, vas deferens) and then *type of procedure* (e.g., incision, excision), or start your search with the *type of procedure*. Let's next review procedures listed in ■ TABLE 28-6.

■ TABLE 28-6 PROCEDURES OF THE MALE GENITAL SYSTEM

Subheading	Category	Procedure(s)	Description
Penis (54000–54450)	*Incision (54000–54015)*	Incision and drainage of penis, deep (54015)	If the penis becomes infected with an abscess that extends *beyond* the skin and subcutaneous tissue, the physician drains it with an incision into the infected area. If the abscess is *at* the skin or subcutaneous level, then you should report this procedure with codes from the Integumentary System subsection, 10060–10160.
	Destruction (54050–54065)	Destruction of lesion(s) (54050–54065)	Procedure to destroy various types of lesions, which you learned about in Chapter 27: condyloma, papilloma, molluscum contagiosum, and herpetic vesicle. Methods of destruction include cryosurgery and laser surgery.
Testis (54500–54699)	*Excision (54500–54535)*	Excision of **extraparenchymal** lesion of testis (54512)	An *extraparenchymal* lesion is located beneath the membranous covering (tunica vaginalis) of the testis and within the testicular capsule (**tunica albuginea**). The physician incises skin and subcutaneous tissue and opens the tunica vaginalis to excise the lesion.
	Exploration (54550–54560)	Exploration for undescended testis (54550–54560)	Undescended testicles are testicles that have not descended into the scrotum, a condition called **cryptorchidism**. The testicles originally form in the back of the abdominal cavity.
			• Near the end of pregnancy, the testes of the fetus begin to descend to the scrotum. If the process is incomplete, a testicle might end up anywhere from inside the abdomen to just above the scrotum.
			• The physician may perform exploration to check the placement of the testicles, which can be done in the inguinal or scrotal area (54550) or with abdominal exploration (54560).
			• Did you notice the CPT guidelines with the exploration codes? They alert you to append modifier -50 (bilateral procedure) if the procedure involves each testis.
			• It is important to note that if during the exploratory procedure, the physician locates the testis and moves it into the scrotal sac, the procedure is no longer an exploration, but is instead a corrective surgery, called an **orchiopexy**. You can find orchiopexy under the Repair category of the Testis subheading (54640–54650).

■ TABLE 28-6   *continued*

Subheading	Category	Procedure(s)	Description
Epididymis (54700–54901)	*Repair (54900–54901)*	**Epididymovasos-tomy** (54900–54901)	An obstruction can block the flow of sperm from the epididymis to the vas deferens. When this occurs, the physician performs an *epididymovasostomy*, removing a portion of the vas deferens and attaching it to the epididymis, placing a drain to assist with healing.

Note that CPT categorizes codes for this procedure by unilateral or bilateral (epididymis). |
| **Tunica Vaginalis** (55000–55060) | *Incision (55000)* | Puncture aspiration of hydrocele (55000) | A hydrocele is a sac of fluid in the tunica vaginalis. Treatment for this condition is aspiration of the fluid with a needle. The physician may also inject medication. |
| **Scrotum** (55100–55180) | *Incision (55100–55120)* | Drainage of scrotal wall abscess (55100) | If an abscess forms in the scrotum, the physician treats it with an incision and drainage (I & D). This procedure is performed by making a cut in the skin over the abscess and expressing the pus or purulent drainage. The area is then packed or left open to heal.

• Notice the CPT guideline directing you to codes in the Integumentary System subsection if the physician debrides infected, necrotizing tissue. |
Vas Deferens (55200–55450)	*Excision (55250)*	Vasectomy, unilateral or bilateral (55250)	A vasectomy is a procedure to sterilize a male so that he cannot reproduce. The physician cuts out a piece of the vas deferens and cauterizes or sutures the ends closed, which stops sperm from entering semen and being ejaculated.
Spermatic Cord (55500–55559)	*Laparoscopy (55550–55559)*	Laparoscopy, surgical, with ligation of spermatic veins or **varicocele** (55550)	A varicocele is a dilated vein in the scrotum, which surrounds the testis. The varicocele could inhibit the production of sperm. The physician ligates the dilated vein(s) to treat the condition, using a laparoscopic approach.
Seminal Vesicles (55600–55680)	*Excision (55650–55680)*	**Vesiculectomy**, any approach (55650)	Removal of one of the seminal vesicles is called a *vesiculectomy*, and physicians may perform it to treat chronic infection or perform it in combination with removal of the prostate to treat prostate cancer.
Prostate (55700–55899)	*Excision (55801–55865)*	**Prostatectomy** (55801–55845)	A prostatectomy is removal of the prostate gland, typically to treat prostate cancer or hypertrophy of the prostate. Problems with the prostate can cause it to restrict urine flow to the urethra.

Take a look at the types of prostatectomies that you can code. Notice that they can also include biopsies of the lymph nodes or removing lymph nodes, along with other variations of the procedure. |
| | *Other Procedures (55870–55899)* | Electroejaculation (55870) | An electroejaculation is an ejaculation stimulated by an electrovibratory device. The patient is placed under general anesthesia. Then the physician places an electrostimulator probe into the patient's rectum next to the prostate and then transmits an electrical current. This causes excitation of the nerves, causing ejaculation, and the physician obtains semen to use in reproductive methods, such as in vitro fertilization.

• This procedure is recommended for men who have conditions that prevent them from ejaculating on their own, such as a spinal cord injury. |

TAKE A BREAK

Nice work! You have finished reviewing all subheadings in the Male Genital System subsection! Let's take a break and then review more about the male genital system.

Exercise 28.7 Male Genital System

Part 1—Theory

Instructions: Fill in the blank with the best answer.

1. Undescended testicles have not descended into the scrotum, a condition called _____.

2. Methods of destruction include _____ and laser surgery.

3. An epididymovasostomy involves removing a portion of the _____ and attaching it to the _____, placing a drain to assist with healing.

4. A(n) _____ is a procedure to sterilize a male so that he cannot reproduce.

5. An extraparenchymal lesion is located beneath the tunica vaginalis of the testis and within the _____.

6. A(n) _____ is a procedure where the physician locates the testis and moves it into the scrotal sac.

Part 2—Coding

Instructions: Review each patient's case, and then assign codes for the procedure(s), appending a modifier when appropriate. Optional: For additional practice, assign the patient's diagnosis code(s) (ICD-9-CM).

1. Robert Wood, age 21, has contracted venereal warts. He previously saw Dr. Suzuki, a urologist, who prescribed a cream to dissolve the warts, but they have not disappeared. He sees Dr. Suzuki again today in his office, and Dr. Suzuki removes them with cryosurgery, using local anesthesia.

   Diagnosis code(s): _____

   Procedure code(s): _____

2. Lou Albina, age 51, had a circumcision almost a month ago due to recurrent **balanoposthitis** (inflammation of the glans penis and foreskin) from *Streptococcus* bacteria. His penis is still partially covered by foreskin. Today at Williton, Dr. Suzuki repairs the incomplete circumcision.

   Diagnosis code(s): _____

   Procedure code(s): _____

3. Rick Wade, age 27, had an **orchiectomy** (testicle removal) several months ago, due to a benign tumor in his right testicle. The area is now healed, and he wants to have a testicular prosthesis inserted to restore the testicle to its normal appearance. Dr. Suzuki performs surgery today at Williton and inserts a prosthesis.

   Diagnosis code(s): _____

   Procedure code(s): _____

4. Dr. Suzuki diagnoses Jose Rodriguez, age 34, with a hydrocele of the tunica vaginalis. He performs a puncture aspiration of the hydrocele without medication injections.

   Diagnosis code(s): _____

   Procedure code(s): _____

5. Tyler Jackson, age 29, has infected seminal vesicles due to E. coli bacteria. Dr. Suzuki performs a **vesiculotomy** (incision of the seminal vesicle) to relieve the pressure.

   Diagnosis code(s): _____

   Procedure code(s): _____

6. Rob Jenner, age 35, father of five, wants a vasectomy. He visits Dr. Suzuki, and today at Williton, Dr. Suzuki performs the procedure bilaterally. He also performs a postoperative semen analysis.

   Diagnosis code(s): _____

   Procedure code(s): _____

balanoposthitis (bal-ə
-nō-päs-thīt′-əs)

orchiectomy (or-kē-ek′-tə
-mē)

vesiculotomy (və-sik-yə-lät′-
ə-mē)

DESTINATION: MEDICARE

In this Medicare exercise, your Medicare destination is a National Coverage Determination (NCD) on Medicare coverage for prostate screenings. Follow the instructions listed next to access the NCD.

1. Go to the website http://www.cms.gov.
2. At the top of the screen on the banner bar, choose *Regulations and Guidance.*
3. Under *Guidance,* choose *Manuals.*
4. Under *Manuals,* choose *Internet-Only Manuals.*
5. Under *Internet-Only Manuals,* choose publication number *100-03 Medicare National Coverage Determinations (NCD) Manual.*
6. Under *Downloads,* choose *Chapter 1 - Coverage Determinations, Part 4.*
7. Press the Ctrl + F keys to access the search function and find the information you need.

   Answer the questions listed next.

1. What two procedures does Medicare cover for prostate cancer screening tests?
2. What is a screening digital rectal exam?
3. Can a nurse practitioner perform a screening digital rectal exam?
4. How frequently will Medicare cover a screening digital rectal exam?
5. How frequently will Medicare cover a screening prostate specific antigen test?

CHAPTER REVIEW

Multiple Choice

Instructions: Circle one best answer to complete each statement.

1. What type of abscess surrounds a kidney and can involve both kidneys?
   a. Coronal
   b. Perineal
   c. Renal
   d. Nephreal

2. Use of electrical current is called
   a. exploration.
   b. fulguration.
   c. cryosurgery.
   d. ablation.

3. The _____ remove(s) urea from the blood through tiny filtering tubules called nephrons.
   a. ureters
   b. bladder
   c. kidneys
   d. urethra

4. Manometric studies are tests that measure the pressure of liquid flowing through the
   a. urethra.
   b. kidneys.
   c. bladder.
   d. ureters.

5. The _____ is a duct at the back and top of each testis where sperm mature.
   a. vas deferens
   b. seminal vesicle
   c. epididymis
   d. spermatic cord

6. How long are ureters?
   a. 1 to 3 inches
   b. 4 to 5 inches
   c. 6 to 7 inches
   d. 8 to 10 inches

7. A _____ is incising a calculus of the bladder.
   a. cystolithotomy
   b. cystoscopy
   c. cystostomy
   d. urethrolithotomy

8. Repair of the ureter to treat a ureteral stricture is called
   a. ureterrhapy.
   b. urethroplasty.
   c. ureteroplasty.
   d. ureterorrhaphy.

9. Medicare guidelines state that if a physician converts a laparoscopic procedure to an open procedure, you may
   a. only code and bill the open procedure.
   b. only code and bill the laparoscopic procedure.
   c. code and bill for both procedures, appending modifier -51 to the open procedure.
   d. code and bill for both procedures, appending modifier -52 or -53 to the laparoscopic procedure.

10. What is the combining form that means kidney?
   a. ren/o
   b. cyst/o
   c. chol/o
   d. nephr/o

Coding Assignments

Instructions: Assign procedure code(s) for the following cases, and append modifiers when appropriate. Optional: For additional practice, assign the patient's diagnosis code(s) (ICD-9-CM).

1. On Saturday night, Larry Hamilton, age 54, has had a painful erection for over five hours (**priapism**). His brother, Jeff, drives him to Williton Medical Center's ED. The ED physician, Dr. Mills, performs an irrigation of the corpus cavernosa, which provides Mr. Hamilton with instant relief because his penis becomes **flaccid** (limp). Dr. Mills instructs the patient to follow up with Dr. Suzuki, a urologist, on Monday.

   Diagnosis code(s): _____

   Procedure code(s): _____

2. While Paul Bell, age 19, was camping in the woods over the weekend, an insect bit him on his penis. Not only did the bite itch, but it also became abscessed. Mr. Bell visits Dr. Hoffman in his office who performs an I & D of the subcutaneous tissue for relief. He also gives the patient a prescription for an antibiotic.

   Diagnosis code(s): _____

   Procedure code(s): _____

3. Dr. Suzuki suspects that Johnathon Kreeman, age 81, has cancer of the testis. Today at Williton, he performs an incisional biopsy and sends the specimen to pathology for analysis. The pathologist determines that the patient has testicular cancer.

   Diagnosis code(s): _____

   Procedure code(s): _____

4. Trent Kozar, age six, has an undescended right testicle. Dr. Hoffman refers the patient to Dr. Thomas, a urologist specializing in treating pediatric conditions. Today, the patient's mother takes him to Dr. Thomas' office for an exam. Dr. Thomas performs an expanded problem-focused history and exam and decides that the best course of action is to intervene surgically. He discusses this option with the patient's mother. She agrees, and later the same day, he performs scrotal exploratory surgery at Williton. Code for Dr. Thomas' office visit and surgery at Williton.

   Diagnosis code(s): _____

   Office visit code(s): _____

   Surgical procedure code(s): _____

5. Jim Burke, age 35, was in an accident involving his ATV, which he drove into a tree in the woods. He received severe lacerations to both testes, along with other injuries. An ambulance transports him to Williton's ED where Dr. Mills examines the patient and calls in Dr. Suzuki to evaluate him. Dr. Suzuki subsequently performs surgery to remove the testes and insert prostheses using an inguinal approach.

   Diagnosis code(s): _____

   Procedure code(s): _____

6. Scott Michael, age nine, has an undescended left testicle. The testicle is located in the abdominal area. Today at Williton, Dr. Thomas performs corrective surgery through an incision in the abdominal area. He places the testis into its correct position.

   Diagnosis code(s): _____

   Procedure code(s): _____

7. Pete Frank, age 30, has endured swelling and redness to his scrotum for several days. He sees Dr. Suzuki in his office, and the physician diagnoses a scrotal wall abscess. The office visit for this new patient includes a comprehensive history and exam with moderate medical decision-making. Dr. Suzuki schedules the patient for outpatient surgery the next day at Williton, in order to perform an incision and drainage of the abscess. Code for both the office visit and the procedure that Dr. Suzuki performs at Williton.

   Diagnosis code(s): _____

   Office visit code(s): _____

   Surgical procedure code(s): _____

8. Brian Rome, age 17, was involved in an altercation at school with three other boys. He received a puncture wound from a pencil to the scrotum. A piece of the lead broke off and remained in his scrotum. His mother picks him up at school and drives him to Williton's ED. Dr. Mills examines the patient and calls in Dr. Suzuki, who subsequently performs surgery to remove the foreign body.

Diagnosis code(s): _____

Procedure code(s): _____

9. Harry Johnston, age 91, has cancer of the prostate. Today at Williton, Dr. Suzuki performs a prostatec-

priapism (prī′-ə-piz-əm)

flaccid (flas′-əd)

tomy, meatotomy, and urethral dilation via a suprapubic (above the pubis) incision. He performs the procedure in two stages.

Diagnosis code(s): _____

Procedure code(s): _____

10. Don Double, age 56, has a severe stricture of his urethra. Dr. Suzuki attempted urethral dilation in the office without success. Today at Williton, Dr. Suzuki performs urethral dilation with sounds under general anesthesia. Code for today's procedure at Williton.

Diagnosis code(s): _____

Procedure code(s): _____

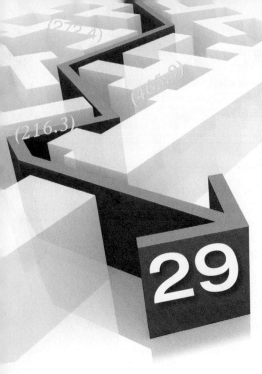

Female Genital System, Maternity Care, and Delivery

29

Learning Objectives

After completing this chapter, you should be able to

- Spell and define the key terminology in this chapter.
- Discuss the functions of the female reproductive system.
- Describe the subheadings and categories of the Female Genital System subsection.
- Discuss procedures in the subheading Vulva, Perineum, and Introitus and how to code them.
- Identify procedures and codes in the Vagina subheading.
- Define procedures and codes in the subheadings Cervix Uteri and Corpus Uteri.
- Explain procedures in the subheadings Oviduct/Ovary and Ovary and how to code them.
- Discuss procedures involved for In Vitro Fertilization.
- Describe procedures of the Maternity Care and Delivery subsection and how to assign codes.

Key Terms

Bishop score
global routine obstetric package

INTRODUCTION

The next stop on your coding journey is to learn about procedures of the female genital and reproductive systems, along with maternity care, and delivery. We will first review the female anatomy, and then you will have the chance to expand on that knowledge by applying it to coding specific procedures. Your coding success will depend on how well you understand female anatomy and the way that the female reproductive system functions. We will not have time to discuss all of the procedures in the Female Genital System subsection, but we will review several of them. So let's get started and continue to broaden your coding skills!

"If you want to be successful, it's just this simple. Know what you are doing. Love what you are doing. And believe in what you are doing."—WILL ROGERS

THE FEMALE REPRODUCTIVE SYSTEM

Before you can begin coding procedures for the female reproductive system, it is important to review the various parts of the reproductive system and understand how they function. You first learned about the female reproductive system (Figure 10-22) in

Chapters 10 and 14. The female reproductive system is made up of the ovaries, uterus, and fallopian tubes. Hormones that the brain and pituitary gland (located at the base of the brain) produce control their functions. These hormones regulate the menstrual cycle, pregnancy, and breast milk production. The ovaries produce *estrogen* and *progesterone,* sex hormones, which are responsible for sexual development and for preparing the uterine wall to hold and nourish a fertilized egg every month. The sex hormones also contribute to the basic health of the heart, bones, liver, and other body tissues.

A woman is born with all of the eggs that she will ever have. If her eggs are damaged or destroyed, she cannot replace them. At puberty, a woman begins to have menstrual cycles, which enable her to release an egg each month from one of her ovaries. Each cycle begins with menstrual flow, and then a new egg starts to grow. After two to three weeks, the ovary releases a mature egg (ovum) into the fallopian tube (also called an oviduct). If a sperm does not fertilize the egg, then it will die and leave the woman's body about two weeks later with the menstrual flow. The cycle repeats until the woman reaches menopause.

If a sperm fertilizes an ovum, then pregnancy occurs, and the ovum is implanted in the uterine lining. The fertilized egg is called a *zygote.* A zygote becomes an *embryo* (Figure 14-1) within two weeks and remains an embryo for up to eight weeks. The embryo is then referred to as a *fetus* from week eight until birth. The *placenta* (membrane) lines the uterine wall and contains the fetus, producing the hormone *human chorionic gonadotropin (hCG),* which causes pregnancy symptoms. The placenta provides blood to the fetus, carrying oxygen and nutrients, through the umbilical cord. The fetus grows within an *amniotic sac* containing amniotic fluid. The temperature inside the sac is higher than the mother's body temperature, and the sac protects the fetus throughout development.

Pregnancy typically lasts about 40 weeks, or 9½ months, called the *period of gestation.* Pregnancies are measured in three-month increments called *trimesters,* which represent continued stages of development.

The **vulva** (■ FIGURE 29-1) includes the external genitals, or genitalia: the **labia majora** (folds of skin, called lips, that protect the internal genitals), **labia minora** (internal folds, also called lips, that cover the vagina), clitoris (which contains erectile tissue, similar to the penis), and **introitus** (entrance) to the vagina, which is also called the birth canal. It connects to the uterus. The **perineum** is the area between the vulva and the anus. The **cervix uteri** is the cervical canal, and the **corpus uteri** is the body of the uterus.

vulva (vŭl′və)—inclusive term referring to the external female genitalia; also referred to as the pudendum; organs that are part of this structure include the mons pubis, labia majora and minora, vestibule (opening between two areas), and clitoris

labia majora (lā′-bē-ə mə-jôr′-ə)

labia minora (lā′-bē-ə mə-nôr′-ə)

introitus (ĭn-trō′ĭ-təs)

perineum (pĕr-ə-nē′-əm)

cervix uteri (sər′-viks yüt′-ə-rī)

corpus uteri (kor′-pəs yüt′-ə-rī)

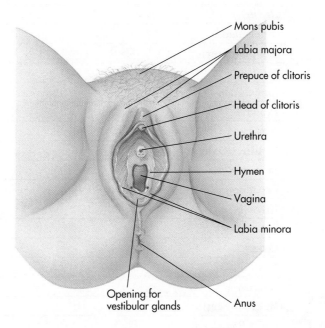

Figure 29-1 ■ The vulva (external female genitalia).

- Mons pubis
- Labia majora
- Prepuce of clitoris
- Head of clitoris
- Urethra
- Hymen
- Vagina
- Labia minora
- Opening for vestibular glands
- Anus

FEMALE GENITAL SYSTEM (56405–58999)

The Female Genital System is a subsection of the Surgery section. CPT divides the female genital system subsection into seven subheadings and then several categories. Subheadings are organized by body site (e.g., vulva, vagina), and categories are organized by the type of procedure (e.g., incision, destruction, excision, repair, endoscopy) (■ TABLE 29-1).

Let's review procedures listed in each of the subheadings and then practice coding them.

■ TABLE 29-1   **FEMALE GENITAL SYSTEM SUBHEADINGS AND CATEGORIES**

Subsection, Subheadings, Categories, and Subcategories	Code Range
FEMALE GENITAL SYSTEM	**56405–58999**
Vulva, Perineum, and Introitus	**56405–56821**
Incision	*56405–56442*
Destruction	*56501–56515*
Excision	*56605–56740*
Repair	*56800–56810*
Endoscopy	*56820–56821*
Vagina	**57000–57426**
Incision	*57000–57023*
Destruction	*57061–57065*
Excision	*57100–57135*
Introduction	*57150–57180*
Repair	*57200–57335*
Manipulation	*57400–57415*
Endoscopy/Laparoscopy	*57420–57426*
Cervix Uteri	**57452–57800**
Endoscopy	*57452–57461*
Excision	*57500–57558*
Repair	*57700–57720*
Manipulation	*57800*
Corpus Uteri	**58100–58579**
Excision	*58100–58294*
Introduction	*58300–58356*
Repair	*58400–58540*
Laparoscopy/Hysteroscopy	*58541–58579*
Oviduct/Ovary	**58600–58770**
Incision	*58600–58615*
Laparoscopy	*58660–58679*
Excision	*58700–58720*
Repair	*58740–58770*
Ovary	**58800–58960**
Incision	*58800–58825*
Excision	*58900–58960*
In Vitro Fertilization	**58970–58976**
Other Procedures	*58999*

VULVA, PERINEUM, AND INTROITUS (56405–56821)

The subheading Vulva, Perineum, and Introitus contains five different categories of codes, depending on the type of procedure that the physician performs (Table 29-1). Common procedures for the categories include I & D, destruction, excision, and repair. You can find procedures in this subheading by searching the index for the *type of procedure* or for the *body site*, and then the *type of procedure*. So let's take a look at the procedures in each category and then practice coding. Turn to each category of codes in your CPT manual as you read more about them next.

Incision (56405–56442)

Remember that an incision and drainage (I & D) is when the physician has to drain fluid, such as pus or blood, from a lesion or mass, like an abscess or cyst. Did you also remember that the physician typically sends the specimen of fluid for testing to identify infections or disease? There are only five codes in the Incision category, and common terms that you will find in code descriptors are listed in ■ TABLE 29-2.

Some common I & D procedures for this section include

- draining of an occluded Bartholin's gland that an acute inflammation causes.
- the surgical formation of a pouch-like sac (marsupialization) on the Bartholin's gland to prevent recurrent cysts or infections.
- lysis of labial adhesion (a common pediatric procedure) to treat adhesions between the labia minor and majora, which often occur as a result of fibrous bands of scar tissue.

Refer to the following example to learn more about coding an I & D procedure. You can try coding this case on your own and checking the answer that is listed, or code along with the steps listed.

> **Example:** Dr. Benton, an OB/GYN, performs an I & D for Ms. McKennon, age 45, at Williton Medical Center. The patient experiences discomfort during intercourse and walking. Dr. Benton diagnoses the patient with a labial abscess, which he excises and debrides.
>
> To code this case, search the index for the main term *vulva*, subterm *abscess*, and subterm *incision and drainage*, which leads you to code **56405**, the final code assignment. The diagnosis code is **616.4** (*abscess, labium*).

■ TABLE 29-2   TERMS IN THE INCISION CATEGORY

Term	Pronunciation	Definition
Bartholin's gland	(bär′-thə-lənz)	One of two small, oval, glands, found on both sides of the base of the vagina, which secrete mucus.
marsupialization	(mär-soo-pē-ə-lĭ-zā′-shən)	To incise a cyst or abscess by cutting a slit into it to drain it and then suturing the edges to surrounding tissue, creating a pouch-like sac for continued drainage and healing.
labial	(lā′-bē-əl)	Pertaining to the labia or lips
hymenotomy	(hĭ-mə-nŏt′-ə-mē)	Incision of the hymen, the fold of mucous membrane that partially covers the external opening of the vagina, to allow for the release of menstrual fluid and sexual intercourse.

Destruction (56501–56515)

The next subheading contains two codes that represent surgical destruction of simple and extensive lesions of the vulva, like vaginal warts. You first learned about destruction in Chapter 22 of this text. Physicians destroy lesions using lasers, electrosurgery, cryosurgery, or chemosurgery. Did you notice that the code descriptors apply to one or more lesions? The codes also represent a simple or extensive procedure. The difference between *simple* and *extensive* destruction generally relates to the number and size of the warts or lesions. Typically, *extensive* destruction means that the physician destroyed several lesions and/or large lesions that required more time and/or chemicals to remove them. Be sure to read the patient's medical documentation carefully to determine if the physician describes the procedure as simple or extensive, or provides detailed information to allow you to assign the correct codes.

Excision (56605–56740)

This subheading contains thirteen codes for surgical excisions of the vulva, perineum, and introitus, including biopsy of a lesion, excision of the Bartholin's gland or cyst, *hymenectomy* (excision of the hymen), and *vulvectomy* (surgical removal of a part of the vulva, typically to treat cancer). CPT categorizes vulvectomies according to whether the procedure was *simple* or *radical* and *partial* or *complete*. Take a look at the definitions of simple, radical, partial, and complete, which CPT defines in your manual before the Incision category. Vulvectomy codes do not represent unilateral or bilateral procedures. However, when the physician performs an **inguinofemoral lymphadenectomy** along with a vulvectomy, you should assign the code that correctly specifies if the lymphadenectomy was bilateral or unilateral.

inguinofemoral lymphadenectomy (ĭng-gwĕn-o-fĕm′-ər-əl lĭm-făd-en-ĕk′-tə-mē)—excision of lymph nodes in the upper leg and groin

Repair (56800–56810)

The next subheading identifies three codes for repairs to the vulva, perineum, and introitus:

- *Plastic repair introitus (56800)*—restores the vaginal opening to its original size after it is enlarged during childbirth
- **Clitoroplasty** *(56805)*—reduces the size of an enlarged clitoris due to a congenital anomaly
- **Perineoplasty** *(56810)*—repairs the tissues of the perineum (between the vagina and anus) that were damaged or torn during childbirth

clitoroplasty (klĭt′er-o-plas-te)

perineoplasty (per-ə-nē′-ō-plas-tē)

colposcopy (kăl-päs′-kə-pē)—visual examination of the vagina and cervix using a colposcope

vulvoscopy (văl-văs′-kə-pē)

colposcope (kŏl′-pə-skōp)—lighted instrument used to magnify and view the vagina and cervix

leukoplakia (loo-kə-plā′kē-ə)—white, thickened spots or patches formed on mucous membranes that tend to become cancerous

mons pubis (monz pyoo′bĭs)

Endoscopy (56820–56821)

The Endoscopy category includes two codes for the **colposcopy** *of the vulva without* and *with biopsy*. This procedure is also called a **vulvoscopy**. The physician examines the vulva using a **colposcope** (colp/o—vagina, scope—instrument to visually examine), which magnifies specific areas of the body to identify benign and malignant lesions, precancerous tissue, **leukoplakia**, ulcers, atrophy, and genital warts. The vulva exam includes the external urethral orifice, **mons pubis** (fatty tissue at the front of the pelvis, covered with pubic hair, also called mons veneris or mound of Venus), labia majora, the rim of labia minora, perineum, and anus.

TAKE A BREAK

That was a lot of information to cover! Let's take a break and practice coding procedures involving the vulva, perineum, and introitus.

Exercise 29.1 **Vulva, Perineum, and Introitus**

Part 1—Theory

Instructions: Fill in the blank with the best answer.

1. An incision of the hymen, the fold of mucous membrane that partially covers the external opening of the vagina, is called a(n) _____.

2. What is a hymenectomy? _____

3. A(n) _____ is the surgical removal of part of the vulva, typically to treat cancer.

TAKE A BREAK *continued*

4. The difference between simple and extensive destruction generally relates to the _____ and _____ of the warts or lesions.

5. A _____ is one of two small, oval glands found on both sides of the base of the vagina, which secrete mucus.

6. What is the name of the entrance to the vagina? _____

Part 2—Coding

Instructions: Review the patient's case, and then assign codes for the procedure(s), appending a modifier when appropriate. Optional: For additional practice, assign the patient's diagnosis code(s) (ICD-9-CM).

1. Janet Miller, age 42, presents to her OB/GYN, Dr. Benton, with vaginal pain and states that she has noticed a lump near her vagina. After examining the patient, Dr. Benton diagnoses her with an abscess of the Bartholin's gland (one of two glands surrounding the vaginal opening). He performs an I & D in his office.

   Diagnosis code(s): _____

   Procedure code(s): _____

2. In his office, Dr. Benton performs extensive cryosurgery on Haley Wilson, age 26, for treatment of multiple genital warts due to human papilloma virus (HPV), confirmed by previous pathology. After surgery, he tells the patient that she will need to have yearly exams because the genital warts increase her risk for developing cancer of the vulva.

   Diagnosis code(s): _____

   Procedure code(s): _____

3. Melanie Watson, age 37, arrives at her gynecologist's office for a scheduled biopsy. Dr. Benton performs biopsies of three vulvar lesions and sends them to Williton Medical Center's pathology department for analysis. The pathology report for all three specimens reveals VIN II (vulvar intraepithelial neoplasia—moderate, abnormal cell growth of the vulva considered to be precancerous). Code for Dr. Benton's services.

   Diagnosis code(s): _____

   Procedure code(s): _____

4. At Williton Medical Center, Dr. Benton performs a bilateral radical vulvectomy, complete with inguinofemoral, iliac, and pelvic lymphadenectomy, on Deborah Jenkins, age 49, due to vulvar cancer. He sends the surgical specimens to the hospital pathologist. The pathologist confirms primary malignancy of the vulva with metastasis to inguinofemoral and iliac lymph nodes. Dr. Benton discusses the findings and further treatment options with the patient. Code for Dr. Benton's services. Mrs. Jenkins will likely undergo a chemotherapeutic treatment plan that an oncologist develops for her.

   Diagnosis code(s): _____

   Procedure code(s): _____

5. At Williton Medical Center, Dr. James, plastic surgeon, performs plastic repair of the introitus for Stephanie Evans, age 23, whom he previously diagnosed with vulvar hypertrophy (overgrowth of fleshy folds of vagina). Dr. Benton referred the patient to Dr. James. The surgery is successful.

   Diagnosis code(s): _____

   Procedure code(s): _____

6. At Williton, Dr. Benton performs colposcopy of the vulva, with multiple biopsies, for Kelly Toman, age 32. The hospital pathology report reveals mild dysplasia (abnormal growth or development of cells, tissue, bone, or an organ) of the labia majora. Ms. Toman will require follow-up exams to ensure that the dysplasia does not progress in severity.

   Diagnosis code(s): _____

   Procedure code(s): _____

VAGINA (57000–57426)

CPT contains seven different categories of codes under the Vagina subheading, arranged by type of procedure (I & D, destruction, excision, introduction, repair). To find codes for these procedures, search the index for the *type of procedure*, or search under *vagina* as the main term and then search for the *type of procedure*. Let's begin by reviewing each category and then practice coding. Turn to each category of codes in your CPT manual as we review them next.

Incision (57000–57023)

The Incision category contains codes for incisions into the vagina, including the following procedures.

colpotomy (käl-pät′-ə-mē)

- **Colpotomy; *with exploration (57000)*—**incision into the wall of the vagina to further examine it for a lesion or abscess. The procedure may also include draining an abscess.

colpocentesis (käl-pō-sen-tē′-səs)

- **Colpocentesis (57020)**—puncturing the vaginal cavity to drain fluid. Do not report a separate code for colpocentesis if the physician performs it with another major procedure.

- **I & D of vaginal hematoma (57022–57023)**—CPT divides the codes by obstetrical and nonobstetrical procedures.

Destruction (57061–57065)

The Destruction category contains two codes for destroying lesions, according to whether the procedure is *simple* or *extensive*. There is no CPT definition for either simple or extensive, so you have to rely on the physician's documentation to guide you to assign the correct code. Always query the physician if you are not sure. Physicians can use lasers, electrosurgery, cryosurgery, and chemosurgery to destroy vaginal lesions.

Excision (57100–57135)

The Excision category has 11 codes for reporting surgical procedures involving the vagina. These procedures include vaginal biopsy, **vaginectomy** (removal of part or all of the vagina), **colpocleisis** (closure of the vaginal canal), removal of a congenital partition within the vagina (vaginal septum), and lesion/cyst removal. CPT divides vaginectomy codes by the extent of the procedure and how much tissue is actually removed, such as partial removal of the vaginal wall or complete removal of the vaginal wall. Before assigning codes from the Excision category, you should be familiar with medical terms that you will find in the code descriptors, including the following terms:

vaginectomy (vaj-ə-nek′-tə-mē)

colpocleisis (käl-pō-klī′-səs)

mucosa (myoo-kō′sə)

- **mucosa**—moist tissue that lines some organs and body cavities
- *para-aortic*—near or next to the aorta
- *paravaginal*—adjacent to the vagina or part of the vagina
- *vaginal septum*—a vertical wall of tissue that divides the vagina into two parts; a congenital anomaly that may need to be removed if it causes health issues

Introduction (57150–57180)

The Introduction category consists of six codes that describe the introduction of a substance or object into the vagina for medicinal or contraception purposes. Review the following examples of procedures from this category for a better understanding of how to assign the codes.

- ***Irrigation of vagina and/or application of medicament (drug) for treatment of bacterial, parasitic, or fungoid disease (57150)*—**The physician places a catheter high in the vaginal canal to flush it with a medicated solution.

- ***Fitting and insertion of pessary or other intravaginal support device (57160)*—**The patient wears the device in the vagina to support a prolapsed (dropped or fallen) uterus or rectum.

diaphragm (dī′-ə-fram)

- ***Diaphragm or cervical cap fitting with instructions (57170)*—**A **diaphragm** or cervical cap is a device that is inserted to prevent pregnancy. It is a contraceptive barrier consisting of a thin flexible dome-shaped disk or cup made of rubber or plastic that fits snugly over the uterine cervix to act as a barrier for sperm. A spermicide is often applied before insertion to kill sperm.

Repair (57200–57335)

This next category contains multiple codes for many types of vaginal surgical repairs. CPT divides several codes by the surgical approach, such as vaginal, abdominal, trans-anal, or transperineal (trans—across or through). So you'll need to review the operative notes carefully before assigning these codes, and query the physician if you are not sure of the type of approach.

Review ■ TABLE 29-3 to become familiar with some of the repair procedures and other medical terms that you will find in the code descriptors for the Repair category.

Manipulation (57400–57415)

The Manipulation category contains three codes to dilate the vagina due to stenosis, per-form a pelvic exam, or remove a foreign body from the vagina (common in children, or in adults who insert objects during sexual encounters). Do not report vaginal dilation when the physician performs it with another vaginal procedure, such as dilation and curettage

■ TABLE 29-3   **REPAIR TERMS AND PROCEDURES**

Term	Pronunciation	Definition
bulbocavernosus	(bəl-bō-kav-ər-nō′-səs)	Muscle that compresses the bulbar portion of the urethra (near the perineum). It divides into lateral halves that extend from immediately behind the clitoris along either side of the vagina, to the central tendon of the perineum.
concomitant	(kən-kom-i′-tənt)	An event that occurs at the same time as another one.
enterocele	(ĕn′-tə-rō-sēl)	Part of the small intestine (small bowel) bulges into the vagina; may also be referred to as a small bowel prolapse.
iliococcygeus	(il-ē-ō-käk-sij′-(ē-)əs)	Muscle of the pelvis.
urethral sphincter	(yoo-rē′-thrəl)	Muscle that controls the retention and release of urine from the bladder.
urethrocele	(yoo-rē′-thrə-sēl)	Protrusion of urethra into the vagina.

Procedure	Pronunciation	Definition
Colporrhaphy (57200)	(kol-pôr-′ə-fē)	Suture of the vagina to repair a defect or weakness in the vaginal wall, often performed to prevent the bladder from protruding (cystocele) or rectum from protruding (rectocele) into the vagina.
Colpoperineorrhaphy (57210)	(käl-pō-per-ə-nē-or′-ə-fē)	Suture of the vagina and perineum.
Colpopexy (57280–57282)	(′käl-pə-pek-sē)	Suture a prolapsed vagina to another structure, such as the abdominal wall, to stabilize and correct vaginal prolapse. Also called vaginofixation.
Insertion of mesh or other prosthesis for repair of pelvic floor defect (+57267)		Repair of tissues that are too weak to be repaired without inserting a mesh or other prosthesis to strengthen it. An add-on code represents this procedure, and you should report it with another primary procedure.
Pereyra procedure (57289)	(pə-ra′-rah)	Surgical technique to correct stress urinary incontinence (weak pelvic floor muscles cause urine leakage) by elevating the bladder by attaching it to abdominal fascia.

POINTERS FROM THE PROS: Interview with a Billing Specialist

Shirley Coccia bills insurances and patients for a chiropractic office. She has worked in the health-care field for 29 years.

What interests you the most about the job that you perform?

Every day is different, and the majority of the patients are nice.

What are the most challenging aspects of your job?

Dealing with the insurance companies on why a code wasn't paid, or when I have to call for benefits and try to get a person to talk to instead of an automated (call system). Some insurance company calls are now rerouted to other countries, and they (customer service representatives) are very hard to understand.

What advice can you give to new coders to help them to communicate effectively with physicians, since physicians can sometimes be intimidating?

Know your codes that are most frequently used, and always have your coding book handy.

What advice would you like to give to coding students about working with different personalities?

Be patient. Think before you react.

(Used by permission of Shirley Coccia.)

dyspareunia (dis-pə-rü′-nē-ə)

(dilation—open the cervix, curettage—scrape away excess uterine tissue). Physicians perform pelvic exams to diagnosis many conditions, including abdominal pain and **dyspareunia** (painful intercourse), which inflammation, infection, neoplasms, or other diseases can cause. A pelvic exam is included in most major and minor gynecological procedures, so you should not report it separately when the physician performs it during the same operative session as the other procedures.

Did you notice that each code descriptor includes anesthesia *other than local?* This means that in order to report these codes, the patient must be anesthetized by general, epidural, or spinal anesthesia, rather than local anesthesia. When the physician performs these procedures without anesthesia or with a local anesthesia only, report instead an evaluation and management (E/M) code for the procedure.

Endoscopy/Laparoscopy (57420–57426)

The Endoscopy/Laparoscopy category includes five procedures for both endoscopic and laparoscopic procedures to the vagina. Physicians conduct endoscopic examinations of the vagina as a result of an abnormal Pap smear. Endoscopy involves using a colposcope to detect cancer and other conditions. Laparoscopic vaginal procedures include:

- *cystocele repair and colpopexy,* to treat uterovaginal prolapse or prolapse of the inside of the vagina, referred to as the vaginal vault, after hysterectomy
- *revision and removal of a prosthetic vaginal graft,* to treat infection. The physician may remove part or all of the graft to excise eroding mesh or revise a tissue graft.

Did you notice that many of the codes in the Endoscopy/Laparoscopy category include CPT guidelines directing you to assign codes for other procedures if the physician performs them? Guidelines also alert you when to append modifier -51 (for multiple procedures) when the physician performs more than one procedure.

TAKE A BREAK

Good job! Let's keep going and take a break to practice coding vaginal procedures.

Exercise 29.2 Vagina

Instructions: Review the patient's case, and then assign codes for the procedure(s), appending a modifier when appropriate. Optional: For additional practice, assign the patient's diagnosis code(s) (ICD-9-CM).

1. Kara Martin, age 44, has a painful vaginal abscess and undergoes colpotomy with drainage of pelvic abscess by Dr. Benton, OB/GYN, in his office. Pathology

TAKE A BREAK *continued*

reveals that an MSSA (methicillin-susceptible *Staphylococcus aureus*) bacterial infection is present. Dr. Benton prescribes antibiotic therapy and advises Ms. Martin to follow up in his office in two weeks.

Diagnosis code(s): _____

Procedure code(s): _____

2. Established patient Amanda Glover, age 27, presents to Dr. Benton for treatment of previously diagnosed vaginal leukoplakia (thickened white patches on the vaginal canal). At Williton Medical Center, Dr. Benton destroys the vaginal lesions using laser surgery.

Diagnosis code(s): _____

Procedure code(s): _____

3. Bearle Liston, age 84, suffers from vaginal prolapse and stress incontinence. After discussing various treatment options with her gynecologist, Dr. Benton, Mrs. Liston decides to undergo colpocleisis (LeForte type procedure) at Williton Medical Center. The surgery is successful and the patient requires no further treatment. Mrs. Liston will follow up with Dr. Benton in six weeks for a routine postoperative examination.

Diagnosis code(s): _____

Procedure code(s): _____

4. Emily Weaver, age 68, sees Dr. Benton in his office for fitting and insertion of an intravaginal pessary (a device made of plastic, rubber, or silicone that supports the pelvic muscles) to aid in the treatment of uterine prolapse.

Diagnosis code(s): _____

Procedure code(s): _____

5. At Williton, Dr. Benton performs posterior colporrhaphy on Mrs. Jordan, age 78, to repair a rectocele. During the procedure, Dr. Benton reinforces the vaginal wall with mesh material. The surgery is successful.

Diagnosis code(s): _____

Procedure code(s): _____

6. After laboratory testing reveals abnormal cells on a Pap smear, Mrs. Swanson, age 47, presents to her gynecologist's office for further testing. Dr. Benton performs colposcopy with biopsy of the vagina/cervix. He sends the specimen to Williton's pathologist for analysis, and the pathology report reveals CA of the cervix. Dr. Benton calls Mrs. Swanson to discuss his findings and recommendations for further surgery.

Diagnosis code(s): _____

Procedure code(s): _____

CERVIX UTERI (57452–57800), CORPUS UTERI (58100–58579)

Before reviewing procedures in the Cervix Uteri and Corpus Uteri subheadings, we should discuss the structure of the uterus (Figure 10-22) in a little more detail to help you understand its anatomy. The *uterus* is a pear-shaped organ that provides a place for the nourishment and development of a fetus during pregnancy. It contracts rhythmically and powerfully to help push out the fetus during birth.

The rounded top of the uterus is called the *fundus*. The *corpus* is the main upper section and the *isthmus* is the lower portion. The narrow neck at the bottom of the uterus is the *cervix*. The lower third, or neck, of the uterus is also known as the *cervix uteri* (uterine cervix) and the upper two-thirds is called the *corpus uteri*.

The wall of the uterus is composed of three layers: *perimetrium*—outer layer; *myometrium*—muscular middle layer, and *endometrium*—mucous membrane lining the inner surface of the uterus. You will also notice a few terms in these two subsections containing the phrase "*with or without fulguration.*" *Fulguration* refers to destruction by electricity.

You can locate codes for procedures of the cervix uteri and corpus uteri by searching the index for *cervix* or *uterus* and then the *type of procedure*, or searching for the *type of procedure* and then searching for the body site. Now let's discuss procedures in these subheadings. Turn to the codes in your CPT manual as you read more about them.

CERVIX UTERI (57452–57800)

This subheading contains four categories of codes for endoscopy, excision, repair, and manipulation of the cervix uteri (uterine cervix), which we will review next.

Endoscopy (57452-57461)

The endoscopy category includes a diagnostic colposcopy of the cervix and therapeutic colposcopies that combine the endoscopy with other procedures. Let's look at an example of a colposcopy with another procedure—code 57460. This procedure is for a colposcopy with loop electrode biopsy of the cervix, where the physician excises cervical tissue for biopsy using a loop electrode (thin wire loop). The loop electrode transmits an electrical current to remove tissue.

Excision (57500–57558)

The excision category codes describe a variety of procedures that include biopsy and lesion excision. Review the following examples of procedures in this category to better understand them.

- *Biopsy of cervix, single or multiple, or local excision of lesion, with or without fulguration (separate procedure) (57500)*—Removal of a small piece of cervical tissue for biopsy to diagnose disorders like cancer
- *Endocervical (within the cervix) curettage (57505)*—Scraping tissue from the endocervical canal (which joins the cervix and uterus) using a curette, and then testing the tissue for diseases
- *Conization of cervix, with or without fulguration, with or without dilation and curettage, with or without repair; cold knife or laser (57520)*—Removal of a cone-shaped piece of tissue from the uterine cervix to diagnose disorders, such as cancer, or to remove precancerous cells

trachelectomy (trak-ə-lek'-tə-mē)

cervicectomy (sər-və-sek'-tə-mē)

- *Trachelectomy (cervicectomy), amputation of cervix (separate procedure) (57530)*—Removal of the uterine cervix, typically to treat cancer. The procedure preserves the uterine body and the patient's fertility and is used in younger women as an alternative to a radical hysterectomy (removal of the uterus and other associated structures like the ovaries and fallopian tubes, typically to treat cancer).

Repair (57700–57720)

There are only two codes covered under the Repair category for repair of the uterine cervix.

cerclage (sār-kläzh')

- **Cerclage** *of uterine cervix, nonobstetrical (not pertaining to childbirth) (57700)*—Extensive suturing using a heavy suture material around the cervix to make the opening smaller; often performed for patients with cervical incompetence (dilated, weakened cervix). To code for cerclage during pregnancy, assign codes from the Maternity and Delivery subsection (59320, 59325).
- *Trachelorrhaphy, plastic repair of uterine cervix, vaginal approach (57720)*—Suture a laceration of the uterine cervix.

Manipulation (57800)

This category contains a single code for *manipulation,* the gradual enlargement of the cervical canal by inserting dilators into the endocervix and through the cervical canal. The procedure treats disorders that occlude the cervical canal or decrease its size, such as vaginal **endometriosis** (when endometrial cells of the uterus spread to other sites), cervix uteri polyps, dysplasia, or absence of menstruation. Notice that "separate procedure" is listed in parentheses after the code descriptor for 57800. Remember that you should not report it separately when it is part of a major procedure.

endometriosis (en-dō-mē-trē-ō'-səs)

CORPUS UTERI (58100-58579)

The Corpus Uteri subheading includes four categories of codes: excision, introduction, repair, and laparoscopy/hysteroscopy, which we will discuss next. Be careful when choosing codes from this category, as CPT divides codes by the approach and whether the physician performs additional procedures during the same encounter. Now let's take a look at some of the codes.

Excision (58100–58294)

Here are some of the procedures included in the Excision category:

- *Endometrial sampling (58100, 58110)*—The physician removes a sample of tissue from the endometrium for a biopsy to diagnose cancer, precancerous cells, and infections. The physician may perform the procedure with a colposcopy.

- *Dilation and curettage (58120)*—This procedure is also called a D & C. The physician dilates the cervix and then scrapes the uterine lining to obtain a tissue sample for biopsy or to treat disorders like retained products of conception or polycystic (many cysts) ovaries. This procedure is performed for nonobstetrical cases. To report a D & C performed due to a postpartum hemorrhage or other postpartum condition, assign code 59160 from the Maternity Care and Delivery subsection.

- *Myomectomy (58140–58146)*—The physician removes **uterine fibroid** tumors without removing healthy uterine tissue. A myomectomy can be a major procedure (abdominal approach, an open myomectomy) or a minor procedure (vaginal approach). Did you notice that CPT divides myomectomy codes by the approach, number of tumors excised, and total tumor weight?

- **Hysterectomy** *(58150–58294)*—This procedure, a subcategory of the Excision category, is the removal of the uterus and/or related structures, such as the ovaries and fallopian tubes. Physicians perform hysterectomies to treat cancer, uterine fibroid tumors (■ FIGURE 29-2), endometriosis, abnormal vaginal bleeding, and uterine prolapse. Note the following points when coding hysterectomies.

> **uterine fibroid** (yoo′tər-ĭn fī′broid)—benign fibrous tumor of the uterus made up of muscle cells and other tissues that grow within the wall of the uterus; also called uterine leiomyoma

> **hysterectomy** (his-tə-rek′-tə-mē)

CPT divides hysterectomy codes by

- approach (abdominal, vaginal—uterus is removed through the vaginal canal)
- associated structures removed

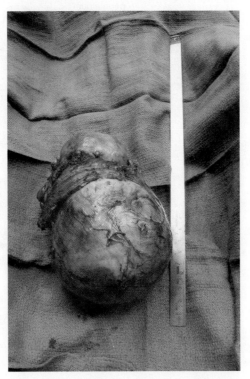

Figure 29-2 ■ Uterus that the physician removed due to uterine fibroid tumors.

Photo credit: Slaven/Custom Medical Stock Photo.

- if the procedure is total, subtotal, radical, or partial. The physician will determine the surgical approach based on the type of disorder that she is treating.

- It is important to review the code descriptors carefully before final code assignment, since there are 19 different codes for hysterectomy procedures.

- Pay close attention to additional procedures listed in code descriptors that physicians perform *with* hysterectomies to ensure that you do not separately code for services that were already included with the hysterectomy. For example, code 58150 is for *Total abdominal hysterectomy (corpus and cervix), with or without removal of tube(s), with or without removal of ovary(s)*. If the physician removes the fallopian tubes and ovaries, then you should *not* report separate codes because these procedures are already part of the total abdominal hysterectomy. On the other hand, if the physician performs a total abdominal hysterectomy *without* removing the fallopian tubes and ovaries, then you should still assign code 58150 because of the wording *with or without* in the code descriptor.

- Vaginal hysterectomy codes (58260–58270, 58290–58294) specify the weight of the uterus, so you should closely review code descriptors before final code assignment.

Refer to the following example to code an excision procedure from the Corpus Uteri subheading. You can try coding this case on your own and checking the answer listed, or code along with the steps listed.

Example: At Williton Medical Center, Dr. Benton, an OB/GYN, excises six uterine fibroid tumors (■ FIGURE 29-3) weighing a total of 280 grams. He uses an abdominal approach. The patient is Mary Shoaff, age 35.

To code this case, search the index for the main term *myomectomy*, subterm *uterus*, which leads you to codes 58140–58146. Assign code **58146**, as it describes the procedure, the number of fibroid tumors, and their total weight. The diagnosis code is **218.9** (*leiomyoma, uterus*).

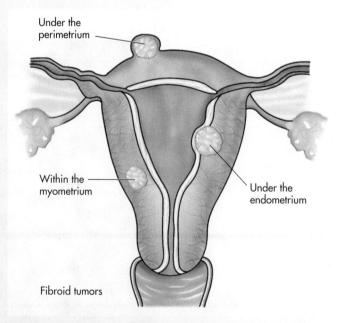

Figure 29-3 ■ Types of uterine fibroid tumors.

Source: Medical Terminology, Jane Rice, 6th edition, Pearson Prentice-Hall (2008) p. 586.

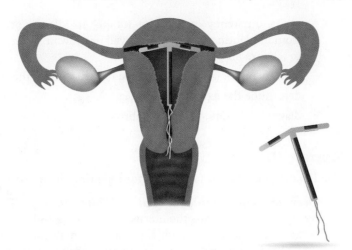

Figure 29-4 ■ An intrauterine device used for contraception.
Source: GRei/Shutterstock.com.

Introduction (58300–58356)

The Introduction category of the Corpus Uteri subheading contains 11 codes that describe the introduction of a substance or object into the uterus for diagnostic, therapeutic, or contraception purposes. Let's review some of the procedures that you will find in the Introduction category so that you can be more familiar with them.

- *Insertion of intrauterine device (IUD) (58300), Removal of intrauterine device (IUD) (58301)*—An IUD is a small device usually made of soft, flexible, lightweight plastic that is placed within the uterus for contraception (to prevent pregnancy) (■ FIGURE 29-4).

- *Artificial insemination; intra-cervical (58321), Artificial insemination; intra-uterine (58322), Sperm washing for artificial insemination (58323)*—Fertility procedures for artificial insemination, the process of artificially (not through sexual intercourse) placing semen into the vagina using a syringe or catheter to reach the cervix or uterus. Conception occurs by the sperm traveling through the fallopian tubes to fertilize an ovum. The sperm donor can be a patient's partner or a known or anonymous donor. Sperm washing involves separating the sperm from seminal fluid (which carries the sperm) and removing chemicals that can be harmful to the uterus.

- *Catheterization and introduction of saline or contrast material for saline infusion sonohysterography (SIS) or hysterosalpingography (58340)*—**Sonohysterography (SIS)** is an ultrasound (technique that uses sound waves to produce images of body structures on a screen) that is performed after a saline solution is infused (introduced) into the uterus. The procedure can diagnose fibroids, polyps, or lesions. The patient receives the saline through a catheter, and the saline expands the uterus to allow for better images.

    sonohysterography (sän-ə-his-tə-räg′-rə-fē)

    - **Hysterosalpingography**—X-ray of the uterus (hyster/o—uterus) and fallopian tubes after injecting contrast material (dye that enhances images of body structures).

    hysterosalpingography (his-tə-rō-sal-pin-gäg′-rə-fē)

- *Transcervical introduction of fallopian tube catheter for diagnosis and/or re-establishing patency (open) (any method), with or without hysterosalpingography (58345)*—Procedure to diagnose disorders of the fallopian tubes or eliminate a tube occlusion or stricture (narrowing).

- Physicians perform procedures represented by codes 58340 and 58345 most often on women with infertility problems who cannot become pregnant or who have had repeated miscarriages. They also perform them on patients who experience painful menstrual periods (**dysmenorrhea**) or recurrent abnormal or unexplained bleeding. Using these procedures, physicians can

    dysmenorrhea (dis-men-ə-rē′-ə)

- evaluate patency of fallopian tube(s) to identify occlusions that prevent an egg from implanting in the uterine wall or prevent sperm from moving through a tube to fertilize an egg.
- identify problems with the shape or structure of the uterus or tube(s).
- determine the extent of an injury.
- diagnose tumors, polyps, or fibroids.

Repair (58400–58540)

The Repair category has four codes for repairing the uterus:

plicating (plī′-kāt-ing)

- *Uterine suspension procedures (58400–58410)*—These procedures shorten the ligament that suspends the uterus by **plicating** (folding) and tacking it back in place to treat uterine or uterovaginal prolapse or malposition of the uterus. The procedure may also include **presacral** sympathectomy to treat dysmenorrhea, with surgical excision or chemical destruction of the presacral nerve in the sympathetic nervous system (the nerve is anterior to the sacrum at the base of spine).

presacral (prē-sak′-rəl)—located anterior to the sacrum

- *Hysterorrhaphy (58520)*—suturing a perforated or ruptured uterus (which trauma can cause) for nonobstetrical cases
- *Hysteroplasty (58540)*—repair of a malformed uterus to treat a congenital anomaly

Laparoscopy/Hysteroscopy (58541–58579)

The Laparoscopy/Hysteroscopy category of the Corpus Uteri subheading contains numerous codes for laparoscopic hysterectomy or myomectomy and for a diagnostic or surgical **hysteroscopy** (insertion of an endoscope through the cervix and into the uterus). CPT divides codes by the approach (laparoscopy, hysteroscopy) and then by additional procedures performed. Did you notice the CPT guidelines at the beginning of this category? The guidelines remind you that a surgical laparoscopy always includes a diagnostic laparoscopy, so you should not report a separate code for diagnostic laparoscopy when it is part of a surgical laparoscopy.

hysteroscopy (his-tə-räs′-kə-pē)

You previously learned that laparoscopic procedures eliminate the need to create a large incision to access body structures. A laparoscopic hysterectomy involves only two or three small incisions into the abdomen, and the physician inserts the laparoscope and other instruments into the patient through the incisions. Laparoscopic surgery is much less invasive and has no sutures, and patients typically recover from laparoscopic procedures faster than from procedures using other approaches. Let's review some of the procedures from the Laparoscopy/Hysteroscopy category:

- *Laparoscopic supracervical hysterectomy (58541–58544)*—removal of the uterus but not the cervix, often performed for larger or multiple fibroids and in cases of severe endometriosis; CPT divides codes based on the weight of the uterus and if the physician also removes fallopian tube(s) and ovary(ies).
- *Hysteroscopy (58555–58565)*—This procedure may be diagnostic or surgical. It allows the physician to visualize the cervix and uterus using a hysteroscope, passing it through the vagina into the cervix and uterine cavity to examine the endometrium and perform other procedures, such as a biopsy or polyp removal. CPT divides hysteroscopy codes by other procedures that the physician performs along with the hysteroscopy.
- *Surgical laparoscopy with total hysterectomy (58570–58573)*—hysterectomy including the removal of both the uterus and the cervix;. CPT divides codes by the weight of the uterus (250 grams or less, greater than 250 grams) and whether the physician removes fallopian tube(s) and/or ovary(ies).

It is important to note that many times, hysterectomies include removing other structures, foreign bodies, and lesions, so you should not separately report codes for additional procedures if they are included with the hysterectomy code descriptor.

TAKE A BREAK

Wow! You have come a long way! Good work! Let's take a break and then practice coding procedures involving the cervix and corpus uteri.

Exercise 29.3 Cervix Uteri, Corpus Uteri

Part 1—Theory

Instructions: Fill in the blank with the best answer.

1. What is the name of the procedure where the physician removes a sample of tissue from the endometrium for a biopsy to diagnose cancer, precancerous cells, and infections?

2. A(n) _____ is a small device usually made of soft, flexible, lightweight plastic that is placed within the uterus for contraception.

3. The procedure where the physician removes uterine fibroid tumors without removing healthy uterine tissue is called a(n) _____.

4. What types of procedures shorten the ligament that suspends the uterus by plicating it and tacking it back in place to treat uterine or uterovaginal prolapse or malposition of the uterus?

5. _____ means to scrape tissue from the endocervical canal using a curette.

6. What three criteria should you review in hysterectomy codes before final code assignment? _____

Part 2—Coding

Instructions: Review the patient's case, and then assign codes for the procedure(s), appending a modifier when appropriate. Optional: For additional practice, assign the patient's diagnosis code(s) (ICD-9-CM).

1. Dr. Benton, an OB/GYN, performs a colposcopy of the cervix with loop electrode biopsies of the cervix on Amy Perkins, age 49. Dr. Benton recently diagnosed her with severe cervical dysplasia. Williton's Medical Center's pathology department's report was negative for carcinoma, and Dr. Benton advises her to return his office in three months for a follow-up Pap smear.

   Diagnosis code(s): _____

   Procedure code(s): _____

2. Nancy Fleming, age 53, has carcinoma of the uterus, which metastasized to the fallopian tubes and ovaries. Dr. Benton performs a vaginal hysterectomy and removes the tubes and ovaries. He uses a laparoscope. The patient's uterus weighs 265 grams.

   Diagnosis code(s): _____

   Procedure code(s): _____

3. Wanda Jackson, age 32, gravida 3, para 0, has suffered multiple miscarriages due to an incompetent cervix. (The official term is cervix uteri, a cervix that is abnormally prone to dilation before termination of the normal period of gestation, resulting in premature expulsion of the fetus). Dr. Benton schedules her for surgery. Today at Williton, Dr. Benton performs cerclage (placement of sutures around a functionally incompetent uterine cervix), nonobstetrical.

   Diagnosis code(s): _____

   Procedure code(s): _____

4. At Williton, Dr. Benton performs a vaginal hysterectomy, with removal of tubes and ovaries, for Sherry Lewis, age 47. Her diagnoses include **menorrhagia** (excessive and frequent menstruation with a regular cycle) and ovarian endometriosis (abnormal uterine tissue creating products of menses and inflamed ovarian tissues). The uterus weighs 62 grams. The surgery is successful.

   Diagnosis code(s): _____

   Procedure code(s): _____

5. Tanasha Lane, age 24, presents to Dr. Benton's office for insertion of an IUD for contraceptive purposes.

   Diagnosis code(s): _____

   Procedure code(s): _____

6. Lee Thorton, age 44, presents to Williton Medical Center to undergo surgical hysteroscopy with removal of leiomyomata to treat uterine fibroids. Dr. Todd, an OB/GYN, performs the surgery.

   Diagnosis code(s): _____

   Procedure code(s): _____

menorrhagia (men-ə-rā′-j(ē-)ə)

OVIDUCT/OVARY (58600–58770)

The Oviduct/Ovary subheading includes four categories, which we will discuss next.

1. Incision
2. Laparoscopy
3. Excision
4. Repair

You can locate procedures for these categories in the index by searching for *oviduct* or *ovary* and then by the *type of procedure*, or start with the *type of procedure* and then search for the *body site*. Turn to the codes in the Oviduct/Ovary subheading to review them as you read more about them in the next sections.

Incision (58600–58615)

Codes from this category describe tubal ligation, also called tubectomy, which is often referred to as "having one's tubes tied." This bilateral or unilateral procedure is a permanent method of birth control (female sterilization) where the physician severs or seals the fallopian tubes so that sperm cannot travel through them to reach an ovum. CPT categorizes tubal ligation codes by the approach—abdominal, vaginal, or suprapubic (above the pubic bone). There is an add-on code for a tubal ligation when the physician performs it with a cesarean delivery or intra-abdominal surgery (+58611).

Laparoscopy (58660–58679)

Codes in the Laparoscopy category includes lysis, fulguration, or excision of lesions and can also include removal of adnexal structures to treat various disorders, such as cancer. One of the CPT guidelines in this category alerts you that codes 58672 and 58673 are unilateral procedures, even though their code descriptors do not specify unilateral. As you learned, you should append modifier -50 (bilateral procedure) to any procedures that are performed on both sides when the code descriptor does not include *bilateral*.

Excision (58700–58720)

salpingectomy (sāl-pĭn-jĕk′ tə-mē)

salpingo-oophorectomy (sāl-pĭng-gō-oo-fə-rĕk′tə-mē)

There are only two procedures in the Excision category: **salpingectomy**, partial or complete removal of one or both fallopian tubes because of infection, endometriosis, or carcinoma or to remove an ectopic pregnancy; and **salpingo-oophorectomy**, partial or complete removal of one or both fallopian tubes *and ovaries* to remove cancerous lesions or to treat endometriosis or infection.

CPT categorizes both of these procedures as a *separate procedure*. Remember that when a physician performs a separate procedure (completely distinct from other procedures performed during the same encounter), you should report it separately and append modifier -59 (separate procedure) to the procedure code. This alerts the insurance to reimburse the procedure without reducing the amount, since it was performed with another procedure. But when a salpingectomy or a salpingo-oophorectomy is *part of another major procedure*, you should not report it separately.

Repair (58740–58770)

salpingolysis (sāl-pĭng-gŏl′-ĭ-sĭs)

ovariolysis (ō-var-ē-ō-lī′sĭs)— lysis of adhesions of the ovary

fimbrioplasty (fĭm′bre-o-plas-te)

fimbriae (fĭm′-brē-ə)

oocyte (ō′ə-sīt)

salpingostomy (sal-pĭŋ-gäs′-tə-mē)

The Repair category in the Oviduct/Ovary subheading contains five codes for the repair of the oviduct/ovary, typically to treat female infertility. Let's look at a few of these procedures.

- *Lysis of adhesions (58740)*—Adhesions are removed from the fallopian tubes, (**salpingolysis**) or from the ovaries (**ovariolysis**).
- **Fimbrioplasty *(58760)***—This procedure treats infertility by opening an obstructed fallopian tube to save the function of the **fimbriae** (border of the fallopian tube entrance) for transporting an **oocyte**.
- **Salpingostomy *(58770)***—This procedure surgically creates an opening in a fallopian tube to restore its patency to treat infection or inflammation.

OVARY (58800–58960)

The Ovary subheading has two categories of codes for Incision and Excision of ovary(ies). Two of the main structures of the ovary include the *cortex*, which contains numerous follicles at various stages of maturation and the *medulla*, which contain lymph channels, nerves, and numerous blood vessels. You can find codes for procedures in this subheading by searching the index for *ovary* and then the *type of procedure* or searching for the *type of procedure* and then the *body site*. Let's review more about incisions and excisions. Turn to the codes in your CPT manual as you read about them next.

Incision (58800–58825)

The Incision category contains only six codes, including I & D of ovarian cysts and abscesses, which can be through a vaginal or abdominal approach. This category also includes *transposition of the ovary(ies)*, which is when the physician moves the ovaries to a higher position so that they are not exposed to radiation the patient receives to treat cervical cancer. Some patients may not regain ovarian function after radiation treatment.

Excision (58900–58960)

The Excision category contains fourteen codes to report procedures such as a biopsy of the ovary(ies), removal of the ovaries (**oophorectomy**), or cystectomy, where the physician excises an ovarian cyst without removing the ovary. CPT divides codes in this category by the type of procedure and whether it involved a malignancy.

IN VITRO FERTILIZATION (58970–58976)

CPT lists three codes in the In Vitro Fertilization (IVF) subheading. IVF is used to treat many causes of infertility, and it is performed to help a woman become pregnant. *In vitro* means "outside the body," and IVF is a form of assisted reproductive technology (ART) performed in a laboratory, where an egg (removed from the female patient—called a follicle puncture) is manually fertilized with sperm and then returned to the female patient. You may have heard of this procedure referred to as a "test tube baby." The procedure involves returning the fertilized embryo, or gamete, to the fallopian tube, a process called **gamete intrafallopian transfer (GIFT)**, or **zygote intrafallopian transfer (ZIFT)**. ZIFT transfers a fertilized egg directly into the fallopian tube, while GIFT transfers a mixture of sperm and eggs to the fallopian tube. The embryo can also be implanted directly into the uterus. You can locate codes for IVF in the index by searching for **in vitro fertilization**.

oophorectomy (oo-fǝ-rĕk'tǝ-mē)

gamete intrafallopian transfer (GIFT) (gām-ēt')—an assisted reproductive procedure involving the removal of a woman's eggs, mixing them with sperm, and immediately placing them into the fallopian tube for fertilization to occur inside the fallopian tubes

zygote intrafallopian transfer (ZIFT) (zī'gōt in-trǝ-fǝ-lō'pē-ǝn—an assisted reproductive procedure where a fertilized embryo is transferred into the fallopian tubes

in vitro fertilization (ĭn-vē'-trō)

TAKE A BREAK

Nice job! Let's take a break and practice coding ovary and oviduct procedures.

Exercise 29.4 Oviduct/Ovary, Ovary, in Vitro Fertilization

Instructions: Review the patient's case, and then assign codes for the procedure(s), appending a modifier when appropriate. Optional: For additional practice, assign the patient's diagnosis code(s) (ICD-9-CM).

1. At Williton Medical Center, Dr. Benton, an OB/GYN, performs bilateral ligation of fallopian tubes, vaginal approach, for established patient Terry Williams, age 41. The patient, gravida 5, para 5, and her husband decided that sterilization would be best.

   Diagnosis code(s): _____

   Procedure code(s): _____

2. Dr. Benton previously diagnosed Janie Marshall, age 26, with tubal occlusion (an obstruction of the fallopian tube) and peritubal adhesions (fibrous scarring abnormally joining structures within the abdomen). He schedules her for surgery at Williton. Today, Dr. Benton performs a surgical laparoscopy with lysis of adhesions and clip occlusion of oviducts.

   Diagnosis code(s): _____

   Procedure code(s): _____

3. Today at Williton, Dr. Todd, an OB/GYN, performs a right-sided salpingo-oophorectomy, open procedure, for Tracy Myers, his 43-year-old established patient. The patient suffers from chronic salpingitis and

continued

TAKE A BREAK *continued*

oophoritis, chronic inflammation of ovary(ies) and fallopian tube(s).

Diagnosis code(s): _____

Procedure code(s): _____

4. Leah McGee is a 28-year-old established patient who sees Dr. Benton for increased lower abdominal pain. After exam and ultrasound, he diagnoses her with a left ovarian cyst. Today at Williton, Dr. Benton drains the cyst by vaginal approach. Code for the patient's surgery.

Diagnosis code(s): _____

Procedure code(s): _____

5. Kiley Cohen, a 21-year-old established patient of Dr. Benton who suffers from polycystic ovarian syndrome (multiple serous-filled cysts on the ovary)

(■ FIGURE 29-5), presents to Williton Medical Center for a wedge resection of her left ovary (removal of part of the ovary).

Diagnosis code(s): _____

Procedure code(s): _____

6. At Williton's IVF clinic, Dr. Todd performs intrauterine embryo transfer (the process of assisted reproduction, in which embryos are placed into the uterus with the intent to establish a pregnancy) for established patient Lisa Smith, age 31. She has been unable to conceive due to **anovulatory** cycle (a menstrual cycle characterized by varying degrees of menstrual intervals and the absence of ovulation).

Diagnosis code(s): _____

Procedure code(s): _____

WORKPLACE IQ

You are working as an office assistant in Dr. Benton's office, which is a large OB/GYN practice. You and five other staff are responsible to assign diagnosis and procedure codes to patients' records and enter the codes into the computer system so that insurances can be billed. Nicole works in the office as an insurance billing and collections specialist. Today, she shows you a Medicare denial for Mrs. Williams and asks for your help. The claim shows that two codes were billed to Medicare: 58291 and 58150. Medicare paid for code 58291 but denied payment for code 58150. The denial reason was "Payment was adjusted because the benefit for this service is included in the payment/allowance for another service/procedure that has already been adjudicated." Nicole asks you if you can help her to understand why Medicare denied payment for the second code.

What would you do?

MATERNITY CARE AND DELIVERY (59000–60699)

anovulatory (an-äv′-yə-lə-tōr-ē)

The Maternity Care and Delivery subsection of Surgery includes services and procedures related to the three stages of pregnancy: antepartum, labor and delivery, and postpartum care. CPT also includes abortion services in this subsection. CPT categorizes codes by the type of service (excision, introduction, cesarean delivery) (■ TABLE 29-4), and arranges procedures by antepartum care, delivery, and postpartum care.

Polycystic Ovaries   Normal Ovaries

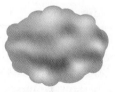 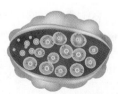 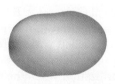 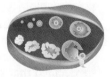

Figure 29-5 ■ Comparison of polycystic ovaries with normal ovaries.
Source: GRei/Shutterstock.com.

■ TABLE 29-4   **MATERNITY CARE AND DELIVERY CATEGORIES**

Subsection and Categories	Code Range
Maternity Care and Delivery	**59000–59899**
Antepartum and Fetal Invasive Services	*59000–59076*
Excision	*59100–59160*
Introduction	*59200*
Repair	*59300–59350*
Vaginal Delivery, Antepartum and Postpartum Care	*59400–59430*
Cesarean Delivery	*59510–59525*
Delivery after Previous Cesarean Delivery	*59610–59622*
Abortion	*59812–59857*
Other Procedures	*59866–59899*

Before you assign codes from the Maternity Care and Delivery subsection, it is important for you to be familiar with terms related to various procedures. In Chapter 14, you learned many different terms related to pregnancy, childbirth, and the puerperium (Table 14-1). It will be helpful to review those terms again to refresh your memory, as you will find many of them in code descriptors for this subsection. You will find additional new terms outlined for you in ■ TABLE 29-5 that you should review before coding from this subsection.

■ TABLE 29-5   **COMMON TERMS RELATED TO MATERNITY CARE AND DELIVERY**

Term	Pronunciation	Definition
cerclage	(sār-kläzh′)	Surgical procedure where the physician sutures the cervix closed during pregnancy due to an incompetent (weak) cervix to reduce the risk of miscarriage; the sutures are removed later in pregnancy when there is no longer a threat of miscarriage.
Cesarean delivery (C-section)	(si-zar′-ē-ən)	Surgical procedure to incise the abdomen and uterus to deliver an infant or infants, typically because a vaginal delivery would harm the mother and/or infant. Physicians may also perform c-sections at the patient's request.
chorionic villus sampling	(kôr-ē-ŏn′ĭk) (vĭl′ŭs)	Prenatal test to determine chromosomal abnormalities and biochemical disorders; often abbreviated as CVS.
cordocentesis	(kor-dō-sēn-tē′-sĭs)	Examine blood from the fetus to detect abnormalities, using ultrasound to detect the umbilical cord and then removing a sample of fetal blood from it. This procedure is also called fetal blood sampling, percutaneous umbilical blood sampling (PUBS), and umbilical vein sampling.
hydatidiform mole	(hī-də-tĭd′ə-fôrm)	Rare mass or abnormal growth that forms inside the uterus at the beginning of a pregnancy. It is caused by an overproduction of the tissue that is supposed to develop into the placenta, and is also known as a molar pregnancy, (natural) missed abortion, or missed miscarriage.
hypertonic solution	(hī-pər-tŏn′-ĭk)	A solution used to induce labor, injected into the amniotic cavity.
interstitial pregnancy	(ĭn-tər-stĭsh′-əl)	An ectopic pregnancy that develops in the small, narrow spaces between the uterus and fallopian tube.
laminaria	(lam-uh-nair′-ee-uh)	Insertion of kelp (seaweed) into the cervix, where it slowly absorbs water and expands to dilate the cervix and induce labor. Also used to dilate the cervix for abortions.
prostaglandins	(prŏs-tə-glăn′-dĭns)	Introduction of a hormone by tablet, gel, or vaginal insert to initiate labor.
trimester	(trī′-mes-tər)	The three segments of three months each of the gestation period. The first trimester begins with the last menstrual period and lasts to 12 weeks; the second trimester continues from weeks 13–27; the third trimester lasts from week 28 to delivery, which usually occurs between the 38th and 40th week.
vesicocentesis	(ves-i-kō-sen-tē′-səs)	Prenatal aspiration of fetal urine for diagnostic purposes (to test for birth defects) or therapeutic purposes (to remove excess urine).

■ TABLE 29-6   COMMON ABBREVIATIONS FOR MATERNITY CARE AND DELIVERY

Abbreviation	Definition
AB, SAB	abortion or spontaneous abortion
C/S, CS	cesarean section
EAB	elective abortion
EDD	estimated date of delivery
LMP	last menstrual period
MLE	**midline (median) episiotomy** (vertical incision along the perineum, from the vagina to the anus), **mediolateral episiotomy** (diagonal incision of the perineum) (■ Figure 29-6)
NSVD, SVD	normal spontaneous vaginal delivery, spontaneous vaginal delivery
VBAC, VBACS	vaginal birth after cesarean section and vaginal births after cesarean section
VTOP	voluntary termination of pregnancy

midline (median) episiotomy
(ĭ-pĭz-ē-ăt′-ə-mē)

mediolateral episiotomy
(mē-dē-ō-lăt′-ər-əl ĭ-pĭz-ē-ŏt′-ə-mē)

You will also need to be familiar with common abbreviations. They will be helpful as you code procedures for maternity care and delivery (■ TABLE 29-6).

Let's discuss the CPT guidelines before reviewing actual services and procedures from the Maternity Care and Delivery subsection.

CPT Guidelines

Turn to your CPT manual to review the guidelines at the beginning of the Maternity Care and Delivery subsection. Let's review these guidelines before we discuss procedures in this subsection because you need to have a solid understanding of how CPT defines procedures and where to search for the codes. A summary of the guidelines is outlined next.

Figure 29-6 ■ The two most common types of episiotomy are mediolateral and midline: (A) Right mediolateral, (B) Midline.

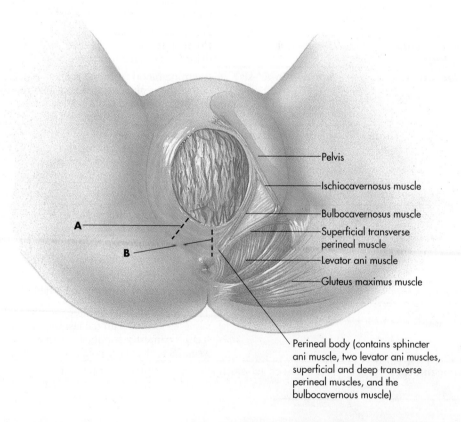

Pelvis

Ischiocavernosus muscle

Bulbocavernosus muscle

Superficial transverse perineal muscle

Levator ani muscle

Gluteus maximus muscle

Perineal body (contains sphincter ani muscle, two levator ani muscles, superficial and deep transverse perineal muscles, and the bulbocavernous muscle)

Antepartum care includes

- Initial and subsequent history
- Physical exams
- Recording weight, blood pressures, fetal heart tones
- Routine chemical urinalysis
- Monthly visits up to 28 weeks gestation
- Biweekly visits from 29–36 weeks gestation
- Weekly visits from 37 weeks until delivery

Delivery care includes

- Hospital admission
- Admission history and physical exam
- Management of uncomplicated labor
- Vaginal delivery (with or without episiotomy, and with or without forceps to guide the baby out of the birth canal). Do not separately code for an episiotomy or the use of forceps when they are performed during a vaginal delivery.
- Cesarean delivery
- Code separately other visits within the antepartum period that are unrelated to the pregnancy. Assign E/M codes or codes from elsewhere in CPT to represent these services.
- Report a delivery code once for each infant delivered. (Append modifier -51, for multiple procedures, to each subsequent delivery code. Remember to report the most complex procedure, a cesarean delivery, first.)

Postpartum care includes

- Inpatient, office, or other outpatient visits after vaginal or cesarean delivery
- Code separately services involving complications or services unrelated to postpartum care.

Complications include

- *Pregnancy complications*—cardiac and neurological disorders, diabetes, hypertension, hyperemesis
- *Surgical complications of pregnancy, labor, and delivery*—appendectomy, hernia, ovarian cyst

    Assign separate codes for procedures and services to treat complications from the E/M or Surgery sections

When Different Physicians Provide Different Aspects of Care

It is important to note that the same physician typically provides antepartum, delivery, and postpartum care to a patient for an uncomplicated pregnancy and delivery. All care is bundled into the **global routine obstetric package**. This package is similar to the global surgical package, where the payer reimburses for all services in the package using only one CPT code. And just like the global surgical package, payers also determine the length of time for and the reimbursement amount of the global routine obstetric package. You will need to check with individual payers for their specific guidelines. There are four CPT codes that represent services within the global routine obstetric care package, based on the type of delivery and if the patient previously delivered by cesarean section.

- Routine obstetric care including antepartum care, vaginal delivery (with or without episiotomy, and/or forceps) and postpartum care (59400)
- Routine obstetric care including antepartum care, cesarean delivery, and postpartum care (59510)

- Routine obstetric care including antepartum care, vaginal delivery (with or without episiotomy, and/or forceps) and postpartum care, after previous cesarean delivery (59610)
- Routine obstetric care including antepartum care, cesarean delivery, and postpartum care, following attempted vaginal delivery after previous cesarean delivery (59618)

There may be occasions when different physicians provide different aspects of the patient's care. For example, let's say Jenny Michaels sees her OB/GYN, Dr. Benton, for routine antepartum care and delivery services. She gives birth vaginally to a healthy baby boy. Her husband then accepts a new job in another town and the family moves, so Mrs. Michaels sees a new physician, Dr. Ryan, who provides the postpartum care services. In this case, Dr. Benton's staff would code and bill the patient's insurance for antepartum care (59425, 59426) and delivery services (59409). Dr. Ryan's staff would code and bill the insurance for postpartum care (59430). Take a look at the CPT guidelines under the Maternity Care and Delivery subheading, which will help you to better understand how to assign codes for antepartum, delivery, and postpartum care only.

Now that you are familiar with the CPT guidelines, let's review procedures and services in the nine categories of the Maternity Care and Delivery subsection. ***Note:*** *Be sure to refer to the terms and abbreviations in Tables 29-5 and 29-6 in this chapter, and refer to terms in Chapter 14 (including Table 14-1) to refresh your memory of terms and definitions pertaining to maternity care and delivery. We will not define terms again that were discussed previously.*

You can locate codes for maternity care and delivery procedures and services by searching the index for *pregnancy, maternity care and delivery, cesarean delivery, or obstetrical care* and then the type of service/procedure, or first search for the type of procedure or the condition *(ectopic pregnancy)*. Turn to the codes in your CPT manual as we review more about them next.

Antepartum and Fetal Invasive Services (59000–59076)

This category contains 13 codes for antepartum care, including diagnostic procedures such as *amniocentesis, cordocentesis,* and *chorionic villus sampling.* These services include the procedure only, not the radiology imaging required to perform the procedure. CPT notes direct you to assign specific radiology codes in addition to the antepartum procedure. On the other hand, *vesicocentesis* includes ultrasound guidance, so you should not code it separately. Let's review some of the procedures in this category so that you can learn more about them.

- ***Therapeutic amniocentesis*** (59001)—This procedure is usually performed after the first 14 weeks of pregnancy to remove excess amniotic fluid. It *includes* ultrasound guidance, so you should not separately code for it. A *diagnostic* amniocentesis involves removing amniotic fluid to test for fetal disorders.
- ***Fetal non-stress test*** (59025)—This test monitors the fetal heartbeat during fetal movement.
- ***Fetal scalp blood sampling*** (59030)—In this procedure, the physician obtains a blood specimen from the scalp (or buttock) of the fetus through the dilated cervix. The procedure helps to identify intrapartum fetal hypoxia (insufficient amount of oxygen during labor and delivery).

Excision, Introduction (59100–59200)

These next two categories, Excision and Introduction, provide codes for the surgical treatment of ectopic pregnancies (■ FIGURE 29-7) and the introduction of a cervical dilator to widen the cervix to perform certain procedures.

Excision procedures include

hysterotomy (hĭs-tə-rŏt'-ə-mē)

- ***Abdominal hysterotomy*** (59100)—a procedure that involves making an incision into the lower portion of the uterus to remove an embryo (an abortion) or a hydatidiform mole (a grape-like cluster which represents a nonviable fetus). A CPT note

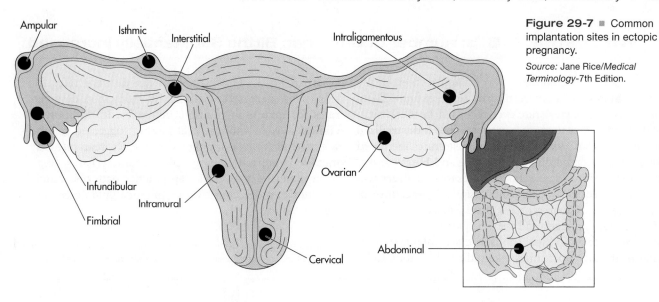

Figure 29-7 ■ Common implantation sites in ectopic pregnancy.

Source: Jane Rice/*Medical Terminology*-7th Edition.

for this procedure directs you to assign code 58611 in addition to code 59100 when the physician also performs a tubal ligation.

- *Surgical and laparoscopic treatment of an ectopic pregnancy* (59120–59151)—Remember that an ectopic pregnancy occurs *outside* the uterus. Report code 59120 when the procedure also requires a salpingectomy and/or oophorectomy.
- *Postpartum curettage* (59160)—removes a retained placenta or clotted blood after delivery.

Introduction procedures include

- *Insertion of cervical dilator* (59200)—catheter insertion of a substance into the cervix to widen (distend) it, called *ripening,* to perform specific procedures, like abortions, or to allow for delivery of a fetus. Substances used in the procedure include prostaglandins, a sticky gel, and laminaria, a sterile rod made of kelp, which both expand when placed inside the cervix and help the uterus to contract.

  - Physicians use a **Bishop score** to assess a patient's condition before inserting a cervical dilator, including measuring the cervix and assessing the position of the fetus's head. The score is based on five criteria (■ FIGURE 29-8). The physician assigns a score to each and then calculates an overall score (the highest possible score is 13). In general, when the Bishop Score is less than 6, the physician inserts a *cervical dilator,* an instrument used to widen the cervix to allow the fetus to pass through it. A score of 9 or more indicates that labor will most likely occur on its own.

Figure 29-8 ■ Example of Bishop Cervical Ripening Scoring System.

Parameter\Score	0	1	2	3	Description
Position	Posterior	Intermediate or mid-position	Anterior	—	The position of the cervix
Consistency	Firm	Intermediate	Soft	—	The hardness of the cervix
Effacement	0–30%	31–50%	51–80%	>80%	Measurement of the stretch (elasticity) of the cervix
Dilation (cm)	0 cm or closed	1–2cm	3–4 cm	>5 cm	Measurement of the diameter of the stretched cervix
Station or fetal position	−3	−2	−1, 0	+1, −2	Position of the fetus' head in relation to the distance from the ischial spines

In 2007, approximately 1.4 million women in the United States had a cesarean birth, representing 32% of all births, the highest rate ever recorded in the United States and higher than rates in most other industrialized countries. From 1996 to 2007, cesarean rates increased for all women, regardless of age, race and Hispanic origin, or state of residence. In 2006, cesarean delivery was the most frequently performed surgical procedure in U.S. hospitals. Cesarean rates also increased for infants of all gestational ages and may be partly related to the increased rate of multiple births, because infants in multiple births are much more likely than singletons to be cesarean births. However, cesarean delivery rates for singletons increased substantially more than cesarean rates for infants in multiple deliveries. In addition to clinical reasons, nonmedical factors suggested for the widespread and continuing rise of the cesarean rate may include maternal demographic characteristics (e.g., older maternal age), physician practice patterns, maternal choice, more conservative practice guidelines, and legal pressures.

(Centers for Disease Control and Prevention, National Center for Health Statistics, http://www.cdc.gov/nchs/data/databriefs/db35.pdf)

Repair (59300–59350)

The next category in the Maternity Care and Delivery subsection includes four codes for repairs during pregnancy, which involve the vagina, cervix, or uterus. The Female Genital System subsection contains codes for these same types of repairs for patients who are *not* pregnant. We already discussed some of these services.

One of the repairs is for an *episiotomy* or vaginal repair (59300) that may be required after delivery. Only a provider of service *other than* the attending physician should report code 59300. When the attending physician performs the repair, it is considered part of the obstetrical care.

polyhydramnios (pol-ē-hī′-dram-nē-äs)

TAKE A BREAK

Wow! You are learning a lot more information! Let's take a break and then code more procedures.

Exercise 29.5 Antepartum and Fetal Invasive Services, Excision, Introduction, Repair

Instructions: Review the patient's case, and then assign codes for the procedure(s), appending a modifier when appropriate. Optional: For additional practice, assign the patient's diagnosis code(s) (ICD-9-CM).

1. Carla Agular, age 29, arrives at Williton Medical Center's radiology department for a diagnostic amniocentesis. Her OB/GYN, Dr. Todd, ordered the test after diagnosing her with **polyhydramnios** (excess amount of amniotic fluid) found on a routine ultrasound. The procedure is performed without incident.

   Diagnosis code(s): _____

   Procedure code(s): _____

2. Dr. Benton, an OB/GYN, performs in his office a fetal nonstress test to monitor fetal heartbeat for Anita Lucas, age 32, due to postterm pregnancy. Mrs. Lucas, gravida 2, para 1, is currently at 42 completed weeks gestation.

The fetal nonstress test (no stress placed on the fetus or mother) was nonreactive, meaning that Dr. Benton cannot determine if the fetus is receiving enough oxygen. He prepares the patient for additional testing.

Diagnosis code(s): _____

Procedure code(s): _____

3. Shelly Farmer, age 30, is from out of town and visiting her family when she experiences preterm labor. She is at 32 weeks gestation. Her husband brings her to Williton's ED, where Dr. Mills, ED physician, admits her for observation. Dr. Benton supervises fetal monitoring, interprets the results, and provides a written report to Mrs. Farmer's OB/GYN in her home town. Despite this episode, Mrs. Farmer's pregnancy progresses to full term without further incident. Code for Dr. Benton's services.

   Diagnosis code(s): _____

   Procedure code(s): _____

4. Today at Williton, Dr. Benton performs a hysterotomy for treatment of a hydatidiform mole on his 38-year-

TAKE A BREAK *continued*

old established patient, Molly Link. Since Mrs. Link wishes no future pregnancies, Dr. Benton also performs tubal ligation at the same session.

Diagnosis code(s): _____

Procedure code(s): _____

5. Melissa Graham, age 33, gravida 2, para 1, is at 42 weeks gestation. Dr. Benton instructs her to go to Williton Medical Center so that he can induce labor. When she arrives, Dr. Benton inserts a cervical dilator, which will help to gradually dilate the cervix before inducing labor.

Diagnosis code(s): _____

Procedure code(s): _____

6. At Williton, Dr. Benton performs a vaginal repair on Sue Robbins, age 27, who suffered a third-degree perineal laceration while giving birth to her son. Dr. Benton is not her attending physician.

Diagnosis code(s): _____

Procedure code(s): _____

Vaginal Delivery, Antepartum and Postpartum Care, Cesarean Delivery, Delivery after Previous Cesarean Delivery (59400–59622)

These categories include codes for antepartum care, postpartum care, vaginal delivery, and cesarean delivery. We already reviewed these services in a previous section, but you should also review the following points for additional coding guidance.

- *Antepartum visits* can vary from patient to patient but on average, a patient has about 13 visits with her OB/GYN before delivery. CPT codes for antepartum care specify the total visits (59425, 59426).

- *Postpartum care* does not include any laboratory or radiology services provided during the postpartum visit (Pap smear, urinalysis, ultrasound). Assign separate codes for these services.

- *Uncomplicated cases*—You can assign code 59400 for most pregnancy cases, which includes antepartum care, delivery, and postpartum care for uncomplicated cases.

- *For cesarean births*—report code 59510 for normal uncomplicated care including the c-section.

Refer to the following example to code a delivery case. You can try coding this case on your own and checking the answer listed next, or code along with the steps listed.

> **Example:** Following his patient's request, Dr. Benton performs a tubal ligation at the time of cesarean delivery for Gina Schmidt, age 37. He performs all routine obstetrical care, including antepartum and postpartum care.
>
> Search the index for *cesarean delivery* and subterm *routine care,* which gives you the correct code for the cesarean delivery, 59510. But if you look further in the index, there is another subterm under *cesarean delivery* for tubal *ligation at time of,* which lists code 58611, a separate procedure. When you cross-reference code 56811, you will find that it is an add-on code that you should report *in addition to* the primary procedure. The final code assignment for this case is code **59510** and code **58611.** The diagnosis code is **669.71** (*delivery, cesarean, delivered, with or without mention of antepartum condition*).

Abortion (59812–59857)

The abortion category includes codes for various types of abortive procedures. An abortion, as you already learned, is when a pregnancy is terminated before the pregnancy reaches full term. Abortions can be *spontaneous* (occurring accidentally), *therapeutic* (performed to protect the health of the mother or to terminate a pregnancy involving a fetus with health disorders), or *voluntary* (when the mother chooses not to continue the pregnancy for various reasons).

An abortion can also be *complete,* meaning that the uterus is completely emptied of the fetus and products of conception, which can happen with a spontaneous abortion or one that is medically induced, or *incomplete,* which requires surgical intervention to remove remaining fetal material. Let's review some of the procedures in this category.

- *Missed abortion* (59820, 59821)—Fetal death occurs sometime early during the pregnancy and the fetus remains in the uterus. Report codes for surgical intervention to remove the fetus and products of conception, and specify the first or second trimester (listed in code descriptors).

- *Septic abortion* (59830)—A septic abortion can be a spontaneous or induced abortion that requires surgical intervention to complete because the fetal material has become infected, creating a life-threatening situation for the mother.

- *Induced abortion* (59840–59741, 59850–59852, 59855–59857)—In an induced abortion, the fetus and placenta are physically removed from the uterus before birth. Complications may lead to the patient having a hysterectomy during the same encounter.

Abortion methods include

- *Evacuation*—suctioning the fetus and placenta out of the uterus with a suctioning instrument placed through the vagina, into the cervix, and into the uterus

- *Dilation and curettage*—scraping away the uterine lining, placenta, and fetus with a **curette** and possibly using evacuation for final removal

- *Drug administration*—use of vaginal suppositories that cause the patient to have premature labor and expulse the fetus and products of conception (**secundines**). If the fetus is alive when expulsed, it will typically expire because it cannot survive outside the uterus. This method can cause violent labor, which may result in serious health risks to the patient.

When you are coding abortions, remember that the correct code depends on the type of abortion and the method used for terminating the pregnancy. You must identify the following information:

- Trimester—Note that some codes do not specify the trimester.
- Type—treatment for abortion or induced abortion
- Method—evacuation, D & C, or drug administration
- Stage of abortion—complete or incomplete

Other Procedures (59866–59899)

The Other Procedures category includes a handful of procedures that are not related to any other categories under Maternity Care and Delivery, such as a *uterine evacuation and curettage for a hydatidiform mole* or removal of a *cerclage suture under anesthesia other than local.* Be sure to thoroughly research these procedures to fully understand their meanings before final code assignment.

curette (kyoo-rĕt')—a surgical instrument designed for scraping biological tissue or debris in a biopsy, excision, or cleaning procedure. At the tip of the curette is a small scoop, hook, or gouge

secundines (sĕ-kun'dīnz)

TAKE A BREAK

You made it! Nice work! You finished reviewing all of the categories in the last CPT subsection covered in this chapter! Let's take a break and then practice coding more procedures.

Exercise 29.6 Vaginal Delivery, Antepartum and Postpartum Care, Cesarean Delivery, Delivery After Previous Cesarean Delivery, Other Procedures

Instructions: Review the patient's case, and then assign codes for the procedure(s), appending a modifier when appropriate. Optional: For additional practice, assign the patient's diagnosis code(s) (ICD-9-CM).

1. At Williton, Kathy Thompson, age 32, gravida 2, para 2, vaginally delivers a healthy baby boy, Bryan, 7 lbs., 2 oz.

TAKE A BREAK *continued*

Dr. Benton, OB/GYN, attends the delivery and performs routine antepartum and postpartum care. Code Dr. Benton's services for both Mrs. Thompson and baby Bryan.

Mother's chart: Diagnosis code(s): _____

Mother's chart: Procedure code(s): _____

Baby's chart: Diagnosis code(s): _____

2. Sarah Collins, age 32, gravida 2, para 1, is pregnant with twins. She sees Dr. Benton in his office for a pregnancy check-up, and he determines that there are no pregnancy complications. Mrs. Collins is moving out of town where she will continue care with a different physician. Dr. Benton provided five antepartum visits.

Diagnosis code(s): _____

Procedure code(s): _____

3. Cindy Higgins, age 28, is 41 weeks pregnant when she experiences labor. Her mother takes her to Williton, where Dr. Todd performs a cesarean section because the baby is large for dates, causing cephalopelvic disproportion (the infant's body is too large to fit through the birth canal). The outcome of delivery is a single liveborn female weighing 10 lbs., 1 oz., named Jocelyn. Dr. Todd also provides antepartum and postpartum care. Code Dr. Todd's services for both Mrs. Higgins and baby Jocelyn.

Mother's chart: Diagnosis code(s): _____

Mother's chart: Procedure code(s): _____

Baby's chart: Diagnosis code(s): _____

4. Dr. Benton guides Heather Moore, age 28, through a successful vaginal delivery after her first and previous delivery by cesarean section. The outcome of this delivery is a single liveborn female. Dr. Benton also provides postpartum care, but another physician provided antepartum care. Code for Dr. Benton's delivery.

Diagnosis code(s): _____

Procedure code(s): _____

5. Kala Ludwick, age 26, arrives at Williton Medical Center, where Dr. Benton provides surgical treatment for her missed abortion (nonviable fetus), which he discovered on ultrasound two days ago. Mrs. Ludwick was in the second trimester of pregnancy. Following surgery, Dr. Benton refers the patient to Dr. Cannon, a psychologist, to counsel her and help her cope with the failed pregnancy. The patient agrees to see Dr. Cannon.

Diagnosis code(s): _____

Procedure code(s): _____

6. Kristy Adams, age 31, undergoes uterine evacuation and curettage for a hydatidiform mole at Williton. Dr. Benton performs the procedure, which is complicated by a urinary tract infection, which *E. coli* caused. Ms. Adams was treated with a course of antibiotics and advised to follow up in his office.

Diagnosis code(s): _____

Procedure code(s): _____

DESTINATION MEDICARE

In this Medicare exercise, your Medicare destination is a National Coverage Determination (NCD) on Medicare coverage for sterilization. Follow the instructions listed next to access the NCD.

1. Go to the website http://cms.gov.
2. At the top of the screen on the banner bar, choose *Regulations and Guidance.*
3. Under *Guidance,* choose *Manuals.*
4. Under *Manuals,* choose *Internet-Only Manuals.*
5. Under *Internet-Only Manuals,* choose publication number *100-03 Medicare National Coverage Determinations (NCD) Manual.*
6. Under *Downloads,* choose *Chapter 1—Coverage Determinations, Part 4.*
7. Press the Ctrl + F keys to access the search function and find the information you need.

continued

Answer the questions listed next.

1. Under what conditions will Medicare pay for sterilization?

_____

2. Will Medicare pay for sterilization at the patient's request?

_____

3. Will Medicare pay for sterilization of a mentally retarded patient?

_____

CHAPTER REVIEW

Multiple Choice

Instructions: Circle one best answer to complete each statement.

1. The procedure used prenatally to remove amniotic fluid from the amniotic sac to detect chromosomal abnormalities or remove excess fluid is called a(n)
   a. lysis.
   b. amniocentesis.
   c. cerclage.
   d. marsupialization.

2. Which procedure is performed to collect blood from the umbilical cord for genetic testing?
   a. Lysis
   b. Amniocentesis
   c. Chorionic villus sampling
   d. Cordocentesis

3. What are the three stages of pregnancy?
   a. Routine, uncomplicated, complicated
   b. First trimester, second trimester, third trimester
   c. Antepartum, labor and delivery, postpartum
   d. Dilation, expulsion, placental

4. A surgical resection of the fallopian tubes is called a
   a. tubectomy.
   b. tubal fulguration.
   c. tubal pregnancy.
   d. tubotubal.

5. Two types of episiotomy mentioned in this chapter are
   a. median and lateral.
   b. mediolateral and midline.
   c. j-shape and mediolateral.
   d. j-shape and lateral.

6. Delivery chart abbreviations include
   a. ABC and ABCD.
   b. NSVD and SVD.
   c. ADHD and ADD.
   d. ID and IQ.

7. A "Bishop Score" is used to calculate
   a. the estimated date of delivery (EDD).
   b. the size of the baby.
   c. whether a cervical ripening agent should be used to induce labor.
   d. if the patient is experiencing a false labor.

8. An episiotomy or other vaginal/cervical repair (59300) that may be required after delivery is only reportable by
   a. a provider of service other than the attending physician.
   b. the attending physician .
   c. either the attending physician or other provider.
   d. both the attending physician and another provider.

9. What are the three components of the global routine obstetric package?
   a. Conception, embryonic care, and delivery
   b. First trimester, second trimester, and third trimester
   c. Before, during, and after pregnancy care
   d. Antepartum care, delivery, and postpartum care

10. To properly code an abortion you must identify
    a. patient condition, trimester, and the type and stage of abortion.
    b. gestation period, type of abortion, complication attributed to the abortion, and stage.
    c. trimester, type of abortion, and method and stage of abortion.
    d. age of patient, type, and stage of abortion.

Coding Assignments

Instructions: Review the patient's case, and then assign codes for the procedure(s), appending a modifier when appropriate. Optional: For additional practice, assign the patient's diagnosis code(s) (ICD-9-CM).

1. Mrs. Goulding, age 21, sees Dr. Hoffman for a follow-up appointment. He diagnosed her with HPV, which

spread warts to her vagina and vulva. The medication he prescribed did not work as well as expected, and only the vaginal warts disappeared. Today, he performs cryosurgery to destroy several warts.

Diagnosis code(s): _____

Procedure code(s): _____

2. After delivering her first child by cesarean section at age 38, Miss Swinderman, now 41 years old, is in labor with her second child. Dr. Benton, her OB/GYN, whom she has seen for both pregnancies, attempts a vaginal delivery at Williton Medical Center. Poor uterine contractions and a pelvic deformity cause obstructed labor, resulting in another cesarean section.

Diagnosis code(s): _____

Procedure code(s): _____

3. In his office, Dr. Benton sees Mary Eddleman, age 57, for pain and incontinence. She is an established patient. Upon examination, he discovers a large urethrovaginal fistula, which he attributes to surgical trauma after recent anterior colporrhaphy. The visit involves an expanded problem-focused history and exam. Later that day, Dr. Benton closes the fistula at Williton. Code for both the office visit and the procedure at Williton.

Diagnosis code(s): _____

Office visit procedure code(s): _____

Williton procedure code(s): _____

4. Kara Nelson, a 22 year-old patient of Dr. Benton, is 10 weeks pregnant. She arrives at Williton Medical Center's ED due to heavy vaginal bleeding. After examination and testing, Dr. Mills, the ED physician, determines that the patient is having a miscarriage. He calls Dr. Benton who performs immediate treatment to surgically complete the miscarriage.

Diagnosis code(s): _____

Procedure code(s): _____

5. At Williton, Dr. Benton performs a bilateral tubectomy for Melanie Mathisen, age 38. The patient recently had her third child and requests a tubectomy for permanent contraception.

Diagnosis code(s): _____

Procedure code(s): _____

6. Dr. Hoffman refers Mrs. Pressnell, a 55-year-old postmenopausal patient, to Dr. Benton for abnormal vaginal bleeding. During the visit, the patient indicates she also has pain in her lower abdomen, which Dr. Hoffman determines is in the left lower quadrant. The exam for this new patient involves a detailed history and exam and moderate medical decision-making. Dr. Benton performs an endometrial biopsy and sends it to pathology for testing.

Diagnosis code(s): _____

Procedure code(s): _____

7. At Williton, Dr. Benton performs a repair of a ruptured uterus on Cindy Keller, age 35, a nonobstetrical patient. The open wound injury was caused by direct trauma from a motor vehicle accident.

Diagnosis code(s): _____

Procedure code(s): _____

8. Ms. Barlowe, an 82-year-old with cervical incompetence, undergoes a cerclage of the uterine cervix at Williton. Dr. Benton performs the procedure.

Diagnosis code(s): _____

Procedure code(s): _____

9. Mandy Nelson, age 41, sees Dr. Benton at Williton to place an occlusion device on her fallopian tubes to ensure that she has no further pregnancies.

Diagnosis code(s): _____

Procedure code(s): _____

10. Dr. Benton performs an abdominal colpopexy for Geraldine Kennedy, age 76, who has a prolapsed vagina.

Diagnosis code(s): _____

Procedure code(s): _____

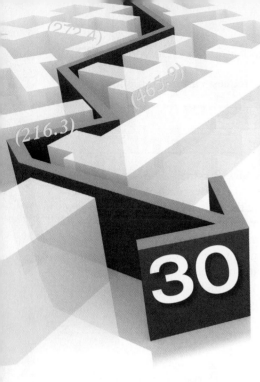

Endocrine and Nervous Systems

Learning Objectives

After completing this chapter, you should be able to

- Spell and define the key terminology in this chapter.
- Describe endocrine system functions and disorders.
- Discuss common terms and procedures for endocrine system codes.
- Describe nervous system functions and neurological disorders.
- Identify functions and areas of the brain and functions of the meninges, cranial, and spinal nerves.
- Review common terms in nervous system code descriptors.
- Describe procedures for the skull, meninges, and brain and how to assign codes.
- Review codes and procedures for the spine and spinal cord.
- Describe procedures for extracranial nerves, peripheral nerves, and autonomic nervous system.

Key Terms

approach procedure
autonomic nervous system
carotid body
definitive procedure
motor system
parasympathetic nervous system

repair/reconstruction procedure
sensory system
shunt
somatic nervous system
sympathetic nervous system
vascular disease

INTRODUCTION

This stop on your journey involves coding procedures for the endocrine and nervous systems. It contains many diagrams and tables to help guide you on your path and help you to better understand anatomy and the types of procedures that you will code. Refer to the diagrams and tables as often as you need to when you review the procedures in your CPT manual and when you perform chapter exercises. Let's press on and keep learning, further expanding your arsenal of coding skills!

"Only as high as I reach can I grow, only as far as I seek can I go, only as deep as I look can I see, only as much as I dream can I be."—KAREN RAVN

ENDOCRINE SYSTEM (60000–60699)

The endocrine system is a subsection of the Surgery section. Recall from Chapter 9 that the endocrine system is made up of glands that secrete hormones into the bloodstream (Figure 9-13). Nine types of endocrine glands may secrete hormones continuously or periodically, depending on the body's need for a specific hormone. Endocrine glands'

■ TABLE 30-1   **ENDOCRINE ORGAN FUNCTIONS**

Endocrine Organ	Hormone Released	Effect
hypothalamus	Numerous hormones that will be discussed in dedicated upcoming section	controls pituitary hormone levels
pineal	melatonin	believed to regulate sleep
pituitary	Numerous hormones that will be discussed in dedicated upcoming section	controls other endocrine organs
thyroid	thyroxine, triiodothyronine	controls cellular metabolism
	calcitonin	decreases blood calcium
parathyroid glands	parathyroid hormone	increases blood calcium
pancreas	insulin	lowers blood sugar
	glucagon	raises blood sugar
adrenal glands	epinephrine, norepinephrine	flight-or-fight response
	adrenocorticosteroids	many different effects
ovaries	estrogen, progesterone	controls sexual reproduction and secondary sexual characteristics, such as pubic and axillary hair, and breast development
testes	testosterone	controls secondary sexual characteristics such as growth of beard or other hair, deepening of voice, increase in musculature, and production of sperm

Source: Colbert, Bruce J.; Ankney, Jeff J.; Lee, Karen, ANATOMY & PHYSIOLOGY FOR HEALTH PROFESSIONS: AN INTERACTIVE JOURNEY, 2nd Ed., © 2011. Reprinted and electronically reproduced by permission of Pearson Education, Inc., Upper Saddle River, New Jersey.

secretions remain *inside* the body and should not be confused with **exocrine** glands, which secrete *outside* the body through ducts, such as sweat glands, mammary glands, and salivary glands. Exocrine glands are *not* part of the ductless endocrine system because their secretions are outside the body.

exocrine ('ek-sə-krən)

The hormones that endocrine glands secrete control different body functions, such as sleep patterns, calcium and sugar levels, male and female sexual characteristics, and the fight-or-flight response, when the body releases adrenaline in response to a threat, causing a person to either run from the situation or fight in self-defense. Refer to Figure 9-13 as you review ■ TABLE 30-1, which lists each endocrine organ, the hormones that it releases, and their effect on the body.

Disorders of the endocrine system occur when the body secretes too little hormones, too much hormones, or secretes no hormones. Endocrine system disorders can be congenital or acquired. Neoplasms and diseases can cause many disorders of the endocrine system, disrupting the body's ability to properly regulate hormones. Endocrinology is the study of diagnosing, treating, and preventing endocrine system disorders, and an endocrinologist specializes in treating disorders of the endocrine system.

The endocrine system subsection is divided into two subheadings organized by glands, and each subheading contains three categories of procedures (■ TABLE 30-2).

Notice that the second subheading in the endocrine system subsection contains the **carotid body**, a small tissue mass of nerves and cells. There are two procedures involving excision of a carotid body tumor with or without the excision of the carotid artery. The

■ TABLE 30-2   ENDOCRINE SYSTEM SUBHEADINGS AND CATEGORIES

Subheadings and Categories	Code Range
Thyroid Gland	**60000–60300**
Incision	*60000*
Excision	*60100–60281*
Removal	*60300*
Parathyroid, Thymus, Adrenal Glands, Pancreas, Carotid Body	**60500–60699**
Excision	*60500–60605*
Laparoscopy	*60650–60659*
Other Procedures	*60699*

bifurcation (bī-fĕr-kā'-shŭn)—the splitting of one body into two parts

paraganglioma (păr-ă-găng-lē-ō'-mă)

adenoma (ăd-ĕ-nō'-mă)

retroperitoneal (rĕt-rō-pĕr-ĭ-tō-nē'-ăl)

peritoneum (pĕr-ĭ-tō-nē'-ŭm)

thyroglossal (thī-rō-glŏs'-săl)

isthmus (ĭs'-mŭs)

tracheostomy (trā-kē-ŏs'-tō-mē)

lobectomy (lō-bek'-tə-mē)

isthmusectomy (is-məs- ek'-tə-mē)

thyroidectomy (thī-roid-ĕk'-tō-mē)

parathyroidectomy (pă-ră-thī-royd-ĕk'-tō-mē)

hyperplasia (hī-pür-plā'-zhä)

hyperparathyroidism (hī-pür-păr ŭ thī' roy-dīzm)

parathyroid (pă-ră-thī'-royd)

thymectomy (thī-mĕk'-tō-mē)

myasthenia gravis (mī-ăs-thē'-nē-ă gră'-vĭs)

thymoma (thī-mō'-mă)—tumor of the thymus gland

adrenalectomy (ĕ-drēn-ăl-ĕk'-tō-mē)

common carotid arteries, located in the right and left sides of the neck, transport blood from the heart to the neck and head. You can feel the pulse of your carotid arteries by running your fingers down the left or right edge of your throat.

The carotid body contains cells that monitor oxygen and carbon dioxide levels in the blood. It is located near the **bifurcation** of the carotid arteries. A **paraganglioma** (a neuro-endocrine neoplasm) can develop in the carotid body; however, paragangliomas are typically benign and rarely occur. If a physician excises a carotid body tumor, then assign a code for one of the two excision procedures (60600, 60605).

Did you notice when you reviewed Table 30-2 that it does not include procedures for all of the endocrine glands? CPT arranges codes for procedures involving the following glands *elsewhere* in the CPT manual because the types of procedures are better described in other Surgery subsections.

- *ovaries*—Female Genital System subsection
- *testes*—Male Genital System subsection
- *pancreas*—Digestive System subsection
- *pineal gland*—Nervous System subsection
- *pituitary gland*—Nervous System subsection

Review codes for procedures of the endocrine system (60000–60699) to gain a better understanding of the types of procedures listed under the subheadings and categories. You should already be familiar with various types of procedures, such as incision and drainage, excision, aspiration of a cyst, biopsy, and laparoscopy. You should also become familiar with additional terms listed in the code descriptors, as well as other types of procedures, which are outlined in ■ TABLE 30-3. You can locate endocrine system procedures by searching the index for the *body site* (thyroid gland, parathyroid gland) and then the *type of procedure* (excision, autotransplant), or start by searching for the *type of procedure*.

Refer to the following example to learn more about coding procedures for the endocrine system.

Example: Dr. Rosa, an otolaryngologist, performs a total thyroidectomy with radical neck dissection at Williton Medical Center for Mr. Warren, a 58-year-old, to treat thyroid cancer.

Search the index for the main term *thyroidectomy*, subterm *total*, subterm *for malignancy,* and subterm *radical neck dissection*, directing you to code **60254**, which is the correct code assignment. The patient's diagnosis code is **193** (main term *neoplasm* and subterm *thyroid (gland)*, *malignant, primary*). Now you try coding endocrine system procedures.

■ TABLE 30-3 **COMMON TERMS AND PROCEDURES FOR ENDOCRINE SYSTEM CODES**

Term	Definition
adenoma	Benign neoplasm originating in a gland
dorsal	Posterior (back) side of a structure
retroperitoneal	Behind the **peritoneum** (membrane lining the abdominal cavity, covering most of the abdominal organs)
thyroglossal duct cyst	A thyroglossal (pertaining to the thyroid gland and tongue) duct cyst is an embryonic congenital anomaly that appears in young children. It occurs after the thyroid gland develops when additional tissue remains that causes a mass to form in the neck.
thyroid lobes	The right and left sides of the thyroid gland, which are shaped like the wings of a butterfly (■ Figure 30-1)
thyroid isthmus	The *center* of the thyroid gland that connects the right and left lobes (Figure 30-1)
transabdominal	Across the abdomen
transcervical	Across the neck
transthoracic	Across the thorax (chest)

Procedure	Definition
transection of thyroid isthmus (60200)	Incision made to divide the isthmus, often to allow the physician to perform a **tracheostomy** (create an opening in the trachea)
thyroid lobectomy (60210–60220)	Excision of all or part of a thyroid lobe, due to neoplasm or other disease, commonly performed with a thyroidectomy
thyroid lobectomy—partial (60210)	Excision of the upper or lower part of a thyroid lobe
thyroid lobectomy—total (60220)	Excision of an entire thyroid lobe
thyroid lobectomy—partial contralateral (opposite side) subtotal (60212)	Excision of an entire thyroid lobe, part of the opposite lobe, and the isthmus
isthmusectomy (performed with other procedures) (60210–60212)	Excision of the thyroid isthmus
thyroidectomy (60240–60271)	Excision of all or part of the thyroid gland, due to carcinoma, hyperthyroidism (overactive thyroid), nodules, Graves disease (most common type of hyperthyroidism), or goiter (enlarged thyroid). The amount of the thyroid gland excised depends upon the extent of the patient's disease or condition. After surgery, many patients must take synthetic hormones to replace the hormones that the thyroid produces. Here are some types of thyroidectomies: *Total or complete*—Excision of the entire thyroid gland, most commonly to treat carcinoma *Subtotal or partial*—Excision of part of the thyroid gland, usually half, to treat carcinoma confined to a smaller area *With limited neck dissection or with radical neck dissection*—Excision of the thyroid gland with neck dissection, which involves excising lymph nodes and surrounding tissue from the neck, most commonly to treat carcinoma. The physician also examines the larynx and additional tissue during a neck dissection. Types of neck dissections include • *Radical neck dissection (RND)*—Excision of lymphatic tissue in the first five regions of lymph nodes of the neck, including the internal jugular vein (IJV), spinal accessory nerve (SAN), and sternocleidomastoid muscle (SCM) • *Modified radical neck dissection (MRND)*—Excision of tissue in the first five regions of lymph nodes of the neck with preservation of the IJV, SAN, and SCM • *Selective neck dissection*—Excision of three regions of cervical lymph nodes • *Limited neck dissection*—Excision of one or two regions of cervical lymph nodes

continued

■ **TABLE 30-3**   *continued*

Procedure	Definition
parathyroidectomy (60500–60505)	Excision of one or more of the four parathyroid glands to remove neoplasms or treat **hyperplasia** (excessive cell production) or **hyperparathyroidism** (excessive production of the parathyroid hormone)
parathyroid autotransplantation (+60512)	Procedure to implant parathyroid tissue after removal of all four parathyroid glands from the neck (Figure 30-1), typically due to disease. Since the patient cannot function properly without the parathyroid hormone, the physician implants parathyroid tissue into muscles in the neck or forearm, and after several weeks, the implanted tissue starts to produce the parathyroid hormone.
thymectomy (60520–60522)	Excision of the thymus gland, which is located in the chest and controls immune system function; thymectomies treat **myasthenia gravis** (weak skeletal muscles), **thymoma**, or thymic carcinoma
adrenalectomy (60540–60545)	Excision of one or both adrenal glands, most commonly to remove neoplasms

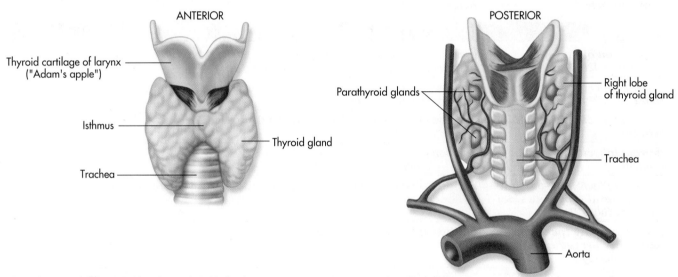

Figure 30-1 ■ The thyroid and parathyroid glands.

Source: Anatomy and Physiology for Health Professions, Colbert, Ankney, Lee, Pearson Prentice-Hall (2007) p. 282.

TAKE A BREAK

Let's take a break and practice assigning codes for the endocrine system.

Exercise 30.1   **Endocrine System**

Instructions: Review each patient's case, and then assign codes for the procedure(s), appending a modifier when appropriate. Optional: For additional practice, assign the patient's diagnosis code(s) (ICD-9-CM).

1. Tina Ferrier, age 56, presents to the office of Dr. Cochran, an endocrinologist, as a new patient, for the aspiration of thyroid cyst.

   Diagnosis code(s): _____

   Procedure code(s): _____

2. Margaret Bingham, age 76, is suffering from myasthenia gravis crisis (severe myasthenia gravis which causes respiratory failure). Dr. Cochran saw her in his office three weeks ago and decided to perform surgery. Today at Williton Medical Center, he removes her thymus using a transthoracic approach.

   Diagnosis code(s): _____

   Procedure code(s): _____

3. During a previous office visit last week, Dr. Cochran diagnosed Bryan Nelson, age 47, with an adrenal adenoma. Today at Williton, Dr. Cochran performs a laparoscopic total adrenalectomy.

   Diagnosis code(s): _____

   Procedure code(s): _____

TAKE A BREAK *continued*

4. Lisa Nicholas, age 27, was diagnosed with a thyroglossal duct cyst by Dr. Cochran two weeks ago. Dr. Cochran excises the cyst today at Williton Medical Center.

   Diagnosis code(s): _____

   Procedure code(s): _____

5. Carson Tomlin, age 23, has been diagnosed with a thyroid lesion by his family physician, who referred the patient to Dr. Cochran. Dr. Cochran saw Mr. Tomlin three days ago and scheduled him for surgery. Dr. Cochran performs a percutaneous core needle biopsy to determine if the lesion is malignant or benign. He sends the specimen to Williton's pathology department for analysis and will follow up with Mr.

Tomlin with the results. Code for Dr. Cochran's services at Williton.

Diagnosis code(s): _____

Procedure code(s): _____

6. Joe Brown, age 39, has been diagnosed with primary hyperparathyroidism during a previous visit, and Dr. Cochran performs a parathyroid exploration but fails to establish a specific cause of the hyperparathyroidism. Dr. Cochran refers the patient to Dr. Anthony, an endocrinologist who specializes in parathyroid surgery. Code for Dr. Cochran's services.

Diagnosis code(s): _____

Procedure code(s): _____

NERVOUS SYSTEM (61000–64999)

The Nervous System is the next subsection of the Surgery section. You first learned about the nervous system in Chapter 9. Recall that the nervous system is made up of a framework of nerves throughout the body that process, receive, and send messages through nerve impulses that tell the body what to do and how to react.

The nervous system consists of the central nervous system (CNS), including the brain and spinal cord, that enable the body to see, hear, touch, taste, and smell, and the peripheral nervous system (PNS), which contains nerves outside the CNS that control voluntary functions (muscle movement) and involuntary functions (cardiac, glands) (Figure 9-18).

Somatic and Autonomic Nervous System

The peripheral nervous system includes the somatic nervous system and the autonomic nervous system (■ FIGURE 30-2). The **somatic nervous system** controls the body's voluntary movements, including movement of skeletal muscles. The **autonomic nervous system** controls involuntary body movements, such as muscles in your organs, heart, and glands (respiration, blood pressure, heart rate).

The autonomic nervous system is made up of two branches, the **parasympathetic nervous system (PSNS)**, which controls body functions, such as digestion, and the **sympathetic nervous system (SNS)**, which controls the body's fight-or-flight response that you learned about earlier in this chapter. The enteric nervous system (ENS) is also part of the autonomic nervous system and controls gastrointestinal functions.

Sensory and Motor Systems

The nervous system is made up of both the sensory and motor systems of nerves. The **sensory system** involves the brain and spinal cord interpreting information that the body senses, such as touching a hot object with your hand, which causes it to react through the motor system. The **motor system** directs the body's muscles and glands to perform specific functions, such as pulling your hand away from the hot object, based on the outside information that the body receives.

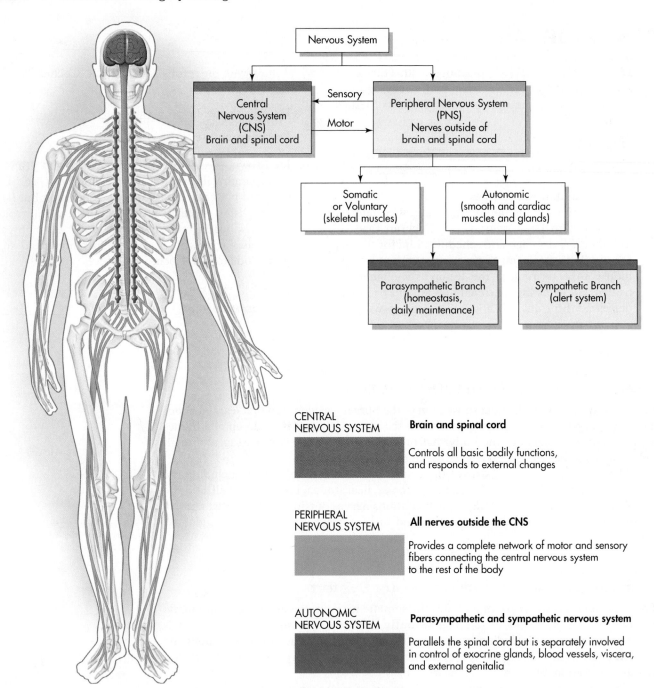

Figure 30-2 ■ Nervous system flowchart.

Source: Anatomy and Physiology for Health Professions, Colbert, Ankney, Lee, Pearson Prentice-Hall (2007) p. 225.

NEUROLOGICAL DISORDERS

Neurology is the study of nerves, and neurologists are physicians specializing in the diagnosis, treatment, and prevention of nervous system disorders. Neurosurgery is the branch of medicine that specializes in surgically correcting nervous system disorders. Nervous system, or neurological, disorders, can have many different causes, including trauma, neoplasms, degenerative diseases, or congenital conditions.

Symptoms of nervous system disorders vary, depending on the patient's specific condition, but common symptoms include headache; muscle weakness; vision, hearing, or memory loss; seizures; and mental impairment. Common disorders of the CNS include bacterial meningitis, Parkinson's disease, and epilepsy. Common disorders of the PNS include Bell's palsy, carpal tunnel syndrome, and polyneuropathy. Pain is also a nervous system disorder.

Just as with any other sections or subsections of CPT, it is also important for you to understand the anatomy involved in procedures that you code for the nervous system to ensure correct code assignment. If you are not sure of a code descriptor's meaning, then you should research the procedure, along with any medical terms that you do not know, before you assign the code. In order to begin coding from the Nervous System subsection, you will need to learn more about its divisions of nerves and their functions. Be sure to refer to this information and corresponding diagrams as you review codes listed under the Nervous System subsection.

BRAIN, MENINGES, CRANIAL, AND SPINAL NERVES

In order to better understand nervous system procedures involving the brain, meninges, cranial nerves, and spinal nerves, it is important to become familiar with the anatomy of the brain and spinal cord. The brain controls the nervous system, and cranial nerves connect the brain to other areas of the body. The cranial nerves receive messages and transmit them to the brain, which represents the sensory system of nerves. The brain's response to those messages represents the motor system of nerves. Refer to ■ TABLE 30-4 to familiarize yourself with various areas of the brain, and refer to ■ FIGURE 30-3 to see the areas in a diagram.

cerebellar (sĕr-ĕ-bĕl′-ĕr)

cerebrum (sĕ-rē′-brŭm)

longitudinal (lŏn-jĭ-tū′-dĭ-năl)

corpus callosum (′kȯr-pǝs ka-′lō-sǝm)

parietal (pǎ-rī′-ĕ-tǎl)

occipital (äk-′sip-ǝt-ǝl)

diencephalon (dī-ǝn-′sef-ǝ-län)

thalamus (thăl′-ă-mŭs)

hypothalamus (hī-pō-thăl′-ă-mŭs)

pineal (pĭn′-ē-ăl)

cerebellum (sĕr-ĕ-bel′-ĕm)

medulla oblongata (mĕ-dŭl′-lă ŏb-lŏng-gŏt′-ă)

■ TABLE 30-4 AREAS OF THE BRAIN

Name	Definition
cortex	Gray matter in the brain that surrounds white matter in the brain. The brain is made up of a cerebral cortex and a **cerebellar** cortex.
nuclei	Areas of the brain composed of deep gray matter surrounded by white matter
ventricles	Cavities throughout the brain filled with cerebrospinal fluid (CSF) (clear fluid that provides shock absorption for the brain and spinal cord, transports nutrients, and eliminates waste)
cerebrum	Largest part of the brain, divided into left and right hemispheres by a **longitudinal** fissure (groove); the **corpus callosum** connects the hemispheres. The cerebrum is divided into four lobes (■ FIGURE 30-4): • frontal (motor movements, speech, conscious thought) • **parietal** (sense, speech) • **occipital** (vision) • temporal (taste, hearing, emotions)
diencephalon	Area of the brain containing the following structures (■ TABLE 30-5): • **thalamus** • **hypothalamus** • **pineal** body • pituitary gland
cerebellum	Area at the back of the brain between the cerebrum and brain stem responsible for balance and motor coordination
brain stem	Stem of the brain connecting it to the spinal cord, which consists of three sections: • **medulla oblongata** (breathing, heartbeat, blood pressure) • pons (breathing) • midbrain (vision, hearing, breathing, heart rate, blood pressure)

Figure 30-3 ■ Anatomy of the brain from three different views.

Source: Anatomy and Physiology for Health Professions, Colbert, Ankney, Lee, Pearson Prentice-Hall (2007) p. 225.

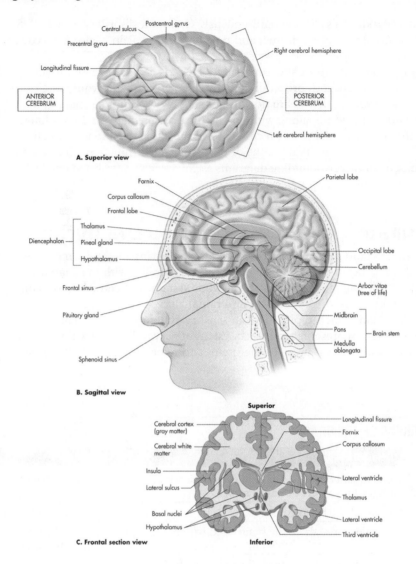

Figure 30-4 ■ Brain anatomy and lobes.

Source: Anatomy and Physiology for Health Professions, Colbert, Ankney, Lee, Pearson Prentice-Hall (2007) p. 221.

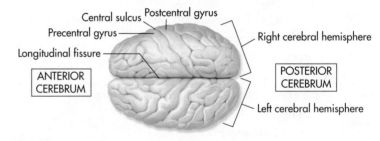

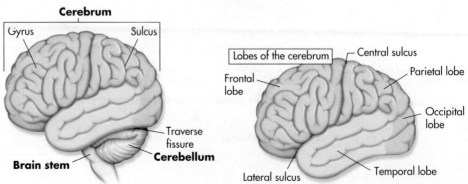

■ TABLE 30-5   DIENCEPHALON

Structure	Function
thalamus	relays and processes information going to the cerebrum
hypothalamus	regulates hormone levels, temperature, water-balance, thirst, appetite, and some emotions (pleasure and fear); regulates the pituitary gland and controls the endocrine system
pineal body	responsible for secretion of melatonin (body clock)
pituitary gland	secretes hormones for various functions

Source: Colbert, Bruce J.; Ankney, Jeff J.; Lee, Karen, ANATOMY & PHYSIOLOGY FOR HEALTH PROFESSIONS: AN INTERACTIVE JOURNEY, 2nd Ed., © 2011. Reprinted and electronically reproduced by permission of Pearson Education, Inc., Upper Saddle River, New Jersey.

The **meninges** is a membrane consisting of three layers of connective tissue that covers the brain and spinal cord (■ FIGURE 30-5):

meninges (mēn-ĭn′-jēz)

- **Dura mater**
- **Arachnoid mater**
- **Pia mater**

dura mater (dū′-ră mă′-ter)

arachnoid mater (ĕ-răk′-noid mā′-ter)

pia mater (pē′-ă mă′-ter)

There are 12 pair of cranial nerves (■ FIGURE 30-6), which direct sensory functions, motor functions, or both (**mixed nerves**) (■ TABLE 30-6).

The spinal cord, located within the vertebral column, contains 31 pair of spinal nerves, located on the left and right sides of the spinal cord. The nerve pairs are named after the area of the vertebrae where they are located (■ FIGURE 30-7):

- cervical (8 pairs)
- thoracic (12 pairs)
- lumbar (5 pairs)
- sacral (5 pairs)
- coccygeal (1 pair)

Spinal nerves are mixed nerves, carrying motor and sensory information. A **plexus** is a group of spinal nerves that connect to other nerves in the body, such as the lumbar

plexus (plĕks′-ŭs)

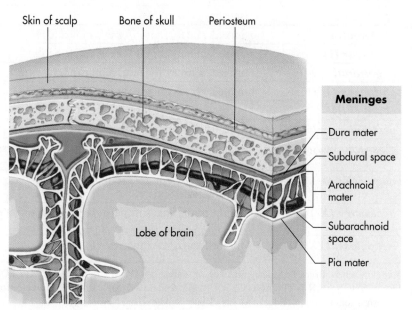

Figure 30-5 ■ The meninges.

Source: Anatomy and Physiology for Health Professions, Colbert, Ankney, Lee, Pearson Prentice-Hall (2007) p. 224B.

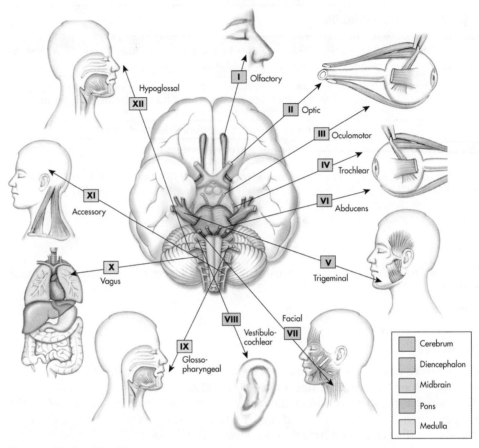

Figure 30-6 ■ Cranial nerves.
Source: Anatomy and Physiology for Health Professions, Colbert, Ankney, Lee, Pearson
Prentice-Hall (2007) p. 228.

■ TABLE 30-6   CRANIAL NERVES AND FUNCTIONS

Nerve	Function
olfactory (I)	sensory (smell)
optic (II)	sensory (vision)
oculomotor (III)	mixed, chiefly motor for eye movements
trochlear (IV)	mixed, chiefly motor for eye movements
trigeminal (V)	mixed, sensory for face, motor for chewing
abducens (VI)	mixed, chiefly motor for eye movements
facial (VII)	mixed; motor for face; sensory for taste
vestibulocochlear (VIII)	sensory, hearing, and balance
glossopharyngeal (IX)	mixed, motor for tongue and throat muscles; sensory for taste and physiology
vagus (X)	mixed, motor for autonomic heart, lungs, viscera; sensory for viscera, taste buds
accessory (XI)	motor for larynx, soft palate, trapezius, and sternocleidomastoid muscles
hypoglossal (XII)	motor for tongue muscles

Source: Colbert, Bruce J.; Ankney, Jeff J.; Lee, Karen, ANATOMY & PHYSIOLOGY FOR HEALTH
PROFESSIONS: AN INTERACTIVE JOURNEY, 2nd Ed., © 2011. Reprinted and electronically reproduced
by permission of Pearson Education, Inc., Upper Saddle River, New Jersey.

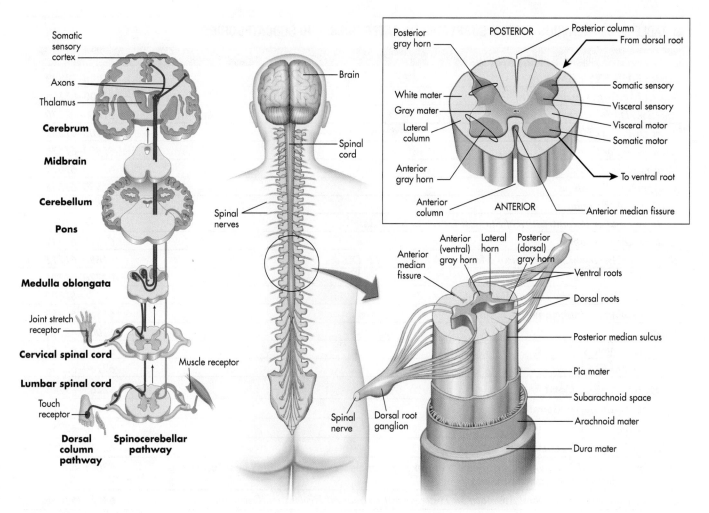

Figure 30-7 ■ The spinal cord and spinal nerves.

Source: Anatomy and Physiology for Health Professions, Colbert, Ankney, Lee, Pearson Prentice-Hall (2007) p. 209.

plexus, with nerves to the abdomen, back, groin, and legs. The **cauda equina**, which looks like a horse's tail, is a group of nerve roots at the end of the spinal cord.

cauda equina (kaw-dŭ′ ē-′kwī-nə)

The nervous system subsection is divided into numerous subheadings organized by body site (skull, spine) and type of procedure (injection, repair), with some procedures divided into subcategories to provide more specific information (somatic nerves, sympathetic nerves) (■ TABLE 30-7).

Assigning codes from the Nervous System subsection can be complex, and it is very important to understand procedures in this subsection. You may already know some of the terms because they were presented in other chapters. To become familiar with medical terms that you will find in the code descriptors, refer to ■ TABLE 30-8 to review many of the terms and their definitions. Some of the terms are part of another term's definition. Use Table 30-8 as a guide as you review procedures from this subsection. Remember that if you find a term or procedure with which you are unfamiliar, then you should always research the definition in your medical dictionary, in anatomy and physiology references, or on the Internet before final code assignment. When you are working in the healthcare field, you can also query the physician for clarification of procedures. To locate codes for nervous system procedures, search for the *body site* (meninges, brain, cranial nerve) and then the *type of procedure* (excision, incision) or start your search with the *type of procedure* or *condition* (cyst, adhesions, tumor).

■ TABLE 30-7 NERVOUS SYSTEM SUBHEADINGS, CATEGORIES, AND SUBCATEGORIES

Subheadings, Categories, and Subcategories	Code Range
NERVOUS SYSTEM	**61000–64999**
Skull, Meninges, and Brain	**61000–62258**
Injection, Drainage, or Aspiration	*61000–61070*
Twist Drill, Burr Hole(s), or Trephine	*61105–61253*
Craniectomy or Craniotomy	*61304–61576*
Surgery of Skull Base	*61580–61619*
• *Approach Procedures*	*61580–61598*
• *Definitive Procedures*	*61600–61616*
• *Repair and/or Reconstruction of Surgical Defects of Skull Base*	*61618–61619*
Endovascular Therapy	*61623–61642*
Surgery for Aneurysm, Arteriovenous Malformation, or Vascular Disease	*61680–61711*
Stereotaxis	*61720–61791*
Stereotactic Radiosurgery (Cranial)	*61796–61800*
Neurostimulators (Intracranial)	*61850–61888*
Repair	*62000–62148*
Neuroendoscopy	*62160–62165*
Cerebrospinal Fluid (CSF) Shunt	*62180–62258*
Spine and Spinal Cord	**62263–63746**
Injection, Drainage, or Aspiration	*62263–62319*
Catheter Implantation	*62350–62355*
Reservoir/Pump Implantation	*62360–62368*
Posterior Extradural Laminotomy or Laminectomy for Exploration/Decompression of Neural Elements or Excision of Herniated Intervertebral Discs	*63001–63051*
Transpedicular or Costovertebral Approach for Posterolateral Extradural Exploration/Decompression	*63055–63066*
Anterior or Anterolateral Approach for Extradural Exploration/Decompression	*63075–63091*
Lateral Extracavitary Approach for Extradural Exploration/Decompression	*63101–63103*
Incision	*63170–63200*
Excision by Laminectomy of Lesion Other Than Herniated Disc	*63250–63295*
Excision, Anterior or Anterolateral Approach, Intraspinal Lesion	*63300–63308*
Stereotaxis	*63600–63615*
Stereotactic Radiosurgery (Spinal)	*63620–63621*
Neurostimulators (Spinal)	*63650–63688*
Repair	*63700–63710*
Shunt, Spinal CSF	*63740–63746*
Extracranial Nerves, Peripheral Nerves, and Autonomic Nervous System	**64400–64999**
Introduction/Injection of Anesthetic Agent (Nerve Block), Diagnostic or Therapeutic	*64400–64530*
• *Somatic Nerves*	*64400–64484*
• *Paravertebral Spinal Nerves and Branches*	*64490–64495*
• *Autonomic Nerves*	*64505–64530*
Neurostimulators (Peripheral Nerve)	*64550–64595*
Destruction by Neurolytic Agent (e.g., Chemical, Thermal, Electrical or Radiofrequency)	*64600–64681*
• *Somatic Nerves*	*64600–64640*
• *Sympathetic Nerves*	*64650–64681*
Neuroplasty (Exploration, Neurolysis, or Nerve Decompression)	*64702–64727*
Transection or Avulsion	*64732–64772*

■ TABLE 30-7   *continued*

Subheadings, Categories, and Subcategories	Code Range
Excision	*64774–64823*
• *Somatic Nerves*	*64774–64795*
• *Sympathetic Nerves*	*64802–64823*
Neurorrhaphy	*64831–64876*
Neurorrhaphy With Nerve Graft, Vein Graft, or Conduit	*64885–64911*
Other Procedures	*64999*

■ TABLE 30-8   **COMMON TERMS IN NERVOUS SYSTEM CODE DESCRIPTORS**

Term	Pronunciation	Definition
bicoronal	(bī-kō-rō′-năl)	Affecting both coronal structures of the skull, the frontal and parietal bones
cerebellopontine	(ser-ĕ-bel′-ō-pŏn-tēn)	Structure at the margin of the cerebellum and the pons (section of the brain stem)
choroid plexus	(ko′-royd plĕk′-sŭs)	Structure that produces cerebrospinal fluid, which is located in the ventricles of the brain
colloid cyst	(kŏl′-oyd sĭst)	Benign brain cyst that typically occurs in the third ventricle area (middle) of the brain
corpus callosum	(kor′-pŭs kă-lō ′-sŭm)	A flat bundle of neural fibers that connect the two cerebral hemispheres and allow communication between the right and left sides of the brain
cortical	(kor′-tĭ-kl)	The outer portion of an organ
costovertebral	(kŏs-tō-vür-tē′-brăl)	The area where the head of the ribs, the end of the rib closest to the vertebral column, connect to the body of the thoracic vertebra, the heart-shaped anterior portion
cranial fossa	(krā′-nē-ăl fŏ′-să)	A hollow or depressed area in the floor of the interior area of the skull
craniofacial	(krā-nē-ō-fā′-shăl)	A term used to describe certain congenital facial malformations
craniomegalic	(krā-nē-ō-meg′-ă-lĭk)	An abnormally large skull
craniopharyngioma	(krānē-ō-fə-rĭn′jē-ō-mă)	A tumor of the brain near the pituitary gland. It is often associated with increased intracranial pressure, and children and young adults are prone to developing it.
craniosynostosis	(krā-nē-ō-sĭn-ŏs-tō′-sĭs)	Premature ossification (forming new bone) of fibrous skull sutures in an infant's skull
dentate ligament	(dĕn′-tāt lĭg′-ĕ-mĕnt)	Scallop-shaped fibrous band of pia mater that extends the length of the spinal cord on each side between the nerves
dura	(dū′-ră)	Outermost of the three layers of meninges surrounding the spinal cord
duraplasty	(dū′-ră -plăs-tĕ)	Repair of the dura
encephalocele	(ĕn-sĕf′-ä-lō-sēl)	Congenital gap in the skull which could cause brain matter to protrude
epidural	(ĕp-ĭ-dö′-räl)	Pertaining to or situated on the dura mater. This term is often used to describe a form of regional anesthesia involving injection of medication into the epidural space.
epileptogenic focus	(ēp·ĭ·lĕp·tō·gĕn′·ĭc fŏ′-kŭs)	Having the capacity to cause an epileptic seizure
extracranial	(ĕks-trä-krā′-nē-ăl)	Situated outside the cranium
extradural	(ĕks-trä-dū′-räl)	On or outside the dura mater

continued

■ **TABLE 30-8**   *continued*

Term	Pronunciation	Definition
gasserian ganglion	(găs′-ĕr-ē-ŏn găn′-glē-ŏn)	A large benign cystic tumor at the root of the trigeminal, or fifth, cranial nerve
infraorbital	(ĭn-fră-ŏr′-bĭ-tăl)	Under the orbit
infratemporal	(ĭn-fră-tĕm′-pō-răl)	Under the temporal fossa of the skull, a broad depression that lies behind the orbit between the temporal line and the **zygomatic** bone (cheekbone)
infratentorial	(ĭn-fră-tĕn′-tōr-e-ăl)	Area of the brain located below the **tentorium cerebelli** (fold of dura mater covering the posterior cranial fossa, which contains the brainstem and cerebellum)
intervertebral	(ĭn-tĕr-vĕr-tē′-brăl)	Area between two adjacent vertebrae
intracavitary	(ĭn-tră-kăv′-ĭ-tā-rē)	Within a cavity
intracerebellar	(ĭn-tră-sĕr-ĕh-bĕl′-ăr)	Within the cerebellum
intracerebral	(ĭn-tră-sĕ-rĕ′-br-ăl)	Within the cerebrum
intracranial	(ĭn-tră-krā′-nĕ-āl)	Within the skull
intradural	(ĭn-tră-dū′-răl)	Within the dura mater
intraparenchymal	(ĭn-tră-păr-ĕn-kī′-măl)	Within the characteristic (normal) tissue of an organ
intraspinal	(ĭn-tră-spī′-năl)	Within the spinal canal
intrathecal	(ĭn-tră-thē′-kăl)	Within the subarachnoid space
meningioma	(mĕn-ĭn-jĭ-ō′-mă)	Tumor of the meninges that originates in the arachnoidal tissue
meningocele	(mĕn-ĭn′-gō-sēl)	Congenital hernia in which the meninges protrude through a defect in the skull or spinal column
mesencephalic	(mĕs-ĕn-sĕf-ăl′-ĭk)	Pertaining to the mesencephalon (midbrain)
myelomeningocele	(mī-ĕ-lō-mĕn-ĭn′-gō-sēl)	A type of **spina bifida**, which is a birth defect where the spinal cord and backbone do not close properly before birth
neuroma	(nū-rō′-mă)	Tumor of nerve cells and fibers
nucleus pulposus	(nū′-klē-ŭs pŭlp′-ŭs)	The gelatinous mass that lies within an intervertebral disc
occipital	(äk-′sip-ət-əl)	Related to or located at the back of the head
optic nerve	(ŏp′-tĭk)	The nerve that carries visual information from the retina to the brain
orbit	(ŏr′-bĭt)	The bony cavity of the skull that contains the eyeball
orbitocranial	(ŏr-bĭt-ō-krā′-nē-al)	Entering the skull through the orbital cavity
paravertebral	(pă-ră-vĕr-tē′-brăl)	Located along the vertebral column
postauricular	(pōst-aw-rĭk′-ū-lăr)	Behind the auricle of the ear
preauricular	(prē-aw-rĭk′-ū-lăr)	In front of the auricle, which is the outer portion of the ear
pseudomeningocele	(sī-dō-mĕn-ĭn′-jĕ-sēl)	Abnormal collection of cerebrospinal fluid contained within a cavity
septum pellucidum	(sĕp′-tŭm pĕ-lū′-si-dŭm)	A thin sheet of nervous tissue connected to the corpus callosum and the fornix, a bundle of fibers that connect the cerebral lobes
spasmodic dysphonia	(spăz-mŏd′-ĭk dĭs-fō′-nē-ă)	Voice disorder caused by involuntary contractions of one or more muscles of the larynx
spasmodic torticollitis	(spăz-mŏd′-ĭk tor-tĭ-kō-lĭt′-əs)	Involuntary neurological movement disorder that causes the neck to move in various directions
spirothalamic tract	(spī-rō-thăl′-a-mĭk)	Sensory pathway, a chain of nerve fibers along which impulses travel. It transmits information to the thalamus, the relay center for all sensory impulses (except olfactory) being transmitted to the sensory areas of the cortex

■ TABLE 30-8 *continued*

Term	Pronunciation	Definition
subarachnoid	(sŭb-ă-răk′-noyd)	The innermost membrane surrounding the central nervous system, between the arachnoid membrane and the pia mater
subcortical	(sŭb-kor′-tĭ-kăl)	Beneath the cerebral cortex
suboccipital	(sŭb-ŏk-sĭp′-ĭ-tăl)	Beneath the occiput or occipital bone
subpial	(sŭb-pī′-ăl)	Beneath the pia mater, a delicate membrane surrounding the brain and spinal column
subtemporal	(sŭb-tĕm′-por-ăl)	Beneath the temples or temporal bones
supraorbital	(sū-pră-or′-bĭ-tăl)	Located above the orbit
supratentorial	(sū-pră-tĕn-tō′-rē-ăl)	Located above the tentorium cerebelli
syrinx	(sĭr′-ĭnks)	Fluid-filled cavity in the spinal cord or brain
temporal lobe	(tĕm′-por-ăl)	One of three lobes of the cerebrum that contains centers for hearing, smell, and language input
tentorium cerebelli	(tĕn-tō′-rē-ŭm sĕr-ĕ-bel′-ă)	A covering of dura mater that supports the occipital lobes and covers the dura mater
thoracolumbar	(thō-răk-ō-′ləm-bər)	Pertaining to the thoracic and lumbar areas of the spinal column
transcochlear	(trăns-kōk′-lē-ăr)	Across or through the cochlea, the auditory portion of the inner ear
transcondylar	(trăns-kŏn′-dĭ-lăr)	Across or through the condyle, the rounded projection at the end of a bone that enters into the formation of a joint
transnasal	(trăns-nā′-zl)	Across or through the nasal bone
transoral	(trăns-ōr′-ăl)	Across or through the mouth or oral region
transpedicular	(trăns-pē-dĭk′-ū-lăr)	Across or through the brain stem
transpetrosal	(trăns-pĕ-trō′-săl)	Across or through the petrous part of the temporal bone, an exceptionally hard and dense portion of the bone that contains the internal auditory organs.
transsphenoidal	(trăns-sfē-noy′-dăl)	Across or through the sphenoid bone, an unpaired, winged, compound bone that is located at the base of the cranium
transtemporal	(trăns-tĕm′-pō-răl)	Across or through the temporal lobe of the cerebrum
vasospasm	(vās′-ō-spăzm)	Spasm of a blood vessel
vertebral interspace	(vĕr-tē′-brăl)	Open area between individual vertebrae
vertebral segment	(vĕr-tē′-brăl)	The bony segments that are stacked on top of one another and act as a support for the spine
vertebrobasilar	(vĕr′-tĭ-brō-bās-ĭ-lăr)	Arterial system that provides blood flow to the posterior (back) of the brain
zygomatic	(zī-gō-măt′-ĭk)	Pertaining to the cheekbone or malar bone (zygoma); paired bone of the human skull (a paired bone is a bone that has a matching, parallel bone on the opposite side)

spina bifida (spī′-nă bĭf′-ĭ-dă)

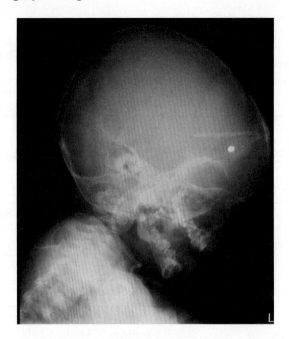

SKULL, MENINGES, AND BRAIN (61000–62258)

The first subheading in the Nervous System subsection is Skull, Meninges, and Brain, which contains 12 different categories of codes, depending on the type of procedure that the physician performs. Let's review more about how to assign codes for procedures in each category and then practice coding.

Injection, Drainage, or Aspiration (61000–61070)

Procedures listed under the category Injection, Drainage, or Aspiration (removal) include removing CSF to test it for specific disorders, such as **meningitis**, or removing excess fluid caused by hydrocephalus (sometimes called water on the brain) or head trauma. The physician orders a CT scan or MRI to first determine the extent of CSF present and then withdraws fluid or directs it elsewhere in the body. Review the codes for this category, which include the following types of procedures:

meningitis (mĕn-ĭn-jī′-tĭs)—inflammation of the meninges of the spinal cord or brain

- *Subdural tap* (fluid collection) (61000–61001)—withdrawal of CSF through a **fontanelle** (a soft spot, or gap, in an infant's skull where bones have not yet formed) to test for disorders (index entry: *subdural tap*)

subdural (sŭb-dū′-răl)—below the dura mater

fontanelle (fŏn′-tă-nĕl)

- *Ventricular puncture* (61020–61026)—withdrawal of CSF from the ventricles of the brain by drilling a hole in the skull to collect CSF to test for disorders (index entry: *ventricular puncture*)

cisternal (sĭs-tĕr′-năl)

- *Cisternal puncture*—withdrawal of CSF from the cisterna magna (space between the pia mater and arachnoid membrane—membrane of brain and spinal cord) to test for disorders (61050–61055) (index entry: *cisternal puncture*)

- *Puncture of shunt tubing or reservoir* (61070)—procedure to test for infection or to withdraw excess CSF after shunt insertion. A **shunt** is a device that includes a catheter (tube) that transports fluid from one area of the body to another (■ Figure 30-8). Hydrocephalus is a condition that physicians can treat with shunts (index entries of main terms and subterms: *skull, puncture, drain fluid* or *skull, shunt, drain fluid*).

Refer the following example to learn more about coding injections, aspirations, and drainage.

LaCrosse encephalitis (lă-krŏs′ ĕn-sĕf-ă-lī′-tĭs)—encephalitis transmitted to humans by the bite of an infected mosquito

Example: Mr. and Mrs. Dixon bring their 2-month-old son, Johnny, to Williton Medical Center's ED with symptoms of seizures, fever, lethargy, and vomiting. His CT scan reveals subdural fluid collections. Dr. Hawkins, a pediatric neurosurgeon, performs a subdural tap. He diagnoses Johnny with **LaCrosse encephalitis**.

To code this case, search the index for the main term *subdural tap*, which then directs you to codes 61000–61001. Assign code **61000** because the documentation states that Dr. Hawkins only performed one subdural tap (initial). The patient's diagnosis code is **062.5** (main term *encephalitis*, subterm *La Crosse*).

Twist Drill, Burr Hole(s), or Trephine (61105–61253)

Procedures in this category involve a physician drilling or cutting into the skull (craniostomy), typically to drain a hematoma or abscess, but they can also perform the procedures to remove part of the bone of the skull in order to gain access to perform further surgery. The procedures are named for the equipment that the physician uses to perform them—a burr and a **trephine** are types of saws, and a twist drill has a drill bit which is twisted.

trephine (trē′-fīn)

Note that some of the procedures also include implanting a catheter, reservoir, EEG electrodes, and pressure recording device. Physicians can implant catheters and reservoirs to deliver chemotherapy to the brain in cancer patients, and catheters can also be used to drain CSF. Implanted EEG electrodes monitor brain functions in patients with seizures and brain damage, and pressure recording devices help physicians to detect intracranial pressure.

Review the procedures under this category to become more familiar with them. Depending on the type of procedure, you can search the index for the main terms *ventricular puncture, burr hole,* and *insertion.*

Refer the following example to learn more about coding burr hole surgery.

Example: Dr. Rice, a neurosurgeon, creates a burr hole to treat a subdural hematoma for Mr. Holmes, an 85-year-old patient, at Williton Medical Center.

To code this case, search the index for the main term *burr hole,* subterm *hematoma,* which then directs you to codes 61154–61156. Assign code **61154** because the procedure includes treatment for a subdural hematoma. The patient's diagnosis code is **852.20** (main term *hematoma,* subterm *brain,* subterm *subdural*).

Craniectomy or Craniotomy (61304–61576)

Recall that a craniectomy is when a physician removes (-ectomy) part of the cranium (crani/o), which is the skull, to drain an abscess, remove neoplasms, or treat swelling of the brain and allow the brain more room to expand. Physicians also perform craniectomies to enable them to access the brain in order to perform procedures on cranial nerves.

A **craniotomy** is an incision (-otomy) into the cranium with an instrument called a craniotome, where the physician removes part of the skull (bone flap) to perform procedures on the brain, such as removing neoplasms, implanting stimulators to treat epilepsy, relieving pressure on the skull and brain swelling, treating a hematoma, or removing a foreign body, such as a bullet. After the procedure, the physician reattaches the bone flap to the skull with screws and plates.

craniotomy (krā-nē-ŏ′-tō-mē)

After a craniectomy or craniotomy, the physician may perform a bone graft to repair the defect. Assign separate codes for bone grafts, as they are not integral parts of a craniectomy or craniotomy.

Sometimes, after a craniectomy, physicians may not be able to replace the patient's bone because of trauma, infection, or edema. Patients are left with a "soft spot" in the skull where there is no bone. The patient wears a protective helmet until his condition improves and he can undergo surgery (cranioplasty) to repair the defect.

Review the procedures listed under this category. CPT arranges procedures by the location where the physician performs them (supratentorial, suboccipital), condition (craniosynostosis, osteomyelitis), and any other procedures performed in addition to the craniectomy or craniotomy (duraplasty, excision of tumor). This is not an easy group of procedures to understand. There are many procedures with which you may not be familiar, and you will need to review their definitions to be able to accurately assign codes from this category.

Refer to ■ TABLE 30-9 to become familiar with some of the procedures that you will find in code descriptors, and use the table as a reference when assigning codes from this category. You can also refer to Table 30-8 for definitions of medical terms.

■ **TABLE 30-9   PROCEDURES INCLUDED IN CODE DESCRIPTORS FOR CRANIECTOMY AND CRANIOTOMY**

Term	Pronunciation	Definition
amygdalohippocampectomy (61566)	(ĕ-mig-dĕ-lō-hĭp-ĕ-kăm-pĕk′-tĕ-mē)	Excision of parts of the brain, the **amygdalae**, which regulates emotions, and the **hippocampus**, which regulates memory. Physicians perform the procedure to treat epilepsy.
cingulotomy (61490)	(sĭn-gū-lŏt′-ō-mē)	Incision into the anterior cingulate cortex, part of the limbic system located at the top of the brain, which controls various body functions, such as the expression of emotions. The procedure treats chronic pain and mental disorders, such as depression.
decompression (61340, 61343–61345, 61450–61458, 61564, 61575)	(dē-kŭm-prĕsh′-ŭn)	Excision of part of the skull or other body site to alleviate pressure, such as excess CSF
electrocorticography (61534, 61536, 61567)	(ĭh-lĕk-trō-kawr-tĭ-kŏg′-ră-fē)	Procedure where the physician implants electrodes on the brain to record electrical impulses and identify areas to surgically remove to treat epilepsy
fenestration (61524)	(fĕn-ĭ-strā′-shĕn)	To pierce to create an opening
hemispherectomy (61542–61543)	(hĕm-ĭ-sfĕr-ĕk′-tō-mē)	Excision of one of the two cerebral hemispheres to treat epilepsy
hypophysectomy (61546, 61548)	(hī-pō-fīz- ĕk′-tō-mē)	Excision of the **hypophysis** (pituitary gland), most commonly to remove a neoplasm
laminectomy (61343)	(lām-ĭ-nĕk′-tō-mē)	Excision of the lamina, the flat part of a vertebra, to remove neoplasms or abnormal intervertebral discs
lobectomy (61323, 61537–61540)	(lō-bĕk′-tō-mē)	Excision of a lobe of the brain to treat epilepsy
pedunculotomy (61480)	(pē-dŭn-kū-lŏt′-ō-mē)	Incision of a cerebral peduncle (brain stem) to stop involuntary body movements
tractotomy (61470–61480)	(trak-′tät-ə-mē)	Procedure where the physician incises a nerve tract (group of nerve fibers) found in the brainstem or spinal cord to treat chronic pain
trephination (61510–61516)	(trē-fĭn-a′-shŭn)	Incision into the skull with a trephine

amygdalae (ĕ-mĭg′-dă-lă)

hippocampus (hĭp-ō-kăm′-pŭs)

hypophysis (hī-′päf-ə-səs)

Refer the following example to learn more about coding a craniectomy.

Example: Dr. Rice, a neurosurgeon, performs a craniectomy at Williton Medical Center for Mrs. Black, a 62-year-old patient. Mrs. Black has acute osteomyelitis (bone infection) in the cranium, which *Streptococcus* bacteria caused.

To code this case, search the index for the main term *craniectomy* and subterm *surgical*, which then directs you to several code ranges in the Craniectomy or Craniotomy category. After reviewing all possible choices, assign code **61501** because Dr. Rice performed the craniectomy to treat osteomyelitis. Diagnosis codes are **730.08** (main term *osteomyelitis*, subterm *acute, other specified sites*) and **041.00** (main term *infection*, subterm *streptococcal*).

Surgery of Skull Base (61580–61619)

Procedures in the category of Surgery of Skull Base include removal of many different types of lesions of the skull base. Surgery to remove lesions from the skull base, the bottom or floor of the skull, is very specialized because the skull base is not easily accessible. The surgery is difficult, involved, and time-consuming. In fact, this type of surgery requires a team of specialized surgeons to perform various components of the surgery. Neurosurgeons must also consider

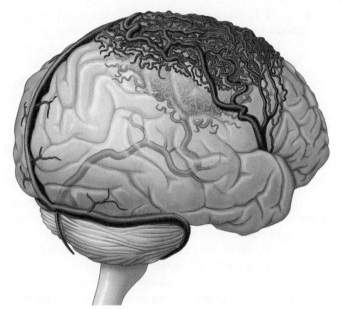

Figure 30-9 ■ Arteriovenous malformation.

Source: Medical-Surgical Nursing Preparation for Practice, Osborn, Wraa, Watson, Pearson Prentice-Hall, (2010), p. 709.

possible problems that could arise during or after surgery and must work with an interdisciplinary team of otolaryngologists, ophthalmologists, plastic surgeons, and physical and occupational therapists to effectively manage patients' care and address their unique needs.

Here are some of the types of lesions that surgeons remove during skull base surgery:

- **aneurysm** (excessive blood vessel dilation, which could lead to a ruptured blood vessel or vein)

  aneurysm (an′-yĕ-rĭz-ŭm)

- **arteriovenous malformation (AVM)** (abnormal connection between arteries and veins) (■ FIGURE 30-9)

  arteriovenous malformation (AVM) (ăr-tē′-rē-ō-vē-nŭs măl-for-mā′-shŭn)

- CSF fistula (abnormal connection between two structures)

- fracture of the skull base

- giant-cell bone tumor

- **neurofibroma** (tumor of nerve fibers and connective tissue)

  neurofibroma (nū-rō-fī-brō′-mă)

- orbital tumor

- pituitary tumor

Review the procedures in this category, and refer to Table 30-8 for definitions of common terms. Did you notice that there are extensive coding guidelines in this category for you to review before assigning codes? The guidelines provide you with detailed information about how CPT categorizes skull base procedures. There are three parts of a skull base procedure, listed as the following subcategories:

1. **Approach procedure (61580–61598)**—The approach procedure is the location where the physician gains access to a lesion in the skull base. Approach procedures are arranged by the location of the skull involved, including the following three areas:

   - anterior cranial fossa—contains the anterior lobe of the brain

   - middle cranial fossa—contains the temporal lobes of the brain

   - posterior cranial fossa—contains the occipital lobes of the brain

   Procedures involving the anterior, middle, and posterior cranial fossa are divided by the type of approach to access the specific part of the cranial fossa, such as craniofacial or infratemporal. Approach procedures can also include other procedures that the physician must perform at the same time, like a **rhinotomy** (incision into the nose).

   rhinotomy (rī-nŏt′-ō-mē)

2. **Definitive procedure (61600–61616)**—After the physician performs the approach procedure, he or another physician performs the definitive procedure, which involves repair, biopsy, resection, or excision of skull base lesions.

transection (trăn-sĕk'-shŭn)—to divide an area by cutting across it

myocutaneous (mī-ō-kū-tān'-ē-ŭs)

CPT arranges definitive procedures by the base of anterior, middle, or posterior cranial fossa and type of approach. Definitive procedures include primary closure of the dura, mucous membranes, and skin. Note the add-on codes for definitive procedures (61609–61612), which include **transection** or ligation of the carotid artery.

3. **Repair/reconstruction procedure (61618–61619)**—This procedure is to repair or reconstruct the dura after a CSF leak. According to CPT guidelines, the physician should only report a repair/reconstruction for extensive dural grafting or skin grafts, cranioplasty, or for local or regional **myocutaneous** pedicle flaps (skin flap with muscle attached). There are only two codes for a repair/reconstruction procedure, 61618 and 61619, which include repair by free tissue graft or repair by pedicle or myocutaneous flap.

To find codes for the *approach* or *definitive* skull base procedure in the index, search under the main term *skull base surgery*, then search for the subterm of the location, including *anterior cranial fossa, middle cranial fossa, or posterior cranial fossa*. Locations are further divided by subterms that identify the type of approach, such as *bicoronal* or *craniofacial*.

To locate a skull base repair/reconstruction procedure, search for the main term *skull base surgery*, subterm *dura*, and subterm *repair of cerebrospinal fluid leak*.

An important point to note in the CPT guidelines for Surgery of Skull Base is that when a separate physician performs each part of a skull base procedure, each physician should report a code for the procedure that he completes. If one physician performs more than one part of a skull base procedure, then he should report a code for each procedure, reporting the most complex procedure first and appending modifier -51 to the lesser procedure(s).

Refer the following example to learn more about coding skull base surgery.

Example: Mr. Nichols, a 45-year-old, arrives unconscious at Williton Medical Center's ED. Dr. Rice is part of a surgical team to treat this emergent case of brain aneurysm. Dr. Rice performs the approach procedure of the anterior cranial fossa, craniofacial approach, extradural, which involves a unilateral craniotomy. Dr. Rice also elevates the frontal lobes and performs an osteotomy of the anterior cranial fossa base.

To code this case, search the index for the main term *skull base surgery*, subterm *anterior cranial fossa*, and subterm *craniofacial approach*, which then directs you to codes 61580–61583. Assign code **61582** because it includes all of the components that Dr. Rice performed in the approach procedure. The diagnosis code is **437.3** (main term *aneurysm*, subterm *brain*).

TAKE A BREAK

Great job! You are doing well! Let's take a break and review more about the skull, meninges, and brain.

Exercise 30.2 Injection, Drainage, or Aspiration, Twist Drill, Burr Hole(s), or Trephine, Craniectomy or Craniotomy, Surgery of Skull Base

Part 1—Theory

Instructions: Fill in the blank with the best answer.

1. A(n) _____ is a procedure where the physician implants electrodes on the brain to record electrical impulses and identify areas to surgically remove to treat epilepsy.

2. The destruction of white matter in the brain to treat chronic pain and mental disorders is called a(n) _____.

3. What is the name of the procedure where the physician incises a cerebral peduncle to stop involuntary body movements? _____

4. A(n) _____ is a procedure where the physician incises a nerve tract found in the brainstem or spinal cord to treat chronic pain.

5. What are the three parts of a skull base procedure? _____

6. A(n) _____ is the withdrawal of CSF through a fontanelle.

TAKE A BREAK *continued*

Part 2—Coding

Instructions: Review the patient's case, and then assign codes for the procedure(s), appending a modifier when appropriate. Optional: For additional practice, assign the patient's diagnosis code(s) (ICD-9-CM).

1. Jennifer Powell, a 23-year-old established patient, has congenital hydrocephalus with a ventricular shunt in place to divert CSF. She recently developed headaches and visual disturbances and Dr. Hill, a neurosurgeon, schedules her for surgery. Today, he punctures the shunt to aspirate the excess CSF, which affords Ms. Powell some relief from the headaches and visual disturbances.

   Diagnosis code(s): _____

   Procedure code(s): _____

2. An ambulance transports, Shelley Moczan, age 22, to Williton Medical Center's ED. She drove into a tree while riding her dirt bike and suffered a severe head injury. She is unconscious. Dr. Mills, the ED physician, examines the patient and orders further workup. He then admits her for a skull fracture with hemorrhage. Dr. Hill, a neurosurgeon, performs emergency surgery, creating multiple burr holes supratentorially to explore for the source of bleeding. Dr. Hill identifies the source of the bleeding and inserts a catheter to close off the hemorrhaging blood vessel.

   Diagnosis code(s): _____

   Procedure code(s): _____

3. 84-year-old Donald Kovak developed a spontaneous subdural hematoma. Dr. Hill meets Mr. Kovak at Williton Medical Center and performs a craniotomy to evacuate the hematoma. Unfortunately, Mr. Kovak does not survive the surgery.

   Diagnosis code(s): _____

   Procedure code(s): _____

4. During an office visit, Dr. Hill diagnoses 48-year-old Sharon Oswald with a primary malignant neoplasm of the cranial fossa. Today, Dr. Hill performs a resection of the posterior cranial fossa, extradural, at Williton Medical Center. His associate, Dr. Walters, also a neurosurgeon, performs the transtemporal approach. Dr. Hill is able to remove the entire tumor. The physicians work as co-surgeons on this case. Assign codes for each physician.

   Diagnosis code(s): _____

   Dr. Hill procedure code(s): _____

   Dr. Walters procedure code(s): _____

5. Today at Williton, Dr. Hill performs a suboccipital craniectomy with incision of the brain stem for Gerald Jones, age 67. He has spasmodic torticollis, a neurological disorder causing involuntary movements of the face, tongue, and left arm.

   Diagnosis code(s): _____

   Procedure code(s): _____

6. Connie Jenkins, age 65, suffers from intractable epilepsy. Today at Williton, Dr. Hill performs a partial hemispherectomy to treat the disorder.

   Diagnosis code(s): _____

   Procedure code(s): _____

ADDITIONAL PROCEDURES FOR THE SKULL, MENINGES, AND BRAIN (61623–62258)

There are other procedures listed under categories for the subsection Skull, Meninges, and Brain with which you will need to be familiar. Categories and their procedures are listed next. Turn to the categories in your CPT manual as you read through the codes and their descriptors, and use Table 30-8 as a reference for definitions of terms that you may not know.

- **Endovascular Therapy (61623–61642)**

  Endovascular therapy involves inserting microcatheters (small catheters) into blood vessels to treat aneurysms, lesions, and neoplasms, including intracranial tumors. Treatment includes inserting balloons and stents into blood vessels or performing embolizations. Recall from Chapter 12 that an embolization is a procedure when the physician purposely inserts an embolus (mass) into an artery to occlude blood flow to a lesion. In endovascular therapy, neurosurgeons work with interventional radiologists to coordinate the patient's treatment and care.

Depending on the type of procedure the physician performs, you can locate codes for endovascular therapy in the index under the following main terms: *endovascular therapy* (subterm *occlusion*), *cerebral vessels* (subterm *angioplasty*), *placement* (subterm *intravascular stent*), and *cerebral vessels* (subterm *dilation*).

- **Surgery for Aneurysm, Arteriovenous Malformation, or Vascular Disease (61680–61711)**

Recall that an aneurysm is excessive blood vessel dilation, which could lead to a ruptured blood vessel or vein, and an *arteriovenous malformation (AVM)* is an abnormal connection between arteries and veins. **Vascular disease** is a broad term that describes various circulatory system diseases, such as peripheral artery disease, that inhibit the ability of blood and lymph vessels to properly circulate blood or lymph.

CPT arranges procedures in this category by treatment for an aneurysm, AVM, or vascular malformation, the type of approach (intracranial, cervical), and whether the procedure is *simple* or *complex.*

Note that there is a CPT note following code 61698 to alert you that codes 61697 and 61698 include aneurysms that are larger than 15 mm. The note also provides additional information about the aneurysm, which you need to review before assigning one of the two codes. Also note that code 61711 is the only code in this category that represents anastomosis of arteries. You should also report code 69990 (Operating Microscope) separately when the physician uses an operating microscope during microsurgery.

To locate codes in the index for these procedures, search for the main terms *aneurysm repair, arteriovenous malformation,* or *anastomosis.*

- **Stereotaxis (61720–61791)**

Stereotaxis involves the use of a computer and radiation to locate specific areas of the body in order to perform specific procedures, such as creating a burr hole, performing a biopsy, performing aspiration, excising a lesion, implanting electrodes to monitor seizures, and placing radiation sources to treat neoplasms. To locate codes for stereotaxis, search under the main term *stereotaxis.*

- **Stereotactic Radiosurgery (Cranial) (61796–61800)**

The Stereotactic Radiosurgery category has extensive coding guidelines that you should review before assigning codes. The surgery uses ionizing radiation to target lesions in the head without making any incision and without affecting surrounding tissue.

A headframe application is when the physician uses pins to attach a stereotactic frame to the patient's head to help direct the radiation treatment. The patient also receives imaging, such as an MRI, CT scan, or angiography, before receiving radiation so that the surgeon can identify the target area(s) before delivering radiation.

CPT arranges radiosurgical procedures according to whether the lesion is single or additional, simple or complex. The application of a stereotactic headframe is a separate procedure (add-on code 61800). To find stereotactic radiosurgical procedures, search the index for the main term *stereotaxis,* subterm *focus beam,* and subterm *radiosurgery.*

- **Neurostimulators (Intracranial) (61850–61888)**

This category includes deep brain stimulator (neurostimulator) implantation. Deep brain stimulation (DBS) is when the physician implants electrodes into the patient's brain to provide electrical stimulation to specific locations in the brain (■ FIGURE 30-10). DBS can reduce or eliminate involuntary movements in patients with Parkinson's disease, essential tremor (hand tremors), **dystonia** (repeated muscle contractions), or **torticollis** (rotation and tilting of neck muscles).

- Codes include twist drill, burr hole, craniectomy, or craniotomy for implanting electrodes and are arranged by cortical or subcortical site of implantation.

- Codes also include revision or removal of intracranial neurostimulator electrodes or pulse generator or receiver (61880, 61888) and insertion or replacement of cranial neurostimulator pulse generator or receiver (61885–61886).

dystonia (dis-tō´-nē-ă)

torticollis (tor-tĭ-kōl´-ĭs)

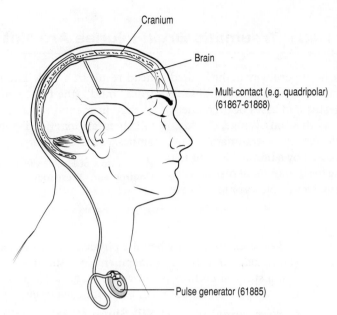

Figure 30-10 ■ Placement of cranial neurostimulator.

Source: From *CPT® Professional Edition*, 2011. Reprinted by permission of American Medical Association.

Cranium

Brain

Multi-contact (e.g. quadripolar) (61867-61868)

Pulse generator (61885)

- Assign HCPCS codes for the implanted device.
- According to CPT guidelines, when a separate physician participates in **neurophysiological mapping** during a DBS implantation procedure, the separate physician should report the following codes:
  - **95961**—Functional cortical and subcortical mapping by stimulation and/or recording of electrodes on brain surface, or of depth electrodes, to provoke seizures or identify vital brain structures; initial hour of physician attendance.
  - **95962**—Functional cortical and subcortical mapping by stimulation and/or recording of electrodes on brain surface, or of depth electrodes, to provoke seizures or identify vital brain structures; each additional hour of physician attendance. (List separately in addition to code for primary procedure).

neurophysiological mapping (nū-rō-fĭz-ē-ō-lŏ′-jĭk-əl)—the use of intraoperative stimulation during brain surgery to identify critical motor pathways, the nerve structures that receive and relay impulses between the central nervous system and the organs and muscles

To locate various procedures involving neurostimulators, search the index for the main term *neurostimulators*, main term *implantation* (subterm *electrode* or subterm *neurostimulators*), or main term *brain* (subterm *removal*, subterm *pulse generator*).

- **Repair (62000–62148)**

  CPT arranges codes in the repair category by type of procedure, including

  - elevation of a depressed skull fracture (fracture where the bone pushes into the brain)
  - craniotomy to repair a CSF leak or encephalocele
  - **cranioplasty** (cranium repair) to repair a skull defect
  - reduction of craniomegalic skull
  - repair of encephalocele
  - removal or replacement of a bone flap or prosthetic plate of the skull
  - incision and retrieval of subcutaneous bone graft for cranioplasty

cranioplasty (krā′-nē-ō-plās-tē)

  To locate codes in this category, search under the main term *skull* in the index, and then search for the subterm of the name of the procedure, or search for fracture.

- **Neuroendoscopy (62160–62165)**

  Neuroendoscopy involves using an endoscope to visualize the CNS and dissect adhesions, remove foreign bodies, and excise tumors. Note that code 62160 is an

neuroendoscopy (nū-rō-ĕn-dŏs′-kō-pē)

TBI is a serious public health problem in the United States. Each year, traumatic brain injuries contribute to a substantial number of deaths and cases of permanent disability. Recent data shows that, on average, approximately 1.7 million people sustain a traumatic brain injury annually. A TBI is caused by a bump, blow, or jolt to the head or a penetrating head injury that disrupts the normal function of the brain. Not all blows or jolts to the head result in a TBI. The severity of a TBI may range from "mild" (the most common type), which is a brief change in mental status or consciousness, to "severe," which is an extended period of unconsciousness or amnesia after the injury.

(Department of Health and Human Services, Centers for Disease Control and Prevention, www.cdc.gov/TraumaticBrainInjury/, accessed 5/29/11.)

add-on code to report when the physician uses neuroendoscopy to place or replace a ventricular catheter and attachment to a shunt system or external drainage. Recall that a surgical endoscopy always includes a diagnostic endoscopy. Locate codes for this category under the main term *neuroendoscopy*.

- **Cerebrospinal Fluid (CSF) Shunt (62180–62258)**

Recall that a shunt is a device that includes a catheter (tube) that transports fluid from one area of the body to another. The purpose of a CSF shunt is to drain CSF from one area of the body into another (such as from the ventricles to the peritoneum). Recall that CSF is present in the brain and spinal cord. A brain tumor or aneurysm, traumatic brain injury (TBI), interventricular hemorrhage, and hydrocephalus are all conditions that can cause excess CSF to build up in the brain.

Procedures in this category include creating, removing, or reprogramming a shunt and replacing or irrigating a catheter. To locate codes, search under the main term *cerebrospinal fluid shunt*.

Refer the following example to learn more about coding additional procedures involving the skull, meninges, and brain.

> **Example:** Dr. Rice inserts a ventriculoperitoneal CSF shunt for Mr. Knight, a 19-year-old patient at Williton Medical Center, to treat excess CSF that viral meningitis caused.
>
> To code this case, search the index for the main term *cerebrospinal fluid shunt* and subterm *creation*, which then directs you to two code ranges: 62180–62192 and 62220–62223. Assign code **62223** because it represents a ventriculoperitoneal shunt. The diagnosis code is **047.9** (main term *meningitis*, subterm *viral*). Now, you try coding the following cases.

TAKE A BREAK

Wow! Keep up the good work! Let's take a break and practice assigning codes for procedures of the skull, meninges, and brain.

Exercise 30.3 Additional Procedures for the Skull, Meninges, and Brain

Instructions: Review each patient's case, and then assign codes for the procedure(s), appending a modifier when appropriate. Optional: For additional practice, assign the patient's diagnosis code(s) (ICD-9-CM).

1. Jennifer Peters, age 27, arrives by ambulance at Williton's ED. Her brother accompanies her. He reports that Ms. Peters fell at home and struck her head on the bathtub. Dr. Mills assesses the patient and after

TAKE A BREAK *continued*

exam and workup, discusses her case with Dr. Hill and the patient's brother. Dr. Mills admits Ms. Peters, and Dr. Hill performs an elevation of a depressed skull fracture with repair of dura. The patient lost consciousness for two hours. Code for Dr. Hill's services.

Diagnosis code(s): _____

Procedure code(s): _____

2. Ray Ransom, 37-years-old, suffers from trigeminal neuropathic pain that has not responded to conservative treatment. Today at Williton, Dr. Hill implants cortical neurostimulator electrodes through a burr hole to help alleviate the pain. Mr. Ransom later reported to Dr. Hill that his pain was relieved.

Diagnosis code(s): _____

Procedure code(s): _____

3. At Williton, Dr. Hill performs a percutaneous balloon dilatation of an intracranial cerebral artery **vasospasm**, a blood vessel spasm leading to constriction, for Frank Angeles, age 78. The surgery is a success; circulation is restored to the ischemic area.

Diagnosis code(s): _____

Procedure code(s): _____

4. Ben Snare, age 18, suffers from temporal lobe epilepsy. Dr. Hill schedules him for surgery at Williton. Today, Dr. Hill stereotactically implants depth electrodes into Mr. Snare's cerebrum for long-term seizure monitoring to try to determine the site of origin. Unfortunately Dr. Hill is not able to establish a definitive site.

Diagnosis code(s): _____

Procedure code(s): _____

5. James Jacobs, age 61, has a 14-mm arteriosclerotic brain aneurysm in the frontal portion of his skull. Dr. Hill performs surgery at Williton to remove the aneurysm by intracranial and cervical occlusion of the carotid artery.

Diagnosis code(s): _____

Procedure code(s): _____

6. Beatrice Fowler, 87-years-old, has cerebral meninges adhesions. Adhesions are bands of fibrous tissue that connect two parts of tissue together that should remain separate. They form in response to trauma or infection as the body attempts to repair itself. Dr. Hill performs an intracranial neuroendoscopy at Williton to dissect the adhesions.

Diagnosis code(s): _____

Procedure code(s): _____

SPINE AND SPINAL CORD (62263–63746)

The subheading Spine and Spinal Cord contains 14 different categories of codes. Refer to ■ TABLE 30-10 for a summary of categories and the procedures listed in each, including definitions of procedures you may not know and explanations of how CPT arranges the codes in each category, including an *anterior* (front) or *posterior* (back) approach. Index entries are also listed to help you locate codes for procedures in specific categories. You should also refer to Table 30-8 to become more familiar with terms you will find in this subheading. It is also important to review any coding guidelines that you find in these categories to better understand how to assign the codes.

As you read through the procedures included in categories of the Spine and Spinal Cord, refer to Figure 30-7, which you reviewed earlier in this chapter. Notice how the vertebrae are identified by a letter, representing the first letter of the vertebrae location—**C**ervical, **T**horacic, **L**umbar, **S**acral—and a number, identifying an individual vertebra, listed in ascending order as the vertebrae move down the spine (C1–C8, T1–T12, L1–L5, S1–S5). These letters and numbers identify the vertebrae involved in procedures, and physicians include them in their documentation. Use Figure 30-7 as a guide to better understand code descriptors that identify procedure locations, such as cervical or lumbar.

lysis (lī'-sĭs)

intervertebral (int-ər-'vərt-ə-brəl)

spondylolisthesis (spŏn-dĭ-lō-lĭs-thē'-səs)—condition in which a vertebrae slips forward or backward onto the vertebrae below it

facetectomy (făs-ĕt-ĕk'-tō-mē)

spinal stenosis (spīn'-əl stĕ-nō'-sĭs)—narrowing of the spinal column

cervical myelopathy (sĕr'-vĭ-kăl mī-ĕ-lŏp'-ă-thē)—gradual loss of nerve function due to pathology of the cervical spine, which may result from a viral process, degeneration, an inflammatory process, an autoimmune response, or trauma

■ **TABLE 30-10   SPINE AND SPINAL CORD CATEGORIES AND PROCEDURES**

Category Name	Code Range	Examples of Procedures	How Procedures Are Arranged
Injection, Drainage, or Aspiration	62263–62319	• Percutaneous **lysis** (*destruction*) of epidural adhesions • Percutaneous aspiration within the **intervertebral** disc (*fibrous tissue/cartilage between vertebrae that allows movement*) • Biopsy of spinal cord, typically performed to diagnose neoplasm behavior • Spinal puncture, lumbar, diagnostic or therapeutic (*Also called a spinal tap. The physician inserts a needle into the lumbar (lower) area of the back to collect a sample of CSF to diagnose conditions, including infections. CSF is normally clear, so if it is another color, like yellow, orange, or pink, it indicates an abnormality.*) • Epidural injection of blood or clot patch (*Recall that a blood patch relieves headache pain that a lumbar puncture caused.*) • Decompression procedure (*Procedure to remove a disc, disc bulges, or bone spurs to relieve pressure on the nerve roots and restore normal spacing between vertebrae.*) **Index entries:** type of procedure (percutaneous lysis), vertebra, or spinal cord	Type of procedure
Catheter Implantation	62350–62355	• Implantation, revision, or repositioning of tunneled intrathecal or epidural catheter for long-term medication administration • Removal of intrathecal or epidural catheter **Index entries:** pain management, spinal cord	Type of procedure
Reservoir/Pump Implantation	62360–62368	• Implantation, replacement, or removal of subcutaneous reservoir or pump for intrathecal or epidural drug infusion • Electronic analysis of programmable implanted pump for intrathecal or epidural drug infusion **Index entries:** pain management, infusion pump	Type of procedure, location (e.g., cervical, thoracic, lumbar, sacral), condition (**spondylolisthesis**)
Posterior Extradural Laminotomy or Laminectomy for Exploration/ Decompression of Neural Elements or Excision of Herniated Intervertebral Discs	63001–63051	• Laminectomy • Laminotomy (incision of the lamina) • Decompression of spinal cord and/or cauda equina • Decompression of nerve root • **Facetectomy** (*excision of the vertebral facet, the connection between vertebrae*) • Excision of a herniated intervertebral disc (*when the fluid inside the disc leaks out, causing bulging; aging and spinal injuries can cause herniated discs*) **Index entries:** type of procedure (laminectomy, excision), spinal cord, intervertebral disc	Type of procedure, location
Transpedicular or Costovertebral Approach for Posterolateral Extradural Exploration/ Decompression	63055–63066	• Decompression of spinal cord, cauda equina, or nerve root **Index entries:** excision, nerve root	Type of approach, location, segment
Anterior or Anterolateral Approach for Extradural Exploration/ Decompression	63075–63091	• Discectomy (*partial or complete removal of an intervertebral disc, such as for a herniated disc*) • Decompression of spinal cord, cauda equina, or nerve root • Osteophytectomy (*excision of osteophytes, bony growths on the vertebrae*)	Type of procedure, location, approach, interspace, segment

■ TABLE 30-10   *continued*

Category Name	Code Range	Examples of Procedures	How Procedures Are Arranged
		• Vertebral corpectomy (*excision of vertebra and vertebral disc to eliminate spinal cord pressure in patients with* **spinal stenosis** *or* **cervical myelopathy**) **Index entries:** type of procedure (decompression), intervertebral disc, vertebral	
Lateral Extracavitary Approach for Extradural Exploration/ Decompression	63101–63103	• Vertebral corpectomy **Index entries:** corpectomy, decompression	Type of procedure, approach, location, segment
Incision	63170–63200	• Laminectomy • Myelotomy (*incision of spinal cord nerve fibers to relieve bilateral pain*) • Cordotomy (*incision of spinal cord nerves to relieve pain; can be performed with a needle, or open, which also includes a laminectomy*) **Index entries:** type of procedure (incision, laminectomy), spinal cord, spinal column	Type of procedure, location, segment, stage
Excision by Laminectomy of Lesion in Other than Herniated Disc	63250–63295	• Laminectomy for excision of lesion, AVM, or neoplasm, biopsy • **Osteoplastic** reconstruction of dorsal spinal elements **Index entries:** type of procedure (laminectomy), condition (AVM)	Type of procedure, condition, location
Excision, Anterior or Anterolateral Approach, Intraspinal Lesion	63300–63308	• Vertebral corpectomy to excise intraspinal lesion **Index entry:** vertebral	Type of procedure, location, segment
Stereotaxis	63600–63615	• Stereotaxis to create lesion • Stereotactic stimulation of spinal cord • Stereotactic biopsy **Index entry:** spinal cord	Type of procedure
Stereotactic Radiosurgery (Spinal)	63620–63621	• Stereotactic radiosurgery for targeting one or more lesions **Index entry:** spinal cord	Type of procedure, number of lesions
Neurostimulators (Spinal)	63650–63688	• Implantation of epidural neurostimulator electrode array • Removal or revision of spinal neurostimulator electrode arrays, plates/paddles • Insertion, replacement, revision, or removal of spinal neurostimulator pulse generator or receiver *Spinal neurostimulators* send electrical impulses in the spine to eliminate **intractable** pain. **Index entries:** type of procedure (implantation), spinal cord	Type of procedure, location, electrode array, pulse generator or receiver
Repair	63700–63710	• Repair of meningocele, myelomeningocele, CSF leak • Dural graft, spinal (*to repair dural defect*) **Index entries:** repair, meningocele, myelomeningocele, spinal cord	Type of procedure, repair size, and other procedures performed at the same time
Shunt, Spinal CSF	63740–63746	• Creation, replacement, removal, irrigation or revision of shunt **Index entries:** cerebrospinal fluid shunt, shunt(s)	Type of procedure, location

osteoplastic (ŏs-tē-ō-plăs´-tĭk)—pertaining to osteoplasty; the repair of a bone

intractable (ĭn-trăk´-tă-b´l)—persisting in spite of therapy (medications, treatments)

claudication (klaw-dĭ-kā´-shŭn)

radicular (ră-dĭ´-kū-lăr)—pain that starts at the nerve root and travels along the nerve

Refer to the following example to learn more about coding procedures involving the spine and spinal cord.

Example: Dr. Hawkins, a pediatric neurosurgeon, repairs a 3.5-cm myelomeningocele for Jean Stone, a newborn at Williton Medical Center, who has cervical spina bifida (a congenital disorder where vertebra do not completely form). After the procedure, the infant is transferred to the neonatal intensive care unit (NICU).

To code this case, search the index for the main term *myelomeningocele*, which then directs you to codes 63704 and 63706. Assign code **63704** because the myelomeningocele was less than 5 cm. The diagnosis code is **741.91** (main term *spina bifida, cervical region*). Now, you try coding the following cases.

TAKE A BREAK

That was a lot of information to remember! Let's take a break and practice assigning codes for procedures involving the spine and spinal cord.

Exercise 30.4 Spine and Spinal Cord

Instructions: Review each patient's case, and then assign codes for the procedure(s), appending a modifier when appropriate. Optional: For additional practice, assign the patient's diagnosis code(s) (ICD-9-CM).

1. Lou Berkibile, age 52, suffers from lumbar spinal stenosis with neurogenic **claudication** (not enough blood flow to blood vessels in the legs or arms, causing pain when walking or exercising). Today at Williton, Dr. Hill implants a tunneled epidural catheter for administration of pain management medication with a laminectomy.

   Diagnosis code(s): _____

   Procedure code(s): _____

2. Debbie Plavok, age 30, has recently experienced pain, numbness, and weakness in her spine. She sees Dr. Hill in his office. After examining her, he orders radiology tests, and Williton's Radiology Department technicians perform them. Dr. Hill reviews the test results and diagnoses Ms. Plavok with nerve root compression of the cervical spine. He calls her to discuss his findings and schedules her for surgery. Today, Dr. Hill performs a cervical neck discectomy on two interspaces to treat the patient's condition. Code for today's surgery.

   Diagnosis code(s): _____

   Procedure code(s): _____

3. Kristy Farisio, age 25, experiences back pain and weakness, and Dr. Hill determines that she has a lesion on her spinal cord. Today, he performs a stereotactic biopsy of the spinal cord lesion. He sends the biopsy to Williton's pathology department for analysis.

   Diagnosis code(s): _____

   Procedure code(s): _____

4. Emma Thorton brings her 10-day-old son, Bobby, to Williton's ED after he develops a fever of 103.2°. The ED physician, Dr. Mills, fails to determine a cause for the fever during his preliminary investigation. The doctor decides to perform a diagnostic lumbar puncture (spinal tap) to rule out meningitis. He sends the CSF sample to the hospital's lab for testing. Lab tests show that the patient does not have meningitis, so Dr. Mills admits him to observation for additional work-up. Assign the code for the lumbar puncture.

   Diagnosis code(s): _____

   Procedure code(s): _____

5. Today at Williton, Dr. Hill performs a thoracic epidural spinal injection of a neurolytic substance, a chemical agent that is used to destroy neural structures involved in the perception of pain, for Ronald James, age 42, who has **radicular** and **visceral** thoracic pain.

   Diagnosis code(s): _____

   Procedure code(s): _____

6. Norma Owens, age 62, suffers from degenerative spondylolisthesis and has exhausted all other treatment options. Dr. Hill performs a Gill **laminectomy** (type of laminectomy that involves a facetectomy) with decompression of lumbar nerve roots.

   Diagnosis code(s): _____

   Procedure code(s): _____

POINTERS FROM THE PROS: Interview with a Chiropractor

You were introduced to Dr. Mock in Chapter 23. He owned a chiropractic medicine and rehabilitation center and now teaches full time. Dr. Mock has more valuable pointers to share with you.

Describe the frequency and types of communication that you had with coders and billing staff.

We had a daily staff meeting in the morning. We would review issues that arose the day before. We also had a weekly production meeting where we would review what was billed and collected. We would check our aging reports (financial report showing how old accounts are that still have not been paid) to see the status of our collections both from insurance companies and private payers.

Did coders and/or billing staff keep you abreast of insurance billing and coding regulatory updates, or did you have to research this information yourself?

Due to the fact my office only had one doctor, we were constantly trying to stay on top of billing and coding changes. I was a member of my state association, and they sent out monthly newsletters with billing and coding updates. My coder would attend at least two weekend seminars per year just to stay ahead of the changes and current issues our field was having with particular insurance carriers.

What advice can you give to coders and billing staff to help them successfully communicate with clinicians?

"Know the talk." As a doctor, it is impossible to work with a coder who isn't able to read your documentation and (know) what "spondylolisthesis in conjunction with osteophytosis at L4/L5 and radiculopathy symptoms into the right lower extremity" is and how to code it.

What should a coding student do to prepare to work successfully in the healthcare field?

Start by understanding the importance of their job. Without excellent coding and collections, the entire doctor's office could be out of business within a few short months. There is always a demand for good coders. To be good takes a lot of effort from the first day of coding class.

(Used by permission of Dr. Bryan R. Mock.)

EXTRACRANIAL NERVES, PERIPHERAL NERVES, AND AUTONOMIC NERVOUS SYSTEM (64400–64999)

The last subheading under the Nervous System section is Extracranial Nerves, Peripheral Nerves, and Autonomic Nervous System. It contains nine different categories of codes. Be sure to review the coding guidelines for these categories to ensure that you understand how to assign the codes. Refer to ■ TABLE 30-11 for a summary of categories and the procedures listed in each, including definitions of procedures you may not know and explanations of how CPT arranges the codes in each category. Index entries are also listed to help you locate codes for procedures in specific categories.

You should also refer to Table 30-8 to become more familiar with terms you will find in this subheading, and refer to anatomy diagrams of the nerves, which you can find at the beginning of this chapter (Figures 30-2, 30-6, and 30-7). It is also very helpful to use anatomy references, including books and Internet searches, if you need further clarification.

Refer to the following example to learn more about coding other procedures involving the nerves.

visceral (vĭs′-ĕr-ăl)—pertaining to the internal organs (viscera)

laminectomy (lăm-ĭ-nĕk′-tō-mē)—surgical excision of a vertebral posterior arch

chemodenervation (kē-mō-dē-nur-vā′-shŭn)

neurolemmoma (nū-rō-lĕ-mō′-mă)

sympathectomy (sĭm-pă-thĕk′-tō-mē)

hyperhidrosis (hī-pŭr-hī-drō′-sĭs)

neurorrhaphy (nū-rŏr′-ă-fē)

Example: Dr. Rice excises a neuroma from the **sciatic** nerve (longest nerve in the body, running down the lower back into the limbs) for Mr. Rose, a 52-year-old patient at Williton Medical Center.

To code this case, search the index for the main term *sciatic nerve*, subterm *lesion*, and subterm *excision*, which then directs you to code 64786. Assign code **64786** because it represents the procedure that Dr. Rice performed. The diagnosis code is **171.3** (main term *neoplasm*, subterm *nerve*, subterm *sciatic, malignant primary*).

sciatic (sī-ăt′-ĭk)

■ **TABLE 30-11   PROCEDURES FOR EXTRACRANIAL AND PERIPHERAL NERVES, AND AUTONOMIC NERVOUS SYSTEM**

Category Name	Code Range	Examples of Procedures	How Procedures Are Arranged
Introduction/Injection of Anesthetic Agent (Nerve Block), Diagnostic or Therapeutic	64400–64530	• Nerve blocks—*Some procedures include imaging guidance (fluoroscopy, CT). Recall that therapeutic nerve blocks treat chronic pain in various locations. A diagnostic nerve block is done to determine the origin of pain by numbing it before administering further treatment.*	Nerve location, imaging guidance performed
		Index entry: nerves	
Neurostimulators (Peripheral Nerve)	64550–64595	• Application of surface neurostimulator	Type of procedure
		• Implantation of neurostimulator electrodes	
		• Neurostimulation, single treatment	
		• Incision for implantation, revision, replacement, removal of neurostimulator electrode array and pulse generator	
		• Incision for implantation, revision, removal of neurostimulator electrodes	
		• Insertion, replacement, revision, removal of neurostimulator pulse generator or receiver	
		Index entries: nerves, neurostimulators	
Destruction by Neurolytic Agent (e.g., Chemical, Thermal, Electrical or Radiofrequency)	64600–64681	• Nerve destruction by neurolytic agent (*type of anesthesia injected in or near nerves, eliminating pain*)	Type of procedure, location
		• **Chemodenervation** of muscles or glands (*injection of a substance, such as botulinum toxin, into a muscle group to stop contractions or spasms, or into glands to stop overproduction, such as excess sweat production*) Report chemodenervation once for one or more injections into the same site.	
		Index entries: destruction, chemodenervation, type of nerve or gland	
Neuroplasty (Exploration, Neurolysis, or Nerve Decompression)	64702–64727	• Neuroplasty (*lysis of nerve scar tissue caused by spinal injury or postsurgical complications*)	Type of procedure, type of nerve(s)
		• Decompression	
		Index entries: neuroplasty, type of nerve(s) (brachial plexus)	
Transection or Avulsion	64732–64772	• Transection (*incision to divide*) of nerves	Type of procedure, type of nerve(s)
		Index entries: type of nerve(s) (phrenic), transection	
Excision	64774–64823	• Excision, implantation, or biopsy of a nerve	Type of procedure, type of nerve(s), number of nerves
		• Excision of neurofibroma (*benign neoplasm of the peripheral nerve*) or **neurolemmoma** (*benign neoplasm of the peripheral nerve sheath*)	
		• **Sympathectomy** (*destruction of sympathetic nerves; commonly performed for patients with pain*) **hyperhidrosis**—*excess palm sweating*—*or axillary* hyperhidrosis—*excess armpit sweating*	
		Index entries: excision, sympathectomy, nerves, neuroma	
Neurorrhaphy	64831–64876	• **Neurorrhaphy** (*suture or anastomosis of nerves*)	Type of procedure, type of nerve(s), number of nerves
		Index entries: neurorrhaphy, suture, type of nerve(s) (tibial)	

■ **TABLE 30-11**   *continued*

Category Name	Code Range	Examples of Procedures	How Procedures Are Arranged
Neurorrhaphy With Nerve Graft, Vein Graft, or Conduit	64885–64911	• Nerve graft, vein graft, conduit (*type of nerve reconstruction using an artificial tube or passageway to fill a nerve gap and promote regrowth*) • Nerve pedicle transfer • Nerve repair **Index entries:** neurorrhaphy, repair, location (neck)	Type of repair, length of repair, location, stage
Other Procedures	64999	• Unlisted procedure, nervous system **Index entry:** unlisted services and procedures	Unlisted procedure

TAKE A BREAK

You made it through the last subheading of codes for the Nervous System! Way to go! Let's take a break and then review more about procedures involving the nerves.

Exercise 30.5   Extracranial Nerves, Peripheral Nerves, and Autonomic Nervous System

Part 1—Theory

Instructions: Fill in the blank with the best answer.

1. A nerve graft, vein graft, or conduit is a type of nerve reconstruction using a(n) _____ or passageway to fill a nerve gap and promote regrowth.

2. A(n) _____ is a type of anesthesia injected in or near nerves, eliminating pain.

3. A(n) _____ is a benign neoplasm of the peripheral nerve, and a(n) _____ is a benign neoplasm of the peripheral nerve sheath.

4. _____ of muscles or glands is the injection of a substance, such as botulinum toxin, into a muscle group to stop contractions or spasms, or into glands to stop overproduction, such as excess sweat production.

5. What is the name of the procedure that destroys sympathetic nerves, commonly performed for patients with pain? _____

6. What is the name of the procedure where the physician divides nerves with incisions? _____

Part 2—Coding

Instructions: Review each patient's case, and then assign codes for the procedure(s), appending a modifier when appropriate. Optional: For additional practice, assign the patient's diagnosis code(s) (ICD-9-CM).

1. Jeff Murphy, age 54, suffers from sciatic pain. Dr. Hill sees Mr. Murphy in his office and administers a therapeutic anesthetic injection of the sciatic nerve.

   Diagnosis code(s): _____

   Procedure code(s): _____

2. An aggressive dachshund bites Nancy Watson, age 50, and she sustains wounds to the fingers of her right hand. She drives herself to Williton's ED, where Dr. Mills determines that she requires surgery to repair two damaged digital nerves. A registered nurse in the ED contacts local police to report the incident. Dr. Hill performs neurorrhaphy to the right thumb and index finger. Code for Dr. Hill's services.

   Diagnosis code(s): _____

   Procedure code(s): _____

3. Charlotte Finn, age 36, develops a neuroma in her left fifth toe. Dr. Hill excises the neuroma in his office.

   Diagnosis code(s): _____

   Procedure code(s): _____

4. Janet Withers, age 72, develops a **blepharospasm** (a spasm of the orbicularis oculi muscle due to eye strain, irritation, and sometimes anxiety). After discussion with Dr. Hill, the patient decides to proceed with surgery. Dr. Hill performs a chemodenervation of the muscle today at Williton.

   Diagnosis code(s): _____

   Procedure code(s): _____

continued

TAKE A BREAK *continued*

5. At his office, Dr. Hill excises a neurofibroma of the femoral nerve for David Pickens, age 45.

Diagnosis code(s): _____

Procedure code(s): _____

6. Jamar Benson, age 17, sustained an injury to his right ulnar nerve from broken glass. He presents to Dr. Hill's office and Dr. Hill sutures the nerve.

Diagnosis code(s): _____

Procedure code(s): _____

WORKPLACE IQ

You are working as a medical coder for Dr. Rice, a neurosurgeon. Today, the office manager, Cheryl, asks you to help a new coder, Rachel, to understand skull base surgical procedures, specifically to explain the three parts of a procedure and when to append modifier -51.

What would you do?

blepharospasm ('blef-ə-rō-spaz-əm)

DESTINATION: MEDICARE

This Medicare exercise will help you to find additional information about deep brain stimulation. Follow the instructions listed next to access Chapter 32 of the Medicare Claims Processing Manual—Billing Requirements for Special Services:

1. Go to the website http://www.cms.gov.
2. At the top of the screen on the banner bar, choose *Regulations and Guidance.*
3. Under *Guidance,* choose *Manuals.*
4. On the left side of the screen, under Manuals, choose *Internet-Only Manuals (IOMs).*
5. Scroll down to Publication *100-04 Medicare Claims Processing Manual,* and click *100-04.*
6. Scroll down to the list of Downloads, and choose *Ch. 32 - Sect. 69 - Medicare Claims Processing Manual.*

Answer the following questions, using the search function (Ctrl + F) to find information that you need.

1. What are the three targets, or body locations, for DBS?
2. Does Medicare cover DBS for essential tremor (ET) or Parkinson's Disease (PD) patients with structural lesions, which caused the movement disorder?
3. Does Medicare allow an Ambulatory Surgical Center (ASC) to report neurostimulator codes 61885 and 61886?
4. Will Medicare reimburse an ASC for implantation of electrodes and a pulse generator?

CHAPTER REVIEW

Multiple Choice

Instructions: Circle one best answer to complete each statement.

1. The endocrine system subsection of CPT contains codes for procedures performed on
   a. all of the endocrine glands.
   b. the endocrine glands that regulate male and female sexual characteristics.
   c. the thyroid, parathyroid, thymus, adrenal glands, pancreas, and carotid body.
   d. the pituitary gland and the pineal gland.

2. The carotid body is a small tissue mass that contains cells that
   a. monitor oxygen and carbon dioxide levels in the blood.
   b. develop when there is a disruption in hormone levels.
   c. secrete hormones that control ovulation.
   d. are part of the circulatory system.

3. Endocrine secretions include
   a. sweat and saliva.
   b. hormones.
   c. urine.
   d. cerebrospinal fluid.

4. The somatic nervous system controls
   a. the heart, organs, and glands.
   b. movement of the skeletal muscles.
   c. involuntary body movements.
   d. digestion.

5. The nerve pairs in the spinal column are named after
   a. the physician who originally documented them
   b. the area of the vertebrae where they are located.
   c. the portion of the brain that controls them.
   d. the functions of the nervous system.

6. CPT codes for spinal injections to control pain are classified according to
   a. the source of the pain.
   b. the site of the injection.
   c. the substance injected.
   d. answers b and c.

7. An epidural blood patch is used to
   a. implant a catheter for long-term medication administration.
   b. decompress a nerve root.
   c. relieve symptoms caused by meningitis.
   d. relieve headache pain caused by a lumbar puncture.

8. Disorders such as Bell's palsy and carpal tunnel syndrome are classified as
   a. orthopedic conditions.
   b. disorders of the circulatory system.
   c. disorders of the peripheral nervous system.
   d. central nervous system conditions.

9. The parietal lobe of the brain is part of the
   a. cerebellum.
   b. cerebrum.
   c. brain stem.
   d. arbor vitae.

10. After a craniotomy or craniectomy is performed, the physician may use a bone graft to repair the defect, and the graft is
   a. considered part of the craniotomy procedure.
   b. assigned a separate code to describe the procedure.
   c. performed by a different physician.
   d. carried out during a separate surgical procedure.

Coding Assignments

Instructions: Assign procedure code(s) for the following cases, and append modifiers when appropriate. Optional: For additional practice, assign the patient's diagnosis code(s).

1. Dr. Hill is treating Milton Herbert, age 65, for back pain. Mr. Herbert's myelogram revealed a displaced thoracic disc with myelopathy (a **myelogram** is an X-ray of the spinal canal after the injection of a radiopaque dye, which enhances body structures on X-ray images). Today at Williton, Dr. Hill performs a laminectomy with surgical decompression to treat the patient's condition.

   Diagnosis code(s): _____

   Procedure code(s): _____

2. Millicent Wick, age 90, has significant degenerative disc disease at L1-L2 and spondylolisthesis at L4-L5. Due to increasing back pain radiating down her left leg, she is having lumbar epidural steroid injections performed by Dr. Hill at his office.

   Diagnosis code(s): _____

   Procedure code(s): _____

myelogram (ˈmī-ə-lə-gram)

3. Dr. Hill diagnoses Joseph Norton, age 74, with stenosis at the L4-L5 and foraminal stenosis at the L5-S1. Dr. Hill performs a hemillaminectomy for each interspace at Williton.

   Diagnosis code(s): _____

   Procedure code(s): _____

4. Dennis Crum, age 67, suffers from cervicocranial syndrome, a condition caused by the misalignment of the cranial bones and/or cervical spine. It often causes dizziness, facial pain, and sinus pain. Today at Williton, Dr. Hill performs surgery on Mr. Crum by implanting electrodes for an occipital nerve stimulator using percutaneous leads.

   Diagnosis code(s): _____

   Procedure code(s): _____

5. Following a motor sensory nerve conduction test Dr. Hill performed in his office on Andrew Casey, age 23, he concludes that the patient suffers from acute radial nerve palsy. He will meet with Mr. Casey next week to discuss his treatment options.

   Diagnosis code(s): _____

   Procedure code(s): _____

6. Kathy Miller, age 35, recently developed left-sided hemiparesis. Dr. Snub, her family physician, diagnoses her with myasthenia gravis. Her surgeon, Dr. Hill, performs a total thymectomy by transcervical approach at Williton.

   Diagnosis code(s): _____

   Procedure code(s): _____

7. After lab and radiology tests, Dr. Hill diagnoses Michael Decker, age 29, with a colloid cyst of the thyroid. Dr. Hill surgically removes the cyst at Williton.

   Diagnosis code(s): _____

   Procedure code(s): _____

8. Dr. Hill reviews radiology tests for Regis Tompkins, age 87, and diagnoses him with an intracranial lesion. He schedules the patient for surgery at Williton, and today Dr. Hill aspirates the lesion stereotactically.

   Diagnosis code(s): _____

   Procedure code(s): _____

9. Marie Main, age 24, sees Dr. Hill in his office to discuss radiology test results. She saw Dr. Hill previously with complaints of intractable headaches. He diagnoses her with a primary malignant bone tumor of the skull and discusses surgical treatment options. Ms. Main decides to proceed with surgery, and today at Williton, Dr. Hill performs a craniectomy and excises the tumor. Code for today's surgery.

   Diagnosis code(s): _____

   Procedure code(s): _____

10. Dorothy Grimley, age 52, has an injection of the paravertebral facet joint at Dr. Hill's office to relieve her chronic neck pain. She later reports to Dr. Hill that the injection relieved her pain.

    Diagnosis code(s): _____

    Procedure code(s): _____

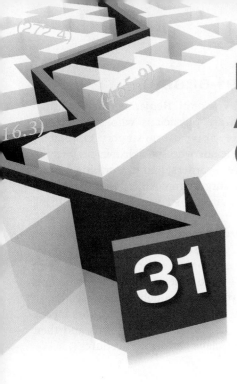

Eye and Ocular Adnexa, Auditory System, and Operating Microscope

31

Learning Objectives

After completing this chapter, you should be able to

- Spell and define the key terminology in this chapter.
- Review the anatomy and functions of the eye.
- Describe procedures performed on the eyeball.
- Discuss the types of procedures listed under the Anterior Segment subheading.
- Explain procedures listed under the subheading of Posterior Segment.
- Review categories and procedures of the Ocular Adnexa.
- Discuss procedures of the conjunctiva.
- Identify the anatomy and functions of the ear.
- Describe procedures of the external ear.
- Identify procedures of the middle ear.
- Discuss procedures of the inner ear.
- Discuss how to code from the subheading Temporal Bone, Middle Fossa Approach.
- Review how to code for the use of an operating microscope.

Key Terms

anterior segment
auditory
external ear
inner ear

middle ear
middle fossa
operating microscope
posterior segment
temporal bone

INTRODUCTION

In Chapter 9, you learned about disorders of the eye and ear and also reviewed eye and ear anatomy. During this stop on your coding journey, you will learn how to code various procedures involving the eye and ear, which will also require you to learn more about the anatomy of both structures so that you understand the procedures that you code. This chapter includes many terms and definitions that you should learn and continue to reference throughout the chapter as you review the procedures in your CPT manual. You will also learn about coding for the operating microscope during microsurgery. Physicians perform many eye and ear procedures in the office or as outpatient procedures at a hospital. This chapter covers the last procedures contained in the Surgery section, so you have traveled a long way to get here! Let's move forward to learn more about eye and ear anatomy and then code procedures!

"It is for us to pray not for tasks equal to our powers, but for powers equal to our tasks, to go forward with a great desire forever beating at the door of our hearts as we travel toward our distant goal."—HELEN KELLER

EYE AND OCULAR ADNEXA (65091–68899)

Eye and Ocular Adnexa is a subsection of the Surgery section. Remember that ophthalmology is the study of the eye. Ophthalmologists are physicians who specialize in diagnosing and treating medical eye disorders, and they also perform surgery. Optometry is the measurement of the eye. Optometrists are physicians who specialize in performing eye examinations, diagnosing and treating certain eye disorders, and prescribing corrective lenses. Optometrists may also perform refractive surgery to correct vision problems. Both ophthalmologists and optometrists examine the internal structures of the eye using a slit lamp (Figure 9-21).

Remember that adnexa means accessory (attached) structures of the eye, such as the extraocular muscles and the eyelid. In order to correctly code diagnoses, it is important not only to become familiar with medical terms related to eye anatomy, but it is also important to understand how the eye functions. Refer to Figure 9-19 to review lacrimal eye structures and Figure 9-20 to review internal eye structures as you read through the next section to become familiar with eye anatomy and terms that you will find in code descriptors for the Eye and Ocular Adnexa subsection. It is very important to review the terms and their definitions so that you can better understand how physicians perform procedures.

ANATOMY OF THE EYE

The external part of the eye contains the *orbit*, a cavity in the skull made up of fatty tissue. The orbit holds the eyeball in place with six muscles that help the eye to move in various directions, which cranial nerves **innervate** (supply nerves to). You first learned about the cranial nerves in Chapter 30. The cranial nerves involved in eye movement are listed as follows and in Figure 30-6:

innervate (ĭn-nĕr′-vāt)

1. *Medial rectus*—cranial nerve III
2. *Superior rectus*—cranial nerve III
3. *Inferior rectus*—cranial nerve III
4. *Lateral rectus*—cranial nerve VI
5. *Inferior oblique*—cranial nerve III
6. *Superior oblique*—cranial nerve IV

canthus kan(t)′-thəs
tarsi (tăr′-sī)
lacrimal (lăk′-rĭm-āl)

The **canthus** is the angle where the upper and lower eyelids meet, and the **tarsi** (singular: tarsus) is tissue that supports the eyelid. The **lacrimal** *apparatus,* or lacrimal system, is made up of the following structures that produce and drain tears:

canaliculi (kăn-ă-lĭk′-ū-lī)

nasolacrimal
(năz-ō- lăk′-rĭm-āl)

- *lacrimal gland*—secretes tears
- *lacrimal* **canaliculi**—drains tears from the surface of the eye
- **nasolacrimal** *duct*—transports tears from the lacrimal sac to the nasal cavity
- *lacrimal sac*—upper part of the nasolacrimal duct
- *lacrimal punctum* (plural: puncta)—lacrimal duct opening

conjunctiva (kŏn-jŭnk-tī′-vă)
palpebral (păl′-pē-brăl)

The **conjunctiva** is a lining that covers the outer surface of eyeball and the inside of the eyelids. The **palpebral** *conjunctiva* lines the eyelids, the *bulbar conjunctiva* covers the eye's outer surface, and the *conjunctiva cul-de-sac* is the area *in between* the palpebral and bulbar conjunctiva.

The eyeball, or globe, contains three layers: outer, middle, and inner. Structures of the *outer layer* of the eye include

sclera (skler′-ə)
collagen (kŏl′-ă-jĕn)

- **sclera**—the white part of the eye, which is made up of **collagen** (protein); it consists of an anterior (front) and posterior (back).
- *cornea*—transparent covering of the anterior portion of the eye, which allows light into the eye. The cornea, which contains the most nerve endings of anywhere in the body, is composed of five layers of tissue:

epithelium (ĕp-ĭ-thē′-lē-ŭm)

1. **epithelium**—outer layer of cells which cover the cornea's surface. When injured, cells can rejuvenate rapidly to repair the injured area.

2. *Bowman's membrane*—located below the epithelium.

3. **stroma**—thickest corneal layer, made of collagen and located below Bowman's membrane.

4. **Descemet's** *membrane*—located between the epithelium and the stroma.

5. **endothelium**—layer located below Descemet's membrane, which keeps the cornea clear by pumping fluid out of the cornea. If this layer is injured, then the cornea may lose some, or all, of its ability to pump fluid, causing cloudy or hazy vision. Any corneal cells lost to injury do not regenerate. Instead, existing cells stretch over the area of dead cells, which can reduce overall vision.

stroma (strō'-mă)

Descemet's (dĕs-ĕ-māz')

endothelium (ĕn-dō-thē'-lē-ŭm)

Structures of the *middle layer* of the eye include

- **choroid**—vascular layer between the retina and sclera.

- *iris*—shows the color of the eye and regulates how much light enters the eye through the pupil.

- *pupil*—opening of the eye that looks like a black dot in the middle of the eye. It dilates (becomes larger) in poorly lit environments and contracts (becomes smaller) when there is more light. A pupil will also dilate when a person becomes excited, is poisoned, or has a traumatic brain injury (TBI).

- *lens*—located behind the pupil and allows focusing of vision, both near and far.

choroid (kō'-royd)

There are fibers, like strings, called **zonules**, which are attached to both the lens and the **ciliary** *body*. The ciliary body is located behind the iris and produces **aqueous** *humor*, a fluid in the eye that provides it with nutrients and eliminates waste products. The ciliary body is composed of the **pars plana** and the **pars plicata**.

When the ciliary muscle relaxes or contracts, the zonules move the lens, bending it or straightening it, allowing the eye to focus vision near or far. You may know someone who has to wear reading glasses, or you may wear them yourself. Having to wear "readers" happens because eyes age (called presbyopia). Researchers speculate that one of the reasons is that as the eye ages, zonules lose their ability to move the lens and focus it near and far. The reading glasses compensate for the lack of the eye's ability to focus.

zonules (zōn'-ūlz)
ciliary (sĭl'-ē-ĕr-ē)
aqueous (ā'-kwē-ŭs)
pars plana (părz plā'-nă)
pars plicata (părz plī'-kă-tă)

Structures of the *inner layer* of the eye include

- **retina**—composed of tissue located at the back of the eye.

- **macula**—part of the central retina.

- *optic nerve* (cranial nerve II)—receives visual signals from the retina and transmits them to the brain.

retina (rĕt'-ĭ-nă)
macula (măk'-ū-lă)

The internal part of the eye contains liquid, called aqueous humor and **vitreous** *humor*, which gives the eyeball a round or elliptical shape. There is much more vitreous humor in the eye than aqueous humor. Without aqueous and vitreous humor, the eyeball would collapse, which sometimes happens when a patient experiences a penetrating eye injury, or ruptured globe.

vitreous (vĭt'-rē-ŭs)

The watery and clear aqueous humor fills the **anterior segment**, which is the front one-third of the eye containing the cornea, anterior chamber, anterior sclera, iris, ciliary body (produces aqueous humor), and lens. The anterior segment is composed of the anterior chamber and posterior chamber. Aqueous humor provides nutrients to the cornea and actually flows from the lens to the iris, then through the pupil to the anterior chamber, finally draining out of the eye into the **trabecular meshwork** (tissue containing canals that drain aqueous humor) and orbital veins.

trabecular meshwork (tră-bĕk'-ū-lăr)

Recall that glaucoma is a disorder where the patient has increased intraocular pressure (IOP), which means that the aqueous humor cannot drain properly and builds up in the eye. The high IOP can place pressure on the patient's optic nerve and cause permanent vision loss. Fortunately, there are many types of medications that physicians use to treat glaucoma patients to avoid surgery, and they can also treat patients with increased IOP who are at risk for developing glaucoma. Advanced age, previous eye trauma, and heredity are all risk factors for developing glaucoma.

hyaloid (hī'-ă-loyd)

The jelly-like vitreous humor fills the back of the eye, from the lens to the retina, which is called the **posterior segment**. The posterior segment is the back two-thirds of the eye, which includes the retina, optic nerve, and anterior hyaloid membrane. The **hyaloid** *membrane* separates vitreous humor from the eye.

Here are some additional terms included in code descriptors for the eye and ocular adnexa:

- *limbal stem cell*—stem cells implanted on the cornea to treat injury or damage from disease.

synechiae (sĭn-ĕk'-ē-ă)

goniosynechiae (gō-nē-ō-sĭ-nĕk'-ē-ă)

retrobulbar (rĕt-rō-bŭl'-băr)

Tenon's (ten'-ənz)

- **synechiae**—adhesion caused by infection, glaucoma, or trauma; types include anterior synechiae (adhesion of the cornea), posterior synechiae (adhesion of the lens), and **goniosynechiae** (adhesion of the iris and cornea).
- **retrobulbar**—behind the eye.
- **Tenon's** capsule—membranous tissue that encloses the eye.
- *muscle cone*—area where the extraocular muscles hold the eyeball.

TAKE A BREAK

Good job! Let's take a break and then review more about eye anatomy.

Exercise 31.1   Anatomy of the Eye

Instructions: Fill in each blank with the best answer.

1. The _____ segment is the front one-third of the eye containing the cornea, anterior chamber, anterior sclera, iris, ciliary body, and lens.

2. Fiber-like strings called _____ are attached to the lens and the ciliary body.

3. When there is an injury to the cornea's surface, _____ cells can rejuvenate rapidly to repair the injured area.

4. The _____ duct transports tears from the lacrimal sac to the nasal cavity.

5. The part of the eye that dilates in low light and contracts in brighter light is called the _____.

6. The _____ transmits visual signals from the retina to the brain.

DIVISIONS OF THE EYE AND OCULAR ADNEXA SUBSECTION

The Eye and Ocular Adnexa subsection is divided into five subheadings, and each represents a specific part of the eye: eyeball, anterior segment, posterior segment, ocular adnexa, and conjunctiva. CPT further divides these subheadings into categories by additional operative sites (vitreous, retina, eyelids) and subcategories for the type of procedure (incision, excision, destruction, repair) (■ TABLE 31-1). To locate codes for eye and ocular adnexa procedures, search the index for the *body site* (e.g., eye, cornea, vitreous) and then the *type of procedure* (e.g., injection, biopsy, aspiration), or start your search with the *type of procedure* or the *condition* (e.g., pterygium, chalazion).

Let's review more about how to assign codes for procedures in subheadings and categories, and then practice coding. Refer to the anatomy diagrams of the eye mentioned earlier in the chapter and to eye anatomy terms and their definitions that we reviewed.

It is important to note that when you assign codes for eye procedures, you should append modifier -LT or -RT to indicate the left or right eye, or modifier -50 for a bilateral procedure. Do not confuse modifiers -LT, -RT, and -50 with abbreviations that physicians use for the left eye (OS), right eye (OD), and both eyes (OU). These abbreviations are not coding modifiers.

EYEBALL (65091–65290)

The subheading Eyeball contains four categories of procedures, including procedures for removing an eyeball and implanting an artificial one.

■ **TABLE 31-1   EYE AND OCULAR ADNEXA SUBHEADINGS, CATEGORIES, AND SUBCATEGORIES**

Subsection, Subheadings, Categories, and Subcategories	Code Range
EYE AND OCULAR ADNEXA	**65091–68899**
Eyeball	**65091–65290**
Removal of Eye	65091–65114
Secondary Implant(s) Procedures	65125–65175
Removal of Foreign Body	65205–65265
Repair of Laceration	65270–65290
Anterior Segment	**65400–66999**
Cornea	65400–65782
• *Excision*	65400–65426
• *Removal or Destruction*	65430–65600
• *Keratoplasty*	65710–65757
• *Other Procedures*	65760–65782
Anterior Chamber	65800–66030
• *Incision*	65800–65880
• *Removal*	65900–65930
• *Introduction*	66020–66030
Anterior Sclera	66130–66250
• *Excision*	66130–66175
• *Aqueous Shunt*	66180–66185
• *Repair or Revision*	66220–66250
Iris, Ciliary Body	66500–66770
• *Incision*	66500–66505
• *Excision*	66600–66635
• *Repair*	66680–66682
• *Destruction*	66700–66770
Lens	66820–66940
• *Incision*	66820–66825
• *Removal*	66830–66940
Intraocular Lens Procedures	66982–66986
Other Procedures	66990–66999
Posterior Segment	**67005–67299**
Vitreous	67005–67043
Retina or Choroid	67101–67229
• *Repair*	67101–67121
• *Prophylaxis*	67141–67145
• *Destruction*	67208–67229
Posterior Sclera	67250–67255
• *Repair*	67250–67255
Other Procedures	67299
Ocular Adnexa	**67311–67999**
Extraocular Muscles	67311–67399
• *Other Procedures*	67399

continued

■ **TABLE 31-1** *continued*

Subsection, Subheadings, Categories, and Subcategories	Code Range
Orbit	*67400–67599*
• *Exploration, Excision, Decompression*	*67400–67450*
• *Other Procedures*	*67500–67599*
Eyelids	*67700–67999*
• *Incision*	*67700–67715*
• *Excision, Destruction*	*67800–67850*
• *Tarsorrhaphy*	*67875–67882*
• *Repair (Brow Ptosis, Blepharoptosis, Lid Retraction, Ectropion, Entropion)*	*67900–67924*
• *Reconstruction*	*67930–67975*
• *Other Procedures*	*67999*
Conjunctiva	**68020–68899**
Incision and Drainage	*68020–68040*
Excision and/or Destruction	*68100–68135*
Injection	*68200*
Conjunctivoplasty	*68320–68340*
Other Procedures	*68360–68399*
Lacrimal System	*68400–68899*
• *Incision*	*68400–68440*
• *Excision*	*68500–68550*
• *Repair*	*68700–68770*
• *Probing and/or Related Procedures*	*68801–68850*
• *Other Procedures*	*68899*

Turn to the categories within the Eyeball subheading in your CPT manual to review the procedures, which we will discuss next. The categories, along with index entries, are as follows.

- Removal of Eye (65091–65114)—index entries: location or type of procedure (evisceration, enucleation)
- Secondary Implant(s) Procedures (65125–65175)—index entry: *ocular implant*
- Removal of Foreign Body (65205–65265)—index entries: location or *removal, foreign body*
- Repair of Laceration (65270–65290)—index entries: location (conjunctiva, cornea, sclera) or *repair*

Removal of Eye (65091–65114)

Physicians remove eyes to ensure complete excision of a neoplasm, alleviate pain in a blind eye, or remove an injured eyeball after trauma. There are three different types of procedures for removing an eye and/or the ocular contents of the orbit, which include blood vessels, nerves, tissue, and fat. After the physician completes the procedure, the patient may receive a prosthetic implant (artificial eye). When the physician attaches extraocular muscles to the implant, the muscles allow the prosthetic implant to move with the other eye. However, not all implants have extraocular muscles attached.

The three types of procedures for removing an eye are

- **Evisceration (65091–65093)**—removal of the ocular contents and removal of the cornea; the sclera and extraocular muscles are not removed. The physician can place an ocular implant over an eviscerated eye.

- **Enucleation (65101–65105)**—removal of the eyeball without removing the ocular contents of the orbit or muscles.

- **Exenteration (65110–65114)** of orbit—removal of the eyeball, including the ocular contents; it can also include removal of bone and muscle or myocutaneous flap.

evisceration
(ē-vĭs-ĕr-ā′-shŭn)

enucleation
(ē-nū-klē-ā′-shŭn)

exenteration
(ĕks-ĕn-tĕr-ā′- shŭn)

Did you notice the CPT guidelines after the category Removal of Eye? The guidelines alert you that if the physician performs a skin graft to the orbit, then you should assign a code from the Integumentary section for a split skin or full-thickness graft. In addition, if the physician repairs the patient's eyelid involving more than skin, you should report a code for reconstruction.

Secondary Implant(s) Procedures (65125–65175)

Did you notice the CPT guidelines for the Secondary Implant(s) Procedures category? They state that an ***ocular implant*** is an implant *inside* the muscular cone, and an ***orbital implant*** is an implant *outside* the muscular cone.

An orbital implant is a small sphere that the physician places into the orbit where the natural eye used to be. The orbital implant does not look like an eye. In fact, you cannot see a patient's orbital implant because an ocular implant, or ocular prosthesis, covers it.

The ocular implant, which is outside the muscle cone, fits directly *over* the orbital implant and under the eyelid (■ FIGURE 31-1). It is made of glass, plastic, or acrylic and is painted to match the color of the patient's eye. An **ocularist** specializes in ocular prosthetic implants, including measuring a patient's orbit in order to fit the patient with a prosthetic eye and customizing the prosthetic to the patient's eye color. The ocularist also educates the patient on caring for the prosthetic implant.

ocularist (ŏk′-ū-lăr-ĭst)

It is important to note that *ocular implant* procedures are categorized under the Eyeball subheading, according to the type of procedure, such as modification of an implant or insertion of an implant. *Orbital implant* insertion, removal, or revision (67550, 67560) procedures are listed as Other Procedures under the Orbit category in the Ocular Adnexa subheading.

Removal of Foreign Body (65205–65265)

The Eyeball subheading also includes the category Removal of Foreign Body for removing a foreign body from the external eye or removing an intraocular foreign body, which may include using a slit lamp. (See Figure 9-21.)

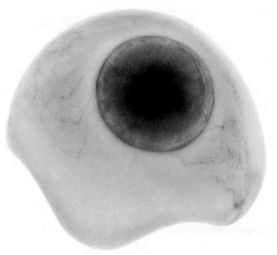

Figure 31-1 ■ Ocular implant made of glass.

Photo credit: © Maximilian Weinzierl/ Alamy.

Repair of Laceration (65270–65290)

The last category under the Eyeball subheading is Repair of Laceration, which includes repairing lacerations and wounds of the conjunctiva, sclera, cornea, extraocular muscle, tendon, and Tenon's capsule. CPT further divides procedures by perforating and nonperforating injuries, if the patient was hospitalized, and the type of repair, including direct closure and application of tissue glue.

There are several CPT coding notes for both Removal of Foreign Body and Repair of Laceration. Some of the coding notes refer you to other codes, depending on the type of procedure the physician performs. It is important to pay close attention to these notes to ensure correct code assignment.

Refer to the following example to learn more about coding an eyeball procedure.

Example: An ambulance transports Mrs. Hudson, a 32-year-old, to Williton Medical Center's ED for a right-eye injury she sustained in a motor vehicle accident. Dr. Fitzpatrick, the on-call ophthalmologist, examines the patient and determines that she sustained a penetrating corneal laceration, which he repairs.

To code this case, search the index for the main term *cornea*, subterm *repair*, subterm *wound*, and subterm *perforating*, which directs you to cross-reference codes 65280–65285. Assign code **65280-RT** because the repair did not involve uveal tissue (part of the eye's middle layer). The patient's diagnosis code is **871.0** (main term *injury*, subterm *eyeball*, subterm *penetrating*, and subterm *without prolapse*).

TAKE A BREAK

You are doing great! Let's take a break and practice assigning codes for the eyeball.

Exercise 31.2   Eyeball

Instructions: Review the patient's case, and then assign codes for the procedure(s), appending a modifier when appropriate. Optional: For additional practice, assign the patient's diagnosis code(s) (ICD-9-CM).

1. Ronald Timmons, age 52, is a new patient who presents to Dr. Moore's office complaining of left-eye pain and tearing. Dr. Moore, a board-certified ophthalmologist, determines that Mr. Timmons has a metal shaving in the conjunctiva of his eye and removes it.

   Diagnosis code(s): _____

   Procedure code(s): _____

2. Molly Stevens, age 27, suffers a perforating laceration to her left cornea when a friend accidentally strikes her with a softball bat during a softball game. She cannot see out of her left eye and has severe eye pain. Dr. Moore repairs the laceration in his office and places her on steroid eye drops and an antibiotic.

   Diagnosis code(s): _____

   Procedure code(s): _____

3. After in-office testing and additional radiology tests, Dr. Moore diagnoses Ranelle Wilkins, age 50, with cancer in her right eyeball. Today at Williton, Dr. Moore performs an exenteration of the eye, including the ocular contents and muscle.

   Diagnosis code(s): _____

   Procedure code(s): _____

4. Mrs. Wilkins returns six weeks later for a follow-up visit, and after Dr. Moore performs the *orbital* implant, he refers the patient to Wendy Gibson, BCO (Board-Certified Ocularist), to insert an ocular implant into the scleral shell. Code for the ocularist's services.

   Diagnosis code(s): _____

   Procedure code(s): _____

5. Three years later, Wendy Gibson, BCO, determines that Mrs. Wilkins' implant has shifted out of place and decides to remove the implant and reinsert another implant at a future date.

   Diagnosis code(s): _____

   Procedure code(s): _____

6. Due to other health issues, Mrs. Wilkins does not return until four months later to see Wendy Gibson and have an ocular implant reinserted with muscle attachment.

   Diagnosis code(s): _____

   Procedure code(s): _____

ANTERIOR SEGMENT (65400–66999)

Remember that the anterior segment is the front one-third of the eye containing the cornea, anterior chamber, anterior sclera, iris, ciliary body, and lens. Turn to the Anterior Segment subheading in your CPT manual to review procedures listed under these seven categories:

1. Cornea
2. Anterior Chamber
3. Anterior Sclera
4. Iris, Ciliary Body
5. Lens
6. Intraocular Lens Procedures
7. Other Procedures

The procedures are discussed in the next sections. You can locate codes in the index by searching for the type of procedure (excision, incision) or location (iris, lens), and then the type of procedure.

Cornea (65400–65782)

Recall that the cornea has five layers that cover the anterior part of the eye. The Cornea category includes four subcategories of procedures.

1. *Excision* (65400–65426)—Procedures include excision of a corneal lesion, biopsy of the cornea, and excision or transposition of a **pterygium**, a growth on the corneal surface. Causes of corneal lesions include disease, injury, and excessive contact lens use.

2. *Removal or Destruction* (65430–65600)—Procedures include
   - Diagnostic corneal scraping to test for infection
   - Removal of corneal epithelium, when a physician removes rust that was left behind (rust ring) from a metal foreign body removed from the cornea
   - Lesion destruction

   Removal or destruction methods include **chemocauterization**, cryotherapy, **photocoagulation** (using a laser to seal tears), and **thermocauterization**.

3. **Keratoplasty** (65710–65757)—A keratoplasty is a corneal repair, including a corneal transplant. Physicians transplant corneas for patients whose corneas are damaged by trauma or disease, which results in corneal scarring or corneal edema that causes partial or complete blindness.

   The corneal endothelium pumps fluid from the cornea, resulting in clear vision. Patients with corneal edema have corneas which are unable to pump fluid, and the fluid accumulates on the cornea, causing hazy, white, cloudy, or smoky vision.

   A corneal transplant, also called a cornea graft, is when the physician removes the damaged or diseased cornea and replaces it with a cadaveric cornea. Penetrating keratoplasty (PKP) is when the physician removes the *entire cornea* and transplants a full-thickness cornea. Lamellar keratoplasty is a partial-thickness transplant, involving a graft of only specific corneal layers.

   For many years, PKP has been the standard corneal transplant that physicians perform, suturing the entire cornea in place (■ FIGURE 31-2).

   Recovery from PKP is a very long process, and it can take several months to two years for a patient to fully recover visually and completely heal from the procedure.

   A newer corneal transplant procedure, called Descemet's Stripping Endothelial Keratoplasty (DSEK), is replacing PKP. It involves stripping Descemet's membrane and removing *only* the corneal endothelium layer, replacing it with a cadaveric endothelium (donor graft). In DSEK surgery, the physician uses an air bubble to hold the new corneal cells in place, instead of using sutures. Patients experience a much shorter recovery time with improved vision relatively quickly.

pterygium (tĕ-rĭj′-ē-ŭm)

chemocauterization (kē-mō-kaw-tĕr-ĭ-zā′-shŭn)—the use of chemicals to destroy tissue
photocoagulation (fō-tō-kō-ăg-ū-lā′-shŭn)
thermocauterization (thĕr-mō-kaw-tĕr-ĭ-zā′-shŭn)—destruction of abnormal tissue by the application of heat
keratoplasty (kĕr′-ă-tō-plăs-tē)

Figure 31-2 ■ An eye with a penetrating corneal transplant, which fine sutures hold in place.

Photo credit: © Medical-on-Line/ Alamy.

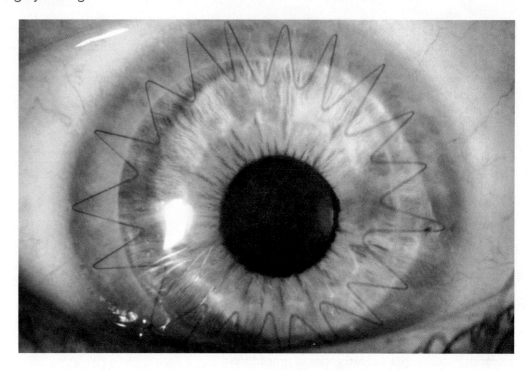

Notice in the Keratoplasty subcategory that there is an add-on code 65757, which represents backbench preparation of corneal endothelial autograft. An eye bank will provide the donor graft for a corneal transplant, and the eye bank may also prepare the graft (separate the endothelium from the rest of the cornea) for the corneal transplant procedure. If the ophthalmologist prepares the graft (backbench preparation), then you can assign add-on code 65757.

4. *Other Procedures* **(65760–65782)**—The Other Procedures subcategory includes procedures to correct refractive errors (inability of the eye to focus near or far) and procedures to treat corneal injuries from infections, burns, and trauma by incising the cornea and transplanting corneal tissue to give the cornea a smooth, round surface.

Many times, payers will *not* reimburse for these procedures unless the patient cannot achieve adequate vision with corrective lenses and has undergone other unsuccessful procedures to correct vision. Other Procedures and their definitions are outlined in ■ TABLE 31-2.

Anterior Chamber (65800–66030)

Recall that the anterior segment consists of both an anterior and posterior chamber. The aqueous humor flows through the anterior chamber. The Anterior Chamber category includes the following three subcategories of procedures, which you can locate in the index under the type of procedure, the body site, or the condition.

INTERESTING FACTS: Many Corneas Are Unsuitable for Transplants

The majority of corneal donors are deceased individuals who chose to donate their corneas for medical purposes, or whose family members consented to donation after the donor's death. An eye bank obtains donated corneas, tests them for diseases, and inspects the corneas to ensure that they are appropriate for transplantation. The eye bank then sends the corneas to hospitals where physicians transplant them. Corneas from donors with HIV, hepatitis, or syphilis are not used because of the risk of infection to the patient who needs the transplant. Corneas from donors who have had previous corneal surgery, including correction of refractive errors, also cannot be used for transplants because the corneas are not shaped normally and are already compromised because of prior surgery.

■ **TABLE 31-2   OTHER PROCEDURES**

Procedure	Pronunciation	Definition
Keratomileusis (65760)	(kĕr-ă-tō-mĭ-lū′-sĭs)	In this type of keratoplasty, the physician removes a slice of the cornea, reshapes it (often with a laser), and places it back onto the cornea.
Keratophakia (65765)	(kĕr-ă-tō-fāk′-ē-ă)	The physician reshapes and transplants donor corneal tissue onto the patient's cornea.
Epikeratoplasty (65767)	(ĕp-ĭ-kĕr′-a-tō-plăs-tē)	The physician transplants donor corneal epithelium onto the patient's cornea.
Keratoprosthesis (65770)	(kĕr′-ă-tō-prŏs-thē-sĭs)	The physician transplants an artificial cornea onto the patient's cornea.
Radial keratotomy (65771)	(kĕr′-ă-tŏt-ō-mē)	The physician creates a pattern of corneal incisions.
Corneal relaxing incision or corneal wedge resection for correction of surgically induced astigmatism (65772–65775)		Some patients experience **astigmatism**, resulting from a cornea that has an irregular shape. Surgically induced astigmatism can happen because the shape of the cornea can change from a corneal transplant or cataract surgery. Physicians treat surgically induced astigmatism by incising the cornea or removing a wedge of the cornea that is shaped irregularly.
Placement of amniotic membrane on ocular surface for wound healing (65778–65779)		Physicians place cells from amniotic membranes on the cornea to heal wounds from injuries or burns, or they can transplant amniotic membrane grafts.
Ocular surface reconstruction—amniotic membrane transplantation—may include a limbal cell allograft or limbal conjunctival autograft (65780–65782)		Physicians place grafted limbal cells from donor eyes on the patient's cornea to treat injuries or disease and restore vision.
		Many times, physicians perform a limbal conjunctival autograft after excising a pterygium to repair the defect and prevent recurrence.

1. *Incision* (65800–65880):
   - Paracentesis of anterior chamber (removal of fluid using a needle) with
     - diagnostic aspiration of aqueous (to diagnose specific conditions)
     - therapeutic release of aqueous (to reduce intraocular pressure—IOP)
     - removal of vitreous and/or discission (incision) of anterior hyaloid membrane
     - removal of blood (*Note: A CPT note directs you to use code 65930 for removal of a blood clot.*)
   - **Goniotomy (65820)**—procedure to treat children with congenital glaucoma. The physician places a **goniolens** (also called a gonioscope) on the patient's cornea to view the iris and cornea. The goniolens allows the physician to see and open the trabecular meshwork to drain aqueous humor and reduce the patient's IOP. (*Note: A CPT note alerts you not to append modifier -63 to a goniotomy. Recall that modifier -63 represents a procedure performed on infants who weigh less than 4 kgs.*)
   - **Trabeculotomy ab externo** (approach from the outside) (65850), **trabeculoplasty** by laser surgery (65855)—incision and repair of the trabecular meshwork to improve aqueous humor outflow and lower IOP in glaucoma patients.
   - Severing adhesions of anterior segment, laser technique (65860)
   - Severing adhesions of anterior segment, incisional technique, for goniosynechiae, anterior and posterior synechiae, and corneovitreal adhesions (65865–65880)
2. *Removal* (65900–65930) of epithelial downgrowth, implanted material, or a blood clot
3. *Introduction* (66020–66030)—injection of air, liquid, or medication to prevent the anterior chamber from collapsing.

astigmatism
(ă-stĭg′-mă-tĭzm)

goniotomy (gō-nē-ŏt′-ō-mē)
goniolens (gō′-nē-ō-lĕnz)

trabeculotomy ab externo
(tră-bĕk′-ū-lŏt-ō-mē ăb ĕks′-ter-nō)
trabeculoplasty
(tră-bĕk′-ū-lō-plăs-tē)

Anterior Sclera (66130–66250)

Remember that the sclera is the white part of the eye and consists of anterior and posterior sections. The Anterior Sclera category contains the following three subcategories of procedures.

1. ***Excision* (66130–66175)**
   - Excision of lesion of sclera (infections can cause scleral lesions) (66130)
   - **Fistulization** (creation of a passageway, or opening) of sclera by incising the iris (iridectomy) to treat glaucoma, infection, or trauma and allow aqueous humor to drain (66150–66170). The physician can perform other procedures with the fistulization, including
     - thermocauterization
     - sclerotomy (incision of the sclera) with punch or scissors
     - iridencleisis or iridotasis (to drain aqueous humor), iridencleisis (implanting part of the iris in the cornea), or iridotasis (stretching the iris)
     - trabeculectomy ab externo
   - **Transluminal** (across a channel) dilation of aqueous outflow canal, without or with a device or stent, to help drain aqueous humor (66174–66175)

2. ***Aqueous Shunt* (66180–66185) *or revision of shunt to extraocular reservoir*—** This procedure helps to drain aqueous humor. Remember that a shunt is a device that includes a catheter (tube) that transports fluid from one area of the body to another. *(Note: A CPT note alerts you to use code 67120 to remove an implanted shunt.)*

3. ***Repair or Revision* (66220–66250)**
   - Repair of scleral **staphyloma** (condition where eye contents protrude through the sclera, many times caused by scleritis—infection/inflammation of the sclera), with or without a graft (66220–66225)
   - Revision or repair of operative wound of anterior segment (66250)

Iris, Ciliary Body (66500–66770)

Remember that the iris is the colored part of the eye, which regulates how much light enters the eye through the pupil. The ciliary body is the tissue inside the eye that is attached to the lens by suspended ligaments and produces aqueous humor. There are four subcategories of procedures listed under Iris, Ciliary Body, many of which include draining aqueous humor for glaucoma patients.

1. ***Incision* (66500–66505)—Iridotomy** (incision of the iris) is performed to drain aqueous humor to treat glaucoma, or to enlarge the pupil. The procedure can include *transfixion* (piercing in order to move a part into a new position) for *iris* **bombé** (protrusion of the iris from excess aqueous humor in the posterior chamber).

2. ***Excision* (66600–66635)—**Excision procedures include an **iridectomy** (excision of the iris) to remove a lesion or drain aqueous humor to treat glaucoma. Iridectomy can also include any of the following procedures:
   - **cyclectomy**—partial excision of the ciliary body
   - peripheral—excision of the peripheral (side) portion of the iris
   - sector—excision of the **pupillary** margin (inner edge of the iris)
   - optical—excision of the center of the iris

3. ***Repair* (66680–66682)—**Repair procedures include repair of the iris, ciliary body, including repair for **iridodialysis** (ruptured iris from trauma) and suture of iris, ciliary body.

4. ***Destruction* (66700–66770)—**These procedures destroy the ciliary body for drainage of aqueous humor which is a procedure of last resort to treat glaucoma after other methods have failed, or a procedure to treat traumatic injuries.

Margin glossary terms:

fistulization
(fĭs-tū-lĭ-zā'-shŭn)

transluminal
(trănz-lū'-mĭn-ăl)

staphyloma (stăf-ĭl-ō'-mă)

iridotomy (ĭr-ĭ-dŏt'-ō-mē)

bombé (bäm'bā)

iridectomy (ĭr-ĭ-dĕk'-tō-mē)

cyclectomy (sī-klĕk'-tō-mē)

pupillary (pyü'-pə-ler-ē)

iridodialysis (ĭr-ĭ-dō-dī-al'ĭ-sis)

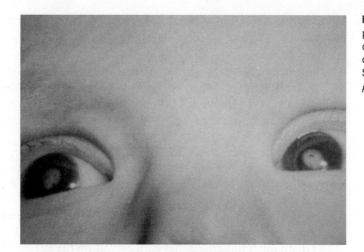

Figure 31-3 ■ This photograph shows the cataracts in a child's eyes due to Congenital Rubella Syndrome (CRS).

Photo credit: CDC.

Lens (66820–66940) and Intraocular Lens Procedures (66982–66986)

Lens procedures involve incision (66820–66825) and removal (66830–66940). Recall that the lens is located behind the pupil and allows focusing of vision both near and far. You learned in Chapter 9 that physicians remove a patient's lens and replace it with an artificial intraocular lens (IOL) during cataract surgery. The lens is encased in a capsular bag. Cataracts, deposits of protein on the lens, cause cloudy or hazy vision because the lens of the eye becomes opaque (white). Advanced age is the most common cause; however, ocular trauma and disease can also result in cataracts (■ FIGURE 31-3).

The most common cataract surgery is a type of extracapsular cataract removal involving **phacoemulsification**, also called phaco, which is an outpatient procedure. During phaco, the physician destroys the cataract with ultrasound and then suctions it out of the eye with an instrument. (Do you remember how physicians removed cataracts in ancient times? They suctioned them out with their mouths!) Phaco eliminates the need to make large incisions, and the patient's recovery time is faster than with any other type of cataract surgery.

When a cataract is too rigid to be broken up by phacoemulsification, physicians may perform conventional *extracapsular cataract extraction* by opening the lens bag to remove all of the cataract in one piece.

Intracapsular cataract extraction is not commonly performed and involves removing both the lens and the capsular bag using several sutures. The patient's recovery time is much longer than with phaco, and the procedure carries greater risks for complications.

Sometimes after cataract surgery, the patient develops a secondary cataract, which happens because the IOL becomes opaque. Physicians typically remove secondary cataracts with a YAG laser, a brief procedure performed in the physician's office. Other times after cataract surgery, the artificial lens displaces, and the patient has to undergo a second surgery to either place the lens in the correct position or replace it with another one.

Procedures listed under the categories Lens and Intraocular Lens Procedures (66982–66986) include removal of a cataract, including a secondary cataract; repositioning or replacement of an IOL; and removal of lens material. Turn to the procedures in your CPT manual to review them, and notice the CPT coding notes under the Removal subcategory (66830–66940) alerting you to other procedures that are bundled into codes for lens extraction.

phacoemulsification
(fāk-ō-ē-mŭl-sĭ-fĭ-kā′-shŭn)

Other Procedures (66900–66999)

The Other Procedures category includes the add-on code 66990 for using an ophthalmic endoscope; however, you can only report it with specific codes, according to the CPT note under code 66990. Code 66999—*Unlisted procedure, anterior segment of eye* is also included in this category.

Refer to the following example to learn more about coding an anterior segment procedure.

> **Example:** Albert Dunn, a 74-year-old, sees Dr. Lindsay, an ophthalmologist, at Williton Medical Center for a senile cataract removal from his left eye. Dr. Lindsay uses phaco to remove the cataract and then inserts an IOL. The surgery is successful without complications, and Mr. Dunn returns to the postoperative recovery room where his wife is waiting. He is later discharged home.
>
> To code this case, search the index for the main term *cataract*, subterm *removal/extraction*, and subterm *extracapsular*, which then directs you to cross-reference codes 66982 or 66984. Code 66982 includes extracapsular cataract removal using phaco but also requires "devices or techniques not generally used in routine cataract surgery." Code 66984 is also for extracapsular cataract removal using phaco but does not require any special techniques, so code **66984-LT** is the correct code, with an -LT modifier indicating that surgery was on the left eye. The patient's diagnosis code is **366.10** (main term *cataract* and subterm *senile*).

TAKE A BREAK

You are doing very well! Let's take a break and review more about the anterior segment.

Exercise 31.3   Anterior Segment

Part 1—Theory

Instructions: Fill in the blank with the best answer.

1. An incision and repair of the trabecular meshwork to improve aqueous humor outflow and lower IOP in glaucoma patients is called _____.

2. During this procedure, the physician reshapes and transplants donor corneal tissue onto the patient's cornea. _____

3. A(n) _____ is the partial excision of the ciliary body.

4. A(n) _____ is a condition where eye contents protrude through the sclera, many times caused by scleritis.

5. A(n) _____ helps to drain aqueous humor.

6. What is another name for a corneal repair, including a corneal transplant? _____

Part 2—Coding

Instructions: Review the patient's case, and then assign codes for the procedure(s), appending a modifier when appropriate. Optional: For additional practice, assign the patient's diagnosis code(s) (ICD-9-CM).

1. At Williton Medical Center, Dr. Moore, an ophthalmologist, performs a penetrating keratoplasty (corneal transplant) for Maria Delacruz, age 26, who developed excessive corneal scarring as the result of a herpes simplex infection. Dr. Moore previously determined that she is not a candidate for DSEK surgery because of the extensive scarring. Mrs. Delacruz will follow up with Dr. Moore in his office and can expect a long recovery before she achieves permanent visual improvement.

   Diagnosis code(s): _____

   Procedure code(s): _____

2. Jacob Anderson, age 65, is an established patient who sees Dr. Moore for management of open-angle glaucoma. Because medications no longer improve the condition, Dr. Moore decides that surgery is the best course of action. Today at Williton, he performs a bilateral laser trabeculoplasty to improve the natural drainage of aqueous humor of the eye. Mr. Anderson will follow up with Dr. Moore tomorrow in his office. Code for the patient's surgery.

   Diagnosis code(s): _____

   Procedure code(s): _____

3. Eugene States, age 48, has a staphyloma of the sclera of his right eye. Dr. Moore repairs it at Williton without the use of a shunt.

   Diagnosis code(s): _____

   Procedure code(s): _____

4. Robert Forsythe, age 52, sees Dr. Moore for destruction of a ciliary body cyst in his left eye.

   Diagnosis code(s): _____

   Procedure code(s): _____

TAKE A BREAK *continued*

5. Following cataract surgery, Janice Williams, age 71, develops a *secondary* membranous cataract in her left eye. Today in his office, Dr. Moore performs a discission by YAG laser, and the patient's vision improves.

Diagnosis code(s): _____

Procedure code(s): _____

6. Today at Williton, Dr. Moore performs phacoemulsification with lens implantation for George Poston, age 72, who has an extracapsular cataract in his right eye. The surgery is successful, and Dr. Moore discharges the patient home with instructions to follow up tomorrow in his office.

Diagnosis code(s): _____

Procedure code(s): _____

POSTERIOR SEGMENT (67005–67229)

Recall that the posterior segment is the back two-thirds of the eye, including the retina, optic nerve and anterior hyaloid membrane, which separates vitreous humor from the eye. Turn to the Posterior Segment subheading in your CPT manual to review procedures listed under the four categories that we will review next:

1. Vitreous
2. Retina or Choroid
3. Posterior Sclera
4. Other Procedures

Be sure to read CPT coding guidelines for procedures in the Posterior Segment subheading. To locate codes for posterior segment procedures, search the index for the type of procedure (repair, diathermy, prophylaxis), or for the body site (vitreous, retina), and then the type of procedure.

Vitreous (67005–67043)

Procedures included under the Vitreous category include a vitrectomy, which is when the physician removes the vitreous from the eye and replaces it with another substance. Reasons for the procedure include the presence of floaters (strands or specks that appear in the field of vision), scar tissue, blood, and distorted or impaired vision, which diabetic retinopathy, cataract surgery, macular holes, and traumatic injuries can all cause. Notice that vitrectomies can also include other procedures, so it is important to carefully read code descriptors for accurate code assignment.

An **intravitreal** injection is when the physician injects medication into the vitreous to treat eye disorders, such as diabetic retinopathy, **macular edema**, and **macular degeneration**. Code 67027 includes intravitreal drug delivery with a ganciclovir implant, which treats **cytomegalovirus retinitis** and slowly releases medication to treat the retinal infection over several months.

Retina or Choroid (67101–67229)

Remember that the retina is the tissue at the back of the eye, and the choroid is the vascular layer between the retina and sclera. Procedures in this category include the subcategory Repair for repair of a retinal detachment, which is an emergent eye condition that needs immediate care.

A retinal detachment is when the retina pulls away from the back of the eye and floats in the vitreous. Diseases or trauma to the eye can cause retinal detachment. Did you notice that there are many different types of procedures for reattaching the retina?

intravitreal (ĭn-tră-vĭt′-rē-ăl)

macular edema (măk′-ū-lăr ĕ-dē′-mă)—swelling of the macula, caused by a build-up of fluid and protein deposits

macular degeneration (măk′-ū-lăr dē-jĕn-ĕ-rā′-shŭn)—loss of vision in the center of the visual field, caused by the degeneration of the macula, the center of the retina

cytomegalovirus retinitis (sī-tō-mĕg′-ă-lō-vī-rŭs rĕ-tĭ-nī′-tĭs)—infection of the eye's retina caused by the cytomegalovirus, which can lead to blindness

Here are two additional subcategories and the types of procedures they contain:

prophylaxis (prō-fĭ-lăk´-sĭs)—preventative care measures taken to preserve health and prevent the spread of disease

- **Prophylaxis** (67141–67145)—procedures for treatment for retinal breaks and degeneration to prevent a detached retina.

- *Destruction* (67208–67229)—procedures that destroy a retinal lesion or choroid lesion using various methods; destruction or treatment of extensive or progressive retinopathy to shrink blood vessels in the retina that cause blood to leak into the eye.

Posterior Sclera (67250–67255) and Other Procedures (67299)

Procedures listed under these categories include posterior scleral repair, including scleral reinforcement, with or without a graft (to treat a thinning sclera from degenerative myopia), and Unlisted procedure, posterior segment. Refer to the following example to learn more about coding a posterior segment procedure.

diathermy (dī´-ă-thĕr-mē)—to heat with an electrical current

Example: Anthony Dunn, age 58, arrives at Williton Medical Center's ED with symptoms of seeing flashes of light and floaters during the past hour. Dr. Lindsay, an ophthalmologist, determines that Mr. Dunn has a total detached retina with retinal defect of the left eye, which he treats with **diathermy**, including drainage of subretinal fluid.

To code this case, search the index for the main term *retina*, subterm *repair*, subterm *detachment*, and subterm *cryotherapy or diathermy*, which directs you to cross-reference code 67101. Assign code **67101-LT**, since it includes all of the elements of the procedure that Dr. Lindsay performed. The patient's diagnosis code is **361.05** (main term *detachment*, subterm *retina*, subterm *with retinal defect*, and subterm *total*).

TAKE A BREAK

Great progress! Let's take a break and practice assigning codes for the posterior segment.

Exercise 31.4 **Posterior Segment**

Instructions: Review the patient's case, and then assign codes for the procedure(s), appending a modifier when appropriate. Optional: For additional practice, assign the patient's diagnosis code(s) (ICD-9-CM).

1. Alfred Jones, age 62, receives a vitreous fluid substitute injection by Dr. Moore, an ophthalmologist, in his office, to treat his macular degeneration.

Diagnosis code(s): _____

Procedure code(s): _____

2. Susan James' husband brings her to Williton's ED. She complains of numerous floaters and what she describes as a black curtain moving down her field of vision. Dr. Daniels, the ED physician, calls Dr. Lindsay, the on-call ophthalmologist, to examine Mrs. James, age 53. Dr. Lindsay determines that Mrs. James developed a partial retinal detachment with multiple defects in her right eye. He performs diathermy retinal repair, and the surgery is successful. Code for Dr. Lindsay's surgery.

Diagnosis code(s): _____

Procedure code(s): _____

3. Jeff Stone, age 43, has a benign lesion on his left retina. Dr. Moore uses cryotherapy in his office to destroy it.

Diagnosis code(s): _____

Procedure code(s): _____

4. Lilly Murphy, a nine-month-old, was born prematurely at 35 weeks and suffers from retinopathy. At Williton, Dr. Lindsay treats the condition with photocoagulation.

Diagnosis code(s): _____

Procedure code(s): _____

5. Ginger Allen, age 67, suffered a spontaneous hemorrhage in her right eye. Dr. Moore performs

TAKE A BREAK *continued*

a mechanical vitrectomy, pars plana approach, to remove the blood that is obscuring her vision.

Diagnosis code(s): _____

Procedure code(s): _____

6. In the office, Dr. Moore severs vitreous face adhesions for John Kelsey, age 32, by laser surgery.

Diagnosis code(s): _____

Procedure code(s): _____

OCULAR ADNEXA (67311–67999)

The subheading Ocular Adnexa includes three categories of procedures involving the extraocular muscles, orbit, and eyelids, which are all adnexa, or accessory structures. Turn to the categories within this subheading in your CPT manual to review the procedures as we discuss them next.

1. Extraocular Muscles
2. Orbit
3. Eyelids

Be sure to review CPT coding guidelines before any final code assignment. You can find codes for ocular adnexa procedures by searching the index for the type of procedure (orbitotomy, tarsorrhaphy, repair), the condition (strabismus, chalazion), or the body site (muscle, orbit, eyelid).

Extraocular Muscles (67311–67399)

Procedures involving the extraocular muscles include **strabismus** correction. Strabismus is a disorder where the eyes do not focus together. Instead, one or both eyes may turn inward (■ FIGURE 31-4), called **esotropia** (the person appears cross-eyed if both eyes turn inward), or an eye may turn out, called **exotropia**. During surgery, the physician adjusts the length of extraocular muscles to change how they move the eye, including making vertical (up and down) or horizontal (side to side) muscles firmer or more flexible.

strabismus (stră-bĭz′-mŭs)

esotropia (ĕs-ō-trō′-pĭ-ă)
exotropia (ĕks-ō-trō′pē-ă)

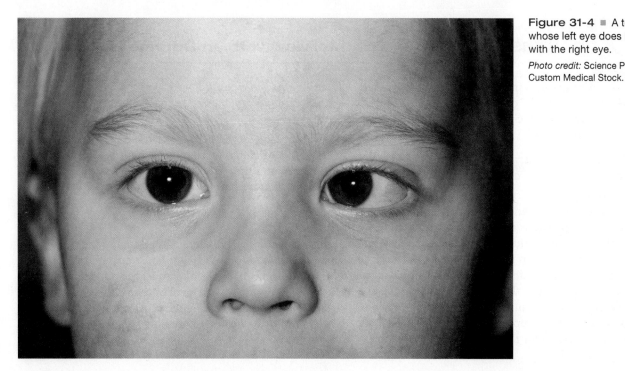

Figure 31-4 ■ A toddler whose left eye does not focus with the right eye.

Photo credit: Science Photo Library / Custom Medical Stock.

Orbit (67400–67599)

The Orbit category is divided into two subcategories:

- Exploration, Excision, and Decompression (67400–67450)
- Other Procedures (67500–67599)

orbitotomy (or-bĭ-tŏt′-ō-mē)

Exploration, Excision, and Decompression includes **orbitotomy** (incision into the orbit, the cavity that holds the eye) to remove a lesion, foreign body, or abscess or to drain fluid. An orbitotomy can also include removing a bone flap to gain access to a specific area of the orbit. CPT arranges orbitotomies by the type of approach the physician uses, such as frontal, transconjunctival (across the conjunctiva), or lateral, and by other procedures performed with the orbitotomy, such as a bone flap or the removal of a lesion.

papilledema (păp-ĭl-ĕ-dē′-mă)—inflammation of the optic nerve at the point where it enters the eyeball in response to increased intracranial pressure

An example of a procedure in the Other Procedures category includes optic nerve decompression. The physician makes an incision into the optic nerve sheath to release CSF and reduce pressure placed on the optic nerve, which is a treatment for **papilledema**.

Eyelids (67700–67999)

The Eyelids category includes six subcategories of procedures:

1. Incision (67700–67715)
2. Excision, Destruction (67800–67850)
3. Tarsorrhaphy (67875–67882)
4. Repair (Brow Ptosis, **Blepharoptosis**, Lid Retraction, Ectropion, Entropion) (67900–67924)
5. Reconstruction (67930–67975)
6. Other Procedures (one unlisted procedure) (67999)

blepharoptosis (blĕf-ă-rō-tō′-sĭs)—drooping of the upper eyelid

There are four eyelids: upper left, lower left, upper right, and lower right. It is important to note that when assigning eyelid procedure codes, you should also append a HCPCS modifier to Medicare claims to show the eyelid involved in the procedure. Other payers may also require these modifiers. Do you remember reviewing these

---

POINTERS FROM THE PROS: Interview with an Optometrist

William K. Vincett, Jr., D.O., has worked for 27 years as a doctor of optometry. He heads several large group practices, which serve over 42,000 patients in many office locations.

Describe your role in determining correct diagnosis and procedure codes for surgeries and office visits.

My role is to take the information provided by my pre-examination technician, and through thorough testing and more direct questions to the patient, go through a differential diagnosis of the patient's signs and symptoms. My examination may indicate the need for further special testing to help confirm my diagnosis or to aid in quantifying the severity of the diagnosis present. We use the Medicare guidelines in regard to a new or previous patient's history and complexity of the case to determine the proper codes for the visits.

Describe any challenges that your office has faced regarding medical documentation correlating to correct diagnosis and procedure codes.

One of the biggest challenges for me is in the constant reassigning of different reimbursement levels for new procedures and the inability of the codes to adequately represent what we have done.

What advice can you give to coders and billing staff to help them successfully communicate with physicians?

I think the biggest challenge is in the nonelectronic (medical) records offices. There must be a set of written communications by the coders to let the physician know the proper way to work a patient up within the guidelines established for treating the most common diseases as required by Medicare regulations.

(Used by permission of William K. Vincett, Jr.)

modifiers in Chapter 18? You can find them in your CPT and HCPCS coding manuals. They are as follows:

- E1—upper left eyelid
- E2—lower left eyelid
- E3—upper right eyelid
- E4—lower right eyelid

It is also important to understand that eyelid surgery can be considered cosmetic, or not medically necessary. Physicians perform cosmetic procedures to improve a patient's physical appearance and reduce or eliminate signs of aging. Insurances do not cover cosmetic procedures but typically reimburse providers for eyelid procedures that are medically necessary. Review examples of procedures under each of the six subcategories outlined next.

Incision subcategory:

- **Blepharotomy**—incision of the eyelid to drain an abscess
- **Cathotomy**—incision into the canthus (angle where eyelids meet), which can be to repair a defect after lesion removal

blepharotomy (blĕf-ă-rŏt′-ō-mē)

cathotomy (kăth-ŏ-tō′-mē)

Excision, Destruction subcategory:

- Excision of **chalazion**—eyelid cyst from a blocked sebaceous gland on the eyelid rim, called the **meibomian** gland, which infection can cause
- Correction of **trichiasis**—eyelashes that grow inward, causing friction on the conjunctiva or cornea. Infection or immune system disorders can cause trichiasis.
- The procedure involves **epilation** (hair removal) by forceps, electrosurgery, cryotherapy, laser surgery, or incision of the lid margin.

chalazion (kă-lā′-zē-ŏn)
meibomian (mī-bō′-mē-ăn)

trichiasis (trĭk-ī′-ăs-ĭs)

epilation (ĕp-ĭ-lā′-shŭn)

Tarsorrhaphy subcategory:

- There are three different procedures for a **tarsorrhaphy** (to partially suture the eyelids together).

tarsorrhaphy (tăr-sor′-ă-fē)

Repair subcategory includes repairs of

- **ectropion**—outward turning of the eyelid or **entropion**—inward turning of the eyelid

ectropion (ĕk-trō′-pē-ŏn)
entropion (ĕn-trō′-pē-ŏn)

Reconstruction subcategory includes

- Suturing of eyelid wounds, removal of foreign bodies, excision and repair of eyelid, and reconstruction of eyelid. Did you notice that CPT includes several guidelines under code 67938 *Removal of embedded foreign body, eyelid*? The notes direct you to use other codes, depending on the procedure that the physician performs.

Refer to the following example to learn more about coding a procedure involving the ocular adnexa.

> **Example:** Leslie Spencer, age 38, sees Dr. Lindsay in his office at Williton Medical Center. She complains of two bumps on her left upper eyelid, redness of the areas, and discomfort. Dr. Lindsay determines that the patient has two chalazions and excises both of them. He sends them to the hospital's lab for analysis, and the lab report reveals that they are both benign.
>
> To code this case, search the index for the main term *chalazion*, subterm *excision*, subterm *multiple*, and subterm *same lid*, which directs you to cross-reference code 67801. Assign code **67801- E1** because it represents multiple chalazion excisions of the same lid (upper left). The patient's diagnosis code is **373.2** (main term *chalazion*).

TAKE A BREAK

Keep up the good work! Let's take a break and practice assigning codes for the ocular adnexa.

Exercise 31.5   Ocular Adnexa

Instructions: Review the patient's case, and then assign codes for the procedure(s), appending a modifier when appropriate. Optional: For additional practice, assign the patient's diagnosis code(s) (ICD-9-CM).

1. Two years ago, Jonathon Ellis, who was one year old at the time, developed accommodative esotropia, crossing of the eyes caused by farsightedness. Today at Williton, Dr. Moore, an ophthalmologist, corrects the strabismus by performing surgery on the inferior oblique muscles and the superior rectus muscles.

   Diagnosis code(s): _____

   Procedure code(s): _____

2. Aubray Masters, age 42, presents to Dr. Moore's office with multiple chalazions on her left upper eyelid, and Dr. Moore excises them.

   Diagnosis code(s): _____

   Procedure code(s): _____

3. Carrie Struthers, age 19, presents to Dr. Moore's office complaining of dryness and tearing of her left eye. Dr. Moore diagnoses her with an ectropian of the left lower lid and performs an excisional tarsal wedge repair.

   Diagnosis code(s): _____

   Procedure code(s): _____

4. Lance Walters, age 83, developed diabetic macular edema in his right eye. Today at his office, Dr. Moore injects triamcinolone acetonide 10 mg into the Tenon's capsule to treat the edema. Code for the procedure and the drug (assign the HCPCS code from the HCPCS Table of Drugs and Chemicals).

   Diagnosis code(s): _____

   Procedure code(s): _____

5. Following Louise Kaufman's blepharoplasty that another physician performed, Dr. Moore diagnoses the 57-year-old with blepharochalasis (eyelid edema and thinning skin). At Williton, he performs a bilateral canthoplasty to strengthen the tissues at the outer corner of the eyes and to better support the lower eyelids.

   Diagnosis code(s): _____

   Procedure code(s): _____

6. Nathan Smothers, age 22, has a foreign body imbedded in his left lower eyelid. He developed pain and swelling after working in his yard on a windy day. Dr. Moore removes the foreign body.

   Diagnosis code(s): _____

   Procedure code(s): _____

CONJUNCTIVA (68020–68999)

The subheading Conjunctiva includes procedures involving the conjunctiva and lacrimal system. Recall that the conjunctiva is a lining that covers the outer surface of the eyeball and inside the eyelids, and the lacrimal system is made up of structures that produce and drain tears.

The subheading Conjunctiva includes six categories of procedures. Turn to the categories within this subheading in your CPT manual to review the procedures. ■ TABLE 31-3 outlines examples of some of these procedures, including some of the reasons that physicians perform them. To locate codes in the index for conjunctiva procedures, search under the body site (conjunctiva), type of procedure (conjunctivoplasty), or condition (cyst).

■ TABLE 31-3   **CONJUNCTIVA CATEGORIES AND PROCEDURES**

Category Name	Code Range	Procedures Included
Incision and Drainage	68020–68040	• **Incision for drainage of cyst** • **Expression** (*evacuation*) **of conjunctival follicles** (*sacs*)**, to treat a trachoma** (*eye infection that can scar the conjunctiva and cornea*) Physicians also perform this procedure to treat conjunctivitis (*conjunctival infection*).
Excision and/or Destruction	68100–68135	• **Biopsy of conjunctiva** • **Excision or destruction of lesion**—codes include lesion size and scleral involvement
Injection	68200	• **Subconjunctival** (*under the conjunctiva*) **injection to treat scleritis** (*scleral infection*) **or other disorders**

continued

■ TABLE 31-3 *continued*

Category Name	Code Range	Procedures Included
Conjunctivoplasty	68320–68340	• **Conjunctivoplasty**—conjunctiva repair
		• **Conjunctivoplasty, reconstruction of cul-de-sac** (*area between the palpebral and bulbar conjunctiva*)
		• **Repair of symblepharon** (*when the palpebral conjunctiva adheres to the bulbar conjunctiva*)
Other Procedures	68360–68399	• **Conjunctival flap** (*procedure to treat a corneal perforation or performed after pterygium excision*)
Lacrimal System	68400–68899	• **Incision, drainage of lacrimal sac—dacryocystotomy** (*incision of lacrimal sac and lacrimal duct*) **or dacryocystostomy** (*creating an opening in the lacrimal sac*) to treat an abscess
		• **Excision of lacrimal sac (dacryocystectomy), or biopsy of lacrimal sac**
		• **Removal of foreign body or dacryolith** (*calculus—hard deposit—in the lacrimal sac or duct*)
		• **Dacryocystorhinostomy** (*fistulization of lacrimal sac to nasal cavity*)—restores tear flow for disorders of the nasolacrimal duct
		• **Conjunctivorhinostomy** (*fistulization of conjunctiva to nasal cavity*)—restores tear drainage stopped by an obstruction
		• **Injection of contrast medium for dacryocystography** (*radiology procedure for visualizing lacrimal system structures*)
		Probing and related procedures involve removal of obstructions and wound exploration.

TAKE A BREAK

That was a lot of information to remember! Good work! Let's take a break and practice assigning codes for the conjunctiva.

Exercise 31.6 Conjunctiva

Instructions: Review the patient's case, and then assign codes for the procedure(s), appending a modifier when appropriate. Optional: For additional practice, assign the patient's diagnosis code(s) (ICD-9-CM).

1. Jimmy Sanders, age 19, has a blocked tear duct in his left eye. Dr. Moore, an ophthalmologist, sees him today in his office and treats the patient by dilating the lacrimal punctum with irrigation.

   Diagnosis code(s): _____

   Procedure code(s): _____

2. During a previous visit, Dr. Moore diagnosed Ron Johnston, age 44, with an everted punctum, an abnormal turning outward of the tear duct, of the left eye. Today at Williton, Dr. Moore performs a cautery correction.

   Diagnosis code(s): _____

   Procedure code(s): _____

3. Today at Williton, Dr. Lindsay, an ophthalmologist, performs conjunctivoplasty with extensive rearrangement to help relieve the pain and tearing that Edna Carey, age 73, is experiencing. Dr. Lindsay previously diagnosed her with bilateral conjunctival chalasis, loose conjunctival tissue.

   Diagnosis code(s): _____

   Procedure code(s): _____

4. Jennifer Cunningham, age 57, has been experiencing visual blurring and has noticed yellow bumps on her left eye. Today in his office, Dr. Moore performs a conjunctival biopsy to screen her for **sarcoidosis** (a chronic granulomatous condition that can involve almost any organ system of the body).

   Diagnosis code(s): _____

   Procedure code(s): _____

5. William Abrams, age 59, has dealt with eye infections for the past year that have been resistant to multiple antibiotic therapies. Today in his office, Dr. Moore expresses conjunctival follicles in both eyes in an attempt to determine the cause.

   Diagnosis code(s): _____

   Procedure code(s): _____

6. Today at Williton, Dr. Moore performs a plastic repair of the lacrimal canaliculi on 30-year-old Chris Murphy's right eye to repair a laceration that she suffered when her cat, Snowball, scratched her.

   Diagnosis code(s): _____

   Procedure code(s): _____

WORKPLACE IQ

You are working as a coder for Dr. Lindsay, who owns a busy ophthalmology practice with nine other physicians and several office employees and technicians. This morning, you are helping Susie, the front desk receptionist, take incoming calls because the employee who normally helps her is out sick.

Mr. Welsh, a current patient, calls to say that his insurance company sent him an explanation of benefits (EOB) for his recent surgery to treat a detached retina. Mr. Welsh states that the EOB shows that he still owes coinsurance for the surgery. The EOB also shows code

67107 along with a description of the code, and he does not understand what the description means. He tells you, "The description mentions buckling, cryotherapy, and photocoagulation. I can't even pronounce these words, let alone know what they mean! I don't mind paying my share of the coinsurance, but I would at least like to know what I'm paying for. I thought I was just having retinal surgery. What is all this other stuff?"

What would you do?

AUDITORY SYSTEM (69000–69979)

symblepharon
(sĭm-blĕf′-ă-rŏn)

dacryocystotomy
(dăk-rē-ō-sĭs-tŏt′-tō-mē)

dacryocystostomy
(dăk-rē-ō-sĭs-tŏs′-tō-mē)

dacryocystectomy
(dăk-rē-ō-sĭs-tĕk′-tō-mē)

dacryolith (dăk′-rē-ō-lĭth)

dacryocystorhinostomy
(dăk-rē-ō-sĭs-tō-rī-nŏs′-
tō-mē)

conjunctivorhinostomy
(kŏn-jŭnk-tī-vō-rī-nŏs′-
tō-mē)

dacryocystography (dăk-
rē-ō-sĭs-tŏg′-ră-fē)

sarcoidosis (sär-koid′-ō-səs)

otologist/neurotologist
(ō-tŏl′-ō-jĭst/n(y)u-rä-təl′-
ə-jəst)

audiologist (aw-dē-ŏl′-ō-jĭst)

pinna (pĭn′-ă)

auricle (aw′-rĭ-kl)

ceruminous
(sə-rü′-mə-nəs)

cerumen (sĕr-ū′-mĕn)

malleus (măl′-ē-ŭs)

incus (ĭng′-kŭs)

The Auditory System, a subsection of Surgery, involves procedures of a body system. (The Operating Microscope is the last subsection under Surgery.) **Auditory** means hearing. You first learned about the ear in Chapter 9. Recall that otolaryngology is the study of the ear and the larynx. Otolaryngologists are physicians who diagnose and treat ear, nose, and throat disorders. An **otologist/neurotologist** is a *board-certified* physician specializing in treating ear and balance disorders, including neoplasms of the bone and hearing device implantation for profoundly deaf patients. An **audiologist** is not a physician but is a healthcare professional with at least a Master's degree who assesses patients' hearing loss, balance problems, and other disorders. An audiologist also fits patients with hearing aids.

Refer to Figure 9-22 to review ear structures as you read through the next section to become familiar with ear anatomy and terms that you will find in code descriptors for the Auditory System subsection.

ANATOMY OF THE EAR

The ear is divided into three parts:

* external ear
* middle ear
* inner ear

The **external ear** is the outer part of the ear that is visible, including the lobe and the **pinna**, or **auricle**, which transmits sounds through the auditory canal, or ***external auditory meatus***. **Ceruminous *glands*** in the auditory canal produce earwax, called **cerumen**, which lubricates the ear.

The **middle ear** contains the eardrum, or ***tympanic membrane***, which receives sound waves transmitted through the auditory canal, resulting in vibrations. There are three bones in the middle ear, called ***ossicles***, which amplify sound waves from the tympanic membrane and transmit them to the inner ear. The bones were named for the shape of the object they resemble:

* *hammer*, or **malleus**
* *anvil*, or **incus**
* *stirrup*, or *stapes*

The ossicles create an *ossicular chain* that transmits sound received from the tympanic membrane. The malleus is attached to the tympanic membrane, and the incus is attached to the malleus. The stapes is attached to the oval window, which receives sound waves from the ossicular chain. The oval window is located in the inner ear (■ FIGURE 31-5).

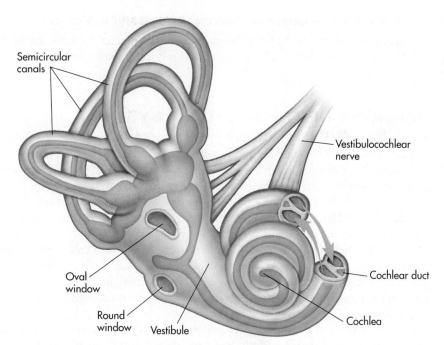

Figure 31-5 ■ The structures of the inner ear.

Source: Anatomy & Physiology for Health Professions, Colbert, Ankney, Lee. 2011, pg. 255.

The **eustachian** *tube,* also called the **otopharyngeal** tube, is also in the middle ear and connects to the pharynx and nasal cavity. It drains fluid from the middle ear and helps to adjust air pressure on both sides of the eardrum. A common condition of the middle ear is otitis media, when the eustachian tube becomes occluded with fluid, which you learned about in Chapter 9. Patients may also suffer from infections or inflammation that cause fluid to build up in the middle ear. The eustachian tube was named after Bartolomeo Eustachi, the Italian anatomist who discovered it in the 1500s.

eustachian (ū-stā′-shŭn)
otopharyngeal
(ō-tō-făr-ĭn′-jē-ăl)

The middle ear also contains two openings, the *oval window* and the *round window.* When the eardrum, or tympanic membrane, vibrates, the stapes *footplate (*flat part) vibrates against the oval window. The membrane of the round window expands, and the fluid in the inner ear then vibrates against the hairlike structures. The hairlike structures transmit messages of sound to the brain through nerve impulses.

The **inner ear,** also called the **labyrinth,** osseous labyrinth, or bony labyrinth, is made up of three bony areas:

labyrinth (lăb′-ĭ-rĭnth)

- **cochlea**—shaped like a snail and contains **perilymph,** a fluid for transmitting sound
- *vestibule chamber*—the center of the inner ear
- *semicircular canals*—help the body to maintain its balance

cochlea (kōk′-lē-ă)
perilymph (pĕr′-ĭ-lĭmf)

The osseous labyrinth consists of many passageways of bones. The ***membranous labyrinth*** refers to periosteum that lines the bones of the osseous labyrinth. There is fluid within the membranous labyrinth called ***endolymph,*** found in the endolymphatic sac, which helps to transmit signals of sound to the brain through the movement of hairlike structures. The **vestibulocochlear** nerve, cranial nerve VIII, carries the signal to the brain.

Here are some additional terms included in code descriptors for the ear that you should know:

vestibulocochlear
(vĕs-tĭb-ū-lō-kōk′-lē-ăr)

- **atticotomy**—incision into the epitympatic recess, a hollow located on the superior aspect of the middle ear, known as the tympanic attic
- **drumhead**—another name for the eardrum, or tympanic membrane
- **geniculate ganglion**—sensory and sympathetic nerve cells of the facial nerve
- **intratemporal**—within the temporal bone
- **postauricular**—behind the auricle (pinna) of the ear
- **temporal bone**—bone located on the side of the skull and at its base. There is a left- and a right-side temporal bone, which connects to the jaw bone (mandible).

atticotomy (ăt-ĭ-kŏt′-ō-mē)
drumhead (drŭm′-hĕd)
geniculate ganglion
(jĕn-ĭk′-ū-lăt găng′-lē-ŏn)
intratemporal
(ĭn-tră-tĕm′-pō-răl)
postauricular
(pōst-aw-rĭk′-ū-lăr)

transcanal approach
(trănz-căn′-ĕl)

translabyrinthine approach
(trănz- lăb′-ĭ-rĭn-thīn)

- **transcanal approach**—to access the middle ear through the external auditory canal
- **translabyrinthine approach**—to access the internal acoustic canal through mastoidectomy and labyrinthectomy, commonly used to remove an acoustic neuroma

DIVISIONS OF THE AUDITORY SYSTEM

The Auditory System is divided first into four subheadings that represent a specific part of the ear: external ear, middle ear, inner ear, and temporal bone. There is a CPT note at the beginning of the Auditory System which alerts you that if you need to assign codes for auditory diagnostic testing, then you should refer to code 92502 *et seq*. *Et seq* means *and the following*. This means that there are also other codes for auditory diagnostic testing besides code 92502. You can find them in the Medicine section under the subsection Special Otorhinolaryngologic Services.

CPT further divides Auditory System subheadings into categories, arranged by type of procedure (■ TABLE 31-4). You can locate codes for auditory system procedures by searching the index for the *body site* (e.g., ear—external, inner, middle) and then the *type of procedure* (e.g., biopsy, incision, insertion), or start your search with the *type of procedure* or the *condition* (e.g., lesion, abscess).

Let's review more about how to assign codes for procedures in subheadings and categories, and then practice coding. Refer to Figures 9-22 and Figure 31-5 to help you to better understand code descriptors. Also be sure to review CPT guidelines before final code assignments.

It is important to note that when you assign codes for ear procedures, you should append modifier -LT or -RT to indicate the left or right ear, or modifier -50 for a bilateral procedure.

■ TABLE 31-4   AUDITORY SYSTEM SUBHEADINGS AND CATEGORIES

Subsection, Subheadings, Categories, and Subcategories	Code Range
AUDITORY SYSTEM	**69000–69979**
External Ear	**69000–69399**
Incision	*69000–69090*
Excision	*69100–69155*
Removal	*69200–69222*
Repair	*69300–69320*
Other Procedures	*69399*
Middle Ear	**69400–69799**
Introduction	*69400–69405*
Incision	*69420–69450*
Excision	*69501–69554*
Repair	*69601–69676*
Other Procedures	*69700–69799*
Inner Ear	**69801–69949**
Incision and/or Destruction	*69801–69840*
Excision	*69905–69915*
Introduction	*69930*
Other Procedures	*69949*
Temporal Bone, Middle Fossa Approach	**69950–69979**
Other Procedures	*69979*

EXTERNAL EAR (69000–69399)

Recall that the external ear is the outer part of the ear that is visible, including the lobe and the pinna, or auricle, which transmits sounds through the auditory canal, or *external auditory meatus*. The subheading External Ear contains five categories of procedures, arranged by type of procedure (incision, excision), with additional codes divided by simple or complicated, simple or complete, and if the patient had general anesthesia for the procedure.

Turn to the categories within the External Ear subheading in your CPT manual to review the procedures as you read more about them in ■ TABLE 31-5.

exostosis (ĕks′-ŏs-tō-sĭs)

otoplasty (ō-tō-plăs′-tē)

meatoplasty (mē-ă′-tō-plăs′-tē)

canalplasty –(kă-năl-plăs′-tē)

atresia (ă-trē′-zē-ă)

■ TABLE 31-5 **EXTERNAL EAR CATEGORIES AND PROCEDURES**

Category Name	Code Range	Examples of Procedures Included
Incision	69000–69090	• **Drainage of an abscess or hematoma of the external ear, simple or complicated**
		Note: The physician's documentation may not specifically state simple or complicated. A complicated procedure would require more time and effort than the physician normally spends for a simple drainage. Always query the physician if you need clarification.
		• **Drainage of an abscess of the external auditory canal**
		• **Ear piercing**—This is a cosmetic procedure that many pediatricians' offices offer, and insurances typically do not reimburse for it.
Excision	69100–69155	• **Biopsy of external ear or external auditory canal** (*to determine behavior of a lesion*)
		• **Excision of external ear—partial with simple repair or excision with complete amputation** (*to remove a neoplasm, infection, or necrosis*)
		Note: There is a CPT note that directs you to see code 15120 and other codes for ear reconstruction.
		• **Excision of exostosis(es) or soft tissue lesion from external auditory canal**
		Exostosis, also called surfer's ear, is when bone grows abnormally in the external auditory canal from continuous exposure to cold water and wind.
Removal	69200–69222	• **Removal of foreign body from external auditory canal, without or with general anesthesia** (*procedure commonly performed for children because they place objects in their ears*)
		• **Removal of impacted cerumen for one or both ears** (*assign the same code, 69210, whether the procedure involves one ear or both*)
		• **Debridement, mastoid cavity, simple** (*routine cleaning*) **or complex** (*with anesthesia, or more than routine cleaning*)
		The mastoid is a protruding bone, located behind the ear, and is part of the temporal bone.
Repair	69300–69320	• **Otoplasty (external ear repair) protruding ear, with or without size reduction** (*treatment for congenital disorders or trauma*). This procedure includes conscious sedation.
		• **Reconstruction of external auditory canal (meatoplasty) for stenosis due to injury or infection**
		• **Reconstruction of external auditory canal** (also called **canalplasty**) **for congenital atresia, single stage**
		Congenital atresia is the congenital absence of external auditory canal, which can result in hearing loss and also anomalies of the middle ear.
Other Procedures	69399	• **Unlisted procedure, external ear**

Refer to the following example to learn more about coding an external ear procedure.

> **Example:** Mr. Spencer, a 43-year-old patient, suffers from surfer's ear, and Dr. Berry, an otolaryngologist, removes the bony growth from the patient's right ear during a scheduled procedure at Williton Medical Center.
>
> To code this case, search the index for the main term *exostosis* and subterm *excision*, which directs you to cross-reference code 69140. Assign code **69140-RT** because it represents the exostosis, also called surfer's ear. The patient's diagnosis code is **380.81** (main term *exostosis* and subterm *ear canal, external*).

TAKE A BREAK

Hang in there! You are doing well! Let's take a break and review more about the external ear.

Exercise 31.7 Anatomy of the Ear, External Ear

Part 1—Theory

Instructions: Fill in the blank with the best answer.

1. The _____ glands in the auditory canal produce earwax, called _____, which lubricates the ear.

2. The _____ drains fluid from the middle ear and helps to adjust air pressure on both sides of the eardrum.

3. When the eardrum, or tympanic membrane vibrates, the stapes _____ vibrates against the oval window.

4. The inner ear is made up of three bony areas: the _____, the _____, and the _____.

5. What is another name for the eardrum, or tympanic membrane? _____

6. What is the name for an external ear repair for a protruding ear that may involve size reduction?
_____

Part 2—Coding

Instructions: Review the patient's case, and then assign codes for the procedure(s), appending a modifier when appropriate. Optional: For additional practice, assign the patient's diagnosis code(s) (ICD-9-CM).

1. Four-year-old Hallee Peters was born with external auditory canal atresia. Today at Williton, Dr. Delgado, an otolaryngologist, reconstructs the external auditory canals.

   Diagnosis code(s): _____

   Procedure code(s): _____

2. Mrs. Murphy brings her two-year-old daughter, Madelynn, to King's Ear Clinic because Madelynn put a pea in her left ear, which her mother could not remove. Dr. Delgado removes it.

   Diagnosis code(s): _____

   Procedure code(s): _____

3. Michael Wilkins, age 35, has a growth in his right auditory canal. He visits Dr. Delgado at King's Ear Clinic, where the physician biopsies the growth. He sends the specimen to Williton's pathologist for analysis and the pathologist finds that the lesion is benign.

   Diagnosis code(s): _____

   Procedure code(s): _____

4. Peggy Lewis, age 56, schedules an appointment with Dr. Delgado because her husband continues to tell her that she cannot hear well. She does not believe it but agrees to see Dr. Delgado anyway. Dr. Delgado examines the patient at the clinic and determines that she has impacted cerumen in both ears, and he removes it. Mrs. Lewis leaves the office a little embarrassed but can hear much better.

   Diagnosis code(s): _____

   Procedure code(s): _____

5. Charles Conner, age 13, was born with macrotia (large, protruding ears). He endures daily teasing on the school bus and wants to quit school. He and his parents meet with Dr. Delgado at King's Ear Clinic to ask for help. Dr. Delgado explains that Charles would greatly benefit from surgery to reduce the size of his ears. Today at Williton, Dr. Delgado performs otoplasty to correct the condition, and the surgery is successful. Code for the patient's surgery.

   Diagnosis code(s): _____

   Procedure code(s): _____

6. Jennifer Anderson, age 42, developed a large abscess in the external canal of her left ear. She meets with Dr. Delgado today at the clinic, where he drains the abscess. He explains to Mrs. Anderson that the condition should resolve on its own but advises her to contact him if any redness, swelling and pain continue after tomorrow.

   Diagnosis code(s): _____

   Procedure code(s): _____

MIDDLE EAR (69400–69799)

Recall that the middle ear contains the tympanic membrane (eardrum), ossicles (three small bones), and the eustachian tube. The *eustachian tube* connects to the pharynx and nasal cavity, draining fluid from the middle ear and helping to adjust air pressure on both sides of the eardrum. A common condition of the middle ear is otitis media, when the eustachian tube becomes occluded. If a patient does not respond to antibiotics to treat otitis media, or has several recurrences of the disorder, then the physician may recommend surgery to correct the problem. Otitis media is one of the most common infections in children. Turn to the Middle Ear subheading in your CPT manual to review procedures listed under the following five categories, which you will learn more about in the next sections:

1. Introduction
2. Incision
3. Excision
4. Repair
5. Other Procedures

Introduction (69400–69405)

The Introduction category contains procedures for eustachian tube inflation, which physicians perform to treat eustachian tube disorders. In these disorders, fluid or a swollen mucous membrane obstructs the eustachian tube and middle ear. They include acute or chronic serous (containing fluid) otitis media, allergies, and sinus infections. The procedure involves blowing air into the middle ear or nose, which moves through the eustachian tube to open the passageway. Introduction may also involve inserting a catheter into the eustachian tube to dilate it, and the procedure can be transnasal (through the nose) or transtympanic (across the tympanic membrane).

Incision (69420–69450)

CPT arranges procedures in this category by the type of procedure, and also arranges some of the procedures according to whether the patient receives general anesthesia, local, or topical anesthesia. Let's review more about procedures in the Incision category:

- **Myringotomy**—to drain fluid or pus from the eardrum to treat disorders such as serous otitis media. During a myringotomy, the physician obtains a sample of the fluid to submit for lab testing. The physician may also insert a ventilating tube during the procedure.

  myringotomy
  (mǐr-ǐn-gǒ′-tō-mē)

- **Tympanostomy**—to create an opening in the eardrum to insert a plastic or metal ventilating tube (also called a pressure equalization tube, or PE tube), which drains fluid from the middle ear. The physician leaves the ventilating tube in the ear, and the eardrum holds it securely in place for several months or several years. The procedure also helps the patient to regain any hearing loss suffered as a result of the fluid build-up. Physicians most commonly perform the procedure for children who typically require general anesthesia to ensure that they do not move during surgery. A PE tube eventually falls out, or the physician removes it, and the eardrum typically heals over the incision that the physician created for the tube.

  tympanostomy
  (tǐm-pǎn-ǒs′-tō-mē)

- *Middle ear exploration*—to investigate lesions and other disorders, including the source of discharged fluid, and to obtain biopsies.

- **Tympanolysis**—to destroy (lysis) tympanic membrane adhesions, granulation tissue, or scar tissue.

  tympanolysis
  (tǐm-pǎn′-ō-lǐ-sǐs)

Excision (69501–69554)

CPT arranges codes in the Excision category by type of procedure, which we will define later in this section, including

- *Transmastoid* **antrotomy** (incision of the mastoid antrum) (simple mastoidectomy)

  antrotomy (ǎn-trǒ′-tō-mē)

- *Mastoidectomy*—complete, modified radical, radical

Figure 31-6 ■
Cholesteatoma, a destructive and expanding keratinizing squamous epithelium in the middle ear and/or mastoid process, excised from an adult's ear.

Photo credit: Biophoto Associates / Photo Researchers, Inc., Enhancement by: Meredith Carlson.

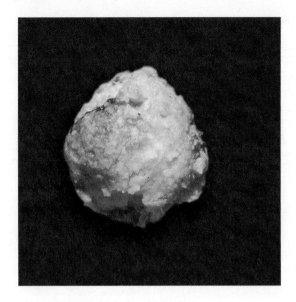

A mastoidectomy (excision of the mastoid process, or bone) is when the physician removes the diseased portion of the mastoid process, the protruding bone behind the ear at the skull base. The mastoid process has air-filled cavities and looks like a honeycomb. It connects to the middle ear through a small passageway in the petrous temporal bone. The *mastoid antrum* is the space between the mastoid cells and the upper part of the middle ear.

Many times, a patient develops *mastoiditis* (inflammation of the mastoid process) from an ongoing middle ear infection, which spreads to the mastoid process and can damage the patient's hearing. On rare occasions when antibiotics do not eliminate infection, the physician must remove part of the mastoid process to treat the infection. Physicians also perform mastoidectomies to treat patients with **chronic otitis**, a **cholesteatoma** (growth in the mastoid process or middle ear) (■ FIGURE 31-6), or a paralyzed facial nerve.

There are four different types of mastoidectomies, depending on the complexity of the procedure:

chronic otitis (ō-tī′-tĭs)— chronic inflammation behind the eardrum

cholesteatoma (kə-les-tē-ə-tō′-mə)

- *Simple*—dissection of the mastoid process, with cultures taken for lab testing
- *Complete*—a simple mastoidectomy with more extensive removal of the mastoid process, especially to treat cholesteatomas
- *Modified radical*—to treat cholesteatomas in patients who may also have suppurative otitis media or in patients where previous surgeries have failed. The procedure includes reconstructing the eardrum (tympanoplasty).
- *Radical*—to treat cholesteatomas and neoplasms of the ear canal, including removing large sections of the mastoid process, middle ear structures, and the eardrum.

Here are some other procedures included in the Excision category:

petrous apicectomy (pĕt′-rŭs ăp-ĭ-sĕk′-tō-mē)

glomus (glō′-mŭs)

- **Petrous apicectomy**—surgical resection (to cut or remove a part) of the petrous apex (part of the temporal bone) due to an infection or neoplasm
- *Resection of temporal bone*—to resect a tumor
- *Excision of aural polyp or aural glomus tumor*—An *aural polyp* is a benign growth of the external auditory canal or the tympanic membrane, and an *aural glomus tumor* is a benign neoplasm of the middle ear.

Repair (69601–69676)

The Repair category for the middle ear contains the following types of procedures:

- *Revision mastoidectomy*—The physician performs a revised mastoidectomy following a previous mastoidectomy that failed to resolve the patient's condition, such as a cholesteatoma or infection.

- *Myringoplasty*—The physician repairs the tympanic membrane, involving the drumhead and donor area, usually with a graft of living tissue (fat, fascia)

- *Tympanoplasty*—The physician performs reconstruction of the tympanic membrane or the ossicles. A graft repair of a perforated eardrum involves using the patient's own tissue to repair the defect.

    CPT arranges tympanoplasty codes by the types of other procedures performed at the same time, including ossicular chain reconstruction, which involves reconstructing at least one of the ossicles and can also include a synthetic prosthesis of one or more ossicles. The two types of prosthetics are

    - Partial ossicular replacement prosthesis (PORP)

    - Total ossicular replacement prosthesis (TORP)

- *Stapedectomy* (excision of the stapes) or *stapedotomy* (incision into the footplate of the stapes)—The physician performs this procedure to treat otosclerosis and it may also involve inserting a prosthesis for hearing loss.

- *Repair of oval window or round window fistula*—A fistula is an abnormal connection between the middle and inner ear. Fistulas of the oval and round window occur as a result of trauma, infection, or other disorder. The physician grafts soft tissue to repair the defect.

Other Procedures (69700–69799)

The Other Procedures category for the middle ear includes implants of hearing devices. In order to better understand these procedures it is helpful to know more about hearing loss. There are three main types of hearing loss.

- *Conductive hearing loss*—A disorder of the external or middle ear that prevents transmission of sound to the inner ear. Causes include otosclerosis, fluid or wax build-up, infection, neoplasms, and perforated eardrum.

- *Sensorineural hearing loss*—This is the most common type of adult hearing loss, when the nerves in the inner ear do not convey hearing signals to the brain. Causes include aging, injury, infection, meningitis, stroke, and exposure to loud noise.

sensorineural
(sĕn-sō-rē-nū′-răl)

- *Mixed hearing loss*—The patient has characteristics of both conductive and sensorineural hearing loss.

    Patients may also experience *functional hearing loss*, when they suffer from emotional or psychological distress and cannot hear, even though there is no physical problem with their hearing. Some patients benefit from *sound therapy*, when they learn to perform various hearing exercises to help them to hear better. For other patients, a hearing device, or hearing aid, is the only solution.

    Hearing aids amplify sounds, and the type of hearing aid that a patient has depends on the patient's condition and the extent of the hearing loss. Types of hearing aids include *air conduction* and *bone conduction*. Air conduction is when sound travels from the external ear through the auditory canal, into the middle ear, and then into the inner ear. Bone conduction is when sound travels through the bones of the ear and does not first travel from the external ear to the middle ear. You can experience bone conduction if you lightly knock your fingers against the side of your head. You can hear a tapping sound, but the sound did not first travel through your external ear. Instead, you heard the sound directly from the knocking against the bone. There are external bone conduction hearing aids, which the patient must wear close to the temporal bone, and implanted bone conduction hearing aids.

    The Other Procedures category contains codes for the implantation, removal, or replacement of an electromagnetic bone conduction hearing device or an **osseointegrated** (integrated with bone) implant. There are also HCPCS codes that represent hearing devices and/or their components. Examples include

osseointegrated
(ŏs-ē-ō-ĭn′-tĕ-grā-tĭd)

- **L8690**—Auditory osseointegrated device, includes all internal and external components

- **L8691**—Auditory osseointegrated device, external sound processor, replacement

Insurances have various guidelines for reimbursing hearing device implants, including specific criteria that patients must meet for medical necessity. It is important to check with each payer to review individual guidelines.

Refer to the following example to learn more about coding a middle ear procedure.

otosclerosis (ō-tō-sklĕ-rō′-sĭs)

Example: Mrs. Matthews, a 33-year-old, suffers from nonobliterative oval window **otosclerosis** (fibrous tissue interfering with the oval window). Dr. Berry, an otolaryngologist, mobilizes the stapes of the patient's right ear at Williton Medical Center during a scheduled procedure.

To code this case, search the index for the main term *mobilization* and subterm *stapes*, which directs you to cross-reference code 69650. Assign code **69650-RT** because it accurately represents the procedure. The patient's diagnosis code is **387.0** (main term *otosclerosis*, subterm *involving*, subterm *oval window*, and subterm *nonobliterative*).

parotid sialectasis
(pă-rŏt′-ĭd sī-ă-lĕk′-tă-sĭs)

TAKE A BREAK

Way to go! Let's take a break and then review more about the middle ear.

Exercise 31.8   Middle Ear

Part 1—Theory

Instructions: Fill in the blank with the best answer.

1. What is the name of the procedure that the physician performs to repair the tympanic membrane, involving the drumhead and donor area, with a graft of living tissue? _____

2. A(n) _____ is a procedure to remove diseased air cells of the mastoid process.

3. A(n) _____ is a benign growth of the external auditory canal or the tympanic membrane.

4. What is the name of the procedure that the physician performs following a previous mastoidectomy that failed to resolve the patient's condition?
_____

5. A(n) _____ is a procedure to drain fluid or pus from the eardrum to treat disorders such as serous otitis media.

6. _____ is a disorder of the external or middle ear that prevents transmission of sound to the inner ear.

Part 2—Coding

Instructions: Review the patient's case, and then assign codes for the procedure(s), appending a modifier when appropriate. Optional: For additional practice, assign the patient's diagnosis code(s) (ICD-9-CM).

1. At King's Ear Clinic, Dr. Delgado sees Mandy Saunders, age 37, who suffers from chronic bilateral **parotid sialectasis** (dilation of salivary ducts). Dr. Delgado, an otolaryngologist, performs a tympanic neurotomy to relieve her symptoms.

Diagnosis code(s): _____

Procedure code(s): _____

2. Dr. Delgado examines Max Winters, age 43, for hearing loss and determines that the cause is otosclerosis of the otic capsule (sac). Today at Williton, he performs a stapedectomy with foot plate (part of the stapes) drill out in an attempt to restore Mr. Winters' hearing.

Diagnosis code(s): _____

Procedure code(s): _____

3. Seven-year-old Rachael Anderson suffered a perforated right eardrum as a result of acute suppurative otitis media. Dr. Delgado performs a myringoplasty to repair the hole.

Diagnosis code(s): _____

Procedure code(s): _____

4. Wilbur Davis, age 87, was diagnosed with a malignancy of the temporal bone. Today at Williton, Dr. Delgado performs a temporal bone resection to treat it.

Diagnosis code(s): _____

Procedure code(s): _____

5. Four-year-old Marissa Allen suffers from chronic otitis media. Dr. Delgado performs a bilateral tympanostomy to help fluid drain from the child's ears.

Diagnosis code(s): _____

Procedure code(s): _____

6. Amy Withers, age 37, has an obstructed eustachian tube. Dr. Delgado inflates the eustachian tube by increasing air pressure in the nasopharynx (upper throat).

Diagnosis code(s): _____

Procedure code(s): _____

INNER EAR (69801–69949)

Recall that the inner ear is also called the osseous labyrinth and is composed of the cochlea, which contains perilymph for transmitting sound; the vestibule chamber; and the semicircular canals, which help the body to maintain its balance. The membranous labyrinth consists of periosteum that lines the bones of the osseous labyrinth, and the endolymphatic sac contains endolymph, which also plays a role in transmitting sound signals to the brain.

The subheading Inner Ear contains four categories of procedures, arranged by type of procedure (excision, introduction). Turn to the categories within the Inner Ear subheading in your CPT manual to review the procedures as you read more about them in ■ TABLE 31-6.

TEMPORAL BONE, MIDDLE FOSSA APPROACH (69950–69979)

Recall that the temporal bone is on the side of the head at the skull base and is connected to the mandible. A **middle fossa** (hollow area or bone cavity) approach is when the physician incises the bone above the ear and removes part of it to gain access to the internal auditory canal. Physicians use the middle fossa approach to treat an acoustic neuroma, meningioma, or skull fracture. Turn to the categories within the Temporal Bone, Middle Fossa Approach subheading in your CPT manual to review the five procedures listed.

■ TABLE 31-6   **INNER EAR CATEGORIES AND PROCEDURES**

Category Name	Code Range	Procedures Included	
Incision and/or Destruction	69801–69840	• **Labyrinthotomy** (*surgical incision into the labyrinth of the ear*), **with perfusion of vestibuloactive drug(s), transcanal; may also include a mastoidectomy**	
		One reason for this procedure is to treat **Meniere's** disease, a disorder with vertigo (dizziness), hearing loss, and tinnitus. The physician injects a medication into the inner ear to treat the patient's symptoms.	Meniere's (mān′-ē-ārz)
		• **Fenestration semicircular canal**—Creation of an opening in the semicircular canal to treat disorders such as otosclerosis	
Excision	69905–69915	• **Labyrinthectomy, transcanal; may also include a mastoidectomy**—procedure to treat vertigo and includes removing the entire inner ear except for the cochlea. The patient loses all hearing in the ear and typically relies on the other ear for maintaining balance.	
		• **Vestibular nerve section, translabyrinthine approach**—procedure to treat vertigo in Meniere's disease and other disorders, involves incising the vestibular nerve fibers but leaving the cochlear nerve fibers intact	
Introduction	69930	• **Cochlear device implantation, with or without a mastoidectomy**—involves implanting a receiver into bone, which sends signals to electrodes implanted in the cochlea. There are also external components of the device that help the patient to hear, including a microphone, speech processor, and transmitter.	cochlear (kōk′-lē-ăr)
		The procedure is for patients who are profoundly deaf or have severe hearing loss. Hospitals purchase the hearing device from a medical supply manufacturer and bill the device to the patient's insurance (Example: HCPCS code L8614—*Cochlear device, includes all internal and external components*).	
Other Procedures	69949	• Unlisted procedure, inner ear	

Refer to the following example to learn more about coding an inner ear procedure.

Example: Shelly Arnold, a 35-year-old, has bilateral sensorineural hearing loss. Dr. Wagner, an otologist, inserts a cochlear implant into the patient's right ear during a scheduled procedure at Williton Medical Center. Williton Medical Center will bill the patient's insurance for the technical portion of the service and for the implanted device purchased from Greencrest Medical Supply.

To code this case for Dr. Wagner's services, search the index for the main term *cochlear device* and subterm *insertion*, which directs you to cross-reference code 69930. Assign code **69930-RT** because it accurately represents the procedure for the right ear. The patient's diagnosis code is **389.18** (main term *deafness*, subterm *sensorineural*, and subterm *bilateral*).

TAKE A BREAK

Wow! You made it through! Give yourself a pat on the back! Let's take a break and practice assigning codes for the inner ear, temporal bone, and middle fossa approach.

Exercise 31.9   Inner Ear, Temporal Bone, Middle Fossa Approach

Instructions: Review the patient's case, and then assign codes for the procedure(s), appending a modifier when appropriate. Optional: For additional practice, assign the patient's diagnosis code(s) (ICD-9-CM).

1. Jerry Benson, a 52-year-old established patient, experiences frequent vertigo as a result of Meniere's disease. Today at King's Ear Clinic, Dr. Delgado, an otolaryngologist, treats the condition with an endolymphatic sac exploration with shunt.

   Diagnosis code(s): _____

   Procedure code(s): _____

2. Vince Mack, a 48-year-old, has an acoustic neuroma. Today at the clinic, Dr. Delgado performs a transcanal labyrinthectomy with mastoidectomy to remove the neuroma.

   Diagnosis code(s): _____

   Procedure code(s): _____

3. Terry Lee, age 61, has recurrent episodes of left-sided facial paralysis. Today at the clinic, Dr. Delgado performs a total facial nerve decompression and repair with graft.

   Diagnosis code(s): _____

   Procedure code(s): _____

4. Maggie Paxton, age five, was born with an oval window malformation and suffers from conductive hearing loss as a result. Dr. Delgado fenestrates (pierces to create an opening) the semicircular canal of her right ear in an attempt to restore some of her hearing.

   Diagnosis code(s): _____

   Procedure code(s): _____

5. Following surgery, Dr. Delgado determines that Ms. Paxton's fenestration did not provide significant improvement in her hearing. Today at the clinic Dr. Delgado performs a revision.

   Diagnosis code(s): _____

   Procedure code(s): _____

6. Today at the clinic, Dr. Delgado removes a benign temporal bone tumor for Molly Stoddard, age 30.

   Diagnosis code(s): _____

   Procedure code(s): _____

OPERATING MICROSCOPE (69990)

The operating microscope is the last subsection of Surgery and contains only one add-on code, 69990—*Microsurgical techniques, requiring use of operating microscope (List separately in addition to code for primary procedure)*. You learned in Chapter 21 that physicians use the **operating microscope** to see small structures, such as in microsurgery. There is an extensive CPT note under the Operating Microscope subsection which you should review.

Medicare's National Correct Coding Initiative (NCCI) bundles the use of the operating microscope with auditory system procedures. This means that Medicare will not separately reimburse for the operating microscope. Check individual payer guidelines to determine which payers will pay for the operating microscope with auditory system procedures.

DESTINATION: MEDICARE

In this exercise, your Medicare destination is to review Medicare's Glaucoma Screening Brochure, which will help you to learn more about glaucoma screening, risk factors, and Medicare reimbursement for services related to glaucoma. Follow the instructions listed next to access the brochure.

1. Go to the website http://www.cms.gov.
2. At the top of the screen on the banner bar, choose *Outreach & Education*.
3. Scroll down to *Medicare Learning Network*, and choose *MLN Products*.
4. On the left side of the screen, choose *Ophthalmology Resource Information*.
5. Scroll down to *Downloads*, and choose *Glaucoma Screening*.

Answer the following questions, using the search function (Ctrl + F) to find information that you need:

1. What services are included with annual glaucoma screening?
2. Will Medicare pay for an annual glaucoma screening for every Medicare beneficiary age 65 or older?
3. When Medicare covers the beneficiary's glaucoma screening, does the beneficiary still have to pay a copayment?

CHAPTER REVIEW

Multiple Choice

Instructions: Circle one best answer to complete each statement.

1. OU, OS, and OD are abbreviations that physicians use to
   a. indicate what modifier should be appended to a code.
   b. document on which eye the procedure is performed.
   c. indicate whether an ophthalmic condition is acute, chronic, or both.
   d. indicate if a procedure is successful, detrimental, or undetermined.

2. Trabecular meshwork
   a. connects the middle ear to the temporal bone.
   b. is used to repair a perforated eardrum.
   c. is no longer indicated for repair of perforated eardrum.
   d. provides canals to drain aqueous humor from the eye.

3. The procedure utilized to remove an eye and the ocular contents is called an
   a. enucleation.
   b. evisceration.
   c. evacuation.
   d. exenteration.

4. _____ may not separately reimburse when a physician uses the operating microscope to perform a procedure.
   a. Private insurances
   b. Medicare and other payers
   c. Medicaid
   d. Workers' Compensation

5. You can find the CPT code for removal of a foreign body from the conjunctiva under the subheading
   a. Ocular adnexa.
   b. Posterior segment.
   c. Eyeball.
   d. Anterior segment.

6. When a physician incises the bone above the ear and removes part of it to gain access to the internal auditory canal, it is considered a
   a. transcranial approach.
   b. transtemporal approach
   c. middle fossa approach
   d. mandibular approach.

7. An orbital implant
   a. is covered by an ocular implant.
   b. is the part that can be seen
   c. improves visual acuity.
   d. restores sight.

8. Strabismus surgery involves
   a. removing the eyeball.
   b. inserting tubes into the ear canal.
   c. adjusting the length of the extraocular muscles.
   d. suctioning out opacities on the lens.

9. Hospitals purchase hearing devices from a medical supply manufacturer and bill the device to the patient's insurance using a
   a. CPT code.
   b. ICD-9-CM Volume 3 procedure code.
   c. HCPCS code.
   d. Status indicator.

10. Mastoiditis is a condition characterized by
   a. ongoing middle ear infection.
   b. tympanic membrane swelling and pain.
   c. an increase in mast cells.
   d. ongoing anterior segment infection.

Coding Assignments

Instructions: Assign procedure code(s) for the following cases, and append modifiers when appropriate. Optional: For additional practice, assign the patient's diagnosis code(s) (ICD-9-CM).

1. Jim Reynolds, age 26, sees Dr. Moore, an ophthalmologist, for an excision of a scleral lesion in his right eye. The lesion is sent for biopsy and it is determined that it is malignant. Dr. Moore refers Mr. Reynolds to an ophthalmic oncologist for further treatment.

   Diagnosis code(s): _____

   Procedure code(s): _____

2. Dr. Moore performs a penetrating keratoplasty today at Williton for Norma Boots, age 32, for acquired **aphakia** (no lens in the eye, caused by cataract surgery, congenital condition, or trauma).

   Diagnosis code(s): _____

   Procedure code(s): _____

3. Nancy McLachlan, age 58, returns to the clinic for a mastoidectomy revision with tympanoplasty that resulted in radical mastoidectomy due to the extensive spread of a cholesteatoma involving the mastoid cavity. Dr. Delgado, an otolaryngologist, performs the procedure.

   Diagnosis code(s): _____

   Procedure code(s): _____

4. Dr. Moore sees established patient Jeremy Kerns, age 49, for chronic mastoiditis. Dr. Moore treats the patient by performing a labyrinthectomy, with mastoidectomy. He uses the operating microscope during the procedure. The patient has Overfield health insurance, which covers both the procedure and the use of the operating microscope.

   Diagnosis code(s): _____

   Procedure code(s): _____

5. Ralph Brown, age 94, sees Dr. Moore today for repair of a senile entropion of his right lower eyelid. Dr. Moore uses thermocauterization to perform the repair.

   Diagnosis code(s): _____

   Procedure code(s): _____

6. Kathy Jewels, age 31, suffers from noise-induced hearing loss. Dr. Delgado implants a cochlear device in an attempt to restore some of Ms. Jewels' hearing. To Ms. Jewels' delight, her hearing is improved significantly.

   Diagnosis code(s): _____

   Procedure code(s): _____

7. Pat Butler, age 22, is being seen today for an abscess on his right upper eyelid. Dr. Moore performs a blepharotomy to drain the abscess.

   Diagnosis code(s): _____

   Procedure code(s): _____

8. Dr. Moore's patient, Nelson Leonard, age 59, is in today for an anterior orbitotomy to remove an infiltrating lesion in Mr. Leonard's right orbital bone. The subsequent pathology reports states that the lesion is a primary malignancy and Dr. Moore refers the patient to an oncologist for further work-up.

   Diagnosis code(s): _____

   Procedure code(s): _____

9. Leslie Summers, age 22, developed trichiasis of her left lower lid. She sees Dr. Moore today in his office, and he is able to correct this condition using only forceps.

   Diagnosis code(s): _____

   Procedure code(s): _____

10. Dr. Delgado implants an electromagnetic bone conduction hearing device in 24-year-old Peter Carl's temporal bone to treat his mixed conductive and sensorineural bilateral hearing loss.

   Diagnosis code(s): _____

   Procedure code(s): _____

aphakia (ă-fā′-kē-ă)

Radiology, Pathology and Laboratory, Medicine, and Coding with HCPCS

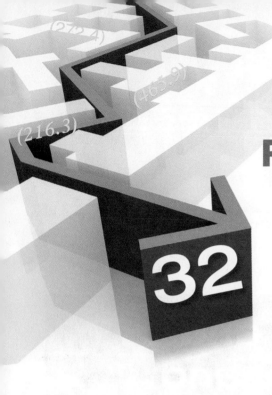

Radiology

Learning Objectives

After completing this chapter, you should be able to

- Spell and define the key terminology in this chapter.
- Define radiology, discuss the types of radiology procedures and clinicians, and describe various radiology coding guidelines.
- Describe subsections and subheadings in the Radiology section.
- Discuss diagnostic radiology procedures and how to code them.
- Explain diagnostic ultrasound procedures and how to assign codes.
- Identify radiologic guidance procedures and how to code them.
- Discuss breast, mammography procedures and codes.
- Describe bone/joint studies and how to code them.
- Explain radiation oncology and how to code procedures.
- Identify nuclear medicine procedures and how to code them.

Key Terms

body position
bone/joint studies
breast mammography
contrast materials
diagnostic radiology
diagnostic ultrasound
minimally invasive

noninvasive
nuclear medicine
radiation oncology
radiography
radiologic guidance
radiological supervision and interpretation
radiology

INTRODUCTION

Roentgen (rent′-gən)

We take X-rays (radiographs) and other radiology tests for granted today because we never lived during the time when they did not exist. A German physicist, Wilhelm Konrad **Roentgen**, actually discovered X-rays over 100 years ago, in 1895. He found that an X-ray (ray of radiation) could pass through human tissue and "see" through it, forming an image of the bones inside. One of his earliest experiments was an X-ray film of his wife's hand, which showed the bones of her hand and a ring that she wore. Roentgen was awarded the Nobel Prize in Physics for his discovery, and in his honor the official name for an X-ray is a roentgenogram (radiograph). The process of taking an X-ray is called **roentgenography**. A roentgen is a unit of measurement for radiation.

roentgenography (rent-gən-äg′-rə-fē)

Early radiographs were made onto glass photographic plates, but in 1928, film was introduced. As time passed, technologies improved, and the image intensifier and X-ray television were developed, allowing the operator to look at a screen to view the image.

These early advancements in imaging technologies have led us to today's CT scans, MRIs, ultrasound (US), and other types of radiology procedures.

Let's learn about the many different types of procedures involving radiology.

"Anyone who stops learning is old, whether at twenty or eighty. Anyone who keeps learning stays young. The greatest thing in life is to keep your mind young."—HENRY FORD

RADIOLOGY

When you think of radiology, you probably first think of X-rays, and you are correct. X-rays are one form of radiology, but there are several other kinds of radiology services. **Radiology** literally means the study of (-ology) X-rays (radi/o). Radiology is a medical specialty that includes many types of tests and therapeutic procedures which involve viewing various internal body structures, like arteries and bones, using radiation, sound waves, magnetic fields, or radio fields. **Radiography** literally means to take a film (-graphy) of X-rays (radio). Radiography is a term that covers a wide range of radiological procedures.

Radiology tests enable physicians to see a clogged artery, a cancerous lesion, or a broken bone. Radiology also includes therapeutic procedures for treating diseases such as cancer (radiation therapy) and treating disorders like uterine fibroids (interventional radiology). You already learned a little about some forms of radiology, including an X-ray, fluoroscopy (live X-ray), US, MRI (Figure 5-3), CT scan (Figure 5-4), positron emission tomography (PET) scan, and interventional radiology.

Radiological procedures can be **noninvasive**, which means the clinician performs the procedure without breaking the skin, such as an X-ray or MRI, or **minimally invasive**, which involves breaking the skin with a small incision and inserting needles, small catheters, balloons, stents, filters, or other devices, and using imaging to guide the surgeon using fluoroscopy or computed tomography. One type of procedure that uses imaging is interventional radiology. (Invasive procedures typically involve larger surgical incisions and more complex treatment.)

All types of imaging require trained healthcare professionals to administer and interpret them. A *radiologist* is a physician with specialized training to obtain and interpret many types of radiological images to determine the patient's diagnosis and recommend additional testing or treatment. Radiologists can also specialize in different areas of medicine, including diagnosing disorders of the cardiovascular system, gastrointestinal system, and breast. They may also provide cancer treatment through radiation (**radiation oncology**) or perform minimally invasive, image-guided surgeries (interventional radiology).

A *radiology technician,* or radiology tech, is specially trained to operate and adjust imaging equipment, explain procedures to patients and answer questions, position patients for imaging, and ensure that the patient's exposure to radiation is limited. A radiology tech may also operate portable (or movable) X-ray equipment to obtain images in the emergency room, operating room, or even at the patient's bedside. A *registered radiologist assistant (RRA)* and a *radiology practitioner assistant (RPA)* are both radiological technologists with advanced education who perform more complex radiological procedures.

A *radiology nurse* can work in diagnostic or therapeutic radiology to assist the radiologist with procedures, assess patients during or after procedures, and administer contrast for procedures. Radiology professionals can work in hospitals, clinics, specialty treatment centers and medical practices. They may also work in sales, research, or education.

Coding Guidelines

Turn to the Radiology section in your CPT manual. Notice the coding guidelines that appear before the radiology codes, just as you have seen with other sections in the CPT manual. You are already familiar with a lot of the information in the guidelines, such as the definition of a separate procedure and the comprehensive list of unlisted services or procedures you can find in the section. Let's take a look at a few areas in these guidelines that you need to understand before assigning codes for radiology procedures: radiological supervision and interpretation, administration of contrast, and written report.

1. **Radiological supervision and interpretation (S & I or RS & I)** describes the radiological portion of a procedure where the physician either supervises radiology clinicians who perform the procedure or performs the procedure directly. The interpretation is the physician's interpretation of the procedure, or the findings. You first learned about S & I in Chapter 18 when you learned about modifiers representing the professional component of a service (physician) and the technical component (equipment, nonphysician staff, supplies). An S & I service, or any radiology service, may have both components, depending on the location where the procedure is performed.

Sometimes, more than one physician is involved in supervision and interpretation, with one physician supervising the procedure and another interpreting the results. In this case, each physician would report the same procedure code to bill insurance, but the codes should include modifier -52 (reduced services) to show that each physician did not perform a complete service.

2. *Administration of contrast*—**Contrast materials**, or contrast agents, are special dyes used to improve the visibility of structures or tissues. The patient receives contrast through various methods, including in a vein or artery, in the subarachnoid space of the spinal cord, through the rectum, or by swallowing. Radiation cannot penetrate body structures containing contrast, so contrast makes certain areas stand out more in an X-ray or other image. When you review codes in the Radiology section, you will find that some code descriptors include the phrase *with contrast material(s)*. This means that clinicians performed the test using contrast, except for oral or rectal contrast. The code includes the radiological procedure, the injection of the contrast, and the contrast material(s). A radiologist, radiologic technologist, or nurse may administer contrast media, subject to the requirements of state law.

Depending on the method of administration, you may also need to assign an injection code from the surgical section in addition to the code for the imaging with contrast service. If the radiological code descriptor does not state *with contrast*, then assign separate codes for injecting the contrast and a HCPCS code for the type of contrast or code 99070 (supplies), depending on the payer's requirements for reporting contrast. Do not assign a code for the type of contrast if it is oral or rectal because these are included in the radiological procedure code.

Some radiology procedures are done without contrast and you will see the phrase *without contrast material(s)* in the code descriptor. Some procedures are first performed without contrast and then performed again with contrast. For these cases, the code descriptor will list *without contrast material(s), followed by contrast material(s)*. Be sure to only assign *one code* for these cases, rather than two separate codes, one for *with contrast material(s)* and another for *without contrast material(s)*.

3. *Written report*—A physician who performs a radiological procedure or interprets findings should document the information in a *written report*, which the physician signs. A written report is a legal document outlining the procedure or interpretation, including the reason for the procedure, the type of procedure, the physician's findings and discussion with the patient and/or family, and the definitive diagnosis. Do not report a separate code for a written report because it is included in a radiology procedure or interpretation.

CPT coding guidelines also appear throughout the Radiology section, before or following various codes. Guidelines alert you to other codes in CPT that you should *not* report with specific radiology codes. They also provide beneficial information about when to assign certain codes. Be sure to carefully read all coding guidelines before final code assignment.

Medicare Edits

Keep in mind that when you report codes for Medicare patients, Medicare may prohibit you from reporting specific radiology codes together, called NCCI edits. You first learned in Chapter 15 that CMS developed NCCI edits to flag procedure codes that should not be reported together. There are NCCI edits that do not allow providers to separately report radiology procedures that are bundled together because they should be performed together. When providers can justify performing radiology procedures separately that are typically bundled, they can append modifiers to specific codes, such as appending modifier -59 (separate procedure). Modifier -59 alerts Medicare that there is a special circumstance which caused the provider to perform a separate procedure that is normally bundled into another one. Appending modifier -59 to a procedure code "bypasses" or "overrides" the NCCI edit and allows Medicare to pay separately for the procedure.

Medicare also created Medically Unlikely Edits (MUEs), which is the maximum number of units of service that a provider would report under most circumstances for the same patient on the same date of service. Not all HCPCS/CPT codes have an MUE. You cannot override an MUE with a modifier. Be sure to check the CMS website for both NCCI edits and MUEs.

Modifiers for Radiology Procedures

As you know, modifiers help to identify special circumstances of procedures. For example, imagine that a clinician takes extra views of the body in addition to the usual number listed in a code descriptor, and there is no other code that represents *additional* views. Append modifier -22 (unusual procedural services) to the code to indicate to the insurance that more work was involved, which may qualify for additional reimbursement. Other modifiers that are common to radiology services, not just diagnostic radiology, include

- **-26**—professional component, includes the physician's work involved in the procedure, including supervision and interpretation
- **-TC**—technical component, includes the use of the equipment, supplies, and the work of nonphysician clinical staff
    - *Remember that when the same provider performs both the professional component and the technical component, it is a global service without any modifier.*
- **-52**—reduced services
- **-50, or -LT, -RT**—bilateral, left, or right
- **-51**—multiple procedures
- **-53**—discontinued procedure
- **-76**—repeat procedure by the same physician
- **-77**—repeat procedure by another physician

Be sure to refer to Chapter 18 for further information about and examples for appending these modifiers.

Body Positions and Projections

One of the most common procedures in the Diagnostic Radiology subsection is an X-ray, which clinicians perform with X-ray equipment that remains stationary or is portable. The *body position,* or the direction of the patient's body during a procedure, is an important part of understanding how a clinician performs a radiology procedure. The description of the body position includes information about what part of the body is closest to the X-ray beam. For example, if the patient is in a *left lateral* position, this means that the patient is lying on her left side, with the left side closest to the X-ray film. Examples of body positions are standing, lying face down (**prone**, or ventral), lying face up (**supine**, or dorsal), or lying on the side (lateral).

prone (prōn)

supine (sù-'pīn)

■ TABLE 32-1   **BODY POSITIONS**

Position	Definition
decubitus	The patient lies down and the X-ray passes through horizontally
distal	Farthest from the trunk of the body
lateral	The patient's right or left side faces the X-ray machine
oblique	The patient's full body or part of the body is rotated and at an angle to the X-ray beam
prone (ventral)	The patient lies face down with the head turned to one side
proximal	Closest to the trunk of the body
recumbent	Lying down
supine (dorsal)	The patient lies on the back, face upward

oblique (oh-bleek′)

anteroposterior projection (AP) (āntə-rō-pŏ-stēr′-ē-ər)

posteroanterior projection (PA) (pŏs-tə-rō-ān-tēr′ē-ər)

In order to correctly code X-rays, you also need to understand the direction of the X-ray beam, called the *projection,* from the location that the X-ray enters the body and the location where it exits. For example, an **anteroposterior projection** (or anterior/posterior, AP) means that an X-ray beam passes into the front of the body (anterior) and out the back of the body (posterior). The front of the body is closer to the X-ray. It is one X-ray beam that passes through the body in one direction, so it is one view. A **posteroanterior projection** (or posterior/anterior, PA) is when the X-ray passes into the back of the body and out the front. The back of the body is closer to the X-ray. A *tangential projection* is when the X-ray touches only one part of a body surface, skimming it. An *axial projection* is when the X-ray passes through the body lengthwise.

A **body position** is the location of the body in relation to the radiology equipment, like the X-ray film. ■ TABLE 32-1 includes various body positions so that you can become more familiar with them.

Examples of body positions and the X-ray projections include

- *Right lateral*—the patient's right side is closest to the X-ray film
- *Left lateral*—the patient's left side is closest to the X-ray film
- *Ventral decubitus*—the patient lies on his stomach, and the X-ray passes from the right side to the left
- *Dorsal decubitus*—the patient lies on his back, and the X-ray passes from the left, but the X-ray view is the right lateral
- *PA chest*—an X-ray passes through the front of the patient's chest and out the back

Not all possible body positions are listed here, so be sure to consult your medical references to ensure that you understand various body positions documented in the patient's record.

In order for you to better understand radiology documentation, it is also important for you to become familiar with the planes of the body (■ FIGURE 32-1):

- *Coronal plane (frontal plane)*—divides the body into anterior and posterior portions (a midcoronal plane divides anterior and posterior portions equally)
- *Sagittal plane (median plane)*—divides the body into left and right portions (a midsagittal plane divides left and right portions equally)
- *Transverse (horizontal) plane*—divides the body into two parts horizontally, with an upper and lower portion; the transverse plane is perpendicular to the coronal or sagittal plane
- *Oblique plane*—any plane that is not coronal, sagittal, or transverse (typically used with MRIs and ultrasounds)

It is important to note that documentation of body planes can also refer to other radiology procedures besides X-rays.

Figure 32-1 ■ Planes of the body. (A) Coronal or frontal plane and a coronal view of the chest and stomach; (B) Transverse or horizontal plane and a cross-sectional view of the upper abdominal region; (C) Midsagittal or median plane and a sagittal view of the head.

Source: Medical Terminology, Jane Rice, Pearson Prentice-Hall (2007) p. 50.

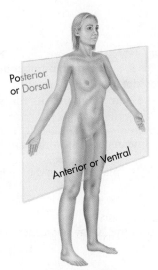

Posterior or Dorsal

Anterior or Ventral

A   Coronal (frontal) plane

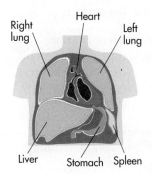

Heart

Right lung

Left lung

Liver

Stomach

Spleen

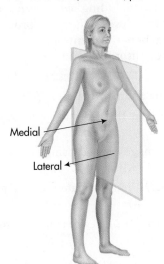

Superior (cranial or cephalic)

Inferior (caudal)

B   Transverse (horizontal) plane

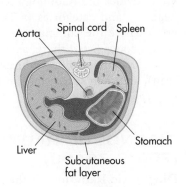

Aorta

Spinal cord

Spleen

Liver

Subcutaneous fat layer

Stomach

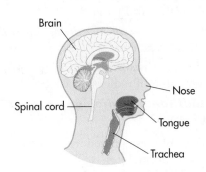

Medial

Lateral

C   Midsagittal (median) plane

Brain

Spinal cord

Nose

Tongue

Trachea

TAKE A BREAK

Wow! That was a lot of information to cover. You are doing great! Let's take a break and then review more about radiology.

Exercise 32.1 Radiology

Instructions: Fill in each blank with the best answer.

1. A(n) _____ procedure involves breaking the skin with a small incision and inserting needles, small catheters, balloons, stents, filters, or other devices, and using imaging to guide the surgeon (fluoroscopy, computed tomography).

2. _____ describes the radiological portion of a procedure when a procedure has *both* a radiology component and a surgery component.

3. _____ is the maximum number of units of service that a provider would report under most circumstances for the same patient on the same date of service.

4. _____ means closest to the trunk of the body.

5. The _____ plane divides the body into left and right portions.

6. The _____ position is when the patient lies on his stomach, and the X-ray passes from the right side to the left.

RADIOLOGY SECTION (70010–79999)

CPT divides the Radiology section codes into seven subsections with additional subheadings and categories (■ TABLE 32-2), divided by the type of procedure and body areas where the clinician performs the procedure. Turn to the Radiology section to review codes listed there, as we discuss procedures in each subsection. You can locate codes for radiology procedures by searching the index for the *type of service* (X-ray, CT scan), and then search for the *body site*, or start your search with the *body site* and then the *type of procedure*.

DIAGNOSTIC RADIOLOGY (DIAGNOSTIC IMAGING) (70010–76499)

Diagnostic Radiology is the first subsection under the Radiology section, which contains most of the standard imaging services, including *noninvasive* and *invasive* diagnostic and therapeutic (interventional) procedures. Common procedures in this subsection involve imaging procedures to view bones and internal structures, such as tissues, organs, and vessels, to diagnose diseases, disorders, and the presence of foreign bodies. They include:

magnetic resonance imaging (MRI) (rez′-uh-nuhns)

magnetic resonance angiography (MRA) (rez′-uh-nuhns an-jee-og′-ruh-fee)

- *Radiologic examination*—an X-ray using a film or plate
- *Computed tomography (CT, or CAT)*—a three-dimensional X-ray using an X-ray tube (■ FIGURE 32-2)
- *Magnetic resonance imaging (MRI)*—image created using strong magnets and radio waves; there is no exposure to radiation (■ FIGURE 32-3)
- *Magnetic resonance angiography (MRA)*—image created using a magnetic field and pulses of radio wave energy (■ FIGURE 32-4)
- *Additional radiologic procedures to image various structures*—see ■ TABLE 32-3

Many of these procedures involve the use of contrast (dye), to view body structures and view abnormalities.

CPT divides the Diagnostic Radiology subsection into subheadings that represent the *anatomic site* of the procedure, such as head and neck or spine and pelvis, and the *type* of procedure, such as X-ray, CT scan, MRI, MRA, and other radiological procedures.

■ TABLE 32-2   **RADIOLOGY SUBSECTIONS AND SUBHEADINGS**

Subsections, Subheadings, and Categories	Code Range
RADIOLOGICAL SERVICES	**70010–79999**
Diagnostic Radiology (Diagnostic Imaging)	**70010–76499**
Head and Neck	*70010–70559*
Chest	*71010–71555*
Spine and Pelvis	*72010–72295*
Upper Extremities	*73000–73225*
Lower Extremities	*73500–73725*
Abdomen	*74000–74190*
Gastrointestinal Tract	*74210–74363*
Urinary Tract	*74400–74485*
Gynecological and Obstetrical	*74710–74775*
Heart	*75557–75574*
Vascular Procedures	*75600–75989*
Other Procedures	*76000–76499*
Diagnostic Ultrasound	**76506–76999**
Head and Neck	*76506–76536*
Chest	*76604–76645*
Abdomen and Retroperitoneum	*76700–76776*
Spinal Canal	*76800*
Pelvis	*76801–76857*
Genitalia	*76870–76873*
Extremities	*76881–76886*
Ultrasonic Guidance Procedures	*76930–76965*
Other Procedures	*76970–76999*
Radiologic Guidance	**77001–77032**
Fluoroscopic Guidance	*77001–77003*
Computed Tomography Guidance	*77011–77014*
Magnetic Resonance Guidance	*77021–77022*
Other Radiologic Guidance	*77031–77032*
Breast Mammography	**77051–77059**
Bone/Joint Studies	**77071–77084**
Radiation Oncology	**77261–77799**
Consultation: Clinical Management	*77261-77799*
Clinical Treatment Planning (External and Internal Sources)	*77261–77299*
Medical Radiation Physics, Dosimetry, Treatment Devices, and Special Services	*77300–77370*
Stereotactic Radiation Treatment Delivery	*77371–77373*
Other Procedures	*77399*
Radiation Treatment Delivery	*77401–77425*
Neutron Beam Treatment Delivery	*77422–77423*
Radiation Treatment Management	*77427–77499*
Proton Beam Treatment Delivery	*77520–77525*
Hyperthermia	*77600–77615*
Clinical Intracavitary Hyperthermia	*77620*
Clinical Brachytherapy	*77750–77799*
Nuclear Medicine	**78000–79999**
Diagnostic	*78000–78999*
Therapeutic	*79005–79999*

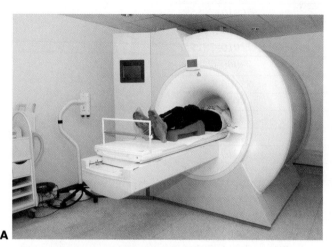

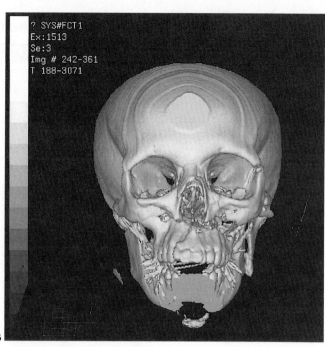

Figure 32-2 ■ (A) A patient undergoes a CT scan of the head, (B) CT scan showing multiple facial fractures.

Photo credits (A): Andrey Ushakov/Shutterstock; (B) Courtesy of Teresa Resch.

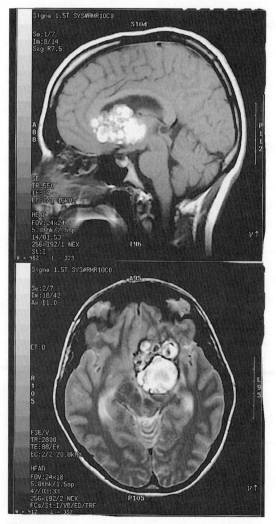

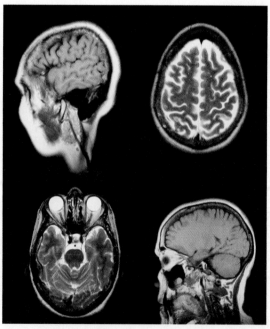

Figure 32-3 ■ MRI of the head showing a large lesion. (Courtesy of Teresa Resch)

Figure 32-4 ■ MRA of the head showing vessels in the brain.

Photo credit: Katrina Brown/Shutterstock.

■ **TABLE 32-3** **EXAMPLES OF ADDITIONAL RADIOLOGIC PROCEDURES IN DIAGNOSTIC RADIOLOGY**

Term	Pronunciation	Definition
angiography	(ăn-ji-ŏg′-ră-fē)	imaging of the inside or lumen of blood vessels by injecting a radiopaque contrast agent into the blood vessel and imaging it using X-ray techniques such as fluoroscopy
aortography	(ā-ôr-tŏg′-rə-fē)	X-ray imaging of the aorta by placing a catheter in the aorta and injecting contrast material to visualize blood flow
bronchography	(brän-käg′-rə-fē)	X-ray of the bronchial tree made visible through the use of a **radiopaque** contrast medium
cephalogram	(sef′-ə-lə-gram)	X-ray of the skull with very precise positioning, used to measure alterations in the growth of skull bones
cholangiography	(kŏ-lăn-jē-ŏg′-ră-fē)	X-ray of the common bile, cystic, and hepatic ducts
cholecystography	(kŏ-lē-sĭs-tŏg′-ră-fē)	X-ray of the gallbladder
cisternography	(sĭs-tər-nŏg′-rə-fē)	images of the spine and brain after injection of a contrast substance into the CSF to determine abnormal CSF flow
cystography	(sĭ-stŏg′-rə-fē)	X-ray of the bladder
discography	(dĭ-skŏg′-rə-fē)	X-ray imaging of the discs of the spinal column
duodenography	(d(y)ú-äd-ən-äg′-rə-fē)	X-ray of the first part of the small intestine
fluoroscopy	(flô -rŏs′-kə-pē)	examination of internal structures by viewing the shadows cast on a fluorescent screen after an X-ray has passed through the body; also known as live X-ray
hysterosalpingography	(hĭs-tĕr-ō-săl-pĭn gə′-grä-fē)	X-ray of the uterus and fallopian tubes
laryngography	(lar-ən-gäg′-rə-fē)	imaging of the internal structures of the larynx
lymphangiography	(lĭm-făn-jē-äg′-rə-fē)	X-ray record of the lymph vessels
myelography	(mi-ĕ-lŏg′-ră-fē)	X-ray recording of the spinal cord
orthopantogram	(ôr-thə-pan′-tə-gram)	X-ray that shows a panoramic view of the teeth, jaw and facial structures of the upper and lower jaw
pelvimetry	(pĕl-vĭm′-ĭ-trē)	X-ray of the pelvis to determine the capacity and diameter of the pelvis
sialography	(sī-ə-läg′-rə-fē)	X-ray of the salivary ducts and glands
spectroscopy, magnetic resonance	(spĕk-trŏs′-kə-pē)	noninvasive imaging used to measure the concentrations of different chemical components within tissues
urography	(y-rŏg′-rə-fē)	imaging of the kidneys and ureters to identify abnormalities of the kidneys and urinary tract
venography	(vē-nŏg′-ră-fē)	X-ray record of veins

There are various aspects of a radiology procedure that you need to know before you can accurately code procedures in this subsection:

radiopaque (rā′dē-ō-pāk)—pertaining to property of obstructing the passage of radiant energy

- anatomical site
- type of procedure
- number of views, including the body position
- unilateral or bilateral
- with contrast or without contrast
- total number of films and number of views
- appropriate modifiers

Diagnostic Radiology Subheadings

The Diagnostic Radiology subsection includes 12 subheadings representing the anatomic site of the procedure and type of procedure:

1. Head and Neck
2. Chest
3. Spine and Pelvis
4. Upper Extremities
5. Lower Extremities
6. Abdomen
7. Gastrointestinal Tract
8. Urinary Tract
9. Gynecological and Obstetrical
10. Heart
11. Vascular Procedures
12. Other Procedures

You can locate codes in the index by searching for the *type of procedure* (X-ray, CT scan) or for the *body site* (head, spine) and then the *type of procedure*. Let's review more about the procedures you will find under the 12 subheadings next.

- *Head and Neck (70010–70599)*—procedures of the head and neck, including the larynx, oral cavity, pharynx, temporal bone, and lymph nodes, to diagnose disorders with symptoms such as vision difficulties, vertigo, tinnitus, dysphagia, pain, numbness, and edema; Images can detect fractures, lesions, and other disorders.

  CPT categorizes some of the codes according to the number of views. You will need to thoroughly review the patient's record before assigning codes, being especially careful of code descriptors that specify the *minimum number of views*. You should only assign this type of code if the service documented *meets* or *exceeds* the minimum number of views listed. For example, if a patient has X-rays involving *seven* views of a patient's skull, choose code 70260—Radiologic examination, skull; complete, *minimum of 4 views*. Code 70260 means that there were *at least* four views, and there could be more.

- *Chest (71010–71555)*—procedures of the chest including areas such as the chest wall, bones of the thorax (trunk), and structures of the thoracic cavity, including the lungs, heart, and airway; Images of the chest are performed for a variety of reasons, ranging from difficulty breathing or a persistent cough to screening for job-related lung conditions. Additional imaging of the chest may be necessary to definitively diagnose the condition or to provide more evidence to support the initial chest X-ray findings.

  Let's look at the following example to learn more about coding a radiological procedure of the chest.

Example: Dr. Davis, an internist, sees Jack Varney, a 56-year-old, who complains of wheezing and shortness of breath. Mr. Varney has a family history of COPD and heart failure. Dr. Davis orders a number of tests including a 4-view chest X-ray with fluoroscopy to evaluate Mr. Varney's condition and determine if there is any diminished movement or paralysis of the diaphragm due to a pulmonary disease. The test results are normal.

To code this case, search the index for the main term *chest*, subterm *x-ray*, and subterm *complete (four views) with fluoroscopy*, which directs you to code 71034 to cross-reference. Code **71034** accurately describes the procedure. The patient's diagnosis codes are **786.05** (*shortness, breath*) and **786.07** (*wheezing*).

INTERESTING FACT: X-rays in Space

The use of X-rays is not just limited to looking at the body. X-rays, believe it or not, also have applications in astronomy. One of the best known X-ray astronomy missions is NASA's Chandra X-ray Observatory, which was launched aboard the Space Shuttle Columbia in 1999. Chandra detects and images X-ray sources that lie within our solar system and beyond. Chandra imaged the remains of exploded stars, observed the area around the giant black hole in the center of our Milky Way, and located other black holes around the universe.

- *Spine and Pelvis (72010–72295)*—procedures of the spine and pelvis; Spinal imaging includes the cervical, thoracic, lumbar, sacral, and coccygeal regions. Spinal imaging can detect injuries or diseases that affect the discs or joints, including spinal fractures, infections, dislocations, tumors, bone spurs, or disc disease.

    It is important to note that there are codes that include more than one procedure, such as a CT scan of the pelvis and a CT scan of the abdomen. You can find codes for variations of this procedure in the *Abdomen* subheading of the Diagnostic Radiology subsection. When a patient receives both CT scans, report *one combination code* for both body sites, using one of the following codes:

    - 74176—Computed tomography, abdomen and pelvis; without contrast material
    - 74177—Computed tomography, abdomen and pelvis; with contrast material(s)
    - 74178—Computed tomography, abdomen and pelvis; without contrast material in one or both body regions, followed by contrast material(s) and further sections in one or both body regions

Do not report two separate codes for a CT scan of each body site. Look for the coding notes in parentheses following these combination codes to guide you to the correct code.

- *Upper Extremities and Lower Extremities (73000–73725)*—procedures of the clavicle, scapula, upper extremity, elbow, wrist, hand, hip, pelvis, lower extremity, knee, ankle, calcaneus, and foot; Imaging of the extremities can be performed to diagnose whether a bone has been fractured or a joint dislocated, to determine the cause of pain, or to find a foreign object. It is also used to check for an injury or damage from conditions such as an infection, arthritis, tumors, or other bone diseases, such as osteoporosis.

- *Abdomen (74000–74190)*—procedures of the abdomen to determine causes of abdominal pain, locate swallowed foreign objects, or locate an obstruction or perforation in the abdomen; A patient may be placed in many different positions to take an abdominal image. Some of them include an upright position (erect abdominal view), lying flat with the exposure made from above the patient (supine abdominal view), or lying flat with the exposure made from the side of the patient (crosstable lateral view).

- *Gastrointestinal Tract (74210–74363)*—procedures of the digestive system including imaging studies (tests) of the pharynx, esophagus, stomach, duodenum, small intestine, colon, gallbladder, bile duct, and pancreas to diagnose disorders such as an ulcer, lesion, or hiatal hernia (condition where part of the stomach protrudes through the diaphragm); Physicians perform radiological procedures of the gastrointestinal tract when patients have symptoms of nausea and vomiting, swallowing difficulty, abdominal pain, and indigestion.

- *Urinary Tract and Gynecological and Obstetrical (74400–74775)*—procedures of the upper urinary tract (kidneys, ureters), lower urinary tract (bladder, urethra), and female reproductive system (uterus, fallopian tubes), which may involve contrast materials administered through a catheter; Procedures are performed to diagnose various disorders and diseases, including lesions, adhesions, and occlusions, such as kidney stones. One example of a procedure in the Urinary Tract subheading includes a KUB, which is an X-ray of the kidneys, ureters, and bladder.

Remember to code injection procedures separately for contrast materials administered for a radiological exam, unless the code descriptor of the radiological exam states *with contrast* (includes injecting the contrast, the contrast material(s), and the radiological procedure).

Codes for injection procedures are from the Surgery section, such as an injection procedure for cystography:

- *51600—Injection procedure for cystography or voiding urethrocystography*

Since code 51600 only covers the injection procedure, you still need to separately report a code for the radiology service:

- *74430—Cystography, minimum of 3 views, radiological supervision and interpretation*

You should also assign a HCPCS code or code 99070 (supplies) for the contrast material(s).

It is important to note that more than one physician may be involved in a procedure, with one physician performing the injection procedure, and the other performing the radiological procedure. If this is the case, each physician should report the code for the procedure she performs.

- *Heart and Vascular Procedures (75557–75989)*—procedures to diagnosis conditions affecting the structures or function of the heart and circulatory system, including measurements of blood flow velocity; Procedures include cardiac magnetic resonance imaging, cardiac computed tomography, angiography (X-ray of blood vessels), aortography (X-ray of the aorta), and venography (X-ray of veins).

There are two components to vascular coding: the imaging component and the surgical procedure component. Any vascular diagnostic or therapeutic procedure may be coded with one or more surgical codes *and* one or more imaging codes (S & I). The surgical component includes catheter placements, which can be selective or non-selective:

- *Nonselective catheterization*—The catheter is inserted directly into a vessel, and no subsequent movement into a branch of that vessel takes place. This procedure also includes placement of the catheter into the aorta or vena cava, by any route, and placement of a catheter directly into the portal vein.

- *Selective catheterization*—The catheter is moved into a main branch (vascular family) off the aorta or vena cava, or off the vessel entered initially. However, any vessels through which the catheter passes in order to be placed into the aorta or vena cava are included in the catheterizing of the aorta or vena cava. Vessels through which the catheter passes in order to reach a higher degree of selectivity are included in the coding for the *highest order* position selected.

Refer to Appendix L in your CPT manual, which outlines vascular families or branches of various vessels. The introductory notes provide additional information for assigning branches to first, second, and third orders, with the aorta as the starting point. You first learned about vascular families in Chapter 25 of this text. You can locate codes for nonselective and selective catheter placement by searching the index for *catheterization*. Take a look at some of these codes in the Cardiovascular System subsection of Surgery (36140, 36215-36218, 36245–36248). Review the code descriptors of these codes to better understand where the catheter is placed. It is not easy to code all catheterizations, and it is important to thoroughly understand vascular anatomy before assigning codes for selective catheterizations.

- *Other Procedures (76000–76499)*—The last subheading under Diagnostic Radiology is Other Procedures, which contains a variety of radiology procedures. Examples of a few of these procedures include:

- *Fluoroscopy, when performed as a separate procedure, up to 1 hour (76000)*

- **Cineradiography/***videoradiography (motion x-ray recordings)* (recorded film of a live x-ray) *(76120–76125)*

- *Consultation on x-ray examination made elsewhere, written report (76140)*

cineradiography (sin-ē-rād-ē-äg′-rə-fē)

cholangiogram (ko-lan′-ji-o-gram)

TAKE A BREAK

Good job! That was a lot of information to cover! Let's take a break and then review more about diagnostic radiology procedures.

Exercise 32.2 Diagnostic Radiology

Part 1—Theory

Instructions: Fill in each blank with the best answer.

1. The two types of contrast that are excluded from the phrase *with contrast material(s)* in a code descriptor are _____ and _____.

2. A(n) _____ is an X-ray of the skull used to measure alterations in the growth of skull bones.

3. What is the name of an X-ray of the uterus and fallopian tubes? _____.

4. _____ is an image created using a magnetic field and pulses of radio wave energy.

5. _____ is when the catheter is inserted directly into a vessel, and no subsequent movement into a branch of that vessel takes place.

6. A KUB is an X-ray of the _____.

Part 2—Coding

Instructions: Review each patient's case, and then assign codes for the procedure(s), appending a modifier when appropriate. Optional: For additional practice, assign the patient's diagnosis code(s) (ICD-9-CM).

1. Dr. Hoffman orders a CT scan of the thyroid without contrast. The patient is Michael Neley, age 14, whose neck is severely swollen. Williton Medical Center's radiology department performs the test. Code for Williton's service.

   Diagnosis code(s): _____

   Procedure code(s): _____

2. Sandy Greg, age 64, is a lifelong smoker. She has a severe cough and hemoptysis. Dr. Hoffman writes an order for her to have a two-view chest X-ray in the radiology department at Williton Medical Center. After the X-ray, the patient waits while Dr. Linguini, the radiologist, interprets the X-ray and finds a dense mass in the lower lobe of the left lung. He calls Dr. Hoffman for approval to complete a CT scan of the chest without contrast, which Dr. Hoffman gives. The radiologist determines from the X-ray and CT scan that the mass is lung carcinoma of the left lower lobe. Code for Dr. Linguini's services.

   Diagnosis code(s): _____

   Procedure code(s): _____

3. John Snyder is a 72-year-old established patient who sees Dr. Hoffman for debilitating back pain. Dr. Hoffman orders an MRI of the lumbar spine. Brandyburg Radiology, Inc., completes the test with contrast. Dr. Rich, the radiologist, diagnoses L-4 radiculopathy and degenerative disc disease at L1 and L2. Code for Brandyburg's global service.

   Diagnosis code(s): _____

   Procedure code(s): _____

4. Dr. Avery, a pediatrician, sees Lisa Lopez, age 16 months, who limps when walking. Her mother is unaware of any reasons for this condition. He orders testing including an X-ray of the pelvis, AP and bilateral frog-leg (or lateral view) of the hips. Williton's radiology department completes the testing. Code for Williton's services.

   Diagnosis code(s): _____

   Procedure code(s): _____

5. Ellie Vince, a 79-year-old, has pain and discomfort under the breastbone, with pain radiating to the back and shoulder. Further workup showed an enlarged gallbladder with cholecystitis. At Williton, Dr. Valencia, a gastroenterologist, performs a laparoscopic cholecystectomy, with a **cholangiogram** (X-ray of the bile ducts) as part of the procedure. Code for Dr. Valencia's services.

   Diagnosis code(s): _____

   Procedure code(s): _____

6. Nancy Smithton, age 52, has mitral valve prolapse: The valve between the left atrium and the left ventricle of her heart does not close properly (regurgitation) but bulges (prolapses) upward, or back, into the atrium. A recent echocardiography suggests that the mitral regurgitation may be moderate to severe. Dr. Woods, a cardiologist, orders a cardiac MRI with and without contrast, including velocity flow mapping to quantify the leak, quantify left ventricular size and function, and serve as a baseline for subsequent follow-up studies. The test is performed at Williton. Code for Williton's services.

   Diagnosis code(s): _____

   Procedure code(s): _____

POINTERS FROM THE PROS: Interview with a Medical Receptionist

Rachel Perkins has an Associate in Science degree in medical office administration and for the past two years has worked as a medical receptionist for an independent living outpatient center.

What interests you the most about the job that you perform?

I like being in a position where I can make an impact on others' lives. I try to keep up with the latest changes in coding, as well as take refresher courses.

What advice can you give to new coders to help them communicate effectively with physicians?

Communicate to physicians the financial impact that correct coding has on their practices.

What advice would you like to give to coding students about working with different personalities?

Remember that they are part of a team of professionals whose ultimate goal is to provide the best possible care to patients and maintain a peaceable work environment.

What should coding students do to prepare to work successfully in the healthcare field?

Keep up-to-date on new coding changes and always strive to improve their skills to make themselves invaluable healthcare professionals.

(Used by permission of Rachel Perkins.)

DIAGNOSTIC ULTRASOUND (76506–76999)

Ultrasound literally means *beyond sound*. Procedures in the subheading **Diagnostic Ultrasound** involve using sound waves, whose frequency is beyond human hearing, to evaluate a patient's internal organs and structures. Ultrasound can be diagnostic (to determine diagnoses) or therapeutic (to guide procedures). It is a noninvasive imaging technology that captures an image of echoes from sound bouncing off structures (like the abdomen, pelvis, heart, vessels, muscles, joints, and tendons). Ultrasound images are in real time, showing movements within the body, such as blood flowing through vessels or a fetus moving in the womb. Ultrasounds can reveal structural abnormalities, show the presence of a lesion and if it is solid or fluid-filled, monitor the growth of a fetus, and identify disorders of the arteries and veins, such as occlusions. Physicians also use ultrasound to image procedures, such as when they obtain biopsies, or for interventional radiology, a minimally invasive procedure that can be performed anywhere in the body using needles and catheters advanced into arteries, including treating vascular disorders like embolisms (occlusions) and aneurysms. Interventional radiologists can use other imaging technology besides ultrasound.

Sonographers are healthcare professionals who perform ultrasound, which a radiologist interprets. However, various types of physicians may also perform ultrasounds. The sonographer or physician applies gel to the body area to be imaged and places a *transducer* on the body area, moving it in various directions, to transfer the image to a screen (■ FIGURE 32-5). You may be interested to know that a transducer can be any device for converting one form of energy into another form. For example, a windmill is a transducer that converts wind energy into electricity.

Turn to the Diagnostic Ultrasound subsection to review codes listed there. Notice that CPT divides the subsection by body site and by type of procedure. There are many different coding guidelines to review in this subsection before final code assignment. Ultrasound, **echography**, and sonography are all terms to describe diagnostic ultrasound. You can locate ultrasound codes in the index by searching for the main term *ultrasound* or *echography* and then searching for the anatomic site, or start with the anatomic site and then search for the type of procedure.

Note that some of the ultrasound code descriptors specify that the procedure is *complete* or *limited*. This means that certain elements of an examination must be included for a scan to be considered *complete*; otherwise, the exam is limited. For example, the guidelines preceding the *Abdomen and Retroperitoneum* subheading state that for an abdominal

echography (ek-og′-ra-fe)— process of using ultrasound as a diagnostic tool by recording the echo produced when sound waves are reflected back through tissues of different density

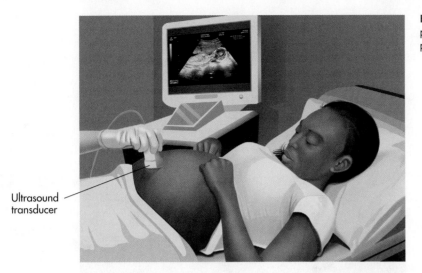

Figure 32-5 ■ A physician performs ultrasound on a pregnant patient.

Ultrasound transducer

ultrasound (76700) to be *complete* it has to include real-time scans of the liver, gall bladder, common bile duct, pancreas, spleen, kidneys, upper abdominal aorta, inferior vena cava, and demonstrated abdominal abnormality.

Ultrasound scans can be one- or two-dimensional (■ TABLE 32-4) or even three-dimensional, called *3-D ultrasound*, which takes multiple two-dimensional scans and combines them using specialized computer software to form 3-D images. There is also *Doppler ultrasound*, which uses high-frequency sound to monitor fetal heartbeat or assess the direction and velocity (speed) of blood flow. Doppler ultrasound can be black and white or use color (color-flow Doppler) (■ FIGURE 32-6).

Refer to ■ TABLE 32-5 to become familiar with some of the terms that you will see as you read through code descriptors in the Diagnostic Ultrasound subsection. Note that some radiological procedures also appear in the Medicine section of CPT, such as duplex scans and *echocardiography* (ultrasound of the heart and great vessels).

CPT divides Diagnostic Ultrasound into nine subheadings:

1. Head and Neck
2. Chest
3. Abdomen and Retroperitoneum
4. Spinal Canal
5. Pelvis
6. Genitalia
7. Extremities
8. Ultrasonic Guidance Procedures
9. Other Procedures

■ TABLE 32-4 **TYPES OF ONE- AND TWO-DIMENSIONAL ULTRASOUND**

Type of Ultrasound	Definition
A-mode (A = Amplitude)	A one-dimensional ultrasonic measurement
M-mode (M = Motion)	A one-dimensional ultrasonic measurement used to display movement of a structure
B-scan (B = Brightness)	A two-dimensional ultrasonic scan that displays movement of tissues and organs, also referred to as gray-scale
Real-time scan (rapid succession of B-mode images producing a moving video)	A two-dimensional ultrasonic scan, with displays of both two-dimensional structures and motion with time

Figure 32-6 ■ Color-flow Doppler of the carotid artery.

Photo credit: Shipov Oleg/Shutterstock.

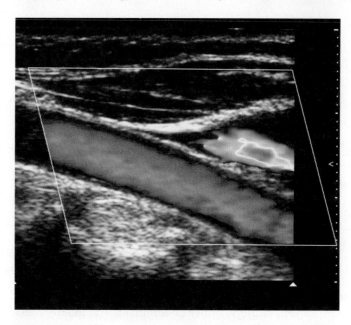

■ TABLE 32-5   **MEDICAL TERMS FOR DIAGNOSTIC ULTRASOUND**

Term	Pronunciation	Definition
amniocentesis	(ăm-nē-ō-sĕn-tē′sĭs)	a prenatal procedure to puncture the amniotic sac and obtain a sample of amniotic fluid containing fetal cells to detect abnormalities
arteriovenous fistulae	(är-tēr′ē-ō-vē-nəs fĭs′chə-lə)	an abnormal connection or passage between an artery and a vein
brachytherapy	(brāk-ē-thĕr′ə-pē)	radioactive seeds or material placed in or near a tumor to administer a high localized dose of radiation
chorionic villus sampling (CVS)	(kôr-ē-ŏn′ĭk)	a prenatal procedure to remove cells from tiny fingerlike projections on the placenta (chorionic villi) to detect chromosomal abnormalities and biochemical disorders (Down's syndrome, cystic fibrosis) (Code 59015 represents the procedure, and code 76945 represents the radiological portion of the procedure)
corneal pachymetry	(pă-kim′-ĕ-trē)	ultrasound to measure the thickness of the cornea
Duplex scan	(doo′-pleks)	ultrasound that uses Doppler and real-time imaging performed either simultaneously or sequentially; you can also find these procedures in the Medicine section of CPT
echocardiography	(ĕk-ō-kär-dē-ŏg′rə-fē)	ultrasound to analyze the size, shape, and movement of structures inside the heart
echoencephalography	(ek-ō-in-sef-ə-lŏg′rə-fē)	ultrasound to study intracranial structures
interstitial	(ĭn-tər-stĭsh′əl)	pertaining to small, narrow spaces (interspaces) of tissue or parts of an organ
ophthalmic biometry	(ŏp-thāl′mĭk hī-ŏm′ĭ-trē)	ultrasound to measure the axial length of the eye for initial cataract surgery
parenchymal	(pə-ren′-kə-məl)	*functioning* tissue of an organ, as opposed to connective tissue, blood vessels, and nerves, which all only give support or serve as a framework
pericardiocentesis	(pĕr-ĭ-kär-dē-ō-sĕn-tē′sĭs)	procedure to remove fluid from the pericardial sac for therapeutic or diagnostic purposes
pseudoaneurysm	(s-dō-ān′yə-rĭz-əm)	a false aneurysm, or hematoma
transvaginal ultrasound	(ŭl′trə-sound)	pelvic ultrasound to view the uterus, ovaries, cervix, and vagina

Let's review the types of procedures listed under each of these subheadings next.

1. *Head and Neck (76506–76536)*—ultrasound procedures performed to
   * study intracranial pathology such as intracranial hemorrhage, fluid collection, masses, or other structural abnormalities
   * measure the axial length of the eye to identify abnormal tissue, measure the power of an IOL lens implant before cataract surgery, or guide the removal of a foreign body in the eye
   * evaluate soft tissues of the head and neck, including the thyroid or parathyroid gland, salivary glands, or lymph nodes; and locate masses, such as cysts and/or lipomas

2. *Chest (76604–76645)*—includes two procedures, for chest imaging to evaluate or determine the presence of fluid within the pleural spaces, and breast imaging to further evaluate abnormalities found on mammograms.

3. *Abdomen and Retroperitoneum (76700–76776)* *(area of the abdomen behind the peritoneum)*—includes procedures that are *complete* or *limited*; used to diagnose gallbladder disorders, appendicitis, calculi, bowel and gynecologic abnormalities, intraabdominal injuries, and inguinal or femoral hernias.

4. *Spinal Canal (76800)*—includes one procedure for ultrasonic imaging of the spinal cord (its canal and contents). It can be used intraoperatively during spinal surgery to diagnose suspected spinal **dysraphism** (incomplete fusion or malformation of the spine), spinal tumors, spinal abnormalities, or birth-related trauma.

   dysraphism (dis-rā′-fiz-əm)

5. *Pelvis (76801–76857)*—includes *obstetrical ultrasounds* to determine the number of gestational sacs and fetuses; closely evaluate fetal anatomy, umbilical cord, and placenta; and assess fetal growth, including testing for fetal abnormalities. Pelvic ultrasounds also include *nonobstetrical ultrasounds* to diagnose endometrial polyps, fibroids, cancer, cysts, lesions, and causes of abnormal vaginal bleeding, or the absence of a monthly cycle (known as **amenorrhea**).

   amenorrhea (ā-men-ə-rē′-ə)

6. *Genitalia (76870–76873)*—includes three codes to evaluate soft tissue masses of the penis, rule out suspected prostatitis, or determine prostate volumes for brachytherapy treatment to plan where the radioactive seeds are to be placed in the prostate.

7. *Extremities (76881–76886)*—includes four codes to evaluate full or partial thickness rotator cuff and bicep tendon tears and diagnose Baker's cyst (behind knee), hip disorders, and causes of leg pain and calf tenderness.

8. *Ultrasonic Guidance Procedures (76930–76965)*—includes using ultrasound to image procedures, such as in an **ultrasound guided biopsy (76932),** to evaluate breast abnormalities without surgically removing tissue. A physician uses ultrasound to guide biopsy *needle* insertion into a mass to remove minimal tissue for testing. Physicians also use ultrasonic guidance to perform:
   * *Thoracentesis,* with ultrasound to guide the needle into the pleural cavity (space between the lining of the outside of the lungs and the wall of the chest) to withdraw fluid
   * *Paracentesis* with ultrasound to guide a needle through the abdominal wall into the *peritoneal cavity* (space between the two layers of membrane (peritoneum) that forms the lining of the abdominal cavity) to drain fluid
   * *Central venous catheter placement* to image the location of the catheter

   Ultrasound guidance can be *static* or *dynamic.* During d*ynamic* guidance, physicians perform the procedure in real time with localization and image-guidance during the procedure. During *static* guidance, they use ultrasound to identify the target, assess it, and mark an appropriate external site, but the physician performs the procedure without using ultrasonic guidance. Other forms of imaging guidance (CT, MRI) are listed under the subheading Radiologic Guidance.

9. *Other Procedures (76970–76999)*—includes five codes for various procedures, including a follow-up ultrasound, and bone mass measurement, and a procedure to diagnose bone diseases and responses to treatment.

   ascites (ə-sīt′-ēz)

   cirrhosis (sə-rō-səs)

TAKE A BREAK

Nice work! You are doing great! Let's take a break and then review more about the Diagnostic Ultrasound category.

Exercise 32.3 Diagnostic Ultrasound

Part 1—Theory

Instructions: Fill in each blank with the best answer.

1. _____ uses high-frequency sound to monitor fetal heartbeat or assess the direction and velocity (speed) of blood flow.

2. A(n) _____ is an abnormal connection or passage between an artery and a vein.

3. An ultrasound to analyze the size, shape, and movement of structures inside the heart is called _____.

4. Spinal canal ultrasound can be used intraoperatively during spinal surgery to diagnose suspected spinal _____, which is incomplete fusion or malformation of the spine.

5. _____ are procedures to determine the number of gestational sacs and fetuses; closely evaluate fetal anatomy, umbilical cord, and placenta; and assess fetal growth, including testing for fetal abnormalities.

6. During _____ guidance, physicians perform the procedure in real time with localization and image-guidance during the procedure.

Part 2—Coding

Instructions: Review the patient's case, and then assign codes for the procedure(s), appending a modifier when appropriate. Optional: For additional practice, assign the patient's diagnosis code(s) (ICD-9-CM).

1. Today at Williton Medical Center, Dr. Drimond, a gastroenterologist, performs an abdominal paracentesis using ultrasonic guidance for Adele Gold, age 59. The patient has **ascites,** a build-up of fluid in the peritoneal cavity. **Cirrhosis** of the liver, a chronic liver disease which resulted from the patient's heavy alcohol use, caused the ascites.

   Diagnosis code(s): _____

   Procedure code(s): _____

2. Tiffany Alleni, age 36, is pregnant and sees Dr. Austin, her OB/GYN, in the Williton OB clinic where Dr. Austin performs a transabdominal ultrasound for fetal and maternal evaluation. The patient is surprised to learn that she is carrying *two* healthy fetuses of 10 weeks gestation.

   Diagnosis code(s): _____

   Procedure code(s): _____

3. Dr. Lindsay, an ophthalmologist, sees Bradley Johnston, age 50, for complaints of poor vision and floaters (opacities) and flashes in his right eye. Dr. Lindsay examines the patient and performs an ophthalmic B-scan (ocular ultrasound) in the office to determine if retinal detachment has occurred. The test is negative. Code for this global service.

   Diagnosis code(s): _____

   Procedure code(s): _____

4. Tasheka Stack, a 32-year-old patient of Dr. Martin, an OB/GYN, complains of abdominal pain and persistent mild vaginal bleeding. After examination and a positive pregnancy test, Dr. Martin sends Mrs. Stack to Williton Medical Center's radiology department for an obstetrical ultrasound, which confirms an ectopic pregnancy without intrauterine pregnancy. Code for Williton's service.

   Diagnosis code(s): _____

   Procedure code(s): _____

5. Dr. Stein, a nephrologist, sends Edwin Watchet, a 15-year-old kidney transplant patient, to Williton's radiology department for a one-year follow-up real-time Doppler ultrasound of the kidneys to assess the current condition of the kidney transplant. Findings indicate a normal functioning kidney. Code for Williton's services.

   Diagnosis code(s): _____

   Procedure code(s): _____

6. Williton's ED physician, Dr. Mills, places a central line under direct dynamic visualization with ultrasound to rapidly establish intravenous access for administration of fluids to Ronald Myers, age 48, who is severely dehydrated.

   Diagnosis code(s): _____

   Procedure code(s): _____

DESTINATION: MEDICARE

In this Medicare exercise, you will learn more about Medicare coverage of radiology services. Follow the instructions listed next to access the Medicare Coverage of Radiology and Other Diagnostic Services Fact Sheet:

1. Go to the website http://www.cms.gov.
2. At the top of the screen on the banner bar, choose *Outreach and Education.*
3. Under *Medicare Learning Network (MLN),* choose *MLN Products.*
4. Under *MLN Products,* choose *MLN Catalog of Products.*
5. Under *Downloads,* choose *MLN Catalog of Products* again.
6. Hold down the Ctrl key and the F key to access the Find box. Type *radiology* into the Find box and hit Enter.
7. You will then see a link to Medicare Coverage of Radiology and Other Diagnostic Services. Click this link to access the Fact Sheet.

Answer the following questions, using the search function (Ctrl + F) to find information that you need:

1. Are hospital outpatient radiology services covered under Medicare Part A, B, C, or D? _____
2. Does Medicare separately pay for the professional component of radiology services for a SNF inpatient? _____
3. What Medicare manual and chapter should you review for information about billing and payment of radiology and other diagnostic services? _____
4. What Medicare manual and chapter should you review for coverage instructions for radiology and other diagnostic tests? _____
5. Does Medicare pay for diagnostic mammography? _____

RADIOLOGIC GUIDANCE (77001–77032)

Physicians use **radiologic guidance** during a procedure to visualize access to an anatomical site in order to direct or guide the placement and/or removal of surgical objects (catheters, needles). Radiologic guidance may be bundled into the code for the surgical procedure, or you may have to report separate codes for the procedure and the radiologic guidance. Be sure to carefully review coding notes and code descriptors to ensure that you correctly assign codes. The Radiologic Guidance subsection includes procedures under four subheadings:

1. Fluoroscopic Guidance
2. Computed Tomography Guidance
3. Magnetic Resonance Guidance
4. Other Radiologic Guidance

Turn to each of the subheadings as we discuss them in the next sections.

1. Fluoroscopic Guidance (77001–77003)

You already learned in this text that fluoroscopy is a live X-ray that physicians use during many types of examinations and procedures, including to guide the placement of a catheter into veins and arteries, such as in an **arteriography**.

Keep in mind that fluoroscopy may be included as part of a major procedure. The CPT manual states that you should not separately report fluoroscopic guidance if it is

arteriography (arte-ri-og′-ra-fe)—process of making an X-ray record of the arteries already included in the code descriptor of a procedure. Code 77001 is an add-on code that represents central venous catheter placement, replacement, or removal. Code 77002 is used to report fluoroscopic guidance of any anatomical area except for the spine, which is represented by code 77003.

2. Computed Tomography Guidance, Magnetic Resonance Guidance (77011–77022)

Computed tomography guidance is the use of CT equipment to visualize body areas during certain procedures. CT guidance can be used for a number of services, from simple interventional procedures, such as a diagnostic tissue biopsy to remove a tissue sample, and fine needle aspirations of superficial lumps or masses, to minimally invasive operations, such as cyst removal or ablation. Diagnostic or therapeutic injections for pain therapy are another example of imaging services that may use CT guidance to visualize the procedure.

3. Magnetic Resonance Guidance (77021–77022)

Magnetic resonance guidance is the use of MRI equipment to visualize body areas during certain procedures, such as biopsies to remove cells in the breast or ablations of liver tumors and uterine fibroids.

4. Other Radiologic Guidance (77031–77032)

There are two additional codes for imaging guidance of the breast not classified elsewhere. These breast localization procedures allow physicians to precisely locate breast lesions for fine needle or puncture aspirations, biopsies, or nodule injections. *Stereotactic guidance* (77031) is a radiological imaging technique which provides 3-dimensional imaging to pinpoint a specific area within the breast. For example, mammography patients can have multiple lesions whose location must be correctly identified before biopsy or surgery. Stereotactic guidance helps to identify the lesions. *Mammographic guidance* (77032) uses mammography to precisely locate lesions. Report these codes for each lesion involved in the procedure.

To locate codes under Radiologic Guidance, search the index for the type of guidance (*fluoroscopy, CT Scan, Magnetic Resonance Imaging (MRI)*) and then the subterm *guidance*.

sciatica (sī-'at-i-kə)

TAKE A BREAK

Way to go! Let's take a break and practice coding from the Radiologic Guidance subsection.

Exercise 32.4   Radiologic Guidance

Instructions: Review the patient's case and then assign codes for the procedure(s), appending a modifier when appropriate. Optional: For additional practice, assign the patient's diagnosis code(s) (ICD-9-CM).

1. Using fluoroscopic guidance, Dr. Hewes, a nephrologist, places a central venous catheter into Devon Martin, a 55-year-old established patient. The implant is a temporary access to provide dialysis to treat Mr. Martin's rapidly advancing kidney disease caused by uncontrolled type 2 diabetic nephropathy. Assign codes for the procedure and fluoroscopic guidance.

Diagnosis code(s): _____

Procedure code(s): _____

2. James Elach, a 68-year-old male with liver metastases, presents for a CT-guided radiofrequency ablation (RFA). Dr. Hewes localizes the liver mass under CT guidance and deploys the RFA probe across the deeper portion and applies radiofrequency energy. Next, he repositions the probe into a smaller lesion and applies radiofrequency energy. Dr Hewes then removes the probe and closes the tract. Assign codes for the procedure and the CT guidance.

Diagnosis code(s): _____

Procedure code(s): _____

3. Dr. Moon, an orthopedic surgeon, performs a sacroiliac (SI) joint injection with fluoroscopic guidance on Alice Stacky, a 46-year-old patient. She suffers from lower back pain with pain radiating down her leg (**sciatica**). Assign codes for the procedure and the fluoroscopic guidance.

Diagnosis code(s): _____

Procedure code(s): _____

TAKE A BREAK *continued*

4. Kristy Delavy, age 27, has a stereotactic-guided vacuum-assisted biopsy of her right breast. Dr. Barnes, a gynecologist, performs the procedure and finds that the patient has irregular calcifications of varying sizes and shapes (pleomorphic) identified in the mid-upper-outer quadrant of her breast. Assign codes for the biopsy and the stereotactic localization.

Diagnosis code(s): _____

Procedure code(s): _____

5. Melissa Verdie, age 52, arrives at Williton Medical Center for radiation treatment planning to treat breast cancer of the lower left breast. Dr. Chan, the radiologist, performs a simulation using CT to gather data for the treatment plan. The next day, Dr. Miles, an oncologist, instills the radiation therapy fields under

CT guidance. Assign a code for the CT guidance that Dr. Miles uses during the instillation of the radiation therapy fields.

Diagnosis code(s): _____

Procedure code(s): _____

6. Candace Jones, age 42, is having a percutaneous breast biopsy procedure performed today under MRI guidance. Dr. Barnes takes the biopsy from the lower-outer quadrant of the right breast. The pathology report reveals carcinoma. Assign a code for Dr. Barnes for the MRI guidance only.

Diagnosis code(s): _____

Procedure code(s): _____

BREAST, MAMMOGRAPHY (77051–77059)

The **Breast, Mammography** subsection includes nine codes for breast imaging services that aid in the early detection of breast cancer or diagnose suspected breast diseases. Standard mammograms are noninvasive medical tests that use low-dose X-rays to examine the breasts, or mammary glands. ■ TABLE 32-6 summarizes procedures you will find in this subsection.

As you code for breast imaging procedures, it is also important to understand the standardized breast imaging grading system that the American College of Radiology (ACR) developed, in cooperation with various government, cancer, and coding organizations. The system is called the *Breast Imaging Reporting and Data System (BIRADS)*. The radiologist uses BIRADS to classify mammogram interpretations. BIRADS is a quality assurance tool designed to standardize mammography reporting. It also reduces discrepancies in imaging interpretation by creating a classification system for mammography, ultrasound, and MRI of the breast.

The ACR defines BIRADS assessment categories or levels as follows:

* Category 0—Need Additional Imaging Evaluation and/or Prior Mammograms for Comparison
* Grade I—Negative
* Grade II—Benign finding(s)
* Grade III—Probably benign finding—Short Interval Follow-Up Suggested
* Grade IV—Suspicious abnormality—Biopsy Should Be Considered
* Grade V—Highly suggestive of malignant neoplasm—Appropriate Action Should Be Taken
* Grade VI—Known Biopsy-Proven Malignancy—Appropriate Action Should Be Taken

The U.S. Food and Drug Administration (FDA) regulations require that each patient's mammographic report include the documentation corresponding to the overall final assessment category, not the numeric code (Grade II, III).

When you are coding for mammography services, it is important to remember that payers, including Medicare, have different guidelines for coding and billing mammography

■ TABLE 32-6   **PROCEDURES IN THE BREAST, MAMMOGRAPHY SUBSECTION**

Procedure	Definition
Computer-aided detection (CAD) (77051–77052)	Computer algorithm analysis of images in order to more accurately detect lesions
Mammary ductogram or galactogram (77053–77054)	Procedure that uses mammography and contrast material to view the inside of the breast's milk ducts (code descriptors are for a single duct or multiple ducts)
Diagnostic mammography (77055–77056)	Procedure furnished to a man or woman with • signs or symptoms of breast disease • dense tissue where the radiologist cannot determine if a lesion is present or needs further information about a suspected lesion • a personal history of breast cancer or benign breast disease • Providers also perform diagnostic mammograms when screening mammogram results are suspicious or inconclusive. • Code descriptors specify unilateral or bilateral.
Screening mammography (77057)	Procedure furnished to a woman without signs or symptoms of breast disease, for the purpose of early detection of breast cancer or other abnormalities (bilateral procedure).
Magnetic resonance breast imaging (77058–77059)	Procedure that uses magnets and radio waves, instead of X-rays, to produce very detailed cross-sectional images of the breast tissue. Breast MRI is most often used to screen for breast cancer in women who are thought to have a very high risk of the disease. It is also used to distinguish between benign (noncancerous) and malignant (cancerous) lesions.

services. For example, according to the ACR's Standard for Diagnostic Mammography, a diagnostic mammogram should be performed on patients with augmented breasts (breast implants). But Medicare will not reimburse for this procedure and will only pay for a *screening* mammogram for a patient with breast implants.

When a Medicare patient without breast implants has a screening mammogram, and the radiologist determines the need for a diagnostic mammogram the *same day*, report *both* mammography procedure codes to Medicare. Append modifier -GG to the diagnostic mammogram code to show that the test changed from a *screening* mammogram to a *diagnostic* mammogram. Medicare requires the –GG modifier for tracking and data collection purposes and will reimburse both procedures. If a patient has the mammograms on different days, you do not need to append modifier -GG to the diagnostic mammogram.

It is also important to note that Medicare and other payers have specific guidelines for approved diagnosis codes submitted with mammography procedures. For example, Medicare requires one of the following diagnosis codes be reported on all *screening* mammography claims:

• V76.11—*Special screening for malignant neoplasm, screening mammogram for high-risk patients*

• V76.12—*Special screening for malignant neoplasm, other screening mammography*

Check each payer's guidelines for specific information on reporting required procedure and diagnosis codes.

To assign codes from the Breast, Mammography section, search the index for the main term *mammography*, and search for the subterm of the *type of imaging* (screening, MRI).

BONE/JOINT STUDIES (77071–77084)

The **Bone/Joint Studies** subsection has **14** different codes covering various imaging techniques to diagnose many conditions. Bone/joint studies are designed to

- identify bone mass
- detect bone loss
- determine bone quality
- identify causes of joint effusion
- conduct a rheumatoid arthritis survey

Here are some examples of bone/joint studies:

- *Bone age studies (77072)*—Evaluates how fast or slow a child's skeleton matures and helps the physician to diagnose conditions that delay or accelerate growth.
- *Bone length studies (77073)*—Diagnoses discrepancies in the lengths of limbs.
- *Dual-energy X-ray absorptiometry (DXA, bone density study)*—Screens patients for osteoporosis (porous bones), which increases the possibility of fractures or osteopenia (deficiency of bone tissue). DXA can also be used to monitor the progress of patients taking FDA-approved osteoporosis drug therapy.

  absorptiometry (əb-sôrp-tē-ŏm´-ĭ-trē)

- *Joint survey (77077)*—Diagnoses rheumatoid arthritis (RA) (arthritis of the joints), through a single PA view of both hands or a single AP view of both feet.

  To locate codes from the Bone/Joint Studies section, search the index for the main term *x-ray* and subterm *bone*, then search for the *type of procedure* (DXA).

TAKE A BREAK

Keep up the good work! Let's take a break and practice coding from the Breast, Mammography, and Bone/Joint Studies subsections.

Exercise 32.5 Breast, Mammography, Bone/Joint Studies

Instructions: Review the patient's case, and then assign codes for the procedure(s), appending a modifier when appropriate. Optional: For additional practice, assign the patient's diagnosis code(s) (ICD-9-CM).

1. Chris Davis, age 53, has her annual screening mammography performed at Williton Medical Center. The mammography radiology technician uses computer-aided detection to assist with lesion identification. Dr. Chan reviews the results and finds no abnormalities. Assign codes for this global service.

   Diagnosis code(s): _____

   Procedure code(s): _____

2. Anne Lavrey, an 89-year-old patient of Dr. Hoffman, complains of muscle and joint stiffness in her feet in the morning and after periods of prolonged inactivity. After examining the patient's joints for inflammation, tenderness, swelling, and deformities, as well as looking for any bumps under the skin (rheumatoid nodules), Dr. Hoffman orders blood work and a joint

X-ray of both feet at Williton Medical Center. The radiology technician performs a single AP view of both feet. The results indicate that the patient has rheumatoid arthritis. Assign codes for Williton's service.

Diagnosis code(s): _____

Procedure code(s): _____

3. Trish McCreary, age 27, presents to Williton's Outpatient Imaging Center with a physician's order for a bilateral diagnostic mammogram with a diagnosis of cystic hypertrophy of the breasts. A radiologist will interpret the results. Code for services at Williton's Outpatient Imaging Center.

   Diagnosis code(s): _____

   Procedure code(s): _____

4. Julie Madden, age 67, a patient of Dr. Hoffman, receives glucocorticoid (steroid) therapy equivalent to 7.5 mg or greater of Prednisone per day because of chronic obstructive airway disease (also known as COPD). Due to Mrs. Madden's age, Dr. Hoffman orders a CT bone mineral density (BMD) scan of the hip to obtain a baseline bone measurement that will help guide therapy. Long-term steroid use is known to cause bone loss,

continued

TAKE A BREAK *continued*

resulting in glucocorticoid-induced osteoporosis and increased fracture. There is a dose-dependent effect, so it is important to monitor the patient closely to ensure that she does not have osteoporosis. Williton's radiology department performs the test.

Diagnosis code(s): _____

Procedure code(s): _____

5. Towanda Emerson, age 52, presents to Williton's Outpatient Imaging Center for a screening mammogram that the mammography radiology technician completes.

Diagnosis code(s): _____

Procedure code(s): _____

6. Lisa Landrey, a 9-month-old baby, is brought to the Williton Medical Center ED with multiple bruises and abrasions over her entire body. Her mother and the mother's boyfriend accompany Lisa. The boyfriend explains at check-in that Lisa fell down the stairs. After examining the patient and questioning her mother in private, Dr. Mills, the ED physician, determines that this is a nonaccidental trauma and is concerned about the extent of her injuries. He orders a complete osseous survey along with several other tests. Code for the osseous survey at Williton.

Diagnosis code(s): _____

Procedure code(s): _____

RADIATION ONCOLOGY (77261–77799)

radiation oncology (ŏn-kŏl′ə-jē)

Radiation Oncology, also called radiation therapy, is a form of cancer treatment that uses high-energy ionizing radiation to shrink or kill malignant neoplasms. It also treats benign neoplasms by shrinking them or stopping their growth. It is a complex, multidisciplinary service that involves a team of radiation experts including radiation oncologist, radiation therapist, radiation oncology **physicist** (who plans resources and selects equipment to use), **dosimetrist** (healthcare professional who measures and administers radiation), nurse, radiotherapy technician, and even social worker and nutritionist.

physicist (fĭz′- ĭ-sĭst)—one who specializes in nature; a scientist who studies the energy, mass, and laws of nature

dosimetrist (dō-sim′-i-trest)

Radiation is usually administered in a precise, calculated dose, on a daily basis and over a period of several days to several weeks. There are two main methods for administering radiation: *External Radiation Therapy (ERT)*, also known as *teletherapy*, the most common form of radiotherapy, and *Internal Radiation Therapy (IRT)*, called *brachytherapy*. In ERT, a machine positioned outside the body delivers the radiation dose by directing beams of high-energy radiation at the cancer site. Brachytherapy involves placing a radioactive source (such as a radioactive seed) directly in a tumor or around the tumor or cancer cells. Before radiation therapy begins, the patient's physician(s) and other healthcare professionals must plan for the patient's individualized treatment and ongoing care.

Take a look at the subheadings under the Radiation Oncology subsection. Did you notice that some of these steps are included in the subheadings for various procedures? The procedures include all phases of radiation therapy, beginning with a preliminary consultation, which is the initial patient evaluation with the radiation oncologist who discusses treatment options with the patient, typically to treat a tumor. A radiation oncologist, along with a radiation therapist, may complete the consultation to determine whether to treat the patient and then plan the details of all phases of radiation therapy.

Once the radiation oncologist and the patient agree to start treatment, the next phase is called *clinical treatment planning*, including professional services to determine all of the details of how and where in or on the body treatment will take place. This phase includes performing a treatment *simulation*, when the oncologist defines where to direct radiation. The oncologist conducts the simulation, placing the patient in the exact position where he will receive treatment, using a virtual-reality–based 3-D simulation system or the standard radiology equipment. The radiation therapy team then uses the simulation data to define the following parameters:

- exact area to be treated
- total radiation dose prescribed

- how much radiation to direct at the tumor
- how much radiation normal tissues and structures surrounding the tumor will absorb
- the safest paths (or angles) to deliver radiation

During treatment planning, the oncologist may mark the patient's skin with tiny temporary markings or permanent tattoos to identify the precise area to be treated. The treatment team may also use body molds, head masks, special radiation-beam–shaping blockers, shields, or other treatment devices to keep the patient in a stable position for administering radiation.

The treatment team checks the patient's treatment plan on the first day of treatment and then on a weekly basis to ensure that treatment is appropriate. The team reevaluates the plan if any changes are to be made. One method which the team uses to ensure that treatments are appropriate is to use X-rays (port films) to verify that the patient is placed in the correct position for treatment delivery. The treatment team evaluates and manages the patient's care and treatment throughout the course of his therapy.

The *treatment planning* phase is generally a one-time-only professional charge for the course of the patient's ongoing radiation therapy. However, the treatment team may decide to change the course of treatment and will then require more simulations, documenting in the patient's medical record the justification for the changes.

Before we take a closer look at the codes listed under Radiation Oncology, let's look at the terms outlined in ■ TABLE 32-7 so that you will better understand them. You will see these terms in the code descriptors for procedures in the Radiation Oncology subsection.

■ **TABLE 32-7   COMMON TERMS FOR THE RADIATION ONCOLOGY SUBSECTION**

Term	Pronunciation	Definition
dose		Amount of radiation administered
dosimetry calculation	(dō-sǐm′-ǐ-trē)	Measurement of internal and external doses of radiation
endocavitary	(en-dō-kav′-ǐ-tar-ē)	Within a (body) cavity
hyperthermia	(hī-pər-thûr′mē-ə)	Treatment in which body tissue is exposed to high temperatures (up to 113°F) to damage and kill cancer cells
intensity modulated radiotherapy		Three-dimensional radiation that conforms to the shape of a tumor
interstitial		Between tissues
intracavitary	(ĭn-trə-cāv′ĭ-tĕr-ē)	Situated or occurring within a body cavity
ionizing radiation	(ī′ə-nīz-ing)	Radiation that can change the structure of a cell
irradiation	(ĭ-rā-dē-ā′shən)	Exposure to radiation
MeV		Mega (million)-electron volt, used to measure the amount of radiation delivered
multileaf collimator (MLC)	(kŏl′ə-mā-tər)	Device made of "leaves" that conform to the three-dimensional shape of a targeted tumor
port, portal (or field)		Interchangeable terms used to refer to the site on the skin where the radiation beam enters the body
radionuclide	(rā′-dē-ō-n(y)ü′-klīd)	An atom with an unstable nucleus
spatially	(spā′shəl-ē)	Relating to, occupying, or having the character of space
stereoscopic	(stĕr-ē-ə-skŏp′-ĭk)	Three-dimensional image
stereotactic radiosurgery (SRS)	(stĕr-ē-ə-tāk′tĭk)	Treatment that delivers a high dose of radiation, often used in treatment of brain tumors
tangential	(tan-jen′-shuhl)	Relating to a targeted point
temporally	(tem′-p(ə-)rəl-ē)	Delivering a precise radiation beam that can adapt to a patient's anatomy

There are 12 subheadings under the Radiation Oncology subsection, which we will review next.

1. Consultation: Clinical Management
2. Clinical Treatment Planning (External and Internal Sources)
3. Medical Radiation Physics, Dosimetry, Treatment Devices, and Special Services
4. Stereotactic Radiation Treatment Delivery
5. Other Procedures
6. Radiation Treatment Delivery
7. Neutron Beam Treatment Delivery
8. Radiation Treatment Management
9. Proton Beam Treatment Delivery
10. Hyperthermia
11. Clinical Intracavitary Hyperthermia
12. Clinical Brachytherapy

CPT has numerous coding guidelines for these subheadings, so be sure to carefully review them before final code assignment.

1. **Consultation: Clinical Management**

   Assign codes for clinical management consultations from the E/M, Medicine, or Surgery sections in CPT, rather than the Radiology section.

2. **Clinical Treatment Planning (External and Internal Sources) (77261–77299)**

   This subheading provides eight codes for both the *treatment planning* phase and the *simulation*. The codes are for professional services only and represent all the services necessary to develop a patient's course of treatment. For both types of services, there are different levels:

   - *Simple (77261)*—involves a single treatment area with a single port or simple parallel opposed ports
   - *Intermediate (77262)*—involves three or more converging ports and two separate treatment areas
   - *Complex (77263)*—involves tangential portals, and three or more treatment areas

   In addition, simulation field setting includes *three-dimensional (3D)* computer-generated reconstruction of the tumor and surrounding tissues from CT scans or MRIs to prepare for therapy directed at the tumor and tissues.

3. **Medical Radiation Physics, Dosimetry, Treatment Devices and Special Services (77300–77370)**

   This subheading has various codes to assign to services for the radiation dose, the exact therapeutic modality that was used (e.g., teletherapy, brachytherapy, hyperthermia, stereotactic radiation), and the detailed delivery planning. CPT divides codes by the type of service, as well as the level of service (simple, intermediate, complex). Also included in this section are the codes for the development of any necessary treatment devices and special services.

4. **Stereotactic Radiation Treatment Delivery (77371–77373)**

   This next subsection covers *Stereotactic Radiosurgery (SRS)*, services which are typically used to treat tumors in the brain, spinal cord, and lungs. SRS involves administering a single, high dose of radiation during one session.

5. **Other Procedures (77399)**

   There is one code under this subheading for an unlisted procedure.

6. **Radiation Treatment Delivery (77401–77425)**

   Radiation treatment delivery procedures measure the amount of radiation administered (MeV) and identify the specific areas treated. CPT divides codes by MeVs, the number of treatment areas targeted, the number of ports, and whether blocks were used to shield healthy tissue from receiving radiation.

7. **Neutron Beam Treatment Delivery (77422–77425)**

This subheading includes only two codes for specialized radiation treatment, which is rarely provided, mostly because of its high cost. Unlike most radiation therapies, neutron beam treatment uses neutrons (particles), which can be more effective in destroying very dense tumors, such as those found in salivary glands. It may also be used for inoperable tumors or those that are very resistant to traditional radiation therapy. Be aware that payers have different guidelines for covering this service, and some may not reimburse for it.

8. **Radiation Treatment Management (77427–77499)**

This subheading contains codes for the management of a patient's radiation therapy services. CPT divides codes in this subheading by the number of treatments within a week, also called fractions. For example, code 77427 represents five treatments. This means that you should report this code when the patient has five treatments within a week, regardless of the specific days when treatments occur. Be sure to read the CPT guidelines for this subheading very carefully before final code assignment.

Professional services bundled into radiation treatment management codes include

• A minimum of one examination of the patient to assess responses to treatment

• Review of port films

• Review of dosimetry, dose delivery, and treatment parameters

• Review of patient treatment set-up

9. **Proton Beam Treatment Delivery (77520–77525)**

Proton beam treatment delivery (PBT), or proton therapy, is a form of noninvasive electromagnetic radiation that is used to treat both in situ benign and malignant tumors. PBT is also effective for treating inoperable tumors or those that do not respond to traditional forms of radiation. It is typically *not* used when cancer has metastasized.

Proton radiation specifically targets and destroys cancer cells but has little effect on healthy tissue surrounding a tumor. Not all providers offer proton therapy, largely due to the fact that it is an expensive treatment.

It is important to note that Medicare covers PBT therapy for many conditions, but other payers may only consider reimbursement on a case-by-case basis. In addition, some Medicare Administrative Contractors (MACs) may require a –GZ modifier *(Item or service statutorily expected to be denied as not reasonable and necessary)* appended to the PBT procedure code if a patient does not have coverage for PBT but PBT is medically necessary.

CPT divides PBT codes by simple, intermediate, and complex, depending on the number of areas treated, number of ports used, and the use of custom blocks.

10. **Hyperthermia (77600–77615) and**

11. **Clinical Intracavitary Hyperthermia (77620)**

The subheadings for Hyperthermia and Clinical Intracavitary Hyperthermia include five codes for hyperthermia that is external, superficial or deep, interstitial, and intracavitary. Hyperthermia, also called thermal therapy or thermotherapy, is used as an adjunct (additional) treatment to radiation therapy or chemotherapy and is reported separately.

Hyperthermia treats cancer, exposing tissue to high temperatures (up to 113°F) in order to damage or kill cancer cells in a localized area. Hyperthermia can also

• make some cancer cells more sensitive to radiation, which helps to eliminate cancer cells

• damage cancer cells when other forms of treatment fail

There are several methods of hyperthermia, but the code descriptors for hyperthermia do not include each specific method:

• ***Local hyperthermia***—Heat, generated by microwave, radiofrequency conduction, ultrasound, or probes, is applied to a small superficial area (depths of 4 cm or less) through external (to the skin) or internal (through a probe) techniques.

- *Regional hyperthermia*—Heat is applied to a part of the body, such as a limb, organ or body cavity. Approaches used include:

- *Deep-tissue hyperthermia*—External applicators are positioned around deep-body sites (greater than 4 cm deep).

- *Regional perfusion*—Some of the patient's own blood is removed, heated, and then perfused (or pumped) back into the affected limb or organ.

- *Continuous hyperthermic peritoneal perfusion (CHPP)*—The abdominal cavity is infused with heated anticancer drugs.

- *Whole-body hyperthermia*—Heat is applied to the entire body through hot water blankets, inductive coils, or thermal chambers, to treat metastatic cancers that have spread throughout the body.

- *Intracavitary hyperthermia*—An intracavitary applicator is placed in close proximity to a tumor to heat it.

- *Interstitial hyperthermia*—This technique treats tumors deep within the body, such as brain tumors. The tumor is heated to higher temperatures than external techniques allow.

12. **Clinical Brachytherapy (77750–77799)**

   Clinical Brachytherapy is the last subheading under the Radiation Oncology subsection. It has codes describing the application of small, encapsulated (within a capsule) radioactive elements (natural or man-made) implanted directly into or near a tumor. Brachytherapy for cancer treatment is administered either continuously, over a short period of time (temporary implants), or over the lifetime of the radioactive source (permanent implants). Like the other forms of radiation oncology, a team of professionals, including radiation oncologists, perform brachytherapy treatment.

   Two examples of brachytherapy treatment application techniques include

- *intracavitary (77761–77763)*—This procedure is generally temporary or of short duration (one to four days). The radioactive sources (e.g., seeds, needles) are placed in an applicator that is positioned in a body cavity close to the tumor.

- *interstitial (77776–77778)*—Either temporary or permanent implants are placed into a tumor. The implants are radioactive sources enclosed in a container, or ribbons, which are radioactive seeds contained on a tape, within the tumor.

   CPT divides brachytherapy codes by simple (1–4 sources/ribbons), intermediate (5–10 sources/ribbons), or complex (more than 10 sources/ribbons), and by the type of service (infusion, intracavitary, interstitial, radionuclide, source application).

   Many payers will reimburse brachytherapy as both a primary treatment or adjunct therapy. You should carefully read the CPT guidelines in this subheading, as they provide very specific information for final code assignment. For example, all codes in this subheading include the patient's admission to the hospital.

   To locate codes for radiation oncology services, search the index for the main term *radiation therapy*, and subterm for the *type of service* (treatment delivery, stereotactic), or search for the *type of service* (brachytherapy).

WORKPLACE IQ

You are working as a reimbursement specialist for Dr. Monjabi, and part of your job is to audit CMS-1500 forms billed to the insurance and compare the services reported with the medical record documentation. Today, you review radiation treatment management services for John Carlisle, an established patient. According to his medical record, he received one treatment session on each of the following days in October: 1, 3, 5, 8, 10, 12, 14, 16, 18, and 20. The CMS-1500 forms for the patient's services show that code 77427 was billed to his insurance for the following dates: October 1–5, October 8–14, and October 16–20. Determine if code 77427 was correctly reported on the CMS-1500 forms. If not, determine the dates of services that should have been reported for code 77427 on the CMS-1500 forms.

What would you do?

TAKE A BREAK

That was a lot of information to remember! Nice job! Let's take a break and then practice coding radiation oncology procedures.

Exercise 32.6   Radiation Oncology

Instructions: Review the patient's case, and then assign codes for the procedure(s), appending a modifier when appropriate. Optional: For additional practice, assign the patient's diagnosis code(s) (ICD-9-CM).

1. Kevin Zimmerman, age 47, has completed his initial interview and simulation with the radiation oncology team at Williton Medical Center. Now the team conducts their treatment planning for the patient, who is suffering from mycosis fungoides (a skin lymphoma). Their decision-making includes a special teletherapy port plan for the use of electrons for total skin irradiation.

   Diagnosis code(s): _____

   Procedure code(s): _____

2. Clarence McElroy, an 85-year-old patient of Dr. Monjabi, a radiation oncologist, receives a superficial voltage radiation treatment to his scalp for basal cell carcinoma today at Williton. Code for Dr. Monjabi's services.

   Diagnosis code(s): _____

   Procedure code(s): _____

3. Janie Gurney, a 46-year-old patient of Dr. Monjabi, receives a 3MeV radiation treatment to her thyroid today at Williton Medical Center. The treatment follows her surgery to kill any thyroid cancer cells that may have not been removed. Code for Dr. Monjabi's services.

   Diagnosis code(s): _____

   Procedure code(s): _____

4. Sally Caperton, a 17-year-old, receives superficial hyperthermia for the treatment of primary superficial subcutaneous tumors of her back at Williton Medical Center. Dr. Monjabi administers the treatment.

   Diagnosis code(s): _____

   Procedure code(s): _____

5. Norman Burbages, age 63, receives radiation therapy five days a week for four weeks due to pancreatic tumors. He has weekly verification port films taken for each of the weeks. Imaging is done of three different ports to identify any changes in the size, shape, or location of the treatment areas for position verification/repositioning needs. Assign the CPT code(s) for the port imaging.

   Diagnosis code(s): _____

   Procedure code(s): _____

6. William Covington, age 56, receives his final nine radiation treatment sessions to end his radiation therapy at Williton Medical Center to treat esophageal cancer. Assign the final treatment management CPT code(s) for these remaining services.

   Diagnosis code(s): _____

   Procedure code(s): _____

NUCLEAR MEDICINE (78000–78099)

The last subsection in the Radiology section is **Nuclear Medicine (NM)**, which uses radioactive elements for two main types of services under the subheadings diagnostic and therapeutic. Nuclear Medicine procedures most often use an extremely small amount of radioactive materials (called radiopharmaceuticals, radiotracers, or tracers) to image the body, diagnose, and treat diseases.

nuclear medicine (noo′-klee-er)

For *diagnostic* services, clinicians administer radioactive substances to the patient through injections, or the patient swallows or inhales the substance. The radioactive substance produces emissions from inside the body that clinicians can image and measure with cameras outside the body.

Therapeutic nuclear medicine can deliver palliative (pain-relieving) or therapeutic doses of radiation to specific tissues or body areas. The procedures found in this subsection are typically used to detect or locate tumor cells, kill the cancerous tissue, reduce the size of a tumor, or reduce pain. They can treat an overactive thyroid, thyroid cancer, treat blood disorders, chronic inflammatory rheumatism, lymphoma, or certain metastatic bone lesions. What makes nuclear medicine procedures different from other procedures in the Radiology section is that nuclear medicine imaging can image *both* structure and function of the anatomy as the radioactive elements are attracted to specific organs, bones, or tissues. Not only can the radiologist see *what* an organ looks like, she can also see it how it functions (physiology). Nuclear medicine procedures are most often performed to image the thyroid, bone, heart, liver, brain, and lungs.

Nuclear medicine imaging is useful for detecting and treating a variety of diseases including cancer, aneurysms (weak spots in blood vessel walls), irregular or inadequate blood flow, and organ disorders.

Let's review some of the procedures included in nuclear medicine under various categories:

positron emission tomography (PET) (tuh-mog′-ruh-fee)

- **Positron emission tomography (PET)**—A PET scan produces a three-dimensional picture of a functioning organ. PET scans detect and stage many cancers and can provide early information about heart disease and neurological disorders, such as Alzheimer's disease.

- *Single photon emission computed tomography (SPECT)*—SPECT is a technique that is similar to PET but it takes two-dimensional cross-section images and combines them to produce a 3D image of the scanned area. SPECT is often used to image the brain, heart, and bones to identify parts of the brain affected by dementia, image occluded blood vessels, and diagnose bone cancer or spinal fractures.

- *Cardiovascular imaging*—This technique uses radioactive substances to image the flow of blood through the heart and blood vessels. Cardiac nuclear medicine diagnoses coronary artery disease and the extent of heart damage from an MI.

- *Bone imaging*—Bone imaging detects the radioactive emissions from radioactive substances that collect in bone tissue, producing bright spots where problems exist. Nuclear medicine bone imaging diagnoses arthritis abnormalities, bone cancer, bone infections, and bone injuries that are undetectable on a standard X-ray.

There are many different types of radiopharmaceuticals (radioactive drugs) used in nuclear medicine, including the following examples:

- Sodium Iodide I-123—for thyroid imaging
- Technetium-99m sestamibi—for various nuclear medicine procedures
- Thallium-201—for myocardial perfusion scans (heart functions)
- Strontium-89—for palliative treatment of pain from metastatic bone cancer

Turn to the codes listed in the Nuclear Medicine subsection. Notice that the first subheading is Diagnostic. CPT divides codes by the body system involved in the procedure and if the imaging involved one or more body areas or the entire body. Review the terms listed in ■ TABLE 32-8 to become more familiar with them as you read them in various code descriptors.

CPT lists various coding guidelines in the Nuclear Medicine subsection, so it is important to review them before final code assignment. For example, there are many codes that you cannot report with specific radiology procedures. In addition, note that the term *limited* in a code descriptor refers to imaging of *only one* body area, while *multiple* can mean two or more areas.

Note that many nuclear medicine services are done only for inpatients, while others are performed for outpatients. Another important point to remember is to report HCPCS codes separately for radiopharmaceuticals so that insurances will reimburse their costs.

To assign codes from the Nuclear Medicine section, search the index for the main term *nuclear medicine*, and search the subterm for the *body site* then *type of service* (imaging, blood loss study), or the subterm for the *type of service* (therapeutic, tumor imaging).

■ TABLE 32-8   **COMMON TERMS IN THE NUCLEAR MEDICINE SUBSECTION**

Term	Pronunciation	Definition
attenuation correction	(ə-tĕn-yoo-ā′-shən)	Process applied to correct measurements and images due to radiation scattering, absorbing and losing power as it travels through the body's deep structures
cisternography	(sĭs-tər-nŏg′rə-fē)	Brain imaging involving injecting the patient with contrast medium
cortex and/or medulla	(kôr′-tĕks) (mĭ-dŭl′-ə)	Outer portion and/or inner portion of an organ or structure
dacryocystography	(dak-rēo-sis-täg′-rə-fē)	Imaging of the tear ducts and associated structures after injection of a contrast medium
ejection fraction		Measurement of blood pumped out of a ventricle with each heartbeat
hemodynamics	(hē-mə-dī-nam′-ĭks)	Study of the heart's function and blood flow
hepatobiliary	(hep-ət-ō-′bil-ē-ar-ē)	The liver, gallbladder, and bile duct
infarct avid	(ĭn′-färkt)	Methods of detecting dead or dying areas of tissue or an organ (heart muscle)
intrinsic factor	(ĭn-trĭn′-zĭk)	Protein produced by cells in the stomach lining that is important for the distribution of vitamin B-12
kinetics	(kə-nĕt′-ĭks)	Rate of change, or movement, and what causes it
radiolabeled monoclonal antibody	(män-ə-klōn′-əl)	Substances that carry a dose of radiation to cancer cells to detect or treat lesions
reticuloendothelial	(rĭ-tĭk′-yə-lō-ĕn-dō-thē-lē-əl)	Cells in the immune system that ingest and destroy abnormal or damaged cells
scintigraphy	(sĭn-tĭg′-rə-fē)	Two-dimensional images of body tissues created by detecting radiopharmaceutical emissions
sequestration	(sē-kwĭ-strā′-shən)	Isolation or singling out
serial images		Series of images taken over intervals of time
tomographic	(tō-mə-grāf′-ik)	Cross-section; such as an X-ray of a selected plane of the body that focuses on one area and eliminates the outline of structures in other planes
uptake	(uhp′-teyk)	Absorption of a substance (like iodine) into a tissue
ventriculography	(vĕn-trĭk-yə-lŏg′-rə-fē)	Imaging of the heart's ventricles after contrast injection
volvulus	(vŏl′-vyə-ləs)	Twisted portion of a bowel, causing an obstruction

TAKE A BREAK

Great work! Congratulations! You made it through the last subsection of Radiology! Let's take a break and practice coding from the Nuclear Medicine section.

Exercise 32.7 Nuclear Medicine

Instructions: Review the patient's case, and then assign codes for the procedure(s), appending a modifier when appropriate. Optional: For additional practice, assign the patient's diagnosis code(s) (ICD-9-CM).

1. Dr. Faulkner, an oncologist, injects Kim Deller, age 43, with sestamibi prior to parathyroid tumor surgery

but does not take any images. He uses a probe for localization during the procedure. The specimen removed is sent to pathology for analysis and it is benign.

Diagnosis code(s): _____

Procedure code(s): _____

2. Dr. Mills, an ED physician at Williton Medical Center, sees Jeremy Johnson, age 11, after the patient is hit by a baseball in the upper abdomen. The patient

continued

TAKE A BREAK *continued*

complains of pain. The area is not distended but is tender to the touch. Dr. Mills orders testing to determine the extent of injury, including a liver/spleen scan to evaluate these organs. The results indicate that there are minor contusions to the spleen but no tears or blood loss.

Diagnosis code(s): _____

Procedure code(s): _____

3. Elnora Nicolson, age 38, has sentinel node injections with lymphoscintigraphy done at Williton Medical Center by Dr. Faulkner, an oncologist, to help identify the first lymph node(s) to which cancer cells are likely to spread from primary breast cancer. The real-time imaging identifies the tracer's flow through the lymphatics and the physician uses static images taken at intervals to mark and locate the sentinel node(s). He then uses multiple images from different directions to identify the exact position.

Diagnosis code(s): _____

Procedure code(s): _____

4. John Duluca, an 81-year-old patient of Dr. Hoffman, sees the doctor with complaints of unexplained shortness of breath, mild chest pain, and a cough that is sometimes bloody. Dr. Hoffman immediately orders tests to identify the underlying problem, including a ventilation-perfusion scan (V/Q scan) that is done at Williton to help identify if there are any blood clots in the lungs. Dr. Hoffman diagnoses the patient with pulmonary artery thrombosis and starts him on a regimen of anticoagulants as an initial treatment to

attempt to dissolve the clots. Code for the radiology procedure at Williton.

Diagnosis code(s): _____

Procedure code(s): _____

5. Melissa Morganfield, a 44-year-old hypertensive patient of Dr. Hoffman, presents to the Williton Nuclear Medicine Department for a renal scan to determine whether she has renal artery stenosis, a narrowing of one or both arteries that carry blood to the kidneys. The department performs the scan with pharmacological intervention but does not administer an ACE inhibitor (angiotensin-converting-enzyme inhibitor, a medication to treat hypertension) because the patient is already taking one. The test is positive and the patient is scheduled for angioplasty.

Diagnosis code(s): _____

Procedure code(s): _____

6. Joseph Warren, a 66-year-old patient of Dr. Hoffman, sees the doctor for follow-up after a visit to Williton Medical Center's ED for an episode of syncope and collapse. Dr. Hoffman orders additional testing, including a myocardial perfusion SPECT scan at rest and stressed, due to the patient's diabetes and worsening cardiac symptoms including palpitations. The test is performed and Mr. Warren is diagnosed with CAD of the native artery.

Diagnosis code(s): _____

Procedure code(s): _____

CHAPTER REVIEW

Multiple Choice

Instructions: Circle one best answer to complete each statement.

1. A procedure or service designated as a "separate procedure" can be reported when
   a. the service is carried out independently (or is unrelated or distinct) from other procedures/services.
   b. a modifier -59 is appended to indicate that the service/procedure is a distinct, independent procedure.
   c. the service or procedure is an integral component of another service/procedure.
   d. both a and b

2. A "complete" ultrasound is
   a. an ultrasound that is discontinued but the radiologist was not forced to stop until close to the end of the procedure.
   b. an ultrasound that meets all of the specific requirements and elements of an anatomical region.

c. a focused ultrasound examination.

d. reported along with a limited exam of the same region.

3. Radiology guidance is used during a procedure
   a. to visualize access to an anatomical site in order to direct or guide the placement and/or removal of objects (e.g., catheters, needles).
   b. as an addition to or in combination with another diagnostic or therapeutic procedure (e.g., endoscope, catheter, graft, shunt or stent placement).
   c. both a and b
   d. none of the above

4. Stereotactic localization is
   a. the use of a real-time movie like an X-ray image of the internal structures of the body to aid with diagnosis and precise targeting of structures.
   b. a one-dimensional ultrasonic measurement procedure used to map a structural outline.
   c. the use of radiographic coordinates provided by medical imaging to visualize targets or detail within the body.
   d. a nuclear imaging technique used to determine the sentinel node.

5. The term contralateral means
   a. to the side, away from the middle.
   b. on the same side.
   c. not advisable.
   d. pertaining to or affecting the opposite side.

6. Absorptimetry, photodensitometry, and radiogrammetry are all types of
   a. imaging processes that make an X-ray record of a joint in motion.
   b. imaging techniques using strong magnets and radio waves to view bones.
   c. bone scan techniques used to measure bone mineral density and/or bone loss.
   d. radiographic add-on processes using computer algorithm analysis of bone/joint images.

7. Computer-aided detection (CAD) is
   a. used at the discretion of the radiologist or facility.
   b. designed to help the radiologist by using the computer to digitally look at and interpret the mammogram image.
   c. obtained from either a conventional film or a digitally acquired mammogram.
   d. all of the above.

8. Teletherapy, stereotactic radiation, hyperthermia, and brachytherapy are all
   a. therapy treatment devices.
   b. therapeutic modalities in radiation oncology.
   c. defined by the levels of service: simple, intermediate and complex.
   d. nuclear medicine imaging techniques.

9. Every nuclear medicine procedure needs at least one of these:
   a. radioimmunoassay.
   b. radiant energy.
   c. radiopharmaceutical.
   d. MeV.

10. To code radiation treatment delivery you need to know
    a. the amount of radiation delivered.
    b. the areas treated.
    c. the number of ports and types of blocks used.
    d. all of the above.

Coding Assignments

Instructions: Assign procedure code(s) to the following cases, appending a modifier when appropriate. Optional: For additional practice, assign the patient's diagnosis code(s) (ICD-9-CM).

1. Dr. Monjabi, a radiation oncologist at Williton Medical Center, performs intra-abdominal placement of 20 interstitial needles to treat 29-year-old Haley Bealls' uterine cancer.

   Diagnosis code(s): _____

   Procedure code(s): _____

2. After obtaining the patient's medical history and performing a complete physical examination, Dr. Hoffman orders a bone marrow survey for Verna Vitello, a new 66-year-old patient who complains of increasing femur pain. The patient receives the test at Williton. The results show that she suffers from aseptic necrosis of the femur.

   Diagnosis code(s): _____

   Procedure code(s): _____

3. Gary Crabtree, a 32-year-old, comes to Williton's Pain Clinic for a trigger point injection of his right thumb. He is experiencing severe pain and his finger is locked in the closed position (called a trigger finger). (Trigger fingers can occur when tendonitis inflames the finger, which may lock in either the open or closed position.) He hopes the injection will relieve his pain and provide mobility again. The injections are performed using fluoroscopic guidance for needle placement.

   Diagnosis code(s): _____

   Procedure code(s): _____

4. Dr. Moon, an orthopedic surgeon, sees Wendy Krulaski, age 50, for arthrocentesis of her right knee for an unexplained joint effusion. Using CT guidance, Dr.

Moon aspirates fluid and injects a corticosteroid (steroid) medication to relieve her pain and the inflammatory pressure on the joint.

Diagnosis code(s): _____

Procedure code(s): _____

5. Edward Vince, an 80-year-old diabetic patient, sees Dr. Fisher, an ophthalmologist, prior to cataract surgery to remove a senile cataract. Dr. Fisher needs to measure the axial length of the eye. He performs an A-scan with IOL power calculation to determine the proper size IOL for the left eye.

Diagnosis code(s): _____

Procedure code(s): _____

6. Dr. Martin, an OB/GYN, sees Patricia Worthington, age 49. An annual mammogram recently revealed a lump in her right breast. An ultrasound of the breast confirmed the presence of a nodule, and the patient and doctor decide to go ahead with an ultrasound-guided core biopsy. The procedure is performed with three separate samples taken and submitted to the pathology department at Williton Medical Center. Code the ultrasonic guided biopsy procedure

Diagnosis code(s): _____

Procedure code(s): _____

7. Kim Wilcox, a 48-year-old female, presents with side pain and gross hematuria. Dr. Hoffman orders a CT of abdomen and pelvis without and with intravenous contrast to assist in identifying the cause of the patient's symptoms. A technician at Williton's radiology department performs the test.

Diagnosis code(s): _____

Procedure code(s): _____

8. Dr. Quan, a vascular surgeon, performs a lower extremity angiography on his 42-year-old diabetic patient, Lucy Kantner, who complains of cramping and leg pain when walking. Dr. Quan accesses the left femoral artery from the groin. He threads the catheter up over the abdominal aorta into the common iliac artery where he injects contrast for the right lower extremity angiography.

Diagnosis code(s): _____

Procedure code(s): _____

9. Dr. Mills treats Bradley Lee, a 10-year-old patient brought to the Williton Medical Center's ED as a result of a slip and fall at his soccer game. The patient complains of left shoulder pain and the shoulder is extremely sensitive to touch. Dr. Mills examines the patient and orders a single-view left shoulder X-ray, along with a 2-view of the left clavicle, which the radiology technician at Williton performs. The results indicate an acromial end clavicle fracture and the physician applies a sling. Code for the radiology procedure at Williton.

Diagnosis code(s): _____

Procedure code(s): _____

10. Raymond Latshaw, a 77-year-old patient, has a whole body PET scan at Williton to determine if his colorectal cancer of the descending colon has metastasized.

Diagnosis code(s): _____

Procedure code(s): _____

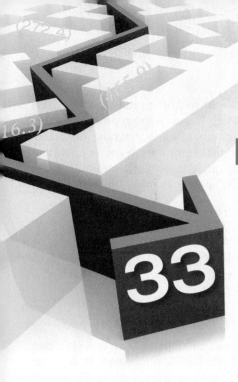

Pathology and Laboratory

Learning Objectives

After completing this chapter, you should be able to

- Spell and define the key terminology in this chapter.
- Differentiate among professional laboratory personnel.
- Define the term specimen.
- Describe the chapter Pathology and Laboratory Services.
- Identify modifiers used with laboratory services.
- List three types of blood draws.
- Summarize lab providers.
- Discuss Clinical Laboratory Improvement Amendments (CLIA).
- Describe the subsection Organ or Disease-Oriented Panel.
- Describe the subsection Drug Testing.
- Describe the subsection Therapeutic Drug Assays.
- Describe the subsection Evocative/Suppression Testing.
- Discuss Consultations.
- Discuss Urinalysis.
- Describe the subsection Chemistry.
- Describe the subsection Hematology and Coagulation.
- Describe the subsection Immunology.
- Describe the subsection Transfusion Medicine.
- Describe the subsection Microbiology.
- Describe the subsection Anatomic Pathology.
- Differentiate among the terms used to describe Cytopathology Procedures.
- Discuss Cytogenetic Studies.
- Describe the subsection Surgical Pathology.
- Define the term In Vivo.
- Identify Other Procedures.
- Identify Reproductive Medicine Procedures.

Key Terms

Clinical Laboratory Improvement Amendments (CLIA)
cytogenetic studies
cytopathology
evocative/suppression test
gross and microscopic examination
gross examination

laboratory test
panel
qualitative test
quantitative test
specimen
surgical pathology services
urinalysis

INTRODUCTION

At this stop along your journey, you will learn about pathology and laboratory services. You learned about pathologists in Chapter 22 when you coded skin procedures that physicians performed, and they sent specimens to pathologists to diagnose disorders. Now, you will code for the services that the pathologist, laboratory technologists, and laboratory technicians perform, in addition to coding office visits. Let's continue on the journey to learn even more new information and then apply it to many different patient situations.

"We have not wings we cannot soar; but, we have feet to scale and climb, by slow degrees, by more and more, the cloudy summits of our time."

—HENRY WADSWORTH LONGFELLOW

PATHOLOGY AND LABORATORY (80047–89398)

Do you remember that pathology is the study of disease, and a pathologist is a physician who studies cells, tissues, and disease behaviors? Pathologists often work in hospital pathology departments and review specimens with and without a microscope. Their findings help to accurately diagnose a patient's condition, such as carcinoma, and help physicians to determine possible treatment options.

The word laboratory comes from the Latin term, *elaborare,* which means *to work through a problem.* You can think of a **laboratory test** as a way to solve a problem, like determining what element is present or absent in a specimen or measuring the body's reaction to a specific substance.

Clinical laboratory technicians and *technologists* work in hospitals or labs and examine and analyze specimens to determine whether various body functions are normal or abnormal, such as cholesterol levels. The lab results help the physician to diagnose a patient's condition, determine further testing, and render treatment. Technicians and technologists review specimens for the presence of bacteria, parasites, and other microorganisms; match donated blood to patients for transfusions; and analyze test results and report results to physicians.

Technologists in small laboratories perform many types of tests, but technologists working for large laboratories specialize in specific areas. For example, *clinical chemistry technologists* prepare specimens and analyze the *chemical and hormonal* contents of body fluids. *Microbiology technologists* examine and identify *bacteria and other microorganisms* in specimens. *Blood bank technologists,* or *immunohematology technologists,* collect, *type* (determine blood type), and prepare blood and its components for blood transfusions.

Clinical laboratory technicians perform less complex tests and laboratory procedures than lab technologists. Technicians prepare specimens, operate automated equipment, and perform manual tests according to detailed instructions. They usually work under the supervision of medical and clinical laboratory technologists or laboratory managers. Like technologists, clinical laboratory technicians can work in several areas of the clinical laboratory or specialize.

A clinical laboratory technologist has a bachelor's degree in medical technology or one of the life sciences, and a clinical laboratory technician has an associate's degree or a certificate. *Phlebotomists* collect blood samples, and **histotechnicians** cut and stain tissue specimens for pathologists to examine microscopically.

histotechnicians (his-tə-tek-ni′-shuns)—technicians who microscopically examine cells in tissues and organs

Specimens

A **specimen** is a collection of fluid or tissue that a physician or clinician examines to determine more about its content. Examples of specimens include tissue from a mass or lesion, urine, vaginal fluid, sputum, blood, stool, semen, saliva, and mucus. Hospitals, physicians' offices, and laboratories can all collect specimens from patients and perform tests on the specimens. Some physicians' offices may only collect specimens and then send them to an outside lab for testing. Recall that an outside lab is a lab that performs tests on specimens and is not associated with the physician's office. Physicians' offices make different arrangements with outside labs for billing the patient's insurance, and you will review more about them later in this chapter. Hospitals may also use outside labs.

CPT Guidelines

Turn to the Pathology and Laboratory section in your CPT manual. Notice that there are CPT section guidelines for pathology and laboratory services, which state that services in the Pathology and Laboratory section are for physicians or technologists whom physicians supervise. There are also additional guidelines within various subsections, and you should review them before assigning codes from any subsections.

DIVISIONS OF THE PATHOLOGY AND LABORATORY SECTION

The Pathology and Laboratory section, or chapter, is divided into 18 subsections, depending on the types of tests performed. CPT divides two of the subsections into subheadings to further specify the type of service (■ TABLE 33-1). There are no categories or subcategories within the Pathology and Laboratory section.

Do you remember that there are specific modifiers for lab services, including modifier -90 (reference (outside) laboratory) and modifier -91 (repeat clinical diagnostic laboratory test), which you learned about in Chapter 18? Modifier -51 is not applicable to laboratory or pathology services because each service requires a specific amount of work. The amount of work does not lessen because the lab performs more than one procedure, so modifier -51 is unnecessary.

■ TABLE 33-1 **PATHOLOGY AND LABORATORY SUBSECTIONS AND SUBHEADINGS**

Subsections and Subheadings	Code Range
ORGAN OR DISEASE-ORIENTED PANELS	80047–80076
DRUG TESTING	80100–80104
THERAPEUTIC DRUG ASSAYS	80150–80299
EVOCATIVE/SUPPRESSION TESTING	80400–80440
CONSULTATIONS (CLINICAL PATHOLOGY)	80500–80502
URINALYSIS	81000–81099
CHEMISTRY	82000–84999
HEMATOLOGY AND COAGULATION	85002–85999
IMMUNOLOGY	86000–86849
Tissue Typing	86805–86849
TRANSFUSION MEDICINE	86850–86999
MICROBIOLOGY	87001–87999
ANATOMIC PATHOLOGY	88000–88099
Postmortem Examination	88000–88099
CYTOPATHOLOGY	88104–88199
CYTOGENETIC STUDIES	88230–88299
SURGICAL PATHOLOGY	88300–88399
IN VIVO (e.g., TRANSCUTANEOUS) LABORATORY PROCEDURES	88720–88749
OTHER PROCEDURES	89049–89240
REPRODUCTIVE MEDICINE PROCEDURES	89250–89398

Now that you know where to find the subsections of the pathology and laboratory codes, let's review what information you should look for in the index that will lead you to the correct codes. Here are the four types of main terms for pathology and laboratory services and procedures:

1. *Name of the test:* blood test, blood cell count, occult blood, drug assay, urinalysis
2. *Substance tested for:* glucose, lipoprotein, iron, insulin
3. *Type of specimen:* bone marrow smear, tissue culture
4. *Method of testing:* fine-needle aspiration, microbiology

Later in this chapter, you will review more about assigning codes from each of the Pathology and Laboratory subsections. You first need to understand more about blood draw services and the types of providers that perform laboratory services, including how they bill for their services.

THREE TYPES OF BLOOD DRAWS (36415, 36416, 36600)

When a patient visits a physician's office to have blood drawn for a lab test, the medical assistant is typically the person who withdraws the blood. Sometimes, the physician, physician's assistant, registered nurse, certified registered nurse practitioner, or phlebotomist withdraws the patient's blood. When a physician or other clinician withdraws the patient's blood for a lab test, the physician's office staff can code for the blood draw and bill the patient's health insurance for the service. The blood draw is a separate service from the lab test.

Keep in mind that some physician offices withdraw the patient's blood and perform specific lab tests in the office. Other offices withdraw the patient's blood but send the specimen to an outside lab for testing, which can include a hospital's lab. When an office performs the blood draw and sends it to an outside lab, code for the blood draw and code for the lab test, appending modifier -90 (reference (outside) laboratory) to the code for the lab test. Still other offices send the patient to a hospital's lab department or to an outside lab for both the blood draw *and* the lab test. You will learn more about these situations in the next section.

Each of the three methods for drawing blood for a lab test requires the clinician to use different skills to perform the service. Physician offices need to report one of the blood draw codes to show how the clinician took the patient's blood. Here are the blood draw codes for lab tests:

venipuncture (ven′-uh-puhngk-cher-)

- 36415—Collection of venous blood by **venipuncture**
- 36416—Collection of capillary blood specimen (e.g., finger, heel, ear stick)
- 36600—Arterial puncture, withdrawal of blood for diagnosis

Review the blood draw codes in your CPT manual. You can find them in the Cardiovascular System subsection of the Surgery section. Notice that code 36415 includes a CPT note that you should not append modifier -63 (procedure performed on infants less than 4 kgs). Code 36415 is considered *routine* venipuncture, and there are other codes that you should assign instead for special circumstances that involve more than routine venipuncture (refer to codes 36400–36410, which represent venipuncture of patients of specific ages). Be sure that you carefully review the documentation in the patient's record to determine the type of venipuncture code that you should assign.

Many insurances will not separately reimburse a blood draw when a patient has an E/M service during the same encounter. The insurances bundle the blood draw into the E/M service. Some insurances will pay separately for the blood draw with an E/M. For these insurances, it is important to append modifier -25 to the E/M code to show that the E/M was separate from the blood draw. In addition, when the office sends a blood specimen to an outside lab, you should append modifier -90 (Reference (outside) laboratory) to the blood draw code.

Offices can also assign code 99000—*Handling and/or conveyance of specimen for transfer from the physician's office to a laboratory* to show that they prepared and sent a blood specimen to an outside lab, including labeling and packaging (index entry: Handling, specimen). Keep in mind that many insurances will not pay separately for this service and may bundle it into other services the patient receives. Other insurances will only pay for this service when the specimen is blood.

TAKE A BREAK

Let's take a break and then review more about blood draw codes.

Exercise 33.1 Three Types of Blood Draws

Instructions: Search the index to determine the main term(s) and subterm(s) for each of the three blood draw codes for lab tests.

1. **36415—Collection of venous blood by venipuncture**

   Index main term(s), subterm(s):

   _____

2. **36416—Collection of capillary blood specimen (e.g., finger, heel, ear stick)**

   Index main term(s), subterm(s):

   _____

3. **36600—Arterial puncture, withdrawal of blood for diagnosis**

   Index main term(s), subterm(s):

   _____

LAB PROVIDERS

Remember that a physician's office can perform both the specimen collection *and* the lab test of the specimen. This type of office is called a Physician Office Laboratory (POL), and a POL codes and bills for services they perform. You will learn more about POLs later in this chapter.

On the other hand, the physician's office may only perform the specimen collection portion of a lab service but send the specimen to an outside lab for testing. In this case, the office can code and bill for *handling* the specimen, which involves the staff time and effort to collect the specimen and send it to an outside lab for analysis. Assign code 99000—*Handling and/or conveyance of specimen for transfer from the physician's office to a laboratory* for specimen collection when the office staff sends the specimen to an outside lab. The outside lab will then code and bill for the lab tests performed on the specimen. Keep in mind that some payers will not separately reimburse physicians' offices for specimen collection or blood draws, or they may bundle the specimen collection and blood draw into the lab test or into an E/M service the patient has during the encounter. It is important to check individual payer guidelines on specific reimbursement information.

If the office staff sends a specimen to an outside lab, then they need to include a lab requisition with the specimen. The lab requisition includes the following information:

- Physician's name, address, and phone number
- Signature of the physician or clinician who ordered the test(s) (required by some payers)
- Patient's name, date of birth, diagnosis to justify the lab test, and medical record number
- Type of test to perform
- Date and time the specimen was collected
- Any pertinent past medical history or past lab results that the lab needs to review

Outside labs can be located anywhere, but a physician's office typically sends specimens to an outside lab located close to the office, especially if the physician needs to review lab results quickly, including sending the specimen to a nearby hospital lab. Hospitals have lab departments where lab technologists and technicians review and analyze specimens.

When the physician's office sends a specimen to an outside lab for testing, either the physician's office or the outside lab bills the patient's insurance for the lab test.

- If the physician's office bills the patient's insurance for the lab test, then office staff must complete the CMS-1500 form for the service, including
  - the date of service
  - CPT-4 code for the lab test
  - charge
  - check YES in block 20 of the CMS-1500 form (Figure 1-1) to show that the specimen went to an outside lab
  - the amount of purchase price for lab services (Block 20 Charges field)
- The physician's office must also reimburse the lab for their services. It is important to note that some payers will not reimburse physicians' offices for lab services that an outside lab performs. They require the lab to bill the insurance directly for lab services.
- If the physician's office *does not* bill the patient's insurance for the lab test, then the outside lab bills the insurance. The physician's office does not need to reimburse the outside lab for their services, since they will receive payment from the patient's insurance.

Many times, instead of collecting specimens in the office, physicians *refer* patients to hospital lab departments where lab staff, such as a phlebotomist, collect the specimen from the patient, and lab technologists or technicians perform lab tests. The physician gives the patient an order for the lab test to take to the hospital lab department so that the staff knows the type of specimen to collect and the specific test to perform.

CLINICAL LABORATORY IMPROVEMENT AMENDMENTS

The Food and Drug Administration (FDA) implemented the **Clinical Laboratory Improvement Amendments (CLIA)** for the federal government to certify labs, including POLs, when they meet certain requirements. These requirements include appropriate training for lab personnel, specific criteria for performing lab services that the lab must meet, and the lab technologists and technicians perform a specific number of lab tests daily.

Depending on the type of tests that the lab offers and the credentials of the individual reviewing and analyzing specimens, CLIA will either issue a *Certificate of Compliance (COC)* or grant a *Certificate of Waiver* to the lab. Review the following information to better understand the requirements for each certificate.

CLIA Certificate of Compliance

If the lab or the POL employs trained lab technicians or technologists to review and analyze test results, then the lab or POL needs a CLIA COC.

- The laboratory must complete an application and pay a registration fee, and must pay a COC fee every two years.
- There are other types of CLIA Certificates, depending on the types of test performed and other criteria, which also include additional fees.
- Labs with a CLIA COC will be issued an individual CLIA number that identifies the lab.

CLIA Certificate of Waiver

CLIA-waived lab tests do not require a trained lab technician or technologist to review and analyze them, such as a urine pregnancy test. If the lab or POL performs these tests, then it can obtain a CLIA Certificate of Waiver instead of a COC.

- The POL must complete an application and pay a Certificate of Waiver fee every two years.

The U.S. Department of Health and Human Services publishes the list of CLIA-waived tests on its website. For some waived tests, Medicare requires providers to append modifier -QW (CLIA-waived test) to the CPT code or to the HCPCS code. There is a limited number of HCPCS codes for lab services (G codes), which Medicare requires providers to submit instead of a CPT code. Refer to the CMS website, where you can find more information about waived tests, including those that require HCPCS codes and modifier -QW.

TAKE A BREAK

Good job! Let's take a break and then review more about lab providers and CLIA.

> **Exercise 33.2** Lab Providers, Clinical Laboratory Improvement Amendments

Instructions: Indicate whether each statement is True or False on the line preceding each statement. For statements marked False, underline the word or words that makes the statement false.

1. _____ Check YES in block 19 of the CMS-1500 form when the physician's office sends a patient's specimen to an outside lab.

2. _____ A POL performs *both* the specimen collection and lab test.

3. _____ Even when a physician's office sends a specimen to an outside lab, the office can still bill the patient's insurance for the lab test.

4. _____ Specimen collection is always bundled into a lab test, and a physician's office cannot separately code and bill for it.

5. _____ CLIA-waived lab tests require a lab technician or technologist to review and analyze specimens.

6. _____ Labs and POLs that perform nonwaived tests require a CLIA COC.

ORGAN OR DISEASE-ORIENTED PANELS (80047–80076)

The first subsection in the Pathology and Laboratory section is Organ or Disease-Oriented Panels. A **panel** is a group of tests performed at the same time, for the same patient, using the same specimen. One CPT code represents *all tests* within a panel, even though each test within the panel has its own CPT code.

Turn to the panel codes at the beginning of the Pathology and Laboratory section in your CPT manual. CPT arranges panel codes by the type of panel. Here are some examples of panel tests:

- 80047—Basic metabolic panel (Calcium, ionized)
- 80050—General health panel
- 80055—Obstetric panel

Notice that each panel lists individual tests included in the panel, and individual tests have their own CPT codes. In order for you to assign a panel CPT code, the provider *must perform all the tests* in the panel. If the provider performs *all but one* test in the panel, then you *cannot* assign the panel code. Instead, you must code each test *individually.* You also cannot assign the panel code with modifier -52 (reduced service) because the provider did not perform all of the tests in the panel. When a provider submits a claim to insurance for a panel, it is because the provider performed *all tests* within that panel.

Physicians order panel tests to help diagnose a patient's condition and to determine if the body is functioning normally, such as with a pregnant patient who receives an obstetric panel (80055). The obstetric panel includes tests commonly performed together to assess the pregnant patient's health. Other panel examples include the hepatic function panel (80076), which assesses a patient's liver function, and the renal function panel (80069), which assesses a patient's kidney function.

Did you notice the CPT guidelines listed before the panel codes? The guidelines state that if a provider performs tests in addition to the tests included in the panel, then the provider should *separately report* codes for the additional tests. The guidelines also state that if a provider performs groups of tests that are included in more than one panel, then the provider should report the code for the panel that contains the *most* tests and report any remaining tests with individual codes.

Panel codes are *bundled* codes. Recall that a bundled code contains more than one service or procedure that you should not code separately. If a patient receives all tests in a panel, then the provider has to code and bill for the panel code. Unbundling the panel code and coding and billing each test in the panel separately to try to obtain more reimbursement would constitute fraudulent billing. Unbundling is also unethical coding. Providers who unbundle codes may have to pay penalties to insurances for overpayments and may also suffer legal consequences.

In addition to panel codes for Organ and Disease-Oriented Panels, there are also panel codes for evocative/suppression testing (80400–80440), which we will review and practice coding later in this chapter. To find panel codes, search the index for the main term *Organ or Disease-Oriented Panel.*

TAKE A BREAK

Let's take a break and then review more about panels with coding exercises. It is important that you understand the following points before completing all lab test coding exercises in this chapter.

- When a lab performs a test, they assign a procedure code for the test and a diagnosis code that justifies the test, such as a specific symptom that the ordering physician documents.
- Assume that in the coding exercises, any physician who orders lab tests will *not* code for the lab test and reimburse the lab later. Only the lab will code for the lab tests and will bill the patient's insurance directly.

Exercise 33.3   Organ or Disease-Oriented Panels

Instructions: Review each case, and then assign codes for the procedure(s), appending a modifier when appropriate. Optional: For additional coding practice, assign the patient's diagnosis code(s) (ICD-9-CM).

1. Brandyburg Laboratory performs the following tests on blood specimens that they received from physicians' offices for various patients:
   a. Patient 1—chloride, glucose, sodium, potassium, creatinine, carbon dioxide, total calcium, and urea nitrogen.
   What procedure code(s) should the lab report for their services? _____
   b. Patient 2—total serum cholesterol, lipoprotein high density cholesterol, and triglycerides
   What procedure code(s) should the lab report for their services? _____
   c. Patient 3—sodium, potassium, chloride, carbon dioxide
   What procedure code(s) should the lab report for their services? _____

2. Ron Willis, a 42-year-old established patient, sees Dr. Hoffman for an office visit with complaints of nausea, vomiting, and darkened urine. Dr. Hoffman performs an expanded problem-focused history and exam with medical decision-making of moderate complexity. Rhonda, the medical assistant, performs venipuncture to obtain a blood specimen, which she then sends to Williton Medical Center's lab department for a hepatic function panel. Code for Dr. Hoffman's services and Williton's services.

   Diagnosis code(s): _____

   Dr. Hoffman's procedure code(s): _____

   Williton's procedure code(s): _____

3. Bella Ray, a 28-year-old established patient, sees Dr. Fulton, a gynecologist/obstetrician, for a pregnancy visit during her first trimester. This is her first pregnancy. She reports that she is not experiencing any problems. He performs a detailed history, detailed exam, and moderate medical decision-making. Dr. Fulton orders an obstetric panel to evaluate the patient's health, and his medical assistant performs venipuncture to obtain the blood specimen, which she sends to Williton Medical Center's lab. Code for Dr. Fulton's services and Williton's services.

   Diagnosis code(s): _____

   Dr. Hoffman's procedure code(s): _____

   Williton's procedure code(s): _____

DRUG TESTING (80100–80104)

There are five codes listed under the Drug Testing subsection for Pathology and Laboratory. Turn to the codes in your CPT manual to review their descriptors and the CPT coding guidelines. Let's review more about the types of tests listed.

A **qualitative test** determines whether or not a substance, or **analyte**, such as a drug, is present in a specimen. Under the Drug Testing heading, note that CPT guidelines list examples of drugs or classes of drugs that lab providers test in specimens. When you think of a drug test, you may only think of an illegal drug. However, qualitative drug screens also test for the presence of any other type of drug, including prescribed medications.

analyte (an′-əl-īt)

A *drug class* represents a group of drugs that have similar properties, and physicians prescribe them to treat the same diagnoses. An **assay** is a test to analyze a substance.

assay (as-ey′)

There are three codes for a qualitative drug screen:

- 80100—Drug screen, qualitative; multiple drug classes chromatographic method, each procedure

- 80101—Drug screen, qualitative; single drug class method (e.g., immunoassay, enzyme assay), each drug class

- 80104—Drug screen, qualitative; multiple drug classes other than chromatographic method, each procedure

Code 80100 represents a screen to determine if multiple drugs are present in a specimen, using the chromatographic method. Chromatographic comes from the word chromatography (*chroma* means color, and *graphein* means to write, literally translated as "color writing"). The process of *chromatography* is actually separating two or more chemical compounds in a solution by removing them from the solution at different rates, a mobile (moving) phase or a stationary (still) phase, in order to detect multiple classes of drugs. Report code 80100 for each multiple drug class chromatographic procedure. Note that the CPT guidelines in this subsection explain how to properly code chromatography and give an example to help you.

Code 80104 also represents a screen to determine if multiple drugs are present in a specimen, but the screen is by a method *other than chromatographic*, such as a multiplexed screening kit. A ***multiplex assay*** can measure several analytes in one assay. Report code 80104 for each multiple drug class screening procedure.

Code 80101 is a screen to test if a single drug class is present in a specimen by immunoassay or enzyme assay. Report code 80101 for each drug class tested.

The remaining codes in the Drug Testing subsection include:

- 80102—Drug confirmation, each procedure—When a qualitative drug screen detects the presence of a substance, the lab will also perform this confirmation test to support the initial findings.

- 80103—Tissue preparation for drug analysis—This commonly applies to postmortem (after death) testing to determine substances present in tissue from various body sites.

A **quantitative test** determines the amount of a substance present in a specimen, and labs only perform a quantitative drug test if the *qualitative* screen detects the *presence* of the substance. CPT categorizes quantitative drug tests to the following subsections:

Therapeutic Drug Assay (80150–80299)

Chemistry (82000–84999)

Refer to ■ TABLE 33-2 to review index entries of main terms and subterms for drug testing and quantitative tests.

THERAPEUTIC DRUG ASSAYS (80150–80299)

A *therapeutic drug* is a drug that a patient takes to treat a specific diagnosis, which can be a long- or short-term condition. For example, digoxin is a medication that physicians use to treat patients with congestive heart failure (CHF). Digoxin helps to regulate heart

■ **TABLE 33-2 DRUG TESTING AND QUANTITATIVE TESTS INDEX ENTRIES**

Service/Procedure	Index Entry
Qualitative drug test	Drug Screen
Confirmation test	Drug, Confirmation
Tissue preparation for drug analysis	Drug, Analysis, Tissue Preparation
Quantitative test	Drug Assay, then search for the name of the analyte, or first search for the name of analyte, such as cyclosporine or aluminum

rhythm, and patients typically take it once a day. Patients continue to take the drug indefinitely because CHF is an ongoing condition that will not disappear.

Therapeutic drugs that patients take for ongoing, or long-term, conditions are also called *maintenance medications*. Sometimes, a patient needs to take a maintenance medication for a couple of weeks before the patient has a high enough level, or concentration, of drugs in the bloodstream for it to become effective. Other maintenance medications may take effect within several hours or a few days. Patients can also take therapeutic drugs for *short-term* conditions, such as taking an antibiotic to treat an infection.

Physicians order *therapeutic drug assays* for different reasons, including to test the amount of medication in a patient's bloodstream because the patient suffers from drug side effects, is also taking another medication, shows signs of problems with specific body functions, or does not show any improvement after taking the medication. The physician wants to know the amount of the drug present to assess whether to increase, decrease, or stop the dosage completely.

The physician will review both peak and trough levels of the therapeutic drug assay.

- The *trough level* is a test on blood that is drawn shortly before it is time for the patient's next dose of medication, which shows the *lowest concentration* of the drug in the bloodstream.

- The *peak level* is a test on blood that is drawn shortly after the patient either takes an oral dose of medication, or shortly after a clinician administers the medication through an IV, which shows the *highest concentration* of the drug in the bloodstream.

Knowing the trough and peak levels allows the physician to assess how well the patient's body absorbs the drug and how effectively the body removes it such as through the kidneys and liver.

Turn to the codes in the Therapeutic Drug Assays subsection to review the types of drugs listed. Notice that the CPT guidelines at the beginning of the subsection alert you that the codes in the subsection are *quantitative*. For qualitative tests, refer to codes under the Drug Testing subsection.

Drugs in the Therapeutic Drug Assays subsection are all listed by their generic names, rather than brand names. A *brand-name drug* is a drug that a **pharmaceutical** company researched, tested, and obtained a patent (exclusive legal right) to manufacture. A *generic drug* is a copy of the brand-name drug, which a different pharmaceutical company manufactures. For the most part, generic drugs and brand-name drugs have the same ingredients, but some ingredients can be different, and some generic drugs may not perform as well as the brand-name drugs. Generic drugs also often cost less than the brand-name drugs.

Did you ever have a prescription filled at the pharmacy, but the drug that you received had a different name from the one that the physician prescribed? This is an example of how the pharmacist will *substitute* the generic drug for the brand-name drug. Typically, it is because insurances will not pay for the brand-name drug and will only reimburse for the generic drug, since it costs less. If patients want the brand-name drug, then they have to pay the full cost of the prescription. Pharmacists do not substitute a generic for a brand-name when the physician includes "brand medically necessary" or "no substitutions" on

pharmaceutical (fahr-muh-soo′-ti-kuhl)—referring to a drug or a chemical

the prescription, which indicates that the patient needs to take the brand-name drug, since it is more effective than the generic version.

If you have to assign a code for a therapeutic drug assay for a brand-name drug, then you will first need to find the name of its *generic* version. You can quickly locate this information on the Internet by accessing websites with drug information, including www. drugs.com, where you can type the brand name of the drug into the search field and find the generic equivalents. You can also use a Physicians' Desk Reference (PDR), a reference manual that you can purchase, which contains brand and generic drug information.

You can find codes for therapeutic drug assays in the index under *Drug Assay,* or search for the name of the drug tested.

TAKE A BREAK

That was a lot of information to remember! Let's take a break and then review more about drug testing and therapeutic drug assays.

| Exercise 33.4 | Drug Testing, Therapeutic Drug Assays

Instructions: Review each case for procedures that Williton's lab performed on specimens that Dr. Hoffman's office submitted. Then assign codes for the procedure(s), appending a modifier when appropriate. Optional: For additional coding practice, assign the patient's diagnosis code(s) (ICD-9-CM).

1. Qualitative drug screen for multiple drug classes using chromatography for a preemployment screen as part of the patient's general medical exam. Lab technicians test three drugs with one stationary phase and three mobile phases:

   Diagnosis code(s): _____

   Procedure code(s): _____

2. Blood theophylline level for a patient with emphysema.

   Diagnosis code(s): _____

   Procedure code(s): _____

3. Digoxin level for a patient with hypertension and congestive heart failure.

   Diagnosis code(s): _____

   Procedure code(s): _____

4. Total dilantin (phenytoin) level for a patient with seizure disorder.

   Diagnosis code(s): _____

   Procedure code(s): _____

5. Lithium level for a patient with bipolar disorder.

   Diagnosis code(s): _____

   Procedure code(s): _____

6. Amitriptyline level for a patient with polyneuropathy secondary to type II diabetes mellitus.

   Diagnosis code(s): _____

   Procedure code(s): _____

EVOCATIVE/SUPPRESSION TESTING (80400–80440)

An *evocative/suppression test* is when the physician administers a pharmaceutical evocative or suppression agent (e.g., drug, steroid) into a patient's body to test the body's response to the agent. Or, the lab introduces an agent into a specimen to *evoke* (stimulate) or to *suppress* (stop) a response. Many evocative/suppression tests reveal information about how the body produces and utilizes hormones. The physician reviews the body's response to the agent compared with normal body responses.

Turn to the codes in the Evocative/Suppression Testing subsection, and you will see that they represent panel tests. You will also see that each analyte in a panel is assigned a quantity for the number of times the test must be performed to be included in the panel. The analyte also has its own CPT code, which you assign individually, if the quantity of tests performed is not the same as the quantity included in the panel.

Review code 80400—*ACTH stimulation panel; for adrenal insufficiency* for an example of an evocative/suppression test that measures cortisol in the body. Code 80400 includes two cortisol tests (82533 × 2). Cortisol, a hormone responsible for various metabolic functions, regulates the level of adrenocorticotropic hormone (ACTH), and the test measures cortisol production in the adrenal glands and pituitary gland.

CPT includes important guidelines for the Evocative/Suppression Testing subsection, which you should carefully follow before assigning codes. You can find a summary of the guidelines next:

1. Assign codes from the Evocative/Suppression subsection only for the lab tests.

2. Assign codes 96360 or 96361 (*Intravenous infusion hydration*), or 96372–96375 (*Therapeutic, prophylactic, or diagnostic injection*) when the physician administers the evocative or suppression agent to the patient. *Note:* Hospitals may report code 96372 when the physician is not present. Facilities, not physicians, report code 96376 (each additional sequential intravenous push of the same substance/drug).

3. Assign code 99070 (*Supplies and materials (except spectacles), provided by the physician over and above those usually included with the office visit or other services rendered*) when the physician provides the drug/agent and/or other supplies involved in the test. *Note:* Some payers may require HCPCS J codes that represent the pharmaceutical agent administered.

4. Assign an E/M code when the physician is in attendance and monitors the patient's testing.

5. Assign an E/M code for prolonged physician care if the physician provides prolonged care. *Note:* Do not report an E/M code for prolonged physician care when the patient receives prolonged infusions reported with 96360 or 96361 (*Intravenous infusion hydration*).

6. Code descriptors for evocative/suppression panel tests include quantities for individual analytes tested. Be sure when you assign an evocative/suppression panel code that all of the tests in the panel were performed.

To find evocative/suppression panel codes in the index, search under the name of the panel, such as *adrenocorticotropic hormone* or *thyrotropin releasing hormone*.

CONSULTATIONS (CLINICAL PATHOLOGY) (80500–80502)

Remember that a consultation, or consult, is when a physician or other agency asks for another physician's opinion about a patient's condition. The physician who performs the consultation writes a report with details of the consult and sends it to the physician who requested the consult.

A *clinical pathology consultation* is when an attending physician (or other physician caring for the patient) asks a pathologist to analyze a specimen, typically because a previous test on the specimen revealed an *abnormal result*. The pathologist writes a report on the findings of the consultation. A clinical pathology consult *does not* include simply reporting a test result without the pathologist's medical interpretative judgment. When a pathologist performs a consultation, she may also review the patient's medical records and history to better understand the patient's condition.

Turn to the subsection of Consultations (Clinical Pathology). Notice that there are only two codes for pathology consults, limited or comprehensive, depending on whether the pathologist reviews the patient's medical records.

Medicare requires providers to meet specific criteria in order to reimburse clinical pathology consultations under the physician fee schedule (Pub. 100-04 Medicare Claims). According to Medicare's requirements, pathology consultations must

1. be requested by the patient's attending physician.

2. relate to a test result that lies outside the clinically significant normal or expected range in view of the condition of the patient.

3. result in a written narrative report included in the patient's medical record.

4. require the exercise of medical judgment by the consultant physician.

Medicare also outlines the following situations that *do not* constitute clinical pathology consultations:

- Routine conversations between a laboratory director and an attending physician about test orders or results unless all four of the previously outlined requirements are met

- Contacts between laboratory personnel, including the lab director, and attending physicians to report test results or suggest additional testing. However, if in the course of the conversation the attending physician requests a consultation from the pathologist, and if the consultation meets the required criteria and is properly documented, Medicare will reimburse the service under the physician fee schedule.

- Information that a nonphysician lab specialist gives to an attending physician

Other payers may have different guidelines for coding and billing clinical pathology consultations, so it is important to check with individual payers for specific information.

Clinical pathology consultations are professional component services only and do not require you to append modifier -26 (professional component) to the consultation code. There is *no technical component* for clinical pathology consultations.

Refer to the following example of a clinical pathology consultation to better understand why a pathologist performs them.

Example: Dr. Warner, an attending physician at Williton Medical Center, telephones Dr. Duncan, a pathologist, to ask if Mr. Olson, a Medicare patient, is stable enough for surgery. Dr. Warner's request requires Dr. Duncan to render a medical judgment and provide a consultation. Dr. Duncan determines that Mr. Olson can withstand surgery, basing her opinion on review of clinical laboratory test results from Williton's lab, the patient's medical history, and additional documentation in the medical record.

An attending physician can request a clinical pathology consultation for various reasons, including consultations on blood specimens to determine why a patient reacted adversely to a blood transfusion. The pathologist examines blood that the patient received and reviews lab test results, including results that indicate infection.

Review the CPT notes following the consultation codes. They state that

- You can also assign the codes for *pharmacokinetic consultations* (how the body absorbs, metabolizes, and excretes drugs).

- If the pathologist *examines the patient* as part of the consultation, then you should instead assign a code from 99241–99255 (Office, Other Outpatient, or Inpatient Consultations).

The Surgical Pathology subsection contains additional codes for pathology consultations, which you will review later in this chapter.

To find clinical pathology consultations in the index, search under *Pathology, Clinical, Consultation.*

URINALYSIS (81000–81099)

A **urinalysis** is a test on a urine specimen to identify abnormalities. It includes reviewing the specimen with or without a microscope. Clinicians obtain urine specimens when the patient urinates into a sterile cup, through a catheter when the patient cannot urinate, or through aspiration of urine from the bladder (commonly performed on infants).

Physicians order urinalyses for patients to determine their overall health; diagnose kidney, endocrine, bladder, or urinary tract conditions; and monitor diabetes. Routine urinalysis includes review of the urine's color, transparency, density and a determination of the presence or levels of pH (acid content), glucose, protein, blood, ketones, nitrite, bilirubin, urobilinogen, and leukocytes (white blood cells). Refer to ■ TABLE 33-3 to become familiar with common terms you will find in urinalysis code descriptors.

To find a urinalysis code in the index, search under *urinalysis.*

ketones (kee'-tohnz)

microscopy (mī-kräs'-kə-pē)

reagent (rē- 'ā-jənt)

■ TABLE 33-3 **COMMON URINALYSIS TERMS**

Term	Definition
Ketones	Substances that are produced when the body breaks down fat for energy.
Bilirubin	Brown/yellow colored fluid in bile, which the liver produces. The test measures liver functioning.
Nitrite	The presence of nitrites in the urine usually indicates a urinary tract infection (UTI).
Urobilinogen	Colorless substance that is produced from the breakdown of bilirubin. Very small amounts can normally be found in the urine. An increased presence of urobilinogen can indicate other diseases such as liver disease.
Nonautomated	A clinician manually reviews the test and checks the specimen for alterations in color and transparency, or abnormal odor.
Automated	An instrument or machine reviews the test for specific analytes and can produce faster and more accurate results than nonautomated, or manual, testing.
Without microscopy	A clinician examines the specimen without a microscope, looking for urinary calculi, blood, and other substances.
With microscopy	A clinician uses a microscope to review the specimen for specific blood cells, yeast, bacteria, cell casts (groups of blood cells whose presence indicates an abnormality), renal epithelial cells, and other analytes.
Dip stick	A plastic strip treated with chemicals that is dipped into a urine specimen. The dip stick changes color when specific analytes are present, such as sugar, protein, or blood (■ FIGURE 33-1). The test is semiquantitative, detecting the presence of a substance through color change but not measuring exact quantities. The quantity can only be estimated because the higher the concentration of the substance, the darker the strip becomes. Only automated testing can provide exact quantity measurements.
Reagent strip, reagent tablet	A reagent is a substance that produces a chemical reaction to identify the presence and amount of another substance. A reagent strip (also called a dip stick) tests urine specimens for various chemical compounds, like glucose, protein, and specific gravity (measurement of urine density). The strip is treated with reagents that cause chemical reactions in the presence of a specific substance. A clinician dips the strip into the urine specimen and reviews its color, which indicates the presence of substances. A reagent tablet also changes color when specific analytes are present in a specimen.
Timed collection	Tests to measure the concentration of specific analytes in urine specimens collected at various times in a given period, such as 2-hour, 6-hour, and 12-hour intervals.
Glass test	Urine test involving more than one specimen, taken in a series, with each specimen in a sterile cup. The excreted urine in each specimen contains substances from different body sites, including the anterior and posterior urethra, bladder, prostate, and seminal vesicles.

Figure 33-1 ■ A physician compares a urine test stick to a reference chart, checking each color against the chart after specific time has elapsed, such as 45 seconds for specific gravity.

Photo credit: Keith A. Frith/ Shutterstock.

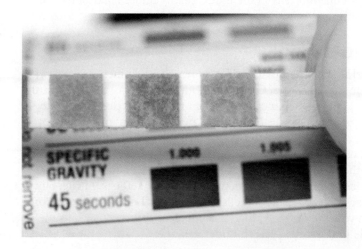

CHEMISTRY (82000–84999)

The Chemistry subsection contains mostly *quantitative* tests for numerous analytes on many different types of specimens. Specimens can be from any source, unless the code descriptor specifies the source, such as blood or urine. Some of the tests in this subsection are *qualitative*, and CPT describes them as qualitative in code descriptors. You already learned that a urinalysis tests for different analytes and cannot provide exact measurements of the quantities of those analytes. Therefore, a physician orders a *chemistry test* on a urine specimen when he wants to determine the *quantity* of an analyte in a specimen.

Turn to the Chemistry subsection in your CPT manual to become familiar with some of the hundreds of codes for analytes tested. Did you notice that some of the code descriptors contain the word *qualitative*, indicating that the test measures the *presence* of an analyte?

The Chemistry subsection contains many CPT guidelines for assigning codes, including guidelines at the beginning of the subsection and guidelines following code descriptors. As you know, it is important to become familiar with the guidelines before final code assignment. Here are some highlights of the guidelines at the beginning of the subsection:

- When a clinician measures an analyte in multiple specimens from different sources, report the code for each analyte separately for each source.

- When a clinician measures an analyte in specimens obtained at different times, report the code for each analyte separately for each specimen.

It is also important to understand that some lab tests provide information about *how* the patient's body functions and if it is functioning normally. For these tests, physicians compare the results of patients' lab tests with what is called the *reference range* or *reference values*, which are the average results of the test for a specific group of patients.

For example, the reference range for a prostate-specific antigen (PSA) test is less than 4 ng/mL (nanograms per milliliter), based on the average range for men who received the PSA test. A male patient with a PSA level of 20 ng/mL is *above* the reference range. There are various meanings for this test result; the lab might need to retest the PSA level, the patient might have prostate cancer, or the patient might have another health problem that is causing the level to increase. Reference ranges are different depending on the type of group of patients tested, and reference ranges *are not called normal ranges* because they represent average ranges of a particular group of people tested, not an entire population.

To find chemistry codes in the index, search under the name of the analyte, such as *acetaminophen* or *amino acids*.

TAKE A BREAK

Nice work! Let's take a break and then practice coding various lab tests.

Exercise 33.5 Evocative/Suppression Testing, Consultations (Clinical Pathology), Urinalysis, Chemistry

Instructions: Review each case, and then assign codes for the procedure(s), appending a modifier when appropriate. Optional: For additional coding practice, assign the patient's diagnosis code(s) (ICD-9-CM).

1. Bob Ducsay, age 62, returns to Dr. Hoffman's office for re-evaluation of his high blood pressure. Dr. Hoffman performs a problem-focused history and a detailed examination of the patient and determines that the patient's antihypertensive medication is not effective. Dr. Hoffman orders an aldosterone (steroid hormone) suppression evaluation panel be performed to rule out primary hyperaldosteronism (overproduction of aldosterone) as the cause for Mr. Ducsay's hypertension. Rhonda, the medical assistant, performs a venipuncture and sends the specimen to Williton's lab for analysis of two aldosterone levels and two levels of renin (an enzyme that the kidneys produce). Code for Dr. Hoffman's services and Williton's services.

Diagnosis code(s): _____

Dr. Hoffman's procedure code(s): _____

Williton's procedure code(s): _____

continued

TAKE A BREAK *continued*

2. Brandyburg Laboratory performs a test on a blood specimen to determine the amount of intrinsic factor (a protein produced by stomach cells to allow vitamin B12 to enter the body). The test is for a patient with complaints of lightheadedness, fatigue, and pallor, and the physician suspects vitamin B_{12}-deficiency anemia.

Diagnosis code(s): _____

Procedure code(s): _____

3. Williton's lab performs an L/S (lecithin-to-sphingo-myelin) ratio test to determine the maturity level of a fetus's lungs. The mother is in prolonged, active labor.

Procedure code(s): _____

4. Alice Roach, age 25, is an established patient who sees Dr. Hoffman and complains of urinary frequency and dysuria. Dr. Hoffman performs an expanded problem-focused history, problem-focused examination, and low-complexity medical decision-making. He asks the patient to submit a urine sample and asks Rhonda, his medical assistant, to perform a urinalysis using the dip stick method to determine what analytes are present. Rhonda reports that leukocytes, nitrates, and a small amount of blood are present. Dr. Hoffman diagnoses the patient with a urinary tract infection.

Diagnosis code(s): _____

Procedure code(s): _____

5. What type of certificate does Dr. Hoffman's office have to allow Rhonda to perform minor laboratory tests, such as dip stick urinalyses?

_____

6. Dr. Dickinson, a surgical pathologist at Williton, receives a written request from Dr. Azoury, a pathologist at Cannon Medical Center, to microscopically review specimens of breast tissue from a lesion. Dr. Azoury observed atypical cells in the specimen. Dr. Azoury also sends the patient's medical records along with the request. Dr. Dickinson reviews the specimens and medical records, calls Dr. Azoury with the results, and also sends a written report indicating that the specimen is benign. Code for Dr. Dickinson's services.

Diagnosis code(s): _____

Procedure code(s): _____

7. Brandyburg Laboratory performs a test on a blood specimen for LDL (low-density lipoprotein) cholesterol, elevated levels of which may cause a myocardial infarction. The patient has chronic angina.

Diagnosis code(s): _____

Procedure code(s): _____

HEMATOLOGY AND COAGULATION (85002–85999)

The Hematology and Coagulation subsection includes hematology tests to determine cell counts of different types of blood cells. Abnormally low or high counts could indicate problems with various organs or body systems. Coagulation tests determine how efficiently the blood clots, and some conditions can cause blood to clot too quickly or too slowly. Tests can be manual or automated. (You can find hematology blood panel tests, such as the basic metabolic panels, in the Organ or Disease-Oriented Panels subsection.)

Turn to the codes listed in this subsection to become familiar with the types of tests included. CPT categorizes codes by the type of test (blood count, heparin assay, thrombin time), including semiquantitative, quantitative, manual, or automated. ■ TABLE 33-4 lists some of these tests. There are also various CPT guidelines throughout the subsection that you should review. When you are coding for tests with which you are unfamiliar, always use medical references, such as a medical dictionary or reputable internet site, to investigate information about the test. You can also query the provider if there is information that you do not understand.

To locate codes for hematology and coagulation tests, search the index for the name of the test (*clotting factor, prothrombin time*).

■ TABLE 33-4 **EXAMPLES OF HEMATOLOGY AND COAGULATION TESTS**

Description	Purpose of Test
Bleeding time	To determine how long it takes blood vessels to clot by cutting the arm and blotting the cuts. A clinician measures the amount of time it takes the cuts to stop bleeding.
Blood count	To measure white blood cells (WBCs), red blood cells (RBCs), platelets, hematocrit (Hct), hemoglobin (Hgb), and reticulocytes (immature red blood cells). Blood count tests include a complete blood count (CBC).
	Clinicians compare test results with reference ranges to diagnose various conditions, including anemia, **thalessemia**, cancer, infections, and bleeding and bone marrow disorders. Blood count tests include automated differential WBC count and manual differential WBC count, which provide measurements about each type of WBC present in a specimen. A buffy coat is a layer of white blood cells.
Blood smear, peripheral	To analyze blood cells for any blood or bone marrow disorders or parasites. A peripheral blood smear is when a provider smears a layer of blood onto a slide, then adds a stain to microscopically visualize blood cells. Many times, providers order blood smears after abnormal CBC results.
Bone marrow, smear interpretation	To diagnose hematologic disorders, anemia, and cancer. The bone marrow **aspirate** is smeared on a microscopic slide for the provider to analyze. It is important to understand that this is a laboratory service for analyzing the smear. The surgical service of aspirating the bone marrow is what the operating physician performs, and his staff codes and bills for the service.
Clotting tests	To determine how quickly or slowly blood clots, including tests of clotting factors (also called coagulation factors), which are proteins in plasma responsible for clotting. Abnormal results can mean clotting time is too fast or too slow.
Prothrombin time (PT)	To determine how long it takes blood to clot, measuring the presence of five different clotting factors: I, II, V, VII, and X. PT tests, or "pro times," also help physicians to determine if blood thinning medications (to prevent clots) are working properly.
	A PT test is also referred to as an INR (international normalized ratio) test, which means that the test results are standard, regardless of the method used to perform the test. An abnormal PT test result may indicate liver disease because the liver manufactures prothrombin (factor II), or it may indicate inappropriate dosage of a blood thinning (**anticoagulant**) medication.
Thromboplastin time, partial (PTT)	To determine how long it takes blood to clot; often performed in conjunction with a PT test. This test helps physicians to determine if anticoagulant medications are working properly and if the patient is receiving the correct dosage.

IMMUNOLOGY (86000–86849)

Remember that immunology is the study of the structure and function of the immune system. The subsection Immunology contains many different tests on antigens, allergens, and antibodies. Turn to the subsection to review the codes listed, and note that there are several CPT guidelines following codes and their descriptors. Refer to ■ TABLE 33-5 to review common terms that you will find in descriptors to better understand various tests. Table 33-5 does not contain all the terms with which you may be unfamiliar, so it is important to refer to your medical resources for additional clarification of terms that you do not know.

Immunology tests on blood or saliva help physicians to diagnose infections and other disorders. The tests identify

- specific antigens that cause a patient to have an adverse reaction, including infections and viruses

- specific antibodies, whose presence shows that the patient suffers from a condition that the antibodies are fighting

To find codes for immunology tests, search the index for the name of the test (*agglutinin*, **Epstein-Barr virus**).

thalessemia (thal-ə-sē'-mē-ə)—a type of anemia in which a patient's hemoglobin forms abnormally

aspirate (as'-pə-rāt)—liquid that has been retrieved using an aspiration procedure and sent for laboratory examination

anticoagulant (an-tee-koh-ag'-yuh-luhnt)

Epstein-Barr virus (ep'-stīn-bär)—virus that causes mononucleosis

■ TABLE 33-5   **COMMON IMMUNOLOGY TERMS**

Term	Definition
allergen	Substance that enters the body and causes an allergic reaction. Common allergens are pollen, mold, dust, pet hair, and specific foods, such as peanuts.
antibody	Proteins that the body's immune system produces to fight off antigens. The antibodies are composed of WBCs (also called B cells or B lymphocytes), which attach to antigens to destroy them or attract other WBCs to antigens to destroy them. An antibody is also called an agglutinin, which is a substance in the body that causes cells to adhere to antigens.
antigen	A protein in bacteria, viruses, and toxins that causes the body to produce antibodies to fight against it.
immunoglobulin	A protein that plasma cells manufacture, which helps the body's immune system defend itself against foreign bodies, like bacteria.
tissue typing	A test that determines whether donor tissue is compatible with recipient tissue before a transplant.
titer	The amount of antibodies in a patient's blood.

TAKE A BREAK

You are doing great! Let's take a break and then practice coding hematology, coagulation, and immunology tests.

Exercise 33.6   Hematology and Coagulation, Immunology

Instructions: Review each case, and then assign codes for the procedure(s), appending a modifier when appropriate. Optional: For additional coding practice, assign the patient's diagnosis code(s) (ICD-9-CM).

1. Williton's lab performs a CBC with differential on a specimen that Dr. Hoffman's office sent for a patient with complaints of right lower quadrant pain, fever of 102°F, and nausea and vomiting for the past six hours.

   Diagnosis code(s): _____

   Procedure code(s): _____

2. Williton's lab performs ANA (antinuclear antibody) testing for immune system disorders on a blood specimen for a patient with complaints of arthralgia (joint pain) and myalgia (muscle pain) for the past two months.

   Diagnosis code(s): _____

   Procedure code(s): _____

3. Marjorie Shear is a long-time patient of Dr. Hoffman's and was in the office last week for a follow-up visit for atrial fibrillation. During that visit, Dr. Hoffman instructed Mrs. Shear to return to the office today to have blood drawn to make sure that her Coumadin level is therapeutic. Rhonda, the medical assistant, reviews Mrs. Shear's electronic health record and determines that Dr. Hoffman ordered a PT/PTT. Rhonda performs a venipuncture and sends the specimen to Williton's lab to perform the tests. Code for Dr. Hoffman's services today and Williton's services.

   Diagnosis code(s): _____

   Dr. Hoffman's procedure code(s): _____

   Williton's procedure code(s): _____

4. Marcia Schlick is a 35-year-old established patient who teaches kindergarten. She tells Dr. Hoffman that one of her students was diagnosed with rubella (German measles), and she wants to know if she still has immunity to rubella or if she needs a booster MMR (measles, mumps, rubella) vaccine. Dr. Hoffman conducts a problem-focused history and exam and asks Rhonda to draw a rubella titer (to measure antibodies present), and she then sends the specimen to Williton's lab for processing. There are no other services performed. Code for Dr. Hoffman's services and Williton's services.

   Diagnosis code(s): _____

   Dr. Hoffman's procedure code(s): _____

   Williton's procedure code(s): _____

5. Brandyburg Laboratory performs an Epstein-Barr virus test for a patient with symptoms of fatigue and a

TAKE A BREAK *continued*

sore throat. The physician who sent the specimen believes that the patient may have mononucleosis.

Diagnosis code(s): _____

Procedure code(s): _____

6. George Miller, age 56, arrives at Williton's lab at Dr. Hoffman's request for a blood draw to test hemoglobin

and hematocrit levels. Mr. Miller was discharged from Williton Medical Center two weeks ago with a diagnosis of acute duodenal ulcer with hemorrhage.

Diagnosis code(s): _____

Procedure code(s): _____

TRANSFUSION MEDICINE (86850–86999)

A blood transfusion is when clinicians replace blood that is lost during surgery or traumatic injury. Blood transfusions also help patients with cancer or other diseases, which can cause internal bleeding or slow blood cell production, causing the patients to require more blood. Before a blood transfusion, providers perform cross-matching, which ensures that the donated blood is compatible with the patient's own blood and that the patient's blood does not contain antibodies that will react to the donor's blood. Before transfusing blood, providers should also ensure that it is free of any bacteria, viruses, or disease, and the Transfusion Medicine subsection includes these services.

A blood bank is a facility (which can be part of a hospital's lab) that collects blood from donors and determines its type (called blood typing) based on whether specific antigens and antibodies are present on RBCs and in plasma (■ FIGURE 33-2). Blood types include

A—The A antigen is present on RBCs, and the B antibody is present in plasma.

B—The B antigen is present on RBCs, and the A antibody is present in plasma.

AB—Both A and B antigens are present on RBCs, but A and B antibodies are not in plasma.

O—A and B antigens are not present on RBCs but A and B antibodies are in plasma. Type O is also called the universal blood type because it is compatible with all other blood types.

The blood bank also checks for presence of other antigens and separates blood products into components of blood cells, plasma, and platelets. Apheresis separates certain components from blood when patients do not need all of them. The blood bank stores blood and its products to distribute to providers for patients who need blood transfusions.

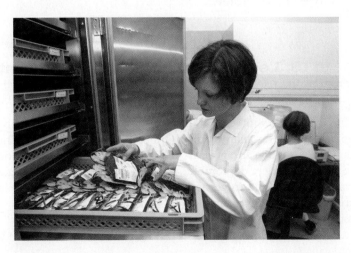

Figure 33-2 ■ A lab technician at a blood bank checks blood types from bags of donated blood.
Photo credit: Lisa S./Shutterstock.

apheresis (a-fə-rē′-səs)

A medical director supervises blood banks and is certfied by the American Board of Pathology in blood banking and transfusion medicine. Medical directors of blood banks can specialize in hematology, pathology, anesthesiology, or other related specialties.

Turn to the codes in the Transfusion Medicine subsection to become more familiar with them. Notice the CPT guidelines at the beginning of the subsection that direct you to codes 36511–36512 to code for **apheresis**. There are additional CPT coding gudielines throughout the subsection.

The Transfusion Medicine subsection includes codes for blood typing, antibody screens, compatibility testing, autologous blood (the patient's own blood) collection processing and storage, thawing plasma, freezing blood, Coombs test (test for autoimmune hemolytic anemia, a condition when the body destroys its own RBCs), and several other services. You should assign a separate code for the blood transfusion from the Surgery section (36430—Transfusion, blood or blood components) and also assign separate HCPCS codes for the blood product transfused. Here are some examples of HCPCS codes:

P9010—Blood (whole), for transfusion, per unit

P9011—Blood, split unit

P9019—Platelets, each unit

To locate codes for transfusion medicine, search the index for the name of the test (*Coombs, blood typing, pooling*).

MICROBIOLOGY (87001–87999)

Microbiology literally means the study of (-ology) small (micro) life (bio), which is the study of *microorganisms* (organisms seen with a microscope). Microbiology lab tests include identifying microorganisms in various types of specimens, as well as tests involving

mycology (mī-käl′-ə-jē)

parasitology (par-ə-sə-täl′-ə-jē)

virology (vī-räl′-ə-jē)

chlamydia (klə-mid′-ē-ə)—a bacterial disease that is spread through sexual contact that causes a pus-like vaginal discharge

tubercle (t(y)ü′-bər-kəl)—a small lump that can grow in tissues

bacteriology —the study of bacteria

mycology —the study of fungi, or fungus

parasitology —the study of parasites

virology —the study of viruses and viral disease

Examples include testing for streptococcus group A, Hepatitis B virus, HIV-1 and HIV-2, **chlamydia**, Human Papillomavirus (HPV), herpes simplex virus, influenza, **tubercle (TB),** yeast, and mold. Physicians can order microbiology tests after an abnormal test result, such as when a patient's urine test result is positive for bacteria, and the microbiology test then determines the specific *type* of bacteria present.

Turn to the Microbiology subsection to review the codes, and refer to ■ TABLE 33-6 to become familiar with common terms associated with microbiology as you read the code descriptors. CPT categorizes codes by the type of test performed, type of specimen, or type of identification.

INTERESTING FACTS: Leprosy Victims Were Forced into Isolation

Hawaiian King Kamehameha V created an isolation law in the late 1800s, forcing people with leprosy to remain in a leper colony on one of the Hawaiian islands because leprosy was contagious. Although the government provided food, living conditions were deplorable, and "lepers" lived in caves. No one wanted to go near them for fear of contracting leprosy. They remained alone on the island for several years before a missionary,

Father Damien, arrived to assist them by building houses, schools, and providing medical care. Gradually, others from the Catholic Church arrived to help him. Father Damien eventually contracted leprosy and died. Surprisingly, the King's isolation law remained effective until the 1960s. Father Damien was canonized as Saint Damien in 2009.

■ **TABLE 33-6   COMMON MICROBIOLOGY TERMS**

Term	Definition
culture	A test to determine if microorganisms are present in a specimen by placing the specimen in a **petri dish** (shallow dish) containing **agar**, a gelatin-like substance that helps bacteria to grow. If bacteria are present in a specimen, then providers will conduct *culture and sensitivity tests*, which identify the type(s) of microorganism present in a specimen and determine which antibiotic can successfully destroy it.
gram stain	A test where the provider stains a specimen to identify bacteria. Gram-positive bacteria retain a purple stain, and gram-negative bacteria retain a red stain.
aerobic bacteria	Bacteria that need oxygen to survive.
anaerobic bacteria	Bacteria that do not need oxygen to survive, commonly found in internal organs.
macroscopic exam of arthropod or parasite	A test that views a parasite or arthropod (flea, tick, lice, worm) with the naked eye (**macroscopic**).
acid fast stain for bacteria	A test to determine the type of bacteria present in a specimen, based on whether the bacteria react to a stain.
mycobacteria	Rod-shaped bacteria that cause tuberculosis and *leprosy* (Hansen's disease). Leprosy is a chronic infectious disease that primarily affects the peripheral nerves, skin, upper respiratory tract, eyes, and nasal mucosa, resulting in skin lesions and permanent scarring (■ FIGURE 33-3). It is no longer contagious because there are medications used to treat it.
ova and parasites, direct smears	A test on stool to determine the presence of parasites and their ova (eggs) for patients with chronic diarrhea. The test is also called an O & P.
wet mount	A technique for viewing specimens on a microscopic slide by adding water, which provides more light to examine the specimen.
KOH slide	A test where the provider adds potassium hydroxide (KOH) to identify the presence of nail or skin fungus.

petri dish (pē′-trē)

agar (äg′-ər)

aerobic bacteria (a(-ə)
r-ō′-bik bak-tir′-ē-ə)

anaerobic bacteria (an-ə-
rō′-bik bak-tir′-ē-ə)

macroscopic (mak-rə-
skäp′-ik)

Notice that there are CPT guidelines at the beginning of and throughout the Microbiology subsection. Before final code assignment, be sure to carefully review these guidelines, consulting your medical references to find information about procedures with which you are unfamiliar. To locate codes for microbiology services, search the index for the name of the test (*bacteria culture, ova*).

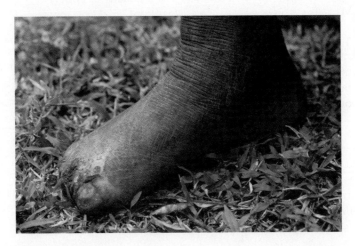

Figure 33-3 ■ The foot of a man suffering from leprosy.

Photo credit: © Nina French/Alamy.

POINTERS FROM THE PROS: Interview with a Coding Manager

Suzan Berman is a Senior Manager for Coding Education and Documentation Compliance for a large teaching hospital medical center. You first read some of her advice in Chapter 17, and she has even more information to share with you.

What interests you the most about the job that you perform?

The clinicians are all very knowledgeable regarding their fields of expertise. They want to be able to bill appropriately; however, a lot of their education doesn't focus on that. I work closely with midlevel providers to make certain they understand their role in the billing and documentation process. I like being their source, their sounding board, as well as their implementer when it comes to electronic medical records details, forms, guidelines, licensure, etc.

What are the most challenging aspects of your job?

The coding guidelines are often cumbersome and carry a lot of detail. I like to be able to appropriately interpret those guidelines for the providers. I often find some of the areas to be confusing myself, and this is a challenge in finding out the correct way to interpret them.

Describe the frequency and types of communication that you have with physicians and/or employees of other departments, organizations, or providers:

I meet with physicians at least yearly. Some will meet with me one-on-one, others in a group setting. When I first started, I made certain to meet with each physician individually to establish a relationship with them. It is important to show the physicians that you understand what they are dealing with on a daily basis with all of the regulations. You are the messenger, and they will come to understand that the more you spend time with them.

What advice can you give to new coders to help them to communicate effectively with physicians, since physicians can sometimes be intimidating?

The best lesson I ever had was spending time shadowing the physicians during clinic, during hospital rounds, and even in the operating room. This gave me an opportunity to see how documentation comes into play during their routine, but also shows me the workflow.

(Used by permission of Suzan Berman.)

TAKE A BREAK

Keep up the good work! Let's take a break and then practice coding transfusion medicine and microbiology services.

Exercise 33.7 Transfusion Medicine and Microbiology

Instructions: Review each case, and then assign codes for the procedure(s), appending a modifier when appropriate. Optional: For additional coding practice, assign the patient's diagnosis code(s) (ICD-9-CM).

1. Brandyburg Laboratory performs an indirect Coombs test for a patient who recently had a miscarriage (complete). She has blood type O, and her ordering physician wanted to be sure that the patient did not develop antibodies that could potentially compromise future pregnancies.

   Diagnosis code(s): _____

   Procedure code(s): _____

2. Dr. Hoffman sees Brittney Plankton, a 2-year-old established patient. Her mother states that Brittney has been scratching her anal area, and states that she also found small worms in Brittney's stool. Dr. Hoffman performs a problem-focused history and examination. He and Rhonda place cellophane tape over Brittney's anus and remove it for a microscopic exam. Dr. Hoffman informs Mrs. Plankton that Brittney has pinworms and prescribes Vermox® (antiworm medication).

   Diagnosis code(s): _____

   Procedure code(s): _____

3. Williton's lab examines cultures for gonorrhea and chlamydia for a patient who complains of yellowish vaginal discharge with a foul odor for the past two weeks.

   Diagnosis code(s): _____

   Procedure code(s): _____

4. Naomi Nixon, age 36, returns to Dr. Hoffman's office with a three-day history of urinary frequency, dysuria, and pelvic cramping. Dr. Hoffman performs an

TAKE A BREAK *continued*

expanded problem-focused history and examination. Dr. Hoffman asks Rhonda, his medical assistant, to collect urine to perform a dip stick urinalysis. Rhonda finds leukocytes, blood, and nitrates in the urine. Dr. Hoffman then diagnoses a UTI. He orders a urine culture with sensitivity from Williton's lab, and Rhonda sends the specimen. Medical decision-making is low complexity. Code for Dr. Hoffman's services and Williton's services.

Diagnosis code(s): _____

Dr. Hoffman's procedure code(s): _____

Williton's procedure code(s): _____

5. Williton's lab tests a stool sample for ova and parasites for a patient with complaints of diarrhea, abdominal pain, and headache.

Diagnosis code(s): _____

Procedure code(s): _____

6. Brandyburg Laboratory performs a bacterial stool culture test with isolation and preliminary exam for a patient who complains of diarrhea, blood in the stool, and abdominal pain.

Diagnosis code(s): _____

Procedure code(s): _____

ANATOMIC PATHOLOGY (88000–88099)

Anatomic pathology services involve an *autopsy* (**necropsy**), also called a postmortem examination. An autopsy is examining a body (cadaver) to determine the cause of death, the victim's overall health at the time of death, circumstances surrounding the death, and if medical treatment or neglect contributed to the death. Not everyone who dies receives an autopsy. Examples of situations requiring an autopsy are suspicious, sudden, accidental, unnatural, or violent deaths, or medical research. Autopsies are typically unnecessary if the deceased suffered from condition(s) that could easily cause death, if the individual was elderly, or if no trauma was involved.

necropsy (nek-răp′-sē)

Providers who perform autopsies include pathologists and *forensic pathologists*, who also collect internal and external evidence during the autopsy, drawing on knowledge of blood analysis, DNA analysis, firearms/ballistics, and toxicology (88040—*Necropsy (autopsy); forensic examination*). Pathologists can work in hospitals, medical schools, or in their own practices. A pathologist can also be a *medical examiner* or *coroner,* a physician elected to or appointed by city, county, state, or the federal government. They perform autopsies to investigate suspicious or unusual deaths to determine the cause (88045—*Necropsy (autopsy); coroner's call*).

An autopsy can be *limited*, where the provider *does not* examine the head or brain, or where she only examines specific organs; or *complete*, where the provider removes and examines *all organs*, including the brain. During an autopsy, a provider may order lab tests and consult with other healthcare professionals to discuss the case. A coroner or medical examiner can also order an *inquest*, which is an investigation to find out more information about the deceased and determine a cause of death.

Are you wondering if a deceased person's medical insurance pays for an autopsy? That is a good question! Insurances, including Medicare, typically do not cover autopsy costs. Medicare considers autopsies to be part of other hospital costs for the patient's care and will not separately reimburse them. If a provider performs an autopsy for legal reasons, then the city, county, state, or federal government pays for it. If the deceased person's family requests the autopsy, then they pay for it. Autopsies can be very expensive to perform, and the specific cost depends on the extent of physician's services.

Turn to the codes in this subsection to review them. CPT divides codes by **gross examination** (examination with the naked eye) and **gross and microscopic examination** (examination with the naked eye and with a microscope). CPT divides gross exams (88000–88016) according to whether the exam *excludes the central nervous system (CNS)* or *includes*

the brain

the brain and spinal cord

an infant with brain

a stillborn or newborn with brain

macerated (ma-sə-rā 'ted) a **macerated** stillborn (stillborn infant with soft or broken skin from continuous exposure to amniotic fluid)

CPT divides gross and microscopic exams (88020–88029) according to whether the exam *excludes the CNS* or *includes*

the brain

the brain and spinal cord

an infant with brain

a stillborn or newborn with brain

To locate codes for anatomic pathology services, search the index for *autopsy*.

CYTOPATHOLOGY (88104–88199)

Cytopathology is the study of (-ology) cellular (cyto/o) diseases (patho/o), including examining cells from anywhere in the body to detect various conditions and determine if neoplasms are benign or malignant. Turn to the Cytopathology subsection to review the codes listed. CPT divides cytopathology services into the following types of services:

- *nongynecological tests*—Beginning with code 88104. Tests include smears from fluids, washings, and brushings, flow cytometry (measuring cells), and other types of tests.
- *gynecological tests*—Beginning with code 88141. Gynecological tests include cervical and vaginal specimens, such as the Papanicolaou (Pap) smear, which is one of the most common cytopathology services.

It is important to become familiar with terms listed in code descriptors to better understand cytopathology services. Refer to ■ TABLE 33-7 for common terms in this subsection, and consult your medical references for further clarification. Also note that there are several different CPT guidelines throughout the Cytopathology subsection.

■ TABLE 33-7 **COMMON CYTOPATHOLOGY TERMS**

Term	Definition
cytopathology washing	Type of specimen obtained from a surgical procedure in which fluid is squirted over a particular body area and then recollected. The fluid is sent to the cytology department of a hospital for microscopic analysis.
cytopathology brushing	A technique in which a surgical brush is swept along an area of tissue in attempt to gather cells. The brush is then sent to the cytology department in a hospital for microscopic analysis.
filter method	A method used in a laboratory in order to collect cells for examination.
morphometric analysis	A type of analysis in which the size and shape of cells are examined.
sex chromatin identification, Barr bodies	A test that is done on amniotic fluid that determines whether the fetus is male or female. A Barr body is an inactive X chromosome that is present in the body cells of normal females.
thin layer preparation	A method used to prepare cells gathered from a women's cervix for examination via Pap smear.
Bethesda System	A system used in reporting diagnosis related to cervical cellular abnormalities.
flow cytometry	A type of technique used in a laboratory that allows a cytologist to examine structures such as cells and chromosomes.

cytometry (sī-täm'-ə-trē)

To locate codes for cytopathology services, search the index for *cytopathology* and then search for the type of test as a subterm, or search for the name of the test (*cervical smears, flow cytometry*).

CYTOGENETIC STUDIES (88230–88299)

Cytogenetic studies are tests involving the structure and function of cells. They may include analyzing chromosomes, which carry genetic material and hereditary traits. Turn to the Cytogenetic Studies subsection to review the codes listed, including tissue cultures for nonneoplastic and neoplastic disorders, cryopreservation (freezing and storage) of cells, thawing and expansion of frozen cells, chromosome analysis, and molecular diagnostic procedures.

Chromosomes consist of protein and DNA in the nucleus of cells, and they carry genes, which are responsible for characteristics of an individual, such as eye, hair, and skin color, along with many other traits. Chromosomes may also carry genetic disorders that a person can inherit from family members. Typically, a person has 46 chromosomes, 23 from his mother, and 23 from his father, received when a sperm fertilizes an egg. The 46 chromosomes include 22 pairs of **autosomal chromosomes** (numbered pairs 1 through 22) and one pair of sex chromosomes (labeled X and Y). Females have two X chromosomes, and males have an X and a Y chromosome. An individual with extra, missing, abnormal, or rearranged chromosomes can have various types of conditions, including leukemia, bone marrow cancer, infertility, Down's syndrome (extra copy of chromosome 21), or may be a carrier of a specific disease.

autosomal chromosomes (ot-ə-sō′-m-əl krō′-mə-sōmz)—all types of chromosomes except for those that determine sex traits

Chromosome analysis is a test that identifies the **karyotype**, or total number, arrangement, size, and shape of chromosomes, to determine chromosomal abnormalities or mutations. *Molecular diagnostic procedures* include testing for inherited disorders and identifying cancer behavior.

Note that the CPT guidelines at the beginning of the Cytogenetic Studies subsection instruct you to refer to Appendix I in your CPT manual for a list of genetic testing modifiers to report with codes for molecular diagnostic and cytogenetic procedures. Review the modifiers listed there to become more familiar with them.

To locate codes for **cytogenetic** studies, search the index for the type of specimen (*tissue*) and then search subterms for the type of test (*culture*), or start by searching for the type of test (*cryopreservation, chromosome analysis*).

cytogenetic (sīt-ə-jen-e′-tik)

TAKE A BREAK

That was a lot to remember! Good job! Let's take a break and then practice coding other types of services.

Exercise 33.8 Anatomic Pathology, Cytopathology, Cytogenetic Studies

Instructions: Review each case, and then assign codes for the procedure(s), appending a modifier when appropriate. *Optional:* For additional coding practice, assign the patient's diagnosis code(s) (ICD-9-CM). Not all of the cases require a diagnosis code.

1. Lucy Matthews, a 46-year-old established patient, sees Dr. Fulton, her gynecologist, for her yearly gynecologic visit and Pap smear. She has no complaints. Dr. Fulton performs Lucy's physical examination and Pap smear. Dr. Fulton's medical assistant, Melissa,

prepares the Pap smear for processing and sends it to Williton Medical Center for evaluation, where it is screened by an automated system with physician supervision. Code for Dr. Fulton's services and Williton's services.

Diagnosis code(s): _____

Dr. Fulton's procedure code(s): _____

Williton's procedure code(s): _____

2. Brandyburg Hospital's cytology department analyzes aspirate from a fine-needle aspiration.

Procedure code(s): _____

continued

TAKE A BREAK *continued*

3. Brandyburg Laboratory received 30 mL of amniotic fluid with a request to perform alpha-fetoprotein analysis.

Procedure code(s):_____

4. Dr. Cline, a pathologist at Williton Medical Center, received a request to perform an autopsy on a 37-year-old male who experienced apparent sudden cardiac death. Dr. Cline received the body with the brain and spinal cord intact and performed a gross and microscopic examination.

Procedure code(s):_____

5. Dr. Cline performed an autopsy on a stillborn infant. Dr. Cline received the specimen with the brain intact and performed a gross examination.

Procedure code(s):_____

6. Brandyburg Laboratory analyzes a Pap smear using the Bethesda System. Manual screening under physician supervision was performed.

Procedure code(s):_____

SURGICAL PATHOLOGY (88300–88399)

Surgical pathology services occur when a pathologist conducts a gross and/or microscopic exam of a specimen that a physician removes from a patient during surgery or during a procedure in the hospital, ambulatory surgery center, or physician's office. The pathologist may also order additional lab tests on the specimen if he needs more information, and will document his findings in a pathology report.

Surgical pathology specimens include

- *biopsies*—removed during surgery to be tested for specific conditions, including a benign or malignant neoplasm

- *surgical resections*—sections of tissue or organs that the surgeon removes from the patient to treat a specific condition

A pathologist examines the biopsy or surgical resection for several purposes: (■ FIGURE 33-4):

- to confirm the initial diagnosis before a procedure

- to confirm that there is no disease present (such as for specimens removed during sterilization procedures)

- to determine the extent of a disease

- to identify any other conditions

Figure 33-4 ■ A pathologist uses ink to determine the orientation and margins of a tumor in breast tissue and lymph nodes removed during a mastectomy.

Photo credit: Boilershot Photo/Photo Researchers, Inc.

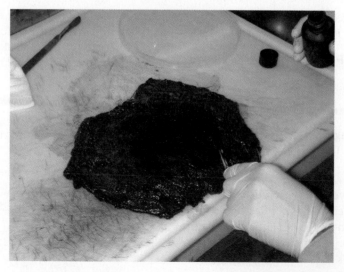

Turn to the Surgical Pathology subsection in your CPT manual. Notice that the first codes listed in this subsection (88300–88309) identify levels of surgical pathology services. CPT categorizes surgical pathology services into six levels, each with a different code, depending on the amount of work the pathologist performs to analyze a specimen. The levels are represented by Roman numerals I–VI, with I as the lowest level service and VI as the highest. The higher the level, the greater the amount of work the pathologist performs. Each level lists the types of specimens the pathologist examines to justify assigning a code from that level. The specimens are listed in alphabetical order, so it is easy to find the type of specimen in order to assign the correct code.

For example, if you read the patient's medical documentation and determine that the pathologist examined a cholesteatoma, you would assign code 88304 *Level III* because *cholesteatoma* is listed as a specimen for code 88304. Note that the pathologist will *not* document that he performed a "Level III" exam of the specimen. He will instead describe the specimen, where it originated, and his findings. The pathologist *does not* have to examine *all* of the specimens listed for a specific code in order for you to assign the code. However, you do need to separately report codes for each specimen examined.

To better understand the various levels of surgical pathology services, review the CPT guidelines at the beginning of the subsection, which include the following information:

1. Report code 88300 (Level I—*Surgical pathology, gross examination only*) for any specimen that the pathologist can accurately diagnose *without* a microscope. Examples include eye lens or foreign bodies, such as a bullet. A physician's assistant may also perform gross exams, but he must work under the pathologist's supervision.

2. Report code 88302 (Level II—*Surgical pathology, gross and microscopic examination*) when the pathologist performs a gross and microscopic exam to confirm the presence or absence of disease. Examples include fallopian tube removal during sterilization, hernia sac, or nerve.

3. Report codes 88304–88309 (Level III–VI—*Surgical pathology, gross and microscopic examination*) for all other specimens where the pathologist performs a gross and microscopic exam. These codes represent ascending levels of physician work. Examples include anus tag (88034), colon biopsy (88305), brain biopsy (88307), or small intestine resection for tumor (88309).

4. If the pathologist examines a specimen that is *not listed* in any of the surgical pathology services, then assign the surgical pathology code that most closely matches the same amount of work that the physician performs to examine other specimens. The physician can clarify this information to better help you to assign the appropriate code.

In addition to understanding the CPT guidelines, it is also important for you to understand how CPT categorizes specimens in the surgical pathology levels. You already know that each level lists specimens that the pathologist must examine in order for you to report a specific code. Be very careful when assigning surgical pathology codes because some specimens are *listed in more than one code level,* but they have differences, depending on the specific exam. You will need to carefully review the pathologist's medical documentation to determine what code level to assign based on these differences. It is also important to understand that you will need to communicate with the physician to clarify information and ensure that she documents information clearly in the patient's record so that you can correctly assign codes.

To better understand these differences, refer to codes 88307 and 88309. Notice that *uterus, with or without tubes and ovaries* is listed under both codes. However, code 88307 includes *uterus, with or without tubes and ovaries, other than neoplastic/prolapse.* Code 88309 includes *uterus, with or without tubes and ovaries, neoplastic.*

Simply knowing that the pathologist examined a uterus after a patient's hysterectomy, is not enough information to report either code. You have to read the documentation to determine *why* the pathologist examined the uterus and determine the *diagnosis* that the pathologist assigned. If the patient underwent a hysterectomy for chronic pelvic pain, and the pathologist does not find evidence of a neoplasm, then assign code 88307 because it represents *other than neoplastic.* If the patient underwent a hysterectomy for

WORKPLACE IQ

You are working as a coder at Williton Medical Center in the Health Information Management Department. Today, your manager asks you to prepare documentation on Surgical Pathology to train new coders. She asks you to address the following list of issues by researching the Surgical Pathology CPT guidelines, and then explain your findings to the coders.

1. Define a unit of service.

2. Identify services that you should report in addition to surgical pathology services.

3. Discuss why code 88300 does not involve a microscope.

4. Review why surgical pathology levels are in ascending order.

What would you do?

---

chronic pelvic pain, and the pathologist finds evidence of carcinoma, then assign code 88309 because it represents *neoplastic*.

To locate codes for surgical pathology, search the index for Pathology, Surgical, Gross Exam, Level I, or Gross and Micro Exam. You will see each of the six levels identified by their Roman numerals. The index *does not* list individual specimens located in each level. You will need to go directly to the surgical pathology codes (88300–88309) and search for the type of specimen in the appropriate level. You may even want to label your CPT manual where these codes begin in the Surgical Pathology subsection so that you can quickly locate them.

Other services listed in the Surgical Pathology subsection include some of the following:

- *Pathology consultation during surgery (88329–88334)*—The pathologist examines a specimen while the patient is still in surgery to determine if the surgeon needs to perform additional procedures. The pathologist may even be present in the operating room. For example, a surgeon excises a malignant neoplasm of the left breast and also excises lymph nodes under the patient's left arm. He provides the pathologist with the excised tissue and lymph nodes. The pathologist determines that the lymph nodes have no evidence of metastasis. Pathology consults can involve

  - *tissue blocks*—a specimen is cut into pieces
  - *frozen section*—a thin layer is cut from a frozen specimen
  - *touch prep*—also called imprint cytology; involves imprinting part of the excised tissue and staining it
  - *squash prep*—squashing a specimen on a slide
- *Additional services (88342–88399)*—Examples of additional services include

  - *immunohistochemistry*—involves tests which analyze cell antigens to diagnose diseases, such as cancer
  - *protein analysis by Western blot*—involves analyzing proteins in a tissue or cell specimen using **electrophoresis**

electrophoresis (ih-lek-troh-fuh-ree´-sis)—a type of test that uses motion to detect pathological conditions

Review the other services in this code range to become more familiar with them, consulting your medical references for clarification. To locate their codes, search the index for *Pathology, Surgical,* or search for the type of test (*smear and stain*).

IN VIVO (e.g., TRANSCUTANEOUS) LABORATORY PROCEDURES (88720–88749)

This subsection contains five codes, including a code for an unlisted procedure. The first four codes represent tests to measure bilirubin and hemoglobin *transcutaneously* (through unbroken skin), most often performed on neonates to avoid painful blood draws. The test uses light to measure wavelengths emitted from the skin and assess values of bilirubin (to diagnose jaundice) and hemoglobin (to diagnose anemia, leukemia, or inherited conditions).

To locate codes for this subsection, search the index for *bilirubin* or *hemoglobin*.

OTHER PROCEDURES (89049–89240)

The Other Procedures subsection contains a variety of 11 different tests, including an unlisted procedure. Review the types of tests in this subsection to become familiar with them. They include some of the following:

- Leukocyte assessment on a fecal specimen
- Nasal smear for **eosinophils** (white blood cells)
- Sweat collection, to assess if the patient has elevated chloride and sodium ions in the sweat, which indicates **cystic fibrosis (CF)**
- Meat fibers or feces, to determine if the body properly digests food; if there are excess meat fibers in the feces, it indicates that the body does not have enough digestive enzymes

To locate codes from the Other Procedures subsection, search the index for the type of test (*fat stain, nasal smear*).

eosinophils (ē-ə-sin′-ə-fils)

cystic fibrosis (CF) (sis′-tik fī-brō′-səs)—a genetic disorder that causes very thick mucus to be produced in the bronchial tree

REPRODUCTIVE MEDICINE PROCEDURES (89250–89398)

Reproductive medicine procedures include testing and preparation for **in vitro fertilization** or **intrauterine insemination (IVF)** and testing on sperm, semen, **oocytes**, and embryos to identify disorders. Also included are services for *cryopreservation* (freezing), storage, and thawing of sperm, oocytes, embryos, and reproductive tissue left over from in vitro fertilization. Once a female patient successfully becomes pregnant, she and her partner may want to freeze reproductive components (sperm, embryos) in case she wants to try to become pregnant again someday.

To locate codes in this subsection, search the index for the type of procedure (*oocyte identification, semen analysis*).

in vitro fertilization (in-vē′-trō fer-til-i-zā ′-shun)—a technique in which the sperm and the egg are brought together in a petri dish and then implanted into a uterus

intrauterine insemination (in-tra-u′-ter-in in-sem-ə-nā′-shun)—a procedure in which semen is brought to the cervix by artificial means

oocytes (ō′-ə-sīts)—female egg cells

TAKE A BREAK

Good job! That was a lot of information to cover! You made it through the last subsections for pathology and laboratory services! Let's take a break and then practice coding other types of pathology and laboratory procedures.

Exercise 33.9   Surgical Pathology, in Vivo Laboratory Procedures, Other Procedures, Reproductive Medicine Procedures

Instructions: Review each case, and then assign codes for the procedure(s), appending a modifier when appropriate. Optional: For additional practice, assign the patient's diagnosis code(s) (ICD-9-CM).

1. Dr. Littleton is an urologist who performs a vasectomy for Kevin Plankton, age 45, today at Williton. Dr. Littleton sends the vas deferens to Williton's pathology department for analysis. Code for the pathologist's services.

   Diagnosis code(s): _____

   Procedure code(s): _____

2. Aimee Sellers is a 46-year-old female who recently found out that she was 6 weeks pregnant. Mrs. Sellers has decided that she does not wish to continue with the pregnancy and sees Dr. Fulton, a gynecologist/obstetrician, who performs an elective abortion at Williton. Dr. Fulton sends the products of conception to Williton's pathology department for analysis. Code for the pathologist's services.

   Diagnosis code(s): _____

   Procedure code(s): _____

3. Sylvia Winters, age 60, has a complete uterine prolapse. She tried using a pessary (internal supportive device used to treat prolapse) but found it very uncomfortable. Mrs. Winters sees Dr. Fulton today, and he performs a total vaginal hysterectomy with a bilateral salpino-oophorectomy. Dr. Fulton sends the uterus, fallopian tubes, and ovaries to Williton's

continued

TAKE A BREAK *continued*

pathology department for analysis. Code for the pathologist's services.

Diagnosis code(s): _____

Procedure code(s): _____

4. One of Williton's pathologists, Dr. Garner, examines part of a patient's colon that was removed due to colon cancer.

Diagnosis code(s): _____

Procedure code(s): _____

5. Dr. Garner examines a specimen from a right lower lobe segmental resection of the right lung for a patient diagnosed with lung cancer.

Diagnosis code(s): _____

Procedure code(s): _____

6. Dr. Garner examines a cervical polyp removed from a patient who has experienced heavy menstrual bleeding for the past three months.

Diagnosis code(s): _____

Procedure code(s): _____

DESTINATION: MEDICARE

In this exercise, you will learn more about the CLIA Certificate of Waiver. Follow the instructions listed next to access one of the CLIA brochures on the CMS website.

1. Go to the website http://www.cms.gov.
2. At the top of the screen on the banner bar, choose *Regulations & Guidance*.
3. In the second column under *Legislation*, choose *Clinical Laboratory Improvement Amendments (CLIA)*.
4. On the left side of the screen, choose *CLIA Brochures*.
5. Scroll down to *Downloads*, and choose *Brochure #6*.

Answer the following questions, using the search function (Ctrl + F) to find information that you need.

1. Can a provider perform tests that are not waived if the provider has a Certificate of Waiver?
2. After applying for a Certificate of Waiver, when can a POL perform waived tests?
3. Are POLs with a Certificate of Waiver routinely inspected?

CHAPTER REVIEW

Multiple Choice

Instructions: Circle one best answer to complete each statement.

1. A pathologist is a physician who specializes in
   a. cells, tissues, and disease behaviors.
   b. skin, hair, and nails.
   c. heart, blood vessels, and blood.
   d. diseases associated with the nervous system.

2. Assign code 99000 for
   a. collection of venous blood by venipuncture.
   b. collection of a capillary blood specimen.
   c. arterial puncture, with withdrawal of blood for diagnosis.
   d. handling and/or conveyance of a specimen to transfer from the physician's office to a laboratory.

3. What organization implemented CLIA?
   a. CMS
   b. The Food and Drug Administration
   c. The U.S. Department of Health and Human Services
   d. The American Medical Association

4. The Pathology section of CPT is divided into
   a. 18 subsections.
   b. 16 subsections.
   c. 14 subsections.
   d. 20 subsections.

5. A _____ test involves administering a pharmaceutical agent (drug, steroid) into a patient's body to monitor the body's response to it.
   a. quantitative/qualitative
   b. evocative/suppression
   c. evocation/suppression
   d. evocative/quantitative

6. Which of the following Medicare requirements does a provider need to meet to code and bill for a pathology consultation?
   a. A consultation is requested by the patient's attending physician.
   b. The consultant generates a written narrative report that will become a part of the patient's permanent medical record.
   c. The consultation involves exercising medical judgment.
   d. All of the above are Medicare requirements to bill pathology consultative services.

7. The CPT subsection that contains codes for blood clotting procedures is
   a. Urinalysis.
   b. Chemistry.
   c. Hematology and Coagulation.
   d. Reproductive Medicine Procedures.

8. An immunoglobulin is
   a. a protein located on a cell's surface that acts as a marker.
   b. a protein located in the plasma that binds to antigens of cells.
   c. a substance contained within a specimen.
   d. the amount of antibodies present in a person's blood.

9. Bacteriology, Virology, Mycology, and Parasitology are types of tests included in which subsection of CPT?
   a. Cytopathology
   b. Microbiology
   c. Chemistry
   d. Immunology

10. Report CPT code 88300 only for a specimen that
    a. a pathologist can accurately diagnose without a microscope.
    b. a pathologist can only diagnose using a microscope.
    c. a pathologist examines.
    d. a physician's office handles and sends to a lab.

Coding Assignments

Instructions: Assign procedure code(s) to the following cases, appending a modifier when appropriate. Optional: For additional coding practice, assign the patient's diagnosis code(s) (ICD-9-CM).

1. Williton's lab performs a CRP (C-reactive protein test for systemic inflammation) and ANA (antinuclear antibodies) on a specimen sent for a patient complaining of joint pain throughout his body. When antinuclear antibodies are present, it may indicate that the patient has an autoimmune disorder.

   Diagnosis code(s):_____

   Procedure code(s): _____

2. Miscinda Lewis is a 22-year-old female who sees Dr. Fulton for her yearly gynecologic exam. Ms. Lewis states that a former sexual partner recently notified her that he was diagnosed with HIV. Ms. Lewis would like to be tested for HIV, so the medical assistant performs venipuncture for a specimen. Dr. Fulton also performs a Pap smear on Ms. Lewis and sends both specimens to Williton's lab. Assign codes for Dr. Fulton and Williton's lab.

   Diagnosis code(s):_____

   Dr. Fulton's procedure code(s): _____

   Williton's procedure code(s):_____

3. Brandyburg Laboratory analyzes a wound culture to isolate specific bacteria causing an infection. The patient has a nonhealing wound with redness, swelling, and pain. The wound is malodorous and has purulent drainage. Results show that *Staphyloccal aureus* bacteria caused the infection.

   Diagnosis code(s):_____

   Procedure code(s): _____

4. Brandyburg Laboratory analyzes a throat culture for a patient with a four-day history of a sore throat.

   Diagnosis code(s):_____

   Procedure code(s): _____

5. Brandyburg Laboratory performs the following tests on specimens from various physicians' offices:
   a. Potassium, creatinine, ionized calcium, carbon dioxide, chloride, glucose, sodium, BUN

      Procedure code(s): _____

   b. Potassium, sodium, chloride—blood specimen

      Procedure code(s): _____

c. Sodium, albumin, total calcium, potassium, inorganic phosphorus, glucose, carbon dioxide, chloride, creatinine, urea nitrogen

Procedure code(s): _____

6. Dr. Hoffman has hired a new biller, Bob, for his practice. Bob asks Rhonda what types of blood collection practices occur at the office and what the codes are for the services. Bob wants to be sure that he is capturing these charges correctly. Code the following procedures:

a. Collection of venous blood by venipuncture

_____

b. Collection of a capillary blood specimen from the finger _____

c. Handling and/or conveyance of specimen for transfer from the physician's office laboratory _____

_____

d. In what section and subsection of the CPT manual is the procedure "venipuncture" located? _____

7. Jason Livengood saw Dr. Hoffman with complaints of right lower quadrant pain. Dr. Hoffman suspected that Mr. Livengood had appendicitis and referred him to Williton Medical Center's ED for evaluation. At the ED, Dr. Daniels determined that Mr. Livengood had appendicitis with perforation. Dr. Nelson, a general surgeon, performed an appendectomy and sent the specimen to the pathology department for analysis.

What are the diagnosis and procedure code(s) for Dr. Nelson's services?

Diagnosis code(s): _____

Procedure code(s): _____

What are the diagnosis and procedure code(s) that the pathology department should report?

Diagnosis code(s): _____

Procedure code(s): _____

8. Williton's lab performs a CBC with diff (differential) for a male patient with complaints of a fever and generalized pelvic pain for three days.

Diagnosis code(s): _____

Procedure code(s): _____

9. Williton's lab received serum from Dr. Hoffman's office with a request to perform a HDL (high-density lipoprotein) cholesterol test. The diagnosis included on the requisition stated hyperlipidemia.

Diagnosis code(s): _____

Procedure code(s): _____

10. Jim Rogers, age 52, sees Dr. Hoffman for a blood draw for a lipid profile. Mr. Rogers started lipid-lowering medication three months ago to treat hyperlipidemia. Dr. Hoffman wants to be sure that the medication is working. Rhonda performs a venipuncture and sends the blood to Williton's lab for total serum cholesterol, HDL cholesterol, and triglyceride tests. Assign codes for Dr. Hoffman and Williton's lab.

Diagnosis code(s): _____

Dr. Hoffman's procedure code(s): _____

Williton's procedure code(s): _____

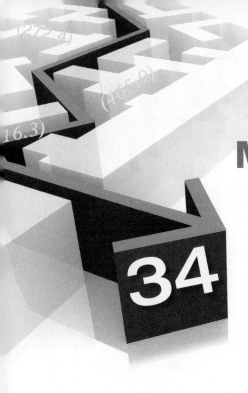

Medicine

Learning Objectives

After completing this chapter, you should be able to

- Spell and define the key terminology in this chapter.
- Explain the types of services and CPT guidelines found in the Medicine section.
- Describe the types of subsections found in the Medicine section.
- Define active and passive immunity.
- Describe immune globulins, serum or recombinant products, and how to code for them.
- Discuss how to assign codes for immunization administration for vaccines/toxoids, and define vaccines/toxoids.
- Explain the types of services found in the Psychiatry subsection and how to code for them.
- Describe biofeedback.
- Discuss the types of dialysis and how to code for them.
- Identify types of gastroenterology services and how to code for them.
- Discuss how to assign codes for ophthalmology services.
- Describe special otolaryngologic services and how to assign codes.
- Identify the types of cardiovascular services and how to assign codes.
- Define noninvasive vascular diagnostic studies and how to code for them.
- Describe how to assign codes for pulmonary services.
- Identify the types of services found in additional medicine subsections.

Key Terms

allergy
biofeedback

immune globulin
immunization
psychotherapy

INTRODUCTION

You have traveled very far on your coding journey, and you are almost finished! You can be proud of what you have accomplished so far, which is quite a lot! In this chapter, you will further expand your skills and learn about many services and procedures in the Medicine section of CPT. Do you remember learning in Chapter 17 that the Medicine section contains a variety of other services and procedures that are not classified to any of the other five sections? Instead of CPT including a separate small chapter for each subsection of services and procedures listed in Medicine, CPT groups them all under one large section. As you can imagine, there are countless codes in the Medicine section, too many for us to discuss in one chapter! So we will concentrate on some of the services and procedures that you will find in Medicine so that you can learn a little more about them. As always, consult your medical references to learn about procedures that we do not review with which you are not familiar. Do not guess when assigning codes because you may assign incorrect ones.

CPT-4 codes in this chapter are from the CPT-4 2012 code set. CPT is a registered trademark of the American Medical Association.

ICD-9-CM codes in this chapter are from the ICD-9-CM 2012 code set from the Department of Health and Human Services, Centers for Disease Control and Prevention.

The Medicine section is the last section in CPT, and a very interesting one, so when you finish this chapter, you will be well-versed in the entire CPT manual! Let's travel forward to discover more about the exciting world of coding different services and procedures and help you to navigate yet another stop along the way!

"Now, voyager, sail thou forth, to seek and find."—WALT WHITMAN

MEDICINE (90281–99607)

The Medicine section contains a variety of tests, services, and procedures from many different specialties of medicine, including some of the following types of services:

- Vaccines
- Psychiatric evaluations
- Ophthalmology exams
- Cardiovascular testing
- Allergy testing
- Physical and occupational therapy

Turn to the Medicine section in your CPT manual, and take a look at the numerous types of services listed there. Because there are so many codes in the Medicine section, we will only review some of them. Be sure to consult your medical dictionary or use Internet searches to find out more information about procedures not discussed in this chapter so that you can better understand how to code them.

CPT Guidelines

There are also CPT coding guidelines that apply to the Medicine section, and you are already familiar with many of them because they also apply to other CPT sections. A summary of the guidelines for the Medicine section are outlined next for you to review:

- *Multiple Procedures*—If more than one provider renders services to the same patient, then each provider should report the service separately.
- *Add-on Codes*—Add-on codes represent procedures that providers perform *in addition to* a primary procedure. You can find them easily because they have a + sign in front of the codes. Add-on codes are exempt from modifier -51 (multiple procedures).
- *Separate Procedures*—Append modifier -59 to identify procedures or services that are distinct or independent from other services, not including E/M services, performed on the same day. Documentation must support a different session or encounter, different procedure or surgery, different site or organ system, separate incision or excision, separate lesion, or separate injury (or area of injury in extensive injuries) *not ordinarily encountered or performed on the same day by the same provider*. You learned about modifier -59 in Chapter 18 of this text.
- *Unlisted Service or Procedure and Special Report*—Unlisted codes appear at the end of specific subsections, subheadings, categories, and subcategories, and you should only assign unlisted codes as a *last resort*, after checking for a more specific Category I or Category III code. Insurances require that you submit additional documentation, or a special report, along with the insurance claim for an unlisted procedure to show what service or procedure the clinician actually provided and to establish medical necessity for providing it.
- *Materials Supplied by Physician*—Assign codes for supplies and materials, including drugs, that the physician or clinician provides (sterile trays/drugs), *over and above* those usually included with the procedure(s). Assign code 99070 to drugs, trays, supplies, and materials provided, or assign a specific supply HCPCS code that the insurance requires for reimbursement.

Keep in mind that there are also numerous CPT guidelines throughout the Medicine section that apply to specific subsections, subheadings, and categories. Be sure to read the guidelines thoroughly before final code assignment.

DIVISIONS OF THE MEDICINE SECTION

The Medicine section, or chapter, is divided into 34 subsections, arranged by the type of service or medical specialty of the service (■ TABLE 34-1).

■ TABLE 34-1   MEDICINE SUBSECTIONS, SUBHEADINGS, CATEGORIES, AND SUBCATEGORIES

Section and Subsections	Code Range
MEDICINE	90281–99607
Immune Globulins, Serum or Recombinant Products	90281–90399
Immunization Administration for Vaccines/Toxoids	90460–90474
Vaccines, Toxoids	90476–90749
Psychiatry	90801–90899
Biofeedback	90901–90911
Dialysis	90935–90999
Gastroenterology	91010–91299
Ophthalmology	92002–92499
Special Otorhinolaryngologic Services	92502–92700
Cardiovascular	92950–93799
Noninvasive Vascular Diagnostic Studies	93800–93999
Pulmonary	94002–94799
Allergy and Clinical Immunology	95004–95199
Endocrinology	95250–95251
Neurology and Neuromuscular Procedures	95800–96020
Medical Genetics and Genetic Counseling Services	96040
Central Nervous System Assessments/Tests (eg, Neuro-Cognitive, Mental Status, Speech Testing)	96101–96125
Health and Behavior Assessment/Intervention	96150–96155
Hydration, Therapeutic, Prophylactic, Diagnostic Injections and Infusions, and Chemotherapy and Other Highly Complex Drug or Highly Complex Biologic Agent Administration	96360–96549
Photodynamic Therapy	96567–96571
Special Dermatological Procedures	96900–96999
Physical Medicine and Rehabilitation	97001–97799
Medical Nutrition Therapy	97802–97804
Acupuncture	97810–97814
Osteopathic Manipulative Treatment	98925–98929
Chiropractic Manipulative Treatment	98940–98943
Education and Training for Patient Self-Management	98960–98962
Non Face-to-Face Nonphysician Services	98966–98969
Special Services, Procedures and Reports	99000–99091
Qualifying Circumstances for Anesthesia	99100–99140
Moderate (Conscious) Sedation	99143–99150
Other Services and Procedures	99170–99199
Home Health Procedures/Services	99500–99602
Medication Therapy Management Services	99605–99607

Let's review the subsections of Medicine, beginning with immunizations, including a discussion of active and passive immunity. Turn to the codes in your CPT manual as we discuss them.

ACTIVE AND PASSIVE IMMUNITY

Active immunity is when the body's immune system produces antibodies to fight off a disease. Active immunity can be:

- *Natural*—A person is exposed to a disease pathogen, becomes ill, and then develops immunity toward the disease.
- *Artificial*—A person is exposed to a disease through an antigen from a vaccine (virus) or toxoid (bacteria). The immune system produces antibodies that attack the antigen, the person does not become ill, and the vaccine or toxoid provides protection against the disease, such as seasonal influenza.

Passive immunity is when the body's immune system receives antibodies to fight off a disease. Passive immunity can be:

- *Natural*—This happens during pregnancy when the mother passes specific antibodies to the fetus, which protect a baby for approximately the first six months of life.
- *Artificial*—A person receives an *immune globulin* that contains antibodies, which help to prevent a disease or lessen the effects of a disease to which a person has already been exposed.

IMMUNE GLOBULINS, SERUM OR RECOMBINANT PRODUCTS (90281–90399)

Turn to this subsection in your CPT manual to review the codes listed there. It is important to understand definitions of specific terms before assigning codes from this subsection.

- **Immune globulins** (passive immunity) consist of serum globulins or recombinant immune globulins to protect a patient against a disease.
- *Serum globulins* are proteins extracted from purified human blood plasma. They contain antibodies that protect an individual against a specific disease, such as rabies.
- **Recombinant** *immune globulin products* are created in a lab from human or animal proteins to protect against disease, such as **hepatitis B**.

recombinant (rē-käm'-bə-nənt)

hepatitis B (hep-ə-tīt'-əs)—inflammation of the liver

Drug companies manufacture immune globulins, and providers purchase them from the manufacturers or from pharmacies to dispense to patients in offices, clinics, hospitals, and other locations. Pharmacies may also bill a patient's insurance directly for supplying an immune globulin to a provider. Patients receive serum globulins and recombinant immune globulin products for protection against a disease, including when they have already been exposed to a disease like hepatitis (called postexposure prophylaxis), or if their immune systems are compromised, called **immunodeficiency**. Immunodeficiency can result from disease, an organ transplant, cancer treatment, or drug side effects. A person with immunodeficiency has a greater risk of becoming ill because his immune system cannot adequately produce antibodies to protect the body from diseases. Immune globulin protection wears off in a short period of time, typically a few months, and an individual could contract a specific disease after the effects of the immune globulin have worn off.

immunodeficiency (im-yoo-nō-di-fish'-ən-sē)

Notice that CPT categorizes the codes for immune globulins by the type of immune globulin (*human, diphtheria, tetanus*) and the route of administration (*intramuscular-IM, subcutaneous, subcutaneous infusion, intravenous*). In addition, codes for Rho(D) immune globulin (which prevents blood disorders during pregnancy or with blood transfusions) also differentiate between a *full dose* and *mini dose*.

The first three codes in this subsection represent human immune globulin (Ig), which providers give to patients with an immunodeficiency disorder to help their bodies produce antibodies necessary to fight off illness.

Coding for immune globulins is a two-part process:

1. Assign a code for the *route of administration* of the immune globulin (intramuscular, subcutaneous, subcutaneous infusion, intravenous, or any route). The route depends on the type of the immune globulin. Codes for the route of administration include 96365–96368, 96372, 96374, and 96375.

2. Assign a code for the immune globulin (serum globulin or recombinant immune globulin). Codes for immune globulins include 90281–90399.

It is important to remember that providers want insurances to pay for *both* the immune globulin *and* the work performed to administer the immune globulin to the patient (route of administration), so you have to be sure to *code for both services.*

The CPT coding guidelines for immune globulins direct you to assign the following codes for the route of administration:

96365—Intravenous infusion, for therapy, prophylaxis, or diagnosis (specify substance or drug); initial, up to 1 hour

+96366—each additional hour (list separately in addition to code for primary procedure)

+96367—additional sequential infusion, up to 1 hour (list separately in addition to code for primary procedure)

+96368—concurrent infusion (list separately in addition to code for primary procedure)

96372—Therapeutic, prophylactic, or diagnostic injection (specify substance or drug); subcutaneous or intramuscular

96373—intra-arterial

96374—intravenous push, single or initial substance/drug

+96375—each additional sequential intravenous push of a new substance/drug (list separately in addition to code for primary procedure)

Do not append modifier -51 when coding for immune globulins and the routes of administration. Also, be very careful to assign additional route of administration and immune globulin codes for *each additional* infusion or intravenous (IV) push of an immune globulin. An IV push enables a provider to quickly administer an immune globulin, rather than through an IV infusion, or drip, which is slower and administered to the patient at regular intervals.

To find procedure codes for the route of immune globulin administration, search the index for *infusion, diagnostic/prophylactic/therapeutic,* or *injection, intramuscular/subcutaneous/ intravenous push.* To find immune globulins, search the index for *immune globulins.*

Diagnosis Codes for Immune Globulin Encounters

When you assign diagnosis codes for patients who receive immune globulins, determine the reason why the patient needs the immune globulin. If it is for an immunodeficiency disorder, then assign a code for the type of immunodeficiency disorder the patient has. If it is because the patient was exposed to a disease but has no symptoms, then search the ICD-9-CM Index under the main term *exposure to,* and search subterms for the type of disease to find code choices.

Refer to the following example to learn more about coding for an immune globulin administration.

Example: Katie Vega, RN, is a home health nurse who visits Mr. Harmon, age 56, in his home to administer a 100-mg weekly dose of human immune globulin IV infusion, using an infusion pump. The patient suffers from **primary immunodeficiency (PID)**. Ms. Vega spends about an hour with the patient administering treatment.

To first code for the route of administration of the immune globulin, search the index for the main term *infusion,* subterm *intravenous unlisted,* and subterm *diagnostic/ prophylactic/therapeutic,* which directs you to codes 96365-96368, and 96379. Assign

primary immunodeficiency (PID)—the immune system does not function properly; primary indicates that another disease did not cause PID

code **96365**, since it represents IV infusion for up to one hour. Did you notice that the code descriptor for 96365 states "specify substance or drug" in parentheses? This means that you still have to assign a code for the immune globulin, which we will do next.

To code for the immune globulin, search the index for the main term *immune globulins*, subterm *human*, which leads you to codes 90281–90284. Assign code **90284**, since it represents a subcutaneous infusion of 100 mg. The patient's diagnosis code is **279.3** (main term *immunodeficiency*).

Codes for this case are as follows:

1. 96372 (route of administration)

2. 90284 (immune globulin)

3. 279.3 (diagnosis of PID)

IMMUNIZATION ADMINISTRATION FOR VACCINES/ TOXOIDS (90460–90474), VACCINES, TOXOIDS (90476–90749)

An **immunization** (active immunity) is when a person receives a vaccine (vaccination) or toxoid that enables the body's immune system to produce antibodies to fight against it. A *vaccine* contains antigens from a *weakened* strain of a *virus* so that the body will fight it, but the person will not become ill. A *toxoid* contains *bacteria* that are nontoxic, so that the immune system will fight them, but the individual will not become ill. Later, if the person is exposed to the active virus or bacteria, then the immune system will recognize the pathogen and attack it.

Examples of vaccines include:

- Hepatitis A
- Influenza virus
- Measles
- Mumps

Examples of toxoids include:

- Diphtheria
- Tetanus

Just like coding for immune globulins, coding for immunizations of vaccines or toxoids is a two-part process:

1. Assign a code for the *immunization administration*, or route of administration, of the vaccine or toxoid: intramuscular, intranasal (in the nose), percutaneous, intradermal (in the skin), subcutaneous, subcutaneous infusion, intravenous, or any route. Codes 90460–90474 are for the route of administration. (index: *administration, immunization*, and then search for the route of administration.)

2. Assign a code for the vaccine or toxoid, also called the *product* or *substance*. Codes 90476–90749 are for the product. (index: *vaccines* and then the type of vaccine or toxoid, or combination of vaccines or toxoids.)

Providers typically purchase the vaccines and toxoids from drug manufacturers or pharmacies. Pharmacies may also bill a patient's insurance directly for supplying a vaccine/ toxoid to a provider, such as a vaccine that requires refrigeration and the provider cannot store it. Pharmacies, which are considered healthcare providers, may also administer vaccines to patients and then bill their insurances for the services.

It is important to remember that providers want insurances to pay for *both* the vaccine or toxoid *and* the work performed to administer the product to the patient (route of administration), so you have to be sure to *code for both services*. Let's review coding for the route of administration first, and then we will review how to code for the vaccine or toxoid.

Immunization Administration

Turn to the subsection Immunization Administration for Vaccines/Toxoids (90460–90474) to review the code choices listed for the route of administration. Notice that CPT categorizes the codes according to the following criteria:

- Whether the physician or other qualified health care professional provides counseling to patients through age 18. *Immunization counseling* includes discussion about the benefits and risks of the vaccine/toxoid and risk of developing a disease without the immunization. A physician and other healthcare clinicians, such as a PA or RN can provide counseling to patients about vaccines/toxoids. Do not assume that each provider counsels every patient who receives a vaccine or toxoid. There must be medical documentation to support assigning a counseling code.
- If the vaccine/toxoid is the *first one* or *an additional* vaccine/toxoid after the first.
- If the immunization is for H1N1.
- The route of administration. Each vaccine or toxoid has a recommended route of administration, based on results of clinical trials and patients' experiences. Drug manufacturers include recommended routes of administration in the information they package with the vaccines/toxoids.

Medicare requires that providers report HCPCS codes (G codes) instead of CPT codes for the following immunization administrations and vaccines:

- *G0008*—Administration of influenza virus vaccine
- *G9141*—Influenza A (H1N1) immunization administration (includes the physician counseling the patient/family)
- *G9142*—Influenza A (H1N1) vaccine, any route of administration
- *G0009*—Administration of pneumococcal vaccine
- *G0010*—Administration of hepatitis B vaccine

Medicare reimburses providers for these services and may also reimburse for other vaccines, depending on specific patient circumstances and Medicare regulations. You can find more information on the Medicare website at http://www.cms.gov.

Vaccines/Toxoids

Now, turn to the vaccines and toxoids (product) codes (90476–90749). CPT arranges codes by the type of product, route of administration, patient's age, and dose schedule. A *dose schedule* means that the patient needs more than one dose of the vaccine or toxoid at specific intervals, such as one dose when the patient is a year old and the second dose when the patient reaches 18 months old.

Did you notice that some of the codes are *combination codes* that contain more than one vaccine or toxoid? Refer to code 90720, which is a combination code that includes diphtheria and tetanus toxoids, along with vaccines for whole-cell **pertussis** and *Hemophilus influenza* B. Some products are available in a combined form, so a provider does not have to administer separate products to a patient. Rather than report four codes for each of the toxoids and vaccines listed in code 90720, you should instead assign *one combination code* (bundled code, 90720) for all of them. You will need to pay close attention to the codes to ensure that you do not assign individual vaccine/toxoid codes if the provider administered a combination product to the patient.

pertussis (pər-təs′-əs)—also called whooping cough; bacterial infection that causes severe coughing lasting several weeks

Remember that you can assign V codes for the patient's diagnosis when the patient has an encounter but is not currently ill. Many times, you will only assign V codes for encounters when patients receive vaccines or toxoids and do not have any other services during the encounter. To find the diagnosis code, search the ICD-9-CM Index for the main term *vaccination*, subterm *prophylactic (against)*, and then search subterms for the type of vaccine or toxoid.

Review the following example to learn how to assign both the immunization administration and the product for a vaccine.

> **Example:** Jacquelyn Moss, a 27-year-old established patient, sees Dr. Hoffman for an intramuscular (IM) hepatitis A vaccine that she needs because her employer is assigning her to work on a temporary project in Mexico. Dr. Hoffman administers the vaccine but does not counsel the patient.
>
> To code for the immunization administration, search the index for the main term *administration*, subterm *immunization*, and subterm *one vaccine/toxoid*, which directs you to codes 90471 and 90473. Assign code **90471**, since it represents an IM injection of *one* vaccine.
>
> To code for the product, search the index for the main term *vaccines* and subterm *hepatitis A*, which leads you to codes 90632–90634. Assign code **90632**, since the medical documentation does not include a 2-dose or 3-dose schedule. The patient's diagnosis code is **V05.3** (main term *vaccination*, subterm *prophylactic*, and subterm *hepatitis, viral*).

Coding Guidelines for Immunizations

The following points are important coding guidelines that you need to review when coding for immunizations:

- Do *not* append modifier -51 when you are coding for vaccines/toxoids and the routes of administration.

- Do *not* assign a code for an E/M service when a patient receives a vaccine/toxoid *unless* the physician performs *separate* E/M services. Just because a patient has an immunization, it does not mean that the patient automatically has an E/M service. The physician/clinician must document components of the E/M service in order for you to code it. If there *is* an E/M along with the vaccine, then be sure to append modifier -25 (significant, separately identifiable E/M) to the E/M code.

  - Medicare's regulations state that if a patient receives reasonable and medically necessary services constituting an *office visit* level of service (E/M), then the physician may bill for the *office visit*, the *vaccine*, and the *administration of the vaccine*. You can check individual payers' regulations for specific coverage for vaccines.

Multiple Immunizations

When a clinician administers multiple immunizations to a patient, assign a code for the route of administration for each immunization and a code for each of the products. If a product is a combination, then you will only need to assign one code. For multiple intramuscular immunizations, search the index for the main term *administration*, subterm *immunization*, and subterm *one vaccine/toxoid*, which directs you to codes 90471 and 90473. Assign code 90471, since it represents one vaccine (the first), and includes intramuscular routes. To code for additional immunizations, search the index for the main term *administration*, subterm *immunization*, and subterm *each additional vaccine/toxoid*, which leads you to codes 90472 and 90474. Assign code 90472 for each additional immunization, since it represents each additional vaccine and is an add-on code to be assigned with 90471. Be sure to review additional codes available for immunization administrations to ensure you choose the correct codes:

- Code 90460 represents the first immunization administration through age 18 with counseling, any route, and code 90461 is for each additional immunization administration.

- Code 90473 represents the first intranasal or oral immunization administration, and code 90474 is for each additional immunization administration.

TAKE A BREAK

Wow! That was a lot of information to absorb! Let's take a break and then review more about immune globulins and vaccines.

Exercise 34.1 Immune Globulins, Serum or Recombinant Products, Immunization Administration for Vaccines/Toxoids, Vaccines, Toxoids

Part 1—Theory

Instructions: Fill in the blank with the best answer.

1. A(n) _____ means that the patient needs more than one dose of a vaccine or toxoid at specific intervals, such as one dose when the patient is a year old and the second dose when the patient reaches 18 months old.

2. A(n) _____ is when a person receives a vaccine or toxoid that enables the body's immune system to produce antibodies to fight against it.

3. Do *not* assign a code for an E/M service when a patient receives a vaccine/toxoid *unless* the physician performs _____ E/M services.

4. Proteins extracted from purified human blood plasma are called _____ .

5. _____ is when the body's immune system produces antibodies to fight off a disease.

6. _____ includes discussion about the benefits and risks of the vaccine/toxoid and risk of developing a disease without the immunization.

Part 2—Coding

Instructions: Review each patient's case, and then assign codes for the procedure(s), appending a modifier when appropriate. Optional: For additional practice, assign the patient's diagnosis code(s) (ICD-9-CM).

1. Mary Killmeyer, age 15, sees Dr. Chico, a family practice physician in the Adolescent Clinic at Williton Medical Center, after being bitten by a rabid squirrel. Dr. Chico administers an IM injection of rabies human immune globulin for preventive care.

   Diagnosis code(s): _____

   Procedure code(s): _____

2. Gene Jeffrey, a 50-year-old established patient, presents to the flu shot clinic at Dr. Wolf's office where the nurse administers the IM split virus injection. Mr. Jeffrey does not see Dr. Wolf, who is an internal medicine physician.

   Diagnosis code(s): _____

   Procedure code(s): _____

3. Timmy Barker, age eight, is an established patient of Dr. John, a pediatrician. He is in the office today with his mother for an injection of DTP (diphtheria, tetanus toxoid, and pertussis) and oral poliovirus. The nurse provides the services, at the direction of the physician.

   Diagnosis code(s): _____

   Procedure code(s): _____

4. Audrey Gordon, an 88-year-old established patient of Dr. Hoffman, comes into the office for split virus influenza and pneumonia 13-Valent vaccines. Dr. Hoffman administers both vaccines by an intramuscular route.

   Diagnosis code(s): _____

   Procedure code(s): _____

5. Dr. John sees established patient Katie Thomas, a 3-year-old, in his office for a well-baby examination. She is healthy and Dr. John administers an IM vaccine for DTP (diphtheria, tetanus toxoid, and pertussis). Dr. John counsels Katie's parents on the vaccines and possible reactions.

   Diagnosis code(s): _____

   Procedure code(s): _____

6. Dr. James, an internal medicine physician, sees Janet Adams, a 73-year-old established patient, in his office for a checkup for insulin-dependent diabetes mellitus that is under control. He performs an expanded problem-focused history and exam. While she is there, Dr. Jones administers an IM split virus influenza vaccine.

   Diagnosis code(s): _____

   Procedure code(s): _____

INTERESTING FACTS: How Are the Viruses Selected To Make Flu Vaccines?

The influenza (flu) viruses that are selected for inclusion in the seasonal flu vaccines are updated each year using information about which influenza viruses are circulating that year, how they are spreading, and how well the previous season's vaccine viruses might protect against any newly identified viruses. Currently, 136 national influenza centers in 106 countries conduct year-round surveillance for influenza viruses and disease activity. These laboratories then send influenza viruses for additional analyses to the five World Health Organization (WHO) Collaborating Centers for Reference and Research on Influenza, located in the U.S., United Kingdom, Australia, Japan, and China.

The seasonal flu vaccine is a trivalent vaccine (a three-component vaccine) with each component selected to protect against one of the three main groups of influenza viruses circulating in humans. Three vaccine viruses are chosen to maximize the likelihood that the influenza vaccine will protect against the viruses which are most likely to spread and cause illness among people during the upcoming flu season. In the U.S., the Food and Drug Administration determines what viruses will be used in U.S.-licensed vaccines.

(Department of Health and Human Services, Centers for Disease Control and Prevention, www.cdc.gov/flu/about/qa/vaccine-selection. htm, accessed 10/29/11)

PSYCHIATRY (90801–90899)

You first learned about the field of psychiatry and common mental health disorders in Chapter 10. Remember that patients with mental health, or psychiatric, disorders can receive treatment in an inpatient or outpatient hospital, other outpatient setting, or a partial hospitalization program. They may also receive services in a residential care setting, where patients live and receive treatment from providers who also live there.

A psychiatrist, psychologist, or social worker treats patients with mental disorders. You may have also heard the terms therapist, psychotherapist, analyst, counselor, or "shrink," which people use to refer to mental health professionals, including psychiatrists. Mental health professionals may also specialize in treating patients who abuse alcohol or drugs or have other behavioral disorders.

Turn to the Psychiatry subsection in your CPT manual to become more familiar with the codes and descriptors listed. Notice that there are several CPT guidelines. It is important to note that one of the guidelines cautions you *not to report a separate E/M service* with specific psychiatric service codes because those services *already include* the E/M component of services. Be sure to review all of the guidelines for the subsection and subheadings before final code assignment.

The Psychiatry subsection is divided into two subheadings: Psychiatric Diagnostic or Evaluative Interview Procedures, and Psychiatric Therapeutic Procedures. During a psychiatric diagnostic interview procedure, or psychiatric exam, the provider assesses a patient's mental status by reviewing the patient's medical history, asking the patient a series of questions, and communicating with family members and other providers involved in the patient's care to determine the patient's diagnosis. The diagnostic interview is typically the first meeting with a patient to diagnose the patient and establish a plan for further treatment options. The interview may also be *interactive*, which many times involves treating children. The provider uses play equipment, such as dolls, to communicate with a patient who cannot or will not communicate verbally.

CPT arranges services in the Psychiatric Therapeutic Procedures subheading by four categories of codes, which are divided by place of service, type of service, and total visit time. The information outlined next explains some of the types of services that you will find under this subheading and its categories.

- *Psychotherapy (90804–90857)*—Psychotherapy treatment involves the provider communicating face-to-face with the patient to determine the cause(s) of a specific condition and develop ways to effectively cope with it. Psychotherapy can also be combined with medication treatment and may be

  - *insight oriented*—The clinician determines motivations behind specific problems.

- *behavior modifying*—The clinician attempts to change a patient's negative or destructive behaviors.
- *supportive*—The clinician helps the patient through active listening, encouragement, and assistance with understanding certain behaviors.
- *interactive*—The clinician uses play equipment, a language interpreter, or nonverbal communication to treat a patient who cannot communicate.

Psychotherapy may also involve

- *medical evaluation and management services*—The physician documents components of an E/M service (history, exam, medical decision-making), along with psychotherapy.
- *family psychotherapy*—Family members meet with the clinician to discuss the patient's condition and how to help the patient. The patient may be present.
- *group psychotherapy*—A group of people with the same disorder meet with the clinician to share information to help one another change their behaviors. An example is group psychotherapy for patients who suffer from anxiety disorders for them to learn techniques to deal with their anxiety. Group psychotherapy may also be interactive.
- *multiple-family group psychotherapy*—A group of families who share the same problems, such as a parenting group made up of parents with children with behavioral problems, meets to discuss the issues they are having. The clinician and families discuss ways to improve the child's behavior and learn effective parenting skills.

- ***Pharmacologic management (90862)***—Also called a *medication check*, pharmacologic management determines the effectiveness of a patient's medication. The clinician administers minimal psychotherapy during the session.
- ***Electroconvulsive therapy (ECT) (90870)***—Also called *shock treatment*, ECT is used to treat conditions like depression when medications and psychotherapy fail. ECT involves placing the patient under anesthesia and attaching electrodes to his head. The electrodes deliver shocks to the brain and cause the patient to seize for a short time. ECT remains a controversial method of treating patients, as many clinicians feel that it causes brain damage or does not improve patients' conditions.
- ***Hypnotherapy (90880)***—This treatment involves hypnotizing the patient to change specific behaviors, such as to stop smoking, lose weight, or cope with anxiety.

You can find codes for psychiatric services by searching the index for the main terms *psychiatric diagnosis* or *psychiatric treatment* and then by the *type of service*.

TAKE A BREAK

Good job! You are continuing to learn more and more! Let's take a break and then practice coding psychiatric services.

Exercise 34.2 Psychiatry

Instructions: Review each patient's case, and then assign codes for the procedure(s), appending a modifier when appropriate. Optional: For additional practice, assign the patient's diagnosis code(s) (ICD-9-CM).

1. Angela Monroe, age 27, sees Dr. Bauer, a psychiatrist, in his office. The visit lasts 30 minutes for individual psychotherapy. The patient's diagnosis is chronic paranoid psychosis, symptoms of which include loss of contact with reality, usually with false beliefs about what is

taking place (delusions) or who is there, as well as seeing or hearing things that are not there (hallucinations).

Diagnosis code(s): _____

Procedure code(s): _____

2. Today in the office, Dr. Bauer sees Ron Corn, a 29-year-old construction worker, for hypnotherapy to quit smoking. Mr. Corn is addicted to nicotine.

Diagnosis code(s): _____

Procedure code(s): _____

continued

TAKE A BREAK *continued*

3. Dr. Bauer reviews the psychiatric evaluation tests and medical records for Tom Gallagher, a 16-year-old male, whom Dr. Bauer previously evaluated for behavioral problems. The patient is not present during the records review. Dr. Bauer confirms his original diagnosis of an overanxious disorder.

Diagnosis code(s): _____

Procedure code(s): _____

4. Dorothy Jane, age 67, sees Dr. Bauer today in his office. Dr. Hoffman referred her to Dr. Bauer for an evaluation, as the patient has been extremely depressed since her husband died. Dr. Bauer performs an initial psychiatric interview examination that includes a history and review of diagnostic and laboratory studies. He diagnoses the patient with a depressive state with tremors.

Diagnosis code(s): _____

Procedure code(s): _____

5. Tommy Jefferson, age 15, sees Dr. Bauer for his weekly psychotherapy session to treat unsocialized conduct disturbance. Tommy is very aggressive and has had outbursts in school. The session lasts 50 minutes.

Diagnosis code(s): _____

Procedure code(s): _____

6. The Miller family sees Dr. Bauer today for family psychotherapy. Jordan, age 5, is not present during the session so that his parents can openly discuss the diagnosis of explosive conduct disturbance. Dr. Bauer's office staff will code and bill the visit under Ralph Miller's insurance plan (Jordan's father).

Diagnosis code(s): _____

Procedure code(s): _____

BIOFEEDBACK (90901–90911)

irritable bowel syndrome (IBS)—disorder that causes abdominal pain, diarrhea, and constipation

Biofeedback teaches patients to regulate certain body functions through mental or physical exercises. For example, patients who suffer from **irritable bowel syndrome (IBS)** or fecal incontinence (inability to control the bowels) can learn to relax or constrict their anal sphincters to manage their disorders. Patients who experience increased heart rate, respirations, and blood pressure in response to stress can learn to control their mental processes to regulate their body functions.

Biofeedback can be offered in a provider setting, and/or the patient can use biofeedback on his own once he receives training for it. Biofeedback involves using some type of equipment to measure body functions, and the equipment provides a reading or sounds an alert (■ FIGURE 34-1).

You may have seen a simplified version of biofeedback if you ever experimented with a stress card, which is a plastic card, similar to a credit card in size and shape, that has a black area where you press your thumb or finger. The black area then changes color in

Figure 34-1 ■ A patient receives biofeedback training to manage stress.

Photo credit: SIU BIOMED COMM Custom Medical Stock

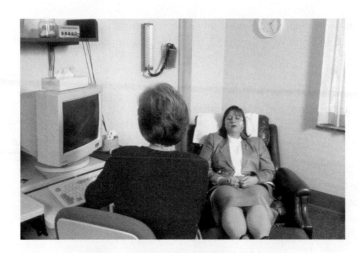

WORKPLACE IQ

You are working as a medical assistant at Dr. Hoffman's office. Part of your job involves assigning diagnosis and procedure codes to patients' encounters. Today, you need to assign codes for immunizations and diagnoses for an established patient, Kim Manning, age 43. She is planning a trip to Jamaica to attend her cousin's wedding and sightsee across the region. She sees Dr. Hoffman to receive the following *four* immunizations:

- intramuscular: hepatitis A, hepatitis B, and tetanus–diphtheria (preservative-free) (total of two injections)

- subcutaneous: yellow fever and measles, mumps, rubella (total of two injections)

Mrs. Manning is a very informed patient, discussing with Dr. Hoffman the results of her research on the benefits and risks of the vaccines. He confirms the information that she found, so he does *not* counsel the patient or provide any other services during the encounter.

What would you do?

---

response to your body's temperature, supposedly indicating your mood and stress level. You may have also had a mood ring or mood earrings, which are also forms of biofeedback because they change color when you wear them, and specific colors are supposed to correlate to specific moods. There are portable biofeedback devices that measure the temperature of the fingers, which a patient can control to eliminate migraine headaches, and other devices that measure heart rate, respirations, and blood pressure to control anxiety and other conditions. The goal is for the patient to eventually regulate his body functions *without* using biofeedback.

Providers may use a **manometric** balloon probe for biofeedback training of patients with rectal disorders, such as fecal incontinence. The clinician inserts a probe with a balloon attached into the rectum and inflates it with air, which creates pressure in the rectum. The probe can measure muscle movement, and the patient can then learn to exercise the anal sphincter muscles. **Electromyelography (EMG)** can also measure muscle movement through electrical activity.

manometric (man-ə-me′-trik)

electromyelography (EMG) (ē-lek-trō-mī-a-läg′-rə-fē)

Many insurances will reimburse providers for biofeedback training because in the long run, biofeedback can successfully resolve many conditions, saving insurances from continuing to cover costs of medications and/or psychotherapy to treat them. There are two codes listed in the Biofeedback subsection, and you can locate them in the index by searching for the main term *training* and subterm *biofeedback*.

DIALYSIS (90935–90999)

Do you remember learning about dialysis in Chapter 10? Dialysis cleanses the body of toxins when the kidneys can no longer separate toxins from the blood. The procedure is done for patients who have CKD, ESRD, or other disorders that inhibit kidney function. Patients can receive temporary or permanent dialysis in hospitals, outpatient clinics, dialysis centers, ESRD clinics, or their own homes and can even learn to *dialyze* (administer dialysis to) themselves.

Nephrologists perform E/M services related to dialysis, along with dialysis administration, and nurses, dialysis technicians, or patient care technicians may also administer dialysis to patients. There are many different variations of dialysis, and depending on a patient's condition, he may need dialysis daily, a few times a week, or just once. Medical supply companies may code and bill for dialysis supplies that patients use, depending on the place of service.

Turn to the codes in the Dialysis subsection, and notice that there are many CPT guidelines for dialysis coding, which include coding examples. You should review them carefully, but we will also review the information from the guidelines as you learn more about coding for dialysis procedures. The subsection contains four subheadings for dialysis procedures, categorized by the place of service, patient's diagnosis, and patient's age.

There are specific codes for dialysis services for patients with ESRD. The subheadings are as follows:

- **Hemodialysis**—inpatient ESRD or non-ESRD, and outpatient non-ESRD
- **Miscellaneous Dialysis Procedures**—inpatient ESRD or non-ESRD, and outpatient non-ESRD
- **End-Stage Renal Disease Services**—outpatient ESRD (hospital, dialysis clinic, ESRD clinic), and home
- **Other Dialysis Procedures**—inpatient or outpatient

Let's review the types of procedures that you will find under each subheading next.

Hemodialysis (90935–90940)

Hemodialysis involves connecting a patient to dialysis equipment through a dialysis access, an opening in the patient. There are several access options:

fistula (fis(h)′-chə-lə)

- inserting an intravenous (IV) catheter
- creating an *arteriovenous (AV)* **fistula**—anastomosis of an artery and vein to create a larger access route for blood
- creating an *arteriovenous (AV) graft*—anastomosis of an artery and vein with a synthetic tube, called a graft, when an AV fistula does not work

A catheter or tubing is connected from the fistula or graft to the dialysis machine. The patient's blood is removed, passed through a dialyzer to filter the blood of toxins, and returned to the body (Figure 10-24), a process that can take several hours or overnight to complete (called *nocturnal hemodialysis*).

Did you notice the coding guidelines under the Hemodialysis subheading? You have to read the guidelines carefully because they can be a bit confusing. Here is a summary:

- The first two codes in the subheading are for hemodialysis procedures when the physician performs either a single evaluation (one time) or a repeat evaluation, so these procedures include E/M services. You should not separately report E/M codes *except* when the physician performs E/M services that are *unrelated* to the patient's dialysis.
- Hemodialysis codes are for
  - Inpatients with ESRD
  - Inpatients with other kidney disorders (non-ESRD)
  - Outpatients with other kidney disorders (non-ESRD)
  - For *outpatient ESRD patients,* refer to the subheading End Stage Renal Disease Services and codes 90951–90970, which you will learn later in this chapter.
- The third code in the subheading is to assess blood flow in AV grafts and AV fistulae.

To find hemodialysis codes in CPT, search the index for *hemodialysis.*

Miscellaneous Dialysis Procedures (90945–90947)

This subheading includes only two codes that cover peritoneal dialysis, hemofiltration, or other continuous renal replacement therapies. Assign these codes for *inpatients,* including ESRD and non-ESRD, and for *outpatients* who are non-ESRD. The coding guidelines state that the codes include E/M services for either a single evaluation or repeated evaluations. Review the guidelines, which contain additional information similar to the Hemodialysis subheading guidelines.

Remember from Chapter 10 that peritoneal dialysis (Figure 10-25) involves introducing a cleansing dialysis solution into the patient's abdomen through a catheter. The peritoneum is a membrane that lines the abdominal cavity and helps to remove toxins from the blood and into the dialysis solution. The solution remains in the abdomen for several hours and is then drained out.

Hemofiltration (90945-90947) works like hemodialysis but is a slower therapy for critically ill patients. The procedure involves removing the patient's blood, filtering it, adding **electrolytes**, and then returning cleansed blood to the patient.

To locate these codes in the CPT index, search for *peritoneal dialysis* or *hemofiltration.*

electrolytes (i-lek′-trə-līts)—substances that regulate metabolic processes

End-Stage Renal Disease Services (90951–90970)

ESRD services in this subheading include monthly hemodialysis or peritoneal dialysis for outpatients in a hospital, ESRD clinic, and dialysis center, or for patients receiving dialysis at home. CPT divides ESRD services into three main groups of codes:

1. Monthly services for outpatients (90951–90962)
2. Monthly services at home (90963–90966)
3. Less than a full month of services for outpatients or home-based patients (90967–90970)

For the first two groups of codes, providers bill insurances for each month (30 days) that a patient receives dialysis and related services, including physician E/M services. A hospital may have a dialysis center, or unit, which initiates and oversees *home* dialysis for patients, and a home dialysis clinic can also perform these services. Monthly services for outpatients and at home include:

• Monitoring the adequacy of nutrition
• Assessing growth and development
• Counseling parents of patients up through age 19

Notice that these codes also state the patient's age and number of face-to-face physician visits each month. CPT guidelines state that physician visits include the following services:

• Establishing a dialyzing cycle (type and frequency of dialysis)
• E/M services
• Phone calls related to the patient's treatment
• Patient management

When patients *do not* receive a full month of services because they recover, are hospitalized, have a kidney transplant, or die, assign codes from the third group listed, 90967–90970 (less than a full month of services). Report the code once for *each day* of dialysis services, based on the patient's age. The CPT guidelines provide an example of this situation.

To locate CPT codes for ESRD dialysis, search the index for *end-stage renal disease services*. Review the following example to code ESRD services for a patient receiving monthly dialysis at home.

> **Example:** Mrs. Townsend, age 52, has ESRD Stage V and requires chronic dialysis. She received dialysis at home from April 1 to April 30. Brandyburg Home Dialysis Clinic oversees her home care.
>
> To code this case for the clinic, search the index for the main term *end-stage renal disease services*, which directs you to codes 90951–90970. Review codes 90963–90966 which represent *a full month of services*, which the patient received. The patient is 52 years old, so assign code **90966** because it is for patients age 20 and older. The patient's diagnosis code is **585.6** (*disease, kidney, chronic, requiring chronic dialysis*).

Other Dialysis Procedures (90989–90999)

This subheading includes codes for dialysis training, hemoperfusion, and an unlisted dialysis procedure for an inpatient or outpatient. Turn to the subheading to review the codes. Notice that CPT divides the dialysis training codes by a completed course or by each session when the patient *does not complete* a training course.

A *dialysis training course (90989-90993)* involves several training sessions where clinicians train patients to dialyze themselves. Services also include training a partner, typically a family member, to assist the patient with dialysis. Providers bill payers for a *completed course* after the patient completes the *last training session* in the course. Providers can also bill payers for *each training session* when the patient attends a training session but *does not complete* all of the sessions required.

Hemoperfusion (90997) is another method to cleanse the patient's blood when the kidneys do not properly function. It can cleanse more blood per treatment than hemodialysis and involves transferring the blood to a device that contains charcoal or resin, which removes toxins. Then the cleansed blood is returned to the patient. A physician is typically present during the therapy in the event that the patient's condition worsens.

Medicare reimburses for dialysis procedures, including dialysis training, but providers must follow very specific guidelines. The CMS website has provider manuals that outline this information. Be sure to check other payers' guidelines for coding and billing dialysis and dialysis training.

TAKE A BREAK

Nice work! Let's take a break and then practice coding biofeedback and dialysis services.

Exercise 34.3 Biofeedback , Dialysis

Instructions: Review each patient's case, and then assign codes for the procedure(s), appending a modifier when appropriate. Optional: For additional practice, assign the patient's diagnosis code(s) (ICD-9-CM).

1. Dr. Hoffman refers Wendell Oliver, age 63, to Dr. Barker, a psychologist, for biofeedback training to help regulate his hypertensive heart disease. Dr. Barker conducts a 45-minute session in his office to train Mr. Oliver in biofeedback techniques, including using equipment.

Diagnosis code(s): _____

Procedure code(s): _____

2. Margie Everest, age 58, sees Dr. Barker today in his office because she has urinary incontinence. Dr. Barker starts biofeedback training exercises for Mrs. Everest so that she can gain control of the related muscles in the urethral sphincter.

Diagnosis code(s): _____

Procedure code(s): _____

3. Johnny Butler, a 10-year-old patient of Dr. Singh, a nephrologist, receives dialysis for ESRD. Dr. Singh sees Johnny at Williton's Dialysis Center and has seen him three times this month.

Diagnosis code(s): _____

Procedure code(s): _____

4. Ebony Ash, age 25, is an inpatient at Williton Medical Center and is currently on the dialysis unit. She is receiving hemodialysis for acute renal failure. Dr. Singh sees Ms. Ash for an initial, single evaluation prior to the start of the hemodialysis.

Diagnosis code(s): _____

Procedure code(s): _____

5. Gary Powers, age 31, is in the inpatient dialysis unit at Williton. He receives peritoneal dialysis for acute renal failure with tubular necrosis (a condition involving the death of tubular cells that form the tubule which transports urine to the ureters). Dr. Singh supervises the peritoneal dialysis and performs repeated evaluations, making changes in the dialysis prescription.

Diagnosis code(s): _____

Procedure code(s): _____

6. Norman Mack, age 72, receives dialysis at home for acute renal failure. Dr. Singh trains Mr. Mack at his residence, instructing him on procedures to perform dialysis. Mr. Mack completes his course today.

Diagnosis code(s): _____

Procedure code(s): _____

GASTROENTEROLOGY (91010–91299)

In Chapter 10, you read about gastroenterology and learned that a gastroenterologist is a physician who specializes in diagnosis, treatment, and prevention of digestive system disorders. You also learned how to code digestive system procedures in Chapter 27. The Gastroenterology subsection includes gastrointestinal tests and imaging. CPT arranges codes in the Gastroenterology subsection by type of procedure. To locate codes in the index, search for *gastroenterology, diagnostic,* or search for the *type of procedure.* Turn to the codes in the subsection to review the descriptors, and we will discuss some of the procedures next:

- *Esophageal motility (manometric) study (91010–91013)*—This test evaluates muscular activity of the esophagus at rest and during swallowing to diagnose esophageal disorders involving motility (movement) or causes of heartburn.

- *Esophagus, acid perfusion (Bernstein) test for esophagitis (91030)*—This test evaluates causes of heartburn. The physician inserts a nasogastric (NG) tube (through the nose and into the esophagus) and introduces hydrochloric acid and then saline solution into the esophagus to determine if the patient experiences pain. No pain indicates a normal esophagus; pain could indicate acid reflux or another disorder, such as esophagitis (esophageal inflammation).

- *Breath hydrogen test (91065)*—This analysis of the patient's breath determines normal levels of hydrogen and methane, followed by levels after introducing another substance, such as fructose (sugar found in fruit) or lactose (sugar found in milk), to determine if the patient can adequately absorb the sugars, or has an overgrowth of intestinal bacteria.

- *Electrogastrography (91132–91133)*—This test uses electrodes to detect electrical activity of the stomach (gastrointestinal contractions) to diagnose stomach disorders.

electrogastrography (ē-lek-trō-gas-trog'rah-fe)

TAKE A BREAK

Way to go! Keep going! Let's take a break and then practice coding gastroenterology services.

Exercise 34.4 Gastroenterology

Instructions: Review each patient's case, and then assign codes for the procedure(s), appending a modifier when appropriate. Optional: For additional practice, assign the patient's diagnosis code(s) (ICD-9-CM).

1. Kim Cortez, age 47, presents to the Gastroenterology Department at Williton Medical Center to evaluate unexplained chest pain that is suspected to be noncardiac in origin. Dr. Burdett, a gastroenterologist, performs an esophageal balloon distension provocation study (a noncardiac test where the physician inserts a balloon into the patient, inflating it with air or water in an attempt to reproduce previously unexplained chest pain).

Diagnosis code(s): _____

Procedure code(s): _____

2. John Peters, 32 years old, presents to the Gastroenterology Department at Williton Medical Center because of gastrointestinal bleeding. Dr. Burdett administers a capsule endoscopy to the patient (a pill that the patient swallows which contains a camera that takes pictures of the esophagus, stomach, and small intestine, sending them to a computer that the physician reviews). Dr. Burdett reviews the photos and diagnoses the patient with irritable bowel syndrome (symptoms of which include chronic constipation, abdominal pain, or diarrhea).

Diagnosis code(s): _____

Procedure code(s): _____

3. Dr. Burdett performs a gastroesophageal reflux test at Williton by placing a nasal catheter with an attached electrode (the electrode transmits acid reflux occurrences to a recorder that the patient wears). The test includes reporting, analysis, and interpretation. The patient is Mark Roberts, age 37, whom Dr. Burdett diagnoses with GERD (gastroesophageal reflux disease, in which stomach contents such as food or liquid leak backward from the stomach into the esophagus).

Diagnosis code(s): _____

Procedure code(s): _____

continued

TAKE A BREAK *continued*

4. Julie Tillman, age 43, suffers from constipation. At Williton, Dr. Burdett initiates a colon motility study (a test in which various stimulants are given to the patient to demonstrate what types of medications can stimulate the colon). The study lasts seven hours.

   Diagnosis code(s): _____

   Procedure code(s): _____

5. Tony Finch, age 48, suffers from fecal incontinence. Dr. Burdett suspects that Mr. Finch suffers from **Hirschsprung's disease** (a congenital medical disorder where part of the nervous system is missing from the end of the bowel). Dr. Burdett performs an anorectal manometry (a technique used to measure contractions in the anus and rectum) in the Outpatient Surgery Department at Williton Medical Center. Dr. Burdett confirms Hirschsprung's disease.

   Diagnosis code(s): _____

   Procedure code(s): _____

6. Heather Mills, age 29, suffers from constant heartburn and indigestion. Dr. Burdett performs a two-hour gastroesophageal reflux test with nasal catheter intraluminal impedance electrode for detection of reflux at the Outpatient Department at Williton Medical Center. Dr. Burdett diagnoses the patient with GERD.

   Diagnosis code(s): _____

   Procedure code(s): _____

Hirschsprung's (hirsh′-sproongz)

OPHTHALMOLOGY (92002–92499)

You already learned about ophthalmology in Chapters 9 and 31, including learning about different types of ophthalmology providers, eye disorders, and surgical procedures. The Ophthalmology subsection contains eye procedures like exams, tests, and imaging. CPT divides the Ophthalmology subsection into four subheadings, depending on the type of service. Turn to the codes in each subheading as we review them next:

- *General Ophthalmological Services (92002–92014)*—Includes a medical exam for a new or established patient, based on the level of service the physician provides (intermediate or comprehensive).

- *Special Ophthalmological Services (92015–92287)*—Includes services that physicians or other clinicians may perform along with an exam, or perform individually *without* an exam. Here are some examples:

gonioscopy (gō-nē-äs′-kə-pē)

- **Gonioscopy (92020)**—The physician views the iris and cornea with a *goniolens*, a magnification lens with an attached mirror, to test for various eye disorders.

topography (tə-päg′-rə-fē)

- Computerized corneal **topography (92025)**—The clinician measures the shape and variations of the cornea when diseases or trauma cause it to be misshapen.

tonometry (tō-näm′-ə-trē)
tonometer (tō-nom′i-tur)

- **Tonometry (92100)**—The clinician measures intraocular pressure (IOP) in the eye with a **tonometer** to test for diseases like glaucoma. An *air-puff tonometer* is a device that measures IOP by assessing the cornea's reaction to a puff of air, and an *impression tonometer* places pressure on the cornea to measure IOP.

ophthalmoscopy (äf-thal-mäs′-kə-pē)

- **Ophthalmoscopy (92225–92226)**—The physician views the inside of the eye with an ophthalmoscope (instrument with a lens and mirror, seen in ■ FIGURE 34-2).

- *Contact Lens Services (92310–92326)*—Includes prescription, modification, and replacement of one or two contact lenses for the cornea or the cornea and sclera (corneoscleral).

- *Spectacle Services (92340–92499)* (eyeglasses) (including a prosthesis for aphakia)—Includes fitting and repair of various types of spectacles, depending on the type of eye disorder that the patient has.

As you can see, these services do not include any type of surgery. To assign surgery codes, review ophthalmology surgical procedures in the Eye and Ocular Adnexa subsection of the Surgery section (Chapter 31).

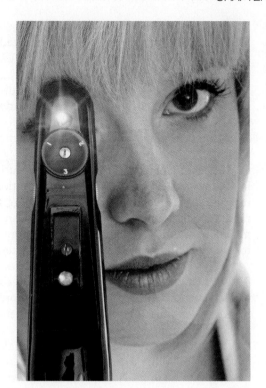

Figure 34-2 ■ An optometrist uses an ophthalmoscope to examine a patient's eyes.

Photo credit: Terence Mendoza/ Shutterstock.

Bilateral and Unilateral

Be sure to review code descriptors, as some state the procedure is for one eye or both eyes (unilateral, bilateral). Append the appropriate modifier for a unilateral, or one-eye procedure, as -LT or -RT. Append modifier -50 if the procedure is bilateral. If the procedure's descriptor states bilateral, and the physician only performed it for one eye, then append modifier -52 (reduced service) to the procedure code. Do not append modifiers for unilateral or bilateral when the code descriptor already includes the words *unilateral* or *bilateral.*

Coding Guidelines for Exams

Refer to CPT's coding guidelines for the Ophthalmology subsection. Did you notice that they are very extensive and include definitions for intermediate and comprehensive services, as well as examples? The general ophthalmological services include intermediate and comprehensive services for a new or established patient. Do you remember the definitions of a new and established patient that you first learned in Chapter 1? Be sure to review the guidelines, including the examples that CPT lists to help you assign the correct codes. An important point to note is that when a physician performs an intermediate or complex exam, you should *not report* an *additional* E/M code or report an E/M code in place of the ophthalmologic exam, unless there is specific documentation to support the E/M code *instead of* an ophthalmologic code.

To locate codes for ophthalmology services, search the index for *ophthalmology, diagnostic,* or search for the type of service (*contact lens services*).

SPECIAL OTORHINOLARYNGOLOGIC SERVICES (92502–92700)

You also learned about otorhinolaryngology in Chapters 9 and 31, including different types of providers; ear, nose, and throat disorders; and surgical procedures. CPT lists a handful of services at the beginning of the subsection and then divides the rest into four subheadings, including tests, evaluations, and therapeutic services. Keep in mind that speech–language pathologists and audiologists, in addition to physicians, may also provide some of these otorhinolaryngological services. Let's discuss these two types of providers next.

Speech–language pathologists (SLPs), also called *speech therapists*, assess, diagnose, treat, and help to prevent disorders related to speech, language, cognitive-communication, voice, swallowing, and fluency. SLPs work with patients who cannot produce any speech or cannot produce sounds clearly, along with patients who have speech rhythm and fluency problems, such as stuttering; voice disorders, such as inappropriate pitch or a harsh voice; problems understanding and producing language; those who want to improve their communication skills by modifying an accent; and those with cognitive communication impairments, such as attention, memory, and problem-solving disorders.

Speech, language, and swallowing difficulties can result from a variety of causes, including stroke, brain injury or deterioration, developmental delays or disorders, learning disabilities, cerebral palsy, cleft palate (congenital disorder where the roof of the mouth is not completely formed, which can be corrected with surgery), voice pathology, mental retardation, hearing loss, or emotional problems. SLPs perform standardized tests to analyze and diagnose the nature and extent of patients' impairments.

SLPs develop an individualized plan of care that is tailored to each patient's needs. They teach patients how to make sounds, improve their voices, or increase their oral or written language skills to communicate more effectively. They also teach individuals how to strengthen muscles or use alternative methods of swallowing without choking or inhaling food or liquid.

Audiologists are healthcare professionals who work with patients with hearing, balance, and related ear problems. They examine patients of all ages and identify those with symptoms of hearing loss and other auditory (hearing) issues, difficulties with balance, and related sensory and neural problems. They then assess the nature and extent of the problems and help the individuals manage them. Using audiometers, computers, and other testing devices, they measure the volume at which a person begins to hear sounds, the ability to distinguish among sounds, and the impact of hearing loss on an individual's daily life. They also use computer equipment to evaluate and diagnose balance disorders. Audiologists interpret these results and may coordinate them with medical, educational, and psychological information to make a diagnosis and determine a course of treatment.

In audiology clinics, audiologists may independently develop and carry out treatment programs. They keep records on the initial evaluation, progress, and discharge of patients. In other settings, audiologists may work with other health and education providers as part of a team in planning and implementing services for children and adults. Audiologists who diagnose and treat balance disorders often work in collaboration with physicians and physical and occupational therapists.

Turn to the codes in the Special Otorhinolaryngologic Services subsection so that you can be more familiar with them. Did you notice the coding guidelines at the beginning of the subsection? You should read these guidelines, along with guidelines listed throughout services in the subsection, before final code assignment. Let's review two services listed in the first group of services in the subsection, and then discuss other types of services listed under the four subheadings:

- *Evaluation of speech, language, voice, communication, and/or auditory processing (92506)*—The clinician evaluates how a patient communicates with others, including receiving and delivering information. It includes assessment and testing of a patient's hearing, which can also affect the ability to communicate.

- *Treatment of speech, language, voice, communication, and/or auditory processing disorder; individual or group (92507)*—The clinician works with patients on various methods and exercises to improve speech, language, voice, and communication, including exercises to strengthen muscles.

- *Vestibular Function Tests (with or without electrical recording) (92531–92548)*—The vestibular system is part of the auditory system that helps a person to maintain balance. Vestibular function tests monitor a patient's ability to balance and can include **electronystagmography (ENG)**, a test in which the physician

electronystagmography
(i-lek-trō-nis-tag-mäg′-
rə-fē)

places electrodes on the face that measure movements of the head and eyes to assess balance disorders like vertigo, dizziness, or involuntary eye movements (**nystagmus**).

nystagmus (nis-tag′-məs)

- *Audiologic Function Tests (92550–92597)*—Includes various types of hearing tests, along with hearing aid checks. Note that the CPT guidelines alert you that all services include testing *both* ears and to append modifier -52 (reduced services) if the test is only for *one* ear.

- *Evaluative and Therapeutic Services (92601–92633)*—Include analysis of a cochlear implant to determine its effectiveness (see Table 31-6 for more information on cochlear implants), swallowing evaluations, and auditory evaluation and rehabilitation.

- *Special Diagnostic Procedures (92640)*—Includes one service for diagnostic analysis with programming of auditory brainstem implant (which uses the brainstem to produce sound), per hour.

- *Other Procedures (92700)*—Includes one code that represents an unlisted otorhinolaryngological service or procedure.

Just like with ophthalmological procedures, you should also carefully review code descriptors for otorhinolaryngological services for unilateral or bilateral to determine if you need to assign modifiers for reduced services (unilateral, one ear, modifier -52), or bilateral services (-50). To locate codes for otorhinolaryngological procedures, search the index for the *type of procedure* (e.g., *speech evaluation, vestibular function tests, audiologic function tests*). To code surgical procedures on the ear, refer to the Auditory System subsection (Chapter 31).

keratoconus (ker-ət-ō-kō′-nəs)

TAKE A BREAK

Great progress! Keep going! Let's take a break and then practice coding eye and ear services.

Exercise 34.5 Ophthalmology, Special Otorhinolaryngologic Services

Instructions: Review each patient's case, and then assign codes for the procedure(s), appending a modifier when appropriate. Optional: For additional practice, assign the patient's diagnosis code(s) (ICD-9-CM).

1. Emily Bender, an 85-year-old established patient, sees Dr. Nickels, an ophthalmologist, for open-angle glaucoma, an eye disorder that damages the optic nerve, permanently diminishing vision in the affected eye(s) and progressing to complete blindness if untreated. It is often, but not always, associated with increased pressure of the fluid in the eye. Dr. Nickels performs a comprehensive ophthalmologic examination in his office.

   Diagnosis code(s): _____

   Procedure code(s): _____

2. Lou Sawyer, age 78, sees Dr. Nickels in his office for fitting of contact lenses for treatment of **keratoconus** (a degenerative eye disorder that changes the shape and structure of the cornea, resulting in a cone shape).

   Diagnosis code(s): _____

   Procedure code(s): _____

3. Dr. Nickels diagnoses Anne Constance, age 63, with a senile cataract of the right eye. Soon, Dr. Nickels will perform a cataract extraction with an intraocular lens implant. In order to implant the correct visual power of the intraocular lens, Dr. Nickels conducts an optical coherence biometry diagnostic test (measures the eye in preparation for cataract surgery and lens implantation) today in his office.

   Diagnosis code(s): _____

   Procedure code(s): _____

4. Ned White, age 72, comes to the Audiology Department at Williton Medical Center for a hearing aid check. He has a sensorineural hearing loss (a disorder of the inner ear, involving the central processing centers of the brain). He wears hearing aids in both ears. Susan Cohen, an audiologist, inspects the hearing aid and battery.

   Diagnosis code(s): _____

   Procedure code(s): _____

continued

TAKE A BREAK *continued*

5. Joey Sanford, age 6, is referred to the Audiology Department at Williton Medical Center by his school nurse. Joey failed a hearing test at school. Susan Cohen conducts a hearing screening test, pure tone, air only (a test that measures responses to both low- and high-pitched sounds).

Diagnosis code(s): _____

Procedure code(s): _____

6. Today in the office, Kelly Brown, age 28, sees Dr. Marks, an otorhinolaryngologist, to evaluate a possible deviated nasal septum. Dr. Marks conducts a nasopharyngoscopy with an endoscope that he introduces through Mrs. Brown's nose to evaluate the nasal passage. Dr. Marks diagnoses Mrs. Brown with a deviated nasal septum and will schedule her for corrective surgery at a later date.

Diagnosis code(s): _____

Procedure code(s): _____

POINTERS FROM THE PROS: Interview with an Optometrist

You first heard from William K. Vincett, Jr., D.O., in Chapter 31. He has even more pointers to share with you.

Describe the types of communication that you have with coders and billing staff.

I think alerts to the doctors of shifts in reimbursement, new code releases, and yearly (updates to) the Medicare fee schedule are mandatory. I also believe that the monthly monitoring of the accounts receivable for both patients and insurance companies is important. There should be an open and friendly exchange at all times between the doctors, billing staff, and coders as they are all on the same team. Failure to do so will cause a less efficient system at best and business failure at worst.

If you could change one aspect of the healthcare field, what would you change?

We should have several of our most common (tests) paid for (by insurances). The equipment (to perform the tests) saves the insurance companies money (because they can detect diseases early before advanced costly treatment is needed). The early detection and education value to the patient justifies the cost of the equipment.

What personal motto do you live by?

Patients deserve the best possible care by the most advanced technology possible and to be educated about their conditions. If I can provide that to them, and they can perceive that is what I am doing, then all the rest will work itself out.

(Used by permission of William K. Vincett, Jr.)

CARDIOVASCULAR (92950–93799)

echocardiography (ek-ō-kärd-ē-äg′-rə-fē)

transesophageal (trans--i-säf-ə-jē′-əl)

claudication (klod-ə-kā′-shən)

bioimpedance (bī- ō-ĭm-pēd′ns)

You are already familiar with different cardiovascular procedures that you learned in Chapter 25. You also learned that the Medicine chapter contains various codes for cardiovascular tests, imaging, and procedures, included in 10 different subheadings. There are too many procedures for us to review in this chapter, so we will only concentrate on some of them. Turn to the procedures in each subheading of the Cardiovascular subsection as you read more about them in ■ TABLE 34-2. Note that many procedures in the Cardiovascular subsection are for diagnosing heart disorders, and the procedures can be complex and involved. Pay attention to the detailed coding guidelines in the Cardiovascular subsection because there are many of them. It is best to consult your medical resources for additional information on any additional procedures that you do not understand to be sure that you assign the correct codes.

SURE that you assign the correct codes.

CPT arranges procedures by the type of service (therapeutic services, cardiovascular monitoring). To locate codes for procedures in the Cardiovascular subsection, search the index for *cardiology* and then the *type of procedure*, or start your search with the *type of procedure*.

■ TABLE 34-2 **PROCEDURES IN THE CARDIOVASCULAR SUBSECTION**

Subheading	Examples of Procedures Included
Therapeutic Services and Procedures (92950–92998)	• *Cardiopulmonary Resuscitation (CPR) (92950)*—This procedure is performed for a patient experiencing cardiac arrest in an attempt to restart the heartbeat, using chest compressions and artificial respiration. • *Cardioversion (92960–92961)*—This procedure attempts to restore normal heart rhythm, using a low electrical current, with the patient under moderate sedation. Patches are placed both over the heart and off to the side of the heart. The procedure is used to treat arrhythmias, such as atrial fibrillation. • *Percutaneous Transluminal Coronary (Balloon) Angioplasty (PTCA) (92982–92984)*—This procedure is performed on a patient with a partially blocked artery in the heart, a condition that contributes to angina. The cardiologist advances a catheter, with a balloon and possibly a stent attached, to the blocked artery and inflates the balloon so that it pushes against the artery wall (Figure 11-17). The physician may also insert a stent to keep the artery open. Plaque can still build up again in the artery with the stent, so the cardiologist places the patient on medication to prevent plaque buildup.
Cardiography (93000–93042)	• *Electrocardiogram (ECG or EKG) (93000–93010)*—This 5–10-minute test measures the electrical activity of the heart, including how fast it beats and its rhythm, using leads placed on the patient's chest, arms, and legs. Results are transmitted to an EKG machine that produces a report of the electrical activity of the heart as well as heart rate and any abnormal rhythm. • *Cardiovascular stress test (93015–93018)*—This test is performed to obtain a better picture of the heart's activity when the patient is exercising and to diagnose the causes of symptoms like chest pain. Multiple leads are placed on the patient's chest and he exercises on a treadmill or bicycle. A cardiologist is present while the patient undergoes the test. The result of the heart's response to activity is recorded, similar to the EKG tracings. • If the patient is unable to exercise, then he can receive medication that mimics the effect of exercise on the heart (called pharmacologic stress) so that he can still undergo the test.
Cardiovascular Monitoring Services (93224–93278), Implantable and Wearable Cardiac Device Evaluations (93279–93299)	Cardiovascular monitoring includes assessments of cardiovascular rhythm, tested remotely or with the patient present, to diagnose various heart disorders. The Implantable and Wearable Cardiac Device Evaluations subheading includes services for evaluating a patient's cardiac devices, such as a pacemaker or other type of monitor. Services can be performed in person or remotely and include the following: • *Programming device evaluation (93279–93285)*—An evaluation where the clinician adjusts the parameters of a monitoring device, such as a pacemaker, to make sure that it is functioning properly. Remember from Chapter 25 that a pacemaker is implanted into a patient to control the heart rate. • *Interrogation device evaluation (93288–93292)*—An evaluation where the clinician does not adjust the parameters of a monitoring device but instead reviews information that the device gathers.
Echocardiography (93303–93352)	• **Echocardiography** *(echo) (93303–93317, 93320–93351)*—A test that uses sound waves to create a moving picture of the heart. It is accomplished by using a transducer on the external chest wall and sending sound waves through the chest. The picture is much more detailed than a plain X-ray image and involves no radiation exposure. Unlike an EKG, the procedure gives a picture of the anatomical structures, and not the electrical activity. Append modifier -26 to the code when the physician performs the S & I. • **Transesophageal** *echocardiography* **(TEE) (93318)**—An endoscopic ultrasound transducer (which transforms one form of energy into another) is introduced into the mouth and then into the esophagus to allow measurements to be taken closer to the chest. A TEE is unlike an echo because it does not have to go through the chest wall and through the ribs.
Cardiac Catheterization (93451–93533)	When patients develop chest pain, many times the physician will perform a cardiac catheterization (also called a cardiac cath or heart cath) to obtain a better picture of the circulation of blood through the heart, as well as potential interruptions to blood flow that plaque or atherosclerosis (plaque buildup in the arteries) can cause. • The physician starts by inserting an IV catheter into the patient's vein. The site that is used most frequently is the femoral vein. Other sites can be used at the discretion of the cardiologist. He advances the catheter through the circulatory system into the right side of the heart and advances to the part of the heart that he wishes to 'see' better. While the catheter is advanced, a contrast dye is injected through the catheter, giving the physician a better picture of the coronary vessel patency. The procedure can detect blockages and narrowed vessels. There are extensive CPT guidelines for cardiac catheterizations, including a table of catheterization codes, so read them carefully to understand the procedures performed before final code assignment.

continued

■ TABLE 34-2 *continued*

Subheading	Examples of Procedures Included
	• **Repair of septal defect (93580)**—The septum is a wall that divides the left and right sides of the heart. It lies between the left and right atria (top), which is called the atrial septum, and also lies between the left and right ventricles (bottom), which is called the ventricular septum. Codes are based on the type of congenital defect repaired.
Intercardiac Electrophys-icological Procedures/ Studies (EP Studies) (93600–93662)	Procedures include invasive diagnostic tests that assess the electrical activity in the heart. The electrical activity for a normal heartbeat starts at the top of the heart and spreads down. A patient may experience cardiac arrhythmias or abnormal heart rhythms when the electrical activity in the heart starts somewhere other than at the top of the heart. • **Bundle of His recording (93600)**—The bundle of His is a group of fibers that carry electrical impulses through the center of the heart. If these signals are blocked, then the patient will have an abnormal heartbeat. • The His bundle electrography is part of an electrophysiology (EP) study. The physician inserts an intravenous catheter (IV line) into the patient's arm to administer medication during the test. • Electrocardiogram (ECG) leads are placed on the patient's arms and legs. The cardiologist makes a small incision in a vein and inserts a catheter and advances it through the vein up into the heart. Fluoroscopy helps guide the physician to the correct location. During the test, the physician monitors the patient's heartbeat for any arrhythmias. The catheter has a sensor on the end, which is used to measure the electrical activity of the bundle of His.
Peripheral Arterial Disease Rehabilitation (93668)	This subheading contains one code for physical exercise for patients with peripheral arterial disease (PAD), a circulatory disorder that prevents the proper amount of blood from flowing through the legs, causing leg pain (called intermittent **claudication**). Rehabilitation to decrease leg pain includes exercise sessions lasting up to an hour, involving a treadmill or track. An exercise physiologist or nurse supervises each patient's program.
Noninvasive Physiologic Studies and Procedures (93701–93790)	Noninvasive procedures measure cardiovascular functions and may include pacemaker services. • **Bioimpedance (93701)-*derived physiologic cardiovascular analysis*—Involves continuous measurement of blood flow, respiration, and other heart functions. *Electronic analysis of antitachycardia pacemaker system (93724)*—Patients with previously implanted pacemakers require periodic analysis of pacemaker functions; The procedure includes the routine analysis of pacemakers used to control irregularly fast heartbeats and includes EKG, programming, tests, and physician interpretation of the tests.
Other Procedures (93797–93799)	*Physician services for outpatient cardiac rehabilitation (rehab) (93797–93798)*—Monitored cardiac rehabilitation is patient exercise for those who suffered an MI or had previous heart surgery. The patient performs exercises under a plan of care that a cardiologist develops and oversees. There is an interdisciplinary team involved in the patient's care, including an exercise physiologist, dietician, and cardiologist, to name a few. *Unlisted cardiovascular service or procedure (93799)*

TAKE A BREAK

Good job! Let's take a break and then review more about cardiovascular procedures.

Exercise 34.6 Cardiovascular

Part 1—Theory

Instructions: Fill in the blank with the best answer.

1. What is the name of an evaluation where the clinician adjusts the parameters of a monitoring device, such as a pacemaker, to make sure that it is functioning properly? _____

2. The _____ is a group of fibers that carry electrical impulses through the center of the heart.

3. This procedure attempts to restore normal heart rhythm, using a low electrical current, with the patient under moderate sedation. _____

4. What is the circulatory disorder that prevents the proper amount of blood from flowing through the legs, causing intermittent claudication? _____

TAKE A BREAK *continued*

5. What is the name of the procedure where multiple leads are placed on the patient's chest and he exercises on a treadmill or bicycle? _____

6. A test that uses sound waves to create a moving picture of the heart is called a(n) _____.

Part 2—Coding

Instructions: Review each patient's case, and then assign codes for the procedure(s), appending a modifier when appropriate. Optional: For additional practice, assign the patient's diagnosis code(s) (ICD-9-CM).

1. Maria Allardo, age 45, arrives by ambulance at Williton's ED. She is in cardiac arrest. Dr. Mills, one of the ED physicians, initiates cardiopulmonary resuscitation. After one hour of resuscitation, he pronounces Mrs. Allardo dead and notifies her family in the waiting room.

   Diagnosis code(s): _____

   Procedure code(s): _____

2. In Williton's Interventional Radiology Department, Gwen Hilton, age 49, sees Dr. Leonard, a cardiologist, to evaluate previously diagnosed coronary artery disease. Dr. Leonard performs a PTCA involving one artery. After the procedure, Miss Hilton remains in post-op recovery and is then discharged home.

   Diagnosis code(s): _____

   Procedure code(s): _____

3. Jodi Innocenti, three years old, has a single-lead pacemaker that was implanted one year ago due to tachycardia. Her mother brings her to Williton where Dr. Leonard conducts a programming device evaluation and testing of the device's function. The pacemaker is in good working order and does not need any adjustment at this time.

   Diagnosis code(s): _____

   Procedure code(s): _____

4. Ed Peters, age 64, is soon scheduled for surgery at Williton Medical Center for a torn rotator cuff (a group of muscles and their tendons that act to stabilize the shoulder) on the left side. Today, Mr. Peters arrives at Williton for surgical clearance. Dr. Leonard performs an ECG using 12 leads. He wants to determine if Mr. Peters can undergo surgery, since he has had previous heart problems. Dr. Leonard also provides the interpretation and report.

   Diagnosis code(s): _____

   Procedure code(s): _____

5. Jason Baird is a 17-year-old basketball player whom Dr. Leonard sees in the Radiology Department at Williton. Dr. Leonard performs a transthoracic echocardiogram (the echocardiography transducer or probe is placed on the chest wall or thorax of the patient, and images are taken through the chest wall). The test is to evaluate a possible congenital heart anomaly because the patient has a family history of heart defects. The test was negative.

   Diagnosis code(s): _____

   Procedure code(s): _____

6. John Macklin, age 72, recently experienced chest pain, so Dr. Leonard schedules a right heart catheterization in the cardiac cath lab at Williton. Dr. Leonard evaluates Mr. Macklin for potential coronary artery disease. The final diagnosis is coronary artery disease in one artery that is 25% blocked. No further treatment will be done at this time. Mr. Macklin will manage his condition with medication.

   Diagnosis code(s): _____

   Procedure code(s): _____

NONINVASIVE VASCULAR DIAGNOSTIC STUDIES (93880–93998)

The subsection Noninvasive Vascular Diagnostic Studies includes specialized services to study veins and arteries, other than the heart and great vessels (e.g., superior vena cava, inferior vena cava, pulmonary artery, aorta). Remember that noninvasive means not breaking the skin to perform a procedure. CPT divides procedures in this subsection into subheadings by body site and whether the study involves an artery, vein, or both. Turn to the codes in this subsection to review them. Notice that this subsection has extensive CPT guidelines for you to read and follow. Let's take a look at a couple of tests to become more familiar with them:

- *Extremity Arterial Studies (93922–93931)*—a test using Doppler ultrasound (sound waves that generate images to a monitor) of the extremities to diagnose circulatory disorders that restrict blood flow to the extremities, like peripheral arterial disease (PAD).

- *Visceral and Penile Vascular Studies (93975–93982)*—a test that measures blood pressures in the legs and at the base of the penis to diagnose vascular problems that could cause impotence (inability to sustain an erection).

To locate codes for noninvasive vascular diagnostic studies, search the index for the main term *vascular studies,* and then search for a subterm for the *type of procedure* or *body site*.

PULMONARY (94002–94799)

The Pulmonary subsection includes two subheadings for Ventilator Management and Pulmonary Diagnostic Testing and Therapies. Turn to the codes in the Pulmonary subsection to become more familiar with them. Ventilator Management includes physician services to initiate ventilator use for patients to breathe, which is intended to rehabilitate the respiratory system so that the patient can return to independent respiration (ventilator weaning). It is performed for inpatients, observation patients, patients at home, in a domiciliary or rest home (assisted living). Services also include ventilator care plan oversight.

Pulmonary Diagnostic Testing and Therapies subheading includes many different diagnostic breathing tests to identify pulmonary and respiratory disorders by assessing lung functions and therapeutic services to help patients to breathe more easily. Here are two tests included in this subheading:

spirometry (spī-rə′-me-trē)

- **Spirometry** (94010)—This pulmonary function test (PFT) measures the ability of the lungs to inhale and exhale as the patient uses a mouthpiece to breathe in and out. The mouthpiece is connected to a spirometer. Spirometry results can help the physician to diagnose disorders like COPD, which includes asthma and emphysema. This test measures the lungs' ability to take oxygen in and the amount the patient is able to exhale and includes many different testing parameters.

- *Continuous inhalation treatment with aerosol medication for acute airway obstruction; first hour and each additional hour (94644, 94645)*—The patient receives medication by aerosol (spray) to treat restrictive airway diseases, like asthma, and congested bronchiole passageways.

plethysmography (pleth-iz-mäg′-rə-fē)

To locate codes for pulmonary procedures, search the index for *pulmonary, diagnostic,* and then the *type of procedure*, or begin your search with the *type of procedure*.

TAKE A BREAK

Way to go! Let's take a break and then practice coding vascular diagnostic studies and pulmonary services.

Exercise 34.7 Noninvasive Vascular Diagnostic Studies, Pulmonary

Instructions: Review each patient's case, and then assign codes for the procedure(s), appending a modifier when

appropriate. Optional: For additional practice, assign the patient's diagnosis code(s) (ICD-9-CM).

1. Irwin Gabby, age 73, is diagnosed with intermittent leg claudication. Dr. Hirsch, a vascular surgeon, sees Mr. Gabby in his office and performs **plethysmography** of the veins of both of Mr. Gabby's legs. The diagnosis is peripheral artery disease of

TAKE A BREAK *continued*

both legs. Mr. Gabby will undergo vascular surgery next month.

Diagnosis code(s): _____

Procedure code(s): _____

2. During an office visit, Dr. Hirsch suspects that patient Jean Marble, age 64, has symptoms of carotid artery occlusion. He decides not to perform an angiogram, due to Miss Marble's age and the risk of complications. Instead, he decides to use a new type of technology, ocular pneumoplethysmography (a noninvasive procedure that measures and records the pressure in the ophthalmic arteries and detects carotid artery disease). Miss Marble presents to the Interventional Radiology department at Williton Medical Center where Dr. Hirsch performs the test. The findings are consistent with carotid artery occlusion.

Diagnosis code(s): _____

Procedure code(s): _____

3. Tonya Robinson, age 13, has sickle cell disease (characterized by abnormal red blood cells, which cause anemia). She was diagnosed at age five. Stroke, especially cerebral infarction, is a major cause of morbidity and mortality in children with sickle cell disease. Since Tonya is in a high-risk group for developing major complications, Dr. Hirsch performs a transcranial Doppler study that is complete (use of ultrasound waves to measure flow velocity—speed—in the large intracranial arteries). He conducts the study in the Radiology Department at Williton Medical Center.

Diagnosis code(s): _____

Procedure code(s): _____

4. Candy Clark, age 57, presents to Dr. Gupta's office with a chronic cough. She has a 20-year smoking habit and is nicotine dependent. Dr. Gupta, a pulmonologist, performs a bronchospasm evaluation with spirometry before and after bronchodilator treatment.

Diagnosis code(s): _____

Procedure code(s): _____

5. Two years ago, Dr. Gupta diagnosed Katie Shaler, age 13, with asthma. Lately, she has been wheezing and having difficulty catching her breath. Dr. Gupta sends her to the Pulmonology Department of Williton Medical Center to have her lung function tested. Dr. Gupta supervises a vital capacity, total evaluation of the volume of gas that can be expelled from the lungs. Dr. Gupta prescribes a rescue inhaler and steroid management of her asthma.

Diagnosis code(s): _____

Procedure code(s): _____

6. Jerry Walker, age 53, a long-time cigarette smoker, suffers from severe COPD. Dr. Gupta performs a simple pulmonary stress test in the Pulmonology Lab at Williton to evaluate Mr. Walker's lungs and pulmonary function. Mr. Walker's COPD continues to worsen, so Dr. Gupta adjusts his medication.

Diagnosis code(s): _____

Procedure code(s): _____

sleep apnea (ap′-nē-ə)—respiration that stops at intervals during sleep
insomnia (in-säm′-nē-ə)—abnormal inability to sleep adequately
narcolepsy (när-kə-lep′-sē)—attacks of deep sleep that occur at various times throughout the day
somnambulism (säm-nam′-byə-liz-əm)—sleep walking
polysomnography (pol-ē-säm-nə′-graf-ē)

ADDITIONAL MEDICINE SUBSECTIONS (95004–99607)

The remaining subsections in Medicine are outlined for you in ■ TABLE 34-3. CPT categorizes each subsection by specific procedures and tests related to each subsection. Turn to the codes in each subsection as you review more about specific services you can find there. Be sure to review CPT guidelines for these subsections because there are many of them which are very detailed. To locate codes for procedures in the Medicine section, search for the name of the *subsection* and then the *type of procedure,* or first search for the *type of procedure.*

■ TABLE 34-3 **ADDITIONAL MEDICINE SUBSECTIONS**

Subsection	Types of Procedures
Allergy and Clinical Immunology (95004–95199)	An **allergy** is an abnormal reaction of the human immune system. It wrongly identifies certain allergens as harmful foreign bodies and produces antibodies against them. When these antibodies are produced in excess, they release histamine and other chemicals in your body, which in turn results in an allergic reaction. • *Allergy Testing (95004–95075)*—A skin or inhalation test to expose a patient to an allergen to determine if it causes an allergic response. • *Allergen Immunotherapy (95115–95199)*—Services to expose a patient to allergenic extracts or insect venoms to increase his immunity to the allergen (desensitization).
Endocrinology (95250–95251)	This subsection contains two codes for ambulatory continuous glucose monitoring of interstitial tissue fluid. A continuous monitoring device is implanted under the abdominal skin (such as a diabetic patient), to measure glucose levels every five minutes for 72 hours. The device transmits the results to a monitor that the patient wears. You can only report codes for these services once a month.
Neurology and Neuromuscular Procedures (95800–96020)	Neurologists typically perform tests and procedures in this subsection, but other healthcare professionals may also assign these codes. Here are some of the procedures: • *Sleep Testing (95803–95811)*—Testing is performed while the patient sleeps to assess various body functions to diagnose sleep disorders such as **sleep apnea**, **insomnia**, **narcolepsy**, and **somnambulism**. Tests include **polysomnography**, which includes multiple measurements of functions and activities of the heart, muscles, brain, and eyes during sleep. • *Evoked Potentials and Reflex Tests (95925–95937)*—These tests are performed to diagnosis neuromuscular diseases, completed by measuring visual, auditory, and automatic nerve reflexes.
Medical Genetics and Genetic Counseling Services (96040)	This subsection includes one code for medical genetics and genetic counseling services, where a genetic counselor meets with patients and their families to discuss the likelihood that the patients' children will inherit genetic diseases. The discussion may also cover family members who already have inherited diseases and various tests for genetic disorders. The service includes counseling for 16–30 minutes, and you cannot code and bill insurance for a service of 15 minutes or less.
Central Nervous System Assessments/Tests (96101–96125)	These procedures are to assess cognitive processes (mental processes including reasoning and memory), mental status, and speech, functions related to the central nervous system. Tests can diagnose disorders such as personality disorders, aphasia, and central nervous system conditions, including damage caused by traumatic injuries.
Health and Behavior Assessment/Intervention (96150–96155)	These assessments include meeting with patients with physical problems to help them to productively handle their illnesses. The patients do not have mental illnesses. Examples include an asthma sufferer who has anxiety about her condition, a cancer patient who cannot manage pain related to cancer treatment, or a child with a chronic illness who needs daily medication but refuses to take it. Psychologists typically perform these assessments and can recommend behavioral therapy, including relaxation techniques.
Hydration, Therapeutic, Prophylactic, Diagnostic Injections and Infusions, and Chemotherapy and Other Highly Complex Drug or Highly Complex Biologic Agent Administration (96360–96549)	This subsection contains numerous CPT guidelines that are complex. It is important for you to review them carefully before assigning codes from this subsection. Let's review what some of these procedures involve: • *Intravenous infusion, hydration (96360–96361)*—IV hydration for patients who are dehydrated and lack the necessary amount of fluid the body requires. This condition is because their bodies have expelled more fluid than they are able to keep in, causing an electrolyte imbalance. Conditions causing dehydration include vomiting, diarrhea, and alcohol-related illnesses. • *Intravenous infusion, for therapy, prophylaxis, or diagnosis (96365–96368)*—IV infusion can involve administering medications to a patient, like an antibiotic for sepsis or a systemic infection. IV infusion provides ongoing introduction of medications using an IV infusion line consisting of a bag and tubing connected to the IV access port, wherever it may be inserted in a vein in the body. The speed at which the clinician delivers the infusion is the IV push. *Prophylactic infusion*—The patient receives an IV antibiotic to prevent infection before an upcoming surgery. • *IV chemotherapy (96413–96417)*—This treatment is administered to cancer patients; the type of medication, frequency with which it is administered, and amount administered varies, depending on each patient's condition. For example, patients may receive one drug or a combination of drugs over a two-day period, then no drugs for two weeks, or they may receive a drug for two weeks, with one week off, then again for two more weeks.

■ TABLE 34-3 *continued*

Subsection	Types of Procedures
Photodynamic Therapy ***(96567–96571)***	Photodynamic therapy involves injecting a patient with a substance that attaches to cancer cells in a tumor. A light is then directed at the tumor, which causes the substance to generate oxygen to kill the cancer cells. A physician can apply the light externally or endoscopically. Different specialties may perform this service, including a dermatologist to destroy a premalignant skin lesion or a gastroenterologist to destroy an esophageal malignancy.
Special Dermatological ***Procedures (96900–96999)***	These are dermatology services, including treatments for skin conditions: • *Actinotherapy (96900)*—This procedure involves applying ultraviolet light to the skin to heal skin disorders like acne, atopic dermatitis, or eczema. • *Photochemotherapy (96910–96913)*—This treatment provides ultraviolet radiation for skin disorders like dermatitis.
Physical Medicine and ***Rehabilitation (97001–97799)***	Physical medicine and rehabilitation includes physical therapy (PT) and occupational therapy (OT), including evaluations, exercises, tests, and wound care management, including debridement. Services are provided for patients with any number of disorders, including physical and neurological conditions. Therapists may treat patients after a stroke or motor vehicle accident to help them to regain their physical and mental strength and abilities.
Medical Nutrition Therapy ***(97802–97804)***	Medical nutrition therapy (MNT) is a service that a registered dietician (RD, a health-care professional specializing in nutrition) provides to patients who need assistance managing their nutritional needs, including patients with diabetes and cancer. The RD meets with the patient to gather information about the patient's condition and current habits and then develops a plan for the patient to follow to ensure that she receives adequate nutrition. There is also follow-up with the patient to determine the progress of the plan and adjust it if necessary.
Acupuncture (97810–97814)	Acupuncture is a form of *alternative medicine*, medical treatment that does not have a basis in scientific research. When you read the word *acupuncture*, images of people with needles all over their bodies probably comes to mind. Acupuncture is used to manage pain from various conditions, including migraine headaches. Acupuncture originated in China and includes inserting needles into the skin of various body sites, and possibly manipulating them. Depending on where the patient experiences pain, there are specific sites to insert the needles to control the pain. Acupuncture may also involve *electrical stimulation* (an electrical current applied to muscles to enable them to strengthen by contracting). An *acupuncturist* is a healthcare professional who is specially trained to administer acupuncture.
Osteopathic Manipulative ***Treatment (98925–98929)***	An osteopathic physician performs osteopathic manipulative treatment (OMT) manually (by hand), which involves moving joints and muscles through various methods, like applying pressure. This treatment can help to alleviate disorders like migraine headaches and carpal tunnel syndrome.
Chiropractic Manipulative ***Treatment (98940–98943)***	A chiropractor, called a doctor of chiropractic (DC), is a healthcare professional who focuses on improving patients' conditions by manipulating body areas, typically the spine, to improve structure and function of specific sites (■ Figure 34-3). Chiropractors manually massage, adjust, and manipulate the spinal column to treat conditions like low back pain. They do not prescribe medications. CPT divides chiropractic manipulative treatment by the total number of *spinal regions* manipulated, including cervical, thoracic, lumbar, and sacral regions. There are also *extraspinal* regions, which include the head, upper and lower extremities, abdomen, and rib cage.
Education and Training for ***Patient Self-Management*** ***(98960–98962)***	Services include educating and training patients on managing their conditions, such as liver disease, cancer, or mental disorders. A physician prescribes services for the patient, and a nonphysician healthcare professional, such as a nurse, performs them using a standardized curriculum (standard plan for what to teach the patient and the frequency of teaching sessions). Education and training can be in individual or group sessions involving patients who suffer from the same condition. CPT divides codes by the number of patients present during a session.
Non-Face-To-Face ***Nonphysician*** ***Services (98966–98969)***	Remember that most E/M codes include face-to-face time between the physician and the patient. These services are for healthcare professionals who are *not* physicians, and the services are provided *without* the patient present. There are two types of services, *telephone* and *online*, where the healthcare professional provides medical assessments and medical discussion to an established patient, the patient's parent(s) or guardian(s), or another healthcare professional. Note that there are extensive CPT guidelines for these services that you should review.

continued

■ **TABLE 34-3** *continued*

Subsection	Types of Procedures
Special Services, Procedures and Reports (99000–99091)	This subsection includes many different types of services, including an emergency office visit, an after-hours office visit, educational supplies given to a patient (books, pamphlets), special reports that an insurance requests that give further information about a patient's case, and travel time spent escorting a patient to another location. Some of the services are provided in addition to another basic service.
Qualifying Circumstances for Anesthesia (99100–99140)	You learned about qualifying circumstances for anesthesia in Chapter 20. , which are codes to report for anesthesia given to patients under special circumstances, like patients who are over age 70 or under age 1, or patients who have an emergent condition. Remember that insurances may reimburse for these codes because they show that the anesthesia case was more complex than with other types of patients.
Moderate (Conscious) Sedation (99143–99150)	You also learned about moderate (conscious) sedation in Chapter 20. Note that codes in this subsection have many related CPT guidelines that you should review.
	• These codes represent moderate (conscious) sedation, other than the codes that you normally assign from the Anesthesia chapter in CPT. They include physician services to administer anesthesia when the same physician also performs the procedure. They can also include a second physician administering sedation while a different physician performs the service.
	• Services may also involve another healthcare professional to assist in monitoring the patient's level of consciousness and physiological status during the procedure.
Other Services and Procedures (99170–99199)	You can find a small variety of services in this subsection, including visual tests and physician attendance when a patient receives oxygen.
Home Health Procedures/ Services (99500–99602)	Nonphysician healthcare professionals report these services rendered to patients in their homes, including mechanical ventilation care, stoma care (care of an opening, such as a colostomy—an opening in the abdomen where stool from the colon drains into a bag), counseling, or fecal impaction (dry feces impacted in the rectum that the patient cannot pass; the healthcare professional can administer enemas or remove the feces manually).
Medication Therapy Management Services (99605–99607)	A pharmacist (healthcare professional specializing in medication use) provides this face-to-face service, including assessing the patient's health history and discussing proper dosage, drug interactions, and the benefits of treatment. CPT divides the codes by a new or established patient and the total visit time.

Figure 34-3 ■ A chiropractor manipulates a patient's spine.

Photo credit: Lisa F. Young/ Shutterstock.

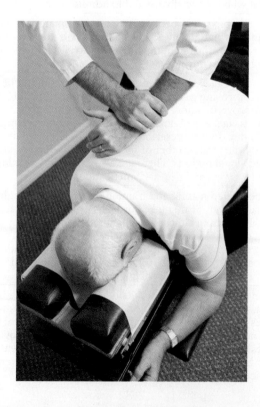

DESTINATION: MEDICARE

In this Medicare exercise, you will learn more about Medicare coverage of speech and medical nutrition therapy. Follow the instructions listed next to access the Medicare National Coverage Determinations Manual:

1. Go to the website http://www.cms.gov.
2. At the top of the screen on the banner bar, choose *Regulations and Guidance.*
3. Under Guidance, choose *Manuals.*
4. On the left side of the screen, under Manuals, choose *Internet-Only Manuals (IOMs).*
5. Scroll down to Publication *#100-03 Medicare National Coverage Determinations (NCD) Manual,* and click *100-03.*
6. Scroll down to the list of Downloads, and choose *Chapter 1—Coverage Determinations Part 3.*

Answer the following questions, using the search function (Ctrl + F) to find information that you need:

1. Does Medicare cover speech language pathology services to treat dysphagia? _____
2. Can speech therapy include modifying the patient's diet? _____
3. Which part of Medicare covers medical nutrition therapy services? _____
4. What diagnoses are covered for medical nutrition therapy? _____
5. What requirements must a patient meet in order for Medicare to cover both MNT and DSMT? _____

TAKE A BREAK

Congratulations! You made it through the Medicine chapter! Give yourself a pat on the back! Let's take a break and then review more about other medicine procedures and services.

> **Exercise 34.8**   Additional Medicine Subsections

Part 1—Theory

Instructions: Fill in the blank with the best answer.

1. These services, which can be provided over the phone or online, involve the healthcare professional providing medical assessments and medical discussion to an established patient, the patient's parent(s) or guardian(s), or another healthcare professional. _____

2. A(n) _____ is the speed at which the clinician delivers an infusion.

3. _____ includes multiple measurements of functions and activities of the heart, muscles, brain, and eyes during sleep.

4. A pharmacist provides this face-to-face service, including assessing the patient's health history and discussing proper dosage, drug interactions, and the benefits of treatment. _____

5. Services to expose a patient to allergenic extracts or insect venoms to increase his immunity to the allergen are called _____ .

6. What is the name of the service that a registered dietician provides to patients who need assistance managing their nutritional needs? _____

Part 2—Coding

Instructions: Review each patient's case, and then assign codes for the procedure(s), appending a modifier when appropriate. Optional: For additional practice, assign the patient's diagnosis code(s) (ICD-9-CM).

1. Jimmy Nino, age 13, presents for allergy testing since he has been sneezing and may have allergies. Dr. Woodley,

continued

TAKE A BREAK *continued*

an allergist, performs percutaneous tests using allergen extracts, immediate type reaction, for 10 tests in the Allergy Clinic at Williton Medical Center. Jimmy is found to be allergic to animal dander.

Diagnosis code(s): _____

Procedure code(s): _____

2. During a previous visit with Dr. North, a neurologist, Dorothy Louis, age 54, states that she has insomnia and feels tired all the time. Dr. North recommends a sleep study. Mrs. Louis presents to the Sleep Lab at Williton Medical Center today for a sleep study that is attended by a technologist. Dr. North interprets the sleep study and diagnoses Mrs. Louis with severe obstructive sleep apnea. He refers Mrs. Louis to Dr. Gupta, a pulmonologist, for further treatment.

Diagnosis code(s): _____

Procedure code(s): _____

3. Maddie Johns, a 10-year-old girl, was referred by her pediatrician to Dr. Schafer, a pediatric psychiatrist for compulsive behavior. Dr. Schafer conducts several limited developmental tests of the patient and today in his office, he discusses the results of the tests with the patient's mother. Code only the developmental testing, which lasts an hour. Dr. Schafer diagnoses Maddie with compulsive disorder.

Diagnosis code(s): _____

Procedure code(s): _____

4. Terence Gordon, age 57, is seen in the Infusion Suite at Williton Medical Center for chemotherapy administration to treat carcinoma of the left lung. Dr. Levy, an oncologist, performs thoracentesis, inserting a catheter into the pleura and injecting chemotherapy into the pleural cavity.

Diagnosis code(s): _____

Procedure code(s): _____

5. Regina Scott, age 83, has had a cerebrovascular accident and has paralysis on the left side. She was an inpatient at Williton but is now at home. Dr. North, her neurologist at Williton, orders physical therapy exercise three times a week to help the patient regain movement on the left side of her body. Today, she arrives at Windy Physical Therapy Clinic for her second treatment. Randy Thomas, a certified physical therapist (PT), provides gait training for 30 minutes.

Diagnosis code(s): _____

Procedure code(s): _____

6. Lisa Lolly, age 38, visits Dr. Wilson, an osteopathic physician, with a chief complaint of low back pain. Dr. Wilson manipulates Mrs. Lolly's lumbar spine and provides partial relief of the pain. Mrs. Lolly will return for another manipulation next week.

Diagnosis code(s): _____

Procedure code(s): _____

CHAPTER REVIEW

Multiple Choice

Instructions: Circle one best answer to complete each statement.

1. This procedure teaches patients to regulate certain body functions through mental or physical exercises.
   a. Photodynamic therapy
   b. Biofeedback
   c. Electroencephalography
   d. Nerve conduction tests

2. _____ treatment involves the provider communicating face-to-face with the patient to determine the cause(s) of a specific condition and developing ways to effectively cope with it.
   a. Medication
   b. Self-management
   c. Psychotherapy
   d. Acupuncture

3. This test evaluates muscular activity of the esophagus at rest and during swallowing to diagnose esophageal disorders involving motility or causes of heartburn.
   a. Esophageal motility study
   b. Esophageal movement study
   c. Gastroesophageal motility study
   d. Gastroesophageal movement study

4. During this procedure, the clinician measures the shape and variations of the cornea when diseases or trauma cause it to be misshapen.
   a. Tonography
   b. Computerized corneal topography
   c. Gonioscopy
   d. Sensorimotor examination

5. What is the name of the test that uses Doppler ultrasound of the extremities to diagnose circulatory disorders that restrict blood flow to the extremities, like PAD?
   a. Extremity venous studies
   b. Visceral vascular studies
   c. Extremity arterial studies
   d. Cerebrovascular arterial studies

6. These tests are performed to diagnose neuromuscular diseases, completed by measuring visual, auditory, and automatic nerve reflexes.
   a. Autonomic function tests
   b. Nerve conduction tests
   c. Muscle and range of motion tests
   d. Evoked potentials and reflex tests

7. What is the name of the test that uses sound waves to create a moving picture of the heart?
   a. Echocardiography
   b. Ultrasonography
   c. Cardiography
   d. Intracardiac electrophysiological study

8. _____ involves connecting a patient to dialysis equipment through a dialysis access such as an AV fistula.
   a. Hemofiltration
   b. Peritoneal dialysis
   c. Hemodialysis
   d. Hemoperfusion

9. What is the name of the healthcare professional who works with patients with hearing, balance, and related ear problems?
   a. Speech language pathologist
   b. Audiologist
   c. Chiropractor
   d. Acupuncturist

10. This pulmonary function test measures the ability of the lungs to inhale and exhale as the patient uses a mouthpiece to breathe in and out.
    a. Thoracic study
    b. Tympanometry
    c. Bekesy audiometry
    d. Spirometry

Coding Assignments

Instructions: Review the patient's case and then assign the appropriate procedure code(s), appending a modifier when appropriate. Optional: For additional practice, assign the patient's diagnosis code(s) (ICD-9-CM).

1. The Landry family meets with Tara Hopley, a genetic counselor at the Genetics Department in Williton Medical Center, for a group session with five other patients. The Landrys' child Lily, age two, has Down's syndrome. Mrs. Landry would like to have another child but is worried that Down's will occur again. Miss Hopley will investigate the family genetic history and assess the risks. The genetic counseling session lasts 30 minutes.

   Diagnosis code(s): _____

   Procedure code(s): _____

2. Tonya Jones, a 10-year-old with sickle cell anemia, is referred by her hematologist to Dr. Knoll, a psychologist in the Behavioral Health Department at Williton Medical Center, for an initial health and behavioral assessment. The patient experiences a lot of pain and is withdrawn. The focus of Dr. Knoll's assessment is on social, biological, and psychological factors related to pain management and managing sickle cell disease. Dr. Knoll assesses the patient with the Pediatric Pain Questionnaire, interviews the child's parents, and interviews Williton Medical Center clinicians who make up the sickle cell and pain treatment teams that care for the patient. Dr. Knoll also measures interactions and behaviors among the child, clinical staff, and parents. The assessment takes 30 minutes, and Dr. Knoll discusses further treatment options with clinical team members and the patient's parents.

   Diagnosis code(s): _____

   Procedure code(s): _____

3. Gina O'Reilly, age 36, has cancer of the left breast with metastasis to the bone of the spinal column. Dr. Levy, an oncologist, sees Mrs. O'Reilly in the Infusion Suite at Williton Medical Center for chemotherapy infusion administered intravenously for 50 minutes.

   Diagnosis code(s): _____

   Procedure code(s): _____

4. Sheilita Crystal, a 34-year-old patient, sees Dr. Lawson, a dermatologist, in his office for a consultation for severe **dermatitis herpetiformis** (skin inflammation). Dr. Wolf, the patient's internal medicine physician, requested the consultation. Dr. Lawson provides a comprehensive history and physical examination with moderately complex medical decision-making. Dr. Lawson determines that Miss Crystal will benefit

from photochemotherapy (ultraviolet light therapy combined with medication). Since Miss Crystal lives more than 50 miles away from Dr. Lawson's office, he starts the treatment on the same day as the consultation. He supervises eight hours of treatment. Dr. Lawson submits medical documentation for the patient's services to Dr. Wolf. Miss Crystal will return to Dr. Lawson's office in three months.

Diagnosis code(s): _____

Procedure code(s): _____

5. Dr. North, a neurologist, refers Brenda Green, age 63, to attend sessions with a chronic disease support group for help with self-managing Parkinson's disease (PD). Mary O'Connor, a certified registered nurse practitioner (CRNP), leads the group at Williton, which consists of individuals with chronic disorders. Today, Mrs. Green attends a 30-minute session with six other patients. The group addresses issues such as medication management, exercise, chronic fatigue, nutrition, and treatment options.

Diagnosis code(s): _____

Procedure code(s): _____

6. Bob Hines, age 37, is an insulin-dependent diabetic who has a nonhealing ulcer on his left ankle. He receives hyperbaric oxygen therapy (oxygen delivered in a closed chamber) today at Williton Medical Center under the direction of Dr. Buck, a pulmonologist.

Diagnosis code(s): _____

Procedure code(s): _____

7. Norma Morgan, age 58, has osteomyelitis (infection of the bone or bone marrow) of the left ankle. She was recently hospitalized for the infection and received intravenous antibiotics in the hospital and is now continuing infusion at home with the help of a home health nurse. The nurse, Anna Martin, RN, sees Ms. Morgan today and administers an antibiotic infusion over 1 hour. She will return each day to evaluate the progress of the infection and administer another dose of the antibiotic.

dermatitis herpetiformis (dər-mə-tī′-tis hər-pə-tə-for′-məs)

Diagnosis code(s): _____

Procedure code(s): _____

8. Dennis Hughes, age 58, is seen in the warfarin clinic at Williton Medical Center. (Warfarin is a medication that helps prevent blood clots and requires extensive medical management and monitoring.) This is the patient's initial visit with Robert Willis, Ph.D., Pharmacy Director, to discuss the medication, side effects, and the patient's concerns about long-term use of an anticoagulant. The visit lasts 30 minutes.

Diagnosis code(s): _____

Procedure code(s): _____

9. Dr. Rheam, a general dentist, sees Don Samir, age five, at King River Dental Clinic. Dr. Rheam diagnoses dental caries in one of the patient's teeth, and the decay is too advanced to be remedied with a filling. Dr. Rheam determines that he should extract the tooth. He discusses his findings with Mrs. Samir, the patient's mother, and schedules Don for the extraction. Because Don is frightened of needles and does not enjoy sitting still, Dr. Rheam recommends conscious sedation during the procedure, and Mrs. Samir agrees. Today, Dr. Rheam performs the extraction, and Dr. Bickel, an anesthesiologist, administers conscious sedation to Don and monitors him throughout the procedure so that he remains comfortable and relaxed. Dr. Bickel assigns a P1 modifier to the patient's case. The sedation lasts 30 minutes. Code only for the conscious sedation for Dr. Bickel.

Diagnosis code(s): _____

Procedure code(s): _____

10. Tyrone Smith, age 48, presents to Dr. Shawn's office with a complaint of pain in his right hip. The chiropractor conducts an assessment and aligns two spinal regions. The alignment brings instant relief of the pain. Mr. Smith is instructed to call the office if the pain returns.

Diagnosis code(s): _____

Procedure code(s): _____

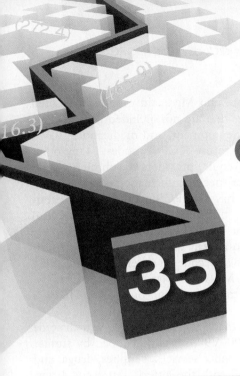

Coding with HCPCS

Learning Objectives

After completing this chapter, you should be able to

- Spell and define the key terminology in this chapter.
- Describe the structure of the HCPCS code set.
- Explain how to code from the HCPCS code set.
- Describe how to use the Table of Drugs.
- Explain when to append HCPCS modifiers.

35

Key Terms

miscellaneous codes
orthotics
permanent national codes

prosthetics
radiopharmaceutical
temporary national codes
transportation services

INTRODUCTION

Congratulations! You have reached the final coding destination of your journey! You have traveled many coding miles, and you are almost to the end of this book. This is the last chapter on coding, and then you will learn more about professionalism in Chapter 36. Your last coding stop is to learn how to assign HCPCS codes. Do you remember learning about HCPCS codes in Chapter 2? The Healthcare Common Procedure Coding System (HCPCS) has two divisions, or levels, of codes:

- Level I—Current Procedural Terminology, Fourth Edition (CPT-4) Codes
- Level II—National Healthcare Common Procedure Coding System (HCPCS) Codes

You already learned about Level I—CPT-4 coding and practiced assigning CPT-4 codes in many different chapters. In this chapter, you will learn how to assign Level II—HCPCS codes. Only providers and insurances in the U.S. utilize Level II—HCPCS codes. They refer to Level II—HCPCS codes simply as *HCPCS codes*, and that is what they are also called in this chapter.

Let's move forward to your last coding stop and learn more about HCPCS codes and how to assign them!

"Success is not final, failure is not fatal; it is the courage to continue that counts."—WINSTON CHURCHILL

HCPCS CODES

Remember that the CMS, which oversees Medicare and Medicaid programs, created HCPCS codes as a classification system for services that are not included in CPT-4, as well as for nonphysician services, medical supplies, equipment, and medications. CMS requires providers who bill Medicare and Medicaid to use HCPCS codes. Many other insurances, including Workers' Compensation, also require providers to submit HCPCS codes, so it is best to check with individual payers for specific information.

Examples of services, supplies, and items that have HCPCS codes include ambulance services, medical and surgical supplies, drugs, nutrition therapy, durable medical equipment, orthotic and prosthetic procedures, hearing and vision services, and many others. CMS maintains HCPCS codes, including quarterly and yearly revisions, additions, and deletions. CMS may also revise, add, and delete codes at other times during the year. You can find current HCPCS codes on the CMS website at http://www.cms.gov/Medicare/Coding/HCPCSReleaseCodeSets/index.html, or you can purchase a HCPCS manual from many different publishers.

There are almost 3,000 HCPCS codes. Each is made up of a letter (A–V, with some letters not used), followed by four numbers (A0000–V9999), and grouped by similar services or items. The letter represents a group of similar services, supplies, drugs, and equipment. For example, HCPCS codes beginning with the letter J represent drugs, called J codes, and codes beginning with the letter D represent dental services. Examples of specific codes and their meanings include

- **A4206**—Syringe with needle, sterile, 1 cc or less, each
- **E0117**—Crutch, underarm, articulating, spring assisted, each
- **G0390**—Trauma response team associated with hospital critical care service
- **J0360**—Injection, hydralazine HCl, up to 20 mg

Providers and insurances refer to HCPCS codes as A codes, B codes, C codes, and so on, depending on the first letter of the code.

It is important to note that the American Dental Association (ADA) created HCPCS dental service codes (D codes), called Current Dental Terminology (CDT) codes, for diagnostic, preventative, and surgical procedures. The ADA holds the copyright of HCPCS D-codes, so CMS no longer publishes them with the other national HCPCS codes. Providers who need to assign a HCPCS code for dental services must obtain the codes from the ADA or purchase them from a publisher that is authorized to reprint them.

Providers Who Assign HCPCS Codes

Recall that providers from various specialties can assign HCPCS codes for patients' encounters, including physicians, hospitals, outpatient clinics, and urgent care centers. Other providers who assign HCPCS codes include pharmacies, ambulance services, and durable medical equipment suppliers.

Categories of HCPCS Codes

HCPCS codes can fall under one of three categories:

1. Permanent national codes
2. Temporary national codes
3. Miscellaneous codes

Let's discuss each category next.

Permanent National Codes   CMS created a HCPCS workgroup, which determines whether to add, revise, or delete HCPCS codes, and some of the workgroup's members include insurance representatives. The HCPCS workgroup oversees **permanent national codes** in the HCPCS code set, that all U.S. providers and insurances can use for billing and statistical purposes.

■ TABLE 35-1 **TEMPORARY NATIONAL CODES**

Type of Code	Description
C codes	Outpatient hospitals that Medicare pays under the Outpatient Prospective Payment System (OPPS) report C codes for new technology procedures, drugs, biologicals, radiopharmaceuticals, magnetic resonance angiography (MRA), and devices. C codes are also called *pass-through codes* because for many of them, Medicare pays hospitals separately from the OPPS payment. C codes have expiration dates for separate reimbursement under Medicare, but hospitals are still required to report C codes on claims, even though Medicare does not pay for them. Non-OPPS hospitals can also report C codes on claims to Medicare or other insurances.
G codes	Identify professional health care procedures and services, such as prostate or colorectal cancer screenings.
H codes	Individual state Medicaid agencies use certain H codes to identify mental health services, such as alcohol and drug treatment.
K codes	Medicare Administrative Contractors (MACs) for durable medical equipment (DME) providers use K codes to identify certain products and supplies when they create coverage policies.
Q codes	Q codes identify drugs, biologicals, and specific types of medical equipment or services.
S codes	Certain insurances and Medicaid use S codes to report drugs, services, and supplies to implement policies, programs, or claims processing. Medicare does not recognize these codes.
T codes	Individual state Medicaid agencies use T codes for specific items and services, and other insurers can also use them.

Temporary National Codes   The HCPCS workgroup also creates **temporary national codes** for services and supplies that do not have a permanent code. The workgroup creates these codes in response to Medicare's needs, but any provider and insurance can use temporary codes. The workgroup can add temporary codes before the scheduled January 1 yearly HCPCS code set update. Temporary codes remain temporary indefinitely until the workgroup decides to replace them with permanent codes. When the workgroup replaces a temporary code with a permanent one, it deletes the temporary code from the code set and provides a cross-reference to the new permanent code. Refer to ■ TABLE 35-1 for the types of temporary national codes.

Miscellaneous Codes   HCPCS permanent national codes include **miscellaneous codes**, or codes that are not otherwise specified, which you will find throughout the HCPCS code set. Providers use miscellaneous codes for items and services for which there is no permanent or temporary national code. Examples of miscellaneous or not-otherwise-specified codes include

- **A9999**—Miscellaneous DME supply or accessory, not otherwise specified
- **J9999**—Not otherwise classified, antineoplastic drugs
- **V5274**—Assistive listening device, not otherwise specified

Miscellaneous codes allow providers to immediately bill insurances for a service or item as soon as the FDA approves its use, even though there is no permanent or temporary code that describes it. When providers report miscellaneous codes, the HCPCS workgroup also avoids creating permanent or temporary codes for items or services that providers rarely furnish.

Medicare and other payers manually review claims with miscellaneous codes, so providers must submit supporting documentation to payers to explain why the patient needs the item or service. Before reporting a miscellaneous code, you should always check with individual payers to ensure that there is not another permanent or temporary code to describe the service that the payer requires instead.

Providers can use a miscellaneous code while the HCPCS workgroup is considering a request for a new temporary or permanent code for the item or service. Any provider or insurance can submit a request to the workgroup for modifying the HCPCS national code set, which involves completing a request to the workgroup with specific information about the new item or service. You can find more information on the CMS website at http://cms.gov/Medicare/Coding/MedHCPCSGenInfo/index.html.

HCPCS Codes with CPT Equivalent Codes

It is also important to remember that a service may have *both* a CPT-4 code and a HCPCS code that represents it. Many of these services are for screening exams. The HCPCS code descriptor may give more detail about the service than the CPT code descriptor. If a patient has *Medicare or Medicaid*, then you should *always report the HCPCS code* for the service, rather than the CPT-4 code. CMS has specific regulations for reimbursing screening exams, including the patient's age (such as age 50 or older) and/or the frequency of exams (such as every four years). When the patient has *another* insurance, then you should *report the CPT-4 code* unless the insurance requires the HCPCS code. Always check individual payer coding guidelines to be sure so that you know whether to report the HCPCS code or the CPT-4 code. Here is an example of a HCPCS code with a CPT equivalent code that describes the same type of service:

G0104—Colorectal cancer screening; flexible sigmoidoscopy

45330—Sigmoidoscopy, flexible, diagnostic; with or without collection of specimen(s) by brushing or washing (separate procedure)

Recall that a provider can enter specific codes for a service into the computer software's chargemaster to bill certain insurances with specific codes. In other words, a provider can enter both a CPT-4 code and a HCPCS code for the same service into the chargemaster's line item. That way, depending on the insurance's coding requirements, the computer will report *either* the CPT-4 or the HCPCS code on the claim form.

As a coder, you would need to assign only the CPT-4 code for any patient because the computer would automatically report the HCPCS code to the insurance if the insurance requires the HCPCS code instead of the CPT. However, you, or an information technology staff member, would first have to identify services that have *both* a CPT and a HCPCS code, enter the codes for the service line item in the chargemaster, and identify insurances that require the HCPCS code. Without this information, the software will not report an equivalent HCPCS code when you assign a CPT code.

TAKE A BREAK

Good job! Let's take a break and review more about HCPCS codes.

Exercise 35.1 HCPCS Codes

Instructions: Fill in each blank with the best answer.

1. _____ created HCPCS codes to provide a classification system for services that are not included in CPT-4, as well as for nonphysician services, medical supplies, equipment, and medications.

2. The _____ of a HCPCS code represents a group of similar services, supplies, drugs, and equipment.

3. The HCPCS workgroup oversees _____, which make up the HCPCS code set that all U.S. providers and insurances can use for billing and statistical purposes.

4. _____ exist for services and supplies that do not have a permanent code.

5. Medicare Administrative Contractors (MACs) for durable medical equipment (DME) providers use _____ to identify certain products and supplies when creating coverage policies.

6. Providers use _____ for items and services for which there is no permanent or temporary national code.

STRUCTURE OF THE HCPCS CODE SET

You may use one of many types of HCPCS coding manuals to assign HCPCS codes or obtain the HCPCS code set from the CMS website, which you can print or access electronically. Regardless of the type of manual that you use, you will need to be familiar with the structure of the code set and know how to locate codes. The HCPCS code set is categorized as follows:

- HCPCS Index
- Tabular List
- Table of Drugs
- Modifiers

HCPCS Index

You can locate the HCPCS Index, also called the Alpha-Numeric Index, at the beginning of the HCPCS coding manual. Turn to the Index in your HCPCS manual. Notice that the Index is arranged alphabetically by main terms, just like the Index for both CPT and ICD-9-CM manuals. Depending on the HCPCS manual that you use, there could be one column of main terms, or several columns. Browse through the Index to become more familiar with the services and items listed there.

Just as in the CPT manual, you may see entries listed on each page in bold at the top left and at the top right. Information printed on the top left appears as the first entry on that page. Information on the top right is the last entry on that page. This placement helps you to quickly navigate through the information you are searching for on that page, or it directs you to move to another page. You may also find code ranges printed on the side of each page.

Notice that main terms in the HCPCS manual are not indented and may appear in bold, depending on the HCPCS manual that you reference. Main terms have corresponding subterms indented underneath. Subterms may also have additional subterms (■ FIGURE 35-1).

The first step in identifying a main term is to locate it in the medical documentation. Then locate it in the HCPCS Index, and identify any subterms that apply to the main term. Keep in mind that there are different ways to locate the same code(s) in the Index, depending on the main term you are searching. You can search for the *name* of an item, the *type of service*, or the *anatomic site* involved.

For example, a patient's medical documentation states that the patient had a prostate specific antigen test (PSA). Let's search for *prostate* as the main term in the Index. Did you notice that *specific antigen test (PSA)* is a subterm under prostate? Did you also notice that the subterm lists code G0103 to cross-reference to the Tabular List? The Tabular List is where you will cross-reference HCPCS codes, and you will learn more about it later in this chapter.

You could have also started your search using *screening* as the main term and then found *prostate specific antigen test (PSA)* as a subterm, which also lists code G0103 to cross-reference to the Tabular. Sometimes the same word can serve as a main term or as a subterm, depending on where you begin your search in the Index. As you continue to practice finding main terms in the Index, you will find faster ways of locating the information that you need.

Code Ranges   When you find a main term and any modifying terms, you will see one of the following types of code choices or ranges:

- one code
- codes separated by a comma
- one or more code ranges separated by a hyphen
- code(s) separated by commas, along with a code range separated by a hyphen

Clamp	◀Main term
dialysis, A4910, A4918, A4920	◀Subterm of Clamp
external urethral, A4356	◀Subterm of dialysis

Figure 35-1 ■ Index entry for the main term clamp, showing subterms.

Figure 35-2 ■ Examples of code choices when referencing main terms in the index.

Nasal application device, K0183

Harness, E0942, E0944, E0945

Heat
    application, E0200-E0239
    lamp, E0200, E0205

Multidisciplinary services, H2000-H2001, T1023-T1028

Hearing devices, V5000-V5299, L8614

Refer to ■ FIGURE 35-2 to review code choices for main terms and subterms. Main terms appear in bold.

Just as with code choices in the CPT Index, when the HCPCS Index provides more than one code choice or code range, it is *not an option* to choose just one of the codes listed. Instead, you must cross-reference *all* of the codes listed to ensure correct code assignment. You learned never to code directly from the Index of ICD-9-CM or CPT-4, and you should never code directly from the HCPCS Index, either. *Always* cross-reference codes in the Index to the Tabular List of the HCPCS manual. Even if there is only one code choice, it does not mean that the code is the correct one. You must cross-reference it, read additional notes, and follow any coding instructions before final code assignment because it may lead you to a completely different code.

Cross-Reference Terms
See and *see also* are cross-reference terms in the HCPCS Index, and you should pay close attention to them to ensure correct code assignment:

- *See*—You are in the wrong place to find the service, supply, drug, or equipment you are searching for, and you must instead look elsewhere, as in the following example from the HCPCS Index:

    RespiGam, see Respiratory syncytial virus immune globulin

- *See also*—You should check an *additional* place in the Index to ensure that you cross-reference the correct code in the Tabular List. Refer to the following example from the HCPCS Index:

    Kartop patient lift, toilet or bathroom (see also Lift), E0625

Depending on the HCPCS manual that you use, you may also find the cross-reference *see* in the *Tabular List,* directing you to another code.

Tabular List

CMS arranges the Tabular List by codes in alphanumeric order, beginning with codes that start with the letter A, followed by four numbers listed in numeric order. Depending on the HCPCS manual that you reference, the Tabular List may include helpful coding notes, CMS coding and billing guidelines, and other information to help you assign the correct code, such as identifying codes with a specific color that represents additional information. You can also find CMS coding guidelines on the CMS website.

Turn to the Tabular List in your HCPCS manual as you refer to ■ TABLE 35-2 to review the code ranges, arranged from A to V, and descriptions of the types of services and supplies they contain.

Notice in the Tabular List that *none* of the code descriptors is indented. Each code has a standalone code descriptor that does not share part of its descriptor with any other code, such as the indented codes that you find in the CPT manual. Review the following examples of HCPCS code descriptors:

- **A4207**—Syringe with needle, sterile 2 cc, each
- **A4208**—Syringe with needle, sterile 3 cc, each
- **L3208**—Surgical boot, each, infant

■TABLE 35-2   **HCPCS CODE RANGES AND DESCRIPTIONS**

HCPCS Code Range	Description
A0021–A9999	Transportation services, such as ambulance; medical and surgical supplies, including supplies for urinary incontinence (loss of urinary bladder control), ostomy, respiratory, and dialysis; and radiopharmaceuticals (radioactive substances used for diagnostic or therapeutic services).
B4000–B9999	Supplies, equipment, and nutritional products for enteral and parenteral nutrition.
C1300–C9899	New technology procedures, drugs, biologicals, radiopharmaceuticals, MRA, and devices for outpatient hospitals to report.
D Codes	The ADA holds the copyright to D-codes. They are not in the HCPCS code set.
E0100–E8002	DME for patients' activities of daily living, including crutches and oxygen equipment.
F	Not in use.
G0008–G9147	Procedures and services that may or may not have equivalent CPT codes, such as screening exams.
H0001–H2037	Mental health services, including treatment for alcohol and drug abuse.
I	Not in use.
J0120–J9999	Drugs that the patient does not self-administer.
K0001–K0899	DME for which there are no other HCPCS codes available, such as power wheelchairs.
L0112–L9900	Orthotics (devices that help to regain functions) (■ FIGURE 35-3) and prosthetics (replacement body parts) (■ FIGURE 35-4), including cervical collars, lumbar support, artificial limbs, or male vacuum erection systems.
M0064–M0301	Six codes in this section represent an office visit for prescription drugs and miscellaneous therapies.
N	Not in use.
O	Not in use.
P2028–P9615	Pathology and laboratory services and blood products.
Q0035–Q9968	Temporary codes for drugs and supplies.
R0070–R0076	Transportation of portable diagnostic radiology equipment to provider locations.
S0012–S9999	Drugs, services, and supplies for Medicaid and other insurances except Medicare.
T1000–T5999	Services and supplies for Medicaid.
U	Not in use.
V2020–V5364	Vision supplies, like eyeglasses; hearing services and supplies; and speech language pathology services.

- **L3209**—Surgical boot, each, child
- **V5210**—Hearing aid, BICROS, in the ear
- **V5220**—Hearing aid, BICROS, behind the ear

Did you notice that *none* of the related codes in the examples shares part of a code descriptor? Each code has its own descriptor. Refer to the following example to learn more about assigning a HCPCS code.

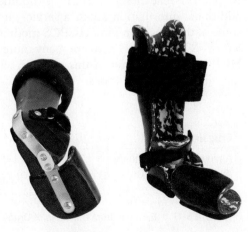

Figure 35-3 ■ Orthotics to correct a clubfoot.

Photo credit: g215/Shutterstock. com.

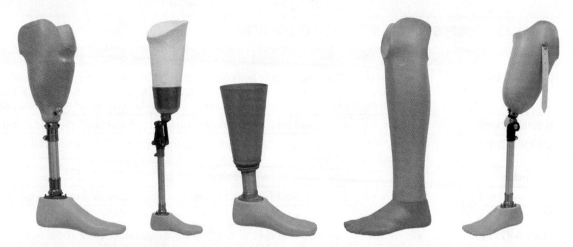

Figure 35-4 ■ Prosthetic legs.

Photo credit: Mayovskyy Andrew/Shutterstock.com.

Example: Mr. Sims, a 42-year-old established patient, returns for a visit with Dr. Avery, a podiatrist, for fitting of a heel wedge in his left shoe to treat plantar fasciitis (inflammation of the plantar fascia on the sole of the foot, which overstretching causes). The patient, who is an athlete, has been suffering from severe heel pain, and Dr. Avery would like him to try the heel wedge to determine if it will help reduce the pain.

Search the Index for the main term *wedges, shoe*, which directs you to codes L3340–L3420. Assign code **L3350-LT**, since it represents a *single heel wedge* that Mr. Sims received for his *left* shoe. The patient's diagnosis code is **728.71** (main term *fasciitis*, subterm *plantar*).

Table of Drugs

Remember that there are HCPCS codes that describe drugs, which include generic or brand name drugs listed alphabetically. Turn to the Table of Drugs to review some of the drugs listed there. Notice that there are four columns with the drug name, quantity, route of administration, and HCPCS code (■ FIGURE 35-5). In the figure, the abbreviation IV is for intravenous administration, and the abbreviation IM is for intramuscular. We will review more about assigning codes from the Table of Drugs later in this chapter.

Modifiers

Remember that there are HCPCS modifiers as well as CPT modifiers to help provide additional information about a service, item, or procedure. You already learned about some of the most common HCPCS modifiers published in the CPT manual, like -LT for left or -RT for right. There are many more HCPCS modifiers that are included with the HCPCS manual. Later in this chapter, we will review more about appending HCPCS modifiers to HCPCS codes.

Drug Name	Unit Per	Route	Code
Aminophylline/Aminophyllin	up to 250 mg	IV	J0280
Amiodarone HCI	30 mg	IV	J0282
Amitriptyline HCI	up to 20 mg	IM	J1320

Figure 35-5 ■ Example from the Table of Drugs from the HCPCS Code Set.

TAKE A BREAK

Keep up the good work! Let's take a break and review more about the HCPCS code set structure.

Exercise 35.2   Structure of HCPCS Code Set

Part 1—Main Terms

Instructions: For each description of services, supplies, equipment, or drugs, identify the main term and subterm(s) to look for in the HCPCS Index. Then list the code(s) to cross-reference to the Tabular.

1. A physician orders a raised toilet seat for a patient to use at home, which the DME supplier provides.

   Main term/subterm(s): _____

   Code(s) to cross-reference: _____

2. A provider gives a female patient a female condom (pouch) for birth control purposes.

   Main term/subterm(s): _____

   Code(s) to cross-reference: _____

3. The physician changes a lead in a patient's pacemaker, which is a transvenous VDD single pass.

   Main term/subterm(s): _____

   Code(s) to cross-reference: _____

4. A primary care physician (PCP) gives a patient an enteral fiber additive to assist the patient in having regular bowel movements.

   Main term/subterm(s): _____

   Code(s) to cross-reference: _____

5. A physician assistant administers the hepatitis B vaccine to a patient.

   Main term/subterm(s): _____

   Code(s) to cross-reference: _____

6. A psychologist conducts a patient assessment for mental health services at an outpatient mental health facility.

   Main term/subterm(s): _____

   Code(s) to cross-reference: _____

Part 2—Theory

Instructions: Fill in each blank with the best answer.

1. What is another name for HCPCS Level II codes?
   _____.

2. What code range contains ambulance and transportation services? _____

3. The HCPCS Index list is arranged in what type of order? _____   _____

4. *True or False*: Once you locate the HCPCS code in the Index, there is no need to verify it in the Tabular list. _____

5. What is the name of the first word or term that you look for in the Index when you are trying to find a HCPCS code? _____

6. What is the HCPCS code range that includes enteral and parenteral nutrition? _____

CODING FROM THE HCPCS CODE SET

You will next learn about coding for services, supplies, equipment, drugs, and screenings in the Tabular List, from A codes to V codes (some letters are not used). You will also practice assigning HCPCS codes from various sections of the code set. Many times, providers assign HCPCS codes for a supply or equipment, in addition to CPT codes for the service related to the supply. An example would be a physical therapist who provides therapy to a patient and also fits the patient with a leg brace. There is a CPT code for the therapy and a HCPCS code for the leg brace. The physical therapist would submit codes for both the service and the supply on the insurance claim form.

When you reviewed the Tabular List of HCPCS codes, you probably noticed that there were hundreds of them! As you can imagine, we will not have time to review all of the codes in complete detail, but we will concentrate on specific types of HCPCS codes so that you can become more familiar with them, including A, B, E, J, and L codes. Turn to the codes in each code range as you read about them in the next sections. You can find all of the HCPCS code ranges with their descriptions in Table 35-2.

A Codes (A0021–A9999)

A codes include transportation services, medical and surgical supplies, and radiopharmaceuticals. Let's review more about these services and how to code for them.

Transportation Services   Ambulance providers use HCPCS codes to bill insurances for **transportation services** for transporting patients to the hospital, skilled nursing facility (SNF), or other destination. Ambulance providers must also append modifiers to HCPCS codes for ambulance services. You may think of an ambulance as the only way to transport patients, but there are other types of services that ambulance providers offer for transportation:

- Air ambulance, including fixed wing (airplane) or rotary wing (helicopter)
- Wheelchair van
- Taxi
- Bus
- Automobile

Ambulance providers can be *institutional-based* or *standalone.* Institutional-based ambulance providers are owned and/or operated by a hospital, critical access hospital (CAH), SNF, comprehensive outpatient rehabilitation facility (CORF), home health agency (HHA), or hospice provider. These providers bill claims on the UB-04.

Standalone ambulance providers, also called suppliers, are *not affiliated* with a healthcare provider. They include independently owned and operated ambulance services, volunteer fire and/or ambulance companies, or local government-run firehouse-based ambulances. They bill claims on the CMS-1500.

According to Medicare's guidelines, any vehicle used as an ambulance must be designed and equipped to respond to medical emergencies. In nonemergency situations, the vehicle must be capable of transporting patients with acute medical conditions. The vehicle must comply with state or local laws governing licensing and certification of an emergency medical transportation vehicle. At a minimum, the ambulance must contain a stretcher, linens, emergency medical supplies, oxygen equipment, and other lifesaving emergency medical equipment and must be equipped with emergency warning lights, sirens, and telecommunications equipment as required by state or local law. The communications equipment should include, at a minimum, a two-way voice radio or wireless telephone.

Ambulances can also offer basic life support (BLS) or advanced life support (ALS). At least two people must be present in a BLS ambulance, including one who is a state or local authority-certified emergency medical technician (EMT). An ALS ambulance must also have two people present, including one who is state- or local authority-certified as an EMT-Intermediate or an EMT-Paramedic.

Each state has guidelines for the type of care that EMTs can render, and EMTs can be certified on different levels (Basic, Intermediate, or Paramedic) depending on the complexity of care they provide. EMTs provide medical care to patients during transport to a hospital's emergency department or other facility, report their observations and actions to emergency department or facility staff, and may provide additional emergency treatment. After each run, EMTs document the trip, replace used supplies, and check equipment. If a transported patient has a contagious disease, then EMTs and paramedics decontaminate the interior of the ambulance and report cases to the proper authorities.

Turn to the transportation codes in your HCPCS manual, beginning with code A0021, to review the services. Here are some examples of transportation services:

- **A0130**—Nonemergency transportation: wheelchair van
- **A0427**—Ambulance service, advanced life support, emergency transport, level I (ALS I-Emergency)
- **A0428**—Ambulance service, basic life support, nonemergency transport (BLS)

Medicare Part B covers ambulance services with a base rate payment and a mileage payment, unless the ambulance transports the patient from one hospital to another, in which case ambulance services are covered under Part A. Always code and bill each ambulance service as *one unit*. A physician may order the ambulance transport, but not in all cases.

For ambulance service claims, providers and suppliers also report an *origin/destination modifier* for each ambulance trip. The first letter of the modifier represents the *origin*, and the second letter represents the *destination*. You have to create the modifier using the following list of origin and destination letters:

- D = Diagnostic or therapeutic site, other than a hospital or physician's office when these are used as origin codes (H or P)
- E = Residential, domiciliary, custodial facility
- G = Hospital-based ESRD facility
- H = Hospital
- I = Site of transfer (airport or helicopter pad) between modes of ambulance transport
- J = Freestanding ESRD facility
- N = Skilled nursing facility
- P = Physician's office
- R = Residence
- S = Scene of accident or acute event
- X = Intermediate stop at physician's office on way to hospital (destination code only)

Refer to the following example to learn more about appending an origin/destination modifier.

Example: You work as a coder for City Ambulance Service, a supplier. You assign HCPCS code A0429—*Ambulance service, basic life support, emergency transport (BLS-emergency)* for Mrs. Oliver, age 83, based on the EMT's documentation (Index entry: *Ambulance*). Mrs. Oliver's son called the ambulance because his mother collapsed on the kitchen floor while she was preparing dinner. The driver picked her up at home and then transported her to Williton Medical Center.

To append the correct modifier to the HCPCS code, refer to the list of origin/destination choices. The letter R represents *residence*, the origin, which is the first letter of the modifier. The letter H represents *hospital*, the destination, which is the second letter. Append modifier -RH to the HCPCS code, **A0429-RH**.

Medicare also requires that institutional-based ambulance providers append one of the following modifiers with every ambulance service *before* they append the origin/destination modifier:

- **QM**—Ambulance service provided under arrangement by a provider of services
- **QN**—Ambulance service furnished directly by a provider of services

Answering the following questions will help you to determine the type of transportation HCPCS code to assign:

- What type of vehicle was used to transport the patient: ground (ambulance), air fixed wing (airplane), or air rotary wing (helicopter)?
- What type of services did the patient need: emergency, nonemergency, ALS, BLS, or Specialty Care Transport (SCT)?
- How many miles did the ambulance have to travel from its origin to its destination?
- Were extra personnel involved?

Medical and Surgical Supplies   You can also find numerous A codes that represent medical and surgical supplies, including supplies to help treat patients with urinary incontinence, ostomies, respiratory problems, and patients receiving dialysis. Here are some examples:

- **A4252**—Blood ketone test or reagent strip, each
- **A4625**—Tracheostomy care kit for new tracheostomy
- **A4653**—Peritoneal dialysis catheter anchoring device, belt, each

Many types of healthcare providers and medical supply companies code and bill insurances for patients' supplies. Providers can purchase supplies directly from supply companies, dispense the supply to a patient, and then bill the patient's insurance. Or the supply company can provide the supply directly to the patient and then bill the patient's insurance.

It is important to note that insurances, including Medicare, have various coding, billing, and reimbursement guidelines for supplies, depending on the type of supply, patient's diagnosis, and circumstances involved when providing the supply. Some insurances will not pay separately for specific supplies that they consider to be a normal part of providing a service. Instead, the insurance issues *one payment* for the service that bundles the supply costs. Recall that insurances may also require healthcare providers to report code 99070 on insurance claims *instead of* a HCPCS code representing the supply.

> 99070—Supplies and materials (except spectacles), provided by the physician over and above those usually included with the office visit or other services rendered (list drugs, trays, supplies, or materials provided)

Because there are so many different coding and billing guidelines among insurances, it is always best to check with individual payers for specific information on their regulations for supplies.

Radiopharmaceuticals   A **radiopharmaceutical** is a radioactive drug that providers, such as hospitals, physicians, and SNFs, administer to patients intravenously and orally for diagnostic and therapeutic radiology procedures, which is called *nuclear medicine*. The radiopharmaceutical, also called *contrast* or a *tracer*, can help diagnose a patient's condition on a radiological scan and can also be used to treat diseases, such as bone cancer. The tracer emits radiation, which shows on a scan and helps physicians and clinicians to determine an organ's structure and function (■ FIGURE 35-6).

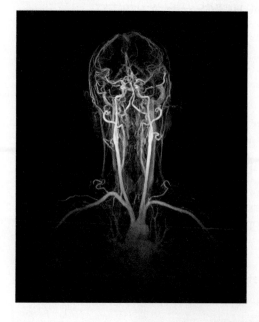

Figure 35-6 ■ Magnetic resonance angiography (MRA) of arteries in the head and neck which can be seen using a tracer.

Photo credit: bendao/Shutterstock.com.

The FDA oversees the approval process of radiopharmaceuticals to determine if they are safe for providers to deliver to patients. There are several A codes that represent radio-pharmaceuticals, including the following codes:

- **A9500**—Technetium tc-99m sestamibi, diagnostic, per study dose
- **A9509**—Iodine I-123 sodium iodide, diagnostic, per millicurie
- **A9546**—Cobalt Co-57/58, cyanocobalamin, diagnostic, per study dose, up to 1 microcurie

The measurements of millicurie and microcurie are based on a *curie (Ci)*, which is a unit of measurement for radioactivity.

Providers assign A codes for pharmaceuticals along with a CPT code for the radiology service. The following example shows the two codes reported for a patient's radiology scan.

- **78491**—Myocardial imaging, positron emission tomography (PET), perfusion; single study at rest or stress
- **A9555**—Rubidium Rb-82, diagnostic, per study dose, up to 60 millicuries

Medicare and other payers have specific guidelines regarding which radiopharmaceuticals providers are permitted to code and bill along with certain radiology services. They also have guidelines for radiopharmaceuticals that *should not be separately reported* because they are included with payment for the CPT code. You should always check individual payer guidelines to ensure that you report correct codes.

B Codes (B4000–B9999)

HCPCS B codes represent supplies, equipment, and nutritional products for parenteral and enteral nutrition. Recall that enteral nutrition therapy is also called tube feeding, where the patient receives nutrients through a tube in the nose (nasogastric, NG tube), stomach (gastrostomy, G tube), or small intestine (jejunostomy, J tube). Parenteral nutrition therapy is when a patient receives nutrients intravenously because the body is unable to take in nutrients orally or by other methods. Patients who need enteral or parenteral therapy suffer from disorders or effects of surgery that prohibit them from taking food by mouth, such as swallowing disorders, neuromuscular diseases, trauma, or reconstructive procedures to treat head, neck, and bowel diseases, like cancer. Patients may experience various types of infections or other complications from receiving enteral and parenteral nutrition.

Patients receive enteral and parenteral therapy at inpatient hospitals, SNFs, and home. DME suppliers can provide enteral and parenteral supplies, equipment, and nutrition to healthcare providers. Medicare and other insurances may reimburse for these items, but payment depends on the place of service, the patient's diagnosis, and whether the condition is short-term or long-term, among other criteria. Typically, insurances will not pay for enteral and parenteral supplies when the patient is an inpatient because the payment is part of the reimbursement for the inpatient stay.

E Codes (E0100–E8002)

E codes represent DME, which includes crutches, wheelchairs, commodes, canes, walkers, hospital beds, oxygen and related respiratory equipment, pacemakers and related

WORKPLACE IQ

You are working as a coder for Brandyburg Supply Company. Today, Mr. Junco calls you to say that he received bills for enteral supplies for his wife, Kit. He tells you that he thought Medicare covered the costs for these supplies. He asks you if you can find out whether Medicare should have paid.

What would you do?

monitoring equipment, patient lifts and other safety equipment, fracture and traction equipment, and artificial kidney machines. Here are two examples of HCPCS E codes:

- **E1130**—Standard wheelchair, fixed full length arms, fixed or swing away detachable foot rests
- **E1170**—Amputee wheelchair, fixed full length arms, swing away detachable elevating leg rests.

As you learned, in order for insurances to pay providers, the services that the provider renders or the equipment or supplies dispensed must meet medical necessity. Examples of diagnoses that would justify the patient's need for a wheelchair include

- Diabetes mellitus, if the patient has severe circulation problems that cause limb amputations
- Cerebrovascular accident (CVA, stroke), if the individual has lost the ability to walk independently

DME suppliers dispense DME *directly* to patients, or sell items to providers who then dispense them to patients. Pharmacies are also providers who dispense some types of DME to patients, such as wound care supplies.

Medicare follows four criteria to assess whether an item is considered DME:

1. The item is able to withstand repeated use.
2. The item is used primarily for medical purposes.
3. The item would not be used if the individual were not ill or injured.
4. The item is used in the patient's residence.

Other payers may also follow these same criteria when determining whether to reimburse providers for DME. Durable Medical Equipment, Prosthetics, Orthotics, and Supplies are known collectively by the acronym DMEPOS. Medical device manufacturers, pharmaceutical companies, medical and supply companies, and providers all are involved in the DMEPOS industry. Refer to the following example to learn more about coding for DME.

Example: Jeff Rohal, a nine-year-old, had his legs severed in a car accident. His power wheelchair's electrical motor has shorted out. Mr. James, an employee of Pittsburgh Medical Supplies and Repairs, has come to Jeff's home to replace the motor. Jeff is insured through Overfield Insurance Company, and his father is the policyholder.

To code this case, search the Index for the main term *wheelchair*, subterm *power*, and subterm *motor*, which leads you to code E2368. Cross-reference code **E2368**—*Power wheelchair component, motor, replacement only* to the Tabular for final code assignment.

TAKE A BREAK

You are doing great! Let's take a break and practice assigning HCPCS and diagnosis codes for patient encounters.

Exercise 35.3 A Codes, B Codes, and E Codes

Instructions: Review the patient's case, and then assign appropriate HCPCS codes for items, equipment, and supplies, using the Index and the Tabular. Append appropriate modifier(s) to the HCPCS code. Do not assign CPT codes for services or procedures. These cases may also include HCPCS codes other than A, B, or E. You can also refer to

Table 35-2 for brief descriptions of each type of code if you need additional assistance. Optional: For additional practice, assign the patient's diagnosis code(s) (ICD-9-CM).

1. Samantha Stone, an 85-year-old, has diabetic polyneuropathy and evidence of callus formation. Dr. Hays, a podiatrist, fits her with a pair of custom molded shoes.

   Diagnosis code(s): _____

   HCPCS code(s): _____

TAKE A BREAK *continued*

2. July Jones, a 73-year-old, has Crohn's disease (enteritis of the large intestine) and must be on total parenteral nutrition (TPN). Williton's SNF provides parenteral nutrition solution, amino acid, 3.5%, home mix (a home mix is a solution that the supplier does not premix).

   Diagnosis code(s): _____

   HCPCS code(s): _____

3. Peter Gonzalez, a 40-year-old, visited his urologist, Dr. Unger, and received an inflatable penile prosthesis because of erectile dysfunction (organic).

   Diagnosis code(s): _____

   HCPCS code(s): _____

4. Williton's DME dispensed a cane to Katherine Jonah, age 70, because she has an unstable back and needs help walking.

   Diagnosis code(s): _____

   HCPCS code(s): _____

5. Brandyburg Supply Company dispensed a rigid adjustable/fixed-height walker to Margaret Viola, an 84-year-old, after she was discharged from Brandyburg Outpatient Rehabilitation Hospital following ankle fracture surgery.

   Diagnosis code(s): _____

   HCPCS code(s): _____

6. Edwin Mock, a 65-year-old Medicare patient, undergoes colorectal cancer screening today at Williton Medical Center. He has a history of malignant neoplasm of the lower GI tract, which was removed four years ago.

   Diagnosis code(s): _____

   HCPCS code(s): _____

7. An ambulance transports Jason Aldridge, age 67, from his home to Williton Medical Center. During the trip, the EMT of Williton Medical Center Ambulance Service provides emergency ALS because the patient is in cardiac arrest. Assign a code for the ambulance transport.

   Diagnosis code(s): _____

   HCPCS code(s): _____

J Codes (J0000–J9999)

J codes include drugs that the patient does not self-administer. They include injections, chemotherapy drugs for cancer treatment, immunosuppressive drugs for treatment of patients whose immune systems are compromised (including AIDS patients), and inhaled solutions. Clinicians administer these drugs to patients, and they closely monitor patients to ensure that there are no contraindications or side effects and that the drugs are administered properly..

Keep in mind that there are also other HCPCS codes for drugs, including A, C, G, K, Q, and S codes. You can find codes for drugs by searching in the Index or going directly to the Table of Drugs, which lists drugs in alphabetical order. We will review more about the Table of Drugs later in this chapter.

In addition, there are HCPCS codes that represent *supplies used to administer drugs*, such as syringes or an IV medication bag. HCPCS codes for drugs and related supplies do not include the actual service that the clinician performs to administer the drug. CPT codes represent these services.

L Codes (L0112–L9900)

L codes represent **orthotics**, devices that help a patient to regain normal functioning, and **prosthetics**, devices that replace a body part lost to disease or trauma. It is important to understand that both orthotics and prosthetics are not only devices, but are also considered to be specialty areas of healthcare, dealing with the design, delivery, and fitting of those devices. Patients with orthotics and prosthetics can include those who have been diagnosed with upper or lower musculoskeletal injuries or conditions, patients

INTERESTING FACTS: Mind Control of Prosthetic Devices

Scientists at the California Institute of Technology have taken an important step in the development of a strategy to use the higher level neural activity of the brain to drive a prosthetic device. Such a strategy would allow paralyzed individuals to use their thoughts to move a device when they cannot move their limbs. A new, innovative approach by Richard Andersen, Sam Musallam, and their colleagues at California Institute of Technology relies on brain signals that initiate movement based on sensory input. Using this method with trained monkeys, the investigators decoded brain signals related to reaching movements to position a cursor on a computer screen. This breakthrough was first conceived in the mid-1990s when Andersen and colleagues discovered a visual area of the brain called the parietal reach region (PRR) in the parietal cortex of monkeys. The discovery of the PRR and its cognitive function led Dr. Andersen to consider creating a neural interface that could decode signals from PRR brain waves, allowing people with paralysis to manipulate prosthetic limbs or robotic devices with their thoughts.

(National Institutes of Health. www.nei.nih.gov/news/scienceadvances/discovery/brain_devices.asp, accessed 1/23/12).)

with amputated limbs, and patients with spinal deformities. Examples of these devices are collars, rib braces and belts, rib aprons with straps to immobilize and support the rib cage, orthotic devices that limit the rotation of the hip, gelatin or silicone breast implants, and molded devices with halo support (a neck and head immobilization device; you learned about cranial halos in Chapter 23).

TAKE A BREAK

Way to go! Let's take a break and practice assigning more HCPCS and diagnosis codes for patient encounters.

Exercise 35.4 J Codes, L Codes

Instructions: Review the patient's case, and then assign appropriate HCPCS codes for items, equipment, and supplies, using the Index and the Tabular. Append appropriate modifier(s) to the HCPCS code. Do not assign CPT codes for services or procedures. These cases may also include HCPCS codes other than J or L. You can also refer to Table 35-2 for brief descriptions of each type of code if you need additional assistance. Optional: Assign the patient's diagnosis code(s) (ICD-9-CM).

1. Wendell Sullivan, age 56, feels that his drinking is out of control. After consuming a fifth of vodka, he visits Williton Outpatient Drug and Alcohol Services for help, where a counselor performs a drug and alcohol screening.

   Diagnosis code(s): _____

   HCPCS code(s): _____

2. Candace Ezzo, age 74, is a type II diabetic who needs administration of Novolin® (insulin) via an insulin pump at her home. Mrs. Ezzo is a patient of Williton Home Health Care. Today, Jan Frank, RN, administers 50 units of insulin to the patient.

   Diagnosis code(s): _____

   HCPCS code(s): _____

3. Brandyburg Supply Company provides Tony Kelso, a 41-year-old morbidly obese patient who weighs 400 pounds, with a new power wheelchair (group 2 heavy-duty, sling/solid seat/back), because his weight prevents him from having full mobility.

   Diagnosis code(s): _____

   HCPCS code(s): _____

4. Kanya Riddle, a 20-year-old college student, experiences neck pain after being involved in a car accident. She goes to the Williton Outpatient Clinic, where Dr. Steele, the clinic physician, provides her with a cervical, flexible, nonadjustable foam collar.

   Diagnosis code(s): _____

   HCPCS code(s): _____

TAKE A BREAK *continued*

5. Rocky Calhoun, age 57, experiences right hand pain due to arthritis. Dr. Derby, an orthopedic medicine specialist, administers prolotherapy injections to the right hand (a solution injection that causes inflammation, resulting in the body's reaction to stimulate natural healing).

   Diagnosis code(s): _____

   HCPCS code(s): _____

6. Twila Orchowski, a 75-year-old Medicare patient, goes to her gynecologist for a Pap screening.

   Diagnosis code(s): _____

   HCPCS code(s): _____

7. Williton Medical Center sets up portable X-ray equipment at the Williton Senior Care Home for residents who are unable to travel to Williton Medical Center.

   HCPCS code(s): _____

8. Janet Newman, a home health aide, works for Williton Home Health Care. She visits Rowland Meyer, age 84, who recently experienced a stroke, a late effect of which caused paralysis of his left side. During her visit, Janet provides an hour of home health services, including training the patient on proper bathing techniques and guidance on appropriate foods to eat.

   Diagnosis code(s): _____

   HCPCS code(s): _____

9. George Rigjay, RN, works for Williton Home Health Care. Today, he visits Norman Kaminski, age 82. The patient has diabetes, and George trains him on techniques for self-administered insulin injections.

   Diagnosis code(s): _____

   HCPCS code(s): _____

10. Vincent Bosco, a 65-year-old, suffered an acute cerebrovascular attack. While he was at Williton Medical Center, Catherine Bell, a speech pathologist, provided a speech assessment noting the irregularities in the patient's speech pattern.

    Diagnosis code(s): _____

    HCPCS code(s): _____

DESTINATION: MEDICARE

In this Medicare exercise, you will learn more about HCPCS codes. Follow the instructions listed to access *Level II Coding Procedures:*

1. Go to the website http://www.cms.gov.
2. At the top of the screen on the banner bar, choose *Medicare.*
3. Scroll down the left column to *Coding,* and choose *HCPCS–General Information.*
4. On the left side of the screen, choose *HCPCS Level II Coding Process & Criteria.*
5. Scroll down to *Downloads,* and choose *Level II Coding Procedures.*

Answer the following questions:

1. Just because a HCPCS code exists for a supply or equipment, does this mean that all insurances will reimburse for it?

2. How many separate categories of like items or services do national codes represent?

3. Who may submit requests for changing codes in the HCPCS code set?

4. When does CMS decide to remove a code from the HCPCS code set?

TABLE OF DRUGS

Remember that the Table of Drugs lists four columns with the drug name, quantity, route of administration, and HCPCS code. Both brand and generic drugs are listed in the first column for the drug name. You first learned about brand and generic drugs in Chapter 33. The HCPCS code set lists some drugs in the Index as well as the Table of Drugs, and lists other drugs only in the Table of Drugs. For example, Torodal® (J9330) is listed in the Table of Drugs but not the Alphabetic Index, but Valium® (J3360) is listed in both the Table of Drugs and the Index. Always cross-reference codes to the Tabular List.

The second column lists the quantity of the drug dispensed. For quantities listed as "up to," this means that the quantity is *up to and including* the amount listed, such as for Draximage® MDP-25 (a radiopharmaceutical); the quantity is "study dose up to 30 mCi (millicurie)."

The third column is for the route of administration, or how the patient receives the drug. The following abbreviations are used to designate the route of administration:

IA	Intra-arterial
IT	Intrathecal (into fluid surrounding the spinal cord)
IV	Intravenous
IM	Intramuscular
SC	Subcutaneous
INH	Inhalant solution
INJ	Injection, not otherwise specified
VAR	Various routes (administered into joints, tissues, and cavities)
ORAL	Oral
OTH	Other routes (including suppositories)

TAKE A BREAK

Great work! Let's take a break and practice assigning HCPCS codes from the Table of Drugs.

Exercise 35.5 **Table of Drugs**

Instructions: Review the patient's case, and then assign appropriate HCPCS codes, using the Table of Drugs and cross-referencing the code to the Tabular. Do not assign CPT codes for services or procedures. Optional: For additional practice, assign the patient's diagnosis code(s) (ICD-9-CM).

1. At Brandyburg Psychiatric Hospital, Dr. Budgie, a psychiatrist, treats Brenda Fish, age 58, with Librium®, 100 mg, IM for an anxiety disorder.

   Diagnosis code(s): _____

   HCPCS code(s): _____

2. Dr. Mills, an ED physician at Williton Medical Center, treats Jessica Reynolds, a 48-year-old, for anthrax. Dr. Mills administers Cipro®, 200 mg, IV, every four hours.

   Diagnosis code(s): _____

   HCPCS code(s): _____

3. Olivia Hann, a 52-year-old, arrives at Williton's ED with complaints of chest pain. Dr. Mills examines her and orders a work-up. He diagnoses her with severe gastroesophageal reflux (GERD). He administers Pepcid®, 20 mg, IV.

   Diagnosis code(s): _____

   HCPCS code(s): _____

TAKE A BREAK *continued*

4. Williton Medical Center Ambulance Service provides emergency transport for Jackson Sobel, a 25-year-old, from his home to Williton's ED because he is experiencing an epileptic seizure. The EMT provides basic life support. Dr. Burns, the ED physician, examines the patient and administers 100 mg of Dilantin®. Code for both the ambulance service and the drug that Dr. Burns administered in the ED.

Williton Medical Center Ambulance Service:

Diagnosis code(s): _____

HCPCS code(s): _____

Williton's ED:

Diagnosis code(s): _____

HCPCS code(s): _____

5. Rhonda Scales drives her husband, Bill, age 62, to Williton's ED because he is nauseated and is having trouble breathing. Dr. Burns examines the patient and orders work-up. He diagnoses the patient with congestive heart failure (CHF), administers a 0.5-mg, IM dose of digoxin, and admits the patient.

Diagnosis code(s): _____

HCPCS code(s): _____

6. Karisha Jones, age 38, drives herself to Williton's ED with complaints of a severe headache and nausea. Dr. Mills examines the patient and diagnoses her with a migraine headache (without aura). He administers 30 mg, IV, of Toradol® and later discharges her home.

Diagnosis code(s): _____

HCPCS code(s): _____

POINTERS FROM THE PROS: Interview with a Reimbursement Specialist

Tammy Haught, CphT (certified pharmacy technician), has worked for five years in the pharmacy industry and is a Reimbursement Specialist for a pharmacy specializing in home infusion.

Please describe your job duties, including whether or not you perform coding.

I do not perform diagnosis coding directly, but it impacts my work dramatically. I bill insurance companies for drugs and services we provide. In order for the insurance company to pay, the right diagnosis code must be in place. I also then pick the right HCPCS code and supplies codes. I must also make sure we have authorization in place from the insurance company before providing services.

What are the most challenging aspects of your job?

Creating a clean claim, having prior authorization in place, submitting correct drug amounts and correct number of days of services.

What advice can you give to new coders to help them to communicate effectively with physicians, since physicians can sometimes be intimidating?

To understand that the physician/pharmacist will always think about the patient's well-being first instead of the claim getting paid.

What advice would you like to give to coding students to help them prepare to work successfully in the healthcare field?

Be confident, organized, compassionate, detail-oriented, and take pride in what you do; it has a great impact not only on yourself but on healthcare professionals and patients.

(Used by permission of Tammy Haught.)

MODIFIERS

Your HCPCS manual lists HCPCS modifiers, which you can append to both HCPCS codes and CPT codes, depending on the specific services a provider performs or items the provider dispenses. You can also find a comprehensive list of HCPCS modifiers in

Appendix D of this text. HCPCS modifiers are either alphanumeric or two letters long. Modifiers range from A1 to VP. The CPT manual lists some of these modifiers, which you reviewed in Chapter 18. There are many HCPCS modifiers, and it takes time to become familiar with them. Be sure to review them so that you have a better idea of the information that they represent. Let's review another example of how to correctly append a HCPCS modifier.

Example: Modifier -RA: On July 6, Dr. Hoffman ordered an electric portable respiratory suction pump for Edna Smith, age 76, who suffers from cystic fibrosis. Brandyburg Supply Company delivered the pump on July 7. About a week later, the patient and her husband observed that the pump seemed to be malfunctioning. So they contacted both Dr. Hoffman and Brandyburg Supply Company. The supply company delivered a replacement respiratory pump on July 15.

Modifier -RA represents *Replacement of a DME, orthotic, or prosthetic item*. The supply company billed the patient's insurance for the first pump using HCPCS code E0600—*Respiratory suction pump, home model, portable or stationary, electric*. Later, the supply company billed the patient's insurance for the second pump by appending modifier -RA to the same HCPCS code, **E0600-RA**. Modifier -RA alerted the insurance that the second pump was medically necessary, so they did not deny reimbursement. If the supply company had not appended modifier -RA to the code for the second pump, then the insurance would have denied the claim as a duplicate.

TAKE A BREAK

Congratulations! You have made it through the last section in this chapter! Give yourself a pat on the back! Let's take a break and practice choosing the correct HCPCS modifiers.

Exercise 35.6 Modifiers

Instructions: Refer to the list of HCPCS modifiers in your HCPCS manual, or turn to Appendix D of this text. Then review each case, and determine the correct HCPCS modifier to assign.

1. The second digit of the patient's left foot was amputated.

   Modifier: _____

2. A nurse midwife delivered baby James Wilbur, 8 pounds, 15½ ounces.

   Modifier: _____

3. A patient receives drug and alcohol counseling. He is an employee of an organization that has a Drug/ Alcohol/Behavioral Assistance program for first-time employees.

   Modifier: _____

4. A single mother received family planning services for raising her newborn infant.

   Modifier: _____

5. An ambulance was called to a home. When the EMTs arrived on the scene, they found that the patient had already expired. No emergency assistance could be given.

   Modifier: _____

6. A hospice nurse dresses a wound for a hospice patient suffering from prostate cancer. The patient lacerated his hand while he was cutting lunchmeat for a sandwich.

   Modifier: _____

Multiple Choice

Instructions: Circle one best answer to complete each statement.

1. _____ report miscellaneous supplies using codes A4206–A4290.
   a. Providers
   b. Facilities
   c. Patients
   d. Ambulance transportation companies

2. DME stands for
   a. diagnostic medical evaluation.
   b. durable medicine equipment.
   c. diagnostic modern equipment.
   d. durable medical equipment.

3. The definition of prosthetics is
   a. the specialty area of healthcare that deals with application of braces to the human body.
   b. the specialty area of healthcare that deals with the production and application of artificial body parts.
   c. the branch of medicine that deals with anesthetizing the body.
   d. the branch of medicine that deals with providing artificial support to the body before surgery.

4. Medicare uses all of the following criteria to determine if an item qualifies as a DME item/supply *except*
   a. the item can be paid for by the patient.
   b. the item can be used primarily for medical purposes.
   c. the item can be used in the patient's residence.
   d. the item can withstand repeated use.

5. What abbreviation is used when the method of administration is insertion directly into the patient's vein?
   a. IM
   b. IT
   c. IA
   d. IV

6. Which of the following considerations are not relevant when you are coding for an ambulance service?
   a. The type of services the patient needs
   b. If extra personnel were needed
   c. The type of insurance reimbursing the services
   d. The type of vehicle used to transport the patient

7. _____ are called _____ terms.
   a. See and code also, cross-reference
   b. Code and code also, cross-reference
   c. See and see also, cross-reference
   d. Code and see also, cross-reference

8. Where in the HCPCS code set are drugs listed in alphabetical order?
   a. Table of Drugs
   b. List of Modifiers
   c. See instructions
   d. Table of Brand Drugs

9. J codes are used for reporting drugs that _____ administers.
   a. the patient
   b. a health care professional
   c. a friend or family member
   d. all of the above

10. The acronym HCPCS stands for
    a. Hospital Care Procedural Coding System.
    b. Hospital Common Procedural Coding System.
    c. Healthcare Common Periodic Coding System.
    d. Healthcare Common Procedure Coding System

Coding Assignments

Instructions: Review the patient's case, and then assign appropriate HCPCS codes for items, equipment, and supplies, using the Index and the Tabular. Append appropriate modifier(s) to the HCPCS code. Do not assign CPT codes for services or procedures. Optional: For additional practice, assign the patient's diagnosis code(s) (ICD-9-CM).

1. Jean Rohal, a 57-year-old, arrives at Williton's ED with complaints of vomiting, nausea, and cramps. Dr. Mills examines her and orders work-up. He diagnoses her with enteritis, due to *Escherichia coli*. He orders ampicillin sodium and sulbactam sodium IV injection 1.5 g every six hours. She receives the drug for 18 hours and then is released.

   HCPCS code(s):_____

   Diagnosis code(s):_____

2. Sonja Stopperich, age 50, arrives at Williton's ED with a badly infected second-degree burn on her scalp that a curling iron caused. She had not taken proper care of the burn. Dr. Mills treated the wound and applied an alginate dressing, 10 square inches, based on the wound's appearance and fluid oozing from it. Dr. Mills gave the patient two additional dressings to change once a week for two weeks and discharged her home.

   HCPCS code(s):_____

   Diagnosis code(s):_____

3. Susan Baroness, a home health nurse, adjusts a colostomy bag for David Connolly, age 62. She fits him with a drainable, rubber colostomy with a faceplate and drain, along with a protective solid skin barrier, size 4 inches square.

   HCPCS code(s):_____

   Diagnosis code(s):_____

4. Susan Baroness reviews Kevin Anderson's diet. Mr. Anderson currently utilizes an enteral feeding supply kit due to malnutrition from neck cancer. Susan determines that the patient needs additional fiber in his diet. She requests an order from his physician for a fiber additive for the enteral formula, which is approved.

   HCPCS code(s):_____

   Diagnosis code(s):_____

5. Gertrude Fisher, an 82-year-old female, was diagnosed with Alzheimer's dementia with behavioral disturbances. For her safety, Dr. Hoffman prescribes a hospital bed with a mattress and variable height side rails (to prevent her from falling out of bed at night).

   HCPCS code(s):_____

   Diagnosis code(s):_____

6. Cal Hobbs, a 68-year-old home health patient whose legs are paralyzed, needs to have his electric wheelchair motor repaired. Brandyburg Supply Company sends Charles Wansworth, a repair technician, to the patient's home. Charles spends 60 minutes on the repair because of multiple problems, which are nonroutine.

   HCPCS code(s):_____

   Diagnosis code(s):_____

7. Jay Seans, a 12-year-old male, has congenital scoliosis. Susie Meckling, a physical therapist at Williton Rehabilitation Center, fits the patient with a cervical-thoracic-lumbar-sacral orthotic (CTLSO) (Milwaukee) brace.

   HCPCS code(s):_____

   Diagnosis code(s):_____

8. On Tuesday morning, Katie Bopper drops off her mother, Mary Daniels, a 100-year-old senile Medicare patient, at Williton Senior Day Care Center. The center provides respite care for Mrs. Daniels for the day. Her daughter, her regular caretaker, needs time to perform some personal errands. She picks up her mother at 4 p.m.

   HCPCS code(s):_____

   Diagnosis code(s):_____

9. James Viola, an 82-year-old Medicare patient, experiences conductive hearing loss in his right ear and visits Dr. Junco, an audiologist, for a hearing assessment.

   HCPCS code(s):_____

   Diagnosis code(s):_____

10. Harry Orchowski, a 72-year-old male, had an open fracture of the neck of his right femur two weeks ago and is an inpatient at Williton. He recovers well enough to be discharged to Williton Nursing and Rehabilitation Center. The rehab center's wheelchair van transports him from Williton Hospital to Williton Nursing and Rehabilitation Center, which is a total distance of 15 miles. There is no emergency equipment on board, and the van attendant documents on his trip ticket that this is a nonemergency transport. Code for both the wheelchair van transport and the mileage for each mile.

   HCPCS code(s):_____

   Diagnosis code(s):_____

Professionalism

(465.9)

(216.3)

(272.4)

(296.22)

(787.91)

(789.07)

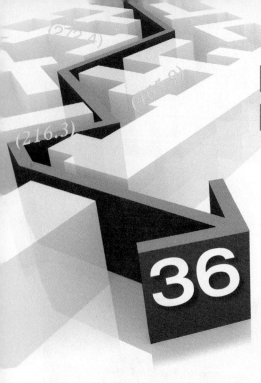

Professionalism and Patient Relations

Learning Objectives

After completing this chapter, you should be able to

- Spell and define the key terminology in this chapter.
- Define the basic traits of a healthcare professional.
- Take the self-assessment to determine if you have professional traits.
- Review real-world professionalism scenarios, and determine the best ways to handle them.
- Identify and define the four areas to know about regarding your employment.
- Discuss why communication is important to professionalism, and identify and define the three types of communication.
- Discuss how to correctly construct emails.
- Explain why working well with others is important to your success.
- Review roadblocks to successful communications with coworkers.
- Identify professionalism rules of the road and roadblocks to avoid.
- Define patient relations and explain why you should treat patients as your customers.
- List common patient complaints about bad service.
- Discuss how you can provide excellent service to patients.
- Name the 12 steps for handling an angry patient, and explain additional tips to remember.

Key Terms

at-will employment
clear speech
enunciating
extraneous
Human Resources Department
insubordination
nonverbal communication
patient relations

phone etiquette
probationary period
professionalism
slang
tone of voice
verbal communication
voice pitch
written communication

INTRODUCTION

You have now come to the last stop, the end of your coding journey in this text, even though your journey will continue on in the healthcare field! Are you wondering what professionalism and patient relations have to do with coding? Everything! Do you remember reading in Chapter 1 that performing coding may become your entire job or only part of your job, depending on your job title and the provider for which you work?

Regardless of how much coding you perform, you will need to possess the qualities of a professional in order to be successful. You can have all the job knowledge in the world, but if you cannot relate well to other people, which is what professionalism and patient relations are all about, you will *not* be successful or be able to advance in your career.

You may be thinking that you already are a professional and wonder what more there is that you could possibly learn. Even the most professional people not only continue to

ICD-9-CM codes in this chapter are from the ICD-9-CM 2012 code set from the Department of Health and Human Services, Centers for Disease Control and Prevention.

expand their current knowledge of *practicing* professionalism, but they also like to continually refresh their existing skills. Professionalism is an art, a learned skill, and people have to deliberately practice it on a daily basis in order to become good at it. It is not something that you are born with or that you "just know." You might say that being a professional is a lifelong endeavor because successfully working with others is a lifelong endeavor. So, no matter how many or how few years of work experience you have, there will be beneficial information for you in this chapter, along with some interesting and fun exercises.

Let's travel forward to the end of this journey and learn more about professionalism and patient relations and how both traits make you successful in your career!

"If it is to be, it is up to me."—WILLIAM H. JOHNSEN

PROFESSIONALISM

When you think of someone who is a professional, what type of person do you think about? What qualities come to mind? Would you say that this person is *successful*? Can you also think of someone whom you feel is unprofessional? What characteristics would you use to describe this person? Would you say that the person you thought of is *unsuccessful*? Professionalism and success go hand-in-hand. Granted, there may be people who seem unprofessional but earn high salaries. But for the most part, someone who is unprofessional is not successful. If you are a professional, then you can expect to succeed in many areas.

Professionalism is possessing the traits necessary to be successful in the workplace, including enthusiasm, dedication, job knowledge, respect for others, and a positive attitude. The most basic traits of a professional are to show

- *Enthusiasm* about your job, even in the midst of negative circumstances. Employer research shows that managers are more likely to hire and promote people with enthusiasm and less experience over those with more experience but are not enthusiastic.
- *Dedication*, demonstrated by arriving for work consistently and on time, even if you do not feel like working
- *Job knowledge*, including a thorough knowledge of your job and an understanding of how your work affects others, even when they may not understand *your* job
- *Respect* for everyone, even when they are rude to you
- *A positive attitude* and a warm smile, even if you feel bad on the inside

Imagine a person who has *one* of these qualities but not the others, like someone who is very enthusiastic but does not know how to perform her job, or maybe someone who has sound job knowledge but disrespects others. It is the combination of these skills that make a person a successful professional. These are certainly not all of the qualities that contribute to being professional. Take a few minutes to jot down a list of what *you feel* are qualities of a professional, and then answer yes or no to each of the following self-assessment questions.

PROFESSIONALISM TRAITS SELF-ASSESSMENT

A professional is someone who is . . .

Honest and Trustworthy		
Do you make sure that you make up any time missed and ensure you record the missed time on your time sheet?	OR	Have you ever arrived late to work but did not make up the time or mark the time missed on your time sheet?
Do you feel that stealing is wrong, no matter what the situation is?	OR	Have you ever made personal copies at work or taken supplies, food, or materials from an employer simply because they would not miss it, they were throwing it away anyhow, or you did not receive that bonus you were promised?

Positive and Friendly		
Do you smile at people you encounter and say "Hello" and "How are you?"	OR	Do you feel that this is not important, so you do not bother?
Do you rise above a negative situation and work through it with a smile on your face?	OR	Do you instantly grumble when something goes wrong, once again believing it is just your bad luck?
Efficient and Accurate		
Do you double-check your work before finalizing it?	OR	Do you "wing it" because you have spent enough time on it already?
Are you organized and able to meet deadlines, keeping a to-do list and following it?	OR	Do you rely on your memory to keep all of your appointments and manage projects, sometimes or frequently missing due dates?
Mature and Reasonable		
Are you able to keep your emotions in check, even when you are angry or upset, and think before you speak?	OR	Do your emotions get the best of you, where you easily become angry or upset, say what you think and raise your voice to others?
Do you give others the benefit of the doubt if they are in a bad mood and try not to take their mood personally?	OR	Do you feel that it is one more time (in a long list of times) that this person has treated you this way?
Motivated and Passionate		
Do you like to work, and does work give you an intrinsic (internal) satisfaction?	OR	Is work something that you do to pay the bills, and that's all?
Do you believe in what you do and feel strongly that you need to do it well?	OR	Do you watch the clock until your work is over, and you can go home?
Respectful and Reliable		
Can you appreciate when someone does not share your religious beliefs or personal interests or just simply disagrees with you?	OR	Do you feel that this person is simply opinionated and hard to get along with?
Do you understand that you have to take orders from your boss, or you could lose your job?	OR	Do you talk back to superiors, enforcing your opinion because you just know you are right?
Flexible and Understanding		
Are you willing to perform work that you have never done before because it needs to be done?	OR	Do you say that you would rather not do the work because you are uncomfortable with it?
Can you understand that when someone else is hurting physically or emotionally, their situation can make them impatient and rude?	OR	Do you think that they are just unhappy and negative?

A professional also...

Shows Good Judgment		
Can your boss/teacher/instructor/ coworker rely on you to perform a task without worrying that you will waste time?	OR	Do you find that surfing the Internet, text messaging, talking on your cell phone, and using other electronic devices are absolutely necessary, even if you are at work or school?
Will you do what someone else needs you to do, regardless of how you are feeling at the moment?	OR	Would you rather do what you want, when you want, regardless of what someone else needs?
Takes Pride in Her Work		
Do you follow up when you say you are going to, in response to someone's question or concern?	OR	Do you follow up when you think of it, even if someone has been waiting for your answer?

Do you feel good about yourself after you complete certain projects?	OR	Is it just another job done, and you are glad that it is over?
Makes Ethical Decisions		
Do you understand the importance of *not* discussing patient information with people who do not need to know it?	OR	Would you share patients' stories with friends and family members?
When you have to make a decision, do you ensure that it does not hurt someone else financially, physically, or emotionally?	OR	Do you make decisions regardless of how they affect others?
Is Fair to Others		
Would you treat everyone the same because they should have to follow the same rules?	OR	Would you bend the rules according to the situation and the person involved?
If you learn that a coworker earns more than you, even though you feel that you perform the same job, would you accept that your boss has valid reasons for paying your coworker more?	OR	Would you assume that your boss favors your coworker over you and angrily confront your boss, demanding to know why she is not paying you more money?
Possesses Excellent Customer Service Skills		
Do you feel that every customer is as important as your family member or best friend?	OR	Are customers people whom you cannot wait to get rid of because they are in your way and wasting your time?
Do you feel that every customer is really your boss, since every customer helps to pay your salary?	OR	Do you feel that even if a customer does not come back, there will always be other customers?
Communicates Well		
Do you listen to others when they speak to you, ensuring that you maintain good eye contact and concentrate on what they say?	OR	Do you find that it is easier to continue working while someone is speaking to you?
Do you double-check written correspondence that you create, including emails, to ensure that there are no grammatical or spelling errors?	OR	Do you write correspondence once and check it as you go without double-checking your work when you finish?

So how did you do on your self-assessment? Do you feel that you have all of the traits needed to be a professional? Count how many times you answered yes in the left column and how many times you answered yes in the right. If you answered yes more on the left, then you handle those situations like a professional. If you answered yes more on the right, then you will need to improve your professionalism and patient relations skills.

Being a professional is not easy! It takes a lot of practice and patience, as well as continuous self-analysis, to review your behavior to determine if you need to improve it. A professional is not a robot, either, and it is important to understand that even the most professional individual will still make mistakes and is always learning! Hopefully, though, the mistakes will be few and minor.

Now that you are familiar with the qualities needed to be a professional, review the following real-world workplace scenarios. Think about how you would handle each situation, drawing from your own experiences and experiences of others you know. If you are unsure how to handle the situation, then remember the professional person you thought of earlier in the chapter. How do you think that person would handle the situation? Sometimes you can think about how someone else would successfully resolve the situation and follow the same methods. Check the recommendations listed after the scenarios to see how you did.

REAL-WORLD PROFESSIONALISM SCENARIOS

You are working at Williton Family Practice, which has three physicians who specialize in primary care. Your job title is Administrative Coding Specialist, and you perform diagnosis and procedure coding. You also assist the billing staff with appealing denied claims and help answer the phones. You report to Katie, the office manager, and you also report to the physicians. Each of the four workplace scenarios that you will read is based on actual events that happened to others in the workplace. Determine how you would handle each situation, and write your answer in the space provided. Then compare your answer with the recommendation listed after the scenario. Keep in mind that there may be several ways to professionally and tactfully handle these situations, which cannot all be mentioned in the recommendations.

Scenario 1: Did you ever hear the saying "Rule No. 1: The Boss Is Always Right?"

Katie asks you to complete a task, and you feel that she used a rude tone of voice when she spoke to you. What should you do? _____

_____

Scenario 2: What about "Rule No. 2: If The Boss Is Wrong, See Rule No. 1?"

You need to explain a situation to Katie. While you are speaking, she keeps interrupting you and tries to finish each one of your sentences. What should you do? _____

_____

Scenario 3: The "That's Just Her" defense

Lori, a billing specialist in the office, has told coworkers that she and her husband have been arguing a lot lately. Lori also seems to frequently be in a bad mood and is often impatient with and disrespectful to her coworkers, including you. If anyone asks Lori if she is all right, then she complains for what seems like forever about everything that is wrong with her husband. One day, Charise, another coworker, talks to you about Lori and says, "She's going through a rough time, and she always handles bad situations this way. She takes it out on others, and then later when she calms down, she's O.K. You just have to tiptoe around her if you sense that she's in a bad mood because *that's just Lori.*" What should you do? _____

_____

Scenario 4: "I Can't Believe That You Would Suggest Such a Thing . . ."

Kelly, a coworker, is trying to pass off her work to you. She is responsible for scheduling all appointments for patients and decides to tell you to do it today, stating that she is "way too busy with other stuff" to handle scheduling on top of everything else that she has to do for the day. She adds, "Since you told me yesterday that you finished your big project, I figured you'd be looking for work to do." Even though you finished the project, your to-do list is full of other projects and other deadlines. What should you do? _____

_____

Scenario 1 Recommendation: Ignore it. Maybe Katie is just having a bad day, and she will later apologize to you. Even though this does not excuse her behavior, you should not take offense. However, if Katie speaks rudely to you on a regular basis, then you should politely ask her if you have done something wrong because you sense that she is upset with you. If there are no problems, then Katie will hopefully realize her actions are counterproductive.

   Because Katie is your boss, you should not report her to one or all of the physicians unless her behavior is abusive, in which case you may also need to find another job. Going over your manager's head, as the saying goes, could cause her to become even more upset and angry.

Scenario 2 Recommendation: Do nothing. Ignore it. Stop talking when she interrupts, and when she finishes talking, continue speaking. Some people interrupt others without realizing it. It is important to not make an issue out of it, and avoid saying something like, "Excuse me, I'd like to finish what I was saying." After all, she is the boss.

Scenario 3 Recommendation: Many people excuse their bad behavior, and others excuse it for them, by saying that it is just the way the person is. However, there are certain job requirements that everyone must meet in order to keep their jobs, including treating other people with respect, regardless of how bad their personal lives are. Imagine if everyone felt that it was acceptable to be impatient with others just because they were in a bad marriage or having a bad day!

No one should have to "tiptoe" around Lori because of her personal problems. It is not appropriate to carry personal problems to work to the point where they affect other employees. This is a situation that Katie should handle because Lori is treating everyone in the office poorly. Charise is defending the bad behavior and further encouraging it by asking you to excuse it, too. The best approach is to avoid interactions with Lori as much as possible, not ask questions about her personal life, and trust that Katie will step in and resolve the situation.

Scenario 4 Recommendation: Tell Kelly that you are sorry but even though you finished your project, you still have other work to do, and if she does not feel that she can keep up with her work, that she should let Katie know. Keep in mind, there will be times that you will help your coworkers with their work, and they will help you with yours. But helping is much different from being asked to complete someone else's entire job for them. It also does not mean that coworkers are permitted to delegate their work to others who do not report to them. Rather, they should *ask* for assistance instead of giving a direct order to someone else to provide it.

Now that you have reviewed workplace scenarios, you can work on the following exercises to further practice your professionalism skills.

TAKE A BREAK

Let's take a break and then analyze additional workplace scenarios.

Exercise 36.1 **Real-World Professionalism Scenarios**

Instructions: Read each scenario, and determine the best way to handle the situation, recording your answer in the space provided.

1. *You Want Me To Do What? When?*

   Today is Wednesday, and Katie gives you three assignments to complete. She tells you that they are all due next Tuesday, so you have a little less than a week to finish them. Because you have other responsibilities and are working on multiple projects, you do not feel that you will have time to finish the new assignments by next Tuesday.

   What should you do?

   _____

   _____

2. *Would Someone Please Answer the Phone?*

   For the first hour every morning, your job is answering incoming phone calls, and it is the busiest time for calls. Debbie, one of your coworkers, works beside you and helps you with the calls. For the past three

   mornings, Debbie has arrived at least 20 minutes late, causing you to handle a lot more phone calls because she is not there to help you.

   What should you do?

   _____

   _____

3. *I Wish I Could Stay and Chat but . . .*

   Gloria is one of your coworkers who has a tendency to talk too much. In fact, once she starts talking to you, it is very hard to break away and get back to work. She talks about what she did the night before, her son's baseball practice, her dog's recent antics, and her latest shopping trips. Today, she has you cornered again, this time in the lunch room. Your lunch ended 10 minutes ago, but you cannot seem to excuse yourself while Gloria is still talking to you.

   What should you do?

   _____

   _____

4. *Ghostly Visits . . .*

   Dr. Singer, one of the physicians in the practice, stops by your desk today to drop off a report. He tells you that the report contains a list of Medicare patients'

continued

TAKE A BREAK *continued*

demographic and insurance information and asks you to enter the patients into the computer system. He also tells you, "Once you've added them, please enter an office visit charge with code 99215." You ask Dr. Singer where the encounter forms are for the patients, since the staff always uses them to enter charges. Dr. Singer says, "Don't worry about it. I'll take care of the encounter forms. Just key the charges, and ask Ashley to submit their claims to Medicare." He then walks away. You check the list of patients and do not recognize any of them as ever having an appointment in the office, let alone a high-level office visit for an established patient.

What should you do?

_____

_____

5. *Are You Talking to Me? . . .*

In the office this morning, one of your coworkers, Gina, raises her voice when she is speaking to you and sounds angry and mean. She questions why you performed a certain task, and she even asks you, "Don't you know *anything*??!!" as she huffs and walks away.

What should you do?

_____

_____

PROFESSIONALISM AND YOUR EMPLOYER

Part of being a professional is also understanding your employer's various departments, policies, and procedures. The four areas with which you should be familiar regarding your employment are

1. Job descriptions
2. At-will employment
3. Probationary period
4. Human Resources Department

Job Descriptions

Recall from Chapter 1 that every position, such as a medical coder or billing specialist, should have a job description. The employer writes the job description and provides each employee with a copy. It is a good idea to ask for a copy of the job description before a scheduled job interview so that you will have a better idea of the job expectations. The job description includes individual job duties; behavior expectations, such as courtesy and respect; shift times; whether professional dress is required; and any other criteria about the job that the employer wants to define for the employee. Being a professional means understanding and following your job description.

Job descriptions will also typically state that the employee will perform "other related duties." This means that your boss can ask you to work on a project or complete a task that is not listed on your job description but does relate to your job. This type of request is not unusual, and it is not appropriate to tell your boss, "That's not my job," or "That isn't on my job description, so I'm not doing it." Failure to perform work that your boss requests is considered **insubordination**, which means not following orders from your boss, and can cost you your job.

At-Will Employment

At-will employment means that your employment is at *your will* or at *your employer's will*, meaning that you can leave your job at any time, for any reason, even without notice, and your employer can terminate your job at any time, for any reason, without notice. Those in favor of at-will employment say that they feel it increases employee productivity because employees never know if or when their employers will terminate their jobs.

At-will employment applies when you *do not* have a written or verbal contract with an employer that protects your job for a specific amount of time, such as a year. Employees who belong to labor unions usually have written contracts. Many federal and state government employees are not at-will employees. They cannot be fired unless there is a very good reason, such as engaging in an illegal activity.

In general, an employer will tell you at the start of a new job if your employment is at-will. They may also include this information in their organization's policy and procedure manual, on your job description, or in an employee handbook. There are exceptions to at-will employment laws; for example, employers cannot fire employees for reasons that violate public policy. In other words, there are state and federal laws that prohibit employers from firing employees because of their race, color, religion, age, gender, national origin, or disability. Employers also cannot fire employees if they refuse to perform work that is illegal or if they take a specific amount of time off for a personal or family medical problem (a situation that for many employers falls under the Family and Medical Leave Act—FMLA—of 1993). There are also other exceptions to at-will employment, which can vary by state.

Under at-will employment, your employer can terminate your job for any reasons that do not violate public policy under state and federal laws. For example, maybe your employer does not feel that you dress professionally and decides to fire you for it. You may think that this is unfair, but if your employment is at-will, then your employer can fire you for violating their dress code policy. Violating a dress code does not fall under public policy. Or maybe your employer feels that you speak disrespectfully to your coworkers and to patients, so they fire you. Again, you may feel it is unfair, and wish you had been given the chance to improve, but your employer can still fire you, and there is nothing legally that you can do to change it and get your job back. Speaking disrespectfully also does not fall under public policy. That is why it is so important to be a true professional at work because you do not want to give your employer any reason to fire you. Instead, you want your employer to see you as a valued employee that they hopefully cannot live without!

Probationary Period

A **probationary period** is the amount of time that an employer allows a new employee to learn all aspects of her job. When you start a new job, it is common for an employer to review the probationary period with you, which typically includes one or more performance reviews to determine your progress. Employers may review new employees every 30 days or some other period of time the employer determines up until the end of the probationary period. Probationary periods can last three months to a year, or a different amount of time, depending on the employer.

An employer can terminate an employee at any time during the probationary period if it appears that the employee will not be successful in the new job. Employers may also reward employees who successfully complete their probationary periods by giving them raises and/or increasing their job responsibilities. You should ensure that you are professional during the probationary period and throughout your employment so that you do not lose your job.

Human Resources Department

Many larger organizations have a **Human Resources Department** whose employees are in charge of hiring and firing employees; overseeing employee benefits (medical, life, and disability insurance); processing the company payroll to ensure that employees are paid correctly and on time, and that appropriate deductions are taken from their pay; and ensuring that all employees follow employment laws, including policies for evaluating and disciplining employees. Often, when you interview for a new job, you first meet with a human resources representative whose job is to screen applicants and choose those who should return to meet with individual department managers. You should treat an interview with human resources as seriously as you would an interview with the department manager.

POINTERS FROM THE PROS: Interview with a Medical Transcriptionist and Former Coder

Nancy Walton works as a medical transcriptionist for an acute care hospital and has also performed coding in previous positions, including emergency department coding and working for a tumor registry where she reported patients' demographic and medical information to the Department of Health. Mrs. Walton has 18 years of healthcare experience and has worked with many types of personalities, including physicians, nurses, medical assistants, billers, and coders.

What advice can you give to someone working in transcription who wants to transition to coding?

Take coding classes. That will help you immensely. Transcription would give you such a leg up because it's easier to understand coding if you are already familiar with the medical terminology.

What advice can you give to coding students about entering the healthcare field?

At all costs, as best as you can, try to disregard 90% of the gossip you hear from coworkers because they'll lead you astray.

What has been the most difficult aspect of any of the positions you have held?

It's tough to read sad charts. The more compassionate you are, the harder time you have if the patient lives in your community. I think it's easier if you are working from home and reading charts from patients from somewhere else, because you don't know them. I've learned that if you can just put the patient's situation out of your mind and try to forget about it, you'll be better off (to handle your duties).

(Used by permission of Nancy Walton.)

It is also important to understand that even though the Human Resources Department handles personnel (people) issues, you should not automatically go to human resources when you have a problem with a coworker or with your boss. Being a professional means understanding that it is best to discuss the problem directly with the person or people involved before you escalate the matter to human resources. Always give others the opportunity to discuss a situation with you before reporting them to a higher authority, unless they ask you to engage in illegal activity or verbally or physically threaten you.

PROFESSIONALISM AND COMMUNICATION

Like it or not, a large part of being a professional is communicating well with others. Your boss, coworkers, patients, families, physicians, and other employees will all judge how well you communicate, and it will affect your job success and opportunities for promotion. Those who communicate well will generally be more successful than those who do not. There are three types of communication: verbal, nonverbal, and written. You should learn how to communicate well using all three methods. You should also understand how others prefer to communicate. For instance, if a coworker prefers email communication, then you should email her, rather than call her. Knowing others' communications preferences will help you to communicate with them quickly and effectively.

Communicating professionally in healthcare also means being sensitive to the specific issues of others with whom you communicate, including patients who

- are deaf, hearing impaired, visually impaired, or blind
- are unable to understand speech because of their medical conditions
- want to talk to you about personal issues
- bring family members with them, in which case you have to address everyone present
- do not speak English well

It is important to be patient and understanding and request assistance when you need it, such as requesting a language interpreter if one is available, or a clinician who has more experience with medical conditions that might make it difficult for a patient to communicate with you.

When you are communicating with patients, always introduce yourself and state your job title to patients and their families because it is not only professional to do so, but they may also meet other people during the visit and may want to remember everyone. Shake hands if you like.

Review the three types of communication next to learn more about how to utilize each one when working with others.

VERBAL COMMUNICATION

Verbal communication means speaking with others. Part of successful communication is knowing the correct amount of information to convey so that you provide enough information, but not too much or too little. Think about this example: You are driving along the highway looking for the nearest grocery store. You stop at a gas station, go in, and ask the clerk for directions. The clerk gives you directions, and on your way out of the station, a male customer stops you and says that he overheard you asking for directions. Before you can say that you already have them, he also gives you directions. Both sets of directions are listed next. Determine which directions you would rather receive and why.

- **The gas station clerk's directions:**   Drive out of the gas station, and turn right at the first stop light. You will be on Highway 12. Then drive about three miles and take the Glen Cove exit, and Sam's Grocery will be on your left.

   OR

- **The customer's directions:**   Drive out of the gas station, oh, I'd say for about a mile. You'll see John's Dairy on the right. They used to be a lot bigger, but they downsized, and now just have milk and juice. Drive for awhile past a couple of farms, and you'll get to an exit; I think it's Glen Cove, but I'm not sure. *[The customer then turns to find his wife.]* Ethel, do you remember if that first exit is for Glen Cove? Oh, she's not listening. I think she's picking out some cookies to take home. I'm pretty sure it's Glen Cove, though. Take that exit, and then almost immediately, you'll see a craft store on the right. It has a big sign out front, but you don't need to worry about that . . .

Did you decide that you would rather have the clerk's directions? Not many people would want the customer's directions, in fact, he is probably still giving them! The customer obviously enjoyed talking to you, but he missed the point of the communication: You wanted directions to the grocery store. He gave too much irrelevant information that you did not need to know.

Know Your Audience

This example illustrates the importance of knowing the *amount* of information that you need to convey, which includes the ability to *know your audience*: know who will receive your message and how much information he needs to have. Ask yourself if the person to whom you are speaking really needs to have *all* of the information that you are about to share. Do not provide unnecessary details; stay focused and only communicate what is pertinent to the listener's needs. You can watch for signs that you may be giving too much information if the listener seems to lose interest, looks at his watch or looks around him, begins talking with someone else, sighs, or interrupts you. You may not be providing enough information if the listener looks confused and/or asks you a lot of follow-up questions. Knowing how much information to convey also applies to written communication, which you will review later in the chapter.

Phone Etiquette

Verbal communication includes face-to-face conversations and conversations over the phone. **Phone etiquette** means showing good manners at work while you talk on the phone. When you work in healthcare, you not only have to talk on the phone with patients, your *external customers*, but you also have to talk with *internal customers*, other employees of the organization, and other external customers from outside organizations such as other providers or insurance companies. It is important to understand that being a professional

■ TABLE 36-1   **PHONE ETIQUETTE TIPS**

If you answer the phone . . .	Be sure to say "Good morning" or "Good afternoon," identify yourself and the organization for which you work, and ask how you may help. Example: *Good morning, Dr. Hoffman's office, this is Joanie, how may I help you?* rather than just saying *Dr. Hoffman's office.*
If you have to place a call on hold . . .	Ask the person if you may do so instead of saying "hold, please" and hanging up. Not everyone can wait on hold and some people would rather have you call them back, or they may prefer to call back later.
When you remove a caller from hold . . .	Thank the caller for holding.
If you cannot understand what the caller says . . .	Say, "Excuse me, can you please repeat that?" rather than saying "What?" "Huh?" or "I can't hear you!"
If you have to take a phone message for someone who is unavailable . . .	Offer the caller the option to leave a message. Do not tell the caller that she will have to call back. This is poor service and inconvenient for the caller.
When you are taking a phone message for someone else . . .	Be sure to include all necessary information, such as the caller's name, phone number, message and best time to reach him. Many software programs and paper message pads have designated areas to list this information.
If you are talking with someone on the phone and need to get back to him with more information . . .	Provide a specific day and time when you will do so. If you do not have the information by that time, then call the person back to at least tell him, and explain when you will have an answer. Not returning the call because you do not have an answer is not professional, and the other person will feel that you forgot about him.
Return phone messages that someone leaves for you . . .	Within 24 hours. Do not use the excuse that you are too busy because most people are busy. Returning phone calls is part of your job requirements.
Say "Goodbye" when you end the call . . .	Rather than just hanging up on the caller. You can also add "Thank you for calling" if it is appropriate for the situation.
Avoid . . .	Eating or chewing gum on the phone. It is distracting to the listener and makes it sound like you do not take your job seriously.
Unless it is an emergency . . .	Do not take a phone call in the middle of a conversation with a patient, other external customer, or another employee.
Do not . . .	Text message while talking with a patient over the phone (or even in person!).
Your voice mail message should . . .	Include your name and job title. Say goodbye when you end the message. Callers should not have to guess that they have reached the correct person.

means treating everyone well and providing excellent service by being mannerly over the phone. Refer to ■ TABLE 36-1 to review tips for good phone etiquette.

Clear Speech

Successful verbal communication, whether it occurs in person or over the phone, includes **clear speech**. If you find that others often ask you to repeat what you say, then it probably means that you are not speaking clearly or loudly enough. You can practice clear speech by

- **Enunciating** (pronouncing) your words correctly
- Ensuring that your **tone of voice** (emotion that your voice conveys when you speak) is even-tempered, rather than upset, anxious, hurried, or mean, which can make it difficult for others to understand you and difficult for you to remain professional.
- Determining that your **voice pitch** (how high or low your voice sounds) does not interfere with your ability to communicate. If your pitch is a whisper, ranges from high to low, or is garbled, then you should improve it.
  - Avoid *up-speak*, which is the tendency to raise the pitch of your voice at the end of a sentence as though you are asking a question, even though you are not. Example: *I will be in early Monday to help with that report? We can work on it together and pull the information from the files if we need it?* Using up-speak makes a person sound unsure of what she is saying and diminishes her credibility.

■ TABLE 36-2   **SLANG WITH PROFESSIONAL TRANSLATION**

Slang Word or Term	Professional Translation . . .
ain't	is not or isn't
y'all or you guys	all of you
gonna	going to
wanna	want to
shoulda	should have
freak out	become upset
grossed out	become disgusted
stuff your face	eat too much
back in the day	a long time ago
run with the big dogs	keep up with the pace and the workload
irregardless	regardless
very unique	unique; the word unique means "one of a kind," so something cannot be *very* one of a kind. It is either one of a kind, or it is not.
cool	great, wonderful, interesting, fascinating
like	Avoid using the word *like* in the following context, "It's like, a busy day at the office." Either it *is* a busy day at the office or it is *not*. It is not *like* a busy day.

- Ensure that you do not make common mistakes, such as consistently pausing when speaking, saying "um," or "ah," swearing, or using **slang**, which are words and phrases that are acceptable to use with friends, but not in a professional environment. Refer to the examples of slang words and terms and the professional translations to say instead in ■ TABLE 36-2.

    Also avoid speaking text messaging jargon, such as LOL (laugh out loud) or OMG (oh my God!). Think about what you are going to say before you say it to ensure that you communicate clearly and professionally.

If you are not sure how you sound to others, then record your voice and determine if you can understand what you are saying and if you sound professional. You can also ask friends and family to critique your voice. Ask them if they can understand you and if they think that others could, too. This will help you to determine the areas that you need to improve. If you need to practice pronouncing words, there are many Internet websites that enable you to listen to correct word pronunciations, and you can practice pronouncing the words yourself. Then ask friends and family to listen to you as you practice to provide feedback.

Listening Skills

Successful verbal communication also depends on how well you listen. Many people appear to be listening to someone when they are really concentrating on something else. Effective listening skills will help you to hear what someone else is telling you, so be sure to concentrate when someone speaks to you to determine what they are trying to say, and you will then be able to ask them pertinent follow-up questions.

    Taking notes while you are listening to someone speak is another technique that will help ensure that you capture pertinent information from the conversation. You can also repeat your notes back to the person talking to be sure you understood the message and ask if you missed anything.

    Avoid interrupting a person when he speaks and finishing his sentences because it is unprofessional and does not allow the speaker to convey the entire message. It also shows that you are not listening effectively. You may think that you know what he is going to say next, but you could be incorrect. Allow the speaker to finish talking before you respond.

NONVERBAL COMMUNICATION

Nonverbal communication involves communicating with others without speaking, and it can be just as important as verbal communication for successfully conveying or responding to a message. Nonverbal communication includes facial expressions, eye contact, body language, and gestures, including pointing.

Body Language

A professional uses body language appropriately when communicating with others, giving the other person his full attention by maintaining eye contact, sitting up straight, and showing an interested facial expression. Unprofessional body language when communicating includes rolling your eyes in disgust, making faces, slouching in your seat, ignoring the other person by working on another task, or having an uninterested facial expression.

An important point to note is that you have to be very aware of your body language even when you think that no one can see you. For example, let's say that Joanie, who works for a primary care physician, has a conversation with a patient whom she thinks is mean. After the patient leaves, Joanie quietly tells a coworker about the conversation, and in the process, she makes a face and rolls her eyes. Even though patients in the waiting room cannot *hear* Joanie's conversation, they can *see* her face, and they wonder if she is talking about them, another patient, or a coworker.

Joanie used poor judgment any way you look at the situation. Her unprofessional body language made the patients wonder why she felt compelled to make faces. Do you think that it would make the patients feel welcome in the office? It actually would have the opposite effect. Joanie also risked being heard by other people even though she thought she was having a private conversation. What if Joanie's office manager saw her making faces? She would then have to explain what she was doing and why. Joanie not only acted unprofessionally but also behaved immaturely. There will always be times when another person makes you angry or upset, and you can think what you choose about that person. But conveying your thoughts through body language is a bad idea. Being professional means rising above a situation with which you do not agree and acting positively anyway, regardless of the negative thoughts you have.

Appearance and Dress

Nonverbal communication also includes taking care of your appearance and dressing appropriately for your position. It is important to follow an employer's dress code policy. Many employers allow casual dress, and clinicians can wear scrubs, but some employers require business dress. Many employers also prohibit their employees from exposing any tattoos or piercings, other than the ears. Tattoos and piercings may be an important part of an individual's self-expression, but they are not appropriate when you are working in healthcare. Part of professional dress also involves maintaining good hygiene, making sure that you are clean, and ensuring that you do not wear too much cologne or perfume. What you think smells good, someone else may find offensive; some people are also allergic to perfumes. Like it or not, people do judge others on their appearance. You could perform outstanding work, but if you show up for work in a strapless dress and flip flops, or a blazer and jacket that are two sizes too small, no one will ever believe that you do your job well. Refer to ■ TABLE 36-3 for appearance dos and don'ts.

The Name Badge

Another form of nonverbal communication is a name badge. Many employers require employees to wear badges that show their names, job titles, and photo. Note that a name badge does not replace introducing yourself and stating your job title to a patient and their family members because not everyone will be able to read your name badge. Name badges also help patients and their families to know that you are an employee, so that they can ask for your assistance when needed.

■ TABLE 36-3   **APPEARANCE DOS AND DON'TS**

Dos	Don'ts
Wear your hair in a clean and neat style, not hanging in the face, over an eye, or big. Hair color should be believable.	Show cleavage or wear miniskirts, tank tops, shorts, cut-off shorts, summer sandals, or clothes that are too tight. Do not go braless.
Wear makeup conservatively.	Wear brightly colored makeup or too much makeup.
Men should be clean shaven or have neatly trimmed facial hair.	Wear to work any outfit that you would wear to a club or party, the beach, to clean out your garage, or out on a date.
Ensure your nails are clean and neatly trimmed—for both men and women. Clinicians should keep their nails short so that they do not injure patients or harbor germs. Wear conservative nail colors—clear, brown, or pink tones. Avoid wearing decals and multicolored nails.	Wear an outfit if you are unsure whether it is appropriate for work. When in doubt, *do not* wear it.
Wear conservative and minimal jewelry. Think in terms of one—one ring, one necklace, and one bracelet. Earrings for men and women should be no longer or wider than one inch.	Wear clothes that are dirty, stained, smell bad, or are wrinkled.

WRITTEN COMMUNICATION

Written communication means communicating with others in writing through various formats, including emails, business letters, memos, reports, phone messages, or notes written to others to ask questions or clarify information. Successful written communication begins with knowing how to write well. Others also judge you and your level of professionalism by how well you communicate in writing. Sloppy and incorrect writing makes an employee appear to be unprepared for work and unable to perform it. It does not make others trust her to do a good job. Writing well does not mean that you have to be a professional writer, but it does mean that you should know the basic rules to follow for clear written communication. You can take a writing class if you need help with your writing skills, or ask someone who writes well to help you. There are also countless articles and books, as well as Internet interactive learning sites, available to assist you. Refer to ■ TABLE 36-4 for tips on successful written communications.

Emails

Emails are a quick and effective way to communicate with other employees, patients, and outside organizations. It is important to treat email communication the same way that you treat all other written communication, following the basic rules for clear writing. Review Example 1, an email that Joanie, a billing specialist, sends to her boss, Ralph. Ralph previously asked Joanie to create a financial report that he could present at the next staff meeting and asks two other employees, Barb and Rob, to assist.

Example 1:

TO: nicotetti.ralph@willitonmedicalcenter.com
FROM: moon.joanie@willitonmedicalcenter.com
CC:
SUBJECT: report

THE REPORT IS ON MY DESK FOR U TO PICK UP AND BQRB WILL MAKE COPIES OF THE HANDOUTS FOR THE MEETING ROB WILL BRING THE POEWR POINT WITH HIM WHEN HE GETS THEIR.

■ **TABLE 36-4   TIPS FOR SUCCESSFUL WRITTEN COMMUNICATIONS**

Spell words correctly	*Spell check* is a function in many software programs that you can use to verify your spelling to avoid mistakes such as spelling "thru" instead of "through" or "nite" instead of "night."
Write clearly and concisely	Ensure that people can understand your writing and that you only convey necessary information. This also includes knowing when to start and end paragraphs.
Use punctuation correctly	The spell check function can find some punctuation errors but not all of them.
Ensure that your writing is grammatically correct	Know basic rules of grammar, such as the differences among "their," "there," and "they're." A common error is the misuse of the word myself, which you should use infrequently. Incorrect use is "If you have any questions, please contact myself." Correct use is "If you have any questions, please contact me." Say sentences out loud as though you are speaking it to someone to determine if they make sense. You would not tell your friend "If you have any questions, please contact myself," because it sounds a little silly.
Explain medical terms in common language that everyone understands	Avoid using medical terminology when you are communicating with people who may not understand it, such as patients and their family members.
Avoid overuse of catch phrases or buzz words that are popular at the moment	Although it is necessary to learn many healthcare abbreviations and common terms used in the industry, it is not appropriate to constantly use words or terms just because they are trendy, such as "At the end of the day. . .," "thinking outside the box," "on the same page," and "win–win situation." The English language is filled with countless words, and it is better to increase your vocabulary to use a variety of words and phrases.
Understand the appropriate amount of information to convey to the person receiving the message	Written communications should only include pertinent information, not **extraneous** information, which is irrelevant and unrelated to the subject.
Know the proper formatting for documents	Business letters, memos, and emails all have standard formats that you should use when composing them. You can also find articles, books, software help functions, and Internet sites that can provide you with formatting assistance.
Type accurately and maintain constant speed of at least 35 words per minute (wpm)	If you do not know how to type, then it is helpful to take a typing course or learn through online tutorials. So much of successful written communication depends on having good typing skills.
Write legibly	If you do not have neat handwriting, then either practice writing neater, or type your messages to others.
Ensure that the document you create is neat and organized	Make it easy for others to read and follow the letters, emails, or reports that you give to them.
Avoid sending written communication if you are upset or angry	You can easily convey your emotions in writing, and it is best to wait to calm down before writing so that you do not later regret it.

Believe it or not, the mistakes that Joanie made in her email are very common in the workplace, although most senders do not make all of them in the same email! Take a few minutes to see how many mistakes you can find, and then compare them with the email tips listed next for Joanie's email:

- **Always be specific on the subject line**—Ralph may have several emails to review and will categorize the order to review them by their subject. He may not instantly remember what information he requested from Joanie when the subject of the email only shows "report."

- **Include a salutation**—Examples include "Hi Ralph" or "Dear Ralph." Joanie should not just start writing without acknowledging the person to whom she is addressing her message.

- **Do not use capital letters in an email because it looks like yelling**—It was unnecessary for Joanie to write in all caps.

- **Use punctuation correctly**—Notice that Joanie does not use *any* punctuation, and her sentences run together, which makes her email difficult to read.

- **Spell correctly**—Joanie used the letter *u* to replace the word *you*. Emailing is not text messaging, and Joanie should not confuse the two. She also misspelled Barb's name as BQRB and misspelled PowerPoint as POEWR POINT.

- **Use grammar correctly**—Note that Joanie incorrectly spelled the word *there* (a place) as *their* (shows possession).

- **Do not give orders to your boss**—Joanie tells Ralph to pick up the report on her desk when she should have delivered it to him.

- **Ask if there is any further information needed or any more that you can do**—It shows courtesy and also ensures that you perform all necessary tasks related to the content of the email. Joanie's email ended abruptly without asking if her boss needed any additional information.

- **Sign your name, and provide your contact information**—This makes it easy for the receiver to know who sent the email without trying to decipher an email address (some addresses do not clearly identify a sender) and identify a quick way to reach her on her phone extension. Joanie failed to list any contact information in her email.

Now review Joanie's corrected email (Example 2) to see how it makes her sound professional:

Example 2:

TO: nicotetti.ralph@willitonmedicalcenter.com
FROM: moon.joanie@willitonmedicalcenter.com
CC:
SUBJECT: Report on unpaid claims from July to December 2010

Hi Ralph,

I finished the unpaid claims report and will drop it off to you today. Barb will make copies of the handouts for the meeting. Rob will bring the PowerPoint explaining the columns of the report. Please let me know if you need anything else.

Joanie Moon
Ext. 5437

Refer to ■ TABLE 36-5 for additional tips for composing emails.

■ TABLE 36-5 **ADDITIONAL TIPS FOR EMAILS**

Never send an email if you are upset or angry.	Avoid writing until you calm down because you can easily convey your emotions in the email, and the receiver can forward it to anyone else at any time.
Avoid using your work email for personal purposes, including sending jokes to others and badmouthing your employer, coworkers, and boss.	Your employer can easily track your emails and read what you wrote, even if you delete them. Think of emails this way: Unless you would be willing to read your email on a billboard along the highway and not be embarrassed, do not send it.
Use the *Reply All* feature on emails only when "all" people on the email list need to read your response.	Some people make it a habit to hit Reply All, even though the message may be irrelevant to all but one person. Only reply to those who need to read your message.
Return emails within 24 hours, even if you do not have an answer to give the sender.	Email anyway and explain why you cannot respond to them and when you expect to respond.
Do not send or receive personal emails while you are at work.	Avoid this use of company resources unless your employer occasionally permits it.

INTERESTING FACT: Private Emails Are Not So Private, After All

Employees often mistakenly believe that their use of the Internet and email at the workplace is private when, in fact, courts have found no reasonable expectation of privacy in such use and have consistently permitted employers to monitor and review employee activity.

Employer and employee myths and legal realities regarding the Internet

Employee Myth: My employer does not have the right to read my personal email or review the Internet sites I visited.

Legal Reality: Employees have no privacy rights in their email and Internet use, and federal law does not prohibit employers from monitoring that use.

Employer Myth: It is no big deal if my employees use email or the Internet for personal reasons on the job. As an employer, I do not need to monitor their use.

Legal Reality: Failure to monitor employees' email and Internet use can lead to legal liability in more ways than one.

(Muhl, Charles J. Bureau of Labor Statistics www.bls.gov/opub/mlr/2003/02/art3full.pdf, February 2003, accessed 8/1/11.)

TAKE A BREAK

Let's take a break and then analyze additional workplace scenarios.

> **Exercise 36.2** **Professionalism and Your Employer, Professionalism and Communication (Verbal, Nonverbal, Written)**

Instructions: Fill in each blank with the best answer.

1. The amount of time that an employer allows a new employee to learn all aspects of her job is called a(n) _____.

2. _____ means speaking with others.

3. _____ is knowing who will receive your message and the amount of information that he needs to know.

4. Avoid overuse of _____ or _____ that are popular at the moment.

5. _____ means that you can leave your job at any time, for any reason, even without notice, and your employer can terminate your job at any time, as long as they do not violate public policy.

6. _____ is the tendency to speak in higher pitch at the end of a sentence as though you are asking a question, even though you are not.

7. Never send _____ if you are upset or angry.

8. _____ means showing good manners at work while you talk on the phone.

9. Employees in the _____ are in charge of hiring and firing employees and overseeing employee benefits.

10. _____ involves communicating with others without speaking.

THE IMPORTANCE OF WORKING WELL WITH OTHERS

It is important to please your boss to be successful, but did you also know that your workplace success depends on how professionally you work with others? This is because everyone works for the same team. Imagine if you were watching a baseball game, and all of the players did whatever they felt like, regardless of how their behavior affected their teammates. Do you think that they would win any games? The team members must work together to achieve a common goal: to win the game, and they understand that they cannot win alone. They need each other to meet their objectives. The same is true in the workplace: Coworkers rely on each other to "win the game," which can be to keep patients satisfied, stay organized, meet deadlines, perform coding and billing, and achieve many other objectives. When one team member does well, the entire team looks good. One of your jobs in healthcare is to support your own team and make each other look good. Follow the tips outlined next for working well with others.

- **Support your coworkers**—Do not resent someone else if he does a good job or earns a promotion. Do not pick on him for making a mistake, and do not openly criticize him in order to get a laugh from others.

- **Congratulate a team member**—Offer congratulations to someone who achieves a goal, and thank him for helping you complete a task or project. It may be easy to forget to say "please" when you are asking for someone's help and "thank you" when she helps you, but using "please" and "thank you" go a long way in ensuring that fellow teammates will support you and assist you in the future.

- **Do not give orders to coworkers**—Only give orders if it is part of your job, like if you are leading a project and have to ask coworkers to complete specific duties. It is the boss's job to delegate work and give orders. Coworkers will resent you if you give them orders and probably will not follow them anyway. This also includes giving orders to your boss, which is inappropriate.

- **Acknowledge coworkers and other people who work in your organization**—Were you ever at work or school, and someone walking toward you simply ignored you by looking the other way or looking down at the floor? Part of professionalism is having the manners to make eye contact, smile, and say "Hello" when you encounter someone else. Not only do you have to acknowledge people whom you know; you should acknowledge everyone you encounter. A smile takes only a second and is well worth the investment. You never know whom you may encounter, including a person who may have the final say on whether you are promoted or not.

- **Use good manners**—Did you know that employers promote mannerly, likeable people over those whom they do not like and who have poor manners? Did you also know that other employees are more willing to work with people whom they like and who have good manners? Set the example that others will want to follow.

- **Get to know other employees**—Ask them how their weekend was or how their day is going. Many people enjoy telling you about themselves, and it helps to build a relationship for working well with others. You should not divulge every personal detail at work or expect your coworkers to be your counselors when they have personal problems. You can get to know someone better without crossing personal boundaries. The best time to do this is before or after your shift or during breaks, so that you are not interrupting your work or someone else's.

- **Be aware of those working around you to avoid offending them**—Awareness includes not talking loudly to others when you are on a phone call, not yelling to other people nearby to get their attention, not taking personal calls at your desk where everyone can hear, and not having loud conversations while you are standing beside someone's work area. You should also monitor the noise level of headphones if you use them—no one else should be able to hear any noise from your headphones. Also avoid playing music at your desk that others may hear.

- **Observe understood departmental traditions**—Traditions may include chipping in money for a coworker's birthday or celebrating a holiday at a local restaurant. If you do not participate with others in regular activities, then they can view you as not wanting to be part of the team. However, if you are asked for money for a birthday or other party, and you do not have it, simply say so because no one should fault you for it.

- **Have a sense of humor**—It is all right to laugh and joke with others at work, as long as it is not at someone else's expense and does not take up much of a day. Having a sense of humor also means not taking yourself or others so seriously that you are incapable of having occasional fun conversations. Many people think that work should not be fun, but this is not true. Having fun does not necessarily mean wasting time. If you enjoy what you do at work, then it is easy to make it fun. Rewarding work should have some component of fun in it. After all, who wants to go to a job where no one ever jokes or laughs?

- **Be a good observer of human nature**—You can learn a lot from others who perform their jobs well and think to yourself "Wow, what a great way to handle that situation. I'll have to remember to do that." You can also learn from the mistakes that others make so that you do not make the same mistakes yourself. You can learn skills for working well with others by reading articles and books, taking classes, and learning from others who have more work experience and who are eager to share it with you.

You will next review roadblocks that coworkers at Williton Medical Center encounter when communicating with one another. Read each roadblock and then the instructions for how the employee can navigate around the roadblock to act more professionally. Then try to navigate around roadblocks on your own in the next exercise.

Roadblocks to Successful Communications with Coworkers

Roadblock 1	*Sam walks up to Christine's desk. She is typing on her computer, and her back is turned. Sam says, "Do you have those totals from the computer report with rejected claims that we printed last week?"*
How to Navigate Around the Roadblock	Sam should say, "Excuse me, Christine, do you have time for a question?" before interrupting her in case she is in the middle of work that she cannot stop. This shows good manners and respect for another person's time and schedule. Just because it was a good time for Sam to discuss the report does not mean that it is also a good time for Christine.
Roadblock 2	*Jeff needs to ask Debbie a question. When he reaches her desk, she is on the phone with a patient. He stands at her desk, waiting for her to finish.*
How to Navigate Around the Roadblock	If Jeff wants to wait a few minutes (not indefinitely) for Debbie to end the call, he should at least move away from her desk to an area nearby, rather than stand at her desk. If he does not have time to wait, then he should come back later. If it is an emergency situation, Jeff can write a quick note to Debbie and place it on her desk directly in front of her so she will read it. It is not polite to stand beside someone while she is on the phone. This same rule would also apply if Debbie were meeting with someone else at her desk.
Roadblock 3	*Kathy and Rita have desks that are side-by-side. Rita has a question for Kathy, so she sends Kathy an email.*
How to Navigate Around the Roadblock	Rita should just ask Kathy the question. She should not email someone sitting right next to her because it diminishes her ability to build rapport with a coworker.
Roadblock 4	*Becky arrives each morning at her desk, which is situated in the middle of the department, along with eight other employees. She always removes her coat and puts her purse in her desk drawer and begins working, without speaking to anyone.*
How to Navigate Around the Roadblock	Becky should say, "Good morning" to her coworkers when she arrives and "Good night" when she leaves. It is courteous to speak to other people at work, rather than walking in and out without talking. If Becky is consistently discourteous to those working around her, then they may not be very eager to assist her if she ever needs help. People are more apt to help those whom they like and who are positive and friendly. In addition, if Becky does not have a good rapport with others, it will adversely affect her ability to succeed at work or be promoted.
Roadblock 5	*After a group project meeting on Monday morning, Ron, the project manager, asked Judy to prepare a report for the next team meeting on Friday morning. Now it's Thursday afternoon, and Judy has not had the chance to even start on the report. She tells Ron that she is sorry, but she will not have the report ready for Friday's meeting.*
How to Navigate Around the Roadblock	Judy should have started preparing the report early in the week, since Ron asked her about it on Monday morning. She did not complete the work that she was required to perform as part of her responsibilities on the team project. The group needed information for Friday's meeting. If Judy did not have time to work on the report, then she should have discussed it with Ron earlier in the week to explain the situation and ask for assistance. She could also have talked with her manager to determine if she could stop working on other tasks in order to complete the report, to ensure that she finished the report on time.

TAKE A BREAK

Let's take a break and then review more roadblocks to working well with others.

| Exercise 36.3 | The Importance of Working Well with Others |

Instructions: Read each roadblock, and determine the best way to navigate around it, recording your answer in the space provided.

Roadblock 1: Every morning, Debbie and Lisa say "Good morning," to each other, but if Lisa asks Debbie how she is, Debbie's only response is "Good."

- What could Debbie do differently to communicate more professionally with Lisa?

_____

Roadblock 2: Nathan and Phil engage in heated debates on a regular basis when they discuss politics at their desks. Nathan's political views are very different from Phil's views, and Nathan becomes upset when Phil disagrees with him. One day, they debate whether abortion should be legal or illegal. The conversations disrupt other coworkers trying to complete their work.

- What could Nathan and Phil do differently to communicate more professionally with each other?

_____

Roadblock 3: Jen has a tendency to attack her coworkers when she feels that they are bothering her. The other day when Debbie asked her a question, she told Debbie, "I'm in the middle of something and can't talk right now. You'll have to wait." Another day she told Phil that he was "getting on her nerves."

- What could Jen do differently to communicate more professionally with Debbie and Phil?

_____

Roadblock 4: When Ashley talks with others, she uses a lot of slang terms and catch phrases. She also overuses the word "like" and has a very high-pitched voice, which almost sounds childlike. Yesterday, she told Phil about a computer problem she had to resolve, stating, "I was like, what now? I can't believe that the computer, like, failed again! But you know what, I got out the manual and was able to find the problem and, like, fix it myself! LOL!"

- What could Ashley do differently to communicate more professionally with her coworkers?

_____

PROFESSIONALISM RULES OF THE ROAD

You have learned a lot of information about professionalism so far, and you are almost finished. Review the rules of the road listed next (■ TABLES 36-6 and 36-7), which will further ensure your success when you are navigating the road to professionalism!

There you have it, many more tips for you to take with you on the new road for your career. You probably already knew some or many of these because you had to follow them somewhere that you worked or are working now. Always remember that a professional strives to constantly improve and continues to learn.

TAKE A BREAK

Let's take a break and review more about professionalism rules of the road.

| Exercise 36.4 | Professionalism Rules of the Road |

Instructions: Read each statement, and determine if it is a way to navigate successfully on the road to professionalism or if it is a roadblock to professionalism.

1. Respect authority and follow your employer's rules.

_____

2. Be inflexible to schedule and shift changes.

_____

3. Bring personal problems to work.

_____

4. Keep confidential information confidential.

_____

5. Arrive late, leave early, or call off on a consistent basis.

_____

6. Overreact to situations and fail to obtain all the facts before formulating an opinion. _____

■ TABLE 36-6   FOURTEEN WAYS TO NAVIGATE SUCCESSFULLY ON THE ROAD TO PROFESSIONALISM

1. Offer to help others . . .	When you have time, or if your help is really needed. You never know when you might need them to help you.
2. If you finish a task or project . . .	Ask your boss for more work. Avoid surfing the web, texting, or making personal calls during time that your employer is paying you to perform work. Show initiative, and make yourself a reliable employee.
3. Find ways to improve processes . . .	If you see that something is not working, then suggest improvements to your boss.
4. Show compassion for others . . .	For example, direct a patient or family members who need help finding their way to specific departments or locations.
5. Take criticism from your boss . . .	Without becoming defensive. Avoid arguing. If you strongly disagree with the criticism, then take time to think before formulating a response, and be sure that your response is valid and based on facts.
6. Stay organized . . .	With a calendar and to-do list, whether you write on paper, use computer software, or use your phone. There are many resources for you to learn organizational skills, including books, articles, and seminars.
7. Go above and beyond . . .	And give more than what your employer or patients expect.
8. Think positively . . .	About your job and others around you, and speak positively. By thinking and acting positively, you will attract positive results.
9. Admit when you make a mistake . . .	And learn from the experience so that you do not make the mistake again. Avoid blaming others for your error or pointing out what *they* always do wrong.
10. Accept new and unfamiliar assignments willingly . . .	Be available to stay later if you are needed to work on projects or last-minute tasks.
11. When in a meeting with others . . .	Allow them to speak without interrupting, and do not be afraid to share your ideas and opinions, but do not take over the meeting. Communicate in a positive, nonthreatening way. Convey the appropriate amount of information.
12. Keep confidential information . . .	Confidential.
13. If you have to tell your boss about a negative situation . . .	Then also suggest possible solutions to resolve the situation.
14. Respect authority and follow your employer's rules . . .	If you disagree with a rule or disagree with your boss, and have a strong reason for your viewpoint, then calmly discuss it with your boss. Do not go above her and talk with the physician or your boss's manager.

WORKPLACE IQ

Lately, Katie, your manager, seems to be giving you more and more work, even more, it seems, than your coworkers are receiving. When you ask Katie why you're receiving so much work, she tells you that she's giving you the work because she trusts that you will be able to finish it on time and finish it correctly. When you mention that your coworkers do not appear to have as much work as you have, Katie tells you not to worry about them. She tells you that she will handle all staffing issues and to worry about your own work.

What would you do?

■ **TABLE 36-7   TWENTY-EIGHT WAYS TO NAVIGATE POORLY ON THE ROAD TO PROFESSIONALISM (THAT MAY COST YOU YOUR JOB)**

1. Argue with your boss, coworkers, and patients.

2. Cry or yell, showing inability to handle stress, maintain your composure, and control your emotions.

3. Refuse to do what your boss asks you, unless it is unethical and/or illegal.

4. Make personal phone calls (unless it is urgent), send text messages, and surf the Internet during scheduled work time when your employer is paying you. Many employers prohibit these activities and terminate employees who violate the rules.

5. Take a longer break than the one to which you are entitled.

6. Arrive late, leave early, or call off on a consistent basis.

7. Refer to patients, your boss, and coworkers using cute names. Many people are offended when they are called "honey," "sweetie," or "dude."

8. Call physicians or other clinicians by their first names, unless they tell you that you can.

9. Talk too much and waste time that should be spent working.

10. Complain—about your boss, coworkers, patients, or family issues—or complain that life is not fair.

11. Give orders to your boss.

12. Bring personal problems to work.

13 Fail to meet deadlines, follow up, and perform accurate work.

14. Swear.

15. Steal, including marking time on your timesheet or time card that you did not work.

16. Complain about your boss and/or your employer on social networking sites that are easy for others to read. Do not become friends with patients on social networking sites. Simply tell patients who request it that it is against your employer's policy.

17. Fail to show up for work and fail to call to let your boss know, or consistently show up late or leave early.

18. Release confidential information to others who do not need to know it.

19. Communicate poorly verbally, nonverbally, or in writing.

20. Overreact to situations and fail to obtain all the facts before formulating an opinion.

21. Fail to learn new job duties or skills by not taking notes or asking questions.

22. Give up easily.

23. Sleep on the job.

24. Fail to give others the benefit of the doubt, taking everything they do and say as a personal attack.

25. Avoid good manners. Neglect to hold the door open for someone walking behind you, allow others to exit an elevator before you step in, or keep your work area neat and organized.

26. Be inflexible to schedule and shift changes, showing unwillingness to help where needed or cover for someone who is off.

27. Date coworkers when it is against the employer's policy. Worse yet, date your boss.

28. Leave a job without giving your boss notice to find a replacement before you go, or give notice but spend the time bad mouthing your employer.

PATIENT RELATIONS

You learned in Chapter 1 that a healthcare provider is a business and needs revenue to survive. Patients, the customers, provide that revenue, and without them, there is no business. Treat patients well, and they will return; treat them poorly, and they will go elsewhere. To lose a patient to poor service hurts everyone: the patient, the employees, and the provider's business. Treat each patient like he is the *most important* patient. Only then will you ensure that the patient is satisfied with the services, you are satisfied that you've done a great job, and all the employees are satisfied that the office will continue to generate revenue. Treat patients with the kindness you would show to your best friend or a family member. Give each patient your attention and time to make him feel important and that you truly care about his well-being. And remember that patients are not diagnoses, like "the shoulder injury," "the mole removal," or "the broken leg." Patients are people, and you should treat them that way, rather than refer to them as a diagnosis. You would not call your mother or best friend by a diagnosis, and you should also avoid doing it with patients.

Patient relations involves interacting with patients and their families to ensure that they receive the best service. Many hospitals have patient relations departments whose employees address patients' questions and concerns and resolve complaints from patients and families regarding the patient's experience at the hospital. Even if you do not work in a patient relations department, you can show excellent patient relations skills because they are the same skills that you should show any customer, including courtesy, respect, sincerity, concern, and compassion. Many customer service skills are also the same as many professionalism skills, such as having excellent communication skills and follow-up abilities. The patient is a customer of healthcare, purchasing services from healthcare providers.

You already learned that you have to follow your employer's rules and perform the work that your boss requests. But your real boss is the patient. Each patient indirectly pays your salary because it is their insurance that pays for their services and procedures, and it is the patient who pays the remaining balances after insurance.

Your job may involve patient interactions on a daily basis, or it may involve only occasional interactions. You may talk with patients in person or over the phone. You may see them in the hallway. You may never see a patient if you have a position working from home or in a separate location where employees perform coding, billing, and collections and where there are no clinicians. But even if you do not see patients you should still appreciate the fact that you work for them.

It is estimated that a dissatisfied customer may tell up to 20 people about his bad experience, and a satisfied customer may tell up to 5 people. You may think that it is unfortunate if one patient has a bad experience, and the only harm in it is that he will not return. After all, there are still other patients! But that one patient can tell many other people not to visit your provider because the same thing might happen to them. A dissatisfied patient may even tell people who are *established* patients. Is it really worth the risk of upsetting one patient? Poor service can also cost healthcare employees their jobs because many jobs require interacting positively with patients. Remember that the customer, the patient, is your boss. Many employers send patients surveys to ask them to rate the service that they received during their encounter, so it is important to keep this fact in mind when working with patients.

For the most part, patients visit providers because they are ill. There are exceptions, such as patients who need yearly exams or work-related physicals. Patients represent a unique customer because they have medical problems. They are not the same customers who vacation at resort hotels on the beach, who are generally healthy, happy, and in a good mood. Those customers are easy to serve.

On the other hand, patients could be in pain, nauseated, dizzy, confused, disabled, terminally ill, or depressed, or they may have several other problems. Many times, a patient's illness also contributes to financial problems. There are patients who have gone bankrupt paying medical bills, and there are patients who cannot afford to pay anything toward their medical bills. Some patients hesitate to visit a physician because they fear that they will not be able to afford care.

Illness can also result in job loss because the patient's condition prohibits him from working. Patients can have family problems because their illness places stress on family members who must care for a patient who can no longer care for himself. Patients can have a host of other problems besides their medical conditions and as a result, they may be angry, tearful, disgusted, resentful, or mean by the time you see them. It does not mean that all patients are this way, but some are, and you have to be prepared for it. That is why it is necessary to take extra care to ensure that you treat all patients with respect, patience, courtesy, and dignity, just like you would treat your best friend or a family member. Patients pay your salary, after all, because they are the real boss!

Poor Service to Patients

Think about a time when you received poor service at a healthcare provider (physician's office, clinic, hospital), restaurant, or store. Did you feel that the people employed there understood that you, the customer, were their boss? Would you ever go back? You most likely will not return for fear of receiving more bad service and because you are unwilling to spend your money at a business where the employees did not appreciate it! Review the following list of common patient complaints about bad service, and avoid repeating these errors at all costs:

- Employee failed to listen to the patient's questions, concerns, and complaints, including failing to acknowledge family members who accompanied the patient.

- Employee failed to acknowledge the patient, such as when the patient arrived for an appointment, or informed the patient of service delays (examples: the physician is running late, the billing specialist is with another patient).

- Employee failed to greet the patient with "Hello," to introduce himself, to say "Good-bye" or to thank the patient for his business.

- Employee showed a lack of interest in the patient's issue, not paying attention, ignoring the patient, or having an uninterested facial expression.

- Employee failed to follow up with a patient after promising to get back to the patient with additional information.

- Employee showed rude behavior toward the patient, including talking down to the patient as though she were a child, interrupting the patient when he was talking, interrupting a conversation with the patient to take personal calls, or using medical terms that the patient did not understand.

- Employee showed lack of interest in the patient's situation and lack of concern for the patient's inability to understand information.

- Employee failed to provide an interpreter for a deaf patient or a patient who speaks another language.

- Employee showed unwillingness to help the patient, failing to direct the patient to the appropriate department or area when he looked lost or asked for directions, failing to help a patient or find someone to help when he was struggling to walk or losing his balance.

- Employee failed to explain required forms to the patient, including patient registration forms, consent to treatment forms, and HIPAA regulations, and simply handed the patient forms to sign.

- Employee assumed that the patient knew all the provider's policies when no one ever explained them or provided the patient with written copies of them, including policies about paying for services and procedures.

Since you now know the common patient complaints about poor service, you can do something about them when you interact with patients to ensure that patients are satisfied with *your* service. You already learned in Chapter 1 that a patient's experience with a provider involves more than just one person. A patient may interact with many types of healthcare professionals from the time she arrives at the provider until the time she leaves. It is crucial that everyone working for the provider ensures that the patient's experience is as comfortable and pleasant as possible, given the patient's circumstances.

Excellent Service to Patients

You can ensure outstanding service just by smiling at and speaking to patients whom you see, even if you are not meeting with them. You might be walking down the hall when you see a patient arriving for an appointment. You can smile and say "Hello, how are you?" or just say "Good morning." When you see a patient leave, say "Good-bye" and "Thank you." "Thank you" is a phrase that many people forget to say to customers or do not know that they should say, and many times, employees tell customers "there you go" instead. Unfortunately, "there you go" is not a substitute for "thank you" and does not mean much because it does not show appreciation for the customer's business. Saying "Thank you" shows a patient that you appreciate his business and the fact that he chose to visit your provider, rather than going somewhere else. Saying "Hello," "Good morning," and "Thank you" may seem like minor activities, but they can have a huge impact in terms of making a patient feel important and appreciated. Imagine if everyone who worked for a provider took the extra *seconds* involved to practice these courtesies; the patient would think that he was visiting a very special place where the people valued him and truly cared. It takes more time for you to pour a cup of coffee or tea in the morning than it takes to stop and say "Hello." Take the extra time, and make the effort to help patients feel important to you and the provider for whom you work.

Many people working in healthcare do not realize that they may be responsible for the only positive interaction a patient has that day. Not all patients have a network of friends and family members to help them, and they may be surrounded by negative people who resent helping them. Maybe it has been a very long time since someone smiled at the patient or greeted him warmly. You could be this person, and it is an important job to have.

Think of a time when you received excellent service. Can you remember what happened that impressed you so much? Could you also employ those same skills to provide patients with excellent service? Professionalism skills that you learned earlier in the chapter also apply when you are providing services to patients. They include having patience, understanding, sympathy, and good manners; listening; and showing kindness.

An important point to note is that it is not advisable to complain to patients about how long you have worked that day, how you are ready to go home, how much you dislike your job, how you just had a fight with your significant other, that your car broke down on the way to work, or any other complaints or issues in your personal life. Remember, patients have their own issues to deal with, and it is not appropriate to complain to them. It is also not part of your job.

The Angry Patient

One of the challenges that healthcare professionals face when they are interacting with patients is handling an angry or frustrated patient who could be unhappy with the services, upset about receiving a bill, disappointed in an employee's inability to follow up on an issue, or upset for any other reason. It is easy to be kind to others and cheerful when they are also kind to you. But it can be especially difficult when you are trying to resolve a problem for an angry patient. It can be very upsetting when someone yells at you, criticizes you, or loudly complains. There are specific techniques that you can use to turn a negative interaction with a patient into a positive one, ensuring that you resolve the patient's problem without making the issue worse.

Review the following case study about an angry patient, and then think about techniques that you could employ to calm the patient and help to resolve her situation.

> You are working as a coder for Dr. Hoffman's office and covering for Judy, the front desk receptionist. Paula, a medical assistant, is working with you. You are busy answering incoming phone calls when a patient walks up to the desk and tells you that she is upset because she received three bills for a $75 service that she says she already paid. She continues to tell you that she does not feel that the office staff is listening to her because she already called twice to say that her bill was paid, but the bills "just keep coming!" Her voice becomes louder, and her face turns red. She points a finger in your face and shouts "*You people* don't know what you're doing, and you don't care how much you've inconvenienced a patient! Why can't you make the corrections and get it right?!" There are other patients in the waiting room who are witnessing her outburst. What should you do?

What techniques did you think about? Would you ask Paula to help you? Would you call your boss and ask her to handle the patient? Would you call the police because you feel threatened? Would you try to talk with the patient, or would you tell the patient to come back when she is calm? Would you insist that the patient calm down before you speak with her?

This situation is a tricky one to handle, first, because the patient is very upset, and second, because she is upset *in the waiting room*, which could easily upset other patients and risk release of her confidential information if you discuss her information in front of others.

Twelve Steps for Handling the Angry Patient   There are many different options for dealing with someone who is upset to help them to *remain calm* and to *resolve the problem*. Your job is to do *both*. In this situation, you will learn additional techniques for ensuring that the patient's confidential information remains confidential. Let's review the steps that you can take to successfully resolve this patient's issue as a true professional.

Step 1: Remain Calm.   It is very difficult *not* to become upset yourself when someone upsets you, but you should not show negative emotions in the workplace. Make sure that you have a calm expression on your face and that you speak calmly to the patient. Remember not to take the situation personally. The patient is upset about a bill that she received. Even if she were upset with you or something that you did, you still do not have to treat it as a personal attack. Remember that you are at work and have to show professionalism. One way to do this is to mentally remove yourself from the situation and pretend that you are another person looking in on it from the outside, someone who has no personal interest in the situation. An observer would remain calm, not become upset.

It is important to note that you should never tell an upset or angry patient to calm down. It will only make the patient more upset and angry because you are telling her what to do. It also does not work—she will not calm down just because you tell her to.

Step 2: Acknowledge the Patient.   As soon as the patient starts talking, look directly at her with a concerned expression on your face. Show interest and sincerity, and make it apparent that you really care about her problem, even if you are busy, even if you are having a bad day, even if you do not feel like it, because you have to act like a professional. Remember, this could be your best friend, mother, father, sister, or brother. What expression would you have if one of them walked up to the desk and said the same thing to you?

Step 3: Apologize, and Say That You Will Help.   As soon as you have the opportunity to speak without interrupting the patient, introduce yourself, and apologize, telling the patient that you will be happy to help her. It does not matter who is to blame for the patient's situation; apologize anyway because you are apologizing that the situation happened. You could say, "I'm sorry that this happened, and I will be happy to investigate the problem and help you," "I'm sorry, and I can understand why you are upset. I'll be glad to help," "I'm sorry, and I would be upset, too. I want to help you," or "I'm very sorry, and I will be glad to help you."

Apologizing and then blaming the patient or someone else is not professional, so do not say things like, "You're wrong," "I find it hard to believe that we billed you when you already paid," or "I'm sorry that this happened. We have had a lot of complaints about Debbie, the billing specialist," and "You're not the first patient to complain about incorrect bills." Remember, everyone works together as a team, and it is a good idea to support your teammates.

Also, apologizing and then saying, "It's not *my* fault," or "That's not *my* job," is not appropriate. When a patient complains to you, it is your job to determine the nature of the problem and help to resolve it, whether it is your fault or not.

Step 4: Allow the Patient to Vent Without Interrupting or Arguing.   To vent means to release anger by talking about it. The patient has a problem and wants to tell you about it. She will eventually stop talking so that you can try to resolve the problem. Do not interrupt her or try to talk over her by saying things like, "Just let me finish," "If you'd just let me talk," or "I'd be happy to help you, if I can only say something." Interrupting her will only upset her more because it makes it appear that you do not care enough about what she has to say to allow her to say it. You are not debating the patient when she complains to you. She has a complaint and needs to be heard. It is not an argument that you need to "win."

Step 5: Listen Carefully, and Take Notes. As the patient is speaking, start taking notes, listening carefully to the information that she provides. This is an important step for a few reasons:

- It helps you ensure that you gather all of the pertinent information related to the patient's problem.
- It helps you to remain calm because you are concentrating on *what* the patient says, rather than *how* she says it.
- It shows the patient that you are concerned enough about her situation to write it down.

Be careful when you are writing not to ignore the patient. Look up at times to make eye contact. If you have the opportunity to speak if the patient pauses, then tell her that you want to be sure that you have all of the necessary information, and that is why you are writing. This helps her to know that you are not ignoring her.

Step 6: Ask the Patient for Her Name. If the patient pauses, you can quickly ask her for her name. Then write it down. If you cannot obtain it, do not worry because you will have the chance later. If she gives her name, then address her by Mrs., Ms., or Miss, and then her last name; never address her by her first name.

Step 7: Ask the Patient to Go to a Private Area with You. Remember that this patient is having an outburst in the waiting area, which can easily upset other patients. In addition, the more that you talk with her about her bill, the greater the risk that other patients will hear you, which violates the patient's confidentiality.

You will have to find an opportunity when the patient pauses to again apologize and say something like, "I'm sorry that this situation happened. I'd like us to go to a private area where we can talk about it." If the patient insists that she does not want to go somewhere else, then you can say, "I would really like to take you to another area where no one can hear us to protect the confidentiality of your information." Note that you do not have to tell the patient that she may be upsetting other patients, that her behavior is disruptive, or that she needs to calm down. You present the fact that you want to protect her information. You should always meet with patients in private when you are discussing their medical or financial information with them.

Notice that you should be the person who takes the patient to a private area to discuss her situation because you are the first person she encountered and the person to whom she told her problem. In order for you to leave the desk, you will also have to tell Paula that you are leaving. If you were working at the front desk alone, then you could ask another employee to work at the front desk for you while you meet with the patient.

If it is not possible to leave the front desk because no one can cover for you, then you will need to find another employee who can meet with the patient, such as Debbie, the billing specialist, or the office manager if Debbie is not available. In this case, you will first want to explain the situation to the other employee, sharing the notes that you took so that the patient does not have to explain the same information to a second person. You will also have to tell the patient that you are calling another person to help her and that you will explain her situation to that person.

Step 8: Buy Some Time. Buying time means giving the patient time alone to calm down. Here is what you can do: Escort the patient to an empty office, conference room, or exam room where there is a comfortable place for her to sit and a computer where you can research her account information. Be sure to ask the patient for her name if you did not have the chance to do so earlier. Also ask the patient, "Would you like to sit down where you will be more comfortable?" as you direct her to a seat, and then ask, "Can I get you something to drink, like coffee, tea, or water?" You want the patient to sit down, but if she does not, that is all right. She can stand while you meet with her and may eventually sit down.

Offering the patient a beverage serves two purposes: It shows the patient that you are concerned about her situation and want her to be more comfortable, and it buys you extra time for her to calm down. This is because if the patient wants a beverage, then you have to get it for her, which will take you a few minutes, and will cause you to be absent for a few minutes. During that few minutes that she waits for you, she may then start to calm down. Note that you do not want to leave her waiting indefinitely because she will then become more upset that she had to wait for you. A few minutes may be just enough time to accomplish your goal. When you return with the beverage, thank the patient for waiting.

If the patient does not want a beverage, then you can still buy time by telling the patient that you need to find her chart, pull a copy of her most recent payment, or get another pen because yours has stopped writing, even if you do not need any of these items. Again, take a few minutes to obtain the item or items that you "need" to allow the patient time alone to calm down, and thank her for waiting when you return.

Step 9: Investigate the Problem. When you sit down to talk with the patient in private,

- Apologize again that the situation happened.
- Thank the patient for bringing the matter to your attention.
- Say that you want to help resolve the problem.

Do not make assumptions without fully investigating the problem, such as assuming that the patient is incorrect or assuming that another employee made a mistake. Your job is to gather all of the facts to determine what happened and how to resolve it.

Continue to speak in a calm tone, and avoid sounding impatient or disgusted, even if you feel that way. Express sincerity on your face. When someone is upset, and you remain calm, it has the tendency to calm the person who is upset. This does not mean that she will calm down immediately, but it will happen gradually.

Gather the notes you already made when the patient began talking to you at the front desk. Tell the patient that you would like to read back your notes to her to ensure that you wrote the information correctly. Then read them, and ask her if there is any information that you missed. She can then provide you with further details or tell you if you made a mistake. If she starts to vent again, then allow her to. Remember, she will stop eventually, and venting will help her to get all of the information out and calm her down. Ask her follow-up questions to find out information that you will need to resolve the problem.

The patient complained that the office billed her three times for a service for $75 for which she already paid. You will need to know the following information to properly investigate the problem in the patient's account on the practice management software:

- The date of service
- If the service is for the patient or a family member
- The date the patient paid $75
- The payment method (cash, check, or credit card)
- The dates of the bills she received

Next, check the patient's account in the software. Tell the patient what you are doing so that she does not wonder what you are typing into the computer or what information you are reading. You can say something like, "I'm going to pull up your account in the computer to make sure we have all of the information you gave to me." Note that you do not want to tell the patient that you are going to pull up her account to determine if she is correct. Remember that your job is to gather all of the facts and then decide how to resolve the problem.

When a patient tells you that she incorrectly received bills, there could be different reasons why. For example, it is possible that she really did pay, and there is no record of payment in the software, or she may have paid for another service, not the service for which she is being billed. How to resolve the problem depends on what the problem is. The main points to remember are that you should

1. Gather all of the facts from the patient.
2. Gather all of the facts from the office's records.
3. Determine what actually happened.
4. Resolve the problem.

Step 10: Ask for Help If You Need It. Maybe you need to find someone else who can assist you because you have additional questions about the bills that you cannot answer. If so, first determine whom you need to ask, and then tell the patient that you need assistance and from whom.

In this case, the problem is with a bill, and Debbie is the billing specialist, so you can ask Debbie to help you. Debbie works in the office with you, so you can call her on the phone and ask her to meet with you and the patient. When she comes into the room, explain to Debbie what the situation is so that the patient will not have to explain again. Then ask Debbie your questions to try to resolve the problem. If you need help from an employee who works outside your office, then you can call her and place the call on speaker so that both you and the patient can hear the call. Again, first explain the situation to the other employee so that patient does not have to do so.

Step 11: Resolve the Problem, and End the Meeting on a Positive Note. Discuss the resolution with the patient (and the other employee if you needed her help). An important point to note is that if the resolution is not obvious, then you can ask the patient what she wants you to do. For example, if a patient complains that there was no parking available, and she had to walk five blocks to your office, you could ask her what she would suggest, rather than give away the store, as they say, and buy her a year's parking pass in the nearest parking garage. Sometimes the patient's solution is simple. She may suggest paying for her parking during her visit to the office.

In this patient's case, if the office did incorrectly bill the patient, the resolution is to note this information on the computer so that she does not receive any more bills. Or if the patient had an additional service that she thought she had already paid for but had not, the resolution is to provide the patient with documentation to show the service and the charge so that she can pay for it.

Maybe you cannot resolve the problem during the meeting with the patient because you or another employee have to further investigate the problem. In that case, you can apologize to the patient, explain why you have to further investigate, and tell her that you will contact her with additional information. Be sure to tell her when she can expect to hear from you. Whatever the resolution is, the goal is to discuss it with the patient so that you can both agree on it.

Then, apologize again for the inconvenience to the patient, whether it was the office at fault or the patient. It does not matter who is to blame; apologize anyway. Thank the patient for bringing the problem to your attention. Give the patient your business card, which will have your name, telephone number, and email address, and tell the patient to call you personally if she needs anything more. If you do not have a business card, then write your contact information on a piece of paper, and give it to the patient.

If you can offer the patient anything more, then do so. You might give her another bottle of water to take with her, validate her parking ticket if she had to pay to park at your office, or give her a pen with the office's name and information—any small gesture that will help her leave the office feeling satisfied with your service. Then personally walk the patient out of the office, and wish her a good day. Say "Good bye" and "Thank you."

Remember how many people an upset customer may tell about their experience, and how many people a satisfied customer may tell? Do not allow the patient to leave without resolving the situation.

Step 12: Document the Meeting, and Perform Necessary Follow-Up.   Many software programs have areas within a patient's account where you can document phone calls, special notes, and meetings with patients. Ensure that you document what happened during the meeting and the steps that were needed to resolve the situation. Documentation is crucial because if another employee has to perform follow-up or talk with the patient again, there will be a record of the details of your meeting, which anyone can refer to when necessary. Perform any follow-up activities required, such as placing the patient's account on hold so that she is not billed again, or researching to find additional records or proof of payment.

Additional Tips for Handling the Angry Patient

Review the following tips for dealing with an angry or upset patient.

- Do not tell the patient that there is nothing that you can do to help.

- Do not say, "It is our policy that . . ." and then say that there is nothing that you can do. People make policies, and people can also review those policies to determine if they make sense and revise them if necessary.

- Do not give the patient orders, such as saying things like, "Your behavior is very rude, and you need to calm down," or "You are being very disrespectful to me, and I am not disrespectful to you." These comments will only make the patient more angry, since the patient will resent you attempting to give her orders regarding her behavior, even if her behavior is inappropriate. She is upset, so allow her the opportunity to tell you about it without policing her behavior.

- Ask for your manager's assistance if you have failed to resolve the problem yourself or with another employee's help. Then, explain the situation to your manager so that the patient does not have to repeat herself. Do not immediately call your manager every time you encounter an angry or upset patient.

- Call your manager, the police, or security (if your provider has a security officer) if a patient threatens you, verbally or physically, and you believe that the patient will harm you. If a patient swears at you, then this does not necessarily mean that she is threatening you. It depends on what she says to you. If she is not threatening you, then you can politely ask her not to swear at you because it makes you feel uncomfortable. If she does not stop, then you can ask for your manager's assistance because you will not be able to successfully resolve the problem if the patient does not stop swearing at you. Sometimes upset customers calm down when they know that they are talking with someone who is a higher authority.

- Avoid labeling patients after negative encounters. This means that after an angry patient leaves, you should not call her names when you are discussing the situation with your manager or other employees, such as calling her a "pain," "psycho," or "old buzzard." Even though it may feel good to complain about her, it serves no purpose and only makes you look unprofessional.

- If the angry patient is on the phone, then you can still employ many of the same techniques for dealing with the patient in person. Apologize, listen without interrupting, introduce yourself, say that you want to help, and take notes and repeat back the information. You can also "buy time" by telling the patient that you need to research her account and with her permission will place her on hold to allow you to find her information. This will give her time to calm down. Do not leave her on hold for more than two to three minutes, but it may be just enough time for her to calm down.

- You may have to meet with, or handle a phone call from, an angry family member if the patient is not present. You can use the same techniques for handling an angry patient. Be sure that you have a signed authorization from the patient allowing you to speak with the family member.

TAKE A BREAK

Let's take a break, and then review more about patient relations.

| Exercise 36.5 | **Patient Relations** |

Instructions: Fill in each blank with the best answer.

1. _____ is interacting with patients and their families to ensure that they receive the best service.

2. It is estimated that a dissatisfied customer may tell up to _____ people about his bad experience, and a satisfied customer may tell up to _____ people.

3. Lack of interest in the patient's issue, displayed by not paying attention, ignoring the patient, or having an uninterested facial expression, are among the _____ about bad service.

4. There are many different options for dealing with someone who is upset to help them to _____ and to _____.

5. To _____ means to release anger by talking about it.

6. An additional tip for _____ is not to say, "It is our policy that . . ." and then say that there is nothing that you can do.

CHAPTER REVIEW

Multiple Choice

Instructions: Circle one best answer to complete each statement.

1. Calming an angry patient involves which of the following?
   a. Telling the patient that you cannot change office policies
   b. Offering the patient a quick solution to the problem
   c. Allowing the patient to vent while you take notes
   d. Telling the patient to calm down

2. Offering an angry or upset patient an empty office or exam room helps because:
   a. it prevents the angry patient from upsetting anyone in the waiting room.
   b. it allows you time to complete other tasks before helping the patient.
   c. it calms the patient because it makes the patient more comfortable.
   d. answers a and c

3. Which of the following should you ALWAYS say to an angry patient?
   a. "Let me finish talking."
   b. "Just calm down."
   c. "I apologize for the mistake."
   d. "You need to more respectful of other people."

4. Any time that a patient comes into a physician's office with a complaint, you should
   a. call the manager to speak with the patient.
   b. call the physician to speak with the patient.
   c. tell the patient that the office was not at fault.
   d. investigate the complaint to determine what happened.

5. An example of INCORRECT behavior when dealing with an angry patient is to
   a. apologize for what happened.
   b. tell the patient that it is not your problem, and you will need to ask someone else.
   c. listen attentively.
   d. tell the patient that you understand why he is upset.

6. The _____ include(s) individual job duties and expected behavior.
   a. time sheet
   b. employer's policies and procedures
   c. job description
   d. practice management software

7. Many larger organizations have a _____ whose employees are in charge of hiring and firing employees, overseeing employee benefits, and processing the company payroll.
   a. Honorary Recruitment Department
   b. Patient Satisfaction Team
   c. healthcare management team
   d. Human Resources Department

8. _____ means to know who will receive your message and how much information he needs to have.
   a. Know your place
   b. Know your audience
   c. Know your job
   d. Know your coworkers

9. _____ means that you can leave your job at any time, for any reason, even without notice, and your employer can terminate your job at any time, for any reason, without notice.
   a. At-will employment
   b. Hire-at-will employment
   c. Fire-at-will employment
   d. All-risk employment

10. _____, _____, and _____ are three types of communication.
   a. Verbal, oral, and written
   b. Nonverbal, written, and email
   c. Verbal, nonverbal, and written
   d. Verbal, nonverbal, and nonspeaking

Workplace Scenarios

Instructions: Read each scenario, and determine the best way to handle the situation, recording your answer in the space provided.

1. You are working for Dr. Hoffman's office, and a coworker, Janine, tells you during a lunch break that another coworker, Ron, has been saying negative things about you. Janine tells you that Ron said that you try to befriend the boss by talking with her all of the time. Janine says that Ron is very insulting when talking about you, including criticisms of your hair style and clothes. What should you do? _____

2. It's Monday, two days before an important staff meeting with all of the office staff, including your manager Chris, and Dr. Hoffman. Chris asks you to create sample form letters for Dr. Hoffman to send to other physicians when they refer new patients to his practice and to give the letters to her before the meeting on Wednesday. You spend about two hours working on the letters. You are very proud of your work because you created a series of four letters, each with a different style, clip art, and creative details. As Chris asked, you give the letters to her before the meeting. During the meeting, Chris distributes copies of the letters in a packet to all in attendance. She then proceeds to tell everyone that she would like to begin using the letters. Dr. Hoffman tells Chris that he is very impressed with the letters, and she smiles brightly and says, "thank you." What should you do? _____

3. You are working at the front desk at Williton Family Practice, scheduling patients' appointments, answering phones, and checking in and checking out patients. You are extremely busy, and there are nine patients in the waiting room scheduled to see either Dr. Young or Dr. Snow. The phone rings, and it's Dr. Reynolds. He is on his way to the office and asks you to order him lunch from the restaurant across the street, proceeds to give you his long lunch order, and then says that after you order his lunch, he needs you to go to the dry cleaner's to pick up two of his suits that his wife dropped off last week. What should you do? _____

4. At Williton Family Practice, Katie calls you into her office after lunch and explains that Bernadette, the billing specialist, told her that you were rude to her this morning and acted very abruptly. Katie tells you that she will not tolerate rudeness to staff and expects you to change this behavior. You are angry because you thought that Bernadette was rude to *you* and talked down to *you*. This morning, when Bernadette stood at the front desk and began criticizing you, you ignored her and took a phone call before she huffed and walked away. What should you do? _____

5. You are the newest employee at Williton Family Practice, starting two months ago. Everyone else has worked there at least three years. It seems that your five coworkers have been giving you the cold shoulder and excluding you from their group lunches in the lunch room. If they order food for pick-up, they never ask you to join them. Recently, they went out after work, talking loudly about it all day, anticipating where they would go for dinner. They did not invite you—AGAIN. What should you do? _____

6. It's 4:30 p.m. on Wednesday at Williton Family Practice. Katie comes to your desk and tells you that she needs your help with a report. She says that she has been working on it all week and has a few more points to include to finish it. Katie tells you that she has to turn in the report tomorrow morning to all three physicians. You made plans after work to have dinner with family members and are supposed to meet them at 5:00 p.m. at the restaurant. What should you do? _____

7. For the past two weeks, you have been off, sick from a gastrointestinal infection. When you return to work at Williton Family Practice, Katie speaks rudely to you, and it seems to you that she is upset that you were off. What should you do? _____

_____

8. You are in charge of sending a letter to Mrs. Klein, a patient at Williton Family Practice, who requests an explanation of how much money she owes to the office. Mrs. Klein said she wants to check the amount the office shows that she owes against her records. You check her balance owed on the computer and find that it's $580. So you write the letter to Mrs. Klein explaining the amount she owes and why. A few days later, Mrs. Klein calls the office and asks to speak with Katie. She is very upset and angry because she received your letter and says that according to her records she only owes $100. Katie checks the computer and finds that Mrs. Klein is correct. She apologizes to Mrs. Klein and explains that she will send her a corrected letter with the balance showing as $100. Katie then tells you that the amount owed in the letter was incorrect and shows you the account in the computer. You instantly see your mistake. What should you do? _____

_____

9. At Williton Family Practice, you work at the front desk with a medical assistant, Kathy, who constantly complains about the office and her work. She says that she does not like the hours or the physicians, and that Katie, the office manager, is too bossy. Kathy has been working at the office for six months. Each time that you see her interact with the physicians or with Katie, Kathy is very nice and gives no indication to them that she hates her job. Kathy's nonstop complaining is getting to you. What should you do? _____

_____

10. At Williton Family Practice, Katie asks you and two coworkers, Annette and Lucy, to complete a project. Each of you has to complete a lengthy section and the team needs to have regular weekly meetings to keep everyone on track. Katie asks you to be in charge of the project. You must make sure that you, Annette, and Lucy all have the work completed accurately and on time for each weekly meeting. You are also in charge of heading the weekly meetings and reporting the team's progress to Katie. The problem is that during your first meeting, Lucy did not have her work completed, not even close. She told you that she had other work to complete and promised to get the work to you by the next week's meeting. You gave her the benefit of the doubt and agreed to wait until the next week. But during the second meeting, Lucy told you the same story. You suspect that Lucy either does not know how to complete the work required or does not want to. Annette has completed all of her work, accurately and on time. She is now complaining to you about Lucy. What should you do? _____

_____

Instructions for Accessing ICD-9-CM and ICD-10-CM Official Guidelines for Coding and Reporting, ICD-10-PCS Coding Guidelines, and 1995 and 1997 Documentation Guidelines for Evaluation and Management Services

- You can find all of the ICD-9-CM and ICD-10-CM Official Guidelines for Coding and Reporting in your coding manual.

- You can also access all of the guidelines through other websites, by following the instructions listed here.

To access the ICD-9-CM Official Guidelines for Coding and Reporting, go to the website for the Centers for Disease Control and Prevention:

1. Go to http://www.cdc.gov/.

2. In the *A–Z Index* on the top banner bar, click the letter I.

3. Click *ICD-9-CM (ICD-9-CM (International Classification of Diseases, Ninth Revision, Clinical Modification)*.

4. You will then see the *International Classification of Diseases, Ninth Revision, Clinical Modification (ICD-9-CM)* page. Scroll down to *ICD-9-CM Addenda, Conversion Table, and Guidelines*, and click on *Guidelines*.

5. On the next page, *ICD-9-CM Addenda, Conversion Table, and Guidelines*, scroll down to *Guidelines*, and click on the link to *ICD-9-CM Guidelines*. The page that loads, a PDF file, will be the guidelines.

6. To view updates to each year's code set, which are published in October of each year, on the *ICD-9-CM Addenda, Conversion Table, and Guidelines* page, scroll down to the year of the addenda or errata that you are searching. Then choose the appropriate Index or Tabular addenda or errata.

To access the ICD-10-CM Official Guidelines for Coding and Reporting, go to the website for the Centers for Disease Control and Prevention:

1. Go to http://www.cdc.gov/.

2. In the *A–Z Index* of the top banner bar, click the letter I.

3. Click *ICD-10-CM (ICD-10-CM International Classification of Disease, Tenth Revision)*.

4. You will then see the *International Classification of Diseases, Tenth Revision, Clinical Modification (ICD-10-CM)* page. Scroll down to the files listed under *2012 release of ICD-10-CM* and click on *ICD-10-CM Guidelines*. The page that loads, a PDF file, will be the guidelines.

5. To view updates to each year's code set, scroll down to the files listed under *2012 release of ICD-10-CM*, and click on *ICD-10-CM 2010 to 2011 Addenda*. On the next page, choose the appropriate file for the addenda.

To access the ICD-10-PCS Coding Guidelines, go to the website for the Centers for Medicare and Medicaid Services:

1. Go to http://cms.gov/.

2. In the *Search* box at the top right of the page, type *ICD-10-PCS coding guidelines*.

3. You will then see search results that include a link to *ICD-10-PCS Coding Guidelines*. Click on the link to view the guidelines.

To access the 1995 and 1997 Documentation Guidelines for Evaluation and Management Services, go to the website for the Centers for Medicare and Medicaid Services:

1. Go to http://cms.gov/.

2. In the *Search* box at the top right of the page, type *1995 1997 guidelines*.

3. You will then see search results that include a link to the *Evaluation and Management Services Guide*. Click on the link to view the guide.

4. In the guide, you will find both 1995 and 1997 Evaluation and Management Documentation Guidelines for Evaluation and Management Services.

Overview of Differences Between ICD-9-CM and ICD-10-CM (Table 6-5 in Chapter 6)

OVERVIEW OF DIFFERENCES BETWEEN ICD-9-CM AND ICD-10-CM

Tabular List Changes	ICD-9-CM	ICD-10-CM
Total Number of Codes	Approximately 14,000	Approximately 70,000
Total Number of Tabular Chapters	17, plus two supplementary classifications (V codes and E codes)	21, with no supplementary classifications Four new chapters were created: • Diseases of the Eye and Adnexa • Diseases of the Ear and Mastoid Process • External Causes of Morbidity • Factors Influencing Health Status and Contact with Health Services
	Chapters are divided into Sections, groups of categories (3 characters). Each chapter *does not* provide a summary of sections within the chapter.	*Chapters are divided into* *Subchapters*, also called *blocks*. Subchapters are divided into groups of categories (3 characters). Each chapter begins with a summary of blocks within the chapter.
	Sections are divided into Categories (3 characters). A category can represent one disease or a group of related diseases or conditions. Category codes (3 characters) are valid codes if they are not further subdivided into 4- or 5-character codes.	*Subchapters are divided into* Categories (3 characters). If a category has no further subdivision, then it is called a code. A category can represent one disease or a group of related diseases or conditions. Category codes (3 characters) are valid as codes if they are not further subdivided into 4-, 5-, or 6-character codes. If they are further subdivided, then you must code them to the highest level of specificity.
	Categories are divided into Subcategories (4 characters).	*Categories are divided into* Subcategories (4, 5, or 6 characters) Each level of a subdivision after a category is called a subcategory.
	Subcategories are divided into Subclassifications (5 characters).	*Subcategories are divided into* Codes (4, 5, 6, or 7 characters) Codes are the *final level* that cannot be further subdivided. Remember that a code can also be 3 characters. Codes that are 7 characters are always called codes because 7 is the maximum number of characters in any code.
Code Ranges	001.0–999.9 (Tabular chapters) V01.0–V91.99 (V code supplementary classification) E000.0–E999.1 (E code supplementary classification)	A00.0–Z99.89 (Tabular chapters) Supplementary classifications were removed.
Code Titles	Code titles can be incomplete. The coder needs to add information from a category title when reading a subcategory or subclassification title.	Code titles are more complete. In many cases, the coder does not need to add information from a category title when reading a subcategory or code title.

OVERVIEW OF DIFFERENCES BETWEEN ICD-9-CM AND ICD-10-CM *continued*

Code Structure Changes	ICD-9-CM	ICD-10-CM
Code Length	Up to 5 alphanumeric characters.	Up to 7 alphanumeric characters.
Use of Letters in Codes	The first character of an ICD-9-CM code is a number or the letter V or E.	The first character of an ICD-10-CM code is always a capital letter and can be any letter except U. The letter U is reserved for additional code expansion and does not currently exist in the ICD-10-CM code set.
		The first character applies to a specific chapter because all codes in the chapter will start with the same letter. However, letters D and H are each used in two chapters.
	The second, third, fourth, and fifth characters are numbers. There is no sixth or seventh character.	The second and third characters are numbers. The fourth, fifth, sixth, and seventh characters can be numbers or any letter except U.
Highest Level of Codes	The highest code level is 5 characters.	The highest code level is 7 characters.
Codes with Five or Six Characters	Many categories show a list of choices for the fifth digit that applies to subcategory codes.	The list of choices for the fifth digit has been eliminated. Codes with five and six characters have code titles that include information that applies to the fifth or sixth character. There is no longer any need to reference a category to find choices for the fifth character.

Changes to Level of Code Detail	ICD-9-CM	ICD-10-CM
Laterality	Not used	Laterality has been added to codes to identify whether the patient's condition affects the left or right side, if it is bilateral, or if the side is unspecified.
Advances in Medicine	Codes reflect limited advances in medicine.	Codes reflect numerous advances in medicine and include conditions that were not previously identified. Codes are more specific regarding anatomy, physiology, pathophysiology, treatments, and updated medical terminology.
Additional Detail	Codes are limited in the amount of detail they provide.	Codes were expanded to further define many disorders and provide more detail about the following conditions: diabetes, postoperative complications, injuries, substance abuse, alcohol abuse, and ambulatory and managed care encounters.
Patient Risk Factors	Limited codes exist for patient risk factors.	Specific codes identify patients' *risk factors*. Risk factors are problems that patients experience which could lead to health issues.
		Examples include tobacco use, lack of exercise, inappropriate diet and eating habits, gambling, and high-risk sexual behavior. All of these risk factors could cause health problems if the patient does not change his or her behavior and lifestyle.
Codes for Pregnancy, Childbirth, and the Puerperium	Codes include a fifth digit to identify the patient's episode of care, the time period when the physician or other clinician treats the patient for a specific condition.	Fifth digits identifying the patient's episode of care were eliminated. Instead, individual code titles identify this information.
	Episodes of care include treating the patient's condition before, during, or after delivery.	
	Codes do not identify if a pregnancy condition is present in a specific trimester.	Codes identify whether a pregnancy condition is present in the first, second, or third trimester.

Changes to Coding Conventions	ICD-9-CM	ICD-10-CM
Use of Codes for Reporting Purposes	This rule does not exist in ICD-9-CM coding conventions. However, it means to report codes to their highest level of specificity, including categories, subcategories, and subclassifications, which has always been a rule for ICD-9-CM coding.	The coding rule "Use of codes for reporting purposes" was added to ICD-10-CM coding conventions. It means to always code to the highest level of specificity when reporting codes to insurances, claims clearinghouses, billing and collection agencies, or any other organizations.

continued

OVERVIEW OF DIFFERENCES BETWEEN ICD-9-CM AND ICD-10-CM *continued*

Changes to Coding Conventions	ICD-9-CM	ICD-10-CM
		In ICD-10-CM, a code that cannot be further subdivided is called a "code." Always report codes, rather than categories or subcategories that can be further subdivided. Also be sure to report applicable seventh characters.
Use Placeholder "x" to fill in a Missing Character	Not used.	Some codes require a seventh character but do not have an applicable fourth, fifth, or sixth character. You are still required to assign the seventh character, even though the characters before the seventh may be missing.
		For example, some codes are five characters long, don't have an applicable sixth character, but require a seventh character to identify encounter information. It is mandatory to fill in the space of the missing sixth character with a placeholder "x" so that the seventh character is in the correct place. The code is invalid if you do not add the "x" to hold the place of the sixth character before adding the seventh.
		ICD-10-CM placeholder "x" was created to allow additional code expansion in case the placeholder "x" is someday replaced by an actual character with a specific meaning.
The Seventh Character Provides Episode of Care and Additional Information	Not used.	The seventh character provides more information about a patient's encounter, including the patient's episode of care, the time period when the physician or other clinician treats the patient. Examples of a seventh character for injuries and external causes of injuries are
		• A—Initial encounter • D—Subsequent encounter • S— Sequela
		Seventh characters can also provide additional information about fractures and other types of encounters.
Not elsewhere classifiable (NEC) and not otherwise specified (NOS)	One code can represent both NEC and NOS.	NEC codes and NOS codes are listed separately. There are no codes that combine NEC and NOS. The meanings of NEC and NOS remain the same as in ICD-9-CM.
Brace }	Used in the Tabular in some coding manuals to connect words written to left of it to words written to the right.	Not used.
Excludes Notes in the Tabular List	There is one type of Excludes Notes which means that the terms listed as excluded should be coded elsewhere.	Excludes Notes were revised to include
		• Excludes1 • Excludes2
		There are two types of Excludes Notes. The Excludes1 note means "NOT CODED HERE!" An Excludes1 note appears under codes in the Tabular. It lists conditions and their corresponding codes that are excluded from the code that you cross-reference. It is similar to the Excludes note in ICD-9-CM.
		The Excludes1 note is a warning that two conditions cannot ever occur together. For example, if you cross-reference a congenital condition, an Excludes1 note would show the acquired form of the same condition. You could not code both conditions together.
		The Excludes2 note means "not included here." When you cross-reference a code to the Tabular, and it has an Excludes2 note, it means that the condition listed in the note is not typically part of the code that you cross-referenced.

OVERVIEW OF DIFFERENCES BETWEEN ICD-9-CM AND ICD-10-CM   *continued*

Changes to Coding Conventions	ICD-9-CM	ICD-10-CM
		The Excludes2 note is a warning that two conditions are not likely to occur together, but they could. For example, a chronic condition typically is not also an acute condition, but it could be.
		When an Excludes2 note appears under a code, it is acceptable to assign both the code and the Excludes2 code together if the patient has both conditions.
Code Also Note	Not used.	A "code also" note is a new convention that you may need to assign two codes to fully describe a condition. The note does not provide you with the order in which to sequence the codes.
Default Codes	Codes are listed next to main terms in the Index, but they are not called default codes.	A default code is a new convention. It is the code listed next to a main term in the Index. The default code represents the condition that is most commonly associated with the main term, or it is the unspecified code for the condition.
		When a physician documents a condition in the medical record but does not provide enough specific information, assign the default code of "unspecified." Always remember to query the physician about the documentation before assigning a code that is unspecified.
Syndromes	Instructions for coding syndromes appear in the Official Guidelines under the General Coding Guidelines.	Instructions for coding syndromes have not changed but were moved from ICD-9-CM General Coding Guidelines to coding conventions in ICD-10-CM.
		When you search for a syndrome, look under the main term *syndrome* and look for the subterm that describes the type of syndrome. In the absence of Index guidance, assign codes for the documented *manifestations* of the syndrome.

Changes to Supplementary Classifications	ICD-9-CM	ICD-10-CM
V codes— Supplementary Classification of Factors Influencing Health Status and Contact with Health Service	V codes are included in their own Supplementary Classification, rather than within a chapter in the Tabular.	There is no separate Supplementary Classification of V codes. Any conditions previously represented by V codes are now included in Chapter 21—Factors Influencing Health Status and Contact with Health Services.
		Chapter 21 includes codes for many conditions that are not in ICD-9-CM. It includes codes for lifestyle problems, such as high-risk behaviors, lack of exercise, and inappropriate diet. Also included are codes for blood types and do not resuscitate (DNR) status.
E codes—Supplementary Classification of External Causes of Injury and Poisoning	E codes are included in their own Supplementary Classification, rather than within a chapter in the Tabular.	There is no separate Supplementary Classification of E codes. Any conditions previously represented by E codes are now included in Chapter 20—External Causes of Morbidity.

Additional Changes	ICD-9-CM	ICD-10-CM
Multiple Codes and Combination Codes	Assign multiple codes for an etiology/manifestation relationship, external cause of poisoning and substance that caused the poisoning, symptoms and related conditions, and when the patient has more than one diagnosis that cannot be represented by a combination code.	In many cases, assign only one combination code that represents both the etiology and manifestation, both the external cause of poisoning and poison substance, and both symptoms and their related conditions.
		In other cases, there can be multiple ICD-10-CM codes that are represented by a single ICD-9-CM code.

continued

OVERVIEW OF DIFFERENCES BETWEEN ICD-9-CM AND ICD-10-CM *continued*

Additional Changes	ICD-9-CM	ICD-10-CM
Morphology Codes	Morphology codes, codes beginning with the letter M, are listed in the Index and cross-referenced to Appendix A—Morphology of Neoplasms.	Codes for morphology of neoplasms are listed in the Index and cross-referenced to the Tabular. They no longer appear in a separate Appendix.
Hypertension Table	Located in the Index, the Hypertension Table separated hypertension into malignant, benign, and unspecified.	The Hypertension Table has been removed. Under the main term *hypertension* in the Index, malignant and benign have been added as nonessential modifiers.
Appendices	There are four Appendices—A, C, D, and E.	Not used.
Hyphen (Dash)	Not used.	A hyphen (dash) can appear after a code in the Index or Tabular to show that you need to add more characters to the code to make it valid.
		Examples are as follows: I87.0—I83.—
		Both of these codes need an additional character in order to be considered valid codes.

Normal Lab Values and Vital Signs

NORMAL LAB VALUES

Tests Performed on Whole Blood, Plasma, or Serum

Note: Test results depend on methods used. Normal ranges and other interpretive data given in this book are intended solely for purposes of orientation and should not be applied to actual test results.

Analyte or Procedure	Normal Range (Metric)	Normal Range (SI)
acid phosphatase	< 0.6 U/L	< 0.6 U/L
ACTH (adrenocorticotropic hormone)	10–50 pg/mL	2.2–11.1 pmol/L
A/G (albumin-globulin) ratio	1.5–3.0	1.5–3.0
albumin	3.5–5.0 g/dL	35–50 g/L
aldolase	2.5 U/L	2.5 U/L
aldosterone, recumbent	3–16 ng/dL	0.08–0.44 nmol/L
upright	7–30 ng/dL	0.19–0.83 nmol/L
alkaline phosphatase (slang "alk phos")	20–120 U/L	20–120 U/L
alpha$_1$-antitrypsin (AAT)	100–300 mg/mL	20–60 mmol/L
alpha fetoprotein (AFP)	< 15 ng/mL	< 15 mcg/L
ALT (alanine aminotransferase) (formerly SGPT)	8–45 U/L	8–45 U/L
ammonia, serum	15–45 mcg/dL	11–32 mcmol/L
amylase	< 125 U/L	< 125 U/L
anion gap	12–20 mEq/L	12–20 mmol/L
AST (aspartate aminotransferase) (formerly SGOT)	< 35 U/L	< 35 U/L
B cells	5–15%	5–15%
bands (banded neutrophils)	4–8%	4–8%
basophils (basos)	0–1%	0–1%
bicarbonate	24–30 mEq/L	24–30 mmol/L
bilirubin, direct	0.1–0.4 mg/dL	0.1–0.5 mg/dL
bilirubin, indirect	0.1–0.9 mg/dL	1.7–6.8 mcmol/L
bilirubin, total	1.7–8.5 mcmol/L	1.7–15.3 mcmol/L
bleeding time	< 4 minutes	< 4 minutes
BNP (brain natriuretic peptide)	< 50 pg/mL	< 50 ng/L
BUN (blood urea nitrogen)	5–20 mg/dL	1.8–7.1 mcmol/L
calcitonin, male	0–15 pg/mL	0–4.20 pmol/L
calcium	8.2–10.2 mg/dL	2–2.5 mmol/L
CD4 cell count	500–1500 cells/mm^3	0.5–1.5 × 10^9 cells/L
CEA (carcinoembryonic antigen)	< 2.5 ng/mL	< 2.5 mcg/L
chloride	100–106 mEq/L	100–106 mmol/L
cholesterol	< 200 mg/dL	< 520 mmol/L
cholinesterase (pseudocholinesterase)	8–18 U/L	8–18 U/L

Source: HEALTH PROFESSIONS INST, MEDICAL TRANSCRIPTION: FUNDAMENTALS AND PRACTICE, 3rd Ed., © 2007. Reprinted and electronically reproduced by permission of Pearson Education, Inc., Upper Saddle River, New Jersey.

continued

Analyte or Procedure	Normal Range (Metric)	Normal Range (SI)
clotting time, Lee-White	6–17 minutes	6–17 minutes
copper	0.7–1.5 mcg/mL	11–24 mmol/L
cortisol, 8 a.m.	5–23 mcg/dL	138-635 nmol/L
4 p.m.	3–16 mcg/dL	83-441 nmol/L
creatinine	0.6–1.2 mg/dL	50–100 mcmol/L
electrolytes: see individual values for sodium, potassium, chloride, and bicarbonate		
eosinophils (eos)	2–4%	2–4%
EPO (erythropoietin)	5–30 mcU/mL	5–30 U/L
erythrocyte sedimentation rate, Westergren	0–20 mm/hr	0–20 mm/hr
Wintrobe	0–15 mm/hr	0–15 mm/hr
erythropoietin (EPO)	5–30 mcU/mL	5–30 mcU/mL
estradiol	24–149 pg/m	90–550 pmol/L
ferritin	20–200 ng/mL	20–200 mcg/L
fibrin degradation products (fibrin split products)	< 3 mcg/mL	< 3 mg/L
5′-nucleotidase	< 12.5 U/L	< 12.5 U/L
follicle-stimulating hormone (FSH), female	1.1–24 ng/mL	5.0–108 U/L
male	0.5–4.5 ng/mL	2.2–20.0 U/L
free fatty acids (FFA)	8–20 mg/dL	0.2–0.7 mmol/L
free T_4 index	0.9–2.1 ng/dL	12–27 pmol/L
FSH (follicle-stimulating hormone), female	1.1–24 ng/mL	5.0–108 U/L
male	0.5–4.5 ng/mL	2.2–20.0 U/L
FSP (fibrin split products)	< 3 mcg/mL	< 3 mg/L
gamma-glutamyl trans-peptidase (GGT)	< 65 U/L	< 65 U/L
gastrin	21–125 pg/mL	10–59.3 pmol/L
GFR (glomerular filtration rate)	90–135 mL/min per 1.73 m²	0.86–1.3 mL/sec per m²
GGT (gamma-glutamyl transpeptidase)	< 65 U/L	< 65 U/L
globulin, total	1.5–3.0 g/dL	15–30 g/L
glomerular filtration rate (GFR)	90-135 mL/min/1.73 m²	0.86–1.3 mL/sec/m²
glucagon	50–200 pg/mL	14–57 pmol/L
glucose	60–115 mg/dL	3.3–64 mmol/L
glycosylated hemoglobin (hemoglobin A_{1C}), normal	4–7%	4–7%
acceptable diabetic control	< 8%	< 8%
haptoglobin	40–180 mg/dL	0.4–1.8 g/L
HDL (high density lipoprotein) cholesterol	35–80 mg/dL	1-2 mmol/L
hematocrit	40–48%	40–48%
hemoglobin	12–16 g/dL	7.5–10 mmol/L
hemoglobin A_{1C} (glycosylated hemoglobin), normal	4–7%	4–7%
acceptable diabetic control	< 8%	< 8%
hexosaminidase A	2.5–9 U/L	2.5–9 U/L
high density lipoprotein (HDL) cholesterol	35-80 mg/dL	1-2 mmol/L
homocysteine	< 1.6 mg/L	< 12 mcmol/L
insulin	5–25 mcU/mL	34–172 pmol/L
iron, males	50–160 mcg/dL	9.0–28.8 mcmol/L
females	45–144 mcg/dL	8.1–26 mcmol/L

Analyte or Procedure	Normal Range (Metric)	Normal Range (SI)
iron-binding capacity	250–350 mcg/dL	45–63 mcmol/L
lactate dehydrogenase (LDH)	< 110 U/L	< 110 U/L
lactic acid	4.5–19.8 mg/dL	0.5–2.2 mmol/L
LDH (lactate dehydrogenase)	< 110 U/L	< 110 U/L
LDL (low density lipoprotein) cholesterol	40–130 mg/dL	1–3 mmol/L
leucine aminopeptidase, serum (SLAP)	< 40 U/L	< 40 U/L
LH (luteinizing hormone), females	0.5–2.7 mcg/mL	4.5–24.3 U/L
males	0.4–1.9 mcg/mL	3.6–17.1 U/L
lipase	< 1.5 U/L	< 1.5 U/L
low density lipoprotein (LDL) cholesterol	40–130 mg/dL	1–3 mmol/L
luteinizing hormone (LH), females	0.5–2.7 mcg/mL	0.4–1.9 mcg/mL
males	4.5–24.3 U/L	3.6–17.1 U/L
lymphocytes	25–40%	25–40%
magnesium	1.5–2.3 mg/dL	0.6–1.0 mmol/L
MCH (mean corpuscular hemoglobin)	27–31 pg/cell	27–31 pg/cell
MCHC (mean corpuscular hemoglobin concentration)	32–36 g/dL	320–360 g/L
MCV (mean corpuscular volume)	82–92 mcm^3	82–92 fL
mean corpuscular hemoglobin (MCH)	27–31 pg/cell	27–31 pg/cell
mean corpuscular hemoglobin concentration (MCHC)	32–36 g/dL	320–360 g/L
mean corpuscular volume (MCV)	82–92 mcm^3	82–92 fL
melatonin, 8 a.m.	0.8–7.7 pg/mL	3.7–23.3 pg/mL
midnight	3.5–33 pmol/L	16–100 pmol/L
methemoglobin	< 3%	< 3%
monocytes	4–6%	4–6%
myeloid/erythroid ratio	2.0–4.0	2.0–4.0
myoglobin	14–51 mcg/L	0.8–2.9 mol/L
osmolality, serum	280–295 mOsm/kg	280–295 mOsm/kg
oxygen saturation	95–100%	95–100%
parathyroid hormone	11–54 pg/mL	1.2–56 pmol/L
partial pressure of carbon dioxide (pCO_2)	35–45 torr	35–45 torr
partial pressure of oxygen (pO_2)	75–100 torr	75–100 torr
partial thromboplastin time (PTT)	22–37 seconds	22–37 seconds
pCO_2 (partial pressure of carbon dioxide)	35–45 torr	35–45 torr
pepsinogen	124–142 ng/mL	124–142 mcg/L
pH	7.35–7.45	7.35–7.45
phenylalanine	2–4 mg/dL	121–242 mcmol/L
phosphorus	2.5–4.5 mg/dL	0.8–1.5 mmol/L
platelets	150,000–400,000/mm^3	150–400 × 10^9/L
pO_2 (partial pressure of oxygen)	75–100 torr	75–100 torr
potassium	3.5–5.0 mEq/L	3.5–5.0 mmol/L
progesterone	0.1–28 ng/mL	0.3–89 nmol/L
prolactin (nonpregnant)	2.5–19 ng/mL	1.1-8.6 nmol/L
PSA (prostate specific antigen)	< 4 ng/mL	< 4 mcg/L
pseudocholinesterase (cholinesterase)	8–18 U/L	8–18 U/L
PT (prothrombin time)	12–14 seconds	12–14 seconds

continued

Analyte or Procedure	Normal Range (Metric)	Normal Range (SI)
PTT (partial thromboplastin time)	22–37 seconds	22–37 seconds
RDW (red cell distribution width)	< 15%	< 15%
red blood cells	4,800,000–5,600,000/mm^3	4.8–5.6 × 10^{12}/L
red cell distribution width (RDW)	< 15%	< 15%
renin, reclining	0.2–2.3 ng/mL	1.6–4.3 ng/mL
upright	4.7–54.5 pmol/L	38–102 pmol/L
reticulocytes	0.5–1.5%	0.5–1.5%
sedimentation rate (see *erythrocyte sedimentation rate*)		
segmented neutrophils	40–70%	40–70%
serum glutamic pyruvic transaminase (SGPT) (now ALT)	8–45 U/L	8–45 U/L
SGGT (see *GGT*)		
SGOT (serum glutamic oxaloacetic transaminase) (now AST)	< 35 U/L	< 35 U/L
SLAP (serum leucine aminopeptidase)	< 40 U/L	< 40 U/L
sodium	136–145 mEq/L	136–145 mmol/L
somatotropin, child	5–10 ng/mL	< 2.5 ng/mL
adult	232–465 pmol/L	< 116 pmol/L
T cells	55–65%	55–65%
T$_3$	70–190 ng/dL	1.1–2.9 nmol/L
T$_3$ uptake	25–38%	0.25–0.38
T$_4$ (thyroxine)	4.5–12.0 mcg/dL	58–154 nmol/L
testosterone, male	300–1200 ng/d	10.5–42 nmol/L
thyroxine (T$_4$)	4.5–12.0 mcg/dL	58–154 nmol/L
transferrin	250–430 mg/dL	2.5–4.3 g/L
triglycerides	< 160 mg/dL	< 1.80 mmol/L
troponin I	< 1.5 ng/mL	< 1.5 mcg/L
troponin T	< 0.029 ng/mL	< 0.029 mcg/L
TSH (thyroid stimulating hormone)	0.4–4.2 mcU/mL	0.4–4.2 mU/L
two-hour (2-hour) postprandial glucose	< 140 mg/dL	< 7.7 mmol/L
uric acid	3.4–7 mg/dL	202–416 mcmol/L
vasopressin	2–12 pg/mL	1.85–11.1 pmol/L
white blood cells	5000–10,000/mm^3	5–10 × 10^9/L
zinc	0.75–1.4 mcg/mL	11.5–21.6 mcmol/L

VITAL SIGNS

Normal Blood Pressure

Systolic measurement (top number):
<120 mm/Hg
Diastolic measurement (bottom number):
<80 mm/Hg

Normal respiratory rate

12–20 breaths per minute

Normal pulse

60–100 beats per minute

Normal temperature

- Oral—98.6°F
- Axillary (armpit)—97.6°F
- Rectal—99.6°F

HCPCS Modifiers

A1	Dressing for one wound
A2	Dressing for two wounds
A3	Dressing for three wounds
A4	Dressing for four wounds
A5	Dressing for five wounds
A6	Dressing for six wounds
A7	Dressing for seven wounds
A8	Dressing for eight wounds
A9	Dressing for nine or more wounds
AA	Anesthesia services performed personally by anesthesiologist
AD	Medical supervision by a physician: more than four concurrent anesthesia procedures
AE	Registered dietician
AF	Specialty physician
AG	Primary physician
AH	Clinical psychologist
AI	Principal physician of record
AJ	Clinical social worker
AK	Non participating physician
AM	Physician, team member service
AP	Determination of refractive state was not performed in the course of diagnostic ophthalmological examination
AQ	Physician providing a service in an unlisted health professional shortage area (HPSA)
AR	Physician provider services in a physician scarcity area
AS	Physician assistant, nurse practitioner, or clinical nurse specialist services
AS	For assistant at surgery
AT	Acute treatment (this modifier should be used when reporting service 98940, 98941, 98942)
AU	Item furnished in conjunction with a urological, ostomy, or tracheostomy supply
AV	Item furnished in conjunction with a prosthetic device, prosthetic or orthotic
AW	Item furnished in conjunction with a surgical dressing
AX	Item furnished in conjunction with dialysis services
AY	Item or service furnished to an ESRD patient that is not for the treatment of ESRD
AZ	Physician providing a service in a dental health professional shortage area for the purpose of an electronic health record incentive payment
BA	Item furnished in conjunction with parenteral enteral nutrition (PEN) services
BL	Special acquisition of blood and blood products
BO	Orally administered nutrition, not by feeding tube
BP	The beneficiary has been informed of the purchase and rental options and has elected to purchase the item
BR	The beneficiary has been informed of the purchase and rental options and has elected to rent the item
BU	The beneficiary has been informed of the purchase and rental options and after 30 days has not informed the supplier of his/her decision

CA	Procedure payable only in the Inpatient setting when performed emergently on an outpatient who expires prior to admission
CB	Service ordered by a renal dialysis facility (RDF) physician as part of the ESRD beneficiary's dialysis benefit, is not part of the composite rate, and is separately reimbursable
CC	Procedure code change (use 'cc' when the procedure code submitted was changed either for administrative reasons or because an incorrect code was filed)
CD	AMCC test has been ordered by an ESRD facility or MCP physician that is part of the composite rate and is not separately billable
CE	AMCC test has been ordered by an ESRD facility or MCP physician that is a composite rate test but is beyond the normal frequency covered under the rate and is separately reimbursable based on medical necessity
CF	AMCC test has been ordered by an ESRD facility or MCP physician that is not part of the composite rate and is separately billable
CG	Policy criteria applied
CR	Catastrophe/disaster related
CS	Item or service related, in whole or in part, to an illness, injury, or condition that was caused by or exacerbated by the effects, direct or indirect, of the 2010 oil spill in the Gulf of Mexico, including but not limited to subsequent clean-up activities
DA	Oral health assessment by a licensed health professional other than a dentist
E1	Upper left, eyelid
E2	Lower left, eyelid
E3	Upper right, eyelid
E4	Lower right, eyelid
EA	Erythropoetic stimulating agent (ESA) administered to treat anemia due to anti-cancer chemotherapy
EB	Erythropoetic stimulating agent (ESA) administered to treat anemia due to anti-cancer radiotherapy
EC	Erythropoetic stimulating agent (ESA) administered to treat anemia not due to anti-cancer radiotherapy or anti-cancer chemotherapy
ED	Hematocrit level has exceeded 39% (or hemoglobin level has exceeded 13.0 g/dl) for 3 or more consecutive billing cycles immediately prior to and including the current cycle
EE	Hematocrit level has not exceeded 39% (or hemoglobin level has not exceeded 13.0 g/dl) for 3 or more consecutive billing cycles immediately prior to and including the current cycle
EJ	Subsequent claims for a defined course of therapy, e.g., epo, sodium
EJ	Hyaluronate, infliximab
EM	Emergency reserve supply (for ESRD benefit only)
EP	Service provided as part of Medicaid early periodic screening diagnosis and treatment (EPSDT) program
ET	Emergency services

EY   No physician or other licensed health care provider order for this item or service

F1   Left hand, second digit

F2   Left hand, third digit

F3   Left hand, fourth digit

F4   Left hand, fifth digit

F5   Right hand, thumb

F6   Right hand, second digit

F7   Right hand, third digit

F8   Right hand, fourth digit

F9   Right hand, fifth digit

FA   Left hand, thumb

FB   Item provided without cost to provider, supplier or practitioner, or full credit received for replaced device (examples, but not limited to, covered under warranty, replaced due to defect, free samples)

FC   Partial credit received for replaced device

FP   Service provided as part of family planning program

G1   Most recent URR reading of less than 60

G2   Most recent URR reading of 60 to 64.9

G3   Most recent URR reading of 65 to 69.9

G4   Most recent URR reading of 70 to 74.9

G5   Most recent URR reading of 75 or greater

G6   ESRD patient for whom less than six dialysis sessions have been provided in a month

G7   Pregnancy resulted from rape or incest or pregnancy certified by physician as life threatening

G8   Monitored anesthesia care (MAC) for deep complex, complicated, or markedly invasive surgical procedure

G9   Monitored anesthesia care for patient who has history of severe cardio-pulmonary condition

GA   Waiver of liability statement issued as required by payer policy, individual case

GB   Claim being re-submitted for payment because it is no longer covered under a global payment demonstration

GC   This service has been performed in part by a resident under the direction of a teaching physician

GD   Units of service exceeds medically unlikely edit value and represents reasonable and necessary services

GE   This service has been performed by a resident without the presence of a teaching physician under the primary care exception

GF   Non-physician (e.g. nurse practitioner (NP), certified registered nurse anesthetist (CRNA), certified registered nurse (CRN), clinical nurse specialist (CNS), physician assistant (PA)) services in a critical access hospital

GG   Performance and payment of a screening mammogram and diagnostic mammogram on the same patient, same day

GH   Diagnostic mammogram converted from screening mammogram on same day

GJ   "Opt out" physician or practitioner emergency or urgent service

GK   Reasonable and necessary item/service associated with a GA or GZ modifier

GL   Medically unnecessary upgrade provided instead of non-upgraded item, no charge, no advance beneficiary notice (ABN)

GM   Multiple patients on one ambulance trip

GN   Services delivered under an outpatient speech language pathology plan of care

GO   Services delivered under an outpatient occupational therapy plan of care

GP   Services delivered under an outpatient physical therapy plan of care

GQ   Via asynchronous telecommunications system

GR   This service was performed in whole or in part by a resident in a Department of Veterans Affairs medical center or clinic, supervised in accordance with VA policy

GS   Dosage of epo or darbepoietin alfa has been reduced and maintained in response to hematocrit or hemoglobin level

GT   Via interactive audio and video telecommunication systems

GU   Waiver of liability statement issued as required by payer policy, routine notice

GV   Attending physician not employed or paid under arrangement by the patient's hospice provider

GW   Service not related to the hospice patient's terminal condition

GX   Notice of liability issued, voluntary under payer policy

GY   Item or service statutorily excluded, does not meet the definition of any Medicare benefit or, for non-Medicare insurers, is not a contract benefit

GZ   Item or service expected to be denied as not reasonable and necessary

H9   Court-ordered

HA   Child/adolescent program

HB   Adult program, non geriatric

HC   Adult program, geriatric

HD   Pregnant/parenting women's program

HE   Mental health program

HF   Substance abuse program

HG   Opioid addiction treatment program

HH   Integrated mental health/substance abuse program

HI   Integrated mental health and mental retardation/developmental disabilities program

HJ   Employee assistance program

HK   Specialized mental health programs for high-risk populations

HL   Intern

HM   Less than bachelor degree level

HN   Bachelors degree level

HO   Masters degree level

HP   Doctoral level

HQ   Group setting

HR   Family/couple with client present

HS   Family/couple without client present

HT   Multi-disciplinary team

HU   Funded by child welfare agency

HV   Funded state addictions agency

HW   Funded by state mental health agency

HX   Funded by county/local agency

HY   Funded by juvenile justice agency

HZ   Funded by criminal justice agency

J1   Competitive acquisition program no-pay submission for a prescription number

J2   Competitive acquisition program, restocking of emergency drugs after emergency

J2   Administration

J3   Competitive acquisition program (cap), drug not available through cap as written, reimbursed under average sales price methodology

J4 DMEPOS item subject to DMEPOS competitive bidding program that is furnished by a hospital upon discharge

JA Administered intravenously

JB Administered subcutaneously

JC Skin substitute used as a graft

JD Skin substitute not used as a graft

JW Drug amount discarded/not administered to any patient

K0 Lower extremity prosthesis functional level 0 - does not have the ability or potential to ambulate or transfer safely with or without assistance and a prosthesis does not enhance their quality of life or mobility.

K1 Lower extremity prosthesis functional level 1 - has the ability or potential to use a prosthesis for transfers or ambulation on level surfaces at fixed cadence. Typical of the limited and unlimited household ambulator.

K2 Lower extremity prosthesis functional level 2 - has the ability or potential for ambulation with the ability to traverse low level environmental barriers such as curbs, stairs or uneven surfaces. Typical of the limited community ambulator.

K3 Lower extremity prosthesis functional level 3 - has the ability or potential for ambulation with variable cadence. Typical of the community ambulator who has the ability to transverse most environmental barriers and may have vocational, therapeutic, or exercise activity that demands prosthetic utilization beyond simple locomotion.

K4 Lower extremity prosthesis functional level 4 - has the ability or potential for prosthetic ambulation that exceeds the basic ambulation skills, exhibiting high impact, stress, or energy levels, typical of the prosthetic demands of the child, active adult, or athlete.

KA Add on option/accessory for wheelchair

KB Beneficiary requested upgrade for ABN, more than 4 modifiers identified on claim

KC Replacement of special power wheelchair interface

KD Drug or biological infused through DME

KE Bid under round one of the DMEPOS competitive bidding program for use with non-competitive bid base equipment

KF Item designated by FDA as class iii device

KG DMEPOS item subject to DMEPOS competitive bidding program number 1

KH DMEPOS item, initial claim, purchase or first month rental

KI DMEPOS item, second or third month rental

KJ DMEPOS item, parenteral enteral nutrition (pen) pump or capped rental, months four to fifteen

KK DMEPOS item subject to DMEPOS competitive bidding program number 2

KL DMEPOS item delivered via mail

KM Replacement of facial prosthesis including new impression/moulage

KN Replacement of facial prosthesis using previous master model

KO Single drug unit dose formulation

KP First drug of a multiple drug unit dose formulation

KQ Second or subsequent drug of a multiple drug unit dose formulation

KR Rental item, billing for partial month

KS Glucose monitor supply for diabetic beneficiary not treated with insulin

KT Beneficiary resides in a competitive bidding area and travels outside that competitive bidding area and receives a competitive bid item

KU DMEPOS item subject to DMEPOS competitive bidding program number 3

KV DMEPOS item subject to DMEPOS competitive bidding program that is furnished as part of a professional service

KW DMEPOS item subject to DMEPOS competitive bidding program number 4

KX Requirements specified in the medical policy have been met

KY DMEPOS item subject to DMEPOS competitive bidding program number 5

KZ New coverage not implemented by managed care

LC Left circumflex coronary artery

LD Left anterior descending coronary artery

LL Lease/rental (use the 'll' modifier when DME equipment rental is to be applied against the purchase price)

LR Laboratory round trip

LS FDA-monitored intraocular lens implant

LT Left side (used to identify procedures performed on the left side of the body)

M2 Medicare secondary payer (MSP)

MS Six month maintenance and servicing fee for reasonable and necessary parts and labor which are not covered under any manufacturer or supplier warranty

NB Nebulizer system, any type, FDA-cleared for use with specific drug

NR New when rented (use the 'nr' modifier when DME which was new at the time of rental is subsequently purchased)

NU New equipment

P1 A normal healthy patient

P2 A patient with mild systemic disease

P3 A patient with severe systemic disease

P4 A patient with severe systemic disease that is a constant threat to life

P5 A moribund patient who is not expected to survive without the operation

P6 A declared brain-dead patient whose organs are being removed for donor purposes

PA Surgical or other invasive procedure on wrong body part

PB Surgical or other invasive procedure on wrong patient

PC Wrong surgery or other invasive procedure on patient

PI Positron emission tomography (pet) or pet/computed tomography (ct) to inform the initial treatment strategy of tumors that are biopsy proven or strongly suspected of being cancerous based on other diagnostic testing

PL Progressive addition lenses

PS Positron emission tomography (pet) or pet/computed tomography (ct) to inform the subsequent treatment strategy of cancerous tumors when the beneficiary's treating physician determines that the pet study is needed to inform subsequent anti-tumor strategy

PT Colorectal cancer screening test; converted to diagnostic test or other procedure

Q0 Investigational clinical service provided in a clinical research study that is in an approved clinical research study

Q1 Routine clinical service provided in a clinical research study that is in an approved clinical research study

Q2 Hcfa/ord demonstration project procedure/service

Q3 Live kidney donor surgery and related services

Q4	Service for ordering/referring physician qualifies as a service exemption	SB	Nurse midwife
Q5	Service furnished by a substitute physician under a reciprocal billing arrangement	SC	Medically necessary service or supply
		SD	Services provided by registered nurse with specialized, highly technical home infusion training
Q6	Service furnished by a locum tenens physician	SE	State and/or federally-funded programs/services
Q7	One class a finding	SF	Second opinion ordered by a professional review organization (pro) per section 9401, p.l. 99-272 (100% reimbursement - no Medicare deductible or coinsurance)
Q8	Two class b findings		
Q9	One class b and two class c findings		
QA	FDA investigational device exemption		
QC	Single channel monitoring	SG	Ambulatory surgical center (ASC) facility service
QD	Recording and storage in solid state memory by a digital recorder	SH	Second concurrently administered infusion therapy
		SJ	Third or more concurrently administered infusion therapy
QE	Prescribed amount of oxygen is less than 1 liter per minute (lpm)	SK	Member of high risk population (use only with codes for immunization)
QF	Prescribed amount of oxygen exceeds 4 liters per minute (lpm) and portable oxygen is prescribed	SL	State supplied vaccine
		SM	Second surgical opinion
QG	Prescribed amount of oxygen is greater than 4 liters per minute (lpm)	SN	Third surgical opinion
		SQ	Item ordered by home health
QH	Oxygen conserving device is being used with an oxygen delivery system	SS	Home infusion services provided in the infusion suite of the iv therapy provider
		ST	Related to trauma or injury
QJ	Services/items provided to a prisoner or patient in state or local custody, however the state or local government, as applicable, meets the requirements in 42 cfr 411.4 (b)	SU	Procedure performed in physician's office (to denote use of facility and equipment)
		SV	Pharmaceuticals delivered to patient's home but not utilized
QK	Medical direction of two, three, or four concurrent anesthesia procedures involving qualified individuals	SW	Services provided by a certified diabetic educator
		SY	Persons who are in close contact with member of high-risk population (use only with codes for immunization)
QL	Patient pronounced dead after ambulance called		
QM	Ambulance service provided under arrangement by a provider of services	T1	Left foot, second digit
		T2	Left foot, third digit
QN	Ambulance service furnished directly by a provider of services	T3	Left foot, fourth digit
		T4	Left foot, fifth digit
QP	Documentation is on file showing that the laboratory test(s) was ordered individually or ordered as a CPT-recognized panel other than automated profile codes 80002-80019, g0058, g0059, and g0060.	T5	Right foot, great toe
		T6	Right foot, second digit
		T7	Right foot, third digit
		T8	Right foot, fourth digit
QR	Item or service provided in a Medicare specified study	T9	Right foot, fifth digit
QS	Monitored anesthesia care service	TA	Left foot, great toe
QT	Recording and storage on tape by an analog tape recorder	TC	Technical component. Under certain circumstances, a charge may be made for the technical component alone. Under those circumstances the technical component charge is identified by adding modifier 'TC' to the usual procedure number. Technical component charges are institutional charges and not billed separately by physicians. However, portable x-ray suppliers only bill for technical component and should utilize modifier TC. The charge data from portable x-ray suppliers will then be used to build customary and prevailing profiles.
QV	Item or service provided as routine care in a Medicare qualifying clinical trial		
QW	CLIA waived test		
QX	CRNA service: with medical direction by a physician		
QY	Medical direction of one certified registered nurse anesthetist (CRNA) by an anesthesiologist		
QZ	CRNA service: without medical direction by a physician		
RA	Replacement of a DME, orthotic or prosthetic item		
RB	Replacement of a part of a DME, orthotic or prosthetic item furnished as part of a repair		
RC	Right coronary artery		
RD	Drug provided to beneficiary, but not administered "incident-to"	TD	RN
		TE	LPN/LVN
RE	Furnished in full compliance with FDA-mandated risk evaluation and mitigation strategy (REMS)	TF	Intermediate level of care
		TG	Complex/high tech level of care
RP	Replacement and repair - RP may be used to indicate replacement of DME, orthotic and prosthetic devices which have been in use for some time. The claim shows the code for the part, followed by the 'RP' modifier and the charge for the part.	TH	Obstetrical treatment/services, prenatal or postpartum
		TJ	Program group, child and/or adolescent
		TK	Extra patient or passenger, non-ambulance
		TL	Early intervention/individualized family service plan (IFSP)
RR	Rental (use the 'RRF' modifier when DME is to be rented)	TM	Individualized education program (IEP)
RT	Right side (used to identify procedures performed on the right side of the body)	TN	Rural/outside providers' customary service area
		TP	Medical transport, unloaded vehicle
SA	Nurse practitioner rendering service in collaboration with a physician	TQ	Basic life support transport by a volunteer ambulance provider

TR	School-based individualized education program (IEP) services provided outside the public school district responsible for the student	UD	Medicaid level of care 13, as defined by each state
TS	Follow-up service	UE	Used durable medical equipment
TT	Individualized service provided to more than one patient in same setting	UF	Services provided in the morning
		UG	Services provided in the afternoon
TU	Special payment rate, overtime	UH	Services provided in the evening
TV	Special payment rates, holidays/weekends	UJ	Services provided at night
TW	Back-up equipment	UK	Services provided on behalf of the client to someone other than the client (collateral relationship)
U1	Medicaid level of care 1, as defined by each state		
U2	Medicaid level of care 2, as defined by each state	UN	Two patients served
U3	Medicaid level of care 3, as defined by each state	UP	Three patients served
U4	Medicaid level of care 4, as defined by each state	UQ	Four patients served
U5	Medicaid level of care 5, as defined by each state	UR	Five patients served
U6	Medicaid level of care 6, as defined by each state	US	Six or more patients served
U7	Medicaid level of care 7, as defined by each state	V5	Vascular catheter (alone or with any other vascular access)
U8	Medicaid level of care 8, as defined by each state	V6	Arteriovenous graft (or other vascular access not including a vascular catheter)
U9	Medicaid level of care 9, as defined by each state		
UA	Medicaid level of care 10, as defined by each state	V7	Arteriovenous fistula only (in use with two needles)
UB	Medicaid level of care 11, as defined by each state	V8	Infection present
UC	Medicaid level of care 12, as defined by each state	V9	No infection present
		VP	Aphakic patient

Glossary

abuse the unintentional act of billing and coding incorrectly

accessory sinuses also called paranasal sinuses; there are four pairs and each pair has a left and right side: the frontal sinuses (located over the eyes), maxillary sinuses (located under the eyes), ethmoid sinuses (located between the eyes and nose), and sphenoid sinuses (located at the center of the base of the skull, at the back of the nose)

Acknowledgement of Receipt of Privacy Practices a form that patients sign to show that they have read the Notice of Privacy Practices and understand how, when, and to whom the provider will release their protected health information (PHI)

activity code an ICD-9-CM code that describes the activity which caused or contributed to the injury or other health condition

admitting diagnosis diagnosis that the physician documents to show why he is admitting the patient

adverse effect also called an adverse reaction or side effect; when a patient's drug or medicinal and biological substance is correctly prescribed and properly administered but the patient has an adverse reaction to it

allergy abnormal reaction of the human immune system, which wrongly interprets certain allergens as harmful foreign bodies and produces antibodies against them

alphabetic filing filing system in which medical records are filed alphabetically by the patient's last name, first name, and middle initial

Alphabetic Index - Volume 2 also known as the Index; contains the names and descriptions for all diagnoses, conditions, diseases, and reasons for encounters, arranged in alphabetical order

ambulatory surgery outpatient surgery when the patient leaves the provider the same day

amniotic sac membrane containing amniotic fluid and the fetus grows inside of it

anesthesia a medical specialty involving administering anesthetic drugs to patients during diagnostic or therapeutic procedures, monitoring their conditions throughout the procedures (by checking their heart rate, blood pressure, respiration, and/or organ functions), ensuring the patients' safety while they are under anesthesia, and providing care before and after the procedures

anesthesia code package one CPT code that includes preoperative, intraoperative, and postoperative anesthesia services

anesthesia time a continuous period when an anesthesia provider is present with the patient which starts when the provider prepares the patient for anesthesia and ends when the provider is no longer furnishing anesthesia services to the patient, and other clinicians, such as nurses, take over the patient's postoperative care

antepartum care maternity care before delivery

anterior segment the front one-third of the eye containing the cornea, anterior chamber, anterior sclera, iris, ciliary body, and lens

Appendix A - Morphology of Neoplasms appendix that contains morphology codes, which specify types of neoplasms

Appendix B - Glossary of Mental Disorders appendix that was deleted October 1, 2004; the American Psychiatric Association instead uses the Diagnostic and Statistical Manual-IV, Text Revision (DSM-IV-TR) to classify mental disorders and help diagnose and research various mental conditions

Appendix C - Classification of Drugs by American Hospital Formulary List Number and Their ICD-9-CM Equivalents a system that pharmacists use to categorize drugs

Appendix D - Classification of Industrial Accidents According to Agency a list of work locations where accidents or injuries occurred, or the type of equipment involved in accidents

Appendix E - list of Three-Digit Categories contains every category, in numeric order, from each of the 17 chapters in the Tabular List

approach the location where the physician gains access to a lesion

arthrodesis surgical fusion of a joint so that it no longer moves

assumption coding coding that happens when the coder reads chart documentation and assumes that the patient has a specific diagnosis, even though the physician did not document it

at-will employment either the employee or the employer can terminate employment at any time, for any reason, with some exceptions

audit the process of insurances reviewing claims to determine if the documentation in the record justified the procedures that were coded and billed on claims

auditory hearing

autonomic nervous system part of the peripheral nervous system that controls involuntary body movements, such as muscles in your organs, and glands

base unit value a number that represents the complexity level of the anesthesia, risk to the patient, and anesthesia provider's skills needed to render services

benign hypertension hypertension that is also described as mild or moderate

benign neoplasm a tumor that is not life-threatening and does not spread

biofeedback a technique that teaches patients to regulate certain body functions through mental or physical exercises

bishop score a score based on five criteria that is used to assess a pregnant patient's condition before inserting a cervical dilator, that involves measuring the cervix and assessing the position of the fetus's head

blood a fluid in the body that maintains homeostasis (stability), by delivering nutrients, eliminating wastes, transporting oxygen and hormones, and fighting infections

body position the direction of the patient's body during a radiology procedure; the description of the body position includes information about what part of the body is closest to the X-ray beam

bone marrow soft, spongy tissue inside bones

bone/joint studies imaging techniques designed to identify bone mass, detect bone loss, determine bone quality, identify causes of joint effusion, and conduct a rheumatoid arthritis survey

breach of confidentiality to break confidentiality of private patient information, an illegal activity

breast mammography breast imaging services that aid in the early detection of breast cancer or diagnose suspected breast diseases

bundled code one code used to represent a group of individual codes

burn a bodily injury resulting from exposure to heat, caustics, electricity, or some forms of radiation

cardiac valves valves of the heart that open and close in response to blood flowing through the atria and ventricles; they include the mitral valve, tricuspid valve, aortic valve, and pulmonary valve

cardiopulmonary bypass (heart–lung machine) a machine that performs the work of the heart and lungs to allow the surgeon to perform procedures in a bloodless surgical field (area of surgery) and to keep the heart from moving during surgery

cardiovascular disease a general description for a disorder affecting the heart and related blood vessels

cardiovascular system also called the circulatory system; the heart and blood vessels

carotid body a small cluster of nerves and capillaries located near the bifurcation of the carotid artery; it contains cells that monitor oxygen and carbon dioxide levels in the blood

carryover line a line of text in the Alphabetic Index that continues to a second line due to lack of space in a column

category (ICD-9-CM diagnosis) a three-digit ICD-9-CM code in the Tabular List representing a single condition; some categories are further subdivided into subcategories

category (ICD-9-CM procedure) a two-digit code in ICD-9-CM that represents the type of inpatient procedure. A category code can never stand alone and will need additional digits before final code assignment.

Category (CPT-4) classification of CPT Category I codes that shows specific methods for completing procedures

Category I codes (five digits)—the largest category in CPT-4; these codes are separated into six sections, starting at the beginning of the coding manual

Category II codes (four numbers and the letter F)—supplemental tracking and performance measurement CPT-4 codes, which providers can assign in addition to Category I codes

Category III codes (four numbers and the letter T)—codes that follow Category II codes in the coding manual, temporary CPT-4 codes representing new technology, services, and procedures

causal relationship a cause-and-effect relationship, where one condition causes another

central nervous system (CNS) the part of the nervous system which contains the brain and spinal cord that enables the body to see, hear, touch, taste, and smell

cervical dilator an instrument used to widen the cervix to allow the fetus to pass through it

chapter a group of two-digit categories that represent related procedures for the same body system(s), or procedures that are not elsewhere classified or miscellaneous

chapters found in the Tabular List; a total of 17 chapters group diagnosis codes in numeric order by body system affected, type of disease, complication, or problem

characters the seven spaces or positions within an ICD-10-PCS code, each of which has a consistent purpose within each section of the ICD-10-PCS coding manual

Charge Description Master (CDM) also called a chargemaster; a database of information in a physician's or hospital's software that contains a list of all the services and procedures that the provider offers, called line items, including the associated CPT or HCPCS code, description of the service/procedure, and current charge for the service/procedure

chart abstracting the process of reviewing medical nomenclature, analyzing its meaning, and then translating it into diagnosis and procedure codes

chief complaint (CC) a concise statement that describes the patient's symptom, problem, condition, diagnosis, or history of present illness (HPI)

circulatory system consists of the heart and blood vessels (arteries and veins); arteries transport blood away from the heart throughout the body, and veins transport blood from body tissues and lungs to the heart

clear speech part of successful verbal communication, including enunciating, being mindful of one's tone of voice and voice pitch, and avoiding frequent pauses or use of slang

Clinical Laboratory Improvement Amendments (CLIA) legislation that requires the federal government to certify labs when they meet certain requirements, including that the lab personnel, meet specific criteria for performing lab services, and complete a specific number of lab tests daily

clinician a person who provides hands-on patient care

code the final level when the classification cannot be further subdivided

Code also note a new convention that alerts you that you may need to assign two codes to fully describe a condition

code descriptions also called descriptors; represent the meaning of a CPT code by describing the service or procedure

coding reading a medical record, interpreting the medical language in it to determine the patient's diagnosis and procedure, and assigning the correct codes

coding conventions found in the ICD-9-CM Official Guidelines for Coding and Reporting; terms, abbreviations, symbols, and punctuation directing you to find the correct code

coding guidelines and instructions specific information about when and how to assign CPT codes, how providers perform procedures, which codes can and cannot be reported together, and many other types of coding information

coding to the highest level of specificity coding diagnoses codes to their highest number of digits available, including assigning a subcategory and subclassification code when available

combination code a single code used to classify two diagnoses, a diagnosis with an associated secondary process (manifestation), or a diagnosis with an associated complication

combination record a record for one patient that includes medical documentation stored in the EMR and the patient's hardcopy forms and test results filed in a manual record

complex repair repair of a wound that requires more than a layered closure, such as scar revision, debridement, extensive undermining, stents, or retention sutures

confidentiality keeping the patient's demographic, insurance, and medical information confidential, or private

continuing education units (CEUs) education necessary to maintain coding credentials; can include monthly local chapter meetings, seminars, teleconferences, web conferences, coursework, and teaching

contraindication a condition that affects another condition; health problem that would make starting or continuing surgery unwise

contrast materials also called contrast agents, special dyes used to improve the visibility of structures or tissues during imaging tests

coordination of care one of the four contributing components of an evaluation and management service when the physician communicates with other providers or agencies to discuss the patient's case and arrange for additional services

coronary artery bypass graft (CABG) a procedure for improving blood flow to the heart

counseling in evaluation and management one of the four contributing components of an evaluation and management service when the physician discusses and educates a patient and/or family regarding test results, the patient's prognosis, benefits and risks of treatment options, treatment instructions, follow-up services that are needed, and reducing risk factors for developing a condition or problem

counseling when a patient or family member receives assistance in the aftermath of an illness or injury, or when the individual receives support to cope with family or social problems

CPT modifier two numbers appended to a CPT or HCPCS code to provide additional information

credentialed coder a coder who passed a national coding certification exam, achieving mastery in the coding field

crosswalk comparison of two different sets of information

Current Procedural Terminology, Fourth Edition (CPT-4) code set codes to classify outpatient medical, surgical, and diagnostic services and procedures

cytogenetic studies tests involving the structure and function of cells, including analyzing chromosomes, which carry genetic material and hereditary traits

cytopathology the process of examining cells from anywhere in the body to detect various conditions and determine if neoplasms are benign or malignant

default code the code listed next to a main term in the Index representing the condition that is most commonly associated with the main term, or the unspecified code for the condition

definitive procedure repair, biopsy, resection, or excision of skull base lesions, performed after the approach procedure

delivery birth of a fetus

diagnosis the patient's problem or condition and reason for the patient's visit

diagnostic examinations/tests exams or tests that are conducted when the patient has a sign or symptom of a suspected condition

diagnostic radiology imaging services including noninvasive and invasive diagnostic and therapeutic (interventional) procedures; common procedures in this subsection involve imaging procedures to view bones and internal structures, such as tissues, organs, and vessels to diagnose diseases, disorders, and the presence of foreign bodies

diagnostic ultrasound imaging test using sound waves, whose frequency is beyond human hearing, to evaluate a patient's internal organs and structures; can be diagnostic (to determine diagnoses) or therapeutic (to guide procedures)

diagnostic workup a series of laboratory and/or radiology tests that the physician orders for the patient to help determine the patient's diagnosis(es)

diaphragm a muscle shaped like half of a dome that is involved in respiration, located between the thoracic and abdominal cavities, which contracts and flattens during inhalation and relaxes during exhalation

digestive system also called the alimentary tract; the body system that begins at the mouth, where food is ingested (taken in), and moves through the stomach, small intestine, and large intestine, and waste products are excreted through the anus

direct laryngoscopy the patient is anesthetized with local or general anesthesia, and the physician looks directly at the larynx through a laryngoscope, inserting it into the mouth or nose to see the larynx

dislocation when a bone or joint moves out of its usual location

downcoding assigning a lower level code for the service than what the physician actually performed

electronic health record (EHR) a comprehensive electronic record for one patient including all of the patient's information that many providers access and share

electronic medical record (EMR) a computerized medical chart; an individual electronic record for one patient including all of the patient's information pertaining to one provider

encounter the date of service or procedure that the patient receives

endocrine system the body system made up of glands that secrete hormones into the bloodstream

enunciate to pronounce words correctly

eponym a disease or condition named after a person

established patient a patient who has seen the physician in the past three years

ethical standards standards for coding that are morally right, correct, and legal

etiology an underlying condition that causes another problem (manifestation)

evocative/suppression test when the physician administers a pharmaceutical evocative or suppression agent (e.g., drug, steroid) into a patient's body to test the body's response to the agent

examination the second of the three key components of an evaluation and management service, which involves objective information that the physician finds during the patient's encounter

Excludes1 note a new convention meaning that the condition listed in the note should never be sequenced with the code that was cross-referenced

Excludes2 note a new convention meaning that the condition listed in the note is not typically part of the code that was cross-referenced, but may be sequenced with it

external cause status the work status and environment of the patient at the time the injury occurred; information found in Appendix D of ICD-9-CM

external ear outer part of the ear that is visible, including the lobe and the pinna, or auricle, which transmits sounds through the auditory canal, or external auditory meatus

external fixation procedure in which the surgeon drills several holes through a bone and inserts wires or pins through the holes with the ends extending outside the skin, which he then attaches to clamps and rods called the frame. The frame helps to align the bone during healing, and the physician can easily adjust the frame to realign the bone at any time.

extraneous irrelevant and unrelated to the subject

False Claims Act qui tam provision regulation that states the whistleblower can sue on behalf of the government and receive part of money recovered from providers who committed fraud

fetus embryo from week eight until birth

fine needle aspiration inserting a fine, or thin, hollow needle under the skin to take a sample of cells

first-listed diagnosis the reason for the patient's encounter with outpatient providers such as physician offices, outpatient surgery centers, urgent care clinics; formerly called the primary diagnosis

flap skin with its blood supply intact; the physician removes the skin and blood vessels and connects them to the recipient site

follow-up care when the patient sees the physician for monitoring after treatment of a disease, condition, or injury is completed

fracture broken bone caused by trauma, disease, or repeated stress to a bone

fraud an intentional act of coding and billing for procedures that did not occur or for higher level procedures than what actually occurred

general coding guidelines found in the ICD-9-CM Official Guidelines for Coding and Reporting; written rules to follow when coding

General Equivalence Mappings (GEMs) protocols that electronically convert ICD-9-CM codes to ICD-10-CM codes

genitourinary system body system that includes the urinary system and the male and female reproductive systems; and disorders of the breast

gestation pregnancy, a period lasting about 40 weeks, or 9½ months

global period a time frame during which the provider must render all of the services related to a surgery, including preoperative, intraoperative, and postoperative services

global routine obstetric package care that includes antepartum, delivery, and postpartum care to a patient for uncomplicated pregnancies and deliveries; all care is bundled into the global routine obstetric package, which is similar to the global surgical package, where the payer reimburses for all services in the package using only one CPT code

global service both the professional and technical components were performed in one provider location, which codes and bills for the service

global surgical package represents a group, or package, of services that all relate to a single surgery and are covered by a single insurance payment, including preoperative, intraoperative, and postoperative services

great vessels the superior vena cava, inferior vena cava, pulmonary artery, and aorta

gross and microscopic examination an examination performed with the naked eye and also with a microscope

gross examination an examination performed with the naked eye

HCPCS modifiers two letters or a letter and a number appended to a CPT or HCPCS code

Health Information Technology for Economic and Clinical Health (HITECH) Act established payment incentives to Medicare- and Medicaid-participating physicians and hospitals to implement Electronic Health Records (EHRs) as part of a nationwide EHR infrastructure

Health Insurance Portability and Accountability Act (HIPAA) federal laws that require providers to notify patients that they will release the patient's medical information to his insurance and other healthcare providers

health status V codes codes which provide additional information about a patient, including if the patient is a carrier of a disease or has another factor influencing her health status, such as an absent organ

Healthcare Common Procedure Coding System (HCPCS) Medicare's classification system for various services not included in CPT-4, as well as nonphysician services, medical supplies, equipment, and medications

healthcare delivery system a network of people and processes working to treat patients' conditions and prevent illnesses

healthcare provider renders healthcare services and procedures to patients; can be a place, such as a physician's office, hospital, nursing home, or clinic, or a person, like a physician, physician assistant, registered nurse, or physical therapist

heart organ with four chambers, two upper and two lower; the heart's upper chambers, the right and left atria, receive and collect blood, while the heart's lower chambers, the right and left ventricles, pump blood out of the heart to other parts of the body

heart disease a general description for any disorder affecting the heart

heart–lung transplant a procedure in which the lung(s) and heart are transplanted

hemic pertaining to the blood

highest level of specificity process of assigning the most specific code available

history the first of the three key components of an evaluation and management service, which consists of subjective information that the patient provides to the physician and other clinicians, that can be verbal, and that can come from the patient's health history form, including past medical, family, and social histories

Human Resources Department department whose employees are in charge of hiring and firing, overseeing employee benefits, processing payroll, and following employment laws

hypertension consistently elevated blood pressure (BP)

Hypertension Table located in the Tabular List, shows various types of hypertension, including malignant, benign, or unspecified

hypertensive heart disease a heart condition that hypertension causes, such as congestive heart failure, coronary artery disease, myocardial infarction, and ischemic heart disease

ICD-9-CM Official Guidelines for Coding and Reporting rules that the Centers for Medicare and Medicaid Services (CMS) and the National Center for Health Statistics (NCHS) created for all three volumes so that providers know how to use the coding manual and follow the same guidelines for coding patients' diagnoses. These are rules and conventions to use when coding diagnoses in the Alphabetic Index and the Tabular List for Volumes 1–3.

ill-defined and unknown causes of morbidity and mortality represent general descriptions of conditions that caused a patient's illness or death but do not provide specific information

immune globulin provides passive immunity, consists of serum globulins or recombinant immune globulins

immunization when a person receives a vaccine (vaccination) or toxoid that enables the body's immune system to produce antibodies to fight against it

indirect laryngoscopy the physician holds a mirror in the back of the patient's throat and shines a light into the throat (attached to the physician's headpiece) to view laryngeal structures, and the patient is not under anesthesia during the procedure

in vitro fertilization (IVF) a technique to help a woman become pregnant that is used to treat many causes of infertility; an egg (removed from the female patient using a follicle puncture) is manually fertilized with sperm and then returned to the uterus of the female patient

incidental to a procedure that is part of another procedure, that should not be coded separately

indented description a partial description of a CPT code that has no meaning by itself but must be combined with a standalone description in order to provide the full description of the code

index found in the last part of the CPT manual, contains procedures and services. Main terms in the index in the CPT manual are arranged alphabetically by procedures and services, body sites, synonyms, eponyms, abbreviations, and some diagnoses.

Index the first portion of ICD-9-CM Volume 3 and ICD-10-PCS, which contains the names and descriptions for all surgical and diagnostic procedures, arranged in alphabetical order

Index to External Causes of Injury (E codes) an alphabetical list of external causes of accidents and injuries, along with their corresponding codes, all beginning with the letter E

infectious disease occurs when a pathogen enters the body, multiplies, and causes illness because the body is not strong enough to defend itself against an attack

inner ear also called the labyrinth, is made up of three bony areas, the cochlea, vestibule chamber, and semicircular canals

inpatient a patient who is typically hospitalized for more than 24 hours, although the inpatient stay can be less than 24 hours, depending on the physician's order

inpatient hospital procedure a therapeutic procedure, such as a surgical operation or a diagnostic service, performed on a patient who has been admitted to an inpatient hospital, including an acute care facility

Inpatient Prospective Payment System (IPPS) Medicare payment system for acute care inpatient hospital stays, which pays after the patient is discharged, based on the diagnosis or diagnoses that a coder assigns to the patient's episode of care

insubordination not following orders from one's boss

integumentary system includes the skin, hair, hair follicles, related glands, and the nails

intermediate repair repair of a wound that involves the epidermis, dermis, and subcutaneous tissues, with layered closure

International Classification of Diseases, Ninth Revision, Clinical Modification (ICD-9-CM) code set diagnosis codes for classifying inpatient and outpatient diagnoses and inpatient procedure codes for classifying inpatient procedures, effective until replaced by ICD-10-CM

International Classification of Diseases, Tenth Revision, Clinical Modification (ICD-10-CM) code set diagnosis codes for classifying inpatient and outpatient diagnoses, not currently effective but will eventually replace ICD-9-CM

jamming coding for diagnoses that do not exist

know your audience knowing who will receive your message and how much information to convey

labor when the cervix dilates (opens) and the uterus contracts to expel a baby

laboratory test a test to determine what element is present or absent in a specimen, or to measure the body's reaction to a specific substance

laterality indication for the side of the body that the condition affects, such as right, left, or bilateral sides

length of stay (LOS) time spent hospitalized

lower respiratory system the lower respiratory tract, or lower respiratory system; contains the lungs, bronchi, and bronchioles, branches of tubes that carry oxygen, and alveoli, air sacs at the ends of bronchioles

lung transplant a procedure to replace all or part of a lung with a healthy donor lung

lymphatic system consists of vessels, nodes, ducts, and organs and moves lymph, a clear fluid containing protein, throughout the body

main term a word in the Alphabetic Index that describes the patient's condition or disease, capitalized and printed in bold, followed by its corresponding code

male genital system body system that contains organs and structures responsible for human reproduction and also includes structures for urination

malignant Ca in situ cancer in which malignant cells are confined to the tissue layer where they originated and have not spread to surrounding tissues within the same organ

malignant neoplasm life-threatening neoplasm or tumor, also called cancer or carcinoma

malignant primary life-threatening neoplasm or tumor that has invaded the tissues within the organ where it started

malignant secondary life-threatening neoplasm or tumor that spread from the primary site

manifestation a problem that develops from an underlying condition or disease, called an etiology

manual medical record also referred to as paper records; a file folder containing various file dividers with labels for specific information, such as progress notes, health history, and lab or radiology test results, filed chronologically

materials supplied by physician materials, such as sterile trays or drugs, that the physician uses in a procedure that are over and above those usually included with the procedure(s)

mediastinum body region located in the thorax and surrounded by connective tissue; separates the lungs and contains the esophagus, heart, superior and inferior vena cava, and aorta

Medicaid a government-sponsored health insurance plan for those with low income, although not everyone with low income qualifies for it

medical decision making (MDM) the third of the three key components of an evaluation and management service, where the physician establishes the patient's diagnosis, treatment, and necessary follow-up tests or exams

medical misadventure any problem that a patient develops which a physician or clinician caused, either directly (through hands-on care) or indirectly (through failure to react to a patient's concerns or symptoms)

medical necessity the patient's diagnosis justified the procedure that the physician performed

medical record also referred to as a medical chart; written descriptions provided by the physician or other clinician, such as a physician assistant, of what happened during a patient's service or procedure and descriptions of the patient's diagnosis

medical/surgical complications unexpected problems from surgery or medical care, which the physician documents; can be the result of medical negligence or incompetence and include infection, illness, disease, pain, or other symptoms

Medicare a federal government-sponsored health insurance plan created in 1965 for people age 65 or older, under age 65 with certain disabilities, and of any age with End-Stage Renal Disease (ESRD)

Medicare Physician Fee Schedule (MPFS) the complete listing of fees that Medicare uses to pay physicians or other providers or suppliers for services and procedures

Medicare Severity Diagnosis Related Groups (MS-DRGs) a system that categorizes a patient's hospital stay into a group based on the principal and secondary diagnoses on the patient's claim

mental disorder a problem with or in the mind

middle ear contains the eardrum, or tympanic membrane, which receives sound waves transmitted through the auditory canal, resulting in vibrations

minimally invasive a procedure that involves breaking the skin with a small incision and inserting needles, small catheters, balloons, stents, or filters or other devices

miscellaneous codes codes that are not otherwise specified in the HCPCS code set

modifier two letters, two numbers, or a letter and a number, appended to a CPT or HCPCS code to provide additional information about the procedure or service

modifiers for anesthesia providers modifiers appended to the anesthesia code that show the type of provider who rendered anesthesia services

motor system part of the nervous system that directs the body's muscles and glands to perform specific functions, such as pulling one's hand away from a hot object, based on the outside information that the body receives

multiple coding assigning more than one code for a single condition or multiple conditions

musculoskeletal system includes both the skeletal and muscular systems

myocardial infarction (MI) also called a heart attack, when plaque and/or a blood clot (thrombus) forms in a coronary artery and occludes blood flow, causing necrosis of heart muscle

nature of presenting problem   one of the four contributing components of an evaluation and management service, which the AMA defines as a "disease, condition, illness, injury, symptom, sign, finding, complaint, or other reason for encounter, with or without a diagnosis being established at the time of the encounter"

neoplasm   abnormal new growth

Neoplasm Table   located in the Alphabetic Index, lists neoplasm by body site and behaviors

nervous system   the body system made of a framework of nerves throughout the body that process, receive, and send messages through nerve impulses that tell the body what to do and how to react

new patient   a patient who has never seen the physician or has not seen the physician in the past three years, or a patient who has never seen a physician of a different specialty in the same group practice

nonessential modifier   found in the Alphabetic Index, a supplementary word or phrase in parentheses ( ) following a main term or subterm; provides additional information but does not need to be present in the diagnosis

noninvasive   a procedure that does not involve breaking the skin, such as an X-ray or MRI

nonspecific abnormal findings   test results that are unusual or irregular, including lab and radiology tests, function studies, blood pressure, and reflex tests

nonverbal communication   communicating with others without speaking

Notice of Privacy Practices   notice that providers give to patients to explain how they will share patient's demographic, insurance, and medical information, as required by regulations in the Health Insurance Portability and Accountability Act of 1996 (HIPAA)

nuclear medicine   use of radioactive elements for diagnostic and therapeutic radiology services

numeric filing   filing of medical records using the terminal digit system, where each record is assigned a series of three pairs of numbers and filed numerically from right to left

nutritional disorders   conditions that occur when the body lacks nutrients for good health or receives too many nutrients

observation   a patient with an unclear diagnosis; the physician does not have enough information about the patient's condition to either admit the patient to the hospital as an inpatient or discharge the patient to home or another facility (such as a skilled nursing facility—SNF)

Office of the Inspector General (OIG) of the Department of Health and Human Services (DHHS)   a department within the federal government that investigates cases of fraud and imposes monetary penalties on providers who are found guilty

open wound   a wound which involves broken skin and can encompass one or more layers of skin or go deeper into muscles, nerves, and organs

operating microscope   a microscope that a physician uses to see small structures, as in microsurgery

orthotics   devices that helps a patient to regain normal functioning; specialty area of healthcare, dealing with the design, delivery, and fitting of those devices

outpatient   a patient who returns home or to another facility the same day after receiving a service or procedure at a hospital or another provider

Outpatient Prospective Payment System (OPPS)   Medicare's payment system for outpatient hospitals, which pays a set amount for a service or procedure based on a specific classification

outpatient provider   includes emergency departments, outpatient hospitals, ambulatory surgery centers (ASCs), clinics, and urgent care centers and clinics

pacemaker   a small device with a battery-operated pulse generator connected to leads (wires), with electrodes attached to the leads, which are then attached to the heart to help control heart rhythms

panel   a group of tests performed at the same time, for the same patient, using the same specimen

parasympathetic nervous system   part of the autonomic nervous system which controls body functions, such as digestion

participating provider   also referred to as a par provider, a provider who signs a contract with insurance; the contract states how much the insurance will pay for specific services rendered to patients with that insurance

patient relations   interacting with patients and their families to ensure that they receive the best service

patient status   the type of patient the physician treats, such as new patient, established patient, inpatient, or outpatient

patient-activated event recorder   a medical device that records the heart's electrical activity

peripheral nervous system (PNS)   the part of the nervous system which contains nerves outside the central nervous system (CNS) that control voluntary functions (muscle movement) and involuntary functions (cardiac, glands)

permanent national codes   codes in the HCPCS code set that all U.S. providers and insurances can use for billing and statistical purposes

personal health record (PHR)   a comprehensive record that the patient creates and owns, containing information about the patient's care, regardless of where he received it

phone etiquette   showing good manners and professionalism during phone conversations

physical status modifier   a HCPCS modifier that starts with the letter P followed by a number from 1 to 6, which describes the patient's overall health status at the time of anesthesia

place of service   location of the facility where the physician provides an evaluation and management service, such as an office, hospital, or nursing facility

placeholder "x"   insertion of a character in an ICD-10-CM code when the code contains less than six characters but requires a seventh character

placenta   a membrane that provides nutrients to the developing fetus

poisoning   a patient's reaction to a drug, medicinal substance, or biological substance that is not properly prescribed or correctly administered

posterior segment   the back two-thirds of the eye, which includes the retina, optic nerve, and anterior hyaloid membrane

postpartum care   maternity care after delivery

pregnancy   condition that results after a male sperm fertilizes a female ovum (egg), and the fertilized egg is implanted in the uterine lining and develops into a baby

prehypertension   blood pressure readings in the at-risk range

prenatal   before birth

preoperative evaluation   examination and testing before surgery or another procedure to ensure that a patient is healthy enough for the surgery or procedure

Present on Admission (POA) Indicator   information about the diagnoses that the patient has at the time of admission

preventive health care   care that prevents illness

principal diagnosis   the condition established after study (e.g., tests, exams) to be chiefly responsible for occasioning the admission of the patient to the hospital, as defined by the Uniform Hospital Discharge Data Set (UHDDS)

principal procedure   the surgical operation or service most closely related to the principal diagnosis

Privacy Rule part of the Health Insurance Portability and Accountability Act (HIPAA) of 1996, which assures that individuals' health information is properly protected, while allowing the flow of health information needed to provide and promote high quality health care and to protect the public's health and well-being

probable/suspected a diagnosis the provider is not sure of yet but believes is likely

probationary period the amount of time that an employer allows a new employee to learn all aspects of her job

problem-oriented medical record (POMR) information in the medical record is grouped according to the patient's specific problem or condition

professional component the physician's supervision and interpretation of the service (also called S and I)

professionalism possessing the traits necessary to be a successful professional, including enthusiasm, dedication, job knowledge, respect for others, and a positive attitude

prosthetics devices that replace a body part lost to disease or trauma; specialty area of healthcare, dealing with the design, delivery, and fitting of those devices

psychotherapy treatment involving the provider communicating face-to-face with the patient to determine the cause(s) of a specific condition and develop ways to effectively cope with it

qualifying circumstances codes CPT codes that describe four different complex anesthesia situations

qualitative test a test that determines whether or not a substance or analyte, such as a drug, is present in a specimen

quantitative test a test that determines the amount of a substance present in a specimen

query to ask the physician to clarify medical documentation

questionable a diagnosis the provider is not sure of yet

radiation oncology cancer treatment using radiation

radiography literally means to take a film (-graphy) of X-rays (radio); covers a wide range of radiological procedures

radiologic guidance technique used during a procedure to visualize access to an anatomical site in order to direct or guide the placement and/or removal of surgical objects (e.g., catheters, needles)

radiological supervision and interpretation describes the radiological portion of a procedure where the physician either supervises radiology clinicians who perform the procedure or performs the procedure directly

radiology literally means the study of (-ology) X-rays (radi/o); medical specialty including many types of tests and therapeutic procedures, which involve viewing various internal body structures, like arteries and bones, using radiation, sound waves, magnetic fields, or radio fields

radiopharmaceutical a radioactive drug that providers, such as hospitals, physicians, and SNFs, administer to patients intravenously and orally for diagnostic and therapeutic radiology procedures which is called nuclear medicine

repair/reconstruction procedure procedure to repair or reconstruct the dura after a CSF leak

replantation to reattach an amputated arm, forearm, hand, digit (finger), thumb, or foot

resource-based relative value scale (RBRVS) a calculation of the cost the physician incurs that includes physician work, practice expense, and malpractice insurance

respiratory system allows the body to inhale oxygen and distribute it throughout the bloodstream to cells in the body to sustain life

revenue cycle also called a billing cycle; all of the steps that take place from the time that a patient calls a provider to schedule an appointment for a service or procedure until the patient's bill is paid in full

routine and administrative examinations exams that patients need for reasons other than illnesses

rule of nines method for calculating the percentage of total body surface area (TBSA) damaged by burns, which divides the body into sections; each section represents a percentage of TBSA divisible by 9

rule out to eliminate the possibility of a particular diagnosis

screening a test or exam for the presence of a disease or for other conditions that may cause a disease

section the first level of classification of CPT Category I codes, a group of three-digit categories within a chapter in the Tabular List in ICD-9-CM; each section represents a group of related conditions or a single condition

Security Rule part of the Health Insurance Portability and Accountability Act (HIPAA) of 1996, which established national standards to protect individuals' electronic protected health information (PHI) that a provider, insurance, or clearinghouse creates, receives, uses, or maintains

sensory system part of the nervous system that involves the brain and spinal cord interpreting information that the body senses (for example, touching a hot object with your hand, which causes it to react through the motor system)

separate procedure a procedure that is performed separately from another major procedure

service treatment, testing, or care to prevent a disease or condition; examples of services and procedures include a physical examination, skin lesion removal, flu shot, or a surgery; also referred to as a procedure

seventh character the last character in a code with seven characters that provides more information about a patient's encounter

shunt a device that includes a catheter (tube) that transports fluid from one area of the body to another

sign objective evidence of disease that the physician discovers

simple repair repair of a superficial wound, which primarily involves the epidermis, dermis, or subcutaneous tissues with simple one-layer closure

skeletal traction (pulling) placing pins and/or wires through broken bones so that the pins or wires are exposed to the outside of the body. Stirrups, ropes, pulleys, or weights are attached to the pins and wires to secure bones in place until they heal.

skin graft when the physician takes skin from one area of the body (donor site) and transfers it to a wound

skull traction applying cranial tongs or calipers to the head for treating cervical spine factures and dislocations. Pins placed in the skull are then attached to ropes and weights on the outside, which secure the spine into place.

slang words and phrases that are acceptable to use with friends, but not appropriate for a professional environment

somatic nervous system part of the peripheral nervous system that controls voluntary movement, including movements of skeletal muscles

source-oriented medical record (SOMR) a medical record in which the information is organized and filed by its type, or source, using filing dividers to create a section for each source

special report medical documentation or letters from clinicians to justify the medical necessity of a procedure and provide greater detail about the procedure performed

specimen a collection of fluid or tissue that a physician or clinician examines to determine more about its content

spinal instrumentation also called fixation, a procedure to stabilize the vertebrae of the spine with metal rods, screws, and pins attached to the vertebrae to align two or more vertebral segments

spinal osteotomy to incise and remove a portion(s) of the vertebral segment(s) to realign the spine to correct a spinal deformity.

spinal vertebrae bones of the spine, located in five separate areas, cervical, thoracic, lumbar, sacral, and coccygeal

spleen organ of the lymphatic system located in the upper left quadrant of the abdomen; produces lymphocytes, creates and stores red blood cells, and filters blood by destroying old red blood cells

sprain a sudden or violent twist or wrench of a joint causing the stretching or tearing of connective tissue and often rupturing of blood vessels

stand alone description a full description of a CPT code that is not indented

strain bodily injury from excessive tension, effort, or use

subcategory (ICD-9-CM) a four-digit code providing further specification for a category, including the site of the body that the condition affects, etiology, and manifestation. Some subcategories are further subdivided into five-digit subclassifications.

subcategory (CPT-4) a further division of some categories of CPT Category I codes, which provides more specific information about the procedure or service

subcategory (ICD-10-CM) each level of a subdivision after a category

subchapter a group of three-character categories in the tabular list

subclassification (ICD-9-CM) a five-digit code that further specifies a subcategory, including body site affected, type of disease, and additional information to describe the condition

subheading a division of CPT Category I codes that groups procedures by location within a body system

subjective, objective, assessment, plan (SOAP) format information that providers document related to a specific encounter

subsection a division of CPT Category I codes that breaks down sections by type and/or anatomic sites

subterm located in the Alphabetic Index, indented under a main term to provide additional information about the main term, such as the body site, cause of the condition, and complications; also referred to as an essential modifier

superficial injury also called surface injury, includes abrasions, blisters, nonvenomous insect bites, splinters, and scratches

Supplementary Classification of External Causes of Injury and Poisoning (E codes) codes found in the Tabular List that represent external causes of injuries and poisonings

Surgery section guidelines guidelines listed at the beginning of the Surgery section that will help you to code surgical procedures correctly

surgical clearance the physician's determination that the patient's medical condition is stable enough for surgery

surgical pathology services services that occur when a pathologist conducts a gross and/or microscopic exam of a specimen that a physician removes from a patient during surgery or during a procedure in the hospital, ambulatory surgery center, or physician's office

sympathetic nervous system part of the autonomic nervous system which controls the body's response to flight-or-fight

symptom subjective evidence of disease that the patient reports to the physician

synchronous procedure a component of another procedure to which you should assign an additional code

Table of Drugs and Chemicals located in the Alphabetic Index, contains an alphabetical list of names of drugs and chemicals responsible for poisonings and injuries, along with their corresponding codes

Tables reference grids that coders use to build ICD-10-PCS codes by selecting the body system, type of procedure, operative approach, body part, and other characteristics

Tabular List - Volume 1 contains all ICD-9-CM diagnosis codes arranged in numeric order, followed by their descriptions

Tabular List - Volume 3 lists all ICD-9-CM procedure codes in numerical order in ICD-9-CM

technical component represents the use of a room to perform a medical service, as well as equipment, supplies, and staff, like a technician, for services performed at hospitals or other facilities where the physician who performed the professional component of the same service is not an employee of the facility or hospital

temporal bone a bone on the side of the head at the skull base that is connected to the mandible.

middle fossa hollow area or bone cavity

temporary national codes HCPCS codes for services and supplies that do not have a permanent code

terrorism the unlawful use of force or violence against persons or property to intimidate or coerce a government, the civilian population, or any segment thereof, to further a political or social objective

time one of the four contributing components of an evaluation and management service; many code descriptors include the average time to complete a service, which includes face-to-face time and non-face-to-face time

time units (anesthesia) increments usually of 15 minutes, used when insurances calculate the amount of time the anesthesia provider spends on a case

tone of voice emotion that your voice conveys when you speak

total body surface area (TBSA) the total skin area of the human body, used in calculations to determine the percentage of the body area that a burn damaged

toxic effect the result when a patient ingests or is exposed to a harmful substance, such as alcohol, gasoline, acid, lead, carbon monoxide, pesticides, soaps, or detergents

transportation services transporting patients to the hospital, skilled nursing facility, or other destination

trimester a three-month increment used to measure pregnancy

tumor new growth of tissue that forms an abnormal mass

Tumor, Nodes, Metastasis (TNM) classification system one of the most common cancer staging systems that classifies the extent of the tumor and if it has spread to the lymph nodes or other body sites

type of service specific service the physician provides, such as an office visit, consultation, hospital admission, or hospital discharge, and whether it was initial or subsequent

ultrasound a radiology imaging method for viewing various structures, including internal organs, muscles, joints, and tendons, using sound waves

unbundling incorrectly coding for each service in a group when they should have been coded with one bundled code

uncertain behavior describes a neoplasm when the pathologist cannot determine whether the neoplasm is malignant or benign

unlisted codes CPT Category I codes used whenever you code a procedure or service for which there is no specific CPT code in either Category I or Category III

unlisted service or procedure a procedure or service for which there is no specific CPT code in either Category I or Category III; report an unlisted Category I code

unspecified (whether malignant or benign) the documentation provides the neoplasm site but does not describe its behavior or histologic type

upcoding incorrectly coding for higher level procedures than what actually occurred

upper respiratory system the upper airway, or upper respiratory system, which includes the nose, larynx (voice box), and pharynx (throat)

up-speak the tendency to speak in higher pitch at the end of a sentence as though you are asking a question, even though you are not

urinalysis a test on a urine specimen to identify abnormalities

urinary system body system that produces and excretes urine, and that consists of two kidneys, two ureters, bladder, sphincter muscles, and urethra

use of codes for reporting purposes a new convention that instructs you to always code to the highest level of specificity when reporting codes to insurances, claims clearinghouses, billing and collection agencies, or any other organizations

V Codes - Supplementary Classification of Factors Influencing Health Status and Contact with Health Services codes found in the Tabular List representing reasons for encounters, other than a disease, condition, or injury

values individual letters and numbers that can occupy the seven positions of an ICD-10-PCS code

vascular disease a broad term that describes various circulatory system diseases, such as peripheral artery disease, that inhibit the ability of blood and lymph vessels from properly circulating blood or lymph

verbal communication speaking with others

vocal cords soft tissue folds in the larynx that, along with certain ligaments, produce sound when air passes through them, to create speech

voice pitch how high or low your voice sounds

working diagnosis a diagnosis that it is not yet definitive, or proven

wound exploration to examine a wound and often enlarge or dissect it in order to determine the wound depth; to remove a foreign body, such as a bullet; to debride the area; and to repair any tissue, fascia, muscle, or blood vessels

written communication communicating with others in writing

zygote fertilized egg

Subject Index